Contents

National Diet and Nutrition Survey:

young people aged 4 to 18 years

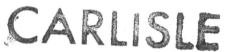
liet

*Iinistry of
'Health by the
s and Medical*

Nutrition

n Research

irch

Robert Wenlock, Department of Health

Melanie Farron, Food Standards Agency[2]

London: The Stationery Office

[1]   Responsibility for this survey and the National Diet and Nutrition Survey programme transferred from the Ministry of Agriculture, Fisheries and Food to the Food Standards Agency on its establishment in April 2000.
[2]   Formerly of Ministry of Agriculture, Fisheries and Food.

ISBN 0 11 621265 9

6 Protein, carbohydrate and alcohol intake

7 Fat and fatty acids intake

Appendices

Foreword

This survey, of a nationally representative sample of young people aged 4-18 years, is one of a programme of national surveys with the aim of gathering information about the dietary habits and nutritional status of the British population. Diet and nutrition have a key role in achieving the targets set out in the White Paper Saving Lives: Our Healthier Nation. The results of this survey, together with a related survey of the oral health of the same group of young people, provide a sound basis for the development of future nutrition policy to enable today's young people to enjoy longer and healthier lives.

This report results from a successful collaboration between the Ministry of Agriculture, Fisheries and Food[1] and the Department of Health with the Office for National Statistics and the Medical Research Council.

We warmly welcome this, the latest report in the National Diet and Nutrition Survey programme and express our thanks to all the respondents who took part.

SIR JOHN KREBS
Chairman
Food Standards Agency

YVETTE COOPER
Minister for Public Health
Department of Health

---

[1] Responsibility for this survey and the NDNS programme has now transferred from the Ministry of Agriculture, Fisheries and Food to the Food Standards Agency on its establishment in April 2000.

Authors' acknowledgements

We would like to thank everyone who contributed to the survey and the production of this Report:

- the young people and their parents without whose co-operation the survey would not have been possible;

- the interviewers of Social Survey Division of ONS who recruited the young people and carried out all the fieldwork stages of the survey;

- colleagues in Social Survey Division of ONS in the Sampling Implementation Unit, Field Branch, Survey Computing Branch, Methodology Unit and Project Support Branch, in particular, Ann Whitby, Marily Troyano, Steve Edwards, Peter Rowswell, Franco Insalaco, Tracie Goodfellow and Kate Foster;

- the ONS nutritionists, Zoe Smith, Melanie Farron (now at FSA), Frankie Robinson and Michael Tumilty;

- staff of the Medical Research Council Human Nutrition Research, particularly Dr Jayne Perks and Ms Adrienne Jennings;

- the professional staff at the Ministry of Agriculture, Fisheries and Food[1] and the Department of Health, in particular Joanne Collins, Gill Marchant, Dr Joyce Hughes and Alison Mills (formerly of MAFF), Michael Day, Dr Clifton Gay, Susan Church, Steven Wearne and Katie Dick (now of Food Standards Agency), Professor Martin Wiseman, Dr Petronella Clarke and Dr Susan Lader (formerly of Department of Health);

- the phlebotomists and local laboratory personnel who were recruited by HNR to take the blood samples, and process and store the blood specimens;

- Professor Elaine Gunter, Chief, NHANES Laboratory, Centres for Disease Control and Prevention, Atlanta, USA, for an independent review of the methodology for the blood sample collection and laboratory analyses;

- Dr Lorraine Cale, Dr Ken Fox and Alison Walker (now of ONS) for advice on the measurements of physical activity in young people.

Further acknowledgements associated with the blood analyses are given in Appendix Q.

---

[1] Responsibility for this survey and the NDNS programme transferred from MAFF to the Food Standards Agency on its establishment in April 2000.

Notes to the tables

Tables showing percentages

In general, percentages are shown if the unweighted base is 30 or more. Where a base number is less than 30, actual numbers are shown within square brackets.

The row or column percentages may add to 99% or 101% because of rounding and weighting.

The varying positions of the percentage signs and bases in the tables denote the presentation of different types of information. Where there is a percentage sign at the head of a column and the base at the foot, the whole distribution is presented and the individual percentages add to between 99% and 101%. Where there is no percentage sign in the table and a note above the figures, the figures refer to the proportion of young people who had the attribute being discussed, and the complementary proportion, to add to 100%, is not shown in the table.

In tables showing cumulative percentages the row labelled 'All' is always shown as 100%. The proportion of cases falling above the upper limit of the previous band can be calculated by subtracting from 100 the proportion in the previous band. Actual maximum values are not shown in tables of cumulative percentages, since they could vary for different subgroups being considered within the same tables.

Unless shown as a separate group, or stated in the text or a footnote to a table, estimates have been calculated for the total number of young people in the subgroup, excluding those not answering. Base numbers shown in the tables are the total number of young people in the subgroup, including those not answering.

The total column may include cases from small subgroups not shown separately elsewhere on the tables, therefore the individual column bases may not add to the base in the total column.

Conventions

The following conventions have been used in the tables:

- no cases
0 values less than 0.5%
[ ] numbers inside square brackets are the actual numbers of cases, when the total number of unweighted cases, that is, the base, is fewer than 30.

Tables showing descriptive statistics – mean, percentiles, standard deviation of the mean

These are shown in tables to an appropriate number of decimal places.

Significant differences

Differences commented on in the text are shown as being significant at the 95% or 99% confidence levels ($p < 0.05$ and $p < 0.01$). Throughout the Report, the terms 'significant' and 'statistically significant' are used interchangeably. Where differences are shown or described as being 'not statistically significant' or 'ns' this indicates $p > 0.05$. The formulae used to test for significant differences are given in Appendix E.

Where differences between subgroups are compared for a number of variables, for example differences between young people in different age groups in their consumption of whole milk, the significance level shown ($p < 0.05$ or $p < 0.01$) applies to all comparisons, unless otherwise stated.

Standard deviations

Standard deviations for estimates of mean values are shown in the tables and have been calculated for a simple random sample design. In testing for the significant difference between two sample estimates, proportions or means, the sampling error calculated as for a simple random design was multiplied by an assumed design factor of 1.5, to allow for the complex sample design. The reader is referred to Appendix E for an account of the method of calculating true standard errors and for tables of design factors for the main variables and subgroups used throughout this Report. In general, design factors were below 1.5 and therefore there will be some differences in sample proportions and means not commented on in the text, which are significantly different at least at the $p < 0.05$ level.

Weighting

Unless otherwise stated, all proportions and means presented in the tables in the substantive chapters in this Report are taken from data weighted to compensate for the differential probabilities of selection and non-response. Base numbers are presented unweighted and represent the actual number of young people in any specified groups. All base numbers are given in italics.

Summary

Introduction

This Report presents the findings of a survey of the diet and nutrition of young people living in private households in Great Britain aged 4 to 18 years, carried out between January and December 1997. The survey forms part of the National Diet and Nutrition Survey programme which was set up jointly by the Ministry of Agriculture, Fisheries and Food[1] and the Department of Health in 1992 following the successful Dietary and Nutritional Survey of British Adults[2]. MAFF's responsibility for the NDNS programme has now transferred to the Food Standards Agency. This cross-sectional study of young people aged 4 to 18 years is part of a planned programme of surveys covering representative samples of defined age groups of the population. The surveys of older adults and pre-school children have been published[3,4], and the next survey in the series will be of adults aged 19 to 64 years. There has been no nationally representative survey of young people aged 4 to 18 years since the government survey, The Diets of British Schoolchildren, carried out in 1983[5].

The young people in the survey

A nationally representative sample of 2672 young people aged 4 to 18 years was identified from a postal sift of addresses selected from the Postcode Address File. Only young people living in private households were eligible to be included and only one child per household was selected. The interview, which was the first stage of the full survey protocol, was completed for 2127 young people (80% of the identified sample). These 2127 young people are referred to as the interview sample. The numbers of young people in the interview sample were 454 aged 4 to 6 years, 581 aged 7 to 10, 570 aged 11 to 14, and 522 aged 15 to 18 years. Data in the Report are shown separately for boys and girls in these age groups. The survey fieldwork covered 12 months to take account of possible seasonal variation in eating habits. *(Chapters 1 and 3 and Appendix D)*

The interview sample of young people was found to be generally representative of the population in terms of social and demographic characteristics as assessed by reference to the 1996-7 General Household Survey[6,7].

The survey design included an interview to provide information about the socio-demographic circumstances of the young person's household, medication and eating and drinking habits; a weighed dietary record of all food and drink consumed over seven consecutive days; a record of bowel movements for the same seven days; physical measurements of the young person (weight, height, mid upper-arm circumference, and for those aged 11 to 18 years, waist and hip circumferences); blood pressure measurements, a request for a sample of blood and urine; and a dental examination. Young people aged 7 to 18 years also kept a seven-day physical activity diary.

Records of weighed dietary intake were obtained for 1701 young people, that is 80% of those completing the interview and 64% of those identified by the sift. Physical measurements were obtained for over 90% of the interview sample. Consent to the request for a blood sample was given for 1284 young people (60% of the interview sample) and blood was obtained from 1193 young people (56%). The final element in the survey was an assessment of oral health by questionnaire and examination. An examination was achieved for 1726 young people, that is 81% of the young people for whom a dietary interview had been obtained. This final element in the survey took place after all the other elements of the survey had been completed. A full Report of this Oral Health Survey is published separately as Volume 2[8]. A description of the oral health survey is at Appendix V. *(Chapter 3)*

The foods and drinks consumed

The proportion of young people consuming the various foods was based on the numbers of consumers during the seven-day period of recording, which would not necessarily be the same as the proportion of these same young people consuming these foods over any longer period. The following foods were consumed by more than 80% of young people during the seven-day recording period; white bread, savoury snacks, potato chips, savoury sauces, pickles, gravies and condiments, biscuits, and other potatoes (boiled, mashed and jacket). All of these foods were as likely to be consumed by boys as by girls. About half of both boys and girls ate wholegrain and high fibre breakfast cereals but boys were more likely than girls to eat 'other' types of breakfast cereals, 74% compared with 64%. Of the meat and meat products food type, chicken and turkey dishes were consumed by the largest proportions of young people (75% of boys and 73% of girls). Chocolate confectionery was also consumed by a large proportion of young people, 84% of boys and 80% of girls. About two thirds of the young people ate sugar confectionery during the dietary recording period.

During the seven-day recording period more than half the young people in the survey had not eaten any citrus fruits, (not eaten by 76% of boys and 72% of girls), any leafy green vegetables, such as cabbage, greens or broccoli (61% and 56%), any eggs (55% and 56%) and any raw tomatoes (68% and 58%).

Polyunsaturated reduced fat spreads were consumed by just over one third of the young people, and non-polyunsaturated reduced fat spreads by about one quarter of boys and girls; over a quarter had used non-polyunsaturated soft margarine, and a similar proportion had used butter during the 7-day dietary recording period. These proportions represent the use of fats as spreads and do not include their use in cooking.

In the interview, it was reported that 43% of boys and 40% of girls usually had whole milk as a drink, while 49% of both sexes usually had semi-skimmed milk and 3% of boys and 4% of girls had skimmed milk to drink. In all 7% of boys and 8% of girls reported not having milk as a drink, although some of these had it mixed with food, for example on cereals and in puddings.

The majority of young people consumed soft drinks. Half of the boys drinking non-low calorie concentrated soft drinks were estimated to be consuming 1516g (about 1 ½ litres) and half of those consuming low calorie concentrated soft drinks were drinking 2250g (about 2 ¼ litres). The comparable amounts for girls were 1332g (about 1 ⅓ litres) of non-low calorie concentrated soft drinks, and about 1867g of low calorie concentrated soft drinks (about 1 ¾ litres). Half the boys drinking non-low calorie carbonated soft drinks were estimated to be drinking 1008g (about 1 litre) and half of those drinking low calorie carbonated soft drinks were drinking 723g (about ¾ litre) over the seven days. The comparable amounts for girls were 816g (about ¾ litre) of non-low calorie carbonated soft drinks, and about 618g of low calorie carbonated soft drinks (about ½ litre). Fruit juice was consumed by 46% of boys and 51% of girls. Tea was consumed by 45% of boys and 48% of girls, and 17% of both sexes drank coffee. *(Chapter 4)*

About one fifth of young people reported in the interview taking vitamin or mineral supplements, including fluoride. Those who reported taking dietary supplements generally had higher intakes of most vitamins from food than those who did not take supplements. *(Chapter 8)*

Overall 2% of boys and 6% of girls reported dieting to lose weight; this increased to 16% for girls aged 15 to 18 years. One per cent of boys and 5% of girls reported in the interview that they were vegetarian or vegan; among girls aged 15 to 18 years this increased to 10%. *(Chapter 3)*

When the age groups were compared, trends in eating patterns with age were identified. For both boys and girls more of the youngest age groups ate breakfast cereals (not high fibre or wholegrain), biscuits, cereal-based milk puddings, whole milk, fromage frais, ice cream, coated and fried white fish, potato products (not fried), savoury snacks, apples and pears, 'other' fruit, preserves, sugar confectionery, concentrated soft drinks, both low calorie and non-low calorie and non-low calorie ready-to-drink soft drinks. Boys and girls in the oldest age group were more likely to have consumed raw tomatoes, tea and coffee.

The quantity of food consumed generally increased with age. However the mean consumption of whole milk decreased with age from 1391g (just under 2 ½ pints) for boys aged 4 to 6 years to 928g (just under 1 ½ pints) for boys aged 15 to 18 years. The comparable amounts for girls were 1333g (about 2 ½ pints) for those aged 4 to 6 years, and 723g (about 1 ⅓ pints) for those aged 15 to 18 years.

For many food items boys ate significantly larger mean amounts than girls. The most marked differences were for pizza, white bread, breakfast cereals, semi-skimmed milk, bacon and ham, sausages, baked beans, potato chips, nuts and seeds, and carbonated soft drinks (not low calorie). In contrast, girls consumed significantly larger mean amounts of 'other' raw and salad vegetables, raw tomatoes, and apples and pears.

There were small differences in the amounts of foods consumed by boys and girls in the older age groups. Compared with girls aged 15 to 18 years, the oldest group of boys had a higher mean consumption of biscuits, beef, veal and dishes made from them, burgers and kebabs, meat pies and pastries, baked beans, potato chips, boiled, mashed and jacket potatoes and potato dishes and beer and lager. Girls were consuming larger mean amounts of 'other' raw and salad vegetables at ages 4 to 6 years than boys, and this difference persisted throughout the age range, except in the 11 to 14 year age group. *(Chapter 4)*

Energy intake
The mean daily energy intakes for young people the survey were, for boys aged 4 to 6 years, 6.39MJ (1520kcal), aged 7 to 10, 7.47MJ (1777kcal), aged 11 to 14, 8.28MJ (1968kcal) and for those aged 15 to 18 years, 9.60MJ (2285kcal). For girls, mean energy intakes were, for those aged 4 to 6 years, 5.87MJ (1397kcal), aged 7 to 10, 6.72MJ (1598kcal), aged 11 to 14, 7.03MJ (1672kcal) and for those aged 15 to 18 years, 6.82MJ (1622kcal).

For each age/sex group the mean energy intakes were below the Estimated Average Requirements (EARs)[9]. For girls aged 15 to 18 years energy intake was 77% of the EAR. These recorded low values of energy intake are likely to be explained at least partly by under-recording. However, other surveys in the NDNS programme have reported energy intakes below the EAR, and young people in this survey were taller and heavier compared with earlier surveys of the same age groups. This suggests that their energy intakes are unlikely to be inadequate.

At all ages cereals and cereal products made the largest contribution to energy intake, about one third, and this was followed by vegetables, potatoes and savoury snacks, 16% for boys and 18% for girls, and meat and meat products, 14% for boys and 13% for girls. The proportion of energy from milk and milk products reduced from 15% and 16% for boys and girls in the youngest age group to 9% for both sexes in the oldest age group.

The amount of energy derived from each of the macronutrients, protein, carbohydrate and fat, and from alcohol for boys and girls in each of the four age groups is shown in the table below.

(Chapter 5 and Appendix J)

Protein

The mean protein intake for boys was 61.6g and for girls 51.2g, which contributed 13.1% to food energy for both sexes. Boys aged 7 to 10 years obtained the lowest proportion of energy from protein and those aged 15 to 18 years, the highest. For girls, there was no significant difference between the three youngest age groups in the proportion of energy obtained from protein, but girls aged 15 to 18 years obtained a significantly higher proportion. Mean intakes of protein for both boys and girls in each age group considerably exceeded the

Reference Nutrient Intake (RNI)[9]. Meat and meat products contributed 32% to protein intake for boys and 30% for girls, cereals and cereal products 26% and 27% respectively, and for both sexes 18% of protein intake came from milk and milk products.

Carbohydrates, including non-starch polysaccharides (dietary fibre)

The mean daily intake of total carbohydrate, excluding non-starch polysaccharides, was 260g for boys and 214g for girls, which contributed about 51% to food energy intake for both sexes. The mean daily total sugars intake was 117g for boys and 97g for girls, and mean daily intake of starch was 143g and 117g for boys and girls respectively. Total sugars have been further divided into non-milk extrinsic sugars and intrinsic and milk sugars. Non-milk extrinsic sugars provided on average 17% of food energy. The main dietary sources of non-milk extrinsic sugars were drinks, which contributed one third of the total, mainly from soft drinks, followed by sugars, preserves and confectionery, which contributed just under one third. Other major contributors were cereals and cereal products (about one quarter).

Of the starch in the diets of these young people, about 60% was obtained from cereals and cereal products and just over one quarter from vegetables, potatoes and savoury snacks. When intrinsic and milk sugars were added to starch they contributed about 35% of the food energy.

(Chapter 6)

The mean daily intake of non-starch polysaccharides was 11.2g for boys and 9.7g for girls. However intakes increased with age; for example the mean daily intake for girls aged 4 to 6 years was 8.0g and for girls aged 15

Macronutrient contribution to total and food energy intake by sex and age of young person

	Sex and age of young person									
	Males aged (years):				All	Females aged (years):				All
	4 -6	7 - 10	11 - 14	15 - 18		4 -6	7 - 10	11 - 14	15 - 18	
Average daily intake:										
Total energy MJ	6.39	7.47	8.28	9.60	8.01	5.87	6.72	7.03	6.82	6.65
Food energy MJ	6.39	7.47	8.27	9.37	7.95	5.87	6.72	7.02	6.69	6.61
Protein (g)	49.0	54.8	64.0	76.5	61.6	44.5	51.2	52.9	54.8	51.2
Carbohydrate (g)	209	248	271	301	260	191	218	228	214	214
Total fat (g)	60.1	69.8	77.2	89.0	74.7	55.9	63.8	67.2	64.0	63.1
Alcohol (g)	0.01	0.01	0.10	6.79	1.79	0.01	0.02	0.11	3.44	0.93
Percentage food energy from:										
Protein (%)	12.9	12.4	13.1	13.9	13.1	12.7	12.8	12.7	13.9	13.1
Carbohydrate (%)	51.6	52.4	51.7	50.5	51.6	51.4	51.3	51.2	50.6	51.1
Total fat (%)	35.5	35.2	35.2	35.9	35.4	35.9	35.9	36.1	35.9	35.9
Percentage total energy from:										
Protein (%)	12.9	12.4	13.1	13.6	13.0	12.7	12.8	12.7	13.6	13.0
Carbohydrate (%)	51.6	52.4	51.7	49.3	51.2	51.4	51.3	51.1	49.7	50.8
Total fat (%)	35.5	35.2	35.2	35.1	35.2	35.9	35.9	36.1	35.2	35.8
Alcohol (%)	<0.1	<0.1	<0.1	1.9	0.5	<0.1	<0.1	<0.1	1.4	0.4
Base	*184*	*256*	*237*	*179*	*856*	*171*	*226*	*238*	*210*	*845*

to 18 years, 10.6g. The main dietary sources of non-starch polysaccharides were vegetables, excluding potatoes, 17% for boys and 18% for girls, all potatoes, 17% for both sexes, high fibre and whole grain breakfast cereals, 10% for boys and 8% for girls, white bread, 10% and 9% and wholemeal bread, 3% and 4%.

(Chapter 6)

Alcohol

About one quarter of boys and girls aged 7 to 18 years reported in the interview that they had consumed an alcoholic drink in the seven days prior to the interview and about one quarter of 11 to 18 year olds recorded consuming items containing alcohol in their seven-day dietary record. Of those who consumed alcohol in the dietary recording period the percentage of total energy from alcohol increased for both boys and girls with age from 0.4% and 0.6% for boys and girls aged 11 to 14 years, to 4.5% and 3.8% for boys and girls aged 15 to 18 years.

(Chapter 6)

Dietary fats and blood lipids

The mean daily intake of total fat was 74.7g for boys and 63.1g for girls, which contributed 35.4% and 35.9% to the food energy of boys and girls respectively.

Saturated fatty acids contributed an average of 14.2% of food energy for boys and 14.3% for girls. The proportion of energy from saturated fatty acids tended to decline with increasing age, for example from 14.8% for boys aged 4 to 6 years, to 13.9% for boys aged 15 to 18 years.

Trans fatty acids provided 1.4% of food energy for boys and 1.3% for girls. Mean daily intakes were 2.87g and 2.36g for boys and girls.

Cis monounsaturated fatty acids provided 11.7% of food energy for boys and 11.8% for girls. *Cis* n-3 polyunsaturated fatty acids provided 0.8% of food energy for both sexes and *cis* n-6 polyunsaturated fatty acids, provided 5.1% for boys and 5.3% for girls.

The contribution made to the intake of total fat and saturated, *trans* and *cis* monounsaturated fatty acids by *milk and milk products,* although not statistically significant, declined steadily as the age of the young person increased. For example, for boys aged 4 to 6 years milk and milk products contributed 20% to the intake of total fat, and 30% to the intake of saturated fatty acids. By age 15 to 18 years, milk and milk products provided only 13% and 20% of the intake for boys of total fat and saturated fatty acids. The same pattern is seen in the data for girls and reflects the fall in milk consumption with age, particularly of whole milk.

Meat and meat products contributed 21% to the intake of total fat for boys and 18% for girls, 19% to the intake of saturated fatty acids for boys and 16% for girls, in a similar range for *trans* fatty acids, 15% for both boys and girls, but slightly higher for *cis* monounsaturated fatty acids, 25% and 22% respectively.

The consumption of vegetables, potatoes and savoury snacks also accounted for a substantial proportion of the intake of total fat for young people, 18% for boys and 20% for girls. This food group contributed 13% and 15% to the intake of saturated fatty acids for boys and girls respectively and 21% and 23% to the intake of *cis* monounsaturated fatty acids.

The main sources of *cis* n-3 polyunsaturated fatty acids were vegetables, potatoes and savoury snacks, cereals and cereal products, and meat and meat products. Vegetables, potatoes and savoury snacks provided over a third of intake for both boys and girls, mainly from roast and fried potatoes and chips.

The main sources of *cis* n-6 polyunsaturated fatty acids in the diets of young people in the survey were vegetables, potatoes and savoury snacks, (27% of intake for boys and 29% for girls) cereals and cereal products (23% for boys and 21% for girls), fat spreads (16% for both boys and girls), and meat and meat products (18% for boys and 16% for girls).

(Chapter 7)

Blood lipid results are reported for plasma total cholesterol, high density lipoprotein (HDL) cholesterol, non-HDL (LDL) cholesterol, and plasma triglycerides. Where possible, fasting blood samples were collected from the young people. Triglycerides concentration is reported only for those young people who provided a fasting sample. Mean plasma total cholesterol concentration was 4.03mmol/l for boys and 4.24mmol/l for girls. For boys there was no association with age, but for girls mean concentration fell from 4.48mmol/l for girls aged 4 to 6 years to 4.08mmol/l for girls aged 15 to 18 years. Overall 8% of boys and 11% of girls had a concentration at or above 5.2mmol/l. Correlation coefficients for plasma cholesterol concentration with dietary intakes of fat and fatty acids were weak and there was no consistent association within sex and age groups.

(Chapter 12)

Vitamins

Vitamin A intakes were derived from an assessment of daily retinol intakes with a contribution from carotenoid precursors of vitamin A combined as 'retinol equivalents'. The mean daily intake from food sources was 537µg for boys and 487µg for girls. The skewed distribution of intakes of vitamin A (retinol equivalents) resulted in the median intakes being lower than the mean intakes, 465µg for boys and 424µg for girls. Mean intakes were 98% and 93% of the RNI[9] for boys and girls respectively and tended to decrease as age increased. For boys between 8% and 13% had a vitamin A intake from food sources below the LRNI[9].

For girls the proportions were 6% of 4 to 6 year olds, 10% of 7 to 10 year olds, and 20% and 12% for girls in the top two age groups. The main food sources of vitamin A were vegetables, potatoes and savoury snacks, milk and milk products, and meat and meat products, of which about half came from liver and liver products. Dietary supplements containing vitamin A increased mean intakes by 7% overall and by about 15% for those in the youngest age groups. *(Chapter 8)*

Blood samples from the young people were analysed for retinol and several carotenoids. Plasma retinol was significantly and positively correlated with dietary intakes of vitamin A, and α- and β-carotene for all boys and girls. Plasma α- and β-carotene were also significantly positively correlated with dietary intakes of α- and β-carotene, though more strongly for α-carotene. *(Chapter 12)*

Mean daily intakes of thiamin from food sources were 1.59g and 1.31mg for boys and girls respectively, of riboflavin, 1.71mg and 1.34mg, of niacin, 29.1mg and 23.6mg, of vitamin B_{12}, 4.4mg and 3.4mg, of vitamin B_6, 2.2mg and 1.8mg, and of folate 240mg and 194mg.

No more than 2% of any age and sex group had intakes of thiamin, niacin, or vitamin B_{12} below the LRNI[9]. Six per cent of boys in the top two age groups had intakes of riboflavin below the LRNI as did 22% of girls aged 11 to 14 and 21% of girls aged 15 to 18 years. For 1% of boys aged 11 to 14 and girls aged 7 to 14 intakes of vitamin B_6 were below the LRNI; 5% of girls in the oldest age group had intakes below the LRNI. Folate intakes were below the LRNI for 1% of boys aged 11 to 14 years, for 2% of girls aged 7 to 10, 3% of girls aged 11 to 14 and 4% of girls aged 15 to 18 years. The range of intakes of vitamin C was wide and the distribution of intakes was skewed, with mean intakes over 200% of the RNI value[9]. The mean daily intake from food sources was 75.2 mg for boys and 71.2mg for girls. Dietary supplements increased mean intakes by about 6% for both sexes. No more than 1% of any age/sex group had a mean intake of vitamin C below the appropriate LRNI[9]. *(Chapter 8)*

Results for blood analyses of the erythrocyte glutathione reductase activation coefficient (EGRAC), a measure of riboflavin status, serum vitamin B_{12}, red cell folate, serum folate, the erythrocyte transketolase activation coefficient (ETKAC), a measure of thiamin status, the erythrocyte aspartate aminotransferase activation coefficient (EAATAC) a measure of vitamin B_6 status, and vitamin C are reported.

Mean EGRAC for boys was 1.42 and for girls, 1.47. The proportion of boys with an EGRAC greater than 1.30, generally considered as the upper limit of normality, rose from 59% of those aged 4 to 6 years, to 78% for 7 to 10 year olds. For girls the proportion rose from 75% of 4 to 6 years olds to 95% of 15 to 18 year olds. The

apparently high proportion of 'deficient' values is a characteristic of the sensitive assay procedure used and moderately raised values are not associated with known functional abnormality. Dietary intake of riboflavin was significantly negatively correlated with EGRAC for each age/sex group.

Mean serum vitamin B_{12} was 403pmol/l for boys and 395pmol/l for girls. There were no young people in the three youngest age groups with levels below 118pmol/l, but 1% of boys and 8% of girls in the oldest age group had levels below this, the lower level of normality for adults[10]. Levels of serum vitamin B_{12} were positively correlated with dietary intakes of vitamin B_{12} for both boys and girls.

Mean red cell folate was 626nmol/l for boys, and 573nmol/l for girls. Levels of less than 230nmol/l, indicative of severe deficiency[11], were found for no more than 1% of any age/sex group. Levels of less than 350nmol/l, indicative of marginal status, were found for 7% of boys and 9% of girls. Red cell folate correlated positively for both boys and girls with dietary intakes of non-haem iron, folate, vitamin C and vitamin B_{12}.

Mean serum folate was 21.7nmol/l for boys and 20.6nmol/l for girls. Levels of less than 6.3nmol/l, indicative of deficiency[10] were found for 1% of the oldest boys and 1% of girls aged 11 to 18 years.

Mean ETKAC was 1.12 for both boys and girls. There were less than 0.5% of boys and 2% of girls with an ETKAC greater than 1.25, which is indicative of biochemical thiamin deficiency[12]. ETKAC was negatively correlated with dietary intake of thiamin for girls, but not for boys.

Mean EAATAC was 1.80 for boys and 1.79 for girls. Levels greater than 2.00, suggesting possible vitamin B_6 deficiency[10], were found for 10% of both boys and girls.

Mean plasma vitamin C was 56.4μmol/l for boys and 58.8μmol/l for girls. No more than 5% of any age/sex group had a plasma vitamin C of less than 11μmol/l, the lower limit of the normal range[13]. There were strong positive correlations between dietary intake of vitamin C and plasma vitamin C concentration for both boys and girls in each age group. *(Chapter 12)*

Mean daily intakes of vitamin D from foods were low, 2.6μg for boys and 2.1μg for girls. Dietary supplements increased mean intakes from food sources by 8% overall for boys and 5% for girls, and by 19% and 22% for boys and girls in the youngest age group. No DRVs are set for vitamin D for children aged 4 years and over because most of the body's requirements for vitamin D in this age group can be synthesised by the skin if they are sufficiently exposed to sunlight.

The largest contribution to mean intake of vitamin D

for both boys and girls was made by cereals and cereal products, accounting for 37% of intake for boys and 35% of intake for girls. Many breakfast cereals are fortified with vitamin D, and breakfast cereals alone contributed one quarter of the intake of vitamin D for boys and one fifth of the intake for girls.

Fat spreads and meat and meat products each contributed about 20% to mean daily intake of vitamin D for both boys and girls[14]. About half the contribution made by fat spreads came from reduced fat spreads. For boys, 7% of vitamin D intake came from eating oily fish, which is a rich source of vitamin D. For girls, oily fish contributed 9% to vitamin D intake. *(Chapter 8)*

Blood levels of plasma 25-hydroxyvitamin D (25-OHD) were determined and mean values of 62.0nmol/l and 60.6nmol/l are reported for boys and girls respectively. For both sexes, mean concentration fell with age. Significant proportions of those in the older age groups had a poor vitamin D status, as shown by a 25-OHD of less than 25.0nmol/l, 11% of boys and girls aged 11 to 14, and 16% of boys and 10% of girls aged 15 to 18 years. There was a strong seasonal variation, with mean levels being highest in blood samples obtained between July and September. From samples from boys aged 15 to 18 between April and June nearly one in four had a mean 25-OHD of less than 25.0nmol/l. Correlations between plasma levels and dietary intakes of vitamin D were very weak. *(Chapter 12)*

The mean daily intake of vitamin E from food sources was 8.6mg for boys and increased with age; for girls, mean daily intake was 7.6mg and increased with age up to the 11 to 14 age group. Dietary supplements increased mean intake from food sources alone by 2% for boys and 3% for girls. *(Chapter 8)*

Plasma α- and γ-tocopherol concentrations were measured. Mean α-tocopherol was 19.8μmol/l and 20.6μmol/l for boys and girls respectively. Mean γ-tocopherol concentration was 1.48μmol/l for boys and 1.50μmol/l girls. For girls, levels of γ-tocopherol decreased as age increased. For boys there were no significant correlations between plasma α-tocopherol levels and dietary intakes of vitamin E. For girls aged 7 to 10 and 15 to 18 years there were significant positive correlations between plasma α-tocopherol and dietary intake of vitamin E. *(Chapter 12)*

Minerals

Iron and zinc were the only minerals to which dietary supplements made a noticeable contribution. Iron in the diets of the young people was assessed as haem iron (mainly found in meat) and non-haem iron. The mean daily intake of total iron from food sources was 10.4mg for boys and 8.3mg for girls. For haem iron mean intakes were 0.4mg and 0.3mg for boys and girls respectively. Dietary supplements increased total iron intake to 10.5mg for boys and 8.5mg for girls. For boys,

mean intakes were above the RNI[9] for all age groups except those aged 11 to 14 years. For girls, mean intake of total iron was above the RNI for those aged 4 to 6 years, and below the RNI for the other three age groups. For the oldest group of girls, mean intake of iron was 58% of the RNI. No more than 3% of boys in any age group or girls aged 4 to 10 years had intakes below the LRNI[9]. Intakes were below the LRNI for 45% of girls aged 11 to 14 years and 50% of girls aged 15 to 18 years. The main food sources of iron were cereals and cereal products, many of which are fortified, vegetables, potatoes and savoury snacks, and meat and meat products. *(Chapter 9)*

Mean haemoglobin concentration was 13.5g/dl for boys, and 12.9g/dl for girls. For boys mean concentration increased significantly with age. For girls, mean levels only increased between the two youngest age groups. Three per cent of boys and 8% of girls aged 4 to 6 years had blood haemoglobin levels below 11.0g/dl, the WHO limit defining anaemia for children aged 6 months to 6 years[15]. Haemoglobin levels for older children and young people are difficult to interpret due to lack of appropriate reference standards. For older boys and girls, mean haemoglobin levels ranged from 13.0g/dl and 12.8g/dl in the 7 to 10 year group to 14.9g/dl and 13.1g/dl in the oldest age group. For boys and girls, haemoglobin concentration correlated positively with dietary intakes of total, haem and non-haem iron and vitamin C, and additionally for boys, with dietary intakes of vitamin B_{12} and folate.

Mean serum ferritin levels were 39μg/l for boys, and 32μg/l for girls. For boys levels rose significantly with age. Serum ferritin concentrations of less than 20μg/l, the lower limit of the normal range for adult males[10], were found for 13% of boys overall, and ranged from 18% for the youngest group to 5% for the oldest age group. For girls, concentrations of less than 15mg/l, the lower limit of the normal range for adult females[10], were found for between 9% of the youngest group, and 27% of the oldest girls. For boys and girls serum ferritin levels positively correlated with dietary intakes of haem iron, and additionally for boys, with dietary intakes of total and non-haem iron and folate. *(Chapter 12)*

Mean daily intakes of calcium were 784mg for boys and 652mg for girls, for phosphorus, 1105mg and 917mg, and for magnesium, 212mg and 178mg for boys and girls respectively. Mean daily intakes of calcium were above the RNI for boys and girls in the two youngest age groups and below the RNI for those in the two oldest age groups[9]. Between 2% and 5% of children aged 4 to 10 years had calcium intakes below the LRNI[9]. Of those aged 11 to 14 years, 12% of boys and 24% of girls had calcium intakes below the LRNI, as did 9% of boys and 19% of girls aged 15 to 18 years. Mean daily intakes of phosphorus were above the RNI for boys and girls in each age group and there were no young people with intakes below the LRNI[9]. For boys and girls aged 4 to 6 years mean daily intakes of magnesium were above the RNI. Three percent of boys and 1% of girls in this age group had intakes below the LRNI[9]. For those aged 11 to 14 years, mean daily intakes of magnesium were below the RNI and 28% of boys and 51% of girls had intakes below the LRNI. In the oldest group, 18% of boys and 53% of girls had intakes of magnesium below the LRNI.

The main source of calcium was milk and milk products which provided 48% of mean intake for boys and 47% for girls; for both sexes the contribution decreased as age increased. *(Chapter 9)*

Mean plasma magnesium concentration was 0.94mmol/l for boys and 0.91mmol/l for girls. *(Chapter 12)*

Mean daily intake of zinc was below the RNI for all age/sex groups[9]. Mean daily intake from food sources was 6.9mg for boys and 5.7mg for girls. The proportions of boys with mean daily zinc intakes below the LRNI[9] in the four age groups were 12% aged 4 to 6 years, 5% aged 7 to 10, 14% aged 11 to 14, and 9% aged 15 to 18 years. For girls, the corresponding proportions with intakes below the LRNI[9] in the four age groups were 26%, 10%, 37%, and 10%.

The mean daily intake of copper was 0.88mg for boys and 0.75mg for girls. For boys, mean daily intakes were above the RNI for each age group[9]. For girls, intakes for those aged 4 to 10 years were above the RNI, and below the RNI for the two oldest age groups[9].

Mean daily intake of iodine was above the RNI for boys and for girls aged 4 to 10 years, and slightly below the RNI for girls aged 11 to 18 years[9]. No more than 3% of boys in any age group had a daily intake of iodine below the LRNI[9]. For girls aged 4 to 6 years 2% had a daily intake below the LRNI[9], increasing to 13% for those aged 11 to 14 years.

Mean daily intake of manganese was 2.20mg for boys and 1.87 mg for girls. *(Chapter 9)*

Blood samples were analysed for plasma zinc, selenium and lead. For boys and girls mean plasma zinc concentration was 14.6µmol/l, and for girls decreased steadily with age. Dietary intakes for selenium were not available, however mean plasma selenium concentration was 0.86µmol.l for boys, and 0.87µmol/l for girls. Levels were significantly higher in the oldest group of boys and girls compared with those aged 4 to 6 years. There were no levels as low as 0.11µmol/l which would correlate with frank selenium deficiency. Mean blood lead levels were low and decreased with age, ranging between 2.4µg/dl for boys aged 15 to 18 and 3.3µg/dl for boys aged 4 to 6 years. For girls in the corresponding age groups mean blood lead levels were 2.0µg/dl and 2.9µg/dl. None of the girls, but 1% of all boys, and 2% of 4 to 6 year-old boys had a blood lead concentration at or above 10µg/dl, the upper tolerable limit. *(Chapter 12)*

Intakes of sodium and chloride, excluding additions during cooking and at the table, were both, on average, about twice the RNI values[9]. Mean daily intake of sodium was 2630mg for boys and 2156mg for girls. For chloride, mean intakes were 3954mg for boys and 3241mg for girls. Mean daily intake of potassium was 2343mg for boys and 2026mg for girls. Mean intakes of potassium were above the RNI for both boys and girls in the two youngest age groups, and below the RNI for those aged 11 to 18 years[9]. No more than 1% of boys or girls aged 4 to 10 years had a mean daily intake of potassium below the LRNI[9]. For those aged 11 to 14 years, intakes were below the LRNI for 10% of boys and 19% of girls, and for those aged 15 to 18 years, were below the LRNI for 15% of boys and 38% of girls.

Single void urine samples were collected from the young people in the survey and analysed for sodium, potassium and creatinine. Sodium and potassium are expressed as ratios to creatinine excretion. The urinary sodium to urinary creatinine ratio was 14.0mol/mol for boys and 14.4mol/mol for girls. The urinary potassium to urinary creatinine ratio was 4.8mol/mol for both boys and girls. Correlations between the urinary sodium to urinary creatinine ratio and dietary intake of sodium were weak. Correlations between the urinary potassium and urinary creatinine ratio and dietary intake of potassium were positive and strongest for those in the youngest age group. Overall, the urinary sodium to urinary creatinine ratio was significantly negatively correlated with Body Mass Index (BMI) for both boys and girls; however for girls aged 15 to 18 years there was a significant positive correlation. *(Chapter 9)*

Anthropometric measurements

Mean height increased with individual year of age for both boys and girls. There were no significant differences in mean height between boys and girls in the three youngest groups. Boys were significantly taller than girls from the age of 14 years.

Mean weight increased with individual year of age for both boys and girls. Boys were significantly heavier than girls from the age of 16 years.

Mean Body Mass Index (BMI) was the same, 16, for boys from ages 4 to 8 years and for girls from ages 4 to 7 years. For both sexes mean BMI increased significantly with grouped age.

For both boys and girls mean mid upper-arm circumference was significantly greater in the oldest compared with the youngest age group. Boys aged 7 to 10 years and 15 to 18 years had a significantly greater mid upper-arm circumference than girls in the same age groups.

Mean waist and hip circumferences increased with grouped age and waist circumference was greater for boys in both age groups (11 to 14 and 15 to 18 years) than for girls.

Mean hip circumference was greater for girls aged 11 to 14 years than for boys in the same age group. Waist to hip ratio did not vary significantly by grouped or individual year of age for boys. For girls, waist to hip ratio was lower for those aged 15 to 18 than for those aged 11 to 14 years.

Measurements of height, weight and BMI were compared with data for young people aged 4 to 15 years in the Health Survey for England carried out in 1995–97[16], and with data for white young people aged 5 to 10 years living in England from the National Survey of Health and Growth carried out in 1994[17]. The measurements for the comparable groups in the NDNS were broadly similar to those from the other surveys and there were no significant differences by sex or age between the three data sets. *(Chapter 10)*

Stage of sexual development in boys

Plasma testosterone concentration was measured in blood samples from boys aged 10 to 16 years, and, as expected, mean concentration increased with age.

There was no significant variation associated with plasma testosterone tertile in mean Body Mass Index (BMI), weight, mid upper-arm circumference, waist or hip circumference or waist to hip ratio for boys aged 10 to 16 years. After adjusting for age, mean haemoglobin and red blood cell count both increased with testosterone concentration, while plasma total and HDL cholesterol concentrations and mean blood lead concentration all decreased with increasing testosterone concentration.

Variation in anthropometric measurements

Because of the strong association between age and the various anthropometric measurements, the technique of multiple regression analysis was used to identify those characteristics, including age, which were independently associated with variation in the measures. The analysis was carried out to examine variation in Body Mass Index and waist to hip ratio.

After controlling for the effects of the other characteristics entered into the model, BMI was positively associated with age for both boys and girls.

Characteristics that were positively associated with BMI for both boys and girls aged 4 to 18 years were systolic blood pressure, average daily total energy intake, and whether the young person reported currently dieting to lose weight.

In addition, for boys aged 4 to 18 years BMI was significantly associated with region, percentage energy from total fat, percentage energy from total sugars, and gross weekly household income. Boys living in London and the South East had, on average, a lower BMI, and those living in Scotland a higher BMI, than the overall average. Boys living in households with a gross weekly household income of less than £160 had, on average, a lower BMI.

Girls aged 4 to 18 years for whom menarché had occurred had a higher BMI than girls for whom menarche had not occurred and there were also inverse relationships between BMI and father's reported height and for those from a manual social class background.

A separate analysis for those aged 7 to 18 years which included the calculated physical activity score found no significant independent association between this measure and BMI for boys or girls.

After controlling for the effects of the other characteristics entered into the model, for both boys and girls aged 11 to 18 years age was inversely associated with waist to hip ratio and positively associated with whether the young person reported currently being on a diet to lose weight.

In addition, boys aged 11 to 18 years living in London and the South East had, on average, a lower waist to hip ratio than the overall average. Those living in Northern England and the Central and South West regions and Wales had a higher waist to hip ratio than average. Boys living in households with two parents and other children had a significantly lower waist to hip ratio than average.

In addition for girls aged 11 to 18 years, those who had reached menarché had a lower waist to hip ratio than other girls as did girls from a non-manual social class background and those who reported being current smokers. There was an inverse relationship between BMI and father's reported height and girls who reported currently being on a diet to lose weight had a significantly greater waist to hip ratio than other girls. *(Chapters 10 and 12)*

Blood pressure

Blood pressure was measured by the automated technique (Dinamap) used in previous surveys and the Health Survey for England (HSE)[16]. Mean systolic pressure was 110mmHg and 108mmHg for boys and girls respectively, and diastolic pressure was 56mmHg for both sexes. Blood pressure increased significantly with age for both boys and girls. Increased systolic pressure was associated with the use of salt at the table for both boys and girls and with use of salt in cooking for girls, with smoking and the consumption of alcohol for boys and with Body Mass Index (BMI) for girls. After adjusting for age, there was no significant association between plasma testosterone tertile and systolic or diastolic blood pressure for boys aged 10 to 16 years.

Both boys and girls had systolic and diastolic measurements which were significantly lower than the measurements obtained from boys and girls of the same age in the Health Survey for England[16]. This is believed to be due to the different field methodologies used in the NDNS and Health Survey for England.

Variation in blood pressure

The technique of multiple regression analysis was used to identify those characteristics which were independently associated with variation in blood pressure for young people. Results are reported for a number of analyses for different sub-groups in the sample, based on whether a physical activity diary was completed and whether, for boys, a blood testosterone sample was obtained.

Overall for boys aged 4 to 18 years the most significant associations with systolic blood pressure were with the physiological measurements included in the analysis, that is with diastolic blood pressure and weight. Age was also independently related to systolic blood pressure for boys. Taking account of all other variables in the model, there was a significant inverse association with systolic blood pressure for boys who were unwell during the 7-day dietary recording period and whose eating was affected and a significant positive relationship with systolic blood pressure for boys who were smokers.

For girls aged 4 to 18 years, as for boys, the most significant associations with systolic blood pressure were with diastolic blood pressure and body weight. There was also a significant inverse relationship for girls living in London and the South East.

An analysis for boys and girls aged 7 to 18 years, which included the calculated physical activity score, showed no significant association between this measure and systolic blood pressure for either sex, and blood testosterone concentration was not associated with variation in systolic blood pressure for boys aged 10 to 16 years.

In the regression analysis to identify characteristics independently related to variation in diastolic blood pressure, for boys aged 4 to 18 years the strongest relationship was between diastolic pressure and systolic pressure. There were also significant inverse independent relationships between diastolic blood pressure and weight, with the urinary potassium to creatinine ratio and for those interviewed in Wave 3 of fieldwork, July to September.

Overall for girls aged 4 to 18 years variation in diastolic pressure was significantly and positively associated with systolic pressure. There were also significant independent associations with fieldwork wave, positively for those interviewed in Wave 1 (January to March) ($p < 0.05$) and inversely for those interviewed in Wave 3 (July to September). Living with one parent and other children, usually adding salt to the food during cooking and body weight were all independently inversely related to diastolic blood pressure for all girls.

The analysis for boys and girls aged 7 to 18 years, which included the calculated physical activity score, showed no significant association between this measure and diastolic blood pressure for either sex, and blood testosterone concentration was not associated with variation in diastolic blood pressure for boys aged 10 to 16 years. *(Chapter 11)*

Physical activity

Level of physical activity was assessed for young people aged 4 to 6 years by questions to their parents in the initial interview. For those aged 7 to 18 years, physical activity information was recorded in a diary for the same seven days as the dietary record. Physical activity was estimated using a number of measures, including a calculated activity score, the total number of activities of at least moderate intensity and mean hours spent in activities of at least moderate intensity per day.

About 50% of young people aged 4 to 18 years walked to school, about one third travelled by car, and about 20% by bus. Between 1% and 6% cycled to school. Boys were significantly more likely than girls to cycle to school. Older children were significantly less likely to travel by car. Of 4 to 6 year olds, 95% were reported by their parents to be fairly or very active. Boys were more likely to be reported as very active than girls.

Of young people aged 7 to 18 years, girls were less active than boys and activity levels fell as age increased.

About 40% of boys and about 60% of girls spent, on average, less than 1 hour a day in activities of at least moderate intensity and they therefore failed to meet the HEA recommendation for young people's participation in physical activity. For boys and girls in the oldest age group the proportions spending less than 1 hour a day in activities of at least moderate intensity were 56% and 69% respectively. Based on a calculated activity score, 3% of boys and girls aged 7 to 18 were classified as 'inactive', 21% and 26% respectively as 'moderately active' and 79% and 74% as 'active'. However, it is suggested that this classification in inappropriate for young people in that it overestimates activity levels. For boys aged 7 to 10 years and girls in all age groups the total number of activities of at least moderate intensity participated in during the seven-day recording period was positively correlated with dietary intake of energy. For all boys and girls aged 7 to 18 years systolic blood pressure was negatively correlated with mean hours spent in all activities of at least moderate intensity.

The proportion of boys and girls who participated in activities of at least moderate intensity was higher at most individual years of age for young people in this NDNS compared with young people of the same age in the Health Survey for England[16]. The mean number of hours in which young people participated in activities of at least moderate intensity were broadly similar between the two surveys for both boys and girls. Taking into account differences between the two surveys in their methodologies, it is concluded that the data on selected measures of physical activity from this NDNS and the Health Survey for England are broadly similar.

Variation in physical activity

The technique of multiple regression was used to identify characteristics with the strongest relationships to the calculated activity score.

For both boys and girls aged 7 to 18 years, the calculated activity score rose significantly with age independently of the other characteristics included in the analysis.

For boys aged 7 to 18 years, the independent socio-demographic and behavioural characteristics that contributed significantly to explaining variation in the calculated activity score, were whether the young person was at school or work, fieldwork wave, age, gross weekly household income and whether they were living with both parents. For girls aged 7 to 18 years, the independent characteristics that contributed significantly to explaining variation in the calculated activity score, were whether the young person was at school or work, percentage energy from total sugars, fieldwork wave, region and average daily alcohol intake.

The data suggest that young people were more active than average in the summer wave (Wave 3, July to September) and the spring wave (Wave 2, April to June) and less active than average in the autumn and winter waves (Wave 1, January to March and Wave 4, October to December). Young people who were attending school only or school and work were less active than average, while those who attending work only or who were not at school or work were more active than average.

For girls aged 7 to 18 years, calculated activity score was independently positively associated with both percentage energy from sugars and average daily intake of alcohol.

For boys aged 7 to 18 years, those from the middle income group were less active than average and those living with a single parent and other children were more active than average. For girls aged 7 to 18 years, those living in the Northern region were significantly less active than average. *(Chapter 13)*

School meals

Among 4 to 10 year olds, school meals provided more than half the total consumption of puddings, fish, vegetables, chips and 'other' potatoes and over one third of meat products. Among 11 to 18 year olds, school meals provided over one half the total consumption of chips and over a third of fish and vegetables. In both age groups, young people who had a free school meal tended to obtain more energy and nutrients from their school meal than those who paid for their school

meal. Those 4 to 10 years olds who took no school meal had significantly lower fat, non-starch polysaccharides and protein intakes than those obtaining a free school meal and higher non-milk extrinsic sugars and vitamin C intakes. Where a school meal was eaten by 4 to 10 year olds, buns, cakes and pastries contributed 30% of non-milk extrinsic sugars intake and 13% to 15% of intakes of energy, fat, saturated fatty acids, carbohydrate, iron and vitamin A. Chips provided 20% of vitamin C intakes and 11% to 15% of energy, fatty acids, carbohydrate, non-starch polysaccharides and folate intakes. Meat pies and pastries also provided 7% of saturated fatty acids intakes.

There were no significant differences between blood cholesterol levels and haematological analytes for 4 to 10 year olds according to the type of school lunchtime meal. *(Appendix X)*

Young people who were unwell

Eighteen per cent of boys and 20% of girls were reported to be unwell on at least one day during the dietary recording period; this included 10% of boys and 11% of girls whose eating was affected by being unwell.

Mean energy intakes were lowest for those whose eating was affected. For boys mean energy intakes were 7.10MJ for those who were unwell and whose eating was affected compared with 8.16MJ, for those who were not unwell. For girls mean energy intakes for the same two groups were 5.63MJ and 6.78MJ respectively. *(Chapter 5)*

Young people who were unwell had lower mean intakes of protein, total carbohydrate, starch, intrinsic and milk sugars and non-starch polysaccharides. However the proportion of food energy derived from total carbohydrates was similar for those who were unwell and not unwell, suggesting that in respect of carbohydrates the reduced intake was due to reduced energy intake and not to any selective avoidance of carbohydrates by the unwell group. There was no difference in mean alcohol intake for boys or girls aged 11 to 18 years between those who reported being unwell, either with or without their eating being affected, and those who were not unwell during the dietary recording period. *(Chapter 6)*

Young people who reported being unwell had lower mean daily intakes of total fat and all fatty acids; however, when intakes were expressed as a percentage of food energy intake there were no significant differences between the well and unwell groups. *(Chapter 7)*

Compared with those who were not unwell, boys who reported being unwell and whose eating was affected had significantly lower absolute mean daily intakes from food sources of pantothenic acid, vitamin E, riboflavin and vitamin B_6. Girls whose eating was affected by being unwell had significantly lower intakes of pre-formed retinol, vitamin A, riboflavin, niacin, vitamins B_6, B_{12}, and C, folate, pantothenic acid, total carotene and biotin. When differences in energy intake were taken into account the only significant differences remaining between those who were unwell and whose eating was affected and those who were not unwell, were, for both boys and girls, intake of pantothenic acid per MJ energy and, additionally for girls, intake of biotin per MJ food energy.

(Chapter 8)

Compared with girls who reported not being unwell during the 7-day dietary recording period, those who said they were unwell and their eating was affected had lower mean daily intakes of all minerals from food sources, except haem iron. For boys mean daily intakes of phosphorus, magnesium and potassium, non-haem iron, sodium, chloride, zinc, copper and iron, were significantly lower for the unwell group.

When differences in mean daily intake of energy were taken into account, none of the differences between those who were unwell and whose eating was affected and those who were not unwell remained. This suggests that the quality of the diet did not change when the young person was unwell, but they simply had a lower energy intake.

(Chapter 9)

There were no differences in mean levels between the unwell and not unwell groups for any of the haematological indices. For girls, mean levels of red cell folate, α-cryptoxanthin and plasma HDL cholesterol were all lower for those whose eating was affected by being unwell, compared with those who were not unwell. For boys, mean levels of γ-tocopherol were higher for those whose eating was affected by being unwell than for boys who were not unwell during the dietary recording period.

(Chapter 12)

Region

The nationally representative sample of young people was sub-divided into four 'regions' for purposes of analysis, based on where the young person was living at the time of interview.

There was considerable variation in the diets of both boys and girls according to the region in which they lived, only some of which was common to both sexes.

Both boys and girls in Scotland were significantly less likely to eat other cereals (not wholegrain or high fibre), other white fish and dishes, green beans, leafy green vegetables, fried and roast potatoes, sauces, pickles, gravies and condiments[18]. Boys and girls living in the Northern region were less likely to have eaten fried and roast potatoes, and those living in the Central and South West regions of England and Wales were less likely to have had soup. In London and the South East

boys and girls who kept a seven-day diary were less likely to have recorded eating other cereals, beef, veal and dishes made from these, non-low calorie carbonated soft drinks, and soup.

(Chapter 4)

Despite there being some significant variation in the types of foods eaten by young people according to the region in which they lived, there was very little difference between the mean energy intakes in each region, and none reached the level of statistical significance. There was almost no variation between young people living in different regions in mean daily intakes of protein, carbohydrate or alcohol. Mean intakes of non-starch polysaccharides were lowest for those living in Scotland, and highest for those in the Central and South West regions and Wales.

(Chapters 5 and 6)

There were no significant regional differences in mean daily intakes of fat or fatty acids for boys or girls. When energy intake was taken into account there were no differences for boys in the percentage of food energy derived from total fat and fatty acids intake. However girls living in Scotland and the Northern region derived significantly more food energy from *cis* monounsaturated fatty acids than girls in the Central and South West regions of England and Wales.

(Chapter 7)

There were very few significant regional differences in the intake of vitamins or minerals. Mean absolute intake of vitamin D and mean intake of vitamin D per MJ food energy were significantly higher for boys living in the Central and South West regions of England and Wales compared with boys living in Scotland, indicating a difference in the quality of the diet between these two groups. The only significant differences for girls were for mean absolute intakes of folate and pantothenic acid which were significantly higher for girls living in the Central and South West regions of England and Wales compared with girls living in Scotland. For girls, after allowing for differences in energy intake, those in Scotland had significantly lower intakes per MJ of energy for thiamin, folate and pantothenic acid than girls who lived in the Central and South West regions and Wales.

There were significant differences for both copper and magnesium intakes between boys in Scotland, who had the lowest mean absolute intakes, and boys in London and the South East who had the highest mean absolute intakes.

There were significant differences for mean absolute intakes of total and non-haem iron and magnesium between girls living in Scotland who had the lowest, and girls living in the Central and South West regions of England and Wales, who had the highest mean intakes. Mean intakes of sodium and chloride were significantly different and highest for girls in the Northern region and lowest for those in London and the South East.

When differences in energy intake were taken into account, for boys, there were significant differences for total and non-haem iron between boys living in Scotland, who had the lowest mean intake per MJ, and boys living in the Central and South West regions of England and Wales, who had the highest mean intake per MJ. Boys in Scotland also had a lower mean intake per MJ of manganese compared with boys living in London and the South East and intake of zinc per MJ energy for boys living in the Northern region was significantly lower than for all other boys except those living in Scotland.

Compared with girls living in the Northern region, girls living in the Central and South West regions of England and Wales had significantly higher mean intakes per MJ of total and non-haem iron and manganese. Girls in the Central and South West regions of England and Wales also had a higher mean intake of potassium per MJ than girls in London and the South East. Compared with girls in London and the South East the diets of girls in Scotland were richer in sodium, since mean intake per MJ, after allowing for variation in energy intake, was significantly higher. *(Chapters 8 and 9)*

The blood results showed very few regional differences. Girls living in London and the South East had a higher mean serum ferritin concentration than other girls. Of the water soluble vitamins the only regional differences were again for girls, those living in the Central and South West regions and Wales having a lower EAATAC than girls in the Northern region, and those in the Northern region having the lowest mean plasma vitamin C concentration. Boys living in the Central and South West regions and Wales had a higher mean plasma total cholesterol than those in Scotland. Mean levels of plasma selenium were lower for boys in Scotland and girls in the Central and South West regions and Wales. *(Chapter 12)*

Socio-economic characteristics

Young people in the survey were classified according to the social class of head of household, based on occupation, which for reporting was described as manual and non-manual backgrounds. Other socio-economic measures were whether the young person's parent(s) were receiving Family Credit, Income Support or Job Seeker's Allowance, and gross weekly household income. In non-benefit households and in households in the higher income groups, the proportion of the older age groups was higher and it is noted that apparent differences in food and nutrient intake by income group and receipt of benefits may therefore, at least in part, be accounted for by these differences in the age distributions.

There were several differences in the proportions of consumers of different foods associated with the socio-economic characteristics considered[19]. Boys from a lower socio-economic background were significantly less likely to have eaten fruit pies, softgrain bread, semi-skimmed milk, cream, other cheese, fromage frais, other dairy desserts, butter, bacon and ham, fruit juice and other beverages. Girls from a lower socio-economic background were significantly less likely to have consumed cream, other cheese, other raw and salad vegetables, green beans, other fruit, fruit juice, and wine. Both boys and girls from a lower socio-economic background were more likely than others to have consumed whole milk and table sugar. *(Chapter 4)*

There were no differences in mean daily intake of energy for boys or girls associated with social class. Among boys, but not girls, there was a marked difference in mean energy intake depending on whether the parents were in receipt of state benefits. Boys living in households receiving benefits had a mean energy intake of 7.22MJ, significantly below that for boys living in non-benefit households, 8.27MJ. Among boys mean energy intake was lowest for boys living in households where the gross income was below £160 a week, and highest for those in households with a gross weekly income of £400 to less than £600 ($p < 0.01$). For girls the pattern was similar although the differences were not statistically significant. *(Chapter 5)*

Mean intakes of protein, total carbohydrate, total sugars, non-milk extrinsic sugars and NSP were significantly lower for young people from households in the lower income groups (gross weekly household income of less than £160 compared with £600 and over) and for those from households that were in receipt of benefits than for other young people. The data suggest that young people from manual households had lower intakes of these nutrients than other young people, although the only significant difference was for total sugars. None of the indicators of lower economic status was associated with either significantly lower starch intakes or significantly lower percentages of food energy from total carbohydrate.

Young people aged 11 to 18 years living in households with the lowest gross weekly household income and those from households receiving benefits were less likely to have consumed alcohol than those from households in the highest income group and those not in receipt of benefits. For the total sample aged 11 to 18 years, mean alcohol intake increased with income, and young people from households that were in receipt of benefits had significantly lower mean alcohol intakes than others. *(Chapter 6)*

There were no significant differences associated with the social class of the head of household for either boys or girls in mean absolute intakes of fat or fatty acids. When fat and fatty acids intake was expressed as a percentage of food energy intake, the data show that the diets of boys, but not girls from a manual home background were richer in *cis* monounsaturated, total *cis* polyunsaturated and *cis* n-6 polyunsaturated fatty acids. The proportion of food energy they derived from these fatty acids was significantly higher than for other boys.

Boys living in households receiving benefits had significantly lower mean intakes of total fat and nearly all fatty acids (except *cis* n-3 polyunsaturated fatty acids) compared with boys living in households not receiving benefits; in contrast for girls there were no significant differences in mean intakes. However, when intakes were expressed as a percentage of food energy intake, there were no significant differences in the fatty acids composition of the diets of boys or girls from households receiving and not receiving benefits.

Mean daily intake of total fat was highest for boys in the middle household income group, £280 to less than £400. For saturated and *trans* fatty acids and cholesterol, mean intakes were highest for boys living in households where the gross weekly household income was between £400 and £600. When intakes were expressed as a percentage of food energy, boys in households where the gross weekly household income was between £400 and £600 had a significantly lower percentage energy from total *cis* and *cis* n-6 polyunsaturated fatty acids than boys in the lowest household income group and boys in households where the gross weekly income was between £280 and £400. For girls there were no significant differences in fat and fatty acids intake associated with household income level. When intakes were expressed as a percentage of energy intake the only difference was the relatively low proportion of food energy derived from *cis* monounsaturated fatty acids for girls in the highest household income group (£600 a week or more) compared with girls in the lowest household income group. *(Chapter 7)*

Although there was a general pattern for young people from manual social class backgrounds to have lower mean daily intakes from food sources of most vitamins than young people from non-manual home backgrounds, there were very few statistically significant differences in mean intake. For both boys and girls mean intakes of vitamin C were markedly lower for those from a manual social class background. Additionally for boys from a manual background, intake of pantothenic acid was lower and for girls from a manual background, mean intake of biotin was lower.

After allowing for differences in energy intake, mean intake of vitamin C from food sources per MJ still varied significantly by social class for both boys and girls, and for boys there also remained a significant difference in intake per MJ energy for pantothenic acid and for girls for intake per MJ energy for biotin.

Absolute mean daily intakes of thiamin, riboflavin, niacin, vitamin B$_6$, folate, biotin and pantothenic acid, vitamin C and vitamin E were lower for boys in households receiving benefits than in households not receiving benefits. There was much less variation in the

intakes of vitamins for girls living in benefit and non-benefit households. For girls, mean intakes were significantly lower for those in benefit households for only vitamin C and biotin. After allowing for differences in energy both boys and girls living in benefit households had significantly lower mean daily intakes of vitamin C from food sources per MJ energy than young people in non-benefit households. Boys in benefit households also had significantly lower intakes per MJ of energy of biotin and pantothenic acid. For girls, but not boys, intakes per MJ of both riboflavin and niacin were also lower for those living in benefit households.

Generally, and before allowing for differences in total energy intake, mean daily intakes from food sources of most vitamins increased as gross weekly household income increased. For boys there were significant differences in mean absolute intakes of vitamins associated with household income for riboflavin, niacin, folate, biotin, pantothenic acid, and vitamin C, total carotene, thiamin and vitamins B$_6$, B$_{12}$ and E. For girls there were differences associated with household income for biotin and vitamin C, total carotene, niacin and folate. After allowing for differences in total energy intake, the only significant differences associated with household income for boys were for biotin and pantothenic acid where the boys in the lowest income households had significantly lower mean daily intakes per MJ than boys in the highest income households. Intakes of vitamin C per MJ energy were significantly lower for boys in households with a gross weekly income of between £280 and £400 than for boys in the highest household income group. Intakes of vitamin D per MJ were significantly lower for boys in households with a gross weekly income of between £400 and £600 than for boys in households with a gross weekly income of up to £280.

For girls, intakes of vitamin C, total carotene and niacin were still significantly lower for the lowest income group compared with the highest income group, after allowing for differences in energy intake. *(Chapter 8)*

For boys intakes of calcium, and for girls intakes of phosphorus, magnesium and manganese, and for both sexes intakes of iodine, were lower for those from a manual background. Most of these differences are likely to reflect differences in the quality of the diet in respect of these minerals, since after allowing for differences in energy intake, boys from a manual background had a lower mean intake of calcium, phosphorus, magnesium and iodine, than boys from a non-manual background. For girls, intakes of phosphorus, magnesium, iodine and manganese per MJ energy were lower for the manual group, while adjusted intakes of sodium were higher for this same group of girls.

Mean daily intakes of all minerals, except haem iron, were significantly lower for boys living in benefit households than for those in non-benefit households.

In contrast there were no significant differences in mean daily intake of minerals between girls living in benefit and non-benefit households. Most of the differences in mineral intake for boys were accounted for by differences between the two groups in energy intake. Only for calcium and haem iron was the mean daily intake significantly lower for boys in benefit households when calculated per MJ energy. For girls, those living in households where neither parent was receiving benefits had diets richer in calcium, phosphorus and iodine, than girls in benefit households, since the mean intake per MJ energy for these minerals was significantly higher for the non-benefit group.

Comparing intakes for boys in the lowest household income group with those for boys in households with an income of between £400 and £600 a week, there were statistically significant differences in the absolute intake of all minerals except haem iron and copper. For girls, mean daily intakes of calcium, phosphorus and magnesium were significantly higher for those in the top compared with the bottom household income group. After allowing for differences in mean energy intake the only difference remaining for boys was for calcium, with boys in households with a weekly income of between £400 and £600 consuming a diet richer in calcium than those in the lowest income group. For girls, mean daily intakes of calcium, phosphorus and magnesium were still significantly higher in the highest income group than in the lowest income group when calculated per MJ energy. *(Chapter 9)*

Of the socio-economic characteristics considered, gross weekly household income was associated with more differences in mean blood analyte levels than receipt of benefits or social class of head of household. Generally, levels of blood analytes were higher for those from a higher socio-economic background and there were more differences for boys than girls.

Boys in households in the highest income group had higher mean levels of mean cell haemoglobin, mean cell volume, plasma iron percentage saturation, plasma iron concentration, plasma vitamin C, plasma zinc, plasma retinol, and α-cryptoxanthin than boys from households in the lowest income group. For girls there were significant differences between those in the highest and lowest income groups for mean levels of plasma vitamin C, plasma retinol, α- and β-cryptoxanthin, α- and β-carotene, and 25-OHD. Mean levels of plasma selenium were lowest for boys in households with a gross weekly household income of £280 to £400 and girls in households with a weekly income of between £160 and £280.

Comparing young people living in households receiving and not receiving benefits, mean levels of vitamin C and α- and β-cryptoxanthin and α- and β-carotene were lower for both boys and girls in benefit households. Additionally for boys, mean levels of haemoglobin concentration, mean cell haemoglobin and plasma retinol was lower for those in benefit households. Girls in households in receipt of benefits had a lower mean lycopene concentration than girls in households not receiving benefits.

Girls from a manual social class background had lower mean concentrations of vitamin C and α-cryptoxanthin and boys from a manual background had a lower mean concentration of serum folate.

Mean blood lead concentration was higher for boys in households in the lowest income group, in households receiving benefits, and for boys from a manual social class background. *(Chapter 12)*

Household type

This classification is based on whether the young person was living with one or both parents, with or without other children. It is noted that there was significant variation in the age distribution for young people by household type, with a much larger proportion of young people aged 15 to 18 years living with both parents and no other children than in other types of household. Any variation associated with differences by household type may therefore be partly accounted for by variation by age.

There were relatively few significant differences in the types of foods eaten by young people living with both parents between those who had other children in their household and those who were the only child at home. There were no clear dietary patterns evident from the data, and the variation was somewhat different for boys and girls. Where the young person was living with both parents and was the only child in the household compared with those living with both parents and other children, both boys and girls were less likely to have eaten fromage frais, apples and pears and sugar confectionery, and to have drunk low calorie concentrated soft drinks and non-low calorie ready to drink soft drinks. Girls from two-parent households with no other children were also less likely to have eaten breakfast cereals, which were not high fibre or whole-grain types. Boys in households with both parents and no other children were more likely than those in two-parent households with other children to have consumed non-polyunsaturated soft margarine, beef, veal and dishes made from them, beer and lager, and coffee, and for girls, semi-skimmed milk, wine, beer and lager, alco-pops and tea. Foods which were less likely to be eaten by young people living with both parents and no other children were also less likely to be consumed by young people living in lone-parent households (with or without other children). For example biscuits, savoury snacks and ready-to-drink soft drinks (not low calorie) were consumed significantly less often both by boys in lone-parent households and in two-parent households with no other children. Girls from lone-parent households were also less likely to have drunk low calorie concentrated soft drinks. *(Chapter 4)*

Boys living with both parents, but with no other children in the household had a significantly higher energy intake than other boys. Their mean energy intake was 8.98MJ (2147kcal) compared with 7.72MJ (1845kcal) for boys living with only one parent. For girls there were no differences in mean energy intake associated with household type.   *(Chapter 5)*

Young people who were living with both parents and no other children had significantly higher mean daily intakes of protein and starch compared with those living with a single parent and those living with both parents and other children. Those living with both parents and no other children also had a significantly higher mean daily intake of non-starch polysaccharides than those living with both parents and other children; the proportion of energy they derived from total carbohydrate was significantly lower. Young people aged 11 to 18 who were living with both parents and no other children had a significantly higher mean daily intake of alcohol and obtained a higher proportion of their energy from alcohol than young people living with both parents and other children.   *(Chapter 6)*

Mean intakes of total fat and each fatty acid were consistently higher for boys living with both parents and no other children than mean intakes for boys living with both parents and other children or in one-parent households, reflecting higher energy intake in this group. Boys living with both parents and no other children and those living in one-parent households, both derived a higher proportion of their food energy from *cis* monounsaturated fatty acids, than did boys living with both their parents and other children.

For girls, the only significant difference in absolute intake was for total *cis* polyunsaturated fatty acids; girls living with both parents and no other children had a higher intake than girls living with both parents and other children. This group also derived a higher proportion of food energy from total *cis* polyunsaturated fatty acids and from *cis* n-6 polyunsaturated fatty acids than girls living with both parents and other children.   *(Chapter 7)*

Comparing mean absolute intakes of vitamins for boys in two-parent, no other children households and boys in single-parent households, there were significant differences in the mean daily intakes of niacin and of vitamins B_6 and B_{12}, folate, biotin and vitamin E. In each case boys from one-parent households had a significantly lower mean daily intake from food sources of the vitamin. There were no differences associated with household type in absolute intake of vitamins for girls. After allowing for differences in total energy intake, mean daily intake of niacin per MJ for boys living in two-parent households with other children, remained lower than for boys living in two-parent households with no other children.   *(Chapter 8)*

Boys living in households with both parents and no other children had the highest mean daily intake of all minerals, including sodium and chloride. For girls, the differences associated with household type were very small and none of the differences in mean intake of any of the minerals reached the level of statistical significance. After allowing for differences in mean energy intake, mean intakes of minerals per MJ energy were still generally highest for boys living in two-parent households with no other children. However, the only differences to reach the level of statistical significance were for mean intakes of phosphorus, potassium and zinc per MJ for boys in two-parent, no other children households, compared with boys in two-parent other children households. There were no significant differences for girls after allowing for differences in mean energy intake.   *(Chapter 9)*

References and endnotes

1 Responsibility for this survey and the National Diet and Nutrition Survey programme transferred from the Ministry of Agriculture, Fisheries and Food to the Food Standards Agency on its establishment in April 2000.

2 Gregory J, Foster K, Tyler H, Wiseman M. *The Dietary and Nutritional Survey of British Adults.* HMSO (London, 1990).

3 Finch S, Doyle W, Lowe C, Bates CJ, Prentice A, Smithers G, Clarke PC. *National Diet and Nutrition Survey: people aged 65 years and over. Volume 1: Report of the diet and nutrition survey.* TSO (London, 1998).

4 Gregory JR, Collins DL, Davies PSW, Hughes JM, Clarke PC. *National Diet and Nutrition Survey: children aged 1½ to 4½ years. Volume 1: Report of the diet and nutrition survey.* HMSO (London, 1995).

5 Department of Health. Report on Health and Social Subjects: 36. *The Diets of British Schoolchildren* HMSO (London, 1989).

6 Thomas M, Walker A, Wilmot A, Bennett N. *Living in Britain. Results from the 1996 General Household Survey.* TSO (London, 1998)

7 1996-7 GHS subsample of households containing at least one young person aged 4 to 18 years.

8 Walker A, Gregory J, Bradnock G, Nunn J, White D. *National Diet and Nutrition Survey: Young people aged 4 to 18 years. Volume 2: Report of the Oral Health Survey.* TSO (London, 2000).

9 Department of Health. *Dietary Reference Values for Food Energy and Nutrients for the United Kingdom.* Report on Health and Social Subjects 41. HMSO (London, 1991).

10 Dacie JV, Lewis SM. *Practical Haematology.* 8th Edition. Churchill Livingstone (Edinburgh, 1995)

11 Sauberlich HE, Skala JH, Dowdy RP. *Laboratory tests for the assessment of nutritional status.* CRC Press (Cleveland, Ohio, 1974)

12 Bates CJ, Thurnham DI, Bingham SA, Margetts BM, Nelson M. Biochemical Markers of Nutrient Intake. In: *Design Concepts in Nutritional Epidemiology.* 2nd Edition. OUP (Oxford, 1997) pp170–240.

13 Sauberlich HE. Vitamin C status: methods and findings. *Ann N Y Acad Sci* 1971; **24**: 444–454

14 Measurable amounts of vitamin D and its metabolites have now been found in meats as a result of new analytical methods. New data for poultry and meat products became available for this survey resulting in higher assessed intakes of vitamin D compared with previous surveys.

15 World Health Organisation. *Nutritional Anaemias.* Technical Report Series: 503. WHO (Geneva, 1972).

16 Prescott-Clarke P, Primatesta P. Eds. *Health Survey for England. The Health of Young People '95–97. Volume 1: Findings.* TSO (London, 1998).

17 The National Study of Health and Growth was set up in 1972 to monitor the growth of primary school children. For example, see Chinn S, Price CE, Rona RJ. The need for new reference curves for height. *Arch Dis Childh* 1989; **64**: 1545–1553.

18 Comparisons are based differences between the reference group, in this case young people living in Scotland, and those living in the region with the highest proportion of consumers of the food.

19 Differences reported here are those which were significantly different on at least two of the three socio-economic measures, that is, social class of head of household, receipt of benefits and gross weekly household income.

1 Background, purpose and research design

This chapter describes the background to the National Diet and Nutrition Survey (NDNS) of young people aged 4 to 18 years, its main aims and the overall sample and research designs and methodologies. The next chapter and its associated appendices give a more detailed account of the various methodologies for the different elements of the survey.

1.1 The National Diet and Nutrition Survey Programme

The National Diet and Nutrition Survey programme is a joint initiative, established in 1992, between the Ministry of Agriculture, Fisheries and Food (MAFF) and the Department of Health (DH) which followed the successful completion and evaluation of the benefits of a survey of the diet and nutritional status of British adults aged 16 to 64 years carried out in 1986/7[1]. MAFF's responsibility for the NDNS programme has now transferred to the Food Standards Agency.

The NDNS programme aims to provide comprehensive, cross-sectional information on the dietary habits and nutritional status of the population of Great Britain. It also contributes to the health improvement programme set out in the Government's White paper, *Saving Lives: Our Healthier Nation*[2].

The NDNS programme is intended to:

- provide detailed quantitative information on the food and nutrient intakes, sources of nutrients and nutritional status of the population under study as a basis for Government policy;
- describe the characteristics of individuals with intakes of specific nutrients that are above and below the national average;
- provide a database to enable the calculation of likely dietary intakes of natural toxicants, contaminants, additives and other food chemicals for risk assessment;
- measure blood and urine indices that give evidence of nutritional status or dietary biomarkers and to relate these to dietary, physiological and social data;
- provide height, weight and other measurements of body size on a representative sample of individuals and examine their relationship to social, dietary, health and anthropometric data as well as data from blood analyses;

- monitor the diet of the population under study to establish the extent to which it is adequately nutritious and varied;
- monitor the extent of deviation of the diet of specified groups of the population from that recommended by independent experts as optimum for health, in order to act as a basis for policy development;
- help determine possible relationships between diet and nutritional status and risk factors in later life;
- assess physical activity levels of the population under study; and
- provide detailed information on the condition and function of the tissues of the mouth in relation to dietary intake and nutritional status.

The NDNS programme is divided into four separate surveys, planned to be conducted at about three-yearly intervals. Each survey is intended to have a nationally representative sample of a different population age group: children aged 1½ to 4½ years; young people aged 4 to 18 years; people aged 65 years and over, and adults aged 19 to 64 years. The reports of the NDNS of children aged 1½ to 4½ years and of people aged 65 and over were published in 1995 and 1998 respectively[3,4].

The next survey in the programme will be of adults aged 19 to 64 years, commissioned jointly by the Food Standards Agency and the Department of Health.

1.2 The need for a survey of young people

The Government's White Paper, *Saving Lives: Our Healthier Nation* set out the key areas and targets for improving health as appropriate to children and young people. For example, in relation to targets for reducing death rates from coronary heart disease (CHD) and stroke, the White Paper noted that "...diet is central to our health throughout life. A balanced diet in childhood helps to ensure that children grow well and do not become overweight as they get older. Good nutrition throughout life, with plenty of fruit and vegetables, cereals, and not too much fatty and salty food, will help protect against coronary heart diseases, stroke and some cancers. Taken together with physical activity a healthy diet enhances not just length but also the quality of life."[2] There is therefore a need for Government to be informed about the diet and nutritional status of young people.

The only large national survey of the diets of school-age children was carried out in 1983[5]. Since then other studies have focused on subgroups of the school-age population, for example, children aged 13 and 14 years living in urban areas, adolescents living in Northern Ireland and adolescents living in the West of Scotland; there have been no further national surveys[6,7,8].

The 1983 survey was commissioned to investigate the effect of the 1980 Education Act, which released Local Authorities from the statutory requirement to provide school meals to prescribed nutritional standards. The survey provided extensive data on the dietary habits of British schoolchildren and the contributions made by school meals at that time. Two age groups were studied; children aged 10 and 11 years, and children aged 14 and 15 years. The survey found that the diets of British schoolchildren were generally adequate but provided more than the recommended amount of energy from fat. The diets of some children, particularly the girls, also fell short in several vitamins and minerals including riboflavin, iron and calcium[5]. Appendix W summarises the main findings of the 1983 schoolchildren's diet survey.

Since the 1983 survey it is likely that the diets of young people, in common with the diets of adults, have changed in response for example to changes in lifestyles, and the variety of foods available. 'Fast food' outlets have become widely available and are popular with young people, as are 'ethnic' foods that are available as 'take-aways' as well as restaurant meals. In schools the type and range of foods offered has changed; nowadays schools provide self-service meals and snacks, as well as more traditional served school lunches. Moreover many secondary-age school children can be seen leaving school premises at lunchtime to eat food taken from home, or items purchased outside school[9]. The contribution of food eaten at school lunchtime to the overall diet and nutrition of young people is of major interest.

One of the major uses of the NDNS data is for food chemical risk assessment. The availability of up-to-date survey data is important to ensure that estimates of dietary exposure to food chemicals are as close to reality as possible. Estimates for young people had been based on the Department of Health survey of the diets of British schoolchildren[5]. However this survey was limited in scope, and had become out of date with respect to the trends in the diets of this age group, particularly teenagers. For these reasons a new survey of this age group was needed.

MAFF and DH therefore commissioned the Social Survey Division of the Office for National Statistics (ONS) and the Medical Research Council (MRC) to carry out this work. The MRC component was conducted by the Micronutrient Status Laboratory, Cambridge, initially at MRC Dunn Nutrition Unit

(DNU), and more recently at MRC Human Nutrition Research[10]. Staff at the DNU were responsible for obtaining ethical approval for the survey from National Health Service Local Research Ethics Committees (LRECs), for recruiting the blood takers and dealing with those aspects of the survey concerned with the venepuncture procedure and urine samples. A Survey Doctor was employed by the DNU principally to liaise with and deal with questions from LRECs, to provide support for ONS fieldworkers and the blood takers in the event of any medical problem arising, to identify abnormal results from blood pressure measurements and blood analyses and bring them to the attention of the young person's GP, and to be available to answer any questions from respondents on the venepuncture and blood pressure procedures[11]. ONS, as the lead contractor, was responsible for all other aspects of the dietary and oral health components of the survey, including sample and survey design, recruitment and training of fieldworkers, data collection and analysis. For the oral health component of the survey, ONS collaborated with, and sub-contracted work to the Dental Schools at the Universities of Birmingham, Newcastle, Dundee and Wales.

1.3 The aims of the survey

The survey was designed to meet the overall aims of the NDNS programme in providing detailed information on the current dietary behaviour, nutritional status and oral health[12,13] of young people living in private households in Great Britain. Additionally the survey was designed to:

- provide data to assist in the development of dietary guidelines for young people, including dietary guidelines for food provided by schools;
- determine the frequency of bowel movement in this age group;
- provide baseline and comparative data for blood pressure and some anthropometric measurements in this age group;
- provide baseline and comparative data for some haematological and biochemical indices in blood and urine in this age group.

The survey design therefore needed to incorporate methods for collecting detailed information on the young person's household circumstances, general dietary behaviour and health status, on the quantities of foods consumed, and on physical activity levels, anthropometric measures, blood pressure levels and blood and urine analytes. Additionally an oral health component was needed to collect information on oral health behaviour and on the number and condition of the teeth, and the condition of the gums and other oral soft tissues[12,13].

1.4 The sample design and selection

A nationally representative sample of young people

aged 4 to 18 years living in private households was required. It was originally estimated that an achieved sample of about 2000 young people was needed for analysis, distributed across four age groups, 4 to 6 years, 7 to 10 years, 11 to 14 years and 15 to 18 years. The age groups were defined to correspond to the age groups for Dietary Reference Values[14]. However, since the youngest age group, 4 to 6 years, only covers three years, rather than four years as in the older age bands, it was agreed that the overall achieved sample should be proportionally adjusted to account for this; hence an achieved sample of about 1880 young people was desired.

As in previous surveys in the NDNS series, fieldwork was required to cover a 12-month period, to cover any seasonality in eating behaviour and in the nutrient content of foods, for example, full fat milk. The 12-month fieldwork period was divided into four fieldwork waves, each of three months duration. The fieldwork waves were:

Wave 1: January to March 1997
Wave 2: April to June 1997
Wave 3: July to September 1997
Wave 4: October to December 1997

Where there was more than one young person between the ages of 4 and 18 years living in the same household, only one was selected to take part in the survey. As well as reducing the burden of the survey on the household, and therefore reducing possible detrimental effects on co-operation and data quality, this reduces the clustering of the sample associated with similar dietary behaviour within the same household and improves the precision of the estimates. For the same reason it was decided that, unlike the earlier survey of the eating habits of school-age children[5], the sample should be household based and <u>not</u> school based, that is the first stage units should be a sample of private addresses and not a sample of schools with young people selected from lists of those attending the school.

The sample was selected using a multi-stage random probability design with postal sectors as first stage units. The sampling frame included all postal sectors within mainland Great Britain, and selections were made from the small users' Postcode Address File. The frame was stratified by 1991 Census variables.

A total of 132 postal sectors was selected as first stage units, with probability proportional to the number of postal delivery points, and 33 sectors were allocated to each of the four fieldwork waves. The allocation took account of the need to have approximately equal numbers of households in each wave of fieldwork, and for each wave to be nationally representative. From each postal sector 210 addresses were randomly selected. To identify households that contained an eligible young person, each selected address was sent a

postal sift form which asked for details of the sex and date of birth of every person living at the address. After two reminder letters, all non-responding addresses together with all multi-household addresses were called on by an interviewer in an attempt to collect the same information as on the sift form. The postal sift was also conducted in four waves, sift forms being sent out to the addresses in the relevant 33 selected postal sectors about five months before the start of the fieldwork wave. Copies of the sift form and accompanying letter are reproduced in Appendix A.

From the postal and interviewer sift returns, households containing an *eligible* young person were identified. Eligibility was defined as being aged between 4 and 18 years on the date of the mid-point of the relevant fieldwork wave. As fieldwork covered a three-month period, at the time of interview eligible young people could have been slightly under 4 years or slightly over 18 years.

One eligible young person was randomly selected from each household identified by the sift procedures as containing an eligible young person. To improve the statistical efficiency of the sample design, by reducing the effects of clustering and re-weighting, only half the households containing just one eligible child were selected. As the resulting sample of young people was larger than needed for fieldwork, sub-sampling was then carried out to reduce the overall set sample size and to achieve the required numbers of male and female young people in the four age groups.

A more detailed account of the sample design and response to the postal sift stages is given in Appendix D. Appendix E gives true standard errors and design factors for the main classificatory variables used in the analysis of the survey data, for intakes of energy and selected nutrients, anthropometric variables, including blood pressures and the biochemical measures, the blood and urine analytes.

1.5 The elements of the survey

These were as follows:

- an initial face-to-face interview using computer assisted personal interviewing methods (CAPI) to collect information about the young person's household, their usual dietary behaviour, smoking and drinking habits (those aged 7 years and over only); their health status, and their use of dietary supplements, herbal remedies and medicines;
- a 7-day weighed intake dietary record of all the food and drink consumed by the young person both in and out of the home;
- a record of the number of bowel movements the young person had over the 7-day dietary recording period;

- a 7-day physical activity diary collected over the same period as the dietary record (those aged 7 years and over only);
- anthropometric measurements: standing height, body weight, mid upper-arm circumference and, for those aged 11 years and over, waist and hip circumferences;
- blood pressure measurements;
- the collection of a spot urine sample;
- if consent was given, a venepuncture procedure to collect a fasting sample of blood;
- a short post-dietary record interview to collect information on any unusual circumstances or illness during the period which might have affected eating behaviour;
- a face-to-face interview, using CAPI, to collect information on the young person's oral health history and oral health behaviour, and an oral health examination[12,13].

While the aim was to achieve co-operation with all the various elements, the survey design allowed for a young person to participate in only some elements.

Depending on the age of the young person the interviews were conducted either with a parent, usually the mother, or were conducted jointly with the parent and young person. For young people who had left the parental home the interviews were conducted with the subject alone.

From age 11 years and over most young people were expected to keep their own dietary, bowel and physical activity record; younger children needed varying levels of help from parents, teachers and other carers. As a token of appreciation a gift voucher for £5 was given to the young person if the dietary record was kept for the full 7 days[15]. Each young person was also given a record of his or her anthropometric and blood pressure measurements.

To help the ONS nutritionists evaluate the quality of the dietary records completed by the young people, interviewers completed a quality assessment questionnaire. This included information on how accurate the interviewers thought the weighing and recording of items eaten in and out of the home had been and whether the diary was an accurate reflection of the young person's actual diet during the recording period.

Copies of the fieldwork documents and the interview questions are given in Appendix A.

Feasibility work carried out in February to April 1996 by the Social Survey Division (SSD) of ONS and the MRC Dunn Nutrition Unit tested all the elements of the survey and made recommendations for revisions for the mainstage[16]. A second fieldwork test, mainly to evaluate changes to the dietary and physical activity recording documents, was carried out in October 1996.

For a sub-group of the initial feasibility study sample the validity of the dietary recording methodology was tested using the doubly-labelled water methodology to compare energy expenditure against reported energy intake[17]. For the same sub-group the physical activity information collected in the diary was validated by directly measuring the young person's activity level using a motion sensor, the Tritrak monitor. Further details of the design and results of the feasibility studies are given in Appendix C.

1.6 Fieldwork

Over the fieldwork period a total of 67 ONS interviewers worked on the survey, the majority working in at least two waves. All the interviewers working on the survey had been fully trained by the Social Survey Division of ONS and most had experience of working on other surveys in the NDNS programme, or of other surveys involving record-keeping such as the Family Expenditure Survey (FES)[18].

Each interviewer attended a five-day personal, residential briefing before starting fieldwork. The briefing was conducted by research and other professional staff from the Social Survey Division of ONS, staff from MAFF and DH, and from the Dunn Nutrition Unit (DNU). Prior to the residential briefing each interviewer was required to keep and code his or her own 3-day weighed intake record.

At the briefing interviewers received individual feedback from the nutritionists on their record-keeping and coding and were trained in all aspects of the survey. The main elements covered by the training were:

- obtaining consents;
- the questionnaire interview, in particular how to deal with certain 'sensitive' topics;
- completing the weighed intake dietary record;
- collecting the physical activity information;
- checking, probing and coding the dietary record;
- techniques for making the anthropometric measurements and measuring blood pressure;
- collecting the spot urine sample;
- the procedures for obtaining a blood sample;
- the oral health interview[12,19].

Emphasis was placed on the need for accuracy in recording and coding and in measurement techniques. Practice in the anthropometric measurements was achieved by measuring a group of young people who joined the briefing for the relevant session. A representative of the company supplying the sphygmomanometers assisted with the training on blood pressure measurement[20].

In addition to the personal briefings, written instructions were provided for all interviewers and for the phlebotomists who would be taking the blood samples. Interviewers working on non-sequential fieldwork waves were recalled for a one-day refresher briefing to maintain the accuracy of dietary coding and anthropometric and blood pressure measurement techniques.

In order that appropriate official bodies and personnel were informed about the nature of the survey, letters were sent by ONS, prior to the start of fieldwork, to Chief Constables of Police, Directors of Social Services, Public Health and Education and to Chief Executives in Health Authorities with responsibility for one or more of the selected fieldwork areas (postal sectors). The letters gave information on when and where the survey would take place, what was involved in the survey and asked that appropriate personnel at a more local level be informed. Copies of these letters are reproduced in Appendix B.

In keeping with SSD normal fieldwork procedures, a letter was sent to each eligible household in the sample in advance of the interviewer calling, telling them briefly about the survey (see *Appendix A*).

1.7 Plan of the report

This report presents data on the dietary, anthropometric, and physiological components of the survey, including physical activity levels. A separate report presents the results from the oral health component, both the interview and the examination[13].

Chapter 2 and its associated appendices describe the methodologies and procedures used in the survey, including the 7-day weighed intake record, the physical activity diary, anthropometry and blood pressure, the urine sample and the venepuncture procedure. Details of the weighing and recording procedures and subsequent coding and editing of the dietary records are given, including details of the procedures for collecting information about items consumed out of the home.

The purpose and choice of anthropometric measurements made and the techniques and instruments used are reported. The reasons for the choice of blood pressure monitor are discussed and the protocol for taking the measurements is described. Chapter 2 also explains the reasons why a 'spot' urine sample was preferred to a 24-hour urine collection, and then gives details of the equipment used. The purpose of the venepuncture procedure and the protocol, including the use of an anaesthetic cream is described. An account of the laboratory processing procedures and the quality control methods and data are given in Appendix Q.

Chapter 3 gives response data for the various elements in the survey and describes the characteristics of the responding sample.

In the subsequent chapters of the report the data presented are based on the samples of young people co-operating with the relevant aspect of the survey rather than those who completed all elements.

The substantive results from the survey are presented in Chapters 4 to 13. Chapters 4 to 9 are primarily concerned with food and nutrient intake data derived from the analyses of the dietary records and the results are presented for different socio-demographic groups in the overall responding sample - for example, by age group, gender, region, social class of head of household and household type.

Chapter 4 reports on the quantities of foods consumed by the different socio-demographic groups. Chapter 5 reports on energy intakes; intakes of carbohydrates, protein and alcohol are given in Chapter 6, and of fats and fatty acids in Chapter 7. In Chapters 8 and 9, data on average daily intakes of vitamins and minerals are given, from food sources alone and from all sources, that is including any dietary supplements being taken. Throughout these chapters, actual intakes are compared with dietary reference values, where appropriate. Chapter 9 also includes results from the analyses of the spot urine samples.

Chapter 10 reports on the anthropometric data – the measurements of height, weight, mid upper-arm circumference, waist and hip circumference, and derived indices. Values are compared with measurements recorded on other surveys. The chapter also considers the associations between the anthropometric measurements and other characteristics of the young people, such as their smoking and drinking behaviour, energy intakes and physical activity levels.

Chapter 11 reports on the results of the blood pressure measurements. The relationships between blood pressure levels and health characteristics, such as smoking and body size are considered. The chapter also examines the relationships between blood pressure and the use of salt and intakes of sodium.

The results from the analyses of the samples of blood are presented in Chapter 12. Where relevant, the associations between dietary intakes and blood levels are examined; for example blood lipid levels with fat and fatty acid intakes.

The final substantive chapter reports on the physical activity information collected in the interview and for the older children in the physical activity diaries.

Inevitably, given the volume of data collected in the survey and the potential range of analyses, this report can only present initial findings. It is therefore largely concerned with providing basic descriptive statistics for the variables measured and their association with social, demographic and behavioural characteristics of the sample population. It has only been possible to present in this report a limited amount of data on the associations between the dietary, physiological, biochemical and activity data.

As noted earlier, the only similar national survey of this age group was carried out in 1983[5], the extent to which comparisons can be made between the results from this present NDNS of young people and other studies is therefore limited and is generally restricted to the dietary intake information.

Like previous surveys in the NDNS programme, a copy of the survey database, containing the full data set will be deposited following publication of this report with The Data Archive at the University of Essex. Independent researchers who wish to carry out their own analyses should apply to the Archive for access[21].

References and endnotes

1   Gregory J, Foster K, Tyler H, Wiseman M. *The Dietary and Nutritional Survey of British Adults.* HMSO (London, 1990).
2   Department of Health. *Saving Lives: Our Healthier Nation.* TSO (London, 1999).
3   Gregory JR, Collins DL, Davies PSW, Hughes JM, Clarke PC. *National Diet and Nutrition Survey: children aged 1½ to 4½ years. Volume 1: Report of the diet and nutrition survey.* HMSO (London, 1995).
4   Finch S, Doyle W, Lowe C, Bates CJ, Prentice A, Smithers G, Clarke PC. *National Diet and Nutrition Survey: people aged 65 years and over. Volume 1: Report of the diet and nutrition survey.* TSO (London, 1998).
5   Department of Health. Report on Health and Social Subjects: 36. *The Diets of British Schoolchildren* HMSO (London, 1989).
6   Hackett AF, Kirby S, Howie M. A national survey of the diet of children aged 13-14 years living in urban areas of the United Kingdom. *J Hum Nutr Dietet* 1997; **10**: 37–51.
7   Strain JJ, Robson PJ, Livingstone MBE et al. Estimates of food and macronutrient intake in a random sample of Northern Ireland adolescents. *Br J Nutr 1994*; **72**: 343–352.
8   Anderson A, Macintyre S, West P. Dietary patterns among adolescents in the West of Scotland. *Br J Nutr* 1994; **71**: 111–122.
9   Gardner Merchant. *What are today's children eating?* The Gardner Merchant School meals survey, Gardner Merchant Ltd (1998).
10 For simplicity and concordance with fieldwork documents (Appendix A), this organisation is referred to throughout as Dunn Nutrition Unit (DNU). However all communications regarding this aspect of the survey should be directed to MRC Human Nutrition Research, Cambridge.
11 Further details of the role and responsibilities of the Survey Doctor are given in Chapter 2.
12 An interview asking about the young person's oral health behaviour was carried out at the last visit to the household in connection with the dietary survey. After the interview the young person was asked to consent to the ONS interviewer calling back with a dentist to carry out an examination of their teeth, gums and other oral soft tissues. The results relating to the oral health component of the survey, including the interview and examination data, are presented in a separate report.
13 Walker A, Gregory J, Bradnock G, Nunn J, White D. *National Diet and Nutrition Survey: Young people aged 4 to 18 years. Volume 2: Report of the Oral Health Survey.* TSO (London, 2000).
14 Department of Health. *Dietary Reference Values for Food Energy and Nutrients for the United Kingdom.* Report on Health and Social Subjects 41. HMSO (London, 1991).
15 Gift vouchers were from WH Smith Ltd.
16 Lowe S. *Feasibility study for the National Diet and Nutrition Survey: young people aged 4 to 18 years.* ONS *(In preparation).*
17 Smithers G, Gregory J, Coward WA, Wright A, Elsom R, Wenlock R. British National Diet and Nutrition Survey of young people aged 4 to 18 years: feasibility study of the dietary assessment methodology. Abstracts of the Third International conference on Dietary Assessment Methods. *Eur. J. Clin. Nutr.* (1998) **52**: S2. S76.
18 Down D. Ed. *Family Spending. A Report on the 1998–99 Family Expenditure Survey.* TSO (London, 1999).
19 Training in the oral examination for interviewers and dentists was provided at a separate residential briefing.
20 The Dinamap 8100 oscillometric blood pressure monitors were supplied by Johnson and Johnson Medical Ltd, Ascot, Berkshire, UK SL5 9EY.
21 For further information about the archived data contact:
The Data Archive
University of Essex
Wivenhoe Park
Colchester
Essex CO4 3SQ
UK
Tel: (UK) 01206 872001
Fax: (UK) 01206 872003
EMAIL: archive@essex.ac.uk
Website: www.data-archive.ac.uk

2 Methodologies and procedures

2.1 The choice of dietary methodology

The survey used a weighed intake methodology since its main aims were to provide detailed quantitative information on the range and distribution of intakes of foods and nutrients for young people aged 4 to 18 years in Great Britain, and to investigate relationships between nutrient intakes, physical activity levels and various nutritional status and health measures.

The advantages and disadvantages of this method and the factors affecting the choice are discussed in Appendix F.

The age range for this NDNS is wide and it was anticipated that the age of the young person would have a bearing on the methodology used. Feasibility work was therefore conducted to determine whether the weighed intake methodology was suitable for use with this age range and to provide information on whether a 7-day recording period would be acceptable (see *Appendix C*)[1]. In particular the feasibility study was designed to determine how to obtain the highest rate of completed diaries in all age groups, 4 to 6 years, 7 to 10 years, 11 to 14 years and 15 to 18 years, and to determine whether it was possible to collect a 7-day diary for all groups, taking account of the effect of the length of the recording period on response and the quality of the dietary information recorded.

For a sub-set of the feasibility survey sample, group estimates of energy expenditure, derived from measurements of the excretion of water labelled with stable isotopes, 'doubly-labelled water', were compared with energy intake, estimated from the weighed intake dietary record[2]. The results showed a sufficient agreement overall for adopting the methodology for the mainstage survey, but also clearly indicated that for the oldest group of girls, those aged 15 to 18 years, there were significant underestimates of energy intake[1,3]. Special attention was paid to this group in the main stage to try to improve the quality of the dietary information.

2.2 Choice of number and pattern of recording days

In deciding to use a weighed intake methodology, the period over which to collect information for an individual needed to be considered. Ideally it needed to be long enough to give reliable information on usual food consumption, but this had to be balanced against the likelihood of poor compliance if the recording period was lengthy.

The feasibility study concluded that it was possible to collect dietary information for a 7-day period from respondents of all ages and that the levels of response and quality of information would be acceptable.

For reasons of interviewer working arrangements, diaries were almost never placed on Saturdays or Sundays and only infrequently on Fridays; this means that the first day of recording was only rarely a Sunday or Monday. Apart from this interviewers were not required to place diaries to a fixed placement pattern, for example placing equal numbers of diaries on each day of the week. The effects of this on the data have not been investigated in this report.

2.3 The questionnaire

Before starting the dietary record, background information about the young person's usual dietary behaviour and about their household was collected, using the computer-assisted personal interviewing method (CAPI). The choice of respondent depended on the age and ability of the young person. Usually the young person and a parent, generally the mother, were interviewed together. Information was also collected on the young person's eating arrangements at lunchtimes on school days; the consumption of artificial sweeteners and herbal teas and drinks; any foods that were avoided and the reasons for doing so, including vegetarianism and dieting behaviours, the use of salt at the table and in cooking, the use of fluoride preparations and dietary supplements, and information on the young person's health status. Information on the frequency of consumption of a number of food types, together with information about the consumption of skin or peel on vegetables and fruit was collected; the respondent was offered the choice of self-completing this information using the interviewer's laptop computer (Computer Assisted Self Interviewing – CASI) or responding to questions from the interviewer.

For all young people aged 7 years and over, the interview also collected information on their smoking and drinking behaviour, and for girls aged 10 years and over on their age at menarché and whether they were taking the oral contraceptive pill. Because these topics were considered sensitive, in that some young people might prefer not to have to answer these questions in front of a parent or the interviewer, the young people were given the option of answering the questions on these topics on either a paper self-completion document or by CASI, entering the answers themselves direct into the interviewer's laptop computer.

The interview questionnaire is reproduced in Appendix A.

Information was also collected which was of use to the interviewer when checking the dietary record, for example, the young person's usual eating pattern on weekdays and at weekends, and on the types of certain commonly consumed food items usually eaten, such as milk, bread and fat spreads, (that is full or low fat milk, white or wholemeal bread, etc).

When the interviewer called back on the household at the end of the seven dietary recording days the main diary keeper was asked if there had been any special circumstances which might have affected the young person's eating behaviour during the period, such as a family celebration. Information was also collected on any illness the young person had during the recording period and any prescribed medication taken.

2.4 The dietary record

The parent and/or young person, depending on the age of the young person, was asked to keep a weighed record of all food and drink consumed by the young person, both in and out of the home, over seven consecutive days. From feasibility work it was expected that young people from about 10 years upwards would be able to keep their own dietary record. Under 10 years the majority of record keeping would need to be done by the young person's mother or other carer. In describing the procedures for weighing and recording the dietary information we have assumed, for clarity, that the young person was the main diary keeper.

Each young person was issued with a set of accurately calibrated Soehnle Quanta digital food scales and two recording diaries; the 'Home Record' diary for use when it was possible for foods to be weighed, generally foods eaten in the home, and a smaller 'Eating and Drinking Away From Home' diary (the 'eating out' diary) for use when foods could not be weighed – generally foods eaten away from home. The 'eating out' diary was also designed for recording information on the young person's physical activities, and for keeping a record of any bowel movements the young person had while they were away from home, over the same 7-day period. The instruction and recording pages from these documents relating to the dietary information are included in Appendix A.

The young person, together with any other household member who might be involved in keeping the diary,

was shown by the interviewer how to use the scales to weigh food and drinks, including how to zero the scales after each item was weighed so that a series of items put on to the same plate could be weighed separately. Instructions were also given on how to weigh and record leftovers, and how to record any food that was spilt or not eaten, which could not be re-weighed.

The 'Home Record' diary was the main recording and coding document. For each item consumed over the seven days a description of the item was recorded, including the brand name of the product, and where appropriate the method of preparation. Also recorded were the weight served and the weight of any leftovers, the time food was eaten, whether it was eaten at home, at school or elsewhere, and whether fruit and vegetables were home grown, defined as being grown in the household's own garden or allotment. Who did the weighing, the young person or someone else, was also recorded for each food item and for each day the young person was asked to indicate whether they were 'well' or 'unwell'.

Young people who completed a full 7-day dietary record were given a £5 gift voucher by the interviewer, as a token of appreciation. It was made clear that receiving the voucher was not dependent on co-operation with any other aspect of the survey, in particular, consenting to provide a blood sample.

2.4.1 The recording procedure

Recording what the young person consumed in the diaries started from the time the interviewer left the home; the interviewer called back approximately 24 hours after placing the diaries in order to check that the items were being recorded correctly, to give encouragement and to re-motivate where appropriate.

Everything consumed by the young person had to be recorded, including medicines taken by mouth, vitamin and mineral supplements and drinks of water. Where a served item could not be weighed, the young person was asked to record a description of the portion size, using standard household measures, such as teaspoons, or to describe the size of the item in some other way.

Each separate item of food in a served portion needed to be weighed separately in order that the nutrient composition of each food item could be calculated. For example, for a sandwich the bread, spread and filling(s) all needed to be weighed and recorded separately. In addition, recipes for all home-made dishes were collected.

The amount of salt used either at the table or in cooking was not recorded, as it would have been very difficult to measure accurately. However questions on the use of salt in the cooking of the young person's food and the young person's use of salt at the table were asked at the interview. All other sauces, pickles and dressings were recorded. Vitamin and mineral supplements and artificial sweeteners were recorded as units consumed, for example, one teaspoon of Canderel Spoonful.

A large amount of detail needed to be recorded in the dietary record to enable similar foods prepared and cooked by different methods to be coded correctly, as such foods will have different nutrient compositions. For example, the nutrient composition of crinkle cut chips made from old potatoes and fried in a poly-unsaturated oil is different from the same chips fried in lard. Therefore, depending on the food item, information could be needed on cooking method, preparation and packaging as well as an exact description of the item before it could be accurately coded.

Young people were encouraged to record details in the diary, including weight information if at all possible, of any leftovers or food that was spilt or dropped. Further details on the recording of leftovers and spillage are given in Appendix F.

The 'eating out' diary was intended to be used only when it was not possible to weigh the food items. In such cases, young people were asked to write down as much information as possible about each food item consumed, particularly the portion size and an estimate of the amount of any left over. To encourage this the diary had a centimetre rule printed around the edge of the diary page. Prices, descriptions, brand names, place of purchase, and the time and place where the food was consumed were all recorded. Check questions to aid completeness of recording asked, for each day, how much the young person had spent on things to eat and drink while they were away from home, and whether they ate or drank anything that they did not have to buy, for example, items they were given, or were free. Duplicate items were bought and weighed by the interviewer where possible.

Where the young person consumed food or drink items provided by their school or college, the interviewer was required to visit the school to collect further information from the school catering manager about, for example, cooking methods, portion sizes, and types of fats used. This information could then be used by the interviewer and nutritionists when coding and allocating weights to items recorded in the 'eating out' diary. The information was recorded on a 'catering questionnaire' (see *Appendix A*) which included standard questions on cooking methods etc, and provision for recording information on specific items that the young person had consumed.

At each visit to the household, interviewers checked the diary entries with the diary keeper(s) to ensure that they were complete and all the necessary detail had been recorded. Reasons for any apparent omission of meals were probed by the interviewers and noted on the

diaries. As the feasibility survey had identified a general problem with the completeness of information in the 'eating out' diaries and under-reporting of food consumed by the oldest group of girls, particular attention was paid to checking information about items consumed out of the home and the diaries of 15 to 18 year old girls.

Before returning the coded diaries to ONS headquarters interviewers were asked to make an assessment of the quality of the dietary record, in particular the extent to which they considered that the diary was an accurate reflection of the young person's actual diet. This information was recorded on an 'assessment questionnaire' (see *Appendix A*).

Further information on recording procedures is provided in Appendix F.

2.4.2 Coding the food record

Interviewers were responsible for coding the food diaries so they could readily identify the level of detail needed for different food items, and probe for missing detail at later visits to the household. They were therefore trained in recognising the detail required for coding foods of different types at the briefing and by exercises they completed before and during the briefing.

A food code list giving code numbers for about 3500 items and a full description of each item was prepared by nutritionists at MAFF and ONS for use by the interviewers. The list was organised into sections by food type, for example milk and cream, soft drinks, breakfast cereals, fruit, vegetables and different types of meat. Interviewers were also provided with an alphabetical index (paper copy) and an electronic version of the food code list that was loaded into their laptop computer to help them find particular foods in the code list. Additional check lists were provided to assist the interviewers when coding fats used for cooking and spreading, soft drinks and savoury snacks.

As fieldwork progressed, further codes were added to the food code list for home-made recipe dishes and new products found in the dietary records; by the end of fieldwork there were approximately 6000 separate food codes. A page from the food code list is reproduced in Appendix G.

Brand information was collected for all food items bought pre-wrapped, as some items, such as biscuits, confectionery and breakfast cereals could not be food coded correctly unless the brand was known. However brand information has been coded only for artificial sweeteners, bottled waters, herbal teas and herbal drinks, soft drinks and fruit juices, to ensure adequate differentiation of these items.

Food source codes were also allocated to each group of

foods in order to identify food eaten at school, including school meals, and other food obtained and consumed outside the home. The contribution to total nutrient intake by foods from different sources could then be calculated.

After the interviewers had coded the entries in the dietary records, ONS headquarters coding and editing staff checked the documents. ONS nutritionists carried out initial checks for completeness of the dietary records, and they and MAFF nutritionists dealt with specific queries from interviewers and coding staff, and advised on and checked the quality of coding. They were also responsible for converting descriptions of portion sizes to weights, and checking that the appropriate codes for recipes and new products had been used.

2.4.3 Editing the dietary information

Computer checks for completeness and consistency of information were run on the dietary and questionnaire data.

Following completion of these checks and calculations the information from the dietary record was linked to the nutrient databank and nutrient intakes were thereby calculated from quantities of food consumed. This nutrient databank, which was compiled by MAFF, holds information on 55 nutrients for each of the food codes. Further details of the nutrient databank are provided in Appendix I.

Most of the dietary analysis presented in this report is based on average daily intakes of nutrients, either including or excluding dietary supplements. Each food code used was also allocated to one of 115 subsidiary food groups; these were aggregated into 57 main food groups and further aggregated into 11 food types (see Appendix H). Information on the quantity of food consumed from each subsidiary group is tabulated in Chapter 4, and data on the contribution of the main food types to intakes of energy and specific nutrients are included in Chapters 5 to 9.

2.5 Physical activity

Information about levels of physical activity was required for all young people aged 4 to 18 years. The main purpose in collecting this information was to allow an investigation of the relationships between dietary intakes (particularly energy intake), body composition (body mass index), and physical activity levels.

If the body does not use all the energy it takes in as food for activity, growth, thermogenesis etc, then it will be stored; over time this will lead to an increase in body weight, which if it continues leads to an increased risk of obesity. The risk of cardio-vascular disease increases with obesity and many other illnesses and conditions are related to overweight[4]. This survey provides the opportunity to relate activity levels to energy intake and body size.

2.5.1 The choice of methodology

In consultation with experts[5] it was agreed that collecting information on physical activities from young people over a 7-day period by retrospective questioning was likely to be unreliable and that record keeping would be likely to provide more complete and accurate information.

Feasibility work tested this methodology and it was recommended that for young people aged 7 years and over, information on physical activities should be collected in a 7-day diary, which the young person should be asked to carry with them and complete during the day; if they were unwilling to do this they were asked to complete the diary at the end of each day (see Appendix C)[1].

For young people aged between 4 and 6 years the feasibility survey found that record keeping was an inappropriate methodology; this youngest group was unable to keep an accurate record of their activities while they were away from home and parents found it difficult to categorise the activities in the way required; physical activity was often unstructured and its duration and intensity difficult to define. It was therefore recommended that for the mainstage survey physical activity information for young people aged 4 to 6 years should be collected in the initial interview principally by asking the parent how active their child was compared with other children.

2.5.2 Outline of methodology

Young people aged 7 to 18 years were asked to keep a diary of their physical activities for seven days, coinciding with the dietary record-keeping period. The recording pages for physical activities were included in the 'Eating and Drinking Away From Home Diary' (see Appendix A).

Since it was considered sufficient for the purposes of the survey to collect information which would allow young people to be classified into broad bands of activity level, for example, very inactive, inactive, moderately active and very active, the diary asked for details of time spent on a list of specified activities. It was felt inappropriate within the context of an already onerous survey to ask young people to provide detailed information on how all their time was spent, for example, by obtaining a 'time use' diary.

Information was therefore collected for each of the seven days on the time spent:

- in bed – lowest energy expenditure;
- watching television, playing computer games, reading and listening to music – very low energy activities;
- on a range of prompted activities which were known to require moderate, high or very high levels of energy expenditure;

- on any other activities which made the young person *"breathe hard, huff and puff and get hot and sweaty"* – high energy activities;
- on any other activities which made the young person *"slightly out of breath and (..feel..) warm, but not exhausted"* – moderate energy activities.

If the young person was at school a further 5½ hours was added for each school day to allow for activities at school which require very low levels of energy expenditure.

For young people in employment their hours worked were recorded and they were asked to categorise their job according to whether it required very low, low or moderate levels of energy expenditure.

By totalling the time spent on all the above and subtracting from 24 hours, the time spent each day on all other activities requiring only low levels of energy expenditure could be obtained, without the need to record each of these activities separately.

Each of the prompted activities has an associated metabolic equivalent value (MET); for example watching television, which is a very low energy activity, has a MET value of 1.5. By multiplying the time spent on an activity by its MET value a score can be calculated each day for a young person which represents their level of energy expenditure that day (see *Appendix K* for MET values for activities). The scores for the seven recording days can then be averaged to give a score which can be categorised into the broad bands described above.

For young people aged 4 to 6 years information was collected for each of the 7 dietary record-keeping days on the hours spent in bed, and time spent watching TV, playing computer games and listening to music. Additionally parents were asked during the initial interview to describe their child's level of activity from prompted categories describing an "inactive" child, a "fairly active" child, and a "very active" child, and to say how active their child was compared with other children of the same age and sex (see *Appendix A*).

2.6 Bowel movements

During the seven days when the dietary record was being kept, young people were asked to keep a record of the number of bowel movements they had each day.

This information was required mainly to determine normative values for young people between the ages of 4 and 18 years, which are not available from other sources, and to be able to relate the information on the number of bowel movements to other information collected, principally dietary data.

The 'eating out' diary included a 7-day chart for recording bowel movements when the young person was away from home. Each day the daily total from the 'eating out' diary was copied onto a second 7-day chart, which was kept at home and used to record bowel movements while at home, and the total number of movements for the day calculated.

2.7 Anthropometry

One of the main aims of this survey is to provide anthropometric data on a representative sample of young people, which can be related to socio-demographic and dietary data.

Anthropometry, the measurement of body size, weight and proportions, is an intrinsic part of any nutritional survey and can be an indicator of health, development and growth. Derived indices, for instance to assess the proportion of body weight that is fat, provide additional information.

2.7.1 Choice of anthropometric measurements

In deciding which measurements should be taken a number of factors needed to be considered; these included the acceptability of the measurement to the young person (and his or her parent), whether equipment suitable for use in the home was available, and whether interviewers could be trained to take the measurements accurately.

Measurements of standing height, weight and mid upper-arm circumference were required for all young people. Additionally waist and hip circumferences were measured for young people aged 11 years and over.

Height and weight can also be used to calculate the Quetelet or Body Mass Index (weight[kg]/height[m]^2) or other indices which control for variations in body weight associated with height. Mid upper-arm circumference was measured to give information on body size. The ratio of waist to hip circumference gives indirect information on the distribution of body fat stores. Several studies in adults have shown that the location of body fat is associated with health risks, in particular cardio-vascular disease [6]. This study provides normative information about body fat distribution in young people. As these measurements are only appropriate post-puberty, waist and hip circumferences were only measured for young people aged 11 and over.

2.7.2 Techniques and instruments used

ONS interviewers have experience of taking height, weight and mid upper-arm circumference measurements on surveys of adults and pre-school children[7,8,9,10]. It is recognised that children and young people are generally more difficult to measure accurately; deciding on appropriate equipment, techniques and training was therefore a requirement of the feasibility study (see *Appendix C*)[1].

At the main stage all interviewers were trained in accurate measurement techniques at personal briefings.

Once trained, any interviewer working on a subsequent, non-consecutive wave of fieldwork attended a one-day refresher briefing where the techniques were checked. Interviewers were able to practice the measurement techniques on young people at the briefings.

Interviewers were allowed to take the measurements at any point after the initial questionnaire had been completed; it was thought that specifying a particular time to take the measurements could affect response, as gaining the co-operation, particularly of the youngest group might be problematic and more than one attempt might be needed. Detailed descriptions of the techniques used to take the measurements are given in Appendix L.

Interviewers recorded the measurement, the date on which it was taken, and if there were any special circumstances which might have affected the accuracy of the measurement. The Department of Health advised on circumstances which were likely to affect the accuracy to such an extent that the measurement should be excluded from the analysis; for example, the young person being unable to keep the correct posture when standing height was being measured, or their hair being arranged in a 'permanent' style which affected the measurement of standing height. For each measurement the measurement protocol was repeated and a second measurement made.

Standing Height: the measurement was taken using the Leicester Height Measure. This is a light-weight, portable stadiometer, which is modular in construction and is produced for the Child Growth Foundation. The Measure has a foot plate, vertical back post with an analogue scale and an adjustable head plate with a friction lock; measurements were made to the nearest millimetre.

The measurement was made with the young person wearing as few clothes as possible; shoes were removed. The young person's head was positioned such that the Frankfort plane was horizontal, and while maintaining this position, he or she was asked to stand as tall as possible. For young people aged between 4 and 6 years who were unable to comply with this instruction without moving their feet off the base plate the interviewer applied gentle traction to the back of the head/neck to attain the maximum unsupported height. For further details on the equipment used and the Frankfort plane see Appendix L.

Weight: Soehnle Quantratronic digital personal weighing scales, calibrated in kilogram and 100 gram units were used, and placed on a hard level surface for taking the measurement. Where no hard level surface was available the interviewer made a note on the recording document. All the scales were checked for accuracy prior to each fieldwork wave before being issued to interviewers.

Young people were asked to wear as little as possible and a record was made of the clothing being worn. The measurement was not made at a standard time of day.

Mid upper-arm circumference: for consistency of technique this measurement was taken from the left side of the young person's body. If for any reason the interviewer was unable to take the measurement on the left side, then the measurement was taken on the right and a note made.

Mid upper-arm circumference was measured in two stages using a standard tape to identify the mid-point of the upper arm, and an insertion tape to measure the circumference.

Interviewers were instructed to take the measurement on bare skin with the young person in a T-shirt or other garment sufficiently loose fitting around the upper arm.

The position of the arm was standardised for each stage of the measurement. The mid-point of the upper arm was identified as halfway between the inferior border of the acromion process and the tip of the olecranon process. In taking the circumference measurement care was taken to ensure that the tape was horizontal and that the tissues of the upper arm were not compressed. Circumference measurements were taken to the nearest millimetre.

Waist and hip circumferences: waist was defined as the mid-point between the iliac crest and the lower rib. Hip circumference was measured at the widest circumference around the buttocks.

The young person was asked to wear only light clothing, and, where possible, to have the same thickness of clothing at both measurement sites. A standard insertion tape was used and interviewers checked the horizontal alignment of the tape before making the measurement. The waist circumference was measured at the end of a normal expiration; interviewers checked that the gluteal muscles were not contracted before measuring the hip circumference. The two measurements were repeated sequentially, and recorded to the nearest millimetre.

Each young person was given a record card with his or her measurements.

2.8 The physiological measurements

2.8.1 Ethical approval

Because this survey, in common with other surveys in the NDNS series, includes physiological procedures which are invasive – venepuncture procedure to take a blood sample – and measurements with possible clinical significance – venepuncture, measurement of blood pressure, and an examination of the teeth and oral soft tissues, it was necessary to obtain approval for the survey protocol from National Health Service Local Research Ethics Committees (LRECs) in the areas where fieldwork would be taking place. In particular approval was sought for the following elements of the survey:

- taking a venepuncture blood sample for nutritional status analyses;
- storing the residue of blood for future analyses;
- flagging the young person's details on the National Health Service Central Register (NHSCR) for subsequent outcome follow up.

However, approval from LRECs for the whole survey package was required, as it would not have been acceptable to proceed only with those aspects of the survey not specifically requiring approval, if approval for some aspects was withheld.

LRECs, in deciding whether to approve the survey, considered not only the measurement and venepuncture protocols, but also needed to be satisfied regarding the adequacy of procedures:

- to ensure that co-operation was voluntary – there was no undue coercion to participate;
- to ensure that the young person was fully informed of the reason for various procedures, and what was involved;
- relating to consent and confidentiality issues.

The Dunn Nutrition Unit sought ethical approval for the survey from the NHS Local Research Ethics Committees covering each of the 132 sampled areas; all gave their approval. Only two Committees required significant changes to the standard survey method, in both cases the Committees required a letter to be sent to the sampled young person in advance of the interviewer calling, allowing the subject to refuse to take part if they so wished. Other changes were minor, mainly alterations to the wording in information leaflets and on consent forms.

A number of LRECs initially requested that the subject be offered the application of a topical anaesthetic cream before venepuncture; this was not part of the original survey protocol. However, immediately prior to the start of the fieldwork in January 1997 we were advised that the Standing Ethics Advisory Committee of the Royal College of Paediatrics and Child Health advocated that an anaesthetic cream should be offered to all subjects for the venepuncture. It was therefore necessary for the Dunn Nutrition Unit to re-contact all the LRECs to inform them of the change to the venepuncture protocol.

If, in the period between the sample being selected and the interviewer calling at the sampled address, the young person had moved, checks were made to ensure that the new address was in an area covered by LREC approval. If the new address was elsewhere then the young person was not approached to take part in the survey and the case was withdrawn (see *Chapter 3* for further details of the sample design and response).

Information about the survey was also sent to Directors of Public Health, Social Services and Education, Chief Constables of Police and Chief Executives of Health Authorities with responsibility for the areas of residence of participant young people; they were asked to inform appropriate local staff (see *Appendix B*).

2.8.2 Consent procedures

GP notification of subject participation
Because the survey included measurements of possible clinical significance, that is blood pressure levels, results for blood analytes and the identification of 'serious oral pathology' during the oral health examination, it was necessary to obtain consent from the subject for their GP to be informed of these by the Dunn Nutrition Unit, and consequently for them to agree for their subject details, name, address, date of birth and gender, to be passed to the Dunn Nutrition Unit.

At the first visit to the young person's home the interviewer therefore sought verbal consent for the young person's GP to be informed that the young person was taking part in the survey and to record the GP details.

If this was given the interviewer immediately sent the GP a standard letter explaining that the young person was taking part in the survey, together with a copy of the survey purpose leaflet, which described the procedures with which the young person would be asked to co-operate. The letter was signed by, and gave a telephone number for the Survey Doctor.

If the young person was not registered with a GP, or consent to pass information to the GP was not given, the young person could not take part in the following aspects of the survey:

- the measurement of blood pressure;
- the venepuncture procedure;
- the oral health examination.

Signed consent
Individual signed consent was required for each of the following elements of the survey:

- the venepuncture procedure; witnessed consent was required;
- reporting blood pressure levels to the young person's GP;
- storing any remaining blood after all the analyses were complete for future nutritional analyses;
- passing information to allow the young person's details to be flagged on the NHSCR;
- reporting any serious oral pathology identified during the oral health examination to the young person's GP.

Consent signatures were obtained according to the age of the young person.

- age 4 to 15 years: signature of person with parental responsibility;
- age 16 and 17 years and living at home: signature of young person and signature of person with parental responsibility;
- age 16 and 17 years and living away from home: signature of young person;
- age 18 years: signature of young person.

For the venepuncture procedure the signature(s) needed to be obtained in the presence of an independent witness (not a member of the survey team or the young person's household) and the signature of the witness was required.

In all cases, even after consent signatures were obtained, the assent of the young person to the procedure was confirmed before it was undertaken.

2.9 Blood pressure

High blood pressure is an important and known risk factor for cardio-vascular disease in adults[11]. The significance of high blood pressure at younger ages is less well understood. Moreover there are no national data available on blood pressure levels for normal, healthy young people.

Blood pressure was measured, with the young person seated, using the Dinamap 8100 oscillometric monitor. This device has previously been used to measure blood pressure on the NDNS of people aged 65 years and over and the latest Health Survey for England, and was the instrument of choice for this NDNS of young people principally for reasons of methodological comparability between all these surveys, instrument reliability and ease of use[12,13]. There has however been some criticism of the validity and reliability of measurements obtained using the Dinamap; a review of studies comparing the Dinamap with other devices, including the standard mercury sphygmomanometer, is given in Appendix L.

Blood pressure could only be taken if all the following were obtained:

- consent to notify the young person's GP of their participation in the survey;
- consent to take the blood pressure measurements;
- signed consent to send a record of the blood pressure readings to the young person's GP.

Interviewers were trained at the personal briefings to make blood pressure measurements following a standardised procedure. Measurements could be made at any visit after the initial questionnaire had been completed and three complete and consecutive cycles of measurement were made at the one visit. The time of day when the measurements were made was not standardised, but interviewers asked that the young person should have been sitting quietly and not eaten or drunk anything for about 30 minutes before they made the first measurement. The three measurements were taken at pre-set one minute intervals. Interviewers recorded from the digital display on the monitor the systolic and diastolic levels, mean arterial pressure and pulse after each measurement cycle. Any unusual circumstances, including any difficulty in wrapping the cuff were noted on the recording document. The young person was given a record of their blood pressure readings. Interviewers were instructed that they should not discuss the blood pressure readings with the respondent or their family. If asked, interviewers suggested that the respondent should contact his or her GP or the survey doctor for advice and information on the interpretation of the measurements.

2.9.1 Reporting blood pressures

Although one of the reasons for making blood pressure measurements in the survey is to establish the normal range of readings for this population, it was a requirement for obtaining approval for the protocol from LRECs that in every case the young person's GP was informed of the blood pressure results and that a procedure for immediate reporting of seriously abnormal blood pressures to the young person's GP was established.

A copy of the blood pressure readings was therefore sent immediately by the interviewer to the Dunn Nutrition Unit where they were scrutinised by the Survey Doctor and then sent with an appropriate covering letter to the young person's GP (see *Appendix N*).

Where the readings obtained by the interviewer were unusually high, defined as all three readings being equal to or above 160mmHg systolic pressure and/or equal to or above 100mmHg diastolic pressure, the interviewer immediately delivered a copy of the results with a standard accompanying letter to the young person's GP. In order that the Survey Doctor was sufficiently informed to discuss the readings with the GP should the need arise, the interviewer also contacted the Survey Doctor by telephone, giving the young person's details, including age and weight.

2.10 The urine sample

2.10.1 The purpose of obtaining urine specimens

The relationship between dietary intakes of sodium, present in salt (sodium chloride) and blood pressure in adults has been investigated in relation to the established association between hypertension and cardio-vascular disease but the evidence regarding the relative importance of dietary sodium intakes remains unclear[14]. Nevertheless the COMA Panel on Dietary Reference Values accepted the possibility that by reducing sodium intakes "public health benefits such as reduced cardiovascular disease mortality might arise..." while acknowledging that "...other interventions such as reduction of obesity, increased potassium, reduced energy intakes, altered quantity and quality of fat intake and reduced alcohol consumption may also have at least as great an impact on such diseases"[15]. In adolescents it has been suggested that obesity may increase the sensitivity of blood pressure to dietary intakes of sodium[16]. Other dietary surveys of young people have reported high consumption levels of snack products, many of which are high in sodium[17]. It was considered important therefore that this survey obtained information on both sodium intakes and blood pressure for young people.

It is not possible to obtain accurate estimates of dietary intake of sodium from weighed food intake information, mainly because it is not possible to assess accurately the amount of salt added to food in cooking or at the table. Estimates of sodium and potassium intakes can be obtained by measuring their urinary excretion, assuming the body is in balance for these minerals.

Since the rate of excretion of both sodium and potassium varies with intake, the best estimate of intake is obtained from the analysis of a urine sample taken from a complete 24-hour collection, which allows for the fluctuations in intake over the collection period.

The Dietary and Nutritional Survey of British Adults included a 24-hour urine collection, but in pilot work for the NDNS of people aged 65 years and over compliance was not sufficiently good, less than 50%, for the procedure to be included in the mainstage survey[7,12]. It was agreed that compliance among young people, who may spend a lot more of their time away from home, either at school or on leisure activities, and who might be embarrassed by the procedure and the need to carry collection equipment with them, would probably be even lower. It was therefore decided that estimates of sodium intake would be obtained from the analysis of a 'spot' urine sample.

2.10.2 The procedure for collecting spot urine samples

All young people taking part in the survey were asked to provide a sample of urine for analysis, if possible during the 7-day dietary recording period. As the sample needed to be taken and despatched on the same day and be with the analytical laboratory the next day, the sample could only be taken on Mondays to Thursdays. The requirement was for approximately a 10ml sample of urine taken from the first void of the day; a first void sample is likely to give a better estimate of 'average'

sodium levels, than a sample taken later in the day after eating and drinking.

The young person was left with the equipment for collecting the sample, together with an instruction card.

The equipment comprised:

- a small disposable urine collection container;
- a Sarstedt 'Urin-stabilisator' syringe; the syringe contains a small amount of boric acid powder as preservative, and has a removable extension tube for withdrawing the urine from the collection container into the syringe. After filling the syringe the extension tube is removed, the end of the syringe sealed with a plastic cap, and the syringe plunger stalk snapped.
- a plastic despatch container; the filled syringe was labelled with the young person's unique survey identifier (serial number) and placed inside the plastic despatch container.

The container with the labelled, filled syringe was then placed inside a padded postal envelope together with completed documentation and immediately posted by the interviewer to the Dunn Nutrition Laboratory in Cambridge to arrive usually the next day.

As well as sodium and potassium, the urine sample was analysed for levels of creatinine. The results from the analysis of the samples of urine are included in Chapter 9.

2.11 Purpose of obtaining a sample of venous blood

One of the main aims of the NDNS programme is to measure haematological and other blood indices that give evidence of nutritional status and to relate these to dietary and social data. As in the earlier pre-school children's survey a main concern was to measure haemoglobin concentrations and other indicators of iron status, since iron deficiency is common among children under 5 years in Britain[10,18]. Blood concentrations of other nutrients and analytes would give valuable information about the nutritional status of young people, and in many cases establish normative ranges for a healthy population of young people in Great Britain (see *Appendix O* for a full list of blood analytes).

Approval from LRECs for blood sampling was subject to a maximum volume of 10ml blood being taken from subjects aged under 7 years and a maximum of 15ml blood from those aged 7 and over. It was expected that the maximum permitted volume would not be obtained in all cases and therefore analytes were prioritised according to nutritional interest for analysis dependent on the volume of blood obtained. The order was as follows:

- haematological indices: including cell counts and haemoglobin

- haematinic indices: serum and red cell folate, serum B_{12}, serum ferritin
- whole blood lead, plasma selenium and magnesium
- plasma 25-hydroxyvitamin D
- plasma cholesterol
- plasma iron
- plasma total iron binding capacity
- all other analytes

Approval was obtained from the LRECs for any unused sample remaining after the above analyses to be stored, subject to consent, and an undertaking was given that neither the original sample nor any stored sample would be tested for viruses, including HIV.

2.11.1 Procedures for obtaining the blood sample

All procedures associated with obtaining and analysing the blood samples were contracted to the Medical Research Council Dunn Nutrition Unit in Cambridge whose staff worked closely with ONS throughout all stages of the survey.

All the procedures were tested in the feasibility study to ensure that they were safe and acceptable to the subjects, their parents, those taking the blood samples and to the medical profession[19] (see *Appendix C* for a report on the feasibility study[1]).

2.11.2 Training and recruitment of the blood takers

As taking blood from young people may be more difficult than bleeding adult subjects it was decided that those recruited to take the blood samples should have recent paediatric experience of taking blood. A total of 80 personnel with appropriate experience was recruited by the Dunn Nutrition Unit to work on the survey. These were mainly phlebotomists, the remainder were nurses and medical laboratory scientific officers; one was a doctor. Some worked on more than one wave of fieldwork, some in more than one area, and some worked in pairs. All received written instructions and attended personal briefings where they were given training in the protocols for obtaining the blood sample and despatching it. For the first two fieldwork waves of the survey the training sessions for blood takers were held as part of the interviewer briefing sessions so that there was the opportunity for the blood taker to meet the interviewer with whom they would be working, and for the roles and responsibilities of the blood taker and interviewer to be clearly defined. Emphasis was placed on the need to standardise procedures and adhere strictly to the protocol that had been presented to and agreed by the LRECs. Further details of the recruitment of blood takers are given in Appendix P.

2.11.3 Laboratory recruitment

For each area covered by the survey a local laboratory was recruited to receive and process a portion of the blood from each respondent. Blood takers delivered samples to these laboratories by hand in a cool box. Great Ormond Street Haematology Department and Southampton University Trace Elements Laboratory were contracted to receive and analyse other portions of the blood, for haematology and trace element analysis respectively, collected from all areas in all waves of the survey.

2.11.4 Outline consent procedures

Explicit formal consent was required for taking the blood sample from the young people. Interviewers were required to tell the young person and their parent(s) at the time they conducted the initial interview that their consent to a blood sample being taken would be sought. This was to avoid the possibility that having built a rapport with the interviewer, respondents might have felt obliged to consent to the venepuncture procedure against their true wishes.

A written statement of the purpose and procedures involved in taking the blood sample was provided and the family was given time to discuss this with others, for example the young person's family doctor, the Survey Doctor or the blood taker. Written, witnessed consent for the procedure was sought, as well as consent for the Dunn Nutrition Unit to inform the young person's GP of the results for the clinically significant analytes.

It should be noted that agreement to this aspect of the survey was independent of agreement to other elements in the survey, and was not associated with the £5 gift voucher given to the young person for completing the full 7-day dietary record.

The young person and their parents were informed that consent to the procedure could be withdrawn at any time, even after written consent had been given, and blood takers were instructed that they should stop the procedure at any point if they felt the young person or family became unduly distressed.

A copy of the consent forms used and information sheets handed to parents is given in Appendix M.

2.11.5 Outline venepuncture procedure

EMLA Cream[20]

It was a condition of approval for the survey from the Royal College of Paediatrics and Child Health that all subjects be offered the option of having a topical anaesthetic cream applied to the venepuncture site. It should be noted that there was no requirement for an anaesthetic cream routinely to be applied in all cases.

EMLA Cream was the product of choice, mainly for reasons of safety and minimal side effects. It is however a prescription-only medicine and individual signed prescriptions were obtained for each young person who requested EMLA Cream, allowing the Survey Doctor individually to assess whether there were any known allergies contraindicating its use.

Interviewers offered the option of EMLA Cream when explaining the purpose and procedures associated with the venepuncture, and before obtaining consent for the procedure. Subjects were provided with an information leaflet and offered the opportunity to discuss the use of EMLA Cream with the Survey Doctor or the blood taker. If EMLA Cream was requested then interviewers asked a check question to screen for any previous allergic reaction to any type of anaesthetic - general or local (including topical creams) which would make the subject unsuitable for EMLA Cream. If the young person had experienced any previous allergic reaction to anaesthetics they were asked if they were still willing to have a blood sample taken without EMLA Cream being applied.

If the young person requested and was suitable for EMLA Cream the interviewer completed their details on a 'prescription' pro-forma which was then sent to the Survey Doctor for signing. After signing the 'prescription' was returned to the interviewer in time for it to be available for the blood taker at the venepuncture visit.

Blood takers were provided with EMLA Cream in single dose units.

In about half the cases the blood taker applied the Cream; in the other cases after explaining how to apply the Cream the blood taker left it with the family or the young person for them to apply themselves. This was decided on consultation with the young person's parent and was at the discretion of the phlebotomist.

Venepuncture
Blood was taken by the phlebotomist in the young person's home with the ONS interviewer present.

If possible, fasting blood samples were collected as the blood analyses included an assessment of triglyceride levels; this measurement is more useful if the sample is taken after fasting. Subjects were therefore asked to comply with the overnight fasting requirements - approximately 8 hours, although a sample could still be taken if they were unwilling to comply. If EMLA Cream was used then the blood taker and interviewer made a preliminary visit to the household to explain the use of the Cream. The Cream was applied to both antecubital fossae and occluded with a small dressing. A minimum of 60 minutes was required to elapse before attempting venepuncture.

Screening questions were asked by the blood takers before attempting to obtain the sample; any young person with epilepsy, or a blood clotting or bleeding disorder was not suitable for the venepuncture procedure.

The approved protocol allowed for a maximum of two attempts at bleeding from the antecubital fossa.

Details of the procedures for taking blood samples and the processing procedures are described in Appendices P and Q.

2.11.6 Procedures for reporting results to parents and General Practitioners

As noted earlier, for many analytes this survey is intended to establish baseline normative values for young people aged 4 to 18 years; for such analytes it was not possible to identify 'abnormal' results nor could General Practitioners be advised on the clinical significance of any particular result.

In respect of the following assays, ranges for young people were defined and any result outside the range was indicated on the letter sent to the subject and to the subject's GP. Subjects were advised to arrange to see their GP if any result was outside the defined range[21] (copies of these letters are given in *Appendix N*).

Results for the following assays were reported:

- full blood count and differential blood count if outside normal range
- haemoglobin
- measures of iron status
- plasma 25-hydroxyvitamin D
- plasma vitamin B_{12}
- plasma cholesterol
- whole blood lead

References and endnotes

[1] Lowe S. *Feasibility study for the National Diet and Nutrition Survey: young people aged 4 to 18 years*. ONS (*In preparation*).

[2] For reasons of cost young people in only four of the six fieldwork areas in the feasibility study took part in the doubly labelled water validation.

[3] Smithers G, Gregory J, Coward WA, Wright A, Elsom R, Wenlock R. British National Diet and Nutrition Survey of young people aged 4 to 18 years: feasibility study of the dietary assessment methodology. Abstracts of the Third International conference on Dietary Assessment Methods. *Eur. J. Clin. Nutr.* 1998; **52**: S2. S76

[4] Royal College of Physicians of London. Obesity. Report. *J Roy Col Phys.* London 1983; **17**: 3–58.

[5] See '*Authors' Acknowledgements*'.

[6] Lapidus L, Bengtsson C, Larsson B, Pennert K, Rybo E, Sjöström L. Distribution of adipose tissue and risk of cardiovascular disease and death: a 12 year follow up of participants in the population study of women in Gothenburg, Sweden. *Br Med J* 1984; **289**: 1257–1260.
Rimm EB, Stampfer MJ, Giovannucci E et al. Body size and fat distribution as predictors of coronary heart disease among middle aged and older US men. *Am J Epid* 1995; **141**: 1117–1127.

[7] Gregory J, Foster K, Tyler H, Wiseman M. *The Dietary and Nutritional Survey of British Adults*. HMSO (London, 1990).

8 White A, Nicolaas G, Foster K, Browne F, Carey S. *Health Survey for England 1991*. HMSO (London, 1993). Breeze E, Maidment A, Bennett N, Flatley J, Carey S. *Health Survey for England 1992*. HMSO (London, 1994). Bennett N, Dodd T, Flatley J, Freeth S, Bolling K. *Health Survey for England 1993*. HMSO (London, 1995).

9 Knight I. *The Heights and Weights of Adults in Great Britain*. HMSO (London, 1984).

10 Gregory JR, Collins DL, Davies PSW, Hughes JM, Clarke PC. *National Diet and Nutrition Survey: children aged 1½ to 4½ years. Volume 1: Report of the diet and nutrition survey.* HMSO (London, 1995).

11 Pickering GW. *High Blood Pressure*. Churchill. (London, 1986).

12 Finch S, Doyle W, Lowe C, Bates CJ, Prentice A, Smithers G, Clarke PC. *National Diet and Nutrition Survey: people aged 65 and over. Volume 1: Report of the diet and nutrition survey.* TSO (London, 1998).

13 Prescott–Clarke P, Primatesta P. Eds *Heath Survey for England 1995*. TSO (London, 1997).

14 Swales JD. Salt saga continued. *Br Med J* 1988; **297**: 307–308.

15 Department of Health. Report on Health and Social Subjects: 41. *Dietary Reference Values for Food Energy and Nutrients for the United Kingdom.* HMSO (London, 1991).

16 Rocchini AP, Key J, Bondie D et al. The effect of weight loss on the sensitivity of blood pressure to sodium in obese adolescents. *New Engl J Med* 1989; **321**: 580–585.

17 Hackett AF, Kirby S, Howie M. A national survey of the diet of children aged 13–14 years living in urban areas of the United Kingdom. *J Hum Nutr Dietet* 1997; **10**: 37–51. Anderson A, Macintyre S, West P. Dietary patterns among adolescents in the West of Scotland. *Br J Nutr* 1994; **71**: 111–122. Strain JJ, Robson PJ, Livingstone MBE et al. Estimates of food and macronutrient intake in a random sample of Northern Ireland adolescents. *Br J Nutr* 1994; **72**: 343–352.

18 Department of Health. Report on Health and Social Subjects: 45. *Weaning and the Weaning Diet*. HMSO (London, 1994).

19 The advice from the Royal College of Paediatrics and Child Health to offer an application of anaesthetic cream in all cases prior to venepuncture was only notified after the completion of the feasibility study; this procedure was therefore not tested prior to the main stage, although anaesthetic cream had been used for some subjects on the *National Diet and Nutrition Survey: children aged 1½ to 4½ years* (ref 10).

20 EMLA® Cream (Astra) lignocaine 2.5%, prilocaine 2.5%. PL 0017/0213.

21 See *Appendix N* for reportable ranges.

3 Response to the survey and characteristics of the responding and non-responding samples

3.1 Introduction

This chapter gives details of response to the various components in the survey, and describes the characteristics of the responding and diary samples, that is those completing the initial dietary interview and those keeping a full seven-day dietary record.

Where possible distributions are compared with data from the 1996/7 General Household Survey (GHS)[1]. The main survey classificatory variables are tabulated against each other to identify interactions which may assist in the interpretation of results in the analysis chapters which follow, where data are generally tabulated by the classificatory variables independently.

The final part of the chapter presents some results from the initial dietary interview.

3.2 Response

Details of the sample selection and response to the postal and interviewer sift stages are given in Chapter 1 and in Appendix D.

Of the 2672 young people selected for interview, 2127 (80%) co-operated with the initial dietary interview and 1701 (64%) with the seven-day dietary record[2,3]. All those who completed a dietary record and went on to co-operate with other aspects of the survey, including the measurements, and urine and blood samples had co-operated with the initial interview. Compared with the NDNS of children aged 1½ to 4½ years, co-operation rates were lower at both the interview and dietary record stages (88% and 80% - p < 0.01)[4]. In respect of the dietary record the record-keeping period was extended from four days on the pre-school children's survey to seven days for this survey of young people, which may have contributed to the lower co-operation rates. However interviewers reported that on this survey co-operation at each stage was needed from the young person and their parent; in the pre-school children's survey co-operation was only needed from the child's mother. If, in this survey of young people, either the young person or their parent was not prepared to take part, that component was not administered. This has undoubtedly contributed to higher non-response than would have been the case had co-operation from only a single person been needed.

Tables 3.1 to 3.3 show response to the dietary interview and dietary record by fieldwork wave[5], age[6,7] and sex of young person and social class of the head of household[8].

There were no significant differences by fieldwork wave or by social class of head of household in the proportions co-operating with either the dietary interview or the dietary record.

As had been identified in the feasibility study[9], in the main stage survey response to both the dietary interview and dietary record was lowest for boys aged 15 to 18 years, despite interviewers making particular efforts to gain co-operation from this age group. As well as the problem of needing the co-operation of both the young person and their parent, there were particular difficulties in contacting and gaining co-operation from the oldest group of boys whose lifestyles were busier and less predictable than those of other young people. Moreover at 16 and 18 years many young people in the sample were taking GCSE or GCE 'A' level examinations, and interviewers reported difficulty in gaining co-operation in the periods leading up to and during these examinations; this is reflected in the lower co-operation rates for both boys and girls in the 15 to 18 year age group.

Without weighting for this differential response effect, estimates for different groups, for example, mean daily intake of energy in different social class groups, would be biased estimates, because in particular they under-represent the oldest group of boys. To correct for this the data presented in the substantive chapters of this report have been weighted using a combined weight based on the weighting factor for differential sampling probabilities and the weighting for differential non-response. Bases in tables are presented unweighted. Further details of the weighting procedures are given in Appendix D. *(Tables 3.1 to 3.3)*

3.2.1 Co-operation with the anthropometric measurements and blood pressure

As described in Chapter 2, each young person taking part in the survey, regardless of whether they completed a dietary record, was asked to consent to having measurements taken of their standing height, body weight, mid upper-arm circumference and blood pressure[10]. Additionally young people aged between 11 and 18 years were asked to consent to their waist and hip circumferences being measured.

Tables 3.4 to 3.6 show response to the various measurements by fieldwork wave, sex and age of young person, and the social class of the head of household. Except for social class, response rates are calculated as percentages of all young people eligible to take part in the survey, *the eligible sample*, and for those who at a minimum co-operated with the initial dietary interview, *the responding sample*[11].

For each of the measurements at least 70% of the eligible sample and 90% of the responding sample consented to their being taken.

Response rates in Wave 4 appeared to be consistently slightly lower than in other waves, but the differences are not statistically significant. Overall girls were no more likely than boys to have consented to the measurements and there was no difference in response by age for girls. For boys, however, the oldest age group, possibly because of embarrassment at being measured, again had lower consent rates, even among those who had agreed to take part in the initial interview. For example for boys aged 15 to 18 years co-operating with the interview, the consent rates for height, weight and mid upper-arm circumference were all 86%, compared with 95% for boys aged 7 to 10 years (p < 0.05).

There were no significant differences in co-operation rates for the anthropometric measurements and blood pressure by social class of head of household. *(Tables 3.4 to 3.6)*

3.2.2 *Co-operation with the urine and blood samples*

All young people taking part in the survey were asked to consent to providing a specimen of urine and to a venepuncture procedure. Details of the consent procedures and procedures for obtaining the samples are given in Chapter 2 and Appendices M and P.

Table 3.7 shows that overall 69% of the eligible sample and 87% of the responding sample agreed to provide a urine sample[12]. As with the anthropometric measurements, there were no significant differences in the proportions consenting to providing a sample of urine by wave, sex, age or social class of head of household. However, boys aged 15 to 18 years were significantly less likely to agree to providing a sample of their urine, again possibly due to embarrassment; 81% of boys aged 15 to 18 years who co-operated with the interview also agreed to provide a urine sample, compared with 90% of those aged between 7 and 14 years (p < 0.05).

It was anticipated that obtaining consent to the venepuncture procedure would be difficult, partly because it was expected that a significant proportion of young people (or their parent) would be apprehensive or fearful and also because given the preference for obtaining a fasting sample, the arrangements for taking the sample were likely to be somewhat inconvenient. The young person was required to have nothing to eat or drink after bedtime on the night before the procedure and the visit to take the sample needed to be made as early as possible in the morning, before the young person had breakfast and before they left for school, college or work. If the young person was willing to provide a sample, but unwilling or unable to comply with the fasting requirements, a non-fasting sample was acceptable.

Table 3.8 shows the proportion of young people consenting to the venepuncture procedure, the proportion of cases where venepuncture was attempted and the proportion of cases where a sample was obtained.

Overall just under half (48%) of the eligible sample, and nearly two-thirds (60%) of the responding sample gave consent for a venepuncture procedure to be attempted. In nearly all cases consent was given for a fasting sample to be obtained; only 1% of those consenting to venepuncture agreed to provide only a non-fasting sample.

There were significant differences in the proportions consenting to the venepuncture in different waves of fieldwork; in Wave 1 consent was obtained for 59% of young people who had taken part in the survey, but this fell to 52% in Wave 2 (ns). This decline in response was identified in the course of Wave 2 fieldwork and efforts were made to identify the reasons and take steps to improve response. In particular interviewers were told about strategies and introductions that had been used successfully by interviewers during Wave 1 of fieldwork, and were given more advice on how to respond positively to objections to or questions about the blood sample. By Wave 3 response had risen to 66% of the responding sample (p < 0.05); in Wave 4 the consent rate fell back slightly to 62% (ns).

Overall (the parents of) boys were no more or less likely than girls to consent to the venepuncture procedure, but for both there were differences according to age. Not surprisingly the (parents of the) youngest group were the least likely to give consent; consent was obtained for 47% of boys and 44% of girls aged 4 to 6 years who were taking part in the survey. This is significantly lower than for the oldest group of children in the pre-school children's survey, where consent was obtained for 64% of those aged 3½ to 4½ years (p < 0.01)[4]. The reasons for this difference may be partly attributable to the age difference between the survey samples; children aged between 4 and 6 years were probably more likely to express their own opinion as to whether they were prepared to have a blood sample taken than those aged

3½ to 4½ years, where the decision largely rested with the child's mother. Other differences in the procedures and content between the two surveys may also have had a negative effect on response to the blood sample, for example, the need for seven-day, rather than four-day dietary records, the measurement of blood pressure in 4 to 6 year olds, and the need for a sample of urine.

The data suggest that for 7 to 10 year olds, (the parents of) boys were more likely to agree to a blood sample being attempted than (the parents of) girls; consent was given for 66% of boys and 57% of girls aged 7 to 10 years (ns). Thereafter the proportions of boys and girls consenting to the procedure were very similar.

There were no differences by social class of the head of household in the proportions consenting to a venepuncture being attempted.

Overall in 3% of cases where consent had been given, venepuncture was not attempted; for the youngest group of children 7% were not subject to the procedure, having previously given their consent (ns). The usual reasons for not attempting venepuncture were that consent was withdrawn at the time of the procedure, generally by the young person themselves, because the young person was unwell or unsuitable for venepuncture, or became distressed and the phlebotomist advised against attempting to obtain a sample.

In 93% of cases where an attempt was made a sample of blood was obtained[13]. The youngest children were the most difficult to bleed, with a success rate of only 81% for boys and 85% for girls aged 4 to 6 years (p < 0.05 for boys, ns for girls). Where venepuncture was abandoned this was generally to avoid distress to the young person.
(Tables 3.7 and 3.8)

3.3   Characteristics of the sample

Table 3.9 shows that the age and sex distributions of the responding and non-responding samples differed significantly. In particular, there was a greater proportion of young people aged 15 to 18 in the non-responding sample than the responding sample.

Table 3.10 shows the age and sex distributions of the responding and diary samples for before and after weighting. There were no significant differences in the sex and age distributions between the responding and diary samples for the unweighted or weighted data.
(Tables 3.9 and 3.10)

3.3.1   Region

In order to provide adequate numbers for analysis the standard government regions were aggregated into four broad regions. A map showing the standard and aggregated regions and a list of the counties they contain is shown in Figure 3.1.

A comparison of the regional distribution of the responding and diary samples with data from the 1996-7 GHS[1] (Table 3.11) shows no significant regional bias[14].

Table 3.12 shows that there was no significant variation in the regional composition of the diary sample by age or sex.   *(Tables 3.11 and 3.12)*

3.3.2   *Social class of head of household*

Social class was derived for the head of household[15] and for the young person's mother from occupation information collected in the interview. The mother was the head of household in 17% of cases (table not shown).

Throughout this Report, analysis using social class information is based on that of the head of household because it is available for the largest number of cases and allows comparisons to be made with other data sources.

Social class could not be derived for 10% of cases; for about one third of these cases this was because the head of household's occupation was inadequately described, they were a member of the armed forces, or they were economically inactive and had never worked. In the remaining two-thirds of cases, social class could not be derived due to a programming error, which resulted in some economically inactive respondents not being asked whether they had ever worked[16].

In order to provide adequate numbers for analysis the standard categories for social class were collapsed into three groups as follows:

Non-manual	Social Classes I and II - professional, managerial and technical professions, and Social Class IIInm - skilled non-manual occupations.
Manual	Social Class IIIm - skilled manual occupations, and Social Classes IV and V - unskilled occupations.
Unclassified	those who were not allocated a social class either because their job was inadequately described, they were a member of the armed forces, had never worked or where it was not known whether they had ever worked.

Table 3.13 shows that there were no significant differences in social class composition between the NDNS responding and diary samples.

There were no significant differences in the proportions of manual and non-manual head of household in the NDNS responding and diary samples compared with the 1996-7 GHS[14].

Figure 3.1   Standard regions of England, Scotland and Wales and aggregated regions for analysis

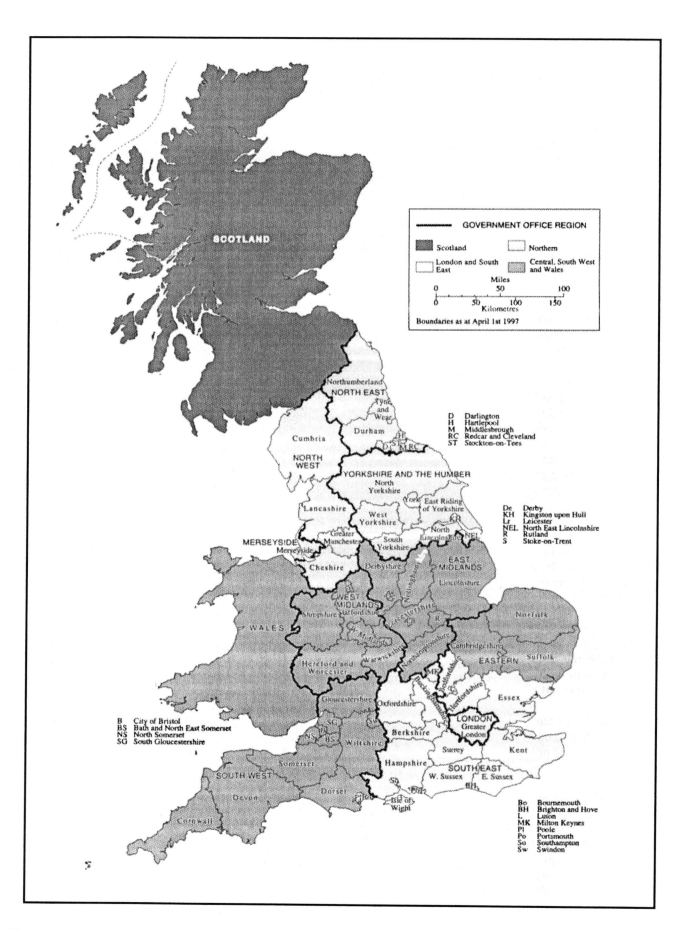

The proportion of manual and non-manual heads of household did not vary significantly with the age or sex of the young person.

Young people living in London and the South East were more likely to come from a non-manual household than young people living elsewhere, although the only significant difference was between London and the South East and the Northern region; in London and the South East 52% of heads of household were in the non-manual group compared with 42% of heads of household in the Northern region (p < 0.05).

(Tables 3.13 to 3.16)

3.3.3 Household type

Household type was derived from information collected on the age and relationship to the young person of each member of the household, and classifies young people into groups depending on whether they were living with one or both parents and with or without other children[17]. In most of the tables in the rest of this report, those who were living with a single parent with and without other children have been grouped together to increase the number of cases for analysis.

Table 3.17 shows that there was almost no difference in the household type distributions for the responding and diary samples. Around three-quarters of the households contained one or more children in addition to the sampled young person, with no significant difference between the responding and diary samples. Overall, around 20% of young people were living in lone-parent households, while around 80% were living with both 'parents', that is a married or cohabiting couple. Compared with young people living with lone-parent households, a higher proportion of those living with both parents were in households containing other children. For example, for the diary sample, 77% of married or cohabiting couples had two or more children compared with 68% of lone parents (p < 0.01).

The young person was living in a household without a parent in less than 1% of cases; most of these young people were living with unrelated others in shared accommodation or with a partner, with or without their own children (table not shown).

Tables 3.18 and 3.19 show that the type of household in which the young person lived varied according to their age. In particular, the proportion of young people living in households with other children decreased as the age of the young person increased. This means that the proportion of young people in different age groups in the different household types differs. Most importantly, the proportion of young people aged 15 to 18 years living in households with both parents and no other children is significantly higher than in the other household types. For example, for boys living with both parents and no other children 51% were aged 15 to 18;

for boys in households with both parents and other children 14% were in the oldest group. This relationship between the age of the young person and household type needs to be borne in mind when interpreting nutrient intake and other data from the survey which appear to show differences associated with household type.

There were no significant differences in the distribution of household types by region (table not shown) or according to whether the social class of the head of household was manual or non-manual. The high proportion of young people living with a lone parent in the 'unclassified' category is an artefact associated with the high proportion of lone parents who were economically inactive some of whom were not asked, in error, the information necessary to derive a social class (see *Table 3.25*). *(Tables 3.17 to 3.20)*

3.3.4 Employment status of head of household

Employment status was derived for the head of household, for the young person's mother and for young people aged 15 to 18 years.

Information was collected about whether the head of household, the young person's mother or the young person was in paid employment during the seven days before the interview. Those not in employment were asked further questions in order to establish whether they were unemployed or economically inactive. Definitions of these categories are given in the Glossary – Appendix U.

Table 3.21 shows that overall, 82% of heads of household in the diary sample were working, 13% were economically inactive and 5% were unemployed. Compared with data from the 1996-7 GHS[1] for a sub-sample of households containing at least one person aged between 4 and 18 years, both the responding and diary samples had significantly greater proportions of heads of household who were working and lower proportions of household heads who were economically inactive, for example 77% of household heads in the GHS sample were working compared with 81% of household heads in the responding sample (p < 0.01). There was no significant difference between the responding and diary samples in the distribution of the employment status of the head of household.

Table 3.22 suggests that the proportion of heads of household who were unemployed decreased with the young person's age, although the only significant difference was between young people aged 4 to 6 years and those aged 15 to 18 years, 7% compared with 2% (p < 0.05).

The employment status of the head of household did not vary significantly by region.

Heads of household who were classified as being in the manual social class group were more likely than those in the non-manual group to be unemployed; 6% of manual heads of household were unemployed compared with 2% of non-manual heads of household ($p < 0.01$).

As would be expected, lone-parent heads of household were significantly more likely to be economically inactive than their married or cohabiting counterparts, for example for households with two or more children, 42% of lone-parent heads of household were economically inactive compared with 8% of married or cohabiting heads of household ($p < 0.01$).

(Tables 3.21 to 3.25)

3.3.5 Household income and receipt of benefits

There is a growing literature which shows income to be an important consideration in an individual's decisions about diet, particularly when resources are limited. Moreover, receipt of certain benefits by the household may entitle a young person to free, reduced price or subsidised school meals.

Detailed information about income was not collected because it might have affected co-operation with other components of the survey; instead, the respondent was asked to choose from a prompt card the range in which the household's gross income fell. Information was also collected on household receipt of certain state benefits - Income support, Family Credit and Job Seeker's Allowance.

Gross weekly household income
Table 3.26 shows that the age distribution between income groups varied, and that generally the proportions of young people in the oldest group increased with income group. For example, of boys living in households in the lowest weekly income group, less than £160, 32% were aged 4 to 6 years and 17% aged 15 to 18 years. For boys living in households in the top income group, £600 a week or more, 20% were aged 4 to 6 years and 25% were aged 15 to 18 years. For girls, the proportions in the bottom and top income groups aged 4 to 6 years were 19% and 15% respectively, and the corresponding proportions aged 15 to 18 years were 14% and 36%.

This relationship between the age of the young person and household income should be borne in mind when interpreting nutrient intake and other data from the survey which appear to show differences associated with household income.

Households where the head was classified as non-manual were significantly more likely than households where the head was classified as manual to have a gross income of £600 per week or more ($p < 0.01$). Non-manual households were also significantly less likely than manual households to have an income below £160 per week ($p < 0.05$). *(Tables 3.26 and 3.27)*

Household receipt of benefits
Overall, 27% of the responding sample and 26% of the diary sample were living in households where their parent(s) were receiving one or more of the prompted state benefits. For those keeping a dietary record, 10% had parents in receipt of Family Credit, 15% Income Support and 2% Job Seeker's Allowance. There were no significant differences between the responding and diary samples in the proportion of young people in households receiving benefits, either overall or by sex.

The proportion of young people living in households in receipt of benefits declined with age, (Table 3.29) from 28% of those aged 4 to 6 years to 17% of those aged 15 to 18 years ($p < 0.05$). This relationship between the age of the young person and receipt of benefits should be borne in mind when interpreting nutrient intake and other data from the survey which appear to show differences associated with the receipt of benefits.

There were no significant differences by region in the receipt of benefits although the data suggest that households in Scotland were the most likely and those in London and the South East of England were the least likely to be in receipt of benefits.

Households where the head was classified as manual were more likely to be in receipt of benefits (31%) than households where the head was classified as non-manual (11%) ($p < 0.01$). The high proportion of households in receipt of benefits in the unclassified category is an artefact associated with some of those who were economically inactive not being asked, in error, the information necessary to derive a social class.

As would be expected, households where the head was unemployed were significantly more likely to be in receipt of benefits (91%) than households where the head was either economically inactive (75%: $p < 0.05$) or working (14%: $p < 0.01$).

Table 3.33 shows that lone-parent households were more likely to be in receipt of benefits than other types of household. For example 50% of lone-parent households with one child were receiving either Income Support, Family Credit or Job Seeker's Allowance compared with 8% of two-parent households with one child ($p < 0.01$). Households containing two or more children were more likely to be receiving benefits than those with one child, for example 72% of lone parents with more than one child were in receipt of benefits compared with 50% of lone parents with one child ($p < 0.01$). *(Tables 3.28 to 3.33)*

3.3.6 Mother's highest educational qualification level

Maternal education may affect nutrition and other aspects of a young person's health behaviour. If there was a 'mother-figure' living in the household, information was collected on the highest educational qualification level she had attained. Foster-mothers and step-mothers, including the father's female partner if the couple were cohabiting as well as if they were married, were defined as the 'mother-figure'.

Overall, 29% of young people who kept a diary had mothers who had obtained at least GCE 'A' level or equivalent; 30% had mothers who had obtained GCSE grades A to C and equivalent, 16% GCSE grades D to G and equivalent and 22% had mothers who had no educational qualification. There was no significant difference between the responding and diary samples by sex of young person in the proportion with mothers who had achieved different qualification levels.

There was no significant difference between regions in the proportion of young people with mothers with different highest educational qualification levels (table not shown).

Although the proportion of young people with mothers with qualifications at or above GCE 'A' level did not vary according to the age group of the young person, there were differences in the proportion with mothers who had no educational qualifications, and in the proportion with mothers whose highest educational qualification was below GCE 'A' level. Table 3.35 shows that 14% of those aged 4 to 6 had mothers who had no formal educational qualifications, compared with 25% of those in the oldest age group (p < 0.05). The oldest group of young people were also less likely to have mothers with qualifications below GCE 'A' level (40%) than those aged 4 to 6 years (53%) (p < 0.05).

Table 3.36 shows the distribution of mother's highest educational qualification level by social class of head of household. Young people in non-manual households were significantly more likely than those from manual households to have mothers with qualifications above GCE 'A' level (33% compared with 10%: p < 0.01). Correspondingly, young people in manual households were more likely to have mothers with no formal educational qualification than those in non-manual households (30% compared with 10%: p < 0.01).

(Tables 3.34 to 3.36)

3.4 Who was the main diary keeper

The young person or a parent could act as the main respondent for the dietary interview and as the main diary keeper, although the person mainly responsible for household food purchase and preparation was required to participate in the dietary interview, irrespective of which member of the household was acting as the main respondent.

In just over half of the cases the main respondent to the dietary interview was the young person's mother, in around 40% of cases the main respondent was the young person and in 4% of cases the main respondent was the young person's father.

Table 3.38 shows that 33% of boys and 44% of girls mainly completed their own dietary record (p < 0.01). Where the young person did not keep their own record, the main diary keeper was generally the mother; this was the case for 61% of boys and 50% of girls (p < 0.01). The proportions of young people mainly keeping their own record increased with age for both boys and girls, rising from 11% for boys aged 7 to 10 years to 69% for boys aged 15 to 18 years (p < 0.01). For girls the corresponding proportions were 15% and 87% (p < 0.01). *(Tables 3.37 and 3.38)*

3.5 Illness and the use of prescribed medicines

The interview included questions about the young person's current and previous health and their current use of dietary supplements and prescribed medicines. In particular, where a full seven-day dietary record had been kept the respondent was asked whether the young person had suffered from diarrhoea, been sick or vomited, or been unwell in any other way during the record-keeping period, and if so, whether this had affected the young person's eating habits.

3.5.1 Illness

Table 3.39 shows that overall, 18% of boys and 20% of girls were reported to have been unwell during the record-keeping period, including 10% of boys and 11% of girls whose eating was affected. There were no significant differences between boys and girls or between age groups in the proportions reporting being unwell.

As would be expected, young people were more likely to report being unwell in the fieldwork waves covering the autumn and winter months (Wave 1, January to March, 23%, and Wave 4, October to December, 20%) than in the spring and summer months (Waves 2, April to June, 15%, and Wave 3, July to September, 17%), although the differences did not reach the level of statistical significance. *(Tables 3.39 and 3.40)*

3.5.2 Prescribed medicines

Information was collected on any prescribed medicines currently being taken by the young person. Information about the use of the contraceptive pill was collected for girls aged 10 to 18 years as part of the self-completion section of the initial dietary interview. The information on prescribed medicines was not coded, but was passed in an anonymised form to the Dunn Nutrition Unit in Cambridge where it was reviewed by staff to see whether any of the medicines were likely to have effects on any of the blood or urine analytes being measured; there were no such effects.

Overall, 13% of boys and 19% of girls reported currently taking one or more prescribed medicine (p < 0.05). For boys and for girls up to the group aged 11 to 14 years, there were no significant differences by age in the proportions taking prescribed medicines. However, 41% of girls aged 15 to 18 years reported taking a prescribed medicine; this was mainly accounted for by the 24% of girls aged 15 to 18 years who reported taking the oral contraceptive pill (table not shown).

There were no significant differences in the proportions of young people taking prescribed medicines by field-work wave.   *(Table 3.41)*

3.6 Dietary and health behaviour of respondents

3.6.1 Smoking

Information was collected about smoking behaviour of young people aged 7 to 18 years and each parent living in the household. In order to ensure confidentiality and improve the quality of the data collected, information about young people's smoking and other sensitive topics such as the consumption of alcohol was collected by self-completion[18]. The young person was offered the choice between entering their answers into the inter-viewer's laptop computer or answering the questions on a paper schedule. The questions about smoking were taken from the Survey of Smoking among Secondary School Children[19] and were designed to identify current smokers, ex-smokers and also those who had tried smoking, even if only a puff or two of a cigarette. Young people who admitted to having tried smoking but who were not current smokers are included in the category of ex-smoker and are classified as having ever smoked in the tables.

Overall, 35% of boys and 36% of girls aged 7 to 18 years reported that they had ever smoked including 12% and 13% respectively who said they were current smokers. Boys were no more likely than girls to report being smokers although the data suggest that girls aged 15 to 18 years were more likely than boys in the same age group to be smoking more than 6 cigarettes per week (ns). As would be expected, the proportion of young people who were both current and ex-smokers increased with age, for example less than 1% of boys aged 7 to 10 years said they were current smokers compared with 6% of boys aged 11 to 14 years and 31% of boys aged 15 to 18 years (p < 0.01).

Table 3.43 shows that significantly fewer young people aged 11 to 14 years reported being current smokers (6%) compared with young people in the same age group surveyed in the 1996 Survey of Smoking among Secondary School Children[20] (16%) (p < 0.01). This difference may be partly explained by differences in the methodology of the two surveys. In this NDNS of young people the questions about smoking (and drinking) were completed in the home, generally with the young person's parent present; in the Survey of

Smoking among Secondary School Children the self-completion questionnaire was completed in the class-room under the supervision of an interviewer but with no teacher present. The classification of smoking behaviour may also differ slightly between the two samples because the Survey of Smoking among Secondary School Children used information from a smoking diary in addition to answers given in the self-completion questionnaire, for example pupils who indicated on the questionnaire that they were not current smokers but who recorded cigarettes in their diary were classified as occasional smokers.

Young people living in households with both parents were more likely to be current smokers if their mothers smoked (21%) than if neither parent (10%), both parents (11%), or just the father smoked (10%). Young people living in households with just one parent were more likely to have ever smoked if their parent was a smoker (45% compared with 36%: p < 0.05). Although the difference did not reach the level of statistical significance, the data suggest that the young person was also more likely to be a current smoker if their parent smoked.   *(Tables 3.42 to 3.44)*

3.6.2 Main activity and arrangements for a lunch-time meal

The age range covered by this survey is broad and included young people who had not yet started school, those who were at school and those who had left school and were working or unemployed. The respondent was asked which of these was the young person's 'main activity'. If the young person was in full-time education or working, the respondent was asked what their usual arrangements were for a lunch-time meal.

Table 3.45 shows that 7% of young people aged 4 to 6 years had not started school and 25% of young people aged 15 to 18 years had left full-time education.

Table 3.46 shows that 84% of boys and 83% of girls aged 15 to 18 years who were no longer in full-time education were working, 13% of boys and 11% of girls were unemployed and the remainder were economically inactive. Of those aged 15 to 18 years still in full-time education, 55% of boys and 51% of girls had done some paid work in the 7 days prior to the interview.

Overall, 45% of boys and 46% of girls attending school or college had a school meal and 44% of boys and 45% of girls took a packed meal from home. For 14% of boys and 15% of girls their school meal was either free or subsidised. For both boys and girls the data suggest that the proportions having a free or subsidised school meal decreased with age. More than half of boys and girls aged 7 to 10 years took a packed lunch to school but by age 15 to 18 years this proportion had fallen to 31% of boys and 35% of girls (both p < 0.01). Compared with young people aged 7 to 10 years the

oldest group of boys and girls were most likely to buy something to eat outside school or college premises (15% of boys and 11% of girls, p < 0.01). Overall less than 5% of both boys and girls had lunch at home (or at the home of a relative). For children aged 4 to 6 years, 8% of boys and 9% of girls were reported to have no lunch-time meal; it is likely that these were small children attending for only part of the day who had lunch at home and should therefore have been included in this category.

Table 3.48 shows that for young people aged 15 to 18 years who had finished full-time education and were working, 9% received a free meal at work, just over one third bought a lunch-time meal and around one third took a packed lunch. The data suggest that girls were more likely to buy their lunch-time meal outside work premises than boys, although perhaps due to the small size of the groups the difference did not reach the level of statistical significance.

Nearly all (94%) of young people receiving a free school meal and 65% of those receiving a reduced price or subsidised school meal were from households that were in receipt of one or more state benefits. Just over half were from one-parent households. Although sufficiently detailed information was not collected to establish eligibility and take-up of free or subsidised school meals, the data show that 47% of young people from households in receipt of benefits were receiving a free or subsidised school meal, as were 37% of young people from lone-parent households (table not shown).

(Tables 3.45 to 3.48)

References and endnotes

1 Thomas M, Walker A, Wilmot A, Bennett N. *Living in Britain. Results from the 1996 General Household Survey.* TSO (London, 1998).

2 Response data are presented and reported on as unweighted data. For an account of the weighting applied to the responding sample to adjust for different sampling probabilities see *Appendix D 'Sample design and response'.*

3 Response to the dietary record is based on those completing a full seven-day diary, which was then included in the dataset for analysis. A small number of young people kept diaries for fewer than seven days and a small number were rejected at the coding and editing stages. The decision to exclude a diary from analysis was based on supplementary information recorded by the interviewer during the diary-keeping period and in a post-record keeping quality assessment, and after scrutiny of the dietary record by ONS nutritionists.

4 Gregory JR, Collins DL, Davies PSW, Hughes JM, Clarke PC. *National Diet and Nutrition Survey: children aged 1½ to 4½ years. Volume 1: Report of the diet and nutrition survey.* HMSO (London, 1995).

5 In response tables (Tables 3.1 to 3.8) 'Fieldwork wave' is defined as the wave (quarter) in which the case w (or reissued) for interview. In the data analysis 'Fieldwork wave' is defined as the wave (period) in which the case was interviewed. See also *Appendix U 'Glossary'.*

6 Eligibility to take part in the survey was defined by age at the mid-point of the fieldwork wave (see *Appendix D*). There were a small number of young people who had not reached their 4th birthday and a small number who had had their 19th birthday at the time they were interviewed. In the analysis these young people are included in the 4 to 6 and 15 to 18 year age groups respectively.

7 In response tables (Tables 3.1 to 3.8) age group for the responding samples is derived from age at the time of the initial dietary interview; for the non-responding samples age is taken as that at the mid-point of the fieldwork wave.

8 Social class information was not collected from the non-responding sample. For details of the derivation of the social class variable see *Section 3.3.2* and *Appendix U.*

9 For details of the feasibility study see *Appendix C* and Lowe, S. *Feasibility study for the National Diet and Nutrition Survey: young people aged 4 to 18 years. Report of the feasibility study.* ONS (*In preparation*).

10 As described in Chapter 2, signed consents to various procedures were required from the young person's parent, (unless the young person was aged 18, or 16 to 17 and living away from home). In this chapter and elsewhere references to the *young person consenting* to a procedure should be taken to include consent being obtained from their parent.

11 The numbers of young people co-operating with each of the anthropometric measurements and blood pressure measurement (may) differ from those shown in the tables in Chapters 10 and 11, since some measurements were excluded at the analysis stage, for example where mid upper-arm circumference was measured over clothing. Details of the reasons for excluding cases from the measurement data are given in Chapters 10 and 11.

12 Response rates are based on those consenting to provide a urine sample; not all those consenting provided a sample, and not all the samples obtained were analysed — some were damaged, or deteriorated in transit. Details of the numbers of urine samples analysed and reported on are given in Chapter 9.

13 Information on the number of samples analysed is given in Chapter 12.

14 1996-7 GHS subsample of households containing at least one young person aged 4 to 18 years.

15 See *Appendix U – 'Glossary'* for the definition of head of household.

16 Within the diary sample social class could not be derived for 10% of heads of household, including 7% who were economically inactive but it was not known whether they had ever worked. Of these 7%, half were male and half female heads of household.

17 Children were defined as siblings, other relatives or non-relatives or the young person's own children aged less than 16 years.

18 Information on the young person's consumption of alcohol, as reported in the interview and recorded in the dietary record, is given in Chapter 6.

19 Diamond A, Goddard E. *Smoking among secondary school children in 1994.* HMSO (London, 1995).

20 Jarvis L. *Smoking among secondary school children in 1996: England.* HMSO (London, 1997).

Table 3.1 Response to the dietary interview and 7-day dietary record by wave of fieldwork*

(Unweighted data)

Response	Wave of fieldwork									
	Wave 1: January to March		Wave 2: April to June		Wave 3: July to September		Wave 4: October to December		All	
	No.	%	No.	%	No.	%	No.	%	No.	%
Eligible sample	557	100	573	100	779	100	763	100	2672	100
Non-contacts	6	1	3	1	5	1	12	2	26	1
Refusals	108	19	107	19	150	19	154	20	519	19
Co-operation with:										
dietary interview	443	80	463	81	624	80	597	78	2127	80
7-day dietary record	379	68	375	65	474	61	473	62	1701	64

* Fieldwork wave is defined as the wave (quarter) in which the case was issued (or reissued) for interview.
See also Appendix U 'Glossary'.

Table 3.2   Co-operation with the dietary interview by sex and age of young person*

(Unweighted data)

Sex and age of young person	Interviews obtained	as % of eligible sample
Males aged:		
4–6 years	230	86
7–10 years	304	82
11–14 years	290	81
15–18 years	258	72
All	1082	80
Females aged:		
4–6 years	224	82
7–10 years	277	80
11–14 years	280	79
15–18 years	264	76
All	1045	79
All	2127	80

*Age group for respondents is derived from age at the time of the initial dietary interview; for the non-responding sample age is taken from the mid-point of the fieldwork wave.

Table 3.3   Co-operation with the 7-day dietary record by sex and age of young person and social class of head of household*

(Unweighted data)

Sex and age of young person and social class of head of household	7-day dietary records	As percentage of:	
		eligible sample	responding sample
Males aged:			
4–6 years	184	68	80
7–10 years	256	69	84
11–14 years	237	67	82
15–18 years	179	50	69
All	856	63	79
Females aged:			
4–6 years	172	63	77
7–10 years	225	65	81
11–14 years	238	67	85
15–18 years	210	61	80
All	845	64	81
Social class of head of household			
Non-manual	815	na**	84
Manual	746	na**	78
All	**1701**	**64**	**80**

* See footnote to Table 3.2.
** not available; social class information is not available for the non-responding sample.

Table 3.4 Co-operation with anthropometric measurements and blood pressure by wave of fieldwork*

(Unweighted data)

Measurement	Wave of fieldwork				All
	Wave 1 Jan to March	Wave 2 Apr to June	Wave 3 July to Sept	Wave 4 Oct to Dec	
Weight					
measurements made	415	423	570	538	1946
as % of eligible sample	*75*	*74*	*73*	*71*	*73*
as % of responding sample	*94*	*91*	*91*	*90*	*91*
Height					
measurements made	415	424	572	538	1949
as % of eligible sample	*75*	*74*	*73*	*71*	*73*
as % of responding sample	*94*	*92*	*93*	*89*	*92*
Mid upper arm circumference					
measurements made	415	424	570	535	1944
as % of eligible sample	*75*	*74*	*73*	*70*	*73*
as % of responding sample	*94*	*92*	*91*	*90*	*91*
Hip and waist circumferences					
measurements made	213	210	297	267	987
as % of eligible sample	*72*	*70*	*71*	*67*	*70*
as % of responding sample	*93*	*89*	*91*	*89*	*90*
Blood pressure					
measurements made	404	412	562	527	1905
as % of eligible sample	*73*	*72*	*72*	*69*	*71*
as % of responding sample	*91*	*89*	*90*	*88*	*90*

* See footnote to Table 3.1.

Table 3.5 Co-operation with anthropometric measurements and blood pressure by sex and age of young person*

(Unweighted data)

Measurement	Males aged (years)					Females aged (years)				
	4–6	7–10	11–14	15–18	All	4–6	7–10	11–14	15–18	All
Weight										
measurements made	213	288	268	222	991	204	251	260	240	955
as % of eligible sample	*79*	*78*	*75*	*62*	*73*	*75*	*72*	*74*	*69*	*72*
as % of responding sample	*93*	*95*	*92*	*86*	*92*	*91*	*91*	*93*	*91*	*91*
Height										
measurements made	213	288	268	223	992	203	251	263	240	957
as % of eligible sample	*79*	*78*	*75*	*62*	*73*	*74*	*72*	*75*	*69*	*73*
as % of responding sample	*93*	*95*	*92*	*86*	*92*	*91*	*91*	*94*	*91*	*92*
Mid upper-arm circumference										
measurements made	208	288	268	222	986	203	251	264	240	958
as % of eligible sample	*77*	*78*	*75*	*62*	*73*	*74*	*72*	*75*	*69*	*73*
as % of responding sample	*90*	*95*	*92*	*86*	*91*	*91*	*91*	*94*	*91*	*92*
Hip and waist circumferences										
measurements made	na	na	268	222	490	na	na	259	238	497
as % of eligible sample			*75*	*62*	*69*			*73*	*69*	*71*
as % of responding sample			*92*	*86*	*89*			*93*	*90*	*91*
Blood pressure										
measurements made	205	282	265	219	971	191	247	260	236	934
as % of eligible sample	*76*	*76*	*74*	*61*	*72*	*70*	*71*	*74*	*68*	*71*
as % of responding sample	*89*	*93*	*91*	*85*	*90*	*85*	*89*	*93*	*89*	*89*

* See footnote to Table 3.2.
na: not applicable; hip and waist circumferences were only measured for young people aged 11 years and over.

Table 3.6 Co-operation with anthropometric measurements and blood pressure by social class of head of household

(Unweighted data)

Measurement	Social class of head of household		
	Non-manual	Manual	All*
Weight			
measurements made	899	876	1946
as % of responding sample	*93*	*91*	*91*
Height			
measurements made	900	878	1949
as % of responding sample	*93*	*91*	*92*
Mid upper-arm circumference			
measurements made	900	874	1944
as % of responding sample	*93*	*91*	*91*
Hip and waist circumferences			
measurements made	440	453	987
as % of responding sample	*91*	*91*	*90*
Blood pressure			
measurements made	882	857	1905
as % of responding sample	*91*	*89*	*90*

* Includes those who could not be allocated to a social class, either because their job was inadequately described, they were a member of the armed forces, had never worked, or it was not known whether they had ever worked.

Table 3.7 Co-operation with the urine sample by wave of fieldwork, sex and age of young person and social class of head of household*

(Unweighted data)

	Samples obtained	As percentage of:	
		eligible sample	responding sample
Fieldwork wave			
Wave 1	400	72	*90*
Wave 2	401	70	*87*
Wave 3	539	69	*86*
Wave 4	511	67	*86*
Sex and age of young person			
Males aged:			
4–6 years	200	74	*87*
7–10 years	273	74	*90*
11–14 years	261	73	*90*
15–18 years	208	58	*81*
All	942	70	*87*
Females aged:			
4–6 years	188	69	*84*
7–10 years	244	70	*88*
11–14 years	249	71	*89*
15–18 years	228	66	*86*
All	909	69	*87*
Social class of head of household			
Non-manual	858	na**	*88*
Manual	829	na**	*86*
All	1851	69	*87*

* See footnotes to Tables 3.1 and 3.2.
** Not available; social class information is not available for the non-responding sample.

Table 3.8 Co-operation with the blood sample by wave of fieldwork, sex and age of young person and social class of head of household*

(Unweighted data)

	Consent obtained			Venepuncture attempted				Blood sample obtained			
	No.	as percentage of:		No.	as percentage of:			No.	as percentage of:		
		eligible sample	responding sample		eligible sample	responding sample	consenting sample		eligible sample	responding sample	consenting sample
Fieldwork wave											
Wave 1	263	47	59	259	46	58	98	254	46	57	97
Wave 2	239	42	52	228	40	49	95	215	38	46	90
Wave 3	410	53	66	401	51	64	98	388	50	62	95
Wave 4	372	49	62	361	47	60	97	336	44	56	90
Sex and age of young person											
Males aged:											
4–6 years	107	40	47	100	37	43	93	87	32	38	81
7–10 years	200	54	66	192	52	63	96	186	50	61	93
11–14 years	190	53	66	186	52	64	98	182	51	63	96
15–18 years	170	47	66	169	47	66	99	168	47	65	99
All	667	49	62	647	48	60	97	623	46	58	93
Females aged:											
4–6 years	99	36	44	92	34	41	93	84	31	38	85
7–10 years	157	45	57	153	44	55	97	144	41	52	92
11–14 years	186	53	66	183	52	65	98	173	49	62	93
15–18 years	175	50	66	173	50	66	99	169	49	64	97
All	617	47	59	601	46	58	97	570	43	55	92
Social class of head of household											
Non-manual	588	na**	61	578	na**	60	98	554	na**	57	94
Manual	586	na**	61	564	na**	59	96	537	na**	56	92
All	1284	48	60	1248	47	59	97	1193	45	56	93

* see footnotes to Tables 3.1 and 3.2.
** not available; social class information is not available for the non-responding sample.

Table 3.9 Comparison of age and sex of sampled young person for responding and non-responding samples

(Unweighted data)

Age of young person (years)	Non-responding sample						Responding sample					
	Male		Female		All		Male		Female		All	
	No.	%	No.	%	No.	%	No.	%	No.	%	No.	%
4–6	39	14	49	18	88	16	230	21	224	21	454	21
7–10	65	24	70	26	135	25	304	28	277	26	581	27
11–14	66	24	73	26	139	26	290	27	280	27	570	27
15–18	100	37	83	30	183	34	258	24	264	25	522	24
Base	*270*	*100*	*275*	*100*	*545*	*100*	*1082*	*100*	*1045*	*100*	*2127*	*100*
All ages		*(49.5%)*		*(50.5%)*		*(100%)*		*(50.8%)*		*(49.2%)*		*(100%)*

Table 3.10 Age and sex of young person for responding and diary samples

Age of young person (years)	Responding sample			Diary sample*		
	Male	Female	All	Male	Female	All
	%	%	%	%	%	%
Unweighted data						
4–6	21	21	21	21	20	21
7–10	28	27	27	30	27	28
11–14	27	27	27	28	28	28
15–18	24	25	25	21	25	23
Base	*1082*	*1045*	*2127*	*856*	*845*	*1701*
All ages	*(50.8%)*	*(49.2%)*	*(100%)*	*(50.3%)*	*(49.7%)*	*(100%)*
*Weighted data**						
4–6	21	21	21	21	21	21
7–10	27	27	27	27	27	27
11–14	26	26	26	26	26	26
15–18	26	26	26	26	26	26

* Young people who kept a dietary record for the full seven days.
** Responding sample is weighted for differential sampling probability; diary sample is weighted for differential sampling probability and differential non-response.

Table 3.11 Regional distribution of responding and diary samples compared with 1996-7 GHS data

Region	Responding sample	Diary sample	1996-7 GHS sample*
	%	%	%
Scotland	**8**	**8**	**10**
North	5	6	7
Yorkshire and Humberside	9	9	9
North West	12	12	12
Northern	**27**	**27**	**28**
East Midlands	8	8	8
East Anglia	4	4	4
West Midlands	9	9	10
South West	9	9	8
Wales	5	5	6
Central, South West and Wales	**35**	**35**	**36**
London	11	11	11
South East	18	18	17
London and South East	**29**	**29**	**27**
Base	*2127*	*1701*	*2638*

*1996-7 GHS subsample of households containing at least one young person aged 4 to 18 years.

Table 3.12 Region by sex and age of young person

Diary sample

Region	Males aged (years)					Females aged (years)				
	4–6	7–10	11–14	15–18	All males	4–6	7–10	11–14	15–18	All females
	%	%	%	%	%	%	%	%	%	%
Scotland	8	9	8	7	8	10	7	8	8	8
Northern	28	28	28	30	28	28	29	25	28	27
Central, South West and Wales	34	36	36	34	35	33	35	37	35	35
London and the South East	31	27	28	29	29	29	29	30	30	29
Base	*184*	*256*	*237*	*179*	*856*	*171*	*226*	*238*	*210*	*845*

Table 3.13 Social class of head of household by sex of young person for responding and diary samples

Social class of head of household	Responding sample			Diary sample*		
	Male	Female	All	Male	Female	All
	%	%	%	%	%	%
I and II	32	32	32	34	34	34
III non-manual	12	12	12	13	11	12
III manual	30	29	29	30	28	29
IV and V	17	15	16	15	15	15
Unclassified*	10	12	11	8	12	10
Base	*1082* *(51.3%)*	*1045* *(48.7%)*	*2127* *(100%)*	*.856* *(50.8%)*	*845* *(49.2%)*	*1701* *(100%)*

*Includes those not assigned a social class because their job was inadequately described, they were a member of the armed forces, had never worked or it was not known whether they had ever worked.

Table 3.14 Social class of head of household for responding and diary samples compared with 1996-7 GHS data*

Social class of head of household	Responding sample	Diary sample	1996-7 GHS sample*
	%	%	%
Non-manual	44	46	47
Manual	45	44	48
Armed forces	1	1	1
Inadequately described	1	1	1
Never worked	2	2	4
Don't know whether ever worked	7	7	–
Base	*2127*	*1701*	*2638*

*1996-7 GHS subsample of households containing at least one young person aged 4 to 18 years.

Table 3.15 Social class of head of household by sex and age of young person

Diary sample

Social class of head of household	Males aged (years)					Females aged (years)				
	4–6	7–10	11–14	15–18	All males	4–6	7–10	11–14	15–18	All females
	%	%	%	%	%	%	%	%	%	%
Non-manual	47	49	46	46	47	47	46	42	47	45
Manual	45	45	44	47	45	44	40	45	42	43
Unclassified*	8	6	10	7	8	8	15	13	11	12
Base	*184*	*256*	*237*	*179*	*856*	*171*	*226*	*238*	*210*	*845*

*Includes those not assigned a social class because their job was inadequately described, they were a member of the armed forces, had never worked or it was not known whether they had ever worked.

Table 3.16   Social class of head of household by region

Diary sample

Social class of head of household	Region				All
	Scotland	Northern	Central, South West and Wales	London and the South East	
	%	%	%	%	%
Non-manual	45	42	45	52	46
Manual	43	50	45	37	44
Unclassified*	13	8	10	11	10
Base	*137*	*460*	*606*	*498*	*1701*

*Includes those not assigned a social class because their job was inadequately described, they were a member of the armed forces, had never worked or it was not known whether they had ever worked.

Table 3.17 Whether young person was living with both parents by sex of young person for responding and diary samples

Whether young person was living with both parents	Responding sample			Diary sample		
	Male	Female	All	Male	Female	All
	%	%	%	%	%	%
Young person living with both parents: married/cohabiting parents and other child(ren)	61	59	60	64	60	62
married/cohabiting parents and no other children	19	18	18	18	18	18
Young person living with lone parent: and other child(ren)	13	14	13	12	14	13
and no other children	7	7	7	6	7	6
Young person living with others, not parent(s)	1	1	1	0	1	0
Base	*1082*	*1045*	*2127*	*856*	*845*	*1701*

Table 3.18   Whether young person was living with both parents by sex and age of young person

Diary sample

Whether young person was living with both parents	Males aged (years)					Females aged (years)				
	4–6	7–10	11–14	15–18	All Males	4–6	7–10	11–14	15–18	All Females
	%	%	%	%	%	%	%	%	%	%
Young person living with both parents: married or cohabiting parents and other child(ren)	70	76	65	40	64	71	70	62	38	60
married or cohabiting parents and no other children	9	7	18	42	18	11	9	16	37	18
Young person lving with lone parent: and other child(ren)	17	12	12	7	12	15	17	13	11	14
and no other children	4	5	5	10	6	3	4	9	11	7
Young person living with others, not parent(s)	–	–	–	1	0	–	–	–	3	1
Base	*184*	*256*	*237*	*179*	*856*	*171*	*226*	*238*	*210*	*845*

Table 3.19 **Age of young person by sex and whether living with both parents**

Diary sample

Age of young person (years)	Sex of young person and whether living with both parents									
	Males: living with				All males*	Females: living with				All females*
	both parents and:		lone parent and:			both parents and:		lone parent and:		
	other children	no other children	other children	no other children		other children	no other children	other children	no other children	
	%	%	%	%	%	%	%	%	%	%
4–6	23	11	31	16	21	23	12	22	9	20
7–10	35	11	29	27	29	32	14	34	16	28
11–14	28	27	28	21	27	29	24	25	35	27
15–18	14	51	13	37	22	16	50	19	41	25
Base	*528*	*169*	*100*	*57*	*856*	*498*	*173*	*105*	*62*	*845*

* Includes 2 boys and 7 girls (unweighted) who were living with others, not parents.

Table 3.20 **Whether young person was living with both parents by social class of head of household**

Diary sample

Whether young person was living with both parents	Social class of head of household			
	Non-manual	Manual	Unclassified*	All
	%	%	%	%
Young person living with both parents:				
married or cohabiting parents and other child(ren)	64	64	45	62
married or cohabiting parents and no other children	19	19	12	18
Young person living with lone parent:				
and other child(ren)	10	12	31	13
and no other children	7	4	12	6
Young person living with others, not parent(s)	0	1	0	0
Base	*815*	*746*	*140*	*1701*

*Includes those who were not assigned a social class either because their job was inadequately described, they were a member of the armed forces, had never worked or where it was not known whether they had ever worked.

Table 3.21 **Employment status of head of household for responding and diary samples compared with 1996-7 GHS data**

Employment status of head of household	Responding sample			Diary sample			1996-7 GHS sample*
	Male	Female	All	Male	Female	All	All
	%	%	%	%	%	%	%
Working	82	79	81	84	80	82	77
Unemployed	5	4	5	5	4	5	6
Economically inactive	13	16	15	11	16	13	17
Base	*1082*	*1045*	*2127*	*856*	*845*	*1701*	*2638*

*1996-7 GHS subsample of households containing at least one young person aged 4 to 18 years.

Table 3.22 Employment status of head of household by age of young person

Diary sample

Employment status of head of household	Age of young person (years)				
	4–6	7–10	11–14	15–18	All
	%	%	%	%	%
Working	81	80	82	85	82
Unemployed	7	5	4	2	5
Economically inactive	12	14	14	12	13
Base	*356*	*481*	*475*	*389*	*1701*

Table 3.23 Employment status of head of household by region

Diary sample

Employment status of head of household	Region				
	Scotland	Northern	Central, South West and Wales	London and the South East	All
	%	%	%	%	%
Working	83	83	80	83	82
Unemployed	5	5	3	6	5
Economically inactive	12	13	16	11	13
Base	*137*	*460*	*606*	*498*	*1701*

Table 3.24 Employment status of head of household by social class of head of household

Diary sample

Employment status of head of household	Social class of head of household			
	Non-manual	Manual	Unclassified*	All
	%	%	%	%
Working	94	86	10	82
Unemployed	2	6	8	5
Economically inactive	4	8	82	13
Base	*815*	*746*	*140*	*1701*

*Includes those not assigned a social class because their job was inadequately described, they were a member of the armed forces, had never worked or it was not known whether they had ever worked.

Table 3.25 Whether young person was living with both parents by employment status of head of household

Diary sample

Employment status of head of household	Young person living with parent(s):				Young person living with others, not parent(s)
	both parents		lone parent		
	and other child(ren)	and no other children	and other child(ren)	and no other children	
	%	%	%	%	No.*
Working	86	92	54	69	[7]
Unemployed	6	1	4	5	[1]
Economically inactive	8	7	42	26	[1]
Base	*1026*	*342*	*205*	*119*	*9*

* Numbers in brackets are absolute (unweighted), not percentages because the cell size is too small to allow a reliable percentage to be calculated.

Table 3.26 Gross weekly household income by sex and age of young person

Diary sample

Sex and age of young person (years)	Gross weekly household income					
	Less than £160	£160 to less than £280	£280 to less than £400	£400 to less than £600	£600 or more	Not answered
	%	%	%	%	%	%
Males aged:						
4–6	32	20	23	15	20	10
7–10	30	34	28	26	30	19
11–14	22	27	28	33	25	31
15–18	17	19	20	26	25	40
Base	*133*	*159*	*157*	*173*	*208*	*26*
Females aged:						
4–6	19	21	22	23	15	17
7–10	35	30	31	22	24	20
11–14	32	27	22	29	25	37
15–18	14	22	25	26	36	26
Base	*131*	*146*	*145*	*192*	*196*	*35*

Table 3.27 Social class of head of household by gross weekly household income

Diary sample

Social class of head of household	Gross weekly household income						
	Less than £160	£160 to less than £280	£280 to less than £400	£400 to less than £600	£600 or more	Not answered	All
	%	%	%	%	%	%	
Non-manual	8	11	14	26	38	3	46
Manual	18	28	23	17	10	4	44
Unclassified*	53	21	11	8	3	4	10
Base	*264*	*305*	*302*	*365*	*404*	*61*	*1701*
All	17%	20%	18%	21%	22%	4%	100%

*Includes those not assigned a social class because their job was inadequately described, they were a member of the armed forces, had never worked or it was not known whether they had ever worked

Table 3.28 Benefits being received by young person's parents for responding and diary samples by sex of young person

Benefits being received by young person's parents	Responding sample			Diary sample		
	Male	Female	All	Male	Female	All
	%	%	%	%	%	%
Receiving:						
Family Credit	12	10	11	11	9	10
Income Support	15	17	16	14	16	15
Job Seeker's Allowance	2	3	3	2	3	2
At least one of the above	27	28	27	25	26	26
Base	*1082*	*1045*	*2127*	*856*	*845*	*1701*

Table 3.29 Whether young person's parents were in receipt of benefits by age of young person

Diary sample

Age of young person (years)	Receiving benefit(s)	Base
4–6	28%	356
7–10	30%	481
11–14	26%	475
15–18	17%	389
All ages	26%	1701

Table 3.30 Whether young person's parents were in receipt of benefits by region

Diary sample

Region	Receiving benefits	Base
Scotland	30%	137
Northern	27%	460
Central, South West and Wales	26%	606
London and the South East	23%	498
All regions	26%	1701

Table 3.31 Whether young person's parents were in receipt of benefits by social class of head of household

Diary sample

Social class of head of household	Receiving benefits	Base
Non-manual	11%	815
Manual	31%	746
Unclassified*	66%	140
All	26%	1701

*Includes those not assigned a social class because their job was inadequately described, they were a member of the armed forces, had never worked or it was not known whether they had ever worked.

Table 3.32 Whether young person's parents were in receipt of benefits by employment status of head of household

Diary sample

Employment status of head of household	Receiving benefits	Base
Working	14%	1428
Unemployed	91%	66
Economically inactive	75%	204
All	26%	1701

Table 3.33 Whether young person was living with both parents by whether parents were in receipt of benefits

Diary sample

Whether young person was living with both parents	Receiving benefits	Base
Young person living with both parents:		
married or cohabiting parents and other child(ren)	19%	1026
married or cohabiting parents and no other children	8%	342
Young person living with lone parent:		
and other child(ren)	72%	205
and no other children	50%	119
Young person living with others, not parent(s)	[2]	9
All cases	26%	1701

[ ] Indicates number, not percentage.

Table 3.34 Mother's highest educational qualification level by sex of young person for responding and diary samples

Mother's highest educational qualification level	Responding sample			Diary sample		
	Male	Female	All	Male	Female	All
	%	%	%	%	%	%
Above GCE 'A' level	19	19	19	21	21	21
GCE 'A' level and equivalent	9	7	8	10	7	8
GCSE grades A-C and equivalent	29	32	30	29	32	30
GCSE grades D-G and equivalent*	15	16	15	15	16	16
No qualifications	26	22	24	23	20	22
No mother in household	3	4	3	2	3	2
Base	1082	1045	2127	856	845	1701

* Includes other qualifications.

Table 3.35 Mother's highest educational qualification level by age of young person

Diary sample

Mother's highest educational qualification level	Age of young person (years)				
	4–6	7–10	11–14	15–18	All
	%	%	%	%	%
Above GCE 'A' level	20	23	19	23	21
GCE 'A' level and equivalent	11	10	7	7	8
GCSE grades A-C and equivalent	37	31	30	24	30
GCSE grades D-G and equivalent*	16	15	16	16	16
No qualifications	14	20	26	25	22
No mother in household	1	2	2	5	2
Base	356	481	475	389	1701

* Includes other qualifications.

Table 3.36 Mother's highest educational qualification level by social class of head of household

Diary sample

Mother's highest educational qualification level	Social class of head of household			
	Non-manual	Manual	Unclassified**	All
	%	%	%	%
Above GCE 'A' level	33	10	16	21
GCE 'A' level and equivalent	12	6	4	8
GCSE grades A-C and equivalent	29	34	22	30
GCSE grades D-G and equivalent*	15	18	12	16
No qualifications	10	30	40	22
No mother in household	2	3	6	2
Base	815	746	140	1701

* Includes other qualifications.
**Includes those not assigned a social class because their job was inadequately described, they were a member of the armed forces, had never worked or it was not known whether they had ever worked.

Table 3.37 Interview respondent by sex and age of young person

Responding sample

Interview respondent was:	Males aged (years)				All males	Females aged (years)				All females	All
	4–6	7–10	11–14	15–18		4–6	7–10	11–14	15–18		
	%	%	%	%	%	%	%	%	%	%	%
young person	6	19	50	83	39	5	12	57	83	41	40
young person's:											
mother	89	74	43	15	56	91	79	39	16	55	55
father	3	6	6	2	4	4	8	2	2	4	4
brother or sister	1	1	1	–	1	–	1	1	–	1	1
grandparent	0	–	–	–	0	1	–	0	–	0	0
Base	*230*	*304*	*290*	*258*	*1082*	*224*	*277*	*280*	*264*	*1045*	*2127*

Table 3.38 Main diary keeper by sex and age of young person

Diary sample

Main diary keeper	Males aged (years)				All males	Females aged (years)				All females	All
	4–6	7–10	11–14	15–18		4–6	7–10	11–14	15–18		
	%	%	%	%	%	%	%	%	%	%	%
Young person	2	11	54	69	33	0	15	68	87	44	39
Young person's:											
mother	90	83	41	30	61	92	76	28	12	50	56
father	6	5	4	0	4	6	7	4	1	5	4
brother or sister	1	2	0	1	1	–	1	–	–	0	1
other relative in household	0	0	–	–	0	0	1	–	–	0	0
Other*	1	0	0	0	0	1	1	0	1	1	0
Base	*184*	*256*	*237*	*179*	*856*	*171*	*226*	*238*	*210*	*845*	*1701*

* Includes nanny or child minder.

Table 3.39 Whether young person was reported as being unwell during the dietary recording period by sex and age of young person

Diary sample

Whether young person was reported as being unwell	Males aged (years)				All males	Females aged (years)				All females	All
	4–6	7–10	11–14	15–18		4–6	7–10	11–14	15–18		
	%	%	%	%	%	%	%	%	%	%	%
Unwell during recording period and:											
eating affected	8	12	9	9	10		13	8	12	11	11
eating not affected	8	8	11	4	8		7	8	11	9	9
Not unwell during recording period	85	80	79	87	82		80	84	77	80	80
Base	*184*	*256*	*237*	*179*	*856*		*171*	*226*	*238*	*210*	*845*

Table 3.40 Whether young person was reported as being unwell during the dietary recording period by fieldwork wave

Diary sample

Whether young person was reported as being unwell	Fieldwork wave*				
	Wave 1	Wave 2	Wave 3	Wave 4	All
	%	%	%	%	%
Unwell during recording period and:					
eating affected	14	7	11	10	10
eating not affected	9	8	6	10	8
Not unwell during recording period	77	85	83	80	81
Base	*379*	*374*	*470*	*478*	*1701*

* Wave 1: January to March 1997
  Wave 2: April to June 1997
  Wave 3: July to September 1997
  Wave 4: October to December 1997

Table 3.41 Percentage of young people taking prescribed medicines by sex and age of young person and wave of fieldwork

Pick-up interview sample*

Sex and age (years) of young person and wave of fieldwork**	Percentage taking prescribed medicines	*Base*
Males aged:		
4–6	12%	*210*
7–10	12%	*281*
11–14	15%	*263*
15–18	15%	*217*
All males	13%	*971*
Females aged:***		
4–6	11%	*200*
7–10	11%	*251*
11–14	11%	*263*
15–18	41%	*239*
All females	19%	*953*
Fieldwork wave:		
Wave 1	18%	*408*
Wave 2	16%	*422*
Wave 3	17%	*556*
Wave 4	15%	*538*
All young people	16%	*1924*

*Including those who answered questions about prescribed medicines but did not complete a dietary record.
** Wave 1: January to March 1997
    Wave 2: April to June 1997
    Wave 3: July to September 1997
    Wave 4: October to December 1997
*** Includes those who reported taking oral contraceptives.

41

Table 3.42   Smoking behaviour of young person by sex and age of young person

Responding sample–young people aged 7 to 18 years

Smoking behaviour of young person	Males aged (years)			All males	Females aged (years)			All females
	7–10	11–14	15–18		7–10	11–14	15–18	
	%	%	%	%	%	%	%	%
Never smoked	86	66	30	61	83	66	27	59
Ex-smoker*	8	25	38	23	6	27	36	23
Current smoker:								
less than 1 cigarette per week	0	3	8	4	–	1	7	3
1 to 6 cigarettes per week	–	1	6	2	–	1	6	2
more than 6 cigarettes per week	–	2	17	6	–	2	22	8
Not answered	6	2	2	3	10	3	2	5
Base	*304*	*290*	*258*	*852*	*277*	*280*	*264*	*821*

* Includes those who said they did once have a puff or two of a cigarette, but never smoke now, those who have only ever tried smoking once, and those who used to smoke sometimes, but never smoke a cigarette now.

Table 3.43   Smoking behaviour of young person compared with data from the 1996 Survey of Smoking among Secondary School Children: England

Smoking behaviour of young person	Responding sample–young people aged 11–14 years– England only	1996 Smoking among Secondary School Children: England*
	%	%
Never smoked	66	56
Ex-smoker**	26	29
Current smoker	6	16
Not answered	2	–
Base	*502*	*2267*

* Subsample of the 1996 Survey of Smoking among Secondary School Children including only children aged 11 to 14 years. Jarvis L. *Smoking among secondary school children in 1996: England.* HMSO (London, 1997)
** Includes those who said they did once have a puff or two of a cigarette, but never smoke now, those who have only ever tried smoking once, and those who used to smoke sometimes, but never smoke a cigarette now.

Table 3.44   Smoking behaviour of young person and parent(s)

Responding sample–young people aged 7 to 18 years

Smoking behaviour of parent(s)		Smoking behaviour of young person			*Base***
		Current smoker	Ever smoked**	Not answered	
Both parents in household					
neither is a smoker	%	10	30	3	*762*
only mother is a smoker	%	21	43	7	*146*
only father is a smoker	%	10	32	4	*174*
both parents are smokers	%	11	38	2	*215*
One parent in household					
smoker	%	18	45	6	*181*
non-smoker	%	10	36	8	*163*
All*	%	12	35	4	*1673*
Number of young people		*198*	*576*	*68*	*1673*

* Includes those living away from parent(s) and cases where parents' smoking behaviour was not known.
** Ever smoked includes current and ex-smokers (see footnote to Table 3.43).
*** Includes those who have never smoked.

Table 3.45 Reported main activity of young person by age and sex of young person

Responding sample

Reported main activity of young person	Age (years) and sex of young person			Male	Female
	4–6	7–10	11–14	15–18	15–18
	%	%	%	%	%
Not yet started school	7	–	–	–	–
At school	93	100	100	49	52
At college or other training	–	–	–	26	22
Working	–	–	–	21	20
Unemployed	–	–	–	4	2
Other*	0	0	0	0	3
Base	356	481	475	258	264

* Includes those excluded from school, those taught at home, those looking after home or family, who were permanently sick or disabled or who had left school but not yet started work or college.

Table 3.46 Employment status of young people aged 15 to 18 years by sex

Responding sample–young people aged 15 to 18 years

Employment status	Whether young person was in full-time education and sex of young person					
	In full-time education		Not in full-time education		All	
	Male	Female	Male	Female	Male	Female
	%	%	%	%	%	%
Working*	55	51	84	83	63	58
Unemployed	–	–	13	11	3	2
Economically inactive	45	49	2	7	34	40
Base	189	200	69	64	258	264

* Includes those who were working while in full-time education. Working includes <u>any</u> paid work (eg paper round).

Table 3.47 Usual week day lunch-time meal by sex and age of young person – those attending school or college

Responding sample – those attending school or college

Usual week day lunch-time meal	Males aged (years)					Females aged (years)				
	4–6	7–10	11–14	15–18	All males	4–6	7–10	11–14	15–18	All females
	%	%	%	%	%	%	%	%	%	%
Free school meal	17	14	13	8	13	13	19	16	6	14
Reduced price or subsidised school meal	–	2	0	1	1	1	0	1	1	1
School meal bought on premises	28	30	34	31	31	25	26	33	39	31
Meal bought outside premises	–	0	3	15	4	0	–	6	11	4
Packed lunch	44	53	45	31	44	48	53	41	35	45
Lunch at home*	3	1	4	7	4	4	0	3	5	3
Other – not specified	–	–	0	1	0	–	–	0	1	0
No lunch time meal	8	–	1	5	3	9	–	1	1	2
Base	222	303	290	186	1001	221	277	280	185	963

* Includes those at nursery school who attended only for half day, those taught at home and those who had lunch at the home of a relative.

Table 3.48   Usual week day lunch-time meal by sex of young person – those aged 15 to 18 years and working*

Responding sample–those aged 15 to 18 and working

Usual week day lunch-time meal	Sex of young person		
	Male	Female	All
	%	%	%
Free meal	10	8	9
Meal bought on premises	13	10	12
Meal bought outside premises	16	34	24
Packed lunch	35	32	34
Lunch at home	7	6	6
Other answers	6	3	5
No lunch-time meal	14	8	11
Base	*58*	*53*	*111*

* Excludes those who were working in addition to being in full-time education.

4 Types and quantities of foods consumed

4.1 Introduction

This chapter presents data on the foods consumed by young people in the survey. Most of the information is taken from the seven-day weighed intake dietary records, but some tables are based on information collected in the interviews; these include tables showing the consumption of artificial sweeteners, dietary supplements and milk, and information on food avoidance.

4.2 Interview data

Nearly all the young people taking part in the survey were living in households with a separate kitchen; only 0.2% were in accommodation with a shared kitchen. Most households had access to a range of amenities for the storage and preparation of food, such as a freezer (99%) and microwave oven (88%). For 85% of the young people the household had the use of a car or van. These proportions are generally close to those for a subsample of households from the General Household Survey (see *Table 4.1*)[1].

On the day of interview most households had available a range of basic food items that would provide the young person with something to eat and drink in an emergency. Of the seven prompted food items over 95% of households had at least six of the items and 76% had all seven available. *(Tables 4.1 and 4.2)*

4.2.1 Current milk consumption

Less than 5% of any age or sex group reported in the interview never having any milk either as a drink or on cereals or in puddings. Most young people in the survey had milk as a drink, although the proportions not drinking milk increased with age for both boys and girls; in the oldest group 15% of girls and 12% of boys reported not drinking milk, compared with 3% of girls and 5% of boys aged 4 to 6 years (p < 0.01). By the age of 11 years over half of boys and girls were drinking semi-skimmed milk, and in the youngest age group semi-skimmed milk was the usual milk for 36% of boys and 41% of girls. This pattern of consumption was broadly similar for milk used other than as a drink, for example, in puddings and on cereals. Boys and girls in the youngest age group were the most likely to have whole milk, but by age 7 years at least 50% of the young people in the survey were having semi-skimmed or skimmed milk in puddings or on cereals. This consumption of semi-skimmed milk is consistent with

current dietary advice that semi-skimmed milk can be introduced from the age of 2 years[2].
(Tables 4.3 and 4.4)

4.2.2 Artificial sweeteners

Respondents were asked in the interview about the young person's use of artificial sweeteners in tea, coffee and cooking. No more than 6% of any age and sex group reported using artificial sweeteners in these ways. The use of artificial sweeteners in tea by girls increased as they got older from 1% in the youngest age group to 5% among girls aged 15 to 18 years (p < 0.01). There were no other age-related trends in the use of artificial sweeteners. *(Table 4.5)*

4.2.3 Dietary supplements

About one fifth of all young people were reported in the interview as taking vitamin and mineral supplements, including fluoride preparations. Among boys the proportions taking supplements declined with age, from 32% in the youngest age group to about 14% among those aged 11 to 18 years (p < 0.01). About one quarter (23%) of the youngest girls were taking dietary supplements, and this fell to 16% among those aged 7 to 14 years (p < 0.05) and then increased again back to 22% among the oldest group (p < 0.05).

The proportions taking supplements were higher among young people from a non-manual than a manual home background for both boys and girls (p < 0.05).

There was little difference in the types of supplements being taken by boys and girls, except that boys were more likely to be taking vitamin A, C and D preparations than girls (p < 0.05). Overall, multivitamins, A, C and D preparations and multivitamin plus multimineral preparations each accounted for about a fifth of the supplements being taken.
(Tables 4.6 and 4.7)

4.2.4 Food avoidance and limitation

The interview included a food frequency questionnaire incorporating 47 items; if a food item was never eaten the reason for its avoidance was asked. The reported reasons included dislike of the food, health reasons, including allergic reactions and weight control, and moral or ethical reasons, including religious beliefs and vegetarian behaviours. All young people were also asked whether they were currently dieting to lose weight and whether they were vegetarian or vegan[3].

Allergic reactions to one or more foods were reported for 9% of the boys and 13% of the girls (p < 0.01); there was no clear pattern by age for either sex. Four per cent of boys and 6% of girls were reported to have allergies that had been diagnosed by a doctor.

Overall, 6% of girls and 2% of boys reported that, at the time of the interview, they were *dieting to lose weight* (p < 0.01). Among the oldest group of girls the proportion rose to 16%, compared with only 3% of the corresponding group of boys (p < 0.01).

At the interview 5% of girls and 1% of boys reported being a *vegetarian or vegan* (p < 0.01). The proportions showed almost no variation by age among the boys, but among girls, increased steadily from 2% among the 4 to 6 year old girls to 10% among those aged 15 to 18 years (p < 0.01). Young people from a non-manual home background were more likely to report being vegetarian or vegan than those from a manual background (p < 0.01).

Young people who reported being vegetarian or vegan were asked what foods they avoided; about one third said they avoided all animal products; of the remainder nearly all said they avoided red meat, about two thirds avoided white meat and about half did not eat fish. (*Table not shown*).

Asked why they became vegetarian or vegan, almost two-thirds said it was for moral or ethical reasons and a third because they did not like the taste of meat. Other less frequently mentioned reasons included religious beliefs, parental vegetarianism, and health reasons. (*Table not shown*)

More than half the young people who were vegetarian or vegan had obtained information about vegetarian and vegan diets from their parents; about one quarter had got information from newspapers, magazines or books and about one fifth from friends. Other less frequently mentioned sources of information included the Vegetarian and Vegan societies, dietitians and nutritionists. About one in seven said they had never obtained any information, possibly because they were being brought up in a vegetarian family or were practising vegetarianism as part of their religion. (*Table not shown*)   (*Tables 4.8 to 4.10*)

4.3 Foods consumed

4.3.1 Deriving food consumption data from the seven-day weighed intake dietary records

Every food item recorded in the dietary record, including those eaten away from home, was allocated an individual food code and hence information on the consumption of food items at the individual food code level can be derived. This level of aggregation separates foods that are nutritionally different, and for some food types, separates at brand level. However the data are more easily presented and interpreted when similar types of foods are grouped.

Each of the approximately 6,000 food codes used in the survey was allocated by MAFF to one of 115 subsidiary food groups; these in turn can be aggregated into 57 food groups, and then into 11 food types. A complete list of food types, food groups and subsidiary food groups, with examples of the foods included in each subsidiary food group is given in Appendix H[4]. Consumption data for artificial sweeteners, dietary supplements and medicines are not shown in the tables since these items were recorded in tablets or teaspoons rather than as gram weights.

For each young person completing a seven-day dietary record, the gram quantity of each food item consumed was calculated from the weight served and the weight, if any, left over. Food item data were then aggregated to subsidiary food group level and the total gram weight of all the items in the subsidiary food group consumed over the seven diary days was calculated. Diaries with fewer than seven days were excluded from the analysis.

Where water was used as a diluent, for example, with fruit squash or instant coffee, the entry for tap water in the diary was coded and assigned to the food group associated with the item being diluted, for example, for fruit squash, to concentrated soft drinks, low calorie or not low calorie as appropriate, and for coffee, to the sub-group 'coffee', in the 'food group tea, coffee and water'[5]. For food items weighed and recorded as dry or concentrate weights, which were subsequently made-up or diluted with water, such as fruit squash, instant coffee or dried milk, the dry/concentrate weight was added to the associated weight of water used as the diluent to give the actual made-up weight. This is used in the tables to show the consumption of concentrated soft drinks, instant coffee and other items made up with water on serving. The consumption of tap water, not used as a diluent, is shown separately in the tables. Thus the total fluid consumption of young people can be estimated from the tables in this report[6].

The tables derived from the dietary records show the mean and median amounts of foods consumed in seven days; in Table 4.12 these averages are based on *all* young people who kept a dietary record, *consumers and non-consumers* of each food item. Other tables show mean and median amounts calculated for *consumers* of the item only and the percentage of young people who consumed each item.

4.3.2 Types of foods consumed by young people and variation by sex

Tables 4.11(a) and (b) show the proportions of boys and

girls consuming different foods during the 7-day dietary recording period. Table 4.11(c) summarises the differences between boys and girls and the reader is referred to this table for the statistical significance levels of the differences commented on below.

The foods consumed by the largest proportions of young people were white bread, by 95% of boys and 96% of girls, savoury snacks (88% and 90%), potato chips (89% and 88%), savoury sauces, pickles, gravies and condiments (89% and 87%), biscuits (both sexes 84%), and 'other' potatoes, that is boiled, mashed and jacket potatoes, and potato dishes (83% and 80%). All of these foods were as likely to be consumed by boys as girls. Of the meat and meat products food type, chicken and turkey dishes were consumed by the largest proportions of young people (75% and 73%). Chocolate confectionery was also consumed by a large proportion of young people, 84% of boys and 80% of girls.

During the seven-day recording period more than half the young people in the survey had not eaten any citrus fruits, (not eaten by 76% of boys and 72% of girls), any leafy green vegetables, such as cabbage, greens or broccoli (61% and 56%), any eggs (55% and 56%) and any raw tomatoes (68% and 58%).

Polyunsaturated reduced fat spreads were consumed by 36% of boys and 38% of girls, and non-polyunsaturated reduced fat spreads by 25% of boys and 22% of girls; over a quarter (27% of boys and 28% of girls) had used non-polyunsaturated soft margarine, and similar proportions, 27% of boys and 31% of girls, had used butter during the 7-day dietary recording period. These proportions represent the use of fats as spreads, and do not include their use in cooking.

Sixty-three per cent of boys and 66% of girls ate sugar confectionery during the dietary recording period, and there were no significant differences between the sexes in the proportions who drank fruit juice (46% and 51%), coffee (both sexes 17%) or tea (45% and 48%). A slightly higher proportion of boys than girls used table sugar (69% and 63%). This may be associated with the differences between the sexes in their reported use of sugar in tea and in coffee (see *Table 4.5*). Similar proportions of boys and girls ate wholegrain and high fibre breakfast cereals (52% and 48%), but boys were more likely than girls to eat 'other' types of breakfast cereals, 74% compared with 64%.

There were very few other significant differences in the foods eaten by boys and girls. Girls were more likely to have eaten raw tomatoes and 'other' raw and salad vegetables, that is apart from raw carrots, and boys were more likely to have consumed sausages and beer.

(Tables 4.11(a), (b) and (c))

4.3.3 *Variation in the foods eaten by age group*

The data clearly show that there were differences in the diets of young people in different age groups (see *Tables 4.11(a) and (b)* and, for a summary of the differences, with significance values, *Table 4.11(c)*).

Younger children were generally more likely to have consumed foods in the cereals and cereals products group. In particular, the youngest group of both boys and girls were significantly more likely than the oldest group of children to have eaten breakfast cereals (not wholegrain or high fibre types) and biscuits. The youngest group of boys was also more likely to have eaten pasta and buns, cakes and pastries than the oldest group of boys, and the youngest group of girls were more likely than the oldest age group to have eaten wholegrain and high fibre breakfast cereals. The only cereal product significantly more likely to have been eaten by the oldest age group was rice which was consumed by 44% of girls aged 15 to 18 years compared with 28% of girls aged 4 to 6 years.

All types of cereal-based and sponge puddings were more likely to have been eaten by the youngest group of boys compared with those aged 15 to 18 years, but for girls the only significant difference was for cereal-based milk puddings. Both fromage frais and ice cream were more likely to have been eaten by the youngest age group of both boys and girls, and the same was true for yogurt for boys but not girls.

The patterns of milk consumption reported in the interview have been described above (*Section 4.2.1*), and the dietary record data confirm the pattern of the proportion of young people using whole milk decreasing as age increased[7]; among those aged 4 to 6 years 75% of boys and 70% of girls had whole milk during the dietary recording period, compared with only 47% of boys and 41% of girls aged 15 to 18 years. However, there were no significant differences in the likelihood of consuming semi or skimmed milk associated with age for either sex.

Among boys but not girls the proportions consuming different types of meat generally increased with age and bacon and ham, and beef, veal and dishes made from them were eaten by a significantly higher proportion of older boys. Only coated chicken was less likely to be eaten by older rather than younger boys. The only significant difference associated with age for girls was for sausages, eaten by 65% of the youngest group and only 37% of those aged 15 to 18 years.

The proportions of both boys and girls eating fried and/or coated white fish (including fish fingers) decreased significantly with age, from 65% and 59% respectively for boys and girls aged 4 to 6 years to 39% and 29% for those aged 15 to 18 years. There was no significant difference by age in the proportions eating potato chips.

There were very few significant differences associated with age for boys or girls in the proportions consuming vegetables, other than potatoes. The youngest group of boys was more likely to have eaten peas, and the youngest group of girls to have eaten baked beans, and for both sexes the youngest groups were less likely to have eaten raw tomatoes. Girls aged 15 to 18 years were more likely to have eaten vegetable dishes, 28% compared with 15% for the youngest group of girls.

For both boys and girls, the proportions who ate potato products which were not fried and crisps and savoury snacks were significantly higher for the youngest than the oldest groups.

The proportions of both boys and girls consuming fruit, and nuts and seeds generally decreased with age, and for both sexes the difference between the proportions in the youngest and oldest age groups were significant for apples and pears and 'other', mainly soft, fruit. The oldest group of girls was also less likely to have eaten bananas and canned fruit in syrup than those aged 4 to 6 years. About one in five boys aged 4 to 6 years had eaten nuts or seeds, which includes peanut butter, during the dietary recording period, compared with about one in ten of boys aged 15 to 18 years.

The proportion of girls consuming chocolate confectionery was fairly constant across the age groups, but among boys there was a marked increase in the proportion eating chocolate confectionery between the ages of 4 to 6 years and 7 to 10 years from 80% to 91% ($p < 0.01$). The proportions of boys and girls eating sugar confectionery and preserves, including jam and honey, were significantly lower for the oldest age group compared with those aged 4 to 6 years. The oldest girls were less likely than the youngest girls to have eaten sweet spreads, fillings and icings.

For soft drinks, the proportions of both boys and girls drinking concentrated and ready-to-drink soft drinks including low calorie types, declined with age. For example, 61% of both boys and girls aged 4 to 6 years drank low calorie concentrated soft drinks compared with 27% of boys and 29% of girls aged 15 to 18 years. The consumption of non-low calorie carbonated drinks increased with age for boys, from 67% of those aged 4 to 6 years to 85% of those aged 15 to 18 years. There was no significant difference by age for girls in the proportions consuming non-low calorie carbonated soft drinks. Not surprisingly, the proportions of both boys and girls consuming tea and coffee increased with age.

Just over one in three (34%) of boys aged 15 to 18 years recorded consumption of beer or lager in their seven-day dietary record, compared with 17% of the oldest group of girls ($p < 0.01$). The consumption of wine was recorded by 10% of girls aged 15 to 18 years, and spirits by 11%; the corresponding proportions for the oldest group of boys were 5% and 7% (ns). Six per cent of

boys and 17% of girls aged 15 to 18 years drank bottled water ($p < 0.05$).

(Table 4.11(a), (b) and (c))

4.3.4 Quantities of foods consumed

Tables 4.12(a) and (b) show the average (mean) quantity of the foods consumed by all young people in the survey; in this table the means are calculated including non-consumers, that is those who did not record consuming any of any item during the seven-day dietary recording period. The data are shown separately for boys and girls within four age bands. Table 4.12(c) summarises the differences between boys and girls in average amounts eaten, and shows significance values.

For many food items boys ate significantly larger mean amounts than girls. The most marked differences were for pizza, white bread, breakfast cereals, semi-skimmed milk, bacon and ham, sausages, baked beans, potato chips, nuts and seeds, and carbonated soft drinks (not low calorie). In contrast, girls consumed significantly larger mean amounts of 'other' raw and salad vegetables, raw tomatoes, and apples and pears.

Differences between boys and girls in the total amount consumed were more apparent in the oldest two age groups, that is from aged 11 years, although the differences for white bread, breakfast cereals, and buns, cakes and pastries were already apparent in the 7 to 10 age group. In the youngest age group, 4 to 6 years, boys were eating larger average amounts of cereal-based milk puddings and sausages than girls. Differences between boys and girls in the mean consumption of biscuits, beef, veal and dishes made from them, burgers and kebabs, meat pies and pastries, baked beans, potato chips, boiled, mashed and jacket potatoes and potato dishes and beer and lager were only apparent for the oldest age group, those aged 15 to 18 years. Girls were consuming larger mean amounts of 'other' raw and salad vegetables at ages 4 to 6 years than boys, and this difference persisted throughout the age range, except in the 11 to 14 year age group.

(Table 4.12(a), (b) and (c))

Tables 4.11(a) and (b) give mean and median consumption figures based only on those consuming the food item 'consumers'.

Generally for boys the mean amounts of foods consumed increased with age. For example comparing the youngest and oldest age groups of boys, the mean amount consumed over seven days at least doubled for the following items; for rice from an average of 181g by boys aged 4 to 6 years, to 510g for boys aged 15 to 18 years; for pizza (from 128g to 376g); for cream (from19g to 40g) for polyunsaturated margarine (from 30g to 90g); for most types of meat and meat products, for example for burgers and kebabs from 99g to 287g; for potato chips (from 265g to 584g); for table sugar (from

37g, about 9 level teaspoons, to 94g, 23$\frac{1}{2}$ level teaspoons); for carbonated soft drinks, not low calorie (from 734g to 2228g, about $\frac{3}{4}$ litre to 2$\frac{1}{4}$ litres); for coffee (from 970g, about 5 cups, to 2053g, about 11 cups) and for tea (from 499g, about 2$\frac{1}{2}$ cups, to 1755g, 9 cups) and for savoury sauces, pickles, gravies and condiments, from 87g to 200g.

The mean amount of whole milk consumed over the seven days was highest among the youngest group of boys, 1391g (just under 2$\frac{1}{2}$ pints) falling to 928g (1$\frac{1}{2}$ pints) by boys aged 15 to 18 years (p < 0.01). Overall, across the whole age range, 50% of boys were drinking at least 1119g (about 2 pints) of semi-skimmed milk a week and 50% were eating at least 77g of cheese, not including cottage cheese, a week. Among the fat spreads median amounts consumed were 26g of butter, 20g of soft margarine, not polyunsaturated, 27g of polyunsaturated margarine, and at least 42g for each of the various types of reduced and low fat spreads.

The mean amounts of fruit consumed by boys increased very little with age; only the mean consumption of citrus fruits increased significantly between ages 4 to 6 and 15 to 18 years from 193g to 294g (p < 0.01).

Overall 50% of boys were eating over 108g in seven days of coated and/or fried white fish (including fish fingers), and over 75g of oily fish. Median amounts for vegetables, (other than potatoes) were quite small, typically less than 70g, except for baked beans where 50% of boys ate more than 181g in seven days. As noted earlier most boys ate savoury snacks (88%), and the median amount consumed was 115g. Fifty per cent of male consumers ate more than 125g of chocolate in seven days and the corresponding figure for sugar confectionery was slightly lower, 87g. Among soft drinks, concentrated soft drinks were drunk in the largest quantities, 50% of male consumers drinking more than 1516g, about 1$\frac{1}{2}$ litres, of non-low calorie versions and 2250g, about 2$\frac{1}{4}$ litres, of low calorie versions (made-up weights). The comparable figures for carbonated soft drinks, non-low calorie and low calorie, were 1008g (1 litre) and 723g (about $\frac{3}{4}$ litre) respectively. Fifty per cent of boys aged 15 to 18 years who recorded drinking beer or lager consumed at least 1800g (about 3 pints) in seven days; for wines and spirits the comparable median amounts were 205g (just over 1$\frac{1}{2}$ average glasses) and 69g (about 3 pub measures) respectively.

For girls the association between age and amount consumed was not as clear as among boys. In the meat and meat products group most items were consumed in the largest quantities by the oldest age group, for example, the mean amount of beef, veal and beef dishes consumed over seven days ranged from 160g for girls aged 4 to 6 years to 318g for those aged 15 to 18 years, for pork and pork dishes from 82g to 171g, and for burgers and kebabs from 96g to 205g.

The pattern was the same for the amounts of most vegetables being consumed, for example, girls aged 4 to 6 years consumed a mean of 77g of leafy green vegetables in seven days compared with a mean of 127g by girls aged 15 to 18 years, and for 'other' raw and salad vegetables the mean amount rose from 91g to 149g.

For girls the mean amounts of fruit consumed, other than canned fruit, also generally rose with age, as did the amounts of coffee and tea consumed.

For many other food items however the data suggest that the quantity consumed increased steadily with age up to the 11 to 14 year age group, and then either remained at a similar level, or appeared to reduce (see *Appendix J* for a discussion of under-reporting in the sample). For example, for rice, wholemeal bread, breakfast cereals which were not wholegrain or high fibre, and buns, cakes and pastries, girls aged 15 to 18 years were, on average, eating no more of these items than girls aged 11 to 14 years. The same pattern appeared for the average amount of sausages eaten over seven days; this increased from 92g for those in the youngest age group, to 141g among those aged 11 to 14 years and then decreased to 125g for the oldest group. There was a decrease in the mean consumption of potato chips, savoury snacks and sugar and chocolate confectionery between those aged 11 to 14 and 15 to 18 years.

As for boys, the mean amount of whole milk consumed by girls in seven days clearly reduced with age from 1333g (about 2$\frac{1}{4}$ pints) by those aged 4 to 6 years to 723g (1$\frac{1}{3}$ pints) by girls aged 15 to 18 years. Average consumption of semi-skimmed milk varied very little with age; 50% of all girls consumed more than 753g (about 1$\frac{1}{4}$ pints) in seven days. Fifty per cent of girls ate at least 80g of cheese, excluding cottage cheese, during the diary-keeping period, and the amounts of fat spreads consumed were only slightly lower than for boys.

The median amount of fruit juice consumed by girls was 521g, about a $\frac{1}{2}$ litre. The median amount of low calorie concentrated soft drinks consumed by girls was 1867g, over 1$\frac{3}{4}$ litres (made-up weight); for non-low calorie versions the median was 1332g (about 1$\frac{1}{3}$ litres); in both cases there was little variation by age. For carbonated soft drinks, low calorie and non-low calorie, the overall median amounts were 618g (over $\frac{1}{2}$ litre) and 816g (over $\frac{3}{4}$ litre) respectively. Consumption of table sugar ranged from a median of 25g for the youngest girls, just over six level teaspoons, to 55g by those aged 15 to 18 years, nearly 14 level teaspoons.

Over the seven dietary recording days the median amounts of beer and lager drunk by girls aged 15 to 18 years who were consumers was 1427g (about 2$\frac{1}{2}$ pints); for wines and spirits the comparable figures were 208g (about $1\frac{1}{2}$ average glasses) and 69g (3 pub measures) respectively, almost identical to the median amounts for boys of the same age.   *(Tables 4.11(a) and (b))*

4.4   Variation in the foods eaten by fieldwork wave

Fieldwork for surveys in the NDNS programme has always been carried out over a 12-month period to ensure that any seasonality in eating behaviour and seasonality in the nutrient composition of certain foods is adequately covered and in reports of the surveys carried out so far, tables have been presented showing the foods eaten by the survey sample analysed according to when they were interviewed, that is by fieldwork wave[8].

Generally speaking there have not been many differences in eating behaviour associated with the time of the year when the subject kept a dietary record, and indeed some of the differences that have been found in the data are not easy to explain in terms of seasonal effects. Certainly the extent to which people's diets are affected by the seasonal availability of different foods is likely to be small. Many of what were previously only seasonal fruits and vegetables, now tend to be widely available for most of the year, either as fresh, imported products or as frozen or chilled items. For example, strawberries, green beans, 'new' potatoes, sweetcorn and melons are generally now available in some form throughout the year, whereas previously they were mainly seasonal produce.

Any seasonality in eating behaviour is therefore more likely to be associated with different food preferences or with traditions associated with different times of the year. For example, the consumption of salad vegetables is likely to be higher in the summer months, not because salad items are only available at that time, but because in warmer weather people are more likely to eat cold meals. Similarly the consumption of cold drinks will increase in warm weather; in the winter months the preference is likely to be for soups, hot beverages, cooked meals with hot meat or fish and vegetables. For the age group covered by this survey, there may also be differences in eating behaviour between school term time and school holidays.

To examine any seasonality in the eating behaviour of young people the data were analysed by fieldwork wave[9]. Tables 4.13(a) and (b) show, for boys and girls separately, the proportion of consumers in each fieldwork wave who ate foods of various types and the mean and median amounts eaten by consumers. Differences between waves, which were statistically significant, are summarised in Table 4.13(c).

In common with previous surveys in the NDNS programme, although some of the patterns were what would be expected in terms of the time of the year when some foods are most popular or available, for other foods it is less easy to account for the apparent

seasonality shown by the survey data. For some of the foods consumed the 'seasonal' patterns were the same for boys and girls, but for others there were differences between the sexes.

There were very few differences between waves in the proportions of young people eating cereals and cereal products; only the consumption of biscuits showed any variation with boys in Wave 1, January to March, being less likely to eat biscuits than boys in Wave 2, April to June, 76% compared with 91%.

There was more variation between the waves in the consumption of milk and milk products, particularly for girls. Cereal-based milk puddings and whole milk were less likely to be consumed by girls in Wave 3, July to September. Not surprisingly both boys and girls were less likely to have eaten ice cream in Waves 1 and 4, January to March and October to December, than between April and September.

There were very few differences in the proportions of consumers of the various types of fats and fat spreads by wave. For boys, the proportion of consumers of reduced fat spreads, not polyunsaturated was significantly higher in Wave 3 than in Waves 1 and 2, and girls in Wave 4 were more likely to have consumed other oils and cooking fats, not polyunsaturated, than girls in Wave 1.

The only type of meat or meat products that varied in consumption by wave, was beef, veal and dishes, which were more likely to be eaten by boys in Wave 3 than in Wave 2, 60% compared with 43%.

The differences between waves in the proportions of young people consuming different types of vegetable are largely associated with seasonal availability and seasonal preference. Thus raw and salad vegetables were more likely to have been eaten in Waves 2 and 3, April to September than at other times of the year.

Boys were more likely to have eaten apples and pears in Wave 2, April to June, than at any other time of the year, but there was no difference for girls. However both boys and girls were more likely to have eaten citrus fruits between October and December than between July and September, and for girls between April and June.

Boys were least likely to have eaten sugar confectionery in Waves 1 and 4, and girls were more likely to have had soup in Wave 4 than in Waves 2 or 3.
          (Tables 4.13(a), (b) and (c))

4.5   Variation in the foods eaten by region

Tables 4.14(a) and (b) show the proportion of boys and girls in each region who consumed different types of food in the seven-day dietary recording period[10]. Table 4.14(c) summarises the data in the main table showing differences between regions which were statistically significant.

There was considerable variation in the diets of both boys and girls according to the region in which they lived, only some of which was common to both sexes.

In the cereals and cereal products food type there were relatively few differences; pasta was least likely to be consumed by boys living in the Northern region. Girls in London and the South East were more likely to have eaten rice and less likely to have eaten white bread. Other cereals were generally consumed by higher proportions of boys and girls from the Northern region than elsewhere.

The proportion of boys having skimmed milk was lowest in Scotland, 1%, as was the proportion of girls in Scotland having cream, 5%. Yogurt and eggs were most likely to have been eaten by girls from the Northern region. Boys from the Northern region were more likely to have eaten egg dishes than boys from London and the South East.

Compared with girls in London and the South East, girls in the Northern region were more likely to have consumed polyunsaturated margarine, and compared with girls in Scotland they were also more likely to have consumed polyunsaturated reduced fat spreads.

Boys in the Northern region were less likely to have consumed beef and veal, lamb and liver than boys in other regions, whereas girls in this region were more likely to have consumed beef, veal and dishes than girls in London and the South East.

Boys in Scotland were generally less likely to have eaten all types of fish except for oily fish. The diets of both boys and girls living in Scotland were clearly characterised by their being less likely to have consumed many types of vegetable, including fried and roast potatoes. For example, during the seven-day recording period only 20% of boys in Scotland consumed leafy green vegetables, 33% ate 'other' raw or salad vegetables and only 30% cooked carrots, compared with 50%, 53% and 53% of boys in London and the South East. Although boys and girls in Scotland were generally less likely to have eaten vegetables than young people in most other regions, they were no less likely than boys or girls living elsewhere to have eaten fruit. Indeed there were few regional differences in the consumption of fruit.

Chocolate confectionery was more likely to have been eaten by boys in Scotland compared with boys in London and the South East (94% compared with 82%).

Both boys and girls in the Northern region were the most likely to have drunk non-low calorie soft drinks.

For example, 83% of boys and 82% of girls in the Northern region had consumed non-low calorie carbonated drinks compared with 71% and 70% of boys and girls in London and the South East. There were also significant regional differences in the proportions of boys drinking tap water; 71% of those in London and the South East drank tap water compared with 56% of boys in the Northern region, 55% of boys in the Central and South West regions of England and Wales, and 52% in Scotland.

The highest proportions of both boys and girls consuming soup, 42% and 60% respectively, were from Scotland while savoury sauces, pickles, condiments and gravies were more likely to be consumed by boys and girls in the Northern region and also by girls in London and the South East. *(Tables 4.14(a), (b) and (c))*

4.6 Variation in the foods eaten by young people by social and economic characteristics of the household

Tables 4.15(a) and (b) to 4.18(a) and (b) show the proportions of young people consuming different types of food and the mean and median amounts consumed according to a range of social and economic characteristics of the household – household type, social class, gross weekly household income and whether the household was in receipt of certain state benefits.

Many of these characteristics are inter-related and tables showing the distributions for the various characteristics and the extent of some of the inter-relationships are given in Chapter 3. For example, whether the household was receiving certain state benefits was related to household income level. In discussing the differences in the types of foods eaten by young people from households with different social and economic characteristics, these inter-relationships need to be borne in mind.

The principal differences in the dietary patterns of young people from different social and economic households are summarised in two tables, Tables 4.15(c) and 4.19, and the reader is referred to these tables for the statistical significance of the differences commented on below.

4.6.1 Variation in the foods eaten by household type

There were relatively few significant differences in the types of foods eaten by young people living with both parents between those who had other children in their household and those who were the only child at home. There were no clear dietary patterns evident from the data, and the variation was somewhat different for boys and girls. It should be noted that some differences between the two household types, particularly in relation to the proportions consuming alcoholic drinks, are probably largely accounted for by age differences between the two groups, the proportion of 15 to 18 year olds being greater in two-parent households where there were no other children in the household, 51%, than when there were other children in the household, 15%, (p < 0.01) (see *Table 3.19*).

Where the young person was living with both parents and was the only child in the household compared with those living with both parents and other children, both boys and girls were less likely to have eaten fromage frais, apples and pears, and sugar confectionery and to have drunk low calorie concentrated soft drinks and non-low calorie ready-to-drink soft drinks. For example, 33% of boys and 38% of girls living in 'two-parent' households[11] with no other children had drunk low calorie concentrated soft drinks compared with 53% of boys and 52% of girls from two-parent households with other children in the household. Girls from two-parent households with no other children were also less likely to have eaten breakfast cereals, which were not high fibre or wholegrain types, 49% compared with 69%, and sausages (45% and 59%).

The tables show that boys in households with both parents and no other children were more likely than those in two-parent households with other children to have consumed non-polyunsaturated soft margarine, beef, veal and dishes made from them, beer and lager, and coffee, and for girls, semi-skimmed milk, wine, beer and lager, alco-pops and tea.

Foods which were less likely to be eaten by young people living with both parents and no other children were also less likely to be consumed by young people living in lone-parent households (with or without other children). For example, biscuits, savoury snacks and ready-to-drink soft drinks (not low calorie) were consumed significantly less often both by boys in lone-parent households and in two-parent households with no other children. Girls from lone-parent households were also less likely to have drunk low calorie concentrated soft drinks (p < 0.01).

(Tables 4.15(a), (b) and (c))

4.6.2 *Variation in the foods eaten by social class, gross weekly household income and receipt of benefits*

Table 4.19 shows the foods which were significantly more and less likely to be eaten by young people from households where the head was classified as manual (compared with those where the head was classified as non-manual); where the gross weekly income was in the lowest band, less than £160 week (compared with those in the highest income band, £600 a week or more) and where the household was in receipt of certain benefits (compared with those not receiving benefits)[12].

Overall, the table shows clearly that there was a comparatively wide range of foods which were less likely to have been eaten by young people from less advantaged households. In contrast there were relatively few foods that they were more likely to eat than young people living in more advantaged households.

It can also be seen from the table that the number of foods which were less likely to have been eaten varied according to which measure of social and economic status was considered, but that many of the foods were common to all measures and that there were generally more differences for boys than girls.

For boys, soft grain bread was significantly less likely to have been eaten by those from households in receipt of benefits and by those from a manual background. Fruit pies were also less likely to have been eaten by boys from benefit households and from households in the lowest income group.

Differences in the types of milk consumed were very clear and consistent across the various measures; for each characteristic considered, apart from for girls from a manual social class background, whole milk was clearly more likely to have been drunk by the young people from the less advantaged households. Semi-skimmed was less likely to have been drunk by boys in low income, benefit and manual social class households. For example, 72% of boys from households with a gross weekly income of less than £160 drank whole milk and 43% drank semi-skimmed milk, compared with 45% and 66% of boys from households with a gross income of over £600 a week. Cream and butter were generally less likely to have been consumed by young people in the less advantaged households, as was cheese, other than cottage cheese, fromage frais and 'other' dairy desserts.

The types of meat eaten showed little variation with socio-economic status although bacon and ham were less likely to have been eaten by boys from the lowest income households and households in receipt of benefits. Boys in the lowest income households were also less likely to have consumed beef, veal and dishes during the recording period.

Boys and girls from less advantaged households were generally less likely to have eaten raw carrots and 'other' raw and salad vegetables; in benefit and the lowest income households girls were also less likely to have eaten green beans.

Young people from less advantaged households measured by most characteristics were generally less likely to have drunk fruit juice or to have eaten any 'other', mainly soft, fruit. The proportion of boys consuming table sugar was significantly higher for boys in the lowest income households, for boys and girls in households receiving benefits and for girls in manual social class households.

(Tables 4.16(a), (b) to 4.18(a), (b) and 4.19)

References and endnotes

[1] 1996/7 General Household Survey subsample of households containing at least one young person aged 4 to 18 years.

[2] Department of Health. Report on Health and Social Subjects: 45. *Weaning and The Weaning Diet*. HMSO (London, 1994).

[3] The interview questionnaire is reproduced in Appendix A.

[4] The subsidiary food groups include infant formula, low alcohol and alcohol-free cider and perry, and commercial toddler's drinks; none of the young people in the survey consumed any of the food items in these sub-groups in the seven-day recording period and therefore these subsidiary food groups are omitted from the tables.

[5] See *Appendix H*.

[6] Other powdered beverages are reported as dry weight, and milk used to make up drinks is reported in the appropriate milk group. See also *Appendix H*.

[7] The dietary record data include the proportion having milk on cereals as well as a drink.

[8] Gregory JR, Collins DL, Davies PSW, Hughes JM, Clarke PC. *The National Diet and Nutrition Survey: Children aged 1½ to 4½ years. Volume 1. Report of the diet and nutrition survey*. HMSO (London, 1995).
Finch S, Doyle W, Lowe C, Bates CJ, Prentice A, Smithers G, Clarke PC. *National Diet and Nutrition Survey: people aged 65 years and over. Volume 1: Report of the diet and nutrition survey*. TSO (London, 1998).

[9] See *Appendix U 'Glossary'* for information on the derivation of fieldwork wave for analysis purposes.

[10] The areas included in each of the four analysis 'regions' are given in Chapter 3.

[11] The term 'two-parent' households is used in the text to describe married or co-habiting couples, one or both of whom was the young person's parent, step parent or foster parent, or, if none of these was present, a grandparent. See *Appendix U 'Glossary'*, for a definition of household types.

[12] Households receiving benefits are those where the young person's parent and/or partner were currently receiving Family Credit or had, in the previous 14 days, drawn Income Support or Job Seeker's Allowance. See also *Appendix U 'Glossary'*.

Table 4.1 Household access to amenities and domestic appliances

Amenities and domestic appliances	NDNS: 4 to 18 years	GHS 1996/7*
With a separate kitchen	100%	100%
Owns or has use of:		
refrigerator	98%	n/a
deep freezer or fridge freezer	99%	97%
microwave oven	88%	86%
car or van	85%	81%
Base	*2127*	*2638*

* 1996/7 GHS; subsample of households containing at least one young person aged 4 to 18 years
n/a Not asked (in the GHS).

Table 4.2 Proportion of households with selected food items in the home at the time of interview

Prompted food item	% with item in the home at time of interview
Milk	100
Bread or bread rolls	99
Breakfast cereal	98
Potatoes	96
A tin of baked beans or spaghetti	95
Eggs	93
Biscuits of any kind	88

Number of items in the home at the time of interview	% of households
All seven items	76
Six items	19
Five items	4
Four items	1
Three items	–
Two items	0
One item	–
None available	0
Base	*2127*

Table 4.3 Type of milk young person usually had as a drink by sex and age of young person

Responding sample

Type of milk young person usually had as a drink	Males aged (years)					Females aged (years)				
	4–6	7–10	11–14	15–18	All	4–6	7–10	11–14	15–18	All
	%	%	%	%	%	%	%	%	%	%
Did not have milk as a drink	5	6	6	12	7	3	12	10	15	8
Whole milk	61	48	34	30	43	60	43	32	27	40
Semi-skimmed milk	36	46	58	54	49	41	43	56	54	49
Skimmed milk	2	2	4	5	3	1	5	6	6	4
Powdered baby milk	–	–	–	–	–	–	–	–	0	0
Soya alternative to milk	–	–	–	–	–	0	–	–	1	0
Other type of milk	0	1	1	0	1	–	0	1	2	1
*Base**	*230*	*304*	*290*	*258*	*1082*	*224*	*277*	*280*	*264*	*1045*

* Percentages add to more than 100 as some young people usually drank more than one type of milk.

Table 4.4   Type of milk young person usually used on breakfast cereal and in puddings by sex and age of young person

Responding sample

Type of milk young person usually had on cereal and in puddings	Males aged (years)					Females aged (years)				
	4–6	7–10	11–14	15–18	All	4–6	7–10	11–14	15–18	All
	%	%	%	%	%	%	%	%	%	%
Did not have any milk	2	1	1	2	1	3	2	2	4	3
Whole milk	59	48	37	35	44	58	44	34	28	40
Semi-skimmed milk	38	50	60	58	52	41	50	61	62	54
Skimmed milk	4	1	4	5	4	1	5	5	6	5
Powdered baby milk	–	–	–	–	–	–	–	–	0	0
Soya alternative to milk	0	0	0	–	0	–	1	–	0	0
Other type of milk	1	2	1	2	1	–	1	0	2	1
*Base**	*230*	*304*	*290*	*258*	*1082*	*224*	*277*	*280*	*264*	*1045*

* Percentages add to more than 100 as some young people usually had more than one type of milk on cereal etc.

Table 4.5   Use of sugar and artificial sweeteners by age and sex of young person

Responding sample

Use of sugar and artificial sweeteners	Males aged (years)					Females aged (years)				
	4–6	7–10	11–14	15–18	All	4–6	7–10	11–14	15–18	All
	%	%	%	%	%	%	%	%	%	%
Tea drinking										
Drinks tea:										
with sugar	37	47	57	62	51	39	49	51	44	46
with artificial sweetener	1	1	2	1	2	1	2	3	5	3
unsweetened	10	14	13	16	13	15	22	21	28	21
Does not drink tea	52	37	27	21	34	46	27	26	22	30
Coffee drinking										
Drinks coffee										
with sugar	13	15	32	48	26	12	13	25	35	21
with artificial sweetener	0	–	2	2	1	0	1	2	2	2
unsweetened	1	2	5	8	4	2	5	6	10	6
Does not drink coffee	87	84	61	42	69	86	82	67	52	71
In cooking										
uses artificial sweeteners	3	3	2	1	2	3	6	4	3	4
Base	*230*	*304*	*290*	*258*	*1082*	*224*	*277*	*280*	*264*	*1045*

Table 4.6   Whether young person reported currently taking vitamin or mineral supplements (including fluoride) by sex and age of young person and social class of head of household

Responding sample

	% taking supplements	*Base*
Sex and age of young person		
Males aged:		
4–6 years	32%	*230*
7–10 years	20%	*304*
11–14 years	14%	*290*
15–18 years	13%	*258*
Females aged:		
4–6 years	23%	*244*
7–10 years	16%	*277*
11–14 years	16%	*280*
15–18 years	22%	*264*
Sex of young person and social class of head of household		
Males:		
Non-manual	22%	*496*
Manual	18%	*496*
All*	19%	*1082*
Females:		
Non-manual	22%	*474*
Manual	16%	*464*
All*	19%	*1045*

Table 4.7 Dietary supplements reported in the interview as being taken by sex of young person

Those reporting in the interview taking supplements

Dietary supplement	Sex of young person		All
	Male	Female	
	%*	%*	%*
Fluoride only	1	–	0
Cod liver oil and other fish-based supplements	7	6	6
Evening primrose oil type supplements	1	2	1
Vitamin C only	11	15	13
Other single vitamins, not vitamin C	1	4	2
Vitamins A, C and D only	24	17	21
Vitamins with iron	6	8	7
Iron only	1	2	1
Multivitamins and multiminerals	21	19	20
Multivitamins, no minerals	18	18	18
Minerals only, not fluoride or iron only	0	1	1
Other	10	9	10
Base, total number of supplements = 100%	*226*	*237*	*463*

*Percentages based on total number of supplements, not young people taking supplements.

Table 4.8 Proportion of young people reported to be allergic to certain foods and the nature of the allergic reaction by sex and age of young person

Responding sample

Whether reported any food allergy and nature of reaction*	Males aged (years):					Females aged (years):				
	4–6	7–10	11–14	15–18	All	4–6	7–10	11–14	15–18	All
	%	%	%	%	%	%	%	%	%	%
Reported being allergic to certain foods, of whom:	8	11	5	10	9	14	9	13	16	13
had allergy diagnosed by doctor	2	7	1	5	4	7	3	6	8	6
Nature of allergic reaction**:										
hyperactivity, behavioural problems	2	5	1	1	3	2	2	2	3	2
rash, blotches	4	1	1	3	2	2	3	4	3	3
eczema	0	1	–	0	1	8	0	–	4	3
asthma, wheezing	0	1	1	0	1	1	1	1	2	1
upset stomach, diarrhoea, vomiting	0	3	1	2	2	1	2	6	1	3
swelling	–	0	0	2	1	1	0	1	–	1
itching	0	–	1	–	0	–	0	–	–	0
allergic rhinitis***	–	–	–	–	–	–	0	0	–	0
migraine	–	1	–	–	0	–	–	1	1	1
other	1	0	1	2	1	0	0	1	1	1
Base	*230*	*304*	*290*	*258*	*1082*	*224*	*277*	*280*	*264*	*1045*

* As reported in response to question why certain foods were not eaten (see Appendix A – interview questionnaire).
** If more than one allergic reaction was reported, all were coded. No order of priority was assigned in coding reactions.
*** Itchy eyes and runny nose or other nasal symptoms.

Table 4.9 Percentage of young people who reported dieting to lose weight by sex and age of young person

Responding sample

Sex and age of young person	% reporting dieting to lose weight	Base
Males aged:		
4–6 years	1%	230
7–10 years	2%	304
11–14 years	4%	290
15–18 years	3%	258
All	2%	1082
Females aged:		
4–6 years	–	224
7–10 years	3%	277
11–14 years	7%	280
15–18 years	16%	264
All	6%	1045

Table 4.10 Percentage of young people who reported being vegetarian or vegan at the time of interview by sex and age of young person and social class of head of household

Responding sample

Sex and age of young person	% reporting being vegetarian or vegan	Base
Sex and age of young person		
Males aged:		
4–6 years	2%	230
7–10 years	1%	304
11–14 years	2%	290
15–18 years	1%	258
All	1%	1082
Females aged:		
4–6 years	2%	224
7–10 years	2%	277
11–14 years	7%	280
15–18 years	10%	264
All	5%	1045
Social class of head of household		
Non-manual	5%	970
Manual	2%	960
All*	2%	2127

*Includes those for whom a social class could not assigned.

Table 4.11(a) Total quantities (grams) of food consumed in seven days by age of young person: male consumers

Type of food	Male consumers aged:												All males		
	4–6 years			7–10 years			11–14 years			15–18 years					
	Mean	Median	% consumers	Mean	Median	% consumers	Mean	Median	% consumers	Mean	Median	% consumers	Mean	Median	% consumers
	g	g	%	g	g	%	g	g	%	g	g	%	g	g	%
Pasta	229	193	75	294	230	65	334	245	53	404	303	49	310	240	60
Rice	181	103	38	282	164	40	397	279	41	510	323	50	362	227	42
Pizza	128	97	37	170	139	46	286	197	48	376	308	47	251	170	45
Other cereals	66	51	29	81	51	32	85	53	30	101	72	32	84	57	31
White bread	378	327	91	470	451	98	522	477	94	641	566	96	510	460	95
Wholemeal bread	172	117	26	194	154	24	254	169	19	234	151	20	211	148	22
Soft grain bread	230	150	2	118	105	2	245	202	4	218	144	4	213	191	3
Other bread	126	82	29	145	90	35	158	108	34	213	185	33	162	108	33
Whole grain and high fibre b'fast cereals	177	134	57	211	157	57	213	152	50	258	202	43	214	154	52
Other b'fast cereals	145	118	83	171	145	84	208	174	69	256	211	61	192	161	74
Biscuits	138	121	93	165	137	92	159	110	84	178	113	70	160	122	84
Fruit pies	99	94	13	135	100	12	117	110	19	133	120	15	122	110	15
Buns, cakes & pastries	186	152	83	227	192	82	229	176	76	228	153	64	218	167	76
Cereal-based milk puddings	214	170	42	211	170	37	251	200	25	234	200	19	224	186	30
Sponge type puddings	102	85	16	106	105	13	183	144	8	131	90	5	123	100	10
Other cereal-based puddings	198	115	40	164	120	31	186	158	24	183	121	17	182	131	28
Whole milk	1391	1153	75	1151	975	58	1134	922	40	928	762	47	1166	934	54
Semi-skimmed milk	997	836	54	1403	1155	53	1480	1243	64	1436	1164	63	1358	1119	59
Skimmed milk	762	601	4	491	292	6	565	373	5	667	457	7	607	369	5
Cream	19	17	12	43	30	13	41	30	10	40	30	14	37	25	12
Other milk	430	336	13	467	335	20	522	432	17	652	430	14	517	402	16
Cottage cheese	76	69	1	48	50	2	162	150	1	193	193	0	101	58	1
Other cheese	76	51	63	78	55	68	93	77	62	148	135	67	100	77	65
Fromage frais	157	110	34	147	121	18	120	98	7	138	94	6	147	108	15
Yogurt	301	203	51	295	250	44	323	196	39	318	200	27	308	228	40
Other dairy desserts	150	89	23	149	111	31	168	126	22	177	131	15	159	119	23
Ice cream	133	120	58	158	129	58	204	128	50	154	108	40	163	122	51
Eggs	111	77	36	117	106	48	134	100	49	144	111	47	128	102	45
Egg dishes	94	64	10	91	80	11	121	118	12	161	143	11	118	97	11
Butter	28	17	27	43	25	32	40	28	26	56	35	24	42	26	27
Block margarine	37	37	0	11	15	1	27	18	1	9	9	2	16	9	1
Soft margarine, not poly-unsaturated	21	14	24	28	16	21	36	24	25	32	20	37	30	20	27
Poly-unsaturated margarine	30	36	4	26	20	7	31	14	8	90	76	4	40	27	6
Poly-unsaturated oils	4	3	1	17	27	1	8	4	2	6	7	2	9	6	1
Other oils and cooking fats, not polyunsaturated	9	3	3	7	5	7	19	14	6	9	10	5	11	9	5
Poly-unsaturated low fat spread	39	22	12	57	53	17	51	46	15	45	27	10	49	43	14
Other low fat spread	37	24	10	45	32	10	65	64	9	70	63	13	56	47	11
Poly-unsaturated reduced fat spread	45	36	41	57	38	35	56	39	37	68	63	32	56	42	36
Other reduced fat spread	42	31	29	71	45	26	65	42	23	75	55	24	64	42	25

Table 4.11(a)   male consumers – continued

Type of food	Male consumers aged:												All males		
	4–6 years			7–10 years			11–14 years			15–18 years					
	Mean	Median	% consumers	Mean	Median	% consumers	Mean	Median	% consumers	Mean	Median	% consumers	Mean	Median	% consumers
	g	g	%	g	g	%	g	g	%	g	g	%	g	g	%
Bacon & ham	82	60	48	82	65	62	114	81	67	165	130	66	114	81	61
Beef, veal and dishes	189	153	43	215	171	52	251	205	48	364	313	63	266	205	52
Lamb & dishes	148	92	24	181	100	30	258	156	28	299	191	25	224	129	27
Pork & dishes	103	71	30	117	85	28	135	83	34	155	115	35	130	92	32
Coated chicken & turkey	118	94	53	125	105	55	175	140	38	243	194	38	159	125	46
Chicken and turkey dishes	143	92	69	161	110	75	258	204	75	346	272	79	234	163	75
Liver, liver products & dishes	41	37	4	63	35	5	65	37	5	70	51	5	61	37	5
Burgers & kebabs	99	100	37	124	94	34	180	117	42	287	200	49	185	124	41
Sausages	138	107	71	146	112	69	142	119	61	202	160	57	156	120	64
Meat pies & pastries	133	96	45	149	120	47	227	151	47	280	230	46	200	142	46
Other meat & meat products	92	59	27	68	41	26	127	71	27	134	101	28	106	71	27
Coated and/or fried white fish	109	91	65	123	88	54	145	128	41	184	140	39	137	108	49
Other white fish & dishes	163	152	9	128	117	11	217	197	13	189	171	9	177	149	10
Shellfish	40	28	4	64	50	2	59	40	6	178	84	9	109	51	5
Oily fish	114	83	18	82	58	24	100	72	26	130	94	23	105	75	23
Raw carrots	101	80	16	79	40	16	59	50	10	131	53	11	92	50	13
Other raw & salad vegetables	71	47	37	80	55	44	100	73	53	124	85	51	97	68	47
Raw tomatoes	57	40	26	85	71	27	76	65	33	104	83	42	84	68	32
Peas	75	57	59	76	61	49	105	78	48	137	88	44	97	70	50
Green beans	44	36	16	56	48	13	78	53	12	112	91	17	76	51	14
Baked beans	208	137	64	197	158	63	261	187	60	325	244	62	248	181	62
Leafy green vegetables	75	60	46	82	60	41	91	69	32	117	95	38	91	67	39
Carrots–not raw	74	56	59	75	61	54	95	80	51	115	84	47	89	70	53
Tomatoes–not raw	45	34	8	87	65	8	76	48	11	106	77	15	85	71	10
Vegetable dishes	203	118	20	164	124	16	252	156	17	262	219	20	222	162	18
Other vegetables	103	79	55	107	93	58	126	105	61	144	99	57	121	95	58
Potato chips	265	210	89	338	290	88	450	380	90	584	500	87	415	330	89
Other fried/ roast potatoes & products	135	97	49	139	113	58	152	130	52	215	188	47	159	127	52
Potato products–not fried	112	90	30	153	100	25	120	100	18	164	147	10	134	100	20
Other potatoes & potato dishes	274	238	81	299	239	86	352	257	84	478	386	80	352	261	83
Savoury snacks	117	106	92	130	117	93	136	114	88	136	120	80	130	115	88
Apples & pears	271	219	70	307	248	59	255	157	48	293	164	39	282	207	53
Citrus fruits	196	160	26	192	166	29	197	160	21	294	242	19	215	160	24
Bananas	232	156	47	232	156	42	221	150	32	254	196	33	234	164	38
Canned fruit in juice	103	100	8	151	121	7	129	98	5	70	40	4	117	100	6
Canned fruit in syrup	127	120	11	120	100	8	123	115	5	219	181	5	142	120	7
Other fruit	159	100	42	214	150	38	191	150	23	185	152	21	189	131	31
Nuts and seeds	43	26	21	53	38	20	88	50	15	75	52	10	62	36	16
Table sugar	37	29	70	48	35	66	68	44	66	94	70	74	63	40	69
Preserves	36	22	42	43	30	35	55	30	29	76	54	20	49	30	31
Sweet spreads, fillings & icings	30	21	22	27	18	28	29	26	15	45	24	13	31	21	20

59

Table 4.11(a)   male consumers – continued

Type of food	Male consumers aged:												All males		
	4–6 years			7–10 years			11–14 years			15–18 years					
	Mean	Median	% consumers	Mean	Median	% consumers	Mean	Median	% consumers	Mean	Median	% consumers	Mean	Median	% consumers
	g	g	%	g	g	%	g	g	%	g	g	%	g	g	%
Sugar confectionery	107	68	71	135	91	77	175	103	67	148	81	39	141	87	63
Chocolate confectionery	108	87	80	148	127	91	183	159	85	208	130	79	164	125	84
Fruit juice	646	405	48	766	449	50	851	559	45	1015	728	43	821	520	46
Concentrated soft drinks– not low calorie, as consumed	2130	1504	61	2572	1483	60	2299	1415	51	3824	2583	37	2626	1516	52
Carbonated soft drinks– not low calorie	734	474	67	1101	676	73	1466	1213	85	2228	1685	85	1456	1008	78
Ready to drink soft drinks– not low calorie	623	382	36	642	382	34	495	382	33	640	396	13	593	382	29
Concentrated soft drinks– low calorie, as consumed	3172	2247	61	3010	2561	56	2961	2034	46	3096	2250	27	3054	2250	47
Carbonated soft drinks– low calorie	777	536	44	1014	715	44	1212	739	49	1045	806	40	1030	723	44
Ready to drink soft drinks– low calorie	691	591	11	644	606	4	498	252	7	695	505	3	623	450	6
Liqueurs	–	–	–	13	20	1	–	–	–	103	69	1	73	28	1
Spirits	–	–	–	–	–	–	3	3	0	159	69	7	153	69	2
Wine	80	80	0	24	24	0	86	89	1	293	205	5	247	144	2
Fortified wine	–	–	–	–	–	–	5	5	0	142	106	2	121	106	1
Low alcohol & alcohol-free wine	80	80	0	–	–	–	–	–	–	–	–	–	80	80	0
Beer & lager	–	–	–	8	8	0	474	504	4	3139	1800	34	2866	1713	10
Low alcohol & alcohol-free beer & lager	150	150	0	–	–	–	–	–	–	–	–	–	150	150	0
Cider & Perry	–	–	–	–	–	–	–	–	–	481	454	4	481	454	1
Alco-pops	–	–	–	–	–	–	337	337	0	959	343	3	894	343	1
Coffee, as consumed	970	1094	6	936	383	7	1615	1231	14	2053	1358	39	1753	1220	17
Tea, as consumed	499	375	29	770	494	40	1093	672	48	1755	1167	61	1166	674	45
Herbal tea, as consumed	–	–	–	57	57	0	266	266	0	569	649	1	370	168	0
Bottled water	763	251	5	443	250	6	584	357	12	1753	965	6	833	426	8
Tap water	767	598	59	1075	750	62	994	571	57	1658	850	60	1142	740	60
Commercial toddler's foods	130	54	3	–	–	–	100	100	0	103	95	1	118	70	1
Other beverages, dry weight	465	280	24	485	317	22	624	414	21	484	240	16	517	322	21
Soup	254	205	21	274	242	25	324	300	20	554	364	21	351	262	22
Savoury sauces, pickles, gravies & condiments	87	65	89	119	98	89	145	111	87	200	186	90	140	104	89
Base = number of young people			184			256			237			179			856

Table 4.11(b) Total quantities (grams) of food consumed in seven days by age of young person: female consumers

Type of food	Female consumers aged:												All females		
	4–6 years			7–10 years			11–14 years			15–18 years					
	Mean	Median	% consumers	Mean	Median	% consumers	Mean	Median	% consumers	Mean	Median	% consumers	Mean	Median	% consumers
	g	g	%	g	g	%	g	g	%	g	g	%	g	g	%
Pasta	215	176	71	301	230	60	311	222	53	333	256	62	291	220	64
Rice	188	94	28	283	142	35	396	225	44	326	230	44	315	180	40
Pizza	113	93	42	142	113	43	176	130	42	223	175	41	165	123	44
Other cereals	61	54	25	82	61	28	104	69	35	97	80	35	90	69	33
White bread	323	281	93	391	359	92	417	365	89	449	395	90	398	359	96
Wholemeal bread	136	93	26	186	110	24	179	115	20	155	108	29	164	109	26
Soft grain bread	153	135	3	231	164	3	212	144	3	135	102	3	185	136	3
Other bread	102	74	33	116	75	29	104	80	37	182	137	41	130	90	37
Whole grain and high fibre b'fast cereals	135	100	59	145	118	47	161	104	45	171	94	33	151	106	48
Other b'fast cereals	119	97	77	128	105	69	156	124	61	151	108	40	137	108	64
Biscuits	142	115	89	158	140	88	135	101	79	100	74	66	136	106	84
Fruit pies	96	103	11	124	85	14	96	74	10	120	110	14	112	94	13
Buns, cakes & pastries	159	147	74	175	145	76	209	165	71	174	133	64	180	147	75
Cereal-based milk puddings	186	146	38	213	176	43	209	179	20	233	195	16	208	171	31
Sponge type puddings	86	73	8	114	96	14	88	100	6	98	89	5	101	95	9
Other cereal-based puddings	143	124	25	179	129	27	165	125	24	176	126	21	167	125	26
Whole milk	1333	1116	70	955	853	51	752	436	38	723	452	41	975	790	51
Semi-skimmed milk	846	771	47	992	721	52	914	784	58	877	723	59	912	753	57
Skimmed milk	287	192	4	388	133	10	926	892	5	563	358	9	536	317	7
Cream	37	26	10	30	19	16	41	27	9	36	30	11	35	27	12
Other milk	370	336	15	399	335	14	430	358	14	317	312	16	378	335	15
Cottage cheese	25	25	1	32	38	2	48	39	2	104	80	3	64	39	2
Other cheese	85	76	72	93	72	63	102	90	61	115	90	69	99	80	69
Fromage frais	144	118	39	153	150	18	148	82	8	98	60	4	144	120	17
Yogurt	320	250	47	302	215	46	286	183	42	269	218	33	296	218	44
Other dairy desserts	138	120	22	146	120	28	133	110	16	128	100	11	139	118	20
Ice cream	132	106	61	167	124	57	147	124	46	131	90	29	147	120	50
Eggs	114	81	44	117	100	44	103	60	41	122	100	40	114	93	44
Egg dishes	81	79	12	104	100	15	118	100	13	137	113	11	110	97	13
Butter	34	22	35	34	22	26	29	18	26	35	23	31	33	22	31
Block margarine	4	3	1	7	7	1	42	15	1	66	49	1	26	7	1
Soft margarine, not poly-unsaturated	25	14	24	32	18	24	28	14	26	28	24	32	29	18	28
Poly-unsaturated margarine	34	27	5	37	14	5	32	25	6	39	28	3	35	27	5
Poly-unsaturated oils	12	10	2	9	5	3	9	10	2	6	5	1	9	6	2
Other oils and cooking fats, not poly-unsaturated	8	9	3	7	5	4	8	7	6	13	10	8	10	8	6
Poly-unsaturated low fat spread	22	19	16	38	32	11	51	34	14	49	42	12	40	28	14
Other low fat spread	39	31	10	47	40	13	50	46	11	32	19	13	42	35	13
Poly-unsaturated reduced fat spread	40	31	41	50	43	37	53	45	32	44	29	38	47	37	38
Other reduced fat spread	45	28	29	41	34	20	53	40	17	60	41	19	49	39	22

61

Table 4.11(b)   female consumers – continued

Type of food	Female consumers aged:												All females		
	4–6 years			7–10 years			11–14 years			15–18 years					
	Mean	Median	% consumers	Mean	Median	% consumers	Mean	Median	% consumers	Mean	Median	% consumers	Mean	Median	% consumers
	g	g	%	g	g	%	g	g	%	g	g	%	g	g	%
Bacon & ham	69	47	58	85	64	59	85	61	52	91	66	48	83	59	57
Beef, veal and dishes	160	134	43	231	161	52	283	214	46	318	229	45	252	180	49
Lamb & dishes	98	57	26	177	119	27	199	118	21	170	153	19	162	115	24
Pork & dishes	82	64	25	114	82	28	131	107	26	171	120	27	127	89	28
Coated chicken & turkey	109	89	53	135	113	49	193	165	39	198	165	42	156	128	48
Chicken and turkey dishes	153	102	69	177	126	71	229	180	65	262	192	69	207	146	73
Liver, liver products & dishes	69	47	4	42	25	5	44	28	4	84	46	3	58	39	4
Burgers & kebabs	96	96	34	124	100	33	164	140	36	205	166	31	149	115	35
Sausages	92	70	65	115	86	62	141	103	48	125	93	37	117	86	55
Meat pies & pastries	115	88	39	143	117	45	181	145	41	175	144	39	155	128	43
Other meat & meat products	51	41	27	102	61	25	90	51	18	125	75	15	90	56	22
Coated and/or fried white fish	106	80	59	107	84	50	135	112	32	161	137	29	122	98	44
Other white fish & dishes	115	77	11	135	120	13	217	133	11	214	142	8	167	124	11
Shellfish	50	33	3	57	46	5	60	28	9	79	60	8	65	43	7
Oily fish	75	45	27	82	62	29	94	65	20	127	104	33	97	65	29
Raw carrots	52	27	19	65	58	16	51	33	13	103	50	19	70	43	18
Other raw & salad vegetables	91	67	52	107	87	49	94	63	56	149	111	66	114	78	59
Raw tomatoes	81	65	30	90	58	35	79	56	37	116	76	54	95	65	42
Peas	64	40	52	93	63	50	84	66	46	96	76	39	85	63	49
Green beans	38	27	15	52	46	12	77	72	12	97	67	12	66	49	13
Baked beans	152	136	62	191	127	60	201	155	50	272	206	44	201	155	57
Leafy green vegetables	77	53	44	84	74	42	117	91	40	127	97	40	102	80	44
Carrots–not raw	69	53	58	76	60	53	86	67	44	89	67	50	80	61	54
Tomatoes–not raw	52	48	5	105	84	8	83	74	8	79	85	9	84	77	8
Vegetable dishes	222	138	15	235	134	16	254	165	21	369	266	28	286	170	22
Other vegetables	97	70	60	116	94	60	154	115	52	179	128	63	138	97	62
Potato chips	232	189	85	301	257	88	452	389	79	408	320	80	351	281	88
Other fried/ roast potatoes & products	111	85	48	141	115	46	179	138	44	144	132	45	145	116	48
Potato products–not fried	98	93	25	122	90	26	128	98	15	148	90	12	121	94	20
Other potatoes & potato dishes	241	201	79	321	270	80	370	287	74	355	300	72	324	261	80
Savoury snacks	110	106	91	127	117	89	143	127	86	110	88	75	124	112	90
Apples & pears	275	209	66	277	196	61	299	224	47	336	210	44	294	210	57
Citrus fruits	204	134	29	226	160	33	225	141	23	286	225	20	233	163	28
Bananas	189	137	50	217	145	38	175	131	28	210	142	30	199	137	38
Canned fruit in juice	126	88	6	156	115	9	173	115	4	157	115	3	154	115	6
Canned fruit in syrup	117	89	13	134	72	10	157	137	6	100	100	1	132	89	8
Other fruit	191	150	42	231	144	42	204	141	28	349	192	24	237	150	35
Nuts and seeds	27	23	14	46	28	15	57	32	14	36	30	10	43	27	14
Table sugar	33	25	62	38	26	61	53	38	60	84	55	59	53	32	63
Preserves	32	23	43	41	28	40	37	26	24	36	30	26	37	27	34
Sweet spreads, fillings & icings	28	20	25	31	23	25	41	25	15	32	20	10	32	20	20

Table 4.11(b) female consumers – continued

Type of food	Female consumers aged:												All females		
	4–6 years			7–10 years			11–14 years			15–18 years					
	Mean	Median	% consumers	Mean	Median	% consumers	Mean	Median	% consumers	Mean	Median	% consumers	Mean	Median	% consumers
	g	g	%	g	g	%	g	g	%	g	g	%	g	g	%
Sugar confectionery	123	92	75	125	75	72	131	82	64	72	42	41	117	75	66
Chocolate confectionery	116	100	76	130	113	80	170	132	76	151	99	72	143	112	80
Fruit juice	617	401	53	737	601	48	741	469	47	899	750	45	750	521	51
Concentrated soft drinks– not low calorie, as consumed	1868	1235	60	2321	1565	56	1798	1081	43	2311	1364	36	2082	1332	51
Carbonated soft drinks– not low calorie	812	600	66	877	590	72	1331	1043	73	1463	1029	73	1141	816	75
Ready to drink soft drinks– not low calorie	582	446	35	616	520	33	550	395	29	543	315	20	577	424	30
Concentrated soft drinks– low calorie, as consumed	2679	1525	61	2935	2234	48	2676	2051	41	2272	810	29	2686	1867	46
Carbonated soft drinks– low calorie	744	521	43	1062	600	47	992	706	44	1075	660	41	983	618	46
Ready to drink soft drinks– low calorie	515	432	11	621	503	8	266	200	3	564	433	4	524	432	7
Liqueurs	–	–	–	–	–	–	–	–	–	63	69	2	63	69	1
Spirits	–	–	–	–	–	–	10	10	0	89	69	11	87	69	3
Wine	54	78	1	141	141	0	210	127	2	401	208	10	339	143	4
Fortified wine	–	–	–	13	8	1	–	–	–	199	124	2	147	73	1
Low alcohol & alcohol-free wine	–	–	–	–	–	–	65	65	0	360	291	1	308	223	0
Beer & lager	–	–	–	95	95	1	317	92	1	1982	1427	17	1803	1386	5
Low alcohol & alcohol-free beer & lager	–	–	–	–	–	–	–	–	–	531	531	0	531	531	0
Cider & Perry	–	–	–	70	70	0	586	533	1	1081	883	3	851	504	1
Alco-pops	–	–	–	–	–	–	673	673	0	884	686	6	874	686	2
Coffee, as consumed	1069	407	6	904	422	11	1069	542	14	2498	1336	32	1766	934	17
Tea, as consumed	528	343	33	720	470	43	1115	705	49	1966	1486	56	1196	698	48
Herbal tea, as consumed	428	277	1	99	140	1	470	204	1	1176	1282	2	634	220	1
Bottled water	800	330	6	401	330	6	705	489	7	748	500	17	681	378	9
Tap water	740	573	54	977	696	63	1145	800	57	1206	720	60	1035	692	62
Commercial toddler's foods	–	–	–	–	–	–	–	–	–	–	–	–	–	–	–
Other beverages, dry weight	429	253	27	554	360	19	352	216	20	462	230	20	449	260	22
Soup	213	190	24	323	267	23	314	288	27	398	345	28	321	257	27
Savoury sauces, pickles, gravies & condiments	87	68	84	118	95	82	160	115	81	183	145	84	140	104	87
Base = number of young people			*171*			*226*			*238*			*210*			*845*

63

Table 4.11(c)   Main differences in the eating behaviour of young people by sex and age group

Foods more likely to be eaten by:

All boys (compared with girls)	Boys aged 4–6 years[1]	Boys aged 15–18 years[2]
breakfast cereals, not high fibre or wholegrain** sausages* beer & lager*	pasta** breakfast cereals, not high fibre or wholegrain** biscuits** buns, cakes & pastries** cereal-based milk puddings** sponge puddings* other cereal-based puddings** whole milk** fromage frais** yogurt** ice cream* coated chicken & turkey* coated &/or fried white fish** peas* potato products, not fried** savoury snacks** apples & pears** other fruit** nuts & seeds* preserves** sugar confectionery** concentrated soft drinks nlc** ready to drink soft drinks nlc** concentrated soft drinks lc** ready to drink soft drinks lc*	bacon & ham* beef, veal & dishes** raw tomatoes* carbonated soft drinks nlc** coffee** tea**

All girls (compared with boys)	Girls aged 4–6 years[1]	Girls aged 15–18 years[2]
other raw and salad vegetables** raw tomatoes**	whole grain & high fibre b'fast cereals** breakfast cereals, not high fibre or wholegrain** biscuits** cereal-based milk puddings** whole milk** fromage frais** ice cream** sausages** coated &/or fried white fish** baked beans* potato products, not fried* savoury snacks** apples & pears** bananas ** canned fruit in syrup** other fruit* preserves* sweet spreads, fillings & icings** sugar confectionery** concentrated soft drinks nlc** ready to drink soft drinks nlc* concentrated soft drinks lc**	rice* raw tomatoes** vegetable dishes* coffee** tea** bottled water* wine**

[1] Compared with same sex aged 15 to 18 years
[2] Compared with same sex aged 4 to 6 years
* p < 0.05
** p < 0.01
pufa: polyunsaturated
nlc: not low calorie
lc: low calorie

Table 4.12(a) Total quantities (grams) of food consumed in seven days by age of young person: males, including non-consumers

Type of food	All males aged:								All males	
	4–6 years		7–10 years		11–14 years		15–18 years			
	Mean	sd	Mean	sd	Mean	sd	Mean	sd	Mean	sd
	g	g	g	g	g	g	g	g	g	g
Pasta	171	189	191	237	179	272	196	282	185	250
Rice	68	152	112	267	163	340	255	481	153	344
Pizza	47	89	79	127	136	212	176	269	112	197
Other cereals	19	44	26	56	26	62	32	71	26	60
White bread	344	262	459	293	492	330	617	419	485	347
Wholemeal bread	45	104	47	120	48	147	47	134	47	128
Soft grain bread	5	44	2	20	11	62	8	47	7	46
Other bread	37	94	50	118	54	115	69	143	53	120
Whole grain and high fibre b'fast cereals	102	148	121	202	106	166	111	229	110	191
Other b'fast cereals	121	103	143	125	144	161	155	193	141	152
Biscuits	128	97	151	126	133	150	124	197	135	149
Fruit pies	12	41	17	58	22	56	20	55	18	54
Buns, cakes & pastries	155	155	186	179	173	217	146	181	166	186
Cereal-based milk puddings	90	145	77	138	64	150	44	107	68	137
Sponge type puddings	16	48	14	41	14	60	6	30	13	46
Other cereal-based puddings	80	157	52	97	44	96	31	90	50	111
Whole milk	1041	1112	672	885	458	803	437	755	632	915
Semi-skimmed milk	536	788	746	1008	951	1152	908	1109	798	1046
Skimmed milk	30	210	27	161	29	156	46	232	33	191
Cream	2	7	6	20	4	18	6	17	4	17
Other milk	57	233	91	264	89	243	90	298	84	263
Cottage cheese	1	7	1	6	2	18	1	11	1	12
Other cheese	48	68	53	65	58	73	99	115	65	86
Fromage frais	54	117	26	73	8	40	9	41	23	74
Yogurt	154	248	131	208	127	227	86	197	123	220
Other dairy desserts	35	87	46	97	37	91	26	82	36	90
Ice cream	77	91	91	112	101	204	62	113	83	140
Eggs	40	76	56	81	65	106	68	103	58	94
Egg dishes	10	37	10	34	14	49	18	68	13	49
Butter	8	19	14	36	10	28	13	40	11	32
Block margarine	0	2	0	1	0	3	0	1	0	2
Soft margarine, not polyunsaturated	5	12	6	15	9	25	12	25	8	21
Polyunsaturated margarine	1	6	2	8	3	13	4	24	2	15
Polyunsaturated oils	0	0	0	2	0	2	0	1	0	2
Other oils and cooking fats, not polyunsaturated	0	0	0	0	0	1	0	0	0	0
Polyunsaturated low fat spread	5	19	9	26	8	24	5	19	7	23
Other low fat spread	4	16	4	17	6	25	9	29	6	23
Polyunsaturated reduced fat spread	2	3	2	4	2	4	2	4	2	4
Other reduced fat spread	12	30	19	63	15	37	18	43	16	46
Bacon & ham	39	69	51	67	77	128	108	146	70	112
Beef, veal and dishes	81	139	111	167	120	196	230	264	138	207
Lamb & dishes	36	112	54	156	73	181	74	225	60	176
Pork & dishes	31	74	33	80	47	96	55	106	42	91
Coated chicken	63	81	69	86	66	111	92	173	73	120
Chicken and turkey dishes	98	130	121	147	194	232	273	276	174	218
Liver, liver products & dishes	2	11	3	24	3	20	4	18	3	19
Burgers & kebabs	37	61	43	82	76	136	140	217	75	146
Sausages	97	112	100	118	87	107	116	156	100	126
Meat pies & pastries	60	93	69	103	106	183	129	189	92	153
Other meat & meat products	25	66	17	45	34	91	38	85	29	75

65

Table 4.12(a) males – continued

Type of food	All males aged:								All males	
	4–6 years		7–10 years		11–14 years		15–18 years			
	Mean	sd	Mean	sd	Mean	sd	Mean	sd	Mean	sd
	g	g	g	g	g	g	g	g	g	g
Coated and/or fried white fish	71	78	66	97	60	89	72	114	67	96
Other white fish & dishes	14	56	14	46	27	103	18	66	18	72
Shellfish	2	12	1	10	3	19	15	72	6	39
Oily fish	21	62	20	50	26	56	30	78	24	62
Raw carrots	17	54	12	53	6	25	14	69	12	53
Other raw & salad vegetables	26	50	35	69	53	87	64	102	45	82
Raw tomatoes	15	33	23	52	25	50	44	73	27	56
Peas	45	57	37	55	51	79	60	105	48	78
Green beans	7	25	7	24	10	32	19	51	11	36
Baked beans	134	175	124	169	156	214	203	284	155	219
Leafy green vegetables	34	56	34	57	30	63	45	80	36	65
Carrots–not raw	44	59	41	56	49	68	54	85	47	68
Tomatoes–not raw	3	16	7	31	8	36	16	48	9	36
Vegetable dishes	42	117	26	89	44	154	54	132	41	126
Other vegetables	56	80	62	81	77	100	82	119	70	97
Potato chips	236	199	299	266	406	327	506	449	367	343
Other fried/roast potatoes & products	66	112	81	111	79	105	101	148	82	121
Potato products–not fried	34	77	39	96	21	56	16	54	27	74
Other potatoes & potato dishes	223	206	257	231	296	283	382	409	293	301
Savoury snacks	107	76	121	91	119	99	109	106	115	94
Apples & pears	191	220	180	238	123	194	115	286	151	240
Citrus fruits	52	118	56	111	42	118	56	152	51	126
Bananas	109	182	97	167	71	154	83	178	89	170
Canned fruit in juice	8	32	10	46	6	31	3	19	7	34
Canned fruit in syrup	14	47	10	41	7	35	11	57	10	46
Other fruit	66	129	82	169	45	125	39	124	58	140
Nuts and seeds	9	26	11	30	13	52	7	29	10	36
Table sugar	26	37	31	42	45	61	69	88	44	64
Preserves	15	34	15	31	16	38	15	45	15	37
Sweet spreads, fillings & icings	7	19	8	20	4	14	6	24	6	20
Sugar confectionery	76	104	104	138	116	181	57	209	89	167
Chocolate confectionery	86	87	134	111	156	133	165	191	138	140
Fruit juice	311	579	380	690	382	679	433	828	380	706
Concentrated soft drinks–not low calorie, as consumed	1290	1869	1547	2354	1179	2055	1418	3090	1365	2413
Carbonated soft drinks–not low calorie	491	669	807	1058	1245	1190	1889	1951	1136	1420
Ready to drink soft drinks–not low calorie	226	427	218	472	161	325	83	316	170	394
Concentrated soft drinks–low calorie, as consumed	1951	2672	1684	2428	1376	2582	842	2081	1441	2471
Carbonated soft drinks–low calorie	341	568	447	830	597	1064	419	759	457	841
Ready to drink soft drinks–low calorie	80	314	26	143	37	185	23	165	39	206
Liqueurs	–	–	0	1	–	–	1	15	0	8
Spirits	–	–	–	–	0	0	11	75	3	39
Wine	0	5	0	2	0	7	16	97	4	50
Fortified wine	–	–	–	–	0	0	3	22	1	11
Low alcohol & alcohol-free wine	0	5	–	–	–	–	–	–	0	2
Beer & lager	–	–	0	0	17	105	1084	2490	285	1352
Low alcohol & alcohol-free beer & lager	1	9	–	–	–	–	–	–	0	4
Cider & Perry	–	–	–	–	–	–	18	99	5	51
Alco-pops	–	–	–	–	1	21	32	244	9	125

Table 4.12(a) males – continued

Type of food	All males aged:								All males	
	4–6 years		7–10 years		11–14 years		15–18 years			
	Mean	sd	Mean	sd	Mean	sd	Mean	sd	Mean	sd
	g	g	g	g	g	g	g	g	g	g
Coffee, as consumed	59	298	65	351	230	749	806	1568	298	963
Tea, as consumed	143	318	311	617	524	1041	1065	1929	527	1219
Herbal tea, as consumed	–	–	0	4	1	14	5	63	1	33
Bottled water	40	262	29	155	68	267	112	647	63	385
Tap water	456	655	666	1090	570	929	993	1830	682	1242
Commercial toddler's foods	4	39	–	–	0	7	1	12	1	19
Other beverages, dry weight	114	303	109	296	133	441	78	262	108	334
Soup	53	145	69	144	65	163	116	308	77	205
Savoury sauces, pickles, gravies & condiments	77	75	105	99	127	122	179	153	124	123
Base = number of young people		*184*		*256*		*237*		*179*		*856*

Table 4.12(b) Total quantities (grams) of food consumed in seven days by age of young person: females, including non-consumers

Type of food	All females aged:								All females	
	4–6 years		7–10 years		11–14 years		15–18 years			
	Mean	sd	Mean	sd	Mean	sd	Mean	sd	Mean	sd
	g	g	g	g	g	g	g	g	g	g
Pasta	159	172	189	248	174	254	218	250	187	237
Rice	56	224	105	259	183	386	150	251	127	293
Pizza	50	72	64	96	78	118	97	148	73	115
Other cereals	16	32	24	52	39	94	36	63	29	66
White bread	314	188	378	240	396	258	425	280	381	249
Wholemeal bread	37	86	47	120	38	103	47	109	42	106
Soft grain bread	4	30	7	48	7	51	4	27	5	41
Other bread	35	72	35	75	41	74	80	136	48	95
Whole grain and high fibre b'fast cereals	84	140	72	114	76	132	59	147	72	133
Other b'fast cereals	97	96	93	103	100	125	64	112	88	111
Biscuits	132	115	147	115	113	110	70	92	115	112
Fruit pies	11	32	18	59	10	37	18	49	15	47
Buns, cakes & pastries	124	115	140	130	156	181	118	138	135	145
Cereal-based milk puddings	74	123	97	143	45	109	41	109	64	124
Sponge type puddings	7	28	17	55	5	23	5	25	9	36
Other cereal-based puddings	38	81	52	100	42	92	39	95	43	93
Whole milk	976	1009	513	709	302	617	312	590	502	777
Semi-skimmed milk	420	631	546	811	561	743	548	722	524	737
Skimmed milk	11	64	40	217	50	278	51	221	39	216
Cream	4	14	5	16	4	16	4	14	4	15
Other milk	59	180	61	167	62	204	52	169	58	180
Cottage cheese	0	3	1	6	1	9	4	30	1	16
Other cheese	64	68	61	78	66	77	84	98	69	82
Fromage frais	58	99	29	69	13	58	4	25	24	69
Yogurt	158	235	146	228	126	211	94	164	130	212
Other dairy desserts	31	74	43	88	22	61	14	49	28	70
Ice cream	85	103	101	128	71	109	40	84	74	110
Eggs	53	86	54	81	44	80	52	92	51	85
Egg dishes	10	35	16	44	16	53	16	58	15	49
Butter	13	29	9	22	8	21	11	26	10	24
Block margarine	0	1	0	1	1	7	0	6	0	5
Soft margarine, not polyunsaturated	6	18	8	22	8	19	9	20	8	20
Polyunsaturated margarine	2	8	2	12	2	10	1	7	2	10
Polyunsaturated oils	0	2	0	2	0	1	0	1	0	2
Other oils and cooking fats, not polyunsaturated	0	0	0	0	0	0	0	1	0	0
Polyunsaturated low fat spread	4	10	4	15	8	24	6	19	5	18
Other low fat spread	4	14	6	18	6	20	4	17	5	18
Polyunsaturated reduced fat spread	2	3	2	4	2	3	2	4	2	3
Other reduced fat spread	13	33	9	21	10	31	12	35	11	30
Bacon & ham	42	62	53	75	47	78	46	77	47	74
Beef, veal and dishes	72	123	126	186	137	211	150	244	124	201
Lamb & dishes	26	64	50	118	44	130	33	84	39	105
Pork & dishes	21	48	34	92	36	78	49	106	36	86
Coated chicken	61	75	70	92	79	126	88	132	75	111
Chicken and turkey dishes	111	161	133	157	159	186	192	215	150	184
Liver, liver products & dishes	3	20	2	12	2	12	3	22	3	17
Burgers & kebabs	34	56	43	85	62	104	67	124	52	98
Sausages	63	71	75	89	72	111	48	88	65	92
Meat pies & pastries	47	77	68	98	79	128	72	121	68	110
Other meat & meat products	15	36	27	77	18	54	20	78	20	65

Table 4.12(b)   females – continued

Type of food	All females aged:								All females	
	4–6 years		7–10 years		11–14 years		15–18 years			
	Mean	sd	Mean	sd	Mean	sd	Mean	sd	Mean	sd
	g	g	g	g	g	g	g	g	g	g
Coated and/or fried white fish	66	78	57	72	46	79	48	89	54	80
Other white fish & dishes	13	47	18	58	25	95	17	71	18	71
Shellfish	2	11	3	17	5	27	7	27	4	22
Oily fish	21	55	25	51	20	50	45	90	28	65
Raw carrots	10	30	11	30	7	26	21	92	12	53
Other raw & salad vegetables	50	77	56	83	56	86	104	135	67	101
Raw tomatoes	26	55	33	71	31	59	67	103	40	77
Peas	35	55	49	71	41	62	39	62	41	64
Green beans	6	19	7	22	9	33	12	51	9	34
Baked beans	98	111	121	168	106	146	127	205	114	164
Leafy green vegetables	36	83	37	57	50	92	54	92	45	82
Carrots–not raw	42	55	43	59	40	60	47	65	43	60
Tomatoes–not raw	3	14	9	35	7	28	7	25	7	27
Vegetable dishes	36	134	41	133	56	154	110	242	62	175
Other vegetables	61	89	73	93	85	158	118	158	85	132
Potato chips	208	178	281	214	379	333	344	325	308	281
Other fried/roast potatoes & products	56	80	68	105	84	129	69	93	70	105
Potato products–not fried	25	49	34	68	20	54	18	68	25	61
Other potatoes & potato dishes	199	189	269	220	291	283	271	252	261	243
Savoury snacks	105	64	119	82	131	92	87	89	111	85
Apples & pears	190	254	179	246	148	218	155	304	167	258
Citrus fruits	62	147	80	147	56	152	60	160	65	152
Bananas	99	149	87	160	52	110	65	132	75	140
Canned fruit in juice	7	37	15	58	8	64	5	37	9	51
Canned fruit in syrup	15	58	14	59	10	49	1	13	10	49
Other fruit	84	151	102	204	60	135	89	303	84	212
Nuts and seeds	4	12	7	25	9	33	4	13	6	23
Table sugar	22	32	25	38	33	50	52	84	33	57
Preserves	14	24	17	30	10	23	10	20	13	25
Sweet spreads, fillings & icings	7	20	8	21	6	23	3	13	6	20
Sugar confectionery	97	134	95	141	89	154	31	64	77	131
Chocolate confectionery	93	90	109	98	137	142	115	137	115	121
Fruit juice	344	587	373	565	373	666	428	696	381	633
Concentrated soft drinks–not low calorie, as consumed	1181	1919	1381	2256	823	1577	890	1803	1068	1923
Carbonated soft drinks–not low calorie	563	660	665	821	1029	1120	1122	1316	856	1050
Ready to drink soft drinks–not low calorie	215	375	211	384	167	345	113	306	175	356
Concentrated soft drinks–low calorie, as consumed	1719	2305	1483	2409	1164	2219	693	2033	1245	2276
Carbonated soft drinks–low calorie	332	600	523	1036	463	755	465	941	453	865
Ready to drink soft drinks–low calorie	62	213	53	225	10	58	22	125	36	169
Liqueurs	–	–	–	–	–	–	2	12	0	6
Spirits	–	–	–	–	0	1	10	35	3	18
Wine	1	6	1	10	5	41	41	240	12	125
Fortified wine	–	–	0	1	–	–	5	38	1	19
Low alcohol & alcohol-free wine	–	–	–	0	0	4	5	50	1	26
Beer & lager	–	–	1	7	5	57	359	1090	94	576
Low alcohol & alcohol-free beer & lager	–	–	–	–	–	–	2	34	1	17
Cider & Perry	–	–	0	5	6	74	31	234	10	125
Alco-pops	–	–	–	0	2	37	54	263	14	137

69

Table 4.12(b) females – continued

Type of food	All females aged:								All females	
	4–6 years		7–10 years		11–14 years		15–18 years			
	Mean	sd	Mean	sd	Mean	sd	Mean	sd	Mean	sd
	g	g	g	g	g	g	g	g	g	g
Coffee, as consumed	64	358	109	483	162	574	852	1918	305	1109
Tea, as consumed	180	437	325	602	575	1009	1156	1662	575	1120
Herbal tea, as consumed	5	56	1	13	4	53	24	206	9	112
Bottled water	46	275	26	123	51	276	134	401	64	288
Tap water	419	728	648	909	686	1109	762	1066	640	982
Commercial toddler's foods	–	–	–	–	–	–	0	3	0	2
Other beverages, dry weight	121	302	112	332	76	238	97	331	101	304
Soup	53	117	77	168	90	161	118	236	86	179
Savoury sauces, pickles, gravies & condiments	76	70	102	98	138	146	162	148	122	126
Base = number of young people		*171*		*226*		*238*		*210*		*845*

Table 4.12(c) Main differences in the total quantity of foods consumed by boys and girls, including non-consumers

Greater quantity eaten by:		
all boys	all girls	
pizza**	raw tomatoes**	* p < 0.05
white bread**	other raw and salad vegetables**	** p < 0.01
wholegrain & high fibre b'fast	apples & pears**	nlc: not low calorie
cereals**	other fruit*	
breakfast cereals, not high fibre		
or wholegrain**		
biscuits*		
buns, cakes & pastries*		
whole milk*		
semi-skimmed milk**		
bacon & ham**		
lamb & dishes*		
burgers & kebabs*		
sausages**		
meat pies & pastries*		
coated &/or fried white fish**		
baked beans**		
potato chips**		
nuts and seeds**		
table sugar*		
chocolate confectionery*		
carbonated soft drinks nlc**		
beer & lager*		

Greater quantity eaten by boys aged (compared with girls in same age group):

4–6 years	7 to 10 years	11–14 years	15–18 years
cereal-based milk puddings*	white bread*	pizza*	pizza*
sausages*	wholegrain & high fibre b'fast	white bread*	white bread**
	cereals*	wholegrain & high fibre b'fast	breakfast cereals, not high fibre
	breakfast cereals, not high fibre	cereals*	or wholegrain**
	or wholegrain**	breakfast cereals, not high fibre	biscuits*
	buns, cakes & pastries*	or wholegrain*	semi-skimmed milk*
		semi-skimmed milk**	bacon & ham**
		bacon & ham*	beef, veal and dishes*
			burgers & kebabs**
			sausages**
			meat pies and pastries*
			baked beans*
			potato chips**
			other potatoes &
			potato dishes*
			beer*

Greater quantity eaten by girls aged (compared with boys in same age group):

4–6 years	7–10 years	11–14 years	15–18 years
other raw and salad vegetables*	other raw and salad vegetables*		other raw and salad vegetables*

Table 4.13(a) Total quantities (grams) of food consumed in seven days by fieldwork wave: male consumers

Type of food	Fieldwork wave											
	Wave 1: January to March			Wave 2: April to June			Wave 3: July to September			Wave 4: October to December		
	Mean	Median	% consumers	Mean	Median	% consumers	Mean	Median	% consumers	Mean	Median	% consumers
	g	g	%	g	g	%	g	g	%	g	g	%
Pasta	300	211	58	312	266	58	333	267	61	300	236	61
Rice	390	207	42	421	225	45	342	230	41	295	228	41
Pizza	252	161	41	238	162	40	275	210	48	241	170	50
Other cereals	87	62	30	93	56	28	79	63	36	81	50	31
White bread	507	436	93	524	465	94	527	482	96	487	438	98
Wholemeal bread	280	200	20	179	140	27	173	106	24	227	158	18
Soft grain bread	358	407	3	189	202	4	115	133	3	205	304	3
Other bread	177	134	32	121	78	31	171	121	30	177	127	37
Whole grain and high fibre b'fast cereals	216	157	49	192	151	52	251	166	53	202	143	51
Other b'fast cereals	195	169	73	195	159	75	188	154	75	189	168	72
Biscuits	166	127	76	155	113	91	163	125	86	158	122	83
Fruit pies	114	110	17	126	110	14	115	103	13	132	110	15
Buns, cakes & pastries	209	163	73	221	171	81	231	164	72	213	169	77
Cereal-based milk puddings	233	196	31	202	170	27	250	202	28	217	180	34
Sponge type puddings	116	97	11	113	85	9	134	109	9	129	100	11
Other cereal-based puddings	200	131	29	182	120	28	173	147	25	173	133	28
Whole milk	1067	925	55	1235	924	59	1169	903	50	1186	1073	53
Semi-skimmed milk	1337	1094	58	1236	909	60	1536	1198	64	1334	1131	54
Skimmed milk	725	269	6	579	373	5	424	306	4	607	466	6
Cream	38	25	12	36	24	15	49	42	13	23	21	9
Other milk	340	300	14	524	432	15	633	432	18	546	400	18
Cottage cheese	113	99	2	58	58	1	114	114	0	96	50	1
Other cheese	98	69	63	86	61	69	103	84	64	113	89	64
Fromage frais	196	124	12	128	109	15	138	100	18	139	100	17
Yogurt	260	196	42	384	300	39	323	254	33	279	198	43
Other dairy desserts	170	142	16	159	100	20	174	131	28	140	100	27
Ice cream	168	120	40	159	120	59	168	125	65	157	130	43
Eggs	139	114	50	126	98	47	120	101	47	125	97	39
Egg dishes	159	120	8	114	85	10	101	94	10	110	103	16
Butter	52	20	29	35	20	26	29	23	26	49	36	27
Block margarine	–	–	–	10	9	3	15	15	1	30	37	1
Soft margarine, not polyunsaturated	33	20	25	28	21	32	31	19	27	28	20	23
Polyunsaturated margarine	29	27	6	46	36	7	88	42	3	30	14	7
Polyunsaturated oils	15	8	2	–	–	–	2	2	1	7	5	3
Other oils and cooking fats, not polyunsaturated	4	2	3	12	10	6	9	10	6	14	8	7
Polyunsaturated low fat spread	56	50	17	53	51	17	38	27	10	44	39	10
Other low fat spread	36	20	12	72	64	10	60	66	11	60	45	10
Polyunsaturated reduced fat spread	62	49	35	60	47	39	61	50	36	43	35	34
Other reduced fat spread	46	37	22	79	40	20	60	42	34	72	52	26

Table 4.13(a)　male consumers – continued

Type of food	Fieldwork wave											
	Wave 1: January to March			Wave 2: April to June			Wave 3: July to September			Wave 4: October to December		
	Mean	Median	% consumers	Mean	Median	% consumers	Mean	Median	% consumers	Mean	Median	% consumers
	g	g	%	g	g	%	g	g	%	g	g	%
Bacon & ham	109	73	61	90	69	55	135	102	67	120	85	63
Beef, veal and dishes	280	231	49	237	169	43	267	205	60	276	213	56
Lamb & dishes	259	113	28	251	172	29	185	103	23	192	123	27
Pork & dishes	139	98	32	119	90	34	114	85	30	145	98	32
Coated chicken & turkey	160	111	44	167	144	50	163	122	47	147	125	43
Chicken and turkey dishes	227	150	76	211	135	77	278	182	75	225	165	72
Liver, liver products & dishes	103	69	6	47	37	7	44	37	3	43	37	5
Burgers & kebabs	196	124	41	143	105	33	207	137	43	188	142	45
Sausages	157	112	58	157	130	62	143	107	70	166	138	67
Meat pies & pastries	183	126	45	195	171	43	215	150	48	206	150	49
Other meat & meat products	117	72	26	92	67	31	95	59	23	120	76	27
Coated and/or fried white fish	122	102	50	128	103	55	154	116	44	148	113	46
Other white fish & dishes	237	192	11	184	193	12	159	150	8	120	96	10
Shellfish	144	50	6	110	60	4	129	88	5	65	50	6
Oily fish	95	58	20	102	80	29	109	92	22	113	80	21
Raw carrots	87	68	9	118	29	13	60	47	18	104	62	14
Other raw & salad vegetables	97	64	41	95	69	56	114	83	50	83	63	41
Raw tomatoes	94	76	23	75	67	41	85	70	34	88	65	30
Peas	94	69	51	98	80	48	108	80	46	92	66	53
Green beans	76	50	15	69	50	12	81	59	17	75	48	14
Baked beans	254	176	62	222	159	68	268	208	61	255	187	59
Leafy green vegetables	100	77	45	76	60	37	79	60	33	103	72	40
Carrots–not raw	86	69	50	87	64	53	86	74	53	96	67	55
Tomatoes–not raw	87	75	8	63	54	9	74	67	10	102	73	14
Vegetable dishes	160	118	20	239	190	24	240	145	13	260	194	16
Other vegetables	115	90	53	119	97	57	131	91	61	120	105	60
Potato chips	417	377	86	375	302	89	458	336	90	416	328	90
Other fried/roast potatoes & products	146	104	55	143	120	52	189	166	45	167	123	53
Potato products– not fried	133	96	17	148	102	22	112	97	22	141	100	20
Other potatoes & potato dishes	372	291	82	348	261	84	316	251	82	366	266	84
Savoury snacks	127	107	87	133	120	94	126	115	88	133	114	84
Apples & pears	338	232	50	251	157	66	284	218	48	269	208	50
Citrus fruits	217	149	27	189	161	21	135	112	16	263	213	29
Bananas	231	190	36	207	158	42	221	128	37	275	185	38
Canned fruit in juice	148	83	4	124	98	6	104	101	7	107	84	7
Canned fruit in syrup	146	120	10	91	47	5	157	144	7	155	131	7
Other fruit	168	109	28	202	150	37	225	189	38	142	82	21
Nuts and seeds	74	50	16	68	40	16	57	34	16	51	29	18
Table sugar	67	42	71	53	35	71	70	41	70	65	42	64
Preserves	58	40	29	44	24	32	44	29	33	52	27	31
Sweet spreads, fillings & icings	35	20	17	29	22	19	29	25	21	32	20	22
Sugar confectionery	85	68	57	154	87	70	205	136	73	114	75	55
Chocolate confectionery	168	137	84	175	133	85	142	113	81	168	126	86

73

Table 4.13(a)   male consumers – continued

Type of food	Fieldwork wave											
	Wave 1: January to March			Wave 2: April to June			Wave 3: July to September			Wave 4: October to December		
	Mean	Median	% consumers	Mean	Median	% consumers	Mean	Median	% consumers	Mean	Median	% consumers
	g	g	%	g	g	%	g	g	%	g	g	%
Fruit juice	909	470	46	725	424	42	839	636	48	808	530	49
Concentrated soft drinks–not low calorie, as consumed	2917	1717	53	2328	1292	53	2918	1483	51	2413	1526	51
Carbonated soft drinks–not low calorie	1305	1001	73	1424	1018	79	1615	1210	83	1485	856	77
Ready to drink soft drinks–not low calorie	706	525	26	586	302	34	562	380	28	529	361	27
Concentrated soft drinks–low calorie, as consumed	2717	2247	45	3065	2634	49	3359	2134	48	3090	1946	47
Carbonated soft drinks–low calorie	1061	739	40	916	525	47	1193	801	45	989	821	45
Ready to drink soft drinks–low calorie	439	323	4	517	406	9	774	378	7	802	788	5
Liqueurs	197	197	1	47	39	1	13	20	1	–	–	–
Spirits	283	69	2	68	69	2	32	24	3	240	138	1
Wine	300	332	2	102	60	2	63	63	0	357	172	3
Fortified wine	106	106	1	–	–	–	188	188	0	107	23	1
Low alcohol & alcohol-free wine	80	80	0	–	–	–	–	–	0	–	–	–
Beer & lager	3035	1143	9	2870	1769	9	3755	3379	15	1358	1354	8
Low alcohol & alcohol-free beer & lager	–	–	–	–	–	–	150	150	0	–	–	–
Cider & Perry	286	286	1	858	858	1	405	454	2	575	575	1
Alco-pops	2860	2860	1	591	337	2	525	343	2	343	343	0
Coffee, as consumed	1883	1620	19	1199	1140	10	1638	1279	20	1977	1140	20
Tea, as consumed	1224	673	48	858	537	46	1086	711	45	1470	756	42
Herbal tea, as consumed	57	57	0	–	–	–	207	168	1	950	950	0
Bottled water	1865	957	5	874	462	6	416	251	14	787	427	6
Tap water	1115	891	59	1170	810	62	1356	653	59	974	590	59
Commercial toddler's foods	181	100	2	20	20	1	–	–	–	102	87	1
Other beverages, dry weight	506	414	19	522	266	24	589	336	25	438	240	17
Soup	447	299	26	241	217	16	380	269	20	310	274	26
Savoury sauces, pickles, gravies & condiments	149	113	88	133	97	91	151	120	91	131	104	85
Base = number of young people			*199*			*176*			*230*			*251*

Table 4.13(b) Total quantities (grams) of food consumed in seven days by fieldwork wave: female consumers

Type of food	Fieldwork wave											
	Wave 1: January to March			Wave 2: April to June			Wave 3: July to September			Wave 4: October to December		
	Mean	Median	% consumers	Mean	Median	% consumers	Mean	Median	% consumers	Mean	Median	% consumers
	g	g	%	g	g	%	g	g	%	g	g	%
Pasta	282	250	62	295	210	66	329	242	60	258	205	67
Rice	351	180	35	358	202	39	263	180	46	301	182	40
Pizza	150	113	43	152	119	42	191	148	41	168	140	51
Other cereals	98	80	38	88	65	35	84	62	26	87	75	32
White bread	385	342	93	388	347	98	417	381	95	401	368	96
Wholemeal bread	144	72	26	177	138	27	191	132	29	130	112	21
Soft grain bread	172	135	5	121	149	1	238	144	4	158	68	2
Other bread	150	112	30	128	89	37	136	90	38	115	82	43
Whole grain and high fibre b'fast cereals	144	94	40	161	104	50	138	108	49	158	108	52
Other b'fast cereals	145	108	62	117	95	69	142	102	65	148	134	61
Biscuits	146	115	84	148	117	86	122	90	81	128	99	87
Fruit pies	96	88	13	122	93	15	106	98	10	118	103	15
Buns, cakes & pastries	170	130	77	185	140	78	173	145	72	192	167	74
Cereal-based milk puddings	228	178	33	223	180	32	182	141	23	193	168	36
Sponge type puddings	109	110	9	137	110	8	74	62	6	81	70	12
Other cereal-based puddings	149	120	27	177	130	27	184	150	20	160	121	30
Whole milk	955	795	52	935	698	58	945	700	42	1069	975	53
Semi-skimmed milk	874	604	51	868	710	56	918	751	63	982	874	60
Skimmed milk	376	194	7	503	324	6	820	366	8	393	262	8
Cream	31	22	12	33	30	16	41	30	11	36	26	10
Other milk	404	350	12	447	335	13	367	335	19	321	335	18
Cottage cheese	34	41	1	47	38	3	53	50	2	101	46	3
Other cheese	100	74	65	94	77	69	101	85	74	103	80	70
Fromage frais	102	79	11	140	100	17	149	150	15	161	143	25
Yogurt	267	150	42	294	246	45	311	247	41	308	244	48
Other dairy desserts	151	122	20	130	109	21	143	102	19	133	120	20
Ice cream	117	88	43	147	120	58	183	143	58	124	95	42
Eggs	134	102	44	110	99	40	102	65	48	112	93	46
Egg dishes	124	100	14	87	95	14	126	111	14	105	92	11
Butter	37	20	35	36	25	30	36	25	30	24	12	28
Block margarine	5	3	1	11	13	1	29	7	2	109	109	0
Soft margarine, not polyunsaturated	25	18	28	38	26	24	31	24	26	23	14	34
Polyunsaturated margarine	43	20	8	22	20	6	37	27	3	40	37	3
Polyunsaturated oils	8	5	1	9	10	2	14	8	2	6	6	2
Other oils and cooking fats, not polyunsaturated	6	5	1	12	10	5	10	9	5	9	7	10
Polyunsaturated low fat spread	38	23	14	34	28	13	50	47	13	49	43	15
Other low fat spread	46	41	11	40	30	14	38	33	13	56	47	12
Polyunsaturated reduced fat spread	49	35	35	47	40	39	49	44	38	42	34	42
Other reduced fat spread	45	24	17	45	30	18	51	40	27	53	43	25

Table 4.13(b)   female consumers – continued

Type of food	Fieldwork wave											
	Wave 1: January to March			Wave 2: April to June			Wave 3: July to September			Wave 4: October to December		
	Mean	Median	% consumers	Mean	Median	% consumers	Mean	Median	% consumers	Mean	Median	% consumers
	g	g	%	g	g	%	g	g	%	g	g	%
Bacon & ham	78	61	58	90	73	53	90	63	62	72	50	56
Beef, veal and dishes	265	169	48	239	151	46	246	175	50	261	200	53
Lamb & dishes	180	119	22	178	124	28	161	122	23	129	78	24
Pork & dishes	140	89	27	118	90	26	119	86	31	135	95	29
Coated chicken & turkey	162	155	48	156	135	50	152	116	44	155	128	49
Chicken and turkey dishes	206	144	72	208	152	71	206	139	74	208	153	73
Liver, liver products & dishes	76	47	4	25	19	5	87	99	5	38	37	3
Burgers & kebabs	141	117	28	161	130	36	155	117	40	135	100	36
Sausages	122	90	56	116	79	51	121	92	55	110	84	60
Meat pies & pastries	163	137	40	149	130	47	141	114	45	173	142	42
Other meat & meat products	82	50	25	101	44	21	87	57	21	92	63	23
Coated and/or fried white fish	123	94	48	117	100	44	124	94	42	125	98	42
Other white fish & dishes	172	142	10	141	101	13	149	128	10	219	156	10
Shellfish	68	63	5	46	17	7	81	73	8	61	46	7
Oily fish	99	87	29	104	62	31	92	58	25	92	64	30
Raw carrots	66	43	16	55	40	19	100	50	23	45	31	13
Other raw & salad vegetables	96	65	52	113	80	64	141	94	67	95	66	51
Raw tomatoes	72	47	32	100	67	45	109	72	47	91	68	42
Peas	74	60	52	87	63	51	92	75	44	86	65	49
Green beans	56	49	14	68	60	11	76	50	17	59	45	11
Baked beans	203	145	61	209	138	56	205	168	52	189	160	58
Leafy green vegetables	117	95	46	89	60	47	91	71	33	109	95	50
Carrots–not raw	75	61	52	76	55	55	84	60	46	85	71	62
Tomatoes–not raw	74	64	10	82	74	5	89	79	11	89	85	7
Vegetable dishes	342	234	23	219	142	22	339	175	20	253	150	21
Other vegetables	164	110	61	115	93	59	141	97	63	137	94	64
Potato chips	351	291	85	338	250	90	353	281	87	363	310	88
Other fried/roast potatoes & products	147	120	53	149	101	39	143	118	49	141	126	52
Potato products– not fried	117	90	22	134	106	17	127	94	23	105	99	19
Other potatoes & potato dishes	339	266	74	350	288	85	275	206	79	331	257	83
Savoury snacks	135	116	88	124	111	89	118	113	91	118	100	90
Apples & pears	286	200	56	268	216	57	300	206	53	322	221	61
Citrus fruits	288	212	30	251	168	19	197	133	19	205	134	44
Bananas	191	136	34	214	150	44	209	134	36	174	131	34
Canned fruit in juice	145	113	6	161	124	7	132	118	3	162	112	7
Canned fruit in syrup	147	100	9	127	72	5	115	89	8	136	93	8
Other fruit	190	90	22	234	130	41	307	195	46	165	116	31
Nuts and seeds	47	25	12	40	15	12	42	32	14	43	32	18
Table sugar	52	30	65	54	39	66	46	27	60	58	30	63
Preserves	35	27	35	38	26	38	35	26	30	39	28	34
Sweet spreads, fillings & icings	42	28	16	34	20	20	28	23	25	29	16	17
Sugar confectionery	79	51	57	122	87	70	162	102	66	97	67	70
Chocolate confectionery	171	140	83	140	103	80	106	82	74	154	133	85

Table 4.13(b)   female consumers – continued

Type of food	Fieldwork wave											
	Wave 1: January to March			Wave 2: April to June			Wave 3: July to September			Wave 4: October to December		
	Mean	Median	% consumers	Mean	Median	% consumers	Mean	Median	% consumers	Mean	Median	% consumers
	g	g	%	g	g	%	g	g	%	g	g	%
Fruit juice	721	553	44	794	557	50	857	747	56	611	401	53
Concentrated soft drinks–not low calorie, as consumed	2296	1541	50	1881	1342	54	2404	1345	50	1797	1290	51
Carbonated soft drinks–not low calorie	979	738	71	1060	726	78	1312	972	78	1190	754	73
Ready to drink soft drinks–not low calorie	574	483	23	565	450	32	568	435	33	603	379	33
Concentrated soft drinks–low calorie, as consumed	2648	2062	46	2403	1757	45	3202	2095	48	2467	1526	46
Carbonated soft drinks–low calorie	941	547	44	1054	765	45	1004	660	51	916	530	44
Ready to drink soft drinks–low calorie	529	502	8	432	263	6	479	263	8	732	716	5
Liqueurs	20	22	1	69	69	0	80	69	1	138	138	0
Spirits	85	69	2	230	230	0	84	69	6	67	55	3
Wine	158	141	2	688	464	4	198	136	5	232	256	4
Fortified wine	–	–	–	39	40	1	289	230	1	136	85	2
Low alcohol & alcohol-free wine	–	–	–	176	223	1	795	795	0	348	348	1
Beer & lager	1529	1136	4	924	1134	3	2594	1428	7	1458	1328	6
Low alcohol & alcohol-free beer & lager	–	–	–	–	–	–	–	–	–	531	531	0
Cider & Perry	226	286	1	1516	1145	1	286	286	0	718	504	2
Alco-pops	746	674	2	343	343	0	792	686	3	1557	1346	1
Coffee, as consumed	1779	673	17	2195	1013	17	1666	1089	19	1365	759	16
Tea, as consumed	1013	492	48	1053	625	52	1337	790	41	1400	958	51
Herbal tea, as consumed	1764	1917	2	194	204	2	249	140	2	506	506	0
Bottled water	860	750	8	514	330	11	853	500	11	509	330	8
Tap water	904	640	61	1066	800	58	1121	703	66	1026	646	62
Commercial toddler's foods	–	–	–	–	–	–	53	53	0	–	–	–
Other beverages, dry weight	440	240	22	389	336	18	377	224	19	538	253	31
Soup	301	251	32	310	285	17	330	257	21	336	254	39
Savoury sauces, pickles, gravies & condiments	143	119	83	147	107	88	130	97	90	139	104	88
Base = number of young people			*180*			*198*			*240*			*227*

77

Table 4.13(c) Main differences in the eating behaviour of young people by sex and fieldwork wave: summary table

Food type and sub-group	Males		Females	
	Less likely to eat in Wave:	Compared with Wave:	Less likely to eat in Wave:	Compared with Wave:
Cereals and cereal products				
biscuits	1	2**		
Milk & milk products				
cereal-based milk puddings			3	4*
whole milk			3	2*
fromage frais			1	4*
ice cream	1	2*, 3**	1	2*, 3*
	4	2*, 3*	4	2*, 3*
other dairy desserts	1	3*		
Fats				
other oil & cooking fats, not pufa			1	4**
other reduced fat spreads	1, 2	3*		
Meat and meat products				
beef, veal & dishes	2	3*		
Vegetables				
other raw & other salad vegetables	1,4	2*	4	3*
raw tomatoes	1	2*	1	3*
leafy green vegetables			3	4*
carrots–not raw			3	4*
savoury snacks	4	2*		
Fruit & nuts				
apples & pears	1, 3, 4	2*		
citrus fruits	3	4*	2, 3	4**
other fruit	4	2*, 3**	1	2**, 3**
			4	3*
Sugars, preserves & confectionery				
sugar confectionery	1	3*		
	4	2*, 3**		
Beverages				
spirits			2	3*
coffee	2	3*		
bottled water	1	3*		
Miscellaneous				
soup			2	1*, 4*
			3	4**
beverages†			2, 3	4*

Wave 1: January–March 1997 Wave 2: April–June 1997 Wave 3: July–September 1997 Wave 4: October–December 1997
* p < 0.05
** p < 0.01
pufa: polyunsaturated
† powdered beverages, except tea and coffee

Table 4.14(a) Total quantities of food consumed in seven days by region: male consumers

Type of food	Region											
	Scotland			Northern			Central, South West and Wales			London and the South East		
	Mean	Median	% consumers	Mean	Median	% consumers	Mean	Median	% consumers	Mean	Median	% consumers
	g	g	%	g	g	%	g	g	%	g	g	%
Pasta	391	301	66	311	226	49	285	221	61	315	252	67
Rice	318	300	52	294	230	36	297	230	43	503	200	45
Pizza	217	162	51	249	166	46	268	183	44	242	165	43
Other cereals	78	64	8	98	64	41	86	53	31	63	45	28
White bread	537	481	97	529	466	96	509	467	95˙	485	404	93
Wholemeal bread	165	106	18	205	140	24	225	169	22	212	151	22
Soft grain bread	134	144	8	193	191	2	218	115	3	264	313	4
Other bread	160	105	27	194	120	31	166	111	37	128	88	31
Whole grain and high fibre b'fast cereals	280	156	43	198	161	53	208	152	51	220	143	53
Other b'fast cereals	193	174	83	189	150	75	205	174	72	178	153	72
Biscuits	149	100	79	154	110	81	157	125	87	173	128	84
Fruit pies	144	113	7	122	110	13	121	95	18	122	110	15
Buns, cakes & pastries	199	175	69	199	167	75	224	169	74	233	167	81
Cereal-based milk puddings	215	198	30	238	177	33	225	190	30	211	186	27
Sponge type puddings	130	93	6	106	89	11	115	92	12	156	136	9
Other cereal-based puddings	188	150	22	204	152	25	158	115	33	198	146	25
Whole milk	1283	934	63	1008	720	59	1199	915	51	1259	1018	52
Semi-skimmed milk	1153	860	55	1339	1096	62	1375	1130	60	1412	1120	55
Skimmed milk	241	241	1	819	852	2	574	370	7	596	245	7
Cream	43	45	9	42	25	12	30	24	11	37	30	14
Other milk	556	430	17	456	285	10	576	428	20	458	362	18
Cottage cheese	50	50	1	102	58	2	99	114	1	120	132	1
Other cheese	118	104	63	103	84	62	100	77	67	93	68	66
Fromage frais	110	100	17	137	100	12	143	100	14	167	125	20
Yogurt	336	286	45	321	252	40	316	203	43	270	175	34
Other dairy desserts	155	124	14	169	130	19	177	120	22	135	100	29
Ice cream	150	127	58	155	120	52	179	130	46	157	120	54
Eggs	129	110	43	129	106	47	129	100	.43	125	97	47
Egg dishes	66	18	8	108	71	6	146	117	12	103	75	15
Butter	24	16	22	50	27	25	41	23	26	41	31	33
Block margarine	–	–	–	22	15	2	9	9	2	–	–	–
Soft margarine, not polyunsaturated	21	14	28	28	16	33	32	24	24	33	20	23
Polyunsaturated margarine	21	22	5	55	27	8	36	27˙	6	24	26	3
Polyunsaturated oils	5	5	1	12	9	1	11	3	2	7	7	2
Other oils and cooking fats, not polyunsaturated	9	10	12	11	8	6	21	13	3	7	8	7
Polyunsaturated low fat spread	39	27	12	42	31	13	56	46	14	50	53	15
Other low fat spread	53	41	18	58	50	11	55	43	10	57	52	9
Polyunsaturated reduced fat spread	57	51	28	58	37	41	51	41	36	60	47	33
Other reduced fat spread	72	55	15	54	41	21	73	46	29	59	40	27

Table 4.14(a) male consumers – continued

Type of food	Region Scotland			Northern			Central, South West and Wales			London and the South East		
	Mean	Median	% consumers	Mean	Median	% consumers	Mean	Median	% consumers	Mean	Median	% consumers
	g	g	%	g	g	%	g	g	%	g	g	%
Bacon & ham	140	100	60	98	75	65	117	79	66	121	85	53
Beef, veal and dishes	232	183	66	252	192	45	289	232	58	258	194	47
Lamb & dishes	191	172	7	239	126	20	156	109	29	286	155	36
Pork & dishes	105	100	23	123	80	33	130	98	32	143	103	33
Coated chicken & turkey	177	165	41	160	133	48	149	113	42	164	123	50
Chicken and turkey dishes	221	151	70	205	155	72	244	173	77	249	163	76
Liver, liver products & dishes	–	–	–	103	44	2	87	74	4	41	35	10
Burgers & kebabs	167	117	47	191	131	36	179	118	43	194	130	41
Sausages	209	129	69	151	111	63	149	115	67	154	125	60
Meat pies & pastries	180	142	48	204	140	53	233	175	46	155	120	40
Other meat & meat products	92	85	33	131	74	29	114	75	26	72	47	24
Coated and/or fried white fish	142	114	37	144	116	59	145	109	47	116	88	45
Other white fish & dishes	133	76	5	178	166	7	162	148	10	192	121	15
Shellfish	90	90	1	94	40	3	186	100	5	62	45	9
Oily fish	102	75	27	112	81	25	107	82	21	96	70	22
Raw carrots	213	58	12	62	40	11	107	54	12	72	48	16
Other raw & salad vegetables	80	50	33	95	60	45	91	69	46	107	82	53
Raw tomatoes	92	76	24	72	59	28	92	75	33	83	68	37
Peas	51	43	37	110	84	51	98	70	53	93	61	47
Green beans	38	30	4	50	40	10	98	60	19	61	43	16
Baked beans	200	171	49	243	188	63	257	182	68	254	165	58
Leafy green vegetables	107	103	20	78	62	31	100	77	40	89	60	50
Carrots–not raw	70	45	30	93	69	51	95	78	59	81	67	53
Tomatoes–not raw	103	81	11	58	54	7	99	67	12	78	73	12
Vegetable dishes	138	165	11	287	200	15	212	179	17	204	145	25
Other vegetables	115	112	45	117	92	55	122	93	63	125	100	58
Potato chips	407	269	94	475	388	93	401	335	86	372	293	86
Other fried/roast potatoes & products	124	97	31	140	111	44	169	130	55	167	144	60
Potato products– not fried	80	92	16	147	100	23	117	100	20	155	103	19
Other potatoes & potato dishes	355	222	86	345	274	82	400	301	87	293	215	79
Savoury snacks	150	136	89	130	119	88	126	108	88	130	113	88
Apples & pears	293	244	52	278	221	47	316	207	58	238	181	54
Citrus fruits	238	164	23	218	170	23	204	149	25	220	166	24
Bananas	177	129	37	239	171	33	225	148	42	259	199	38
Canned fruit in juice	147	84	3	138	136	2	97	92	8	137	100	7
Canned fruit in syrup	103	118	12	154	130	7	130	100	8	176	137	5
Other fruit	164	136	27	156	112	28	170	118	26	231	169	40
Nuts and seeds	93	92	12	48	34	12	64	38	18	63	38	20
Table sugar	54	37	67	51	32	68	69	48	65	70	42	75
Preserves	57	24	43	49	25	29	46	39	27	50	29	35
Sweet spreads, fillings & icings	55	25	16	32	22	19	30	20	22	27	22	19
Sugar confectionery	127	107	68	171	103	59	119	85	62	146	80	66
Chocolate confectionery	196	172	94	183	135	82	154	121	85	149	118	82

Table 4.14(a) male consumers – continued

Type of food	Region											
	Scotland			Northern			Central, South West and Wales			London and the South East		
	Mean	Median	% consumers	Mean	Median	% consumers	Mean	Median	% consumers	Mean	Median	% consumers
	g	g	%	g	g	%	g	g	%	g	g	%
Fruit juice	748	553	37	785	530	46	901	530	47	774	506	48
Concentrated soft drinks–not low calorie, as consumed	2455	1098	39	2567	1425	51	2508	1507	53	2850	1698	55
Carbonated soft drinks–not low calorie	1759	1026	81	1527	1255	83	1498	1012	79	1226	694	71
Ready to drink soft drinks–not low calorie	566	459	33	647	391	32	601	410	28	526	263	25
Concentrated soft drinks–low calorie, as consumed	2738	2278	57	2641	1874	46	3209	2291	46	3359	2397	47
Carbonated soft drinks–low calorie	861	402	47	1045	806	48	1106	739	46	961	647	39
Ready to drink soft drinks–low calorie	547	631	7	435	370	9	726	500	6	876	591	4
Liqueurs	–	–	–	2	2	0	84	58	1	–	–	–
Spirits	–	–	–	37	41	1	142	69	2	178	69	3
Wine	–	–	–	185	186	2	352	238	2	186	108	2
Fortified wine	5	5	1	188	188	0	250	250	0	71	106	1
Low alcohol & alcohol-free wine	–	–	–	–	–	–	–	–	–	80	80	0
Beer & lager	3699	442	4	3445	1882	12	2085	1805	9	2909	1327	11
Low alcohol & alcohol-free beer & lager	–	–	–	–	–	–	150	150	0	–	–	–
Cider & Perry	454	454	2	589	858	1	379	402	1	575	575	1
Alco-pops	–	–	–	1048	537	3	343	343	0	337	337	0
Coffee, as consumed	1792	1573	18	1550	1094	17	1480	1161	17	2270	1509	17
Tea, as consumed	714	370	46	1312	639	45	1235	716	44	1072	768	46
Herbal tea, as consumed	–	–	–	–	–	–	395	163	1	266	266	0
Bottled water	219	230	5	900	602	5	614	259	7	1037	500	12
Tap water	833	310	52	1212	710	56	1030	756	55	1258	820	71
Commercial toddler's foods	–	–	–	–	–	–	197	126	1	53	33	2
Other beverages, dry weight	521	330	12	502	290	18	579	406	22	459	300	25
Soup	431	269	42	323	240	26	297	275	17	402	262	18
Savoury sauces, pickles, gravies & condiments	95	71	73	144	111	92	146	104	90	140	105	89
Base = number of young people	*68*			*243*			*300*			*245*		

Table 4.14(b) Total quantities of food consumed in seven days by region: female consumers

Type of food	Region											
	Scotland			Northern			Central, South West and Wales			London and the South East		
	Mean	Median	% consumers	Mean	Median	% consumers	Mean	Median	% consumers	Mean	Median	% consumers
	g	g	%	g	g	%	g	g	%	g	g	%
Pasta	373	256	68	265	215	63	288	220	62	295	225	67
Rice	269	180	55	243	153	35	295	185	33	391	202	51
Pizza	142	112	44	162	120	44	165	125	44	175	136	45
Other cereals	57	55	15	84	80	45	108	73	32	76	56	26
White bread	364	369	99	413	368	97	419	371	98	366	321	91
Wholemeal bread	131	99	25	128	108	23	171	104	26	194	124	28
Soft grain bread	91	72	6	123	114	1	213	169	3	220	136	4
Other bread	124	59	32	134	84	42	134	104	36	123	90	34
Whole grain and high fibre b'fast cereals	170	71	38	144	108	52	156	127	51	147	86	43
Other b'fast cereals	128	85	63	122	93	63	149	121	66	139	116	64
Biscuits	100	82	82	138	101	85	143	117	87	136	108	82
Fruit pies	149	88	5	100	94	13	128	94	14	99	95	14
Buns, cakes & pastries	145	131	67	177	143	74	172	142	76	201	169	78
Cereal-based milk puddings	189	132	22	215	164	34	224	181	32	182	160	29
Sponge type puddings	105	110	5	90	85	11	114	110	10	94	62	6
Other cereal-based puddings	121	115	23	141	119	28	171	150	23	199	142	28
Whole milk	778	582	53	1032	853	57	1041	975	51	884	629	46
Semi-skimmed milk	957	710	48	837	695	61	1024	873	56	848	682	59
Skimmed milk	522	334	6	414	226	8	603	500	8	577	324	7
Cream	30	32	5	27	20	16	42	35	12	37	20	11
Other milk	449	336	19	359	336	13	368	335	18	383	335	14
Cottage cheese	2	2	2	75	38	4	80	75	2	32	39	1
Other cheese	105	92	71	95	74	67	102	82	72	98	81	68
Fromage frais	111	83	14	137	129	14	139	119	17	160	129	20
Yogurt	286	244	42	315	243	50	300	236	46	266	175	36
Other dairy desserts	158	66	14	133	120	21	145	120	16	135	117	25
Ice cream	146	119	52	143	120	46	146	120	52	151	103	53
Eggs	106	71	43	116	97	51	119	96	45	106	84	37
Egg dishes	125	142	6	118	95	13	108	104	14	104	100	15
Butter	27	20	30	35	23	26	33	23	30	34	20	36
Block margarine	–	–	–	32	15	1	60	66	1	5	7	1
Soft margarine, not polyunsaturated	35	27	28	28	20	34	29	14	27	28	18	23
Polyunsaturated margarine	18	14	9	33	27	9	48	58	4	24	28	1
Polyunsaturated oils	–	–	–	5	5	1	14	8	1	8	8	4
Other oils and cookingfats, not polyunsaturated	8	10	5	8	7	5	10	6	4	10	8	9
Polyunsaturated low fat spread	36	23	20	41	28	16	45	37	13	34	19	10
Other low fat spread	29	25	13	40	26	11	45	40	14	43	36	12
Polyunsaturated reduced fat spread	55	57	25	44	34	44	47	40	40	46	37	36
Other reduced fat spread	29	21	18	54	39	20	47	34	20	51	44	26

Table 4.14(b)   female consumers – continued

Type of food	Region											
	Scotland			Northern			Central, South West and Wales			London and the South East		
	Mean	Median	% consumers	Mean	Median	% consumers	Mean	Median	% consumers	Mean	Median	% consumers
	g	g	%	g	g	%	g	g	%	g	g	%
Bacon & ham	93	48	63	82	58	58	83	63	60	80	57	52
Beef, veal and dishes	262	169	54	243	159	57	278	191	47	226	179	43
Lamb & dishes	115	82	15	136	113	22	149	120	25	202	124	28
Pork & dishes	138	124	18	110	85	29	144	90	31	120	89	27
Coated chicken & turkey	150	125	52	166	135	49	155	137	45	152	117	49
Chicken and turkey dishes	186	156	85	197	130	71	192	143	69	240	162	75
Liver, liver products & dishes	194	194	2	27	24	4	54	37	5	75	56	5
Burgers & kebabs	155	110	47	152	121	36	144	100	33	148	112	34
Sausages	146	118	62	124	93	57	106	86	56	114	82	50
Meat pies & pastries	139	117	47	173	145	49	157	128	40	138	120	42
Other meat & meat products	54	55	16	116	72	31	73	44	21	79	50	17
Coated and/or fried white fish	114	91	33	137	113	46	120	94	49	108	91	38
Other white fish & dishes	137	110	5	180	139	16	185	100	5	151	120	15
Shellfish	62	8	6	56	41	9	84	50	6	54	43	6
Oily fish	121	86	30	92	76	28	93	65	34	102	54	23
Raw carrots	70	57	17	62	40	21	65	51	15	85	45	18
Other raw & salad vegetables	124	100	59	98	70	55	111	80	60	127	68	61
Raw tomatoes	95	68	40	85	54	39	98	68	46	101	67	39
Peas	48	45	34	100	80	54	84	66	53	74	60	44
Green beans	67	32	5	48	40	11	72	59	13	71	49	18
Baked beans	174	135	51	185	148	60	224	172	61	195	130	49
Leafy green vegetables	99	70	28	90	80	44	110	81	44	103	80	49
Carrots–not raw	58	50	40	85	65	56	92	68	59	63	54	50
Tomatoes–not raw	57	54	4	73	74	8	100	85	8	78	60	9
Vegetable dishes	241	203	15	273	131	17	288	172	24	298	211	25
Other vegetables	113	68	58	131	101	60	133	94	63	158	97	63
Potato chips	404	307	91	384	322	93	366	305	89	277	208	80
Other fried/roast potatoes & products	136	84	32	127	100	41	141	108	56	166	149	50
Potato products– not fried	85	82	18	113	90	24	137	94	19	121	115	20
Other potatoes & potato dishes	317	252	81	329	287	81	365	280	82	270	219	77
Savoury snacks	129	117	94	128	113	91	122	113	88	119	104	89
Apples & pears	329	224	57	283	224	55	284	210	59	307	187	56
Citrus fruits	212	181	30	200	143	28	284	192	26	214	153	30
Bananas	224	172	33	191	133	44	206	145	38	192	124	32
Canned fruit in juice	69	40	5	112	86	4	161	128	6	184	120	8
Canned fruit in syrup	131	77	7	102	60	8	153	115	8	135	60	6
Other fruit	326	152	34	190	116	31	226	173	32	258	152	44
Nuts and seeds	40	30	7	54	32	11	42	23	14	37	28	19
Table sugar	34	17	47	53	30	65	58	35	66	49	35	63
Preserves	39	27	30	38	25	39	35	28	34	39	27	32
Sweet spreads, fillings & icings	32	17	20	31	20	20	34	20	18	33	23	20
Sugar confectionery	110	82	64	125	77	70	116	72	67	112	74	62
Chocolate confectionery	147	112	88	158	127	81	133	104	80	139	109	78

Table 4.14(b)   female consumers – continued

Type of food	Region											
	Scotland			Northern			Central, South West and Wales			London and the South East		
	Mean	Median	% consumers	Mean	Median	% consumers	Mean	Median	% consumers	Mean	Median	% consumers
	g	g	%	g	g	%	g	g	%	g	g	%
Fruit juice	618	382	49	775	599	51	793	553	49	713	424	53
Concentrated soft drinks–not low calorie, as consumed	1451	1055	36	1773	1304	58	2606	1787	52	1886	1222	48
Carbonated soft drinks–not low calorie	1156	751	84	1279	943	82	1061	700	72	1080	847	70
Ready to drink soft drinks–not low calorie	741	604	36	561	419	30	500	290	29	628	551	31
Concentrated soft drinks–low calorie, as consumed	2439	1312	47	2047	1292	45	2714	1882	44	3271	2645	50
Carbonated soft drinks–low calorie	1193	974	61	870	470	47	972	650	45	1032	600	43
Ready to drink soft drinks–low calorie	768	633	9	374	253	9	565	451	6	601	508	5
Liqueurs	46	46	1	44	23	1	138	138	0	69	69	1
Spirits	168	216	4	94	92	3	69	55	3	65	46	3
Wine	502	356	3	521	222	4	139	125	3	278	125	4
Fortified wine	–	–	–	–	–	–	147	124	2	146	58	1
Low alcohol & alcohol-free wine	348	348	2	223	223	1	65	65	0	795	795	0
Beer & lager	771	899	4	2055	1427	6	1506	1051	6	2229	1450	4
Low alcohol & alcohol-free beer & lager	–	–	–	531	531	0	–	–	–	–	–	–
Cider & Perry	504	504	2	487	286	1	968	286	1	1239	1007	1
Alco-pops	515	515	3	1135	905	2	973	858	2	375	286	1
Coffee, as consumed	1643	1106	16	2022	684	21	1858	905	18	1279	992	14
Tea, as consumed	1052	474	35	1105	745	52	1373	849	51	1081	650	44
Herbal tea, as consumed	753	753	1	213	211	2	965	552	1	811	150	1
Bottled water	817	675	8	646	465	6	789	500	10	573	330	13
Tap water	774	398	50	919	600	64	1020	660	60	1214	915	66
Commercial toddler's foods	–	–	–	53	53	0	–	–	–	–	–	–
Other beverages, dry weight	598	300	17	359	266	19	576	336	25	331	225	25
Soup	376	325	60	298	220	25	290	251	27	354	280	19
Savoury sauces, pickles, gravies & condiments	117	73	70	146	104	92	158	136	87	116	85	88
Base = number of young people			*69*			*217*			*306*			*253*

Table 4.14(c)   Main differences in the eating behaviour of young people by sex and region – summary table

Food type and sub-group	Males		Females	
	Less likely to eat in:	Compared with:	Less likely to eat in:	Compared with:
Cereals and cereal products				
pasta	N	L & SE**		
rice			CSW & W	Sc*, L & SE**
			N	L & SE*
white bread			L & SE	S*, N*, CSW & W*
other cereals	Sc	N**, CSW & W**, L & SE**	Sc	N**, CSW & W*
	L & SE	N*	L & SE	N**
			CSW & W	N*
Milk, milk products, eggs & egg dishes				
skimmed milk	Sc	CSW & W*, L & SE*		
cream			Sc	N*
yogurt			L & SE	N*
eggs			L & SE	N*
egg dishes	N	L & SE*		
Fats				
pufa margarine			L & SE	N*
pufa reduced fat spread			Sc	N*
Meat and meat products				
bacon & ham	L & SE	CSW & W*		
beef, veal & dishes	N	Sc*, CSW & W*	L & SE	N*
	L & SE	Sc*		
lamb & dishes	N	L & SE**		
	Sc	N*, CSW & W**, L & SE**		
chicken & turkey dishes			CSW & W	Sc*
liver, liver products & dishes	N	L & SE*		
other meat & meat products			L & SE	N*
Fish & fish dishes				
coated &/or fried white fish	Sc, L & SE	N*		
other white fish & dishes	Sc	L & SE*	Sc	N*
			CSW & W	L & SE**, N**
shellfish	Sc	L & SE*		
Vegetables				
other raw & salad vegetables	Sc	L & SE*		
peas			Sc	N*, CSW & W*
green beans	Sc	CSW & W**, L & SE*	Sc	L & SE*
leafy green vegetables	Sc	CSW & W**, L & SE**	Sc	L & SE*
	N	L & SE**		
carrots–not raw	Sc	N*, CSW & W**, L & SE*		
vegetable dishes	Sc	L & SE*		
potato chips			L & SE	N*
other fried & roast potatoes & products	Sc	CSW & W**, L & SE**	Sc, N	CSW & W*
	N	L & SE**		
Fruit & nuts				
canned fruit in juice	N	CSW & W*		
other fruit	CSW & W	L & SE*		
nuts & seeds			Sc	L & SE*
Sugars, preserves & confectionery				
chocolate confectionery	L & SE	Sc*		
Drinks				
carbonated soft drinks nlc	L & SE	N*	L & SE	N*
concentrated soft drinks nlc			Sc	N*
tap water	N	L & SE*		
	CSW & W	L & SE**		
Miscellaneous				
soup	CSW & W	Sc**	N, CSW & W, L & SE	Sc**
	L & SE	Sc*		
savoury sauces, pickles, gravies & condiments	Sc	N*	Sc	N**, L & SE*

Sc Scotland N Northern CSW & W Central, South West & Wales L & SE London & South East
* $p < 0.05$.   ** $p < 0.01$.   pufa: polyunsaturated.   nlc: not low calorie

Table 4.15(a) Total quantities (grams) of foods consumed in seven days by whether young person was living with both parents: male consumers

Type of food	Both parents: and other children			and no other children			Single parent: with/without other children		
	Mean	Median	% consumers	Mean	Median	% consumers	Mean	Median	% consumers
	g	g	%	g	g	%	g	g	%
Pasta	286	220	64	371	300	56	343	265	52
Rice	357	200	42	314	273	42	423	232	42
Pizza	228	155	45	332	298	49	230	165	41
Other cereals	85	56	30	81	62	37	88	62	29
White bread	507	470	95	565	472	95	457	380	94
Wholemeal bread	204	151	21	246	171	21	203	136	28
Soft grain bread	208	202	4	269	135	3	118	102	2
Other bread	153	105	32	208	187	37	136	79	32
Whole grain and high fibre b'fast cereals	211	158	54	222	125	48	212	151	48
Other b'fast cereals	191	171	76	217	161	68	168	137	74
Biscuits	155	127	89	176	115	78	166	111	73
Fruit pies	130	110	16	114	108	16	97	100	11
Buns, cakes & pastries	216	167	79	232	173	75	212	170	67
Cereal-based milk puddings	223	181	31	212	200	29	243	170	29
Sponge type puddings	124	100	10	115	104	8	125	92	12
Other cereal-based puddings	173	129	29	201	142	24	200	144	27
Whole milk	1130	924	56	1285	1176	44	1189	834	58
Semi-skimmed milk	1390	1153	59	1466	1120	63	1107	955	56
Skimmed milk	489	307	4	641	369	9	870	1082	6
Cream	37	25	13	42	39	15	23	20	7
Other milk	520	419	15	564	430	16	472	336	22
Cottage cheese	119	100	1	94	58	1	33	27	1
Other cheese	90	66	66	127	103	68	105	82	59
Fromage frais	153	114	18	141	102	9	120	108	12
Yogurt	293	237	43	368	228	41	297	160	30
Other dairy desserts	145	111	23	169	126	27	207	142	17
Ice cream	164	121	54	170	146	44	148	124	48
Eggs	125	99	43	125	102	53	139	115	47
Egg dishes	102	80	11	148	95	15	132	116	9
Butter	41	26	27	38	26	26	50	22	28
Block margarine	14	9	2	37	37	0	–	–	–
Soft margarine, not polyunsaturated	28	16	23	35	23	37	28	26	31
Polyunsaturated margarine	35	22	6	47	40	4	54	20	7
Polyunsaturated oils	10	6	2	8	6	1	–	–	–
Other oils and cooking fats, not polyunsaturated	11	10	5	9	5	6	15	7	5
Polyunsaturated low fat spread	48	43	15	69	63	11	38	26	12
Other low fat spread	52	41	11	83	70	12	36	14	9
Polyunsaturated reduced fat spread	56	42	36	66	51	32	45	31	37
Other reduced fat spread	65	41	26	74	58	23	51	38	25
Bacon & ham	91	69	61	159	115	71	140	92	53
Beef, veal and dishes	245	191	50	349	296	63	222	160	45
Lamb & dishes	206	124	29	242	172	25	285	113	22
Pork & dishes	128	88	30	142	98	39	124	92	32
Coated chicken & turkey	147	118	47	183	165	44	170	104	44
Chicken and turkey dishes	207	144	74	301	239	78	245	160	73
Liver, liver products & dishes	45	37	5	79	58	7	102	40	4
Burgers & kebabs	174	115	38	217	194	42	187	117	48
Sausages	146	112	64	173	132	67	172	138	63
Meat pies & pastries	196	142	45	215	181	50	190	129	46
Other meat & meat products	100	60	26	117	96	30	115	75	26
Coated and/or fried white fish	129	100	52	156	127	42	149	112	46
Other white fish & dishes	171	134	10	169	119	8	198	193	13
Shellfish	78	50	5	111	62	9	288	104	3
Oily fish	100	75	22	99	82	25	129	75	24

Table 4.15(a)   male consumers – continued

Type of food	Young person living with*:								
	Both parents:						Single parent:		
	and other children			and no other children			with/without other children		
	Mean	Median	% consumers	Mean	Median	% consumers	Mean	Median	% consumers
	g	g	%	g	g	%	g	g	%
Raw carrots	97	53	15	76	50	9	81	39	10
Other raw & salad vegetables	82	56	47	132	96	50	105	83	42
Raw tomatoes	74	64	30	105	83	42	87	63	29
Peas	90	66	52	118	89	42	104	70	48
Green beans	68	50	14	92	60	15	81	59	13
Baked beans	236	179	63	253	182	59	287	190	64
Leafy green vegetables	84	60	40	109	79	38	98	80	36
Carrots–not raw	82	61	54	109	89	50	94	82	51
Tomatoes–not raw	79	67	9	79	60	16	116	100	9
Vegetable dishes	203	158	20	279	162	14	246	157	19
Other vegetables	115	92	58	137	99	58	121	100	56
Potato chips	380	328	88	486	357	89	458	347	89
Other fried/roast potatoes & products	151	114	54	197	172	51	147	127	43
Potato products–not fried	130	100	23	129	97	16	163	116	16
Other potatoes & potato dishes	317	240	82	441	362	86	375	279	84
Savoury snacks	130	117	92	134	112	82	123	106	79
Apples & pears	260	200	57	346	205	41	308	240	54
Citrus fruits	192	160	24	300	248	21	221	160	26
Bananas	220	156	38	296	217	37	222	160	39
Canned fruit in juice	143	134	5	90	75	7	73	80	6
Canned fruit in syrup	142	120	8	168	144	5	105	86	5
Other fruit	196	148	30	173	147	30	180	107	34
Nuts and seeds	61	38	17	77	36	15	49	29	16
Table sugar	57	38	71	82	49	62	66	42	69
Preserves	44	25	32	76	54	27	43	34	33
Sweet spreads, fillings & icings	30	20	21	35	28	15	33	20	19
Sugar confectionery	141	87	67	163	79	52	126	95	61
Chocolate confectionery	166	130	88	172	131	78	145	110	76
Fruit juice	806	520	47	962	653	46	667	415	43
Concentrated soft drinks–not low calorie, as consumed	2619	1520	54	2799	1523	48	2462	1383	48
Carbonated soft drinks–not low calorie	1334	862	77	1794	1355	84	1483	991	76
Ready to drink soft drinks–not low calorie	591	382	34	521	273	21	687	572	20
Concentrated soft drinks–low calorie, as consumed	3166	2334	53	3269	2317	33	2362	1772	42
Carbonated soft drinks–low calorie	1010	723	45	1143	870	46	980	604	41
Ready to drink soft drinks–low calorie	523	491	6	457	332	5	921	375	7
Liqueurs	45	45	0	117	151	1	2	2	0
Spirits	49	24	1	216	69	4	172	94	3
Wine	119	71	1	343	205	4	221	121	2
Fortified wine	150	250	0	104	106	2	–	–	–
Low alcohol & alcohol-free wine	80	80	0	–	–	–	–	–	–
Beer & lager	2125	1037	5	3665	2138	22	2339	1143	13
Low alcohol & alcohol-free beer & lager	150	150	0	–	–	–	–	–	–
Cider & Perry	538	402	1	445	454	3	–	–	–
Alco-pops	343	343	0	1444	1122	2	339	337	2
Coffee, as consumed	1652	1094	14	1767	1282	27	1924	1253	17
Tea, as consumed	1061	594	44	1634	1122	52	927	380	45
Herbal tea, as consumed	143	57	0	163	163	0	950	950	1
Bottled water	572	426	6	1449	801	11	607	250	7
Tap water	1032	611	62	1292	891	58	1404	804	53
Commercial toddler's foods	166	100	1	151	151	1	36	20	2
Other beverages, dry weight	518	322	20	444	280	23	615	408	21
Soup	329	270	22	451	281	21	326	246	21
Savoury sauces, pickles, gravies & condiments	128	98	89	178	156	89	144	110	85
Base = number of young people		528			169			157	

Table 4.15(b) Total quantities (grams) of foods consumed in seven days by whether young person was living with both parents: female consumers

Type of food	Young person living with*:								
	Both parents:						Single parent:		
	and other children			and no other children			with/without other children		
	Mean	Median	% consumers	Mean	Median	% consumers	Mean	Median	% consumers
	g	g	%	g	g	%	g	g	%
Pasta	271	206	65	320	300	61	324	228	63
Rice	333	180	39	267	180	47	314	198	38
Pizza	153	116	47	212	160	44	158	123	38
Other cereals	80	63	31	93	80	37	111	63	33
White bread	396	363	96	411	352	95	396	348	94
Wholemeal bread	169	123	24	159	103	30	153	87	26
Soft grain bread	230	150	3	170	192	2	111	99	4
Other bread	128	87	38	124	100	38	145	103	34
Whole grain and high fibre b'fast cereals	146	110	47	156	81	44	161	94	54
Other b'fast cereals	141	111	69	121	101	49	136	116	65
Biscuits	143	113	88	109	79	78	138	106	82
Fruit pies	101	88	13	117	103	15	144	110	10
Buns, cakes & pastries	179	147	78	184	142	70	180	154	73
Cereal-based milk puddings	204	161	33	206	146	26	227	192	30
Sponge type puddings	93	87	10	99	104	9	160	110	5
Other cereal-based puddings	166	125	26	163	121	25	174	161	26
Whole milk	1058	906	53	730	580	41	922	759	58
Semi-skimmed milk	959	784	55	803	548	70	911	858	53
Skimmed milk	617	346	8	374	231	7	329	314	5
Cream	38	20	11	28	25	17	36	30	12
Other milk	329	335	13	402	336	20	426	358	18
Cottage cheese	49	46	2	122	70	3	28	38	2
Other cheese	98	79	71	108	85	70	96	72	66
Fromage frais	154	125	21	117	100	9	113	120	12
Yogurt	281	180	46	324	247	34	317	250	47
Other dairy desserts	136	115	22	166	128	15	130	103	19
Ice cream	152	122	54	140	95	43	137	106	48
Eggs	108	84	46	132	85	42	117	99	43
Egg dishes	112	97	15	110	111	16	102	95	8
Butter	32	20	31	36	24	32	34	23	28
Block margarine	28	7	1	30	30	1	15	15	1
Soft margarine, not polyunsaturated	29	18	27	24	19	34	33	17	25
Polyunsaturated margarine	41	28	4	38	39	5	27	22	9
Polyunsaturated oils	8	7	2	16	5	1	9	5	1
Other oils and cooking fats, not polyunsaturated	7	6	5	16	10	8	8	5	5
Polyunsaturated low fat spread	40	28	14	36	34	16	45	43	12
Other low fat spread	41	35	12	40	33	13	44	40	13
Polyunsaturated reduced fat spread	50	41	37	47	34	36	39	32	46
Other reduced fat spread	50	41	22	45	34	20	42	30	21
Bacon & ham	82	54	57	93	64	60	75	65	57
Beef, veal and dishes	233	175	48	317	233	48	229	157	52
Lamb & dishes	174	116	27	124	81	17	149	139	24
Pork & dishes	124	89	29	168	124	30	97	80	26
Coated chicken & turkey	138	115	46	211	165	49	161	135	51
Chicken and turkey dishes	198	144	72	228	154	79	207	150	67
Liver, liver products & dishes	59	39	4	54	46	6	59	20	4
Burgers & kebabs	146	109	34	159	126	34	151	114	40
Sausages	111	82	59	120	105	45	133	91	53
Meat pies & pastries	144	111	43	201	169	42	146	130	47
Other meat & meat products	75	56	21	106	55	22	114	50	25
Coated and/or fried white fish	122	97	47	131	120	35	116	91	43
Other white fish & dishes	178	125	12	163	139	9	147	90	11
Shellfish	60	43	5	74	60	12	60	36	6
Oily fish	92	62	28	117	104	32	88	60	27

Table 4.15(b) female consumers – continued

Type of food	Young person living with*:								
	Both parents:						Single parent:		
	and other children			and no other children			with/without other children		
	Mean	Median	% consumers	Mean	Median	% consumers	Mean	Median	% consumers
	g	g	%	g	g	%	g	g	%
Raw carrots	74	40	20	67	37	19	54	57	11
Other raw & salad vegetables	115	78	58	122	88	68	103	68	53
Raw tomatoes	95	65	39	108	69	50	83	58	42
Peas	82	61	48	89	73	58	86	60	46
Green beans	62	46	15	74	49	12	70	60	9
Baked beans	192	150	59	218	176	53	217	161	55
Leafy green vegetables	98	77	44	121	95	45	93	75	43
Carrots–not raw	81	63	52	77	60	61	80	60	54
Tomatoes–not raw	84	64	8	73	85	9	93	85	9
Vegetable dishes	283	173	22	315	170	26	254	170	16
Other vegetables	140	94	60	147	110	68	124	100	61
Potato chips	329	257	87	366	308	86	394	320	91
Other fried/roast potatoes & products	145	120	48	162	125	52	127	106	45
Potato products–not fried	116	91	22	160	124	16	106	94	19
Other potatoes & potato dishes	306	251	80	351	280	82	349	305	79
Savoury snacks	123	114	93	122	92	87	129	113	86
Apples & pears	311	224	61	275	187	46	255	183	58
Citrus fruits	245	180	30	183	138	26	224	160	23
Bananas	188	133	38	188	132	37	240	191	37
Canned fruit in juice	160	115	6	84	70	3	162	115	7
Canned fruit in syrup	118	72	9	168	101	7	163	180	4
Other fruit	244	155	40	247	192	29	201	105	29
Nuts and seeds	46	25	16	38	25	13	35	35	10
Table sugar	45	28	63	56	29	60	70	45	66
Preserves	36	27	35	37	34	28	39	23	38
Sweet spreads, fillings & icings	31	20	21	38	21	18	32	20	16
Sugar confectionery	127	85	70	116	58	49	91	59	71
Chocolate confectionery	142	110	82	137	85	80	153	130	77
Fruit juice	766	542	55	723	499	47	720	496	43
Concentrated soft drinks–not low calorie, as consumed	1951	1332	54	2015	1338	47	2571	1419	49
Carbonated soft drinks–not low calorie	1000	735	74	1485	1137	76	1227	862	76
Ready to drink soft drinks–not low calorie	562	446	32	680	505	27	545	420	28
Concentrated soft drinks–low calorie, as consumed	2886	1994	52	2028	973	38	2548	1893	38
Carbonated soft drinks–low calorie	951	530	49	1050	705	46	1030	685	39
Ready to drink soft drinks–low calorie	538	432	8	675	715	5	367	285	6
Liqueurs	59	63	0	63	23	2	69	69	0
Spirits	85	69	2	93	69	8	55	45	2
Wine	214	141	2	435	195	10	175	125	2
Fortified wine	91	19	1	202	124	2	–	–	–
Low alcohol & alcohol-free wine	239	348	0	–	–	–	795	795	0
Beer & lager	2230	1428	3	1541	1134	14	1949	2008	4
Low alcohol & alcohol-free beer & lager	–	–	–	–	–	–	531	531	0
Cider & Perry	420	202	1	1318	1144	2	–	–	0
Alco-pops	699	698	0	1008	829	6	580	582	2
Coffee, as consumed	1238	655	14	2259	1224	24	2390	1685	19
Tea, as consumed	1059	650	47	1497	964	60	1156	654	41
Herbal tea, as consumed	253	204	1	1081	932	1	971	140	2
Bottled water	635	377	8	698	500	14	799	330	9
Tap water	1025	758	61	1146	710	64	990	598	60
Commercial toddler's foods	–	–	–	53	53	1	–	–	–
Other beverages, dry weight	441	266	22	379	201	22	531	356	24
Soup	318	261	25	310	222	30	329	260	28
Savoury sauces, pickles, gravies & condiments	134	102	86	156	121	90	141	100	88
Base = number of young people			498			173			167

89

Table 4.15(c) Main differences in the eating behaviour of young people by whether young person was living with both parents

	Living with both parents and no other children (compared with living with both parents and other children)		Living with lone parent, with/without other children (compared with living with both parents and other children)	
	Boys	Girls	Boys	Girls
Foods less likely to be eaten	biscuits* fromage frais* savoury snacks* apples & pears* sugar confectionery* ready-to-drink soft drinks nlc* concentrated soft drinks lc** concentrated soft drinks lc*	breakfast cereals, not high fibre or wholegrain** fromage frais** sausages* apples & pears* sugar confectionery** ready-to-drink soft drinks nlc*	biscuits** savoury snacks** chocolate confectionery* ready-to-drink soft drinks nlc*	concentrated soft drinks lc**
Foods more likely to be eaten	soft margarine, not pufa* beef, veal & dishes* beer & lager** coffee* tea*	semi-skimmed milk* wine* beer & lager** alco-pops*		

* p < 0.05
** p < 0.01
nlc: not low calorie
lc: low calorie
not pufa: not polyunsaturated

Table 4.16(a) Total quantities (grams) of foods consumed in seven days by social class of head of household: male consumers

Type of food	Social class of head of household*					
	Non manual			Manual		
	Mean	Median	% consumers	Mean	Median	% consumers
	g	g	%	g	g	%
Pasta	312	245	61	297	229	60
Rice	293	218	39	349	221	44
Pizza	269	187	51	236	165	40
Other cereals	77	54	31	91	59	33
White bread	483	443	95	551	485	96
Wholemeal bread	212	151	24	206	146	21
Soft grain bread	219	191	5	192	148	1
Other bread	178	112	36	147	108	31
Whole grain and high fibre b'fast cereals	218	166	55	215	143	50
Other b'fast cereals	189	148	73	200	181	74
Biscuits	157	125	86	169	125	83
Fruit pies	125	107	18	121	110	11
Buns, cakes & pastries	238	187	81	199	150	72
Cereal-based milk puddings	235	200	31	211	170	30
Sponge type puddings	114	90	11	135	100	10
Other cereal-based puddings	187	145	29	174	130	27
Whole milk	1226	975	46	1165	975	61
Semi-skimmed milk	1407	1230	66	1331	1073	53
Skimmed milk	674	457	7	438	287	4
Cream	39	30	17	32	22	9
Other milk	504	347	19	535	402	14
Cottage cheese	116	58	1	69	75	1
Other cheese	108	85	68	94	69	63
Fromage frais	168	124	18	128	100	13
Yogurt	312	200	46	313	250	35
Other dairy desserts	155	100	27	162	125	19
Ice cream	166	127	55	155	120	48
Eggs	128	105	43	119	86	45
Egg dishes	106	89	13	136	120	9
Butter	43	28	32	44	20	22
Block margarine	22	14	1	14	9	2
Soft margarine, not polyunsaturated	30	21	25	31	20	30
Polyunsaturated margarine	29	16	4	42	28	7
Polyunsaturated oils	4	3	1	8	6	2
Other oils and cooking fats, not polyunsaturated	6	5	4	15	10	7
Polyunsaturated low fat spread	52	50	14	48	38	13
Other low fat spread	68	56	11	43	24	10
Polyunsaturated reduced fat spread	53	36	37	60	44	35
Other reduced fat spread	54	37	25	78	55	25
Bacon & ham	112	81	64	114	75	63
Beef, veal and dishes	265	210	53	270	202	52
Lamb & dishes	172	102	25	227	129	25
Pork & dishes	137	91	34	119	88	30
Coated chicken & turkey	162	132	47	158	116	48
Chicken and turkey dishes	233	167	76	241	165	73
Liver, liver products & dishes	46	36	4	63	37	6
Burgers & kebabs	198	139	39	174	124	42
Sausages	142	110	64	172	136	67
Meat pies & pastries	195	140	46	201	151	48
Other meat & meat products	104	65	25	111	74	28
Coated and/or fried white fish	139	112	46	137	103	51
Other white fish & dishes	159	134	10	152	120	9
Shellfish	103	48	6	120	60	4
Oily fish	102	72	24	100	80	22

Table 4.16(a)   male consumers – continued

Type of food	Social class of head of household*					
	Non manual			Manual		
	Mean	Median	% consumers	Mean	Median	% consumers
	g	g	%	g	g	%
Raw carrots	78	60	15	100	38	13
Other raw & salad vegetables	103	72	52	93	63	43
Raw tomatoes	95	76	34	78	68	32
Peas	100	63	50	95	75	49
Green beans	73	47	18	81	60	12
Baked beans	250	176	60	246	189	63
Leafy green vegetables	84	60	40	98	68	38
Carrots–not raw	85	64	55	92	76	53
Tomatoes–not raw	101	75	10	73	61	11
Vegetable dishes	226	145	19	223	168	18
Other vegetables	125	104	56	117	90	59
Potato chips	370	279	87	456	367	90
Other fried/roast potatoes & products	151	128	48	166	120	55
Potato products–not fried	134	106	19	128	90	22
Other potatoes & potato dishes	339	254	84	370	284	82
Savoury snacks	128	112	86	136	121	90
Apples & pears	295	208	59	273	168	47
Citrus fruits	207	160	26	224	170	23
Bananas	261	175	44	205	158	33
Canned fruit in juice	129	120	8	101	80	4
Canned fruit in syrup	142	120	8	141	130	6
Other fruit	204	147	39	163	115	22
Nuts and seeds	53	30	18	70	50	16
Table sugar	55	36	65	73	48	73
Preserves	50	30	34	48	30	29
Sweet spreads, fillings & icings	29	22	24	32	18	16
Sugar confectionery	147	84	68	136	91	58
Chocolate confectionery	164	127	87	167	120	83
Fruit juice	842	544	56	811	484	37
Concentrated soft drinks–not low calorie, as consumed	2699	1520	52	2620	1528	54
Carbonated soft drinks–not low calorie	1408	873	77	1587	1172	76
Ready to drink soft drinks–not low calorie	589	355	30	590	393	28
Concentrated soft drinks–low calorie, as consumed	3203	2274	50	2866	2334	44
Carbonated soft drinks–low calorie	1069	692	44	1011	750	47
Ready to drink soft drinks–low calorie	665	421	7	622	591	6
Liqueurs	86	69	1	20	20	0
Spirits	113	69	2	209	69	2
Wine	174	121	2	460	375	1
Fortified wine	142	106	1	5	5	0
Low alcohol & alcohol-free wine	80	80	0	–	–	-
Beer & lager	2475	1330	12	3425	1882	10
Low alcohol & alcohol-free beer & lager	–	–	–	150	150	0
Cider & Perry	584	575	1	403	440	1
Alco-pops	340	337	1	1110	1011	2
Coffee, as consumed	1946	1280	16	1526	1220	17
Tea, as consumed	1324	654	41	1116	742	48
Herbal tea, as consumed	504	506	0	163	163	0
Bottled water	807	462	10	988	500	5
Tap water	1122	690	62	1098	690	57
Commercial toddler's foods	87	70	1	256	151	1
Other beverages, dry weight	472	309	27	568	308	16
Soup	324	257	20	366	275	21
Savoury sauces, pickles, gravies & condiments	135	103	90	148	105	88

Base = number of young people			414			385

Table 4.16(b) Total quantities (grams) of foods consumed in seven days by social class of head of household: female consumers

Type of food	Social class of head of household*					
	Non manual			Manual		
	Mean	Median	% *consumers*	Mean	Median	% *consumers*
	g	g	%	g	g	%
Pasta	305	230	68	267	215	64
Rice	244	160	41	322	199	39
Pizza	171	125	46	162	121	46
Other cereals	88	69	30	91	65	35
White bread	393	356	95	406	365	99
Wholemeal bread	184	134	26	141	85	25
Soft grain bread	215	216	3	146	136	2
Other bread	137	98	41	112	80	33
Whole grain and high fibre b'fast cereals	162	111	51	137	85	47
Other b'fast cereals	135	102	61	134	114	67
Biscuits	139	111	87	137	106	82
Fruit pies	120	103	15	95	90	11
Buns, cakes & pastries	197	160	77	165	139	70
Cereal-based milk puddings	194	157	29	213	171	31
Sponge type puddings	96	95	9	92	80	7
Other cereal-based puddings	161	126	31	173	125	21
Whole milk	999	822	46	954	780	54
Semi-skimmed milk	926	743	61	910	784	56
Skimmed milk	531	346	8	535	231	7
Cream	38	30	16	31	26	8
Other milk	357	335	16	341	336	14
Cottage cheese	82	46	2	58	39	3
Other cheese	105	87	74	94	78	68
Fromage frais	142	119	21	145	129	14
Yogurt	318	250	46	285	200	43
Other dairy desserts	141	113	21	146	120	21
Ice cream	149	120	55	145	110	47
Eggs	122	96	45	112	96	43
Egg dishes	110	99	14	112	98	12
Butter	35	24	35	27	17	27
Block margarine	34	12	1	40	8	1
Soft margarine, not polyunsaturated	23	14	26	31	20	30
Polyunsaturated margarine	43	39	5	20	14	5
Polyunsaturated oils	11	8	2	6	7	1
Other oils and cooking fats, not polyunsaturated	11	9	8	9	7	4
Polyunsaturated low fat spread	37	27	11	45	36	15
Other low fat spread	45	44	12	41	33	12
Polyunsaturated reduced fat spread	47	42	34	50	40	43
Other reduced fat spread	52	40	24	49	41	21
Bacon & ham	79	64	59	91	59	57
Beef, veal and dishes	248	175	47	252	191	52
Lamb & dishes	149	120	23	143	86	24
Pork & dishes	144	107	30	111	87	26
Coated chicken & turkey	161	135	48	147	116	49
Chicken and turkey dishes	195	139	76	208	151	73
Liver, liver products & dishes	66	40	5	59	45	4
Burgers & kebabs	141	110	32	161	117	40
Sausages	123	92	53	112	86	60
Meat pies & pastries	150	118	38	155	120	51
Other meat & meat products	69	44	20	98	64	25
Coated and/or fried white fish	118	93	45	127	100	42
Other white fish & dishes	168	123	9	176	130	11
Shellfish	69	46	7	69	45	5
Oily fish	100	65	32	96	66	25

Table 4.16(b)   female consumers – continued

Type of food	Social class of head of household*					
	Non manual			Manual		
	Mean	Median	% consumers	Mean	Median	% consumers
	g	g	%	g	g	%
Raw carrots	71	51	18	75	40	18
Other raw & salad vegetables	125	90	63	104	72	57
Raw tomatoes	110	78	41	82	57	43
Peas	78	64	47	91	68	51
Green beans	64	55	16	65	40	12
Baked beans	169	135	52	226	182	58
Leafy green vegetables	97	82	50	103	74	39
Carrots–not raw	80	60	56	82	67	54
Tomatoes–not raw	75	64	10	91	84	6
Vegetable dishes	274	184	23	300	145	19
Other vegetables	146	97	66	124	89	58
Potato chips	309	234	86	392	333	91
Other fried/roast potatoes & products	145	110	53	139	113	45
Potato products–not fried	118	93	20	130	96	20
Other potatoes & potato dishes	309	245	81	345	291	81
Savoury snacks	117	106	88	130	118	91
Apples & pears	337	257	58	261	175	53
Citrus fruits	245	184	33	194	160	25
Bananas	201	134	43	192	138	34
Canned fruit in juice	154	115	8	120	92	4
Canned fruit in syrup	138	100	8	124	89	7
Other fruit	240	155	43	256	150	29
Nuts and seeds	40	25	18	46	26	12
Table sugar	47	27	57	52	30	68
Preserves	37	25	36	35	25	31
Sweet spreads, fillings & icings	35	23	22	27	16	17
Sugar confectionery	107	78	63	132	74	69
Chocolate confectionery	141	105	83	149	123	81
Fruit juice	828	621	58	663	424	46
Concentrated soft drinks–not low calorie, as consumed	2158	1323	50	1991	1332	54
Carbonated soft drinks–not low calorie	1168	736	71	1169	858	80
Ready to drink soft drinks–not low calorie	604	446	29	561	420	34
Concentrated soft drinks–low calorie, as consumed	2847	1935	49	2572	1648	47
Carbonated soft drinks–low calorie	923	521	46	1082	730	48
Ready to drink soft drinks–low calorie	481	379	8	544	490	6
Liqueurs	95	112	1	23	23	0
Spirits	70	61	4	108	92	2
Wine	242	127	4	468	143	3
Fortified wine	146	58	1	150	210	0
Low alcohol & alcohol-free wine	–	–	0	293	223	1
Beer & lager	2076	1427	6	1601	1246	5
Low alcohol & alcohol-free beer & lager	–	–	0	531	531	0
Cider & Perry	1029	202	1	728	1007	1
Alco-pops	696	686	1	985	686	2
Coffee, as consumed	1556	916	16	1793	898	18
Tea, as consumed	1392	849	46	1060	552	49
Herbal tea, as consumed	631	506	1	17	17	0
Bottled water	697	500	12	711	465	7
Tap water	1133	753	65	912	616	58
Commercial toddler's foods	53	53	0	–	–	–
Other beverages, dry weight	481	253	25	453	286	19
Soup	322	252	25	337	270	27
Savoury sauces, pickles, gravies & condiments	137	103	89	146	110	86
Base = number of young people			*401*			*361*

* Excludes those for whom a social class could not be assigned.

Table 4.17(a) Total quantities (grams) of foods consumed in seven days by gross weekly household income: male consumers

Type of food	Gross weekly household income																	
	less than £160			£160 to less than £280			£280 to less than £400			£400 to less than £600			£600 and over			All*		
	Mean	Median	% consumers	Mean	Median	% consumers	Mean	Median	% consumers	Mean	Median	% consumers	Mean	Median	% consumers	Mean	Median	% consumers
	g	g	%	g	g	%	g	g	%	g	g	%	g	g	%	g	g	%
Pasta	338	266	55	278	220	57	292	214	62	385	300	61	279	230	65	310	240	60
Rice	572	287	50	345	239	51	352	227	36	282	185	32	259	202	41	362	227	42
Pizza	179	128	41	232	155	42	214	160	46	265	206	49	295	203	47	251	170	45
Other cereals	102	61	32	98	62	26	67	45	29	79	63	37	71	41	31	84	57	31
White bread	448	394	97	517	475	95	554	492	96	566	497	95	440	400	94	510	460	95
Wholemeal bread	165	144	18	265	200	19	214	136	27	250	218	22	178	139	28	211	148	22
Soft grain bread	–	–	–	166	144	4	150	150	1	237	257	3	229	138	7	213	191	3
Other bread	112	76	29	136	105	23	150	107	29	184	137	42	184	95	39	162	108	33
Whole grain and high fibre b'fast cereals	232	152	47	175	142	53	205	125	55	235	162	52	222	170	52	214	154	52
Other b'fast cereals	161	137	77	193	172	80	194	163	77	219	193	71	190	148	68	192	161	74
Biscuits	151	89	80	138	110	83	173	135	88	191	151	88	147	120	86	160	122	84
Fruit pies	118	95	7	114	91	8	123	110	17	112	101	17	118	107	23	122	110	15
Buns, cakes & pastries	196	166	72	202	151	69	191	146	76	216	154	80	248	190	85	218	167	76
Cereal-based milk puddings	223	160	37	197	180	25	212	198	25	233	156	33	242	205	32	224	186	30
Sponge type puddings	140	102	14	94	85	10	153	122	6	132	90	11	107	104	10	123	100	10
Other cereal-based puddings	210	115	28	173	144	24	149	131	23	160	120	32	178	137	31	182	131	28
Whole milk	1059	805	72	1032	899	66	1271	1029	52	1379	1057	41	1230	1085	45	1166	934	54
Semi-skimmed milk	1046	876	43	1229	998	52	1238	1052	64	1625	1502	66	1425	1184	66	1358	1119	59
Skimmed milk	601	542	2	870	919	4	642	179	3	473	373	8	579	307	9	607	369	5
Cream	21	20	7	67	50	6	29	25	10	48	32	16	29	27	22	37	25	12
Other milk	413	392	19	396	251	13	592	545	16	531	418	17	592	431	17	517	402	16
Cottage cheese	33	27	1	–	–	0	42	42	1	154	114	2	98	58	2	101	58	1
Other cheese	71	45	51	90	79	64	104	69	70	109	89	74	114	87	68	100	77	65
Fromage frais	125	111	11	139	111	11	132	100	15	129	100	16	179	116	24	147	108	15
Yogurt	298	151	28	325	151	28	305	250	42	340	281	48	282	200	42	308	228	40
Other dairy desserts	158	133	15	177	120	18	185	172	20	145	111	29	150	100	32	159	119	23
Ice cream	141	123	42	162	107	42	173	125	57	176	145	59	153	120	56	163	122	51
Eggs	139	110	44	150	120	44	93	75	51	118	97	49	132	98	40	128	102	45
Egg dishes	108	100	10	125	118	9	175	120	9	105	86	11	97	61	16	118	97	11
Butter	26	16	23	53	39	21	33	20	18	35	27	28	41	26	41	42	26	27
Block margarine	14	14	1	13	9	4	42	42	1	5	5	1	–	–	–	16	9	1
Soft margarine, not polyunsaturated	–	–	–	–	–	–	–	–	–	–	–	–	–	–	–	–	–	–
Polyunsaturated margarine	26	14	24	34	28	28	32	20	28	26	14	20	29	21	29	30	20	27
Polyunsaturated oils	65	28	6	21	–	9	51	44	8	18	9	3	36	42	2	40	27	6
Other oils and cooking fats, not polyunsaturated	–	–	–	–	–	–	14	8	3	7	6	3	6	4	2	9	6	1
Polyunsaturated low fat spread	16	10	8	8	9	3	15	10	5	14	10	3	6	5	9	11	9	5
Other low fat spread	38	17	12	51	59	12	51	35	12	62	53	19	42	35	15	49	43	14
Polyunsaturated reduced fat spread	43	29	41	58	55	34	48	67	38	58	39	32	52	36	37	56	42	36
Other reduced fat spread	54	38	31	65	51	21	69	96	27	62	42	29	46	35	21	64	42	25

95

Table 4.17(a) male consumers – continued

Type of food	Gross weekly household income															All*		
	less than £160			£160 to less than £280			£280 to less than £400			£400 to less than £600			£600 and over					
	Mean	Median	% consumers	Mean	Median	% consumers	Mean	Median	% consumers	Mean	Median	% consumers	Mean	Median	% consumers	Mean	Median	% consumers
	g	g	%	g	g	%	g	g	%	g	g	%	g	g	%	g	g	%
Bacon & ham	122	74	44	107	71	60	104	91	66	119	84	67	107	75	67	114	81	61
Beef, veal and dishes	207	157	41	230	181	50	282	200	52	293	207	50	274	220	62	266	205	52
Lamb & dishes	390	165	33	206	165	27	173	84	27	193	115	30	153	100	25	224	129	27
Pork & dishes	105	87	29	109	90	27	158	107	34	119	82	39	138	102	30	130	92	32
Coated chicken & turkey	160	100	46	141	126	37	169	130	51	133	113	42	165	136	55	159	125	46
Chicken and turkey dishes	217	149	73	226	157	71	220	150	75	242	185	86	250	163	73	234	163	75
Liver, liver products & dishes	102	35	3	107	80	3	66	44	5	36	31	7	50	53	6	61	37	5
Burgers & kebabs	162	123	45	175	109	42	195	123	42	189	139	40	207	152	35	185	124	41
Sausages	176	130	63	163	116	66	155	119	66	145	117	66	148	115	67	156	120	64
Meat pies & pastries	177	123	54	193	141	44	231	197	44	216	150	44	172	141	46	200	142	46
Other meat & meat products	96	65	27	131	74	26	92	73	26	134	76	24	85	44	32	106	71	27
Coated and/or fried white fish	135	109	48	135	112	54	157	104	43	134	108	48	130	107	51	137	108	49
Other white fish & dishes	237	193	17	192	195	7	121	76	9	161	148	8	148	117	11	177	149	10
Shellfish	55	28	2	63	84	2	131	60	7	63	43	6	93	60	7	109	51	5
Oily fish	122	62	22	106	69	20	89	60	28	100	77	25	97	78	20	105	75	23
Raw carrots	215	114	7	61	39	8	67	51	14	93	47	17	89	60	19	92	50	13
Other raw & salad vegetables	84	64	39	88	63	41	87	51	48	109	58	47	100	77	59	97	68	47
Raw tomatoes	73	60	26	90	75	33	73	68	29	95	80	31	82	66	41	84	68	32
Peas	85	56	51	101	80	50	85	70	48	100	69	53	102	70	46	97	70	50
Green beans	90	60	11	83	84	10	75	45	14	75	55	19	67	43	16	76	51	14
Baked beans	252	209	68	211	132	68	211	185	68	312	216	55	246	194	59	248	181	62
Leafy green vegetables	95	75	33	86	67	38	78	65	39	75	60	41	103	67	41	91	67	39
Carrots–not raw	98	60	47	89	67	52	88	75	54	85	71	55	87	64	55	89	70	53
Tomatoes–not raw	121	100	8	78	72	9	83	58	14	88	48	12	78	73	10	85	71	10
Vegetable dishes	278	190	19	193	178	20	193	125	17	198	147	17	230	138	18	222	162	18
Other vegetables	135	119	57	100	83	57	111	82	59	132	97	57	120	92	59	121	95	58
Potato chips	495	377	95	425	349	88	397	319	88	371	308	85	388	287	87	415	330	89
Other fried/roast potatoes & products	161	120	51	164	137	46	134	103	53	172	137	54	146	134	55	159	127	52
Potato products–not fried	182	160	12	125	85	19	142	100	22	111	85	22	137	120	25	134	100	20
Other potatoes & potato dishes	336	280	85	329	222	75	366	295	86	317	250	91	367	295	82	352	261	83
Savoury snacks	120	108	85	125	116	90	152	129	91	132	120	88	123	105	87	130	115	88
Apples & pears	281	251	51	261	147	53	279	169	56	271	233	55	320	207	53	282	207	53
Citrus fruits	200	160	25	214	170	26	204	149	20	205	150	26	211	160	22	215	160	24
Bananas	223	164	30	172	124	45	245	207	40	249	161	33	284	219	42	234	164	38
Canned fruit in juice	107	100	3	71	80	6	81	72	6	160	144	7	132	133	5	117	100	6
Canned fruit in syrup	109	100	7	142	120	5	172	181	5	94	55	10	204	140	5	142	120	7
Other fruit	129	107	31	201	148	20	154	109	19	223	190	38	191	147	43	189	131	31
Nuts and seeds	54	27	16	62	50	16	79	86	19	47	30	15	66	30	18	62	36	16
Table sugar	62	42	79	73	54	67	66	41	73	63	34	64	52	33	62	63	40	69
Preserves	36	22	32	60	38	27	34	29	28	59	30	35	53	30	35	49	30	31
Sweet spreads, fillings & icings	36	15	19	39	16	14	29	18	14	25	20	24	32	25	25	31	21	20

Table 4.17(a) male consumers – continued

Type of food	Gross weekly household income																		All*		
	less than £160			£160 to less than £280			£280 to less than £400			£400 to less than £600			£600 and over								
	Mean	Median	% consumers	Mean	Median	% consumers	Mean	Median	% consumers	Mean	Median	% consumers	Mean	Median	% consumers	Mean	Median	% consumers	Mean	Median	% consumers
	g	g	%	g	g	%	g	g	%	g	g	%	g	g	%	g	g	%			
Sugar confectionery	150	102	62	121	83	59	132	87	65	155	95	67	152	80	68	141	87	63			
Chocolate confectionery	134	110	76	176	127	82	179	137	87	176	134	89	150	123	85	164	125	84			
Fruit juice	645	326	35	702	416	29	906	563	51	667	456	53	971	710	62	821	520	46			
Concentrated soft drinks–not low calorie, as consumed	2615	1383	49	1821	893	56	2946	1586	54	3070	1655	57	2687	1703	48	2626	1516	52			
Carbonated soft drinks–not low calorie	1343	926	79	1370	864	80	1679	1299	73	1375	831	86	1547	965	73	1456	1008	78			
Ready to drink soft drinks–not low calorie	633	416	21	569	382	31	600	382	29	407	272	25	687	459	33	593	382	29			
Concentrated soft drinks–low calorie, as consumed	2237	1711	38	3256	2219	43	2846	2291	58	3552	2678	50	3199	2316	47	3054	2250	47			
Carbonated soft drinks–low calorie	823	604	37	1150	817	40	1060	739	51	1140	815	47	904	604	46	1030	723	44			
Ready to drink soft drinks–low calorie	749	323	7	686	631	4	498	244	9	444	252	5	732	491	7	623	450	6			
Liqueurs	2	2	0	20	20	1	47	39	1	–	–	0	197	197	1	73	28	1			
Spirits	–	–	–	42	46	2	285	263	1	92	92	0	169	63	5	153	69	2			
Wine	21	21	1	77	60	1	132	121	2	203	187	1	338	218	4	247	144	2			
Fortified wine	–	–	–	–	–	–	–	–	0	–	–	–	121	106	2	121	106	1			
Low alcohol & alcohol-free wine	–	–	–	–	–	–	–	–	–	–	–	–	80	80	0	80	80	0			
Beer & lager	4364	3824	3	3269	2000	6	2122	886	11	1351	570	9	3633	1916	17	2866	1713	10			
Low alcohol & alcohol-free beer & lager	–	–	1	–	–	–	–	–	0	150	150	0	–	–	–	150	150	0			
Cider & Perry	454	454	1	504	504	0	–	–	0	548	575	3	–	–	–	481	454	1			
Alco-pops	–	–	–	625	343	2	1757	2860	2	343	343	1	607	337	1	894	343	1			
Coffee, as consumed	1598	1140	15	1664	1358	18	1479	1059	12	1167	686	20	2358	2072	19	1753	1220	17			
Tea, as consumed	844	562	47	1062	641	47	924	650	46	1603	1147	49	1262	527	37	1166	674	45			
Herbal tea, as consumed	–	–	–	163	163	0	950	950	1	266	266	1	57	57	1	370	168	0			
Bottled water	429	250	5	208	230	2	533	357	4	674	314	12	1210	500	12	833	426	8			
Tap water	1242	820	64	1181	810	48	808	410	52	1179	800	65	1205	720	68	1142	740	60			
Commercial toddler's foods	20	20	1	151	151	1	33	33	0	219	100	2	89	56	1	118	70	1			
Other beverages, dry weight	685	488	14	436	300	15	439	280	22	659	504	28	381	220	24	517	322	21			
Soup	333	242	23	382	254	16	270	224	24	450	282	23	313	286	20	351	262	22			
Savoury sauces, pickles, gravies & condiments	134	102	89	130	99	84	129	97	89	161	137	89	141	108	92	140	104	89			
Base = number of young people	133			159			157			173			208			856					

97

Table 4.17(b)   Total quantities (grams) of foods consumed in seven days by gross weekly household income: female consumers

Type of food	Gross weekly household income															All*		
	less than £160			£160 to less than £280			£280 to less than £400			£400 to less than £600			£600 and over					
	Mean	Median	% consumers	Mean	Median	% consumers	Mean	Median	% consumers	Mean	Median	% consumers	Mean	Median	% consumers	Mean	Median	% consumers
	g	g	%	g	g	%	g	g	%	g	g	%	g	g	%	g	g	%
Pasta	269	201	59	303	217	59	291	209	67	281	217	67	316	247	70	291	220	64
Rice	465	225	45	327	200	30	316	260	37	245	190	38	229	150	47	315	180	40
Pizza	142	113	37	138	101	45	159	120	39	168	118	44	188	155	52	165	123	44
Other cereals	109	55	28	97	80	31	89	62	36	77	59	38	87	69	30	90	69	33
White bread	390	338	95	377	344	97	444	386	98	414	376	97	374	355	93	398	359	96
Wholemeal bread	126	76	21	161	92	24	142	88	22	144	125	27	197	131	31	164	109	26
Soft grain bread	115	99	3	123	135	3	187	216	2	217	229	2	247	136	5	185	136	3
Other bread	129	81	30	120	80	38	127	98	35	143	111	31	133	80	50	130	90	37
Whole grain and high fibre b'fast cereals	151	132	44	166	98	44	113	82	48	146	108	50	169	108	51	151	106	48
Other b'fast cereals	146	129	65	152	133	76	131	90	65	131	86	66	119	98	52	137	108	64
Biscuits	137	102	82	139	100	83	152	117	88	137	117	85	128	100	85	136	106	84
Fruit pies	160	113	9	103	80	10	104	102	17	107	93	11	111	103	17	112	94	13
Buns, cakes & pastries	187	155	74	162	144	70	166	127	78	162	133	79	220	189	78	180	147	75
Cereal-based milk puddings	215	180	31	236	185	31	181	132	37	204	161	30	193	139	28	208	171	31
Sponge type puddings	151	110	8	81	87	9	84	64	9	101	102	9	95	86	10	101	95	9
Other cereal-based puddings	170	150	23	168	121	22	164	120	24	159	125	27	178	130	32	167	125	26
Whole milk	843	623	67	1054	929	67	966	927	44	1142	1008	49	821	581	39	975	790	51
Semi-skimmed milk	925	784	50	924	780	52	853	627	56	884	802	56	969	790	74	912	753	57
Skimmed milk	374	315	3	285	163	4	520	452	8	737	334	10	518	346	9	536	317	7
Cream	30	22	10	27	23	10	47	35	10	27	25	8	38	30	22	35	27	12
Other milk	435	336	21	417	358	12	397	336	13	353	335	14	301	300	18	378	335	15
Cottage cheese	61	39	2	1	1	1	28	22	4	67	76	1	100	50	4	64	39	2
Other cheese	88	71	60	83	65	65	115	91	71	95	84	72	111	88	80	99	80	69
Fromage frais	130	123	10	140	150	15	161	100	18	155	118	21	128	120	20	144	120	17
Yogurt	294	206	50	273	175	34	287	163	46	330	250	43	286	250	50	296	218	44
Other dairy desserts	119	118	16	137	120	20	153	118	23	150	120	23	129	110	20	139	118	20
Ice cream	123	80	48	161	117	41	143	120	55	134	125	54	169	122	56	147	120	50
Eggs	117	100	43	121	97	39	111	97	51	125	76	48	98	85	42	114	93	44
Egg dishes	99	95	9	121	97	11	103	119	14	134	91	11	102	95	21	110	97	13
Butter	36	26	24	26	14	26	35	20	23	35	28	35	35	24	39	33	22	31
Block margarine	56	15	2	7	7	3	—	—	—	3	3	1	66	49	1	26	7	1
Soft margarine, not polyunsaturated	44	24	31	25	14	28	36	28	31	22	20	23	20	14	27	29	18	28
Polyunsaturated margarine	22	14	7	47	32	6	38	60	4	33	27	5	39	39	3	35	27	5
Polyunsaturated oils	8	5	2	6	7	1	13	7	3	10	10	1	7	6	3	9	6	2
Other oils and cooking fats, not polyunsaturated	8	5	3	8	7	4	7	8	3	10	6	5	11	10	12	10	8	6
Polyunsaturated low fat spread	39	24	11	54	52	15	41	39	17	28	18	9	39	32	15	40	28	14
Other low fat spread	39	40	12	38	26	9	38	33	14	47	39	19	43	33	10	42	35	13
Polyunsaturated reduced fat spread	42	37	42	43	31	43	55	41	35	47	41	37	48	45	36	47	37	38
Other reduced fat spread	30	30	14	52	37	24	59	43	27	50	34	23	48	41	22	49	39	22

Table 4.17(b) female consumers – continued

Type of food	Gross weekly household income																	
	less than £160			£160 to less than £280			£280 to less than £400			£400 to less than £600			£600 and over			All*		
	Mean	Median	% consumers	Mean	Median	% consumers	Mean	Median	% consumers	Mean	Median	% consumers	Mean	Median	% consumers	Mean	Median	% consumers
	g	g	%	g	g	%	g	g	%	g	g	%	g	g	%	g	g	%
Bacon & ham	67	60	52	84	56	51	77	53	64	93	64	61	86	57	60	83	59	57
Beef, veal and dishes	242	179	44	263	184	52	292	176	50	218	144	52	252	208	51	252	180	49
Lamb & dishes	227	180	30	154	122	24	140	86	15	128	70	20	154	122	27	162	115	24
Pork & dishes	119	84	27	85	75	25	136	90	31	129	89	29	153	120	32	127	89	28
Coated chicken & turkey	153	114	44	136	123	52	158	142	50	165	131	45	160	128	53	156	128	48
Chicken and turkey dishes	222	154	71	200	126	62	198	160	78	176	140	71	223	146	80	207	146	73
Liver, liver products & dishes	42	19	4	58	37	4	54	57	4	63	38	5	66	47	5	58	39	4
Burgers & kebabs	129	106	33	152	117	43	110	96	41	184	145	36	145	117	25	149	115	35
Sausages	127	92	55	114	83	61	121	102	66	120	86	52	107	77	49	117	86	55
Meat pies & pastries	168	138	48	146	120	51	169	128	52	155	121	39	136	102	32	155	128	43
Other meat & meat products	156	89	24	78	48	24	82	42	24	69	45	26	75	47	17	90	56	22
Coated and/or fried white fish	120	96	53	137	112	41	117	91	43	126	97	45	108	92	41	122	98	44
Other white fish & dishes	151	119	18	136	65	7	188	110	12	165	130	7	170	128	12	167	124	11
Shellfish	51	36	9	62	45	2	39	40	7	64	36	4	85	60	12	65	43	7
Oily fish	94	68	28	86	60	23	85	65	33	85	50	29	125	105	34	97	65	29
Raw carrots	50	50	11	54	21	10	105	52	21	58	45	24	73	36	23	70	43	18
Other raw & salad vegetables	89	62	54	100	77	42	114	66	55	97	69	66	154	111	72	114	78	59
Raw tomatoes	82	57	38	87	63	31	82	64	43	91	63	45	125	77	49	95	65	42
Peas	88	60	57	99	79	46	88	61	49	80	68	45	76	58	53	85	63	49
Green beans	71	26	7	69	49	10	79	55	14	52	43	16	68	51	19	66	49	13
Baked beans	200	152	63	244	166	59	189	153	64	197	152	54	177	150	48	201	155	57
Leafy green vegetables	114	81	42	81	72	32	99	70	46	97	83	49	111	88	51	102	80	44
Carrots–not raw	85	69	50	91	67	50	74	58	59	77	60	56	79	63	56	80	61	54
Tomatoes–not raw	100	78	10	120	128	4	109	85	7	71	77	6	59	43	13	84	77	8
Vegetable dishes	251	140	20	304	146	17	239	165	13	257	153	21	307	200	30	286	170	22
Other vegetables	147	115	55	112	86	57	141	97	64	139	99	61	148	97	71	138	97	62
Potato chips	375	300	92	432	364	88	347	281	92	330	293	87	264	210	82	351	281	88
Other fried/roast potatoes & products	147	128	44	141	118	50	122	100	47	161	135	53	145	108	49	145	116	48
Potato products–not fried	97	90	21	138	115	18	113	98	23	111	91	18	141	113	23	121	94	20
Other potatoes & potato dishes	333	287	81	382	305	76	318	288	82	300	233	82	307	240	84	324	261	80
Savoury snacks	142	114	92	135	131	89	123	110	94	119	113	94	105	86	84	124	112	90
Apples & pears	220	177	58	292	185	56	332	224	62	326	265	62	303	176	60	294	210	57
Citrus fruits	260	160	25	210	183	20	218	146	31	258	194	31	226	163	35	233	163	28
Bananas	195	137	37	244	167	25	178	140	37	179	112	37	202	135	43	199	137	38
Canned fruit in juice	108	100	8	298	362	4	132	114	7	185	133	7	134	91	8	154	115	6
Canned fruit in syrup	175	150	6	146	163	6	130	96	8	124	72	10	91	69	7	132	89	8
Other fruit	221	130	30	251	147	26	242	120	32	195	124	40	279	200	48	237	150	35
Nuts and seeds	28	20	10	70	44	10	34	15	10	45	23	18	39	32	22	43	27	14
Table sugar	54	34	71	70	42	70	47	27	63	49	27	59	41	27	58	53	32	63
Preserves	46	28	34	34	26	34	29	25	35	40	25	33	37	25	37	37	27	34
Sweet spreads, fillings & icings	38	27	17	32	16	16	29	17	19	23	20	24	38	23	21	32	20	20
Sugar confectionery	116	74	73	135	74	69	106	65	70	109	83	62	116	77	60	117	75	66
Chocolate confectionery	153	112	75	159	133	76	137	123	84	153	119	86	115	75	80	143	112	80

99

Table 4.17(b) female consumers – continued

Type of food	Gross weekly household income																		All*		
	less than £160			£160 to less than £280			£280 to less than £400			£400 to less than £600			£600 and over								
	Mean	Median	% consumers	Mean	Median	% consumers	Mean	Median	% consumers	Mean	Median	% consumers	Mean	Median	% consumers	Mean	Median	% consumers			
	g	g	%	g	g	%	g	g	%	g	g	%	g	g	%	g	g	%			
Fruit juice	664	450	35	619	380	46	529	366	48	793	519	53	948	801	69	750	521	51			
Concentrated soft drinks–not low calorie, as consumed	2151	1421	47	2141	1332	57	2415	1409	52	1808	1235	50	2168	1290	48	2082	1332	51			
Carbonated soft drinks–not low calorie	1010	754	77	1177	834	81	1211	881	75	1200	847	72	1090	724	71	1141	816	75			
Ready to drink soft drinks–not low calorie	529	435	28	537	345	29	547	422	38	496	332	28	797	726	30	577	424	30			
Concentrated soft drinks–low calorie, as consumed	2000	1562	38	2781	1887	46	3108	2412	49	2963	2116	53	2477	1437	44	2686	1867	46			
Carbonated soft drinks–low calorie	1114	743	38	945	562	38	879	580	55	1003	530	56	1027	660	42	983	618	46			
Ready to drink soft drinks–low calorie	514	260	5	920	631	4	476	263	9	392	379	10	542	346	6	524	432	7			
Liqueurs	–	–	–	–	–	–	67	23	1	69	69	0	59	52	2	63	69	1			
Spirits	23	23	1	64	46	2	90	92	3	102	69	3	88	66	6	87	69	3			
Wine	208	208	1	335	342	1	635	176	5	165	127	2	258	125	9	339	143	4			
Fortified wine	–	–	–	–	–	–	327	242	1	19	19	0	106	58	3	147	73	1			
Low alcohol & alcohol-free wine	–	–	–	–	–	–	–	–	–	–	–	–	–	–	–	–	–	–			
Beer & lager	402	209	1	308	223	3	2017	1425	4	1512	1386	5	1923	1389	11	1803	1386	5			
Low alcohol & alcohol-free beer & lager	–	–	–	2270	2280	4	–	–	–	–	–	–	–	–	–	308	223	0			
Cider & Perry	1145	1145	1	531	531	1	856	286	2	234	202	1	1702	1070	1	531	504	1			
Alco-pops	552	337	2	291	322	1	1651	2266	2	662	858	3	752	674	2	851	686	2			
Coffee, as consumed	1284	651	16	2255	1088	16	1956	1326	20	1990	957	18	1451	890	19	1766	934	17			
Tea, as consumed	1027	527	54	1398	866	42	1069	647	49	1194	704	46	1337	965	51	1196	698	48			
Herbal tea, as consumed	232	140	2	17	17	1	753	753	1	910	220	2	824	204	1	634	220	1			
Bottled water	836	340	8	496	250	6	875	428	10	647	500	5	597	377	17	681	378	9			
Tap water	1026	764	64	982	758	55	937	587	61	857	609	55	1248	813	73	1035	692	62			
Commercial toddler's foods	–	–	–	–	–	–	–	–	–	–	–	–	53	53	0	53	53	0			
Other beverages, dry weight	427	297	20	600	286	17	509	359	21	394	240	21	424	253	31	449	260	22			
Soup	349	288	23	314	253	33	308	250	29	299	226	30	344	280	21	321	257	27			
Savoury sauces, pickles, gravies & condiments	132	102	86	162	137	84	124	101	88	148	104	90	139	104	90	140	104	87			
Base = number of young people	131			146			145			192			196			845					

Table 4.18(a) Total quantities of foods consumed in seven days by whether young person's 'parents' were receiving certain benefits: male consumers

Type of food	Whether receiving benefits					
	Receiving benefits			Not receiving benefits		
	Mean	Median	% consumers	Mean	Median	% consumers
	g	g	%	g	g	%
Pasta	307	240	52	311	240	62
Rice	537	300	48	295	208	41
Pizza	198	140	38	265	186	47
Other cereals	99	75	28	80	55	32
White bread	458	398	94	526	476	96
Wholemeal bread	162	144	18	223	151	24
Soft grain bread	202	202	1	214	150	4
Other bread	109	80	25	173	121	35
Whole grain and high fibre b'fast cereals	224	166	49	211	154	53
Other b'fast cereals	161	143	77	202	170	73
Biscuits	144	95	78	165	130	86
Fruit pies	104	81	8	125	110	17
Buns, cakes & pastries	208	158	69	221	170	79
Cereal-based milk puddings	227	170	33	223	191	29
Sponge type puddings	128	100	14	121	90	9
Other cereal-based puddings	227	120	23	171	131	29
Whole milk	1107	834	70	1193	987	49
Semi-skimmed milk	1029	888	45	1438	1197	63
Skimmed milk	565	306	2	604	342	6
Cream	31	20	6	37	30	14
Other milk	416	336	17	552	426	16
Cottage cheese	33	27	0	112	99	1
Other cheese	76	55	51	106	81	69
Fromage frais	127	111	8	151	108	18
Yogurt	324	226	33	304	228	42
Other dairy desserts	159	126	13	159	117	26
Ice cream	154	110	42	165	126	54
Eggs	135	120	43	126	97	46
Egg dishes	110	100	9	120	94	12
Butter	38	17	21	43	28	29
Block margarine	27	18	1	12	9	1
Soft margarine, not polyunsaturated	29	19	29	30	20	26
Polyunsaturated margarine	33	36	7	40	21	5
Polyunsaturated oils	27	27	1	6	5	2
Other oils and cooking fats, not polyunsaturated	14	10	7	10	8	5
Polyunsaturated low fat spread	41	31	12	52	44	14
Other low fat spread	43	24	8	59	52	11
Polyunsaturated reduced fat spread	40	28	35	61	46	36
Other reduced fat spread	52	36	26	68	45	25
Bacon & ham	121	70	44	113	83	67
Beef, veal and dishes	198	153	47	285	220	53
Lamb & dishes	379	195	29	168	100	26
Pork & dishes	107	92	29	137	92	33
Coated chicken & turkey	157	116	39	159	125	48
Chicken and turkey dishes	215	156	70	239	163	76
Liver, liver products & dishes	112	37	4	48	38	5
Burgers & kebabs	167	113	42	191	127	40
Sausages	184	130	64	147	116	64
Meat pies & pastries	188	126	51	204	149	45
Other meat & meat products	111	67	24	105	71	28
Coated and/or fried white fish	141	114	49	135	104	49
Other white fish & dishes	222	200	15	151	120	9
Shellfish	59	51	3	116	56	6
Oily fish	125	82	19	99	75	24

101

Table 4.18(a)   male consumers – continued

Type of food	Whether receiving benefits					
	Receiving benefits			Not receiving benefits		
	Mean	Median	% consumers	Mean	Median	% consumers
	g	g	%	g	g	%
Raw carrots	184	103	5	82	50	16
Other raw & salad vegetables	74	63	38	103	69	49
Raw tomatoes	78	47	30	86	73	33
Peas	101	70	50	96	70	50
Green beans	105	84	9	70	48	16
Baked beans	245	182	68	250	180	60
Leafy green vegetables	96	77	35	90	65	40
Carrots–not raw	88	60	52	90	72	53
Tomatoes–not raw	94	67	8	83	73	11
Vegetable dishes	259	168	16	212	156	19
Other vegetables	123	90	60	121	96	57
Potato chips	474	379	92	394	313	88
Other fried/roast potatoes & products	171	126	49	155	126	53
Potato products–not fried	142	80	15	133	100	22
Other potatoes & potato dishes	375	280	81	344	261	84
Savoury snacks	124	106	85	132	118	89
Apples & pears	286	237	47	281	201	55
Citrus fruits	202	170	21	219	160	25
Bananas	223	166	31	237	161	40
Canned fruit in juice	110	115	4	119	98	6
Canned fruit in syrup	136	120	7	143	120	7
Other fruit	142	107	24	200	147	33
Nuts and seeds	60	32	15	63	38	17
Table sugar	59	42	77	65	39	66
Preserves	49	24	30	50	30	31
Sweet spreads, fillings & icings	34	15	16	31	22	21
Sugar confectionery	123	87	56	147	90	65
Chocolate confectionery	145	115	76	170	127	86
Fruit juice	611	320	33	864	566	50
Concentrated soft drinks–not low calorie, as consumed	1986	1135	52	2837	1669	52
Carbonated soft drinks–not low calorie	1267	914	78	1522	1030	78
Ready to drink soft drinks–not low calorie	602	408	25	590	382	30
Concentrated soft drinks–low calorie, as consumed	2581	1998	38	3182	2316	50
Carbonated soft drinks–low calorie	908	699	38	1066	727	46
Ready to drink soft drinks–low calorie	630	591	6	621	375	6
Liqueurs	13	20	1	103	69	0
Spirits	46	46	1	163	69	2
Wine	21	21	0	264	186	2
Fortified wine	–	–	–	121	106	1
Low alcohol & alcohol-free wine	–	–	–	80	80	0
Beer & lager	3294	1769	3	2837	1713	12
Low alcohol & alcohol-free beer & lager	–	–	–	150	150	0
Cider & Perry	454	454	1	487	466	1
Alco-pops	340	341	1	1048	537	1
Coffee, as consumed	1738	1620	15	1765	1220	18
Tea, as consumed	850	530	49	1285	768	44
Herbal tea, as consumed	–	–	–	370	168	1
Bottled water	438	250	3	878	432	9
Tap water	1203	893	59	1126	619	60
Commercial toddler's foods	20	20	1	149	100	1
Other beverages, dry weight	571	408	14	506	300	23
Soup	389	243	21	340	270	22
Savoury sauces, pickles, gravies & condiments	142	104	84	140	105	90
Base = number of young people			*189*			*666*

Table 4.18(b)   Total quantities of foods consumed in seven days by whether young person's 'parents' were receiving certain benefits: female consumers

Type of food	Whether receiving benefits					
	Receiving benefits			Not receiving benefits		
	Mean	Median	% consumers	Mean	Median	% consumers
	g	g	%	g	g	%
Pasta	272	205	58	297	227	66
Rice	433	199	40	274	180	40
Pizza	136	100	41	175	140	45
Other cereals	104	80	34	84	62	32
White bread	376	337	97	406	364	95
Wholemeal bread	145	81	22	170	123	27
Soft grain bread	113	99	3	215	136	3
Other bread	132	80	33	130	96	39
Whole grain and high fibre b'fast cereals	156	119	45	150	103	49
Other b'fast cereals	143	120	71	135	100	62
Biscuits	148	105	81	132	106	86
Fruit pies	146	110	9	104	93	14
Buns, cakes & pastries	176	155	75	182	145	75
Cereal-based milk puddings	236	195	34	197	150	30
Sponge type puddings	139	110	7	91	86	9
Other cereal-based puddings	169	125	24	166	125	27
Whole milk	889	749	64	1018	822	47
Semi-skimmed milk	902	707	52	915	780	59
Skimmed milk	487	261	3	556	346	9
Cream	32	26	10	36	27	13
Other milk	398	336	18	369	335	15
Cottage cheese	50	39	1	66	42	3
Other cheese	92	72	60	101	84	73
Fromage frais	162	150	13	139	100	18
Yogurt	238	175	44	316	250	44
Other dairy desserts	130	120	18	141	115	21
Ice cream	132	103	45	152	120	52
Eggs	120	99	45	111	91	44
Egg dishes	113	96	10	110	97	15
Butter	32	20	28	34	22	32
Block margarine	32	14	2	22	7	1
Soft margarine, not polyunsaturated	40	18	31	24	17	27
Polyunsaturated margarine	35	24	8	35	28	4
Polyunsaturated oils	8	5	2	9	7	2
Other oils and cooking fats, not polyunsaturated	7	7	5	10	9	6
Polyunsaturated low fat spread	39	23	11	41	32	14
Other low fat spread	35	26	11	44	36	13
Polyunsaturated reduced fat spread	42	35	46	49	37	36
Other reduced fat spread	34	30	18	53	41	23
Bacon & ham	73	57	56	86	59	58
Beef, veal and dishes	268	184	51	247	177	49
Lamb & dishes	195	141	30	147	113	22
Pork & dishes	103	79	25	135	93	29
Coated chicken & turkey	144	114	47	161	132	49
Chicken and turkey dishes	204	123	66	209	150	75
Liver, liver products & dishes	55	20	3	58	40	5
Burgers & kebabs	132	106	41	156	117	33
Sausages	128	92	58	113	84	54
Meat pies & pastries	167	140	51	150	120	40
Other meat & meat products	133	88	25	72	45	21
Coated and/or fried white fish	126	96	47	120	98	43
Other white fish & dishes	167	120	12	168	125	11
Shellfish	51	35	6	69	45	7
Oily fish	94	78	26	98	63	30

Table 4.18(b) female consumers – continued

Type of food	Whether receiving benefits					
	Receiving benefits			Not receiving benefits		
	Mean	Median	% consumers	Mean	Median	% consumers
	g	g	%	g	g	%
Raw carrots	101	50	9	65	42	21
Other raw & salad vegetables	98	63	47	118	84	63
Raw tomatoes	86	60	37	98	67	43
Peas	96	62	52	80	64	48
Green beans	97	56	7	61	49	16
Baked beans	203	155	62	202	155	55
Leafy green vegetables	110	80	37	99	80	46
Carrots–not raw	86	61	54	78	61	54
Tomatoes–not raw	109	102	8	75	67	8
Vegetable dishes	279	163	20	290	179	22
Other vegetables	140	107	55	138	94	64
Potato chips	410	344	92	327	264	86
Other fried/roast potatoes & products	137	118	49	148	116	48
Potato products–not fried	113	100	21	124	93	20
Other potatoes & potato dishes	341	286	79	319	253	81
Savoury snacks	131	113	92	121	111	89
Apples & pears	249	183	58	310	221	57
Citrus fruits	212	140	20	237	180	31
Bananas	200	141	31	199	137	40
Canned fruit in juice	158	115	7	152	113	6
Canned fruit in syrup	143	115	6	128	89	8
Other fruit	239	121	25	236	160	39
Nuts and seeds	54	26	12	39	27	15
Table sugar	54	39	72	52	29	60
Preserves	41	29	35	36	26	34
Sweet spreads, fillings & icings	36	20	16	31	20	21
Sugar confectionery	120	74	74	115	75	63
Chocolate confectionery	151	116	76	140	110	82
Fruit juice	597	430	41	795	553	54
Concentrated soft drinks–not low calorie, as consumed	2223	1355	57	2023	1291	49
Carbonated soft drinks–not low calorie	1081	837	79	1163	778	74
Ready to drink soft drinks–not low calorie	510	297	32	608	505	29
Concentrated soft drinks–low calorie, as consumed	2197	1562	39	2827	1935	49
Carbonated soft drinks–low calorie	918	660	41	1005	610	48
Ready to drink soft drinks–low calorie	607	298	5	502	443	7
Liqueurs	–	–	–	63	69	1
Spirits	99	23	1	85	69	4
Wine	313	313	0	340	143	5
Fortified wine	–	–	–	147	73	1
Low alcohol & alcohol-free wine	–	–	–	308	223	1
Beer & lager	1369	1134	3	1867	1393	6
Low alcohol & alcohol-free beer & lager	–	–	–	531	531	0
Cider & Perry	70	70	0	946	723	1
Alco-pops	485	343	2	999	858	2
Coffee, as consumed	1517	1073	15	1840	902	18
Tea, as consumed	1064	548	50	1246	808	47
Herbal tea, as consumed	971	140	2	482	220	1
Bottled water	817	465	7	646	377	10
Tap water	985	758	60	1052	668	63
Commercial toddler's foods	–	–	–	53	53	0
Other beverages, dry weight	559	297	21	414	260	23
Soup	336	257	25	316	256	28
Savoury sauces, pickles, gravies & condiments	136	104	84	141	104	88
Base = number of young people			*199*			*645*

Table 4.19 Main differences in the eating behaviour of young people by social class, income and receipt of benefits – summary table

Foods less likely to be eaten by:	HOH's classified as manual (compared with non-manual HOHs)	Gross weekly h'hld income less than £160pw (compared with £600pw and over)	Households in receipt of benefits (compared with those not receiving)
Boys	pizza* soft grain bread* semi skimmed milk * cream * yogurt* butter* apples & pears* bananas* other fruit** sweet spreads, fillings & icings* fruit juice** other beverages**	fruit pies** buns, cakes & pastries* semi skimmed milk** cream** other cheese* fromage frais* other dairy desserts* butter* bacon & ham** beef, veal & dishes* other raw & salad vegetables* raw carrots* raw tomatoes* fruit juice**	soft grain bread* fruit pies** semi skimmed milk** cream** other cheese** fromage frais* other dairy desserts** bacon & ham** raw carrots** chocolate confectionery* fruit juice** beer & lager** bottled water* other beverages*
Girls	other cereal-based puddings* cream* other fruit* fruit juice*	other bread* semi skimmed milk** cream* other cheese* egg dishes* other oils & cooking fats, not pufa* other raw & salad vegetables* green beans* other vegetables* other fruit* nuts & seeds* fruit juice** spirits* wine* beer & lager**	other cheese* skimmed milk* raw carrots** other raw & salad vegetables** green beans* citrus fruits* other fruit** fruit juice* wine**

Foods more likely to be eaten by:	HOH's classified as manual (compared with non-manual HOHs)	Gross weekly h'hld income less than £160pw (compared with £600pw and over)	Households in receipt of benefits (compared with those not receiving)
Boys	whole milk**	whole milk** table sugar*	whole milk** table sugar*
Girls	white bread* meat pies & pastries* table sugar* carbonated soft drinks nlc*	whole milk**	whole milk** table sugar* sugar confectionery*

* p < 0.05
** p < 0.01
not pufa: not polyunsaturated

105

5 Energy intake

5.1 Introduction

In this and the following four chapters, data are presented on the intakes of energy and nutrients by young people in the survey who kept a dietary record for the full seven days, a total of 1701 young people (unweighted). Intakes of energy and nutrients are presented separately for boys and girls in each of the four age groups, 4 to 6 years, 7 to 10 years, 11 to 14 years, and 15 to 18 years. Variation in intake of energy and various nutrients according to the main socio-demographic characteristics of the young people and their households is also discussed, and for energy and selected nutrients the percentage of the total intake derived from different food types is shown.

Where appropriate, intakes for groups of young people are compared with the Dietary Reference Values (DRVs) as defined by the Department of Health in the report *Dietary Reference Values for Food Energy and Nutrients for the United Kingdom*[1].

Intake data are presented as average daily amounts, that is the 7-day intake derived from the dietary record averaged to produce a daily intake. For energy and each nutrient the mean and standard deviation of the intakes are given, together with selected points in the cumulative distribution, the 2.5^{th}, 50th (median) and 97.5^{th} percentiles. All the data shown in the tables in this and subsequent chapters have been weighted to adjust both for the differing sample selection probabilities and differential non-response (see *Chapter 1: Section 1.4* and *Appendix D*). Base numbers to tables are shown as unweighted numbers[2].

For energy, the majority of tables show intakes expressed as megajoules (MJ); key tables and textual figures also give kilocalorie values (kcal)[3].

Intake of energy from food eaten during school hours is presented and discussed in Appendix X.

5.2 Intake of energy

As Table 5.3 shows, mean daily energy intake increased with age for boys from 6.39MJ (1520kcal) for those aged 4 to 6 years to 9.60MJ (2285kcal) for those aged 15 to 18 years (p < 0.01). Among girls there was an increase in mean energy intake with age from 5.87MJ (1397kcal) for 4 to 6 year olds to 7.03MJ (1672kcal) for 11 to 14 year olds (p < 0.01), but there was no further increase

for girls aged 15 to 18 years, whose mean energy intake was 6.82MJ (1622kcal), close to that for 7 to 10 year olds 6.72MJ (1598kcal).

In each age group the mean daily energy intake for boys was higher than for girls, the difference increasing with increasing age.

Median energy intakes for both sexes and in all age groups were close to the mean values. However, there was a wide range of intakes in each age and sex group. For example, for those aged 4 to 6 years, intakes at the lower 2.5 percentile were 3.54MJ (841kcal) for boys, and 3.90MJ (927kcal) for girls, while at the upper 2.5 percentile intakes were 8.68MJ (2072kcal) (boys) and 8.58MJ (2038kcal) (girls). In the oldest group of boys, 15 to 18 years, intakes at the lower and upper 2.5 percentiles were 5.57MJ and 13.91MJ (1331kcal and 3303kcal) respectively. Among girls, intakes at the lower and upper 2.5 percentiles showed much less variation by age, indeed, at the lower 2.5 percentile girls aged 15 to 18 years had energy intakes at 3.53MJ (841kcal), lower than the comparable figure for 4 to 6 year-old girls. At the upper 2.5 percentile intakes were 10.08MJ (2399kcal) for girls from the age of 11 years.

(Tables 5.1 and 5.2)

5.2.1 Energy intake and estimated average requirements

Estimates of energy requirements of different population groups are termed 'Estimated Average Requirements' (EARs)[1] and are defined as the energy intake estimated to meet the *average* requirements of the population group. It is expected therefore that approximately 50% of the population group will have requirements above, and 50% requirements below the EAR. Table 5.3 shows the EARs for the eight sex and age groups in the survey, together with the mean energy intakes for each group derived from the dietary record data. Actual intake as a percentage of the appropriate EAR was calculated for each young person and the mean percentages are shown in the table.

Mean energy intakes were below EARs for each sex and age group. Apart from girls aged 15 to 18, mean energy intakes were at least 83% of the appropriate EAR. For example, for the youngest boys mean energy intake was 6.39MJ (1527kcal) compared with an EAR of 7.16MJ (1711kcal), lower by almost 0.77MJ (184kcal), and 89%

of the EAR. For girls aged 15 to 18 years the mean energy intake was 6.82MJ (1630kcal) compared with an EAR of 8.83MJ (2110kcal), and only 77% of the EAR. The low energy intakes of the oldest girls are commented on in Section 5.2.2 below.

Mean energy intakes below EARs have been found for other populations surveyed in the NDNS programme, all of which have used the same dietary methodology. For example, in the survey of pre-school children the mean energy intake expressed as per kilogram body weight for boys and girls aged 3½ to 4½ years was 82% of the EAR for the group, and in the survey of people aged 65 years and over, the mean energy intakes for free-living men and women were 85% and 76% respectively of the EAR[4,5]. As was noted in the reports of these previous surveys, the difference between estimated intakes and EARs could arise from an inadequate energy intake, a biased low estimate of intake, arising from mis-reporting or modifying the diet during the recording period, or an overestimate of energy requirements. In the pre-school children's survey it was suggested that the difference between the EARs for the different age and sex groups and the estimated energy intakes could not be ascribed to methodological errors in assessing the children's intakes, since measures of energy intake and energy expenditure, compared using the doubly-labelled water technique at the stage of the feasibility study, were extremely close and also below the EARs.

In the feasibility study for this survey of young people, estimates of energy intake using the same dietary methodology as in the main stage, were compared with measurements of energy expenditure using the doubly-labelled water methodology[6]. The data showed that the estimates of energy intake for both sexes and most age groups were below both the EARs and measures of energy expenditure; the difference was particularly marked for the oldest group of girls[7]. As a result particular attention was paid in the mainstage survey to improving the quality of the dietary information by probing and checking. However it is likely that the estimates of energy intake particularly for the oldest group of girls are underestimates. This is discussed further in Appendix J (*Under-reporting*) in which a method is used to identify those energy intakes which are implausibly low and likely to be under-reported. This analysis indicates that a substantial proportion of both boys and girls were under-reporting their food consumption and that the proportions increased with age. However it is important to bear in mind the limitations of the method used (see *Appendix J* for further details). *(Table 5.3)*

5.2.2 Energy intakes for girls aged 15 to 18 years

It was noted in Chapter 2 that the feasibility study had highlighted a problem of getting complete and accurate dietary records from the oldest girls and that in the mainstage survey interviewers paid particular attention

to this group in probing and checking their records for completeness and accuracy. The extent to which the reported relatively low energy intakes by the oldest girls may be the result of under-reporting or changed dietary behaviour during the record-keeping period or whether they are, for the most part, accurate estimates of actual intakes during the dietary recording period which also reflect habitual diet, is discussed in Appendix J.

In Chapter 13 the association between energy intake and level of physical activity in both boys and girls is discussed[8]. Others have reported low energy intakes associated with smoking and slimming behaviours[9,10,11,12], and the survey data were therefore examined to see to what extent these behaviours might help explain the particularly low energy intakes for girls aged 15 to 18 years.

Table 5.4 and 5.5 show energy intakes for girls aged 15 to 18 years according to their reported smoking behaviour and whether they were currently dieting to lose weight (as reported in the initial interview).

Mean energy intake was lower for girls who reported usually smoking at least one cigarette a week, 6.61MJ (1580kcal) compared with 7.12MJ (1702kcal) for those reporting never having smoked, although the difference did not reach the level of statistical significance (p > 0.05). There was a similar pattern at the lower and upper extremes of the distribution, with energy intakes being lower for the usual smokers, compared with those who said they had never smoked.

The difference in mean energy intake between girls who reported they were dieting to lose weight and other girls was small, 6.40MJ (1530kcal) compared to 6.89MJ (1647kcal) and not statistically significant, although this may be partly due to the relatively small number of girls reporting dieting to lose weight. The difference was more marked at the lower 2.5 percentile; energy intake was 0.77MJ (184kcal) lower for those dieting than for those not dieting to lose weight. At the upper 2.5 percentile girls aged 15 to 18 years who reported dieting had a slightly higher energy intake than those not dieting – 10.39MJ (2483kcal) compared with 9.90MJ (2366kcal). Appendix J presents the results of a separate analysis of those reporting dieting to lose weight in relation to under-reporting. *(Tables 5.4 and 5.5)*

5.2.3 Young people who were unwell

In the interview at the end of the 7-day dietary recording period 18% of boys and 20% of girls reported being unwell on at least one of the record-keeping days. Of these, about half said that on the day or days when they had been unwell their eating had been affected.

Table 5.6 shows the energy intakes of young people who reported being unwell according to whether their eating was affected, together with intakes for those who had not been unwell.

As might be expected, the mean energy intakes of those who reported being unwell were lower than those who had not been unwell, and for those whose eating had been affected, intakes were the lowest. Among boys mean energy intakes ranged from 7.10MJ (1697kcal) for those whose eating was affected by being unwell to 8.16MJ (1950kcal) for the not unwell group (p < 0.01). Among girls there was a difference of 1.15MJ (275kcal) between the mean intakes of those who were not unwell 6.78MJ (1620kcal) and those whose eating had been affected by being unwell at some time over the 7-day period 5.63MJ (1346kcal) (p < 0.01).   (Table 5.6)

5.3   Macronutrient contribution to energy intake

Chapters 6 and 7 give detailed information on intakes of protein, carbohydrates, alcohol and fat. The average contribution of these macronutrients to intake of food energy and total energy, that is including alcohol, for young people in the survey is shown in Table 5.7.

Among boys just over half, 52%, of their food energy on average was derived from carbohydrate, just over a third, 35%, from total fat and 13% from protein. Among girls, the proportions were very similar, on average 51% of their food energy came from carbohydrate, 36% from total fat and 13% from protein.

There was very little variation by age for either boys or girls in the contribution made by macronutrients to food energy; the data suggest the contribution of protein to food energy intake increased slightly with increasing age (ns), the contribution of carbohydrate decreased slightly with increasing age (ns), and the contribution from total fat showed no clear association with age.

Not surprisingly the contribution of alcohol to the total energy intake of boys and girls between the ages of 4 and 14 years was negligible, less than 0.5%. In the top age band, 15 to 18 years, alcohol contributed about 2% to the total energy intake of boys and about 1% to the total energy intake of girls.   (Table 5.7)

5.4   Variation in energy intake

Caveat
In this section and in other chapters which look at variation in intake of nutrients, inter-relationships between the main classificatory variables, for example, between gross weekly household income and whether the young person's parents were receiving benefits, need to be borne in mind when interpreting the results. It should also be remembered that there is significant variation in the age distribution of young people by household type and by gross weekly household income and any variation associated with these characteristics may be partly accounted for by variation by age[13]. Because of the limited overall achieved sample size it has not been possible to present tables of distributions and

descriptive statistics for the various socio-demographic and other sub-groups within sex and age group. However in the later chapters dealing with variation in the physiological measures, blood pressure and anthropometry and in Chapter 13 on physical activity, the technique of multiple regression is used to identify characteristics independently associated with variation in the main outcome measure.

Tables 5.8 to 5.13 show the distribution of energy intake for different sub-groups in the sample of young people.

Region
Despite there being considerable variation in the types of foods eaten by young people according to the region in which they lived, there was very little difference between the mean energy intakes in each region, and none reached the level of statistical significance.

For boys mean energy intake ranged from 7.88MJ (1883kcal) for those living in Scotland to 8.07MJ (1929kcal) for those living in the Central and South West regions of England and in Wales. At the lower 2.5 percentile boys from London and the South East had the lowest energy intake, 4.17MJ (997kcal), compared with 4.91MJ (1174kcal) for boys in Scotland.

For girls mean energy intake ranged from 6.36MJ (1520kcal) per day for girls in Scotland to 6.78MJ (1620kcal) for girls in the Northern region (ns).
        (Table 5.8)

Fieldwork wave[14]
It was noted in Chapter 4 (see *Section 4.4*) that there were very few clear patterns associated with fieldwork wave in the types of foods eaten by young people and hence it is not surprising that energy intakes also showed no significant variation by fieldwork wave. Indeed for girls mean energy intake varied by no more than 0.13MJ (31kcal) between waves.

Boys who kept dietary records during Wave 3 of fieldwork, July to September, had a somewhat higher mean energy intake than other boys, 8.33MJ (1991kcal) compared with, for example, 7.89MJ (1886kcal) in Wave 4 (ns). Boys in Wave 3 also had higher energy intakes at the lower and upper 2.5 percentiles. However there were no obvious differences in the types of foods eaten by boys in Wave 3 that would account for this.
        (Table 5.9)

Household type
Boys living with both parents, but with no other children in the household had a significantly higher energy intake than other boys. Their mean energy intake was 8.98MJ (2147kcal) compared with 7.72MJ (1845kcal) for boys living with only one parent (p < 0.01). This difference existed also at the lower and upper 2.5 percentile levels, for example at the lower 2.5 percentile level boys living with one parent had an

energy intake of 3.54MJ (846kcal) compared with 5.34MJ (1276kcal) for boys living with both parents and no other children. However it should be noted that this difference is more likely to be associated with differences in the age structure of the groups than differences in eating behaviour, since over half the boys living with both parents and no other children were aged 15 to 18 years, whereas only about a quarter of the boys in single-parent families were aged 15 to 18 years (see *Table 3.19*).

Although there were the same differences in the age structure of the household types for girls in the sample, the effect on the mean energy intakes is less apparent, since it has already been shown that there was not a consistent rise in mean energy intake throughout the age range for girls. Table 5.10 shows that mean energy intake varied by only 0.14MJ (34kcal) between girls living with both parents and no other children 6.76MJ (1616kcal) and girls living with both parents and other children 6.62MJ (1582kcal) (ns).   *(Table 5.10)*

Social class
Mean energy intakes for young people from non-manual and manual home backgrounds were very similar; for example for boys mean intake was 8.14MJ (1946kcal) for those from a non-manual home background and 8.01MJ (1914kcal) for those from a manual home background (ns). At the upper 2.5 percentile of the distribution energy intake for boys from a manual background was 13.32MJ (3183kcal), compared with 12.60MJ (3011kcal) for boys from a non-manual background.   *(Table 5.11)*

Measures of income level
Among boys, but not girls, there was a marked difference in mean energy intake depending on whether the family was in receipt of state benefits. Boys living in households receiving benefits had a mean energy intake of 7.22MJ (1726kcal), significantly below that for boys living in non-benefit households, 8.27MJ (1976kcal) (p < 0.01).

Similar differences were found at the lower end of the distribution for both boys and girls, with those living in benefit households having lower energy intakes than others. However, at the upper end of the distribution for girls, those in benefit households had a higher energy intake than those in non-benefit households, 10.09MJ (2411kcal) compared with 9.47MJ (2263kcal).

The pattern was similar in relation to energy intake and household income in that there was a general increase in mean energy intake for both boys and girls associated with an increase in the gross weekly household income level. As noted above, this may be partly associated with differences in the age distribution between income groups, the proportion of the oldest group of boys and girls being significantly higher in the top compared with the bottom income group (see *Table 3.26*).

Among boys mean energy intake ranged from 7.39MJ (1766kcal) for boys living in households where the gross income was below £160 a week, to 8.50MJ (2031kcal) for boys in households with a gross weekly income of £400 to less than £600 (p < 0.01). For girls mean energy intake ranged from 6.53MJ (1561kcal) for girls in the lowest household income group to 6.77MJ (1618kcal) for those in households with a gross weekly income of £600 or more (ns). For boys, but not girls, there was a similar pattern at the lower 2.5 percentile of the distribution, with the lowest intake being for boys in households with the lowest income, 3.54MJ (846kcal) and the highest energy intake by those in the highest income households, 5.33MJ (1274kcal). At the upper 2.5 percentile the relationship between energy intake and household income was less clear for boys and girls. Among girls, the data show that intakes were higher for girls in the lowest income households, 10.37MJ (2478kcal) compared with 9.27MJ (2215kcal) for girls in households where the gross income was over £600 a week.   *(Tables 5.12 and 5.13)*

5.5 Contribution of main food types to intake of energy
Table 5.14 shows the average contribution of the major food types to the energy intake for young people by age group; data are shown separately for boys and girls.

For boys and girls in each age group the largest contribution to energy intake came from the consumption of cereals and cereal products, providing about one third of the average intake (35% for boys and 33% for girls). This is a slightly higher proportion than was found for pre-school children in the 1992/93 NDNS, where cereals and cereal products provided about 30% of mean energy intake[4]. There were no significant differences in the contribution of cereals and cereal products by age group for either boys or girls. The main contributors to energy intake within the cereals and cereal products group were bread, which provided 11% of energy intake for all young people, and biscuits, buns, cakes and pastries (10%). Breakfast cereals contributed 7% to the energy intake of boys and 5% to the energy intake of girls.

Overall boys obtained 16%, and girls 18%, of their energy intake from the consumption of vegetables, including 6% from potato chips and about 5% from savoury snacks. Among boys the contribution made by vegetables, potatoes and savoury snacks was fairly similar for each age group. Among girls the contribution appeared to increase with age up to the 11 to 14 age group, although this trend did not reach statistical significance (p > 0.05).

Overall boys obtained 14% and girls 13% of their energy from meat and meat products and the data suggest a steady increase for boys in this contribution with increasing age. For example among boys, those aged 4 to 6 years obtained 11% of their energy from meat and meat products compared with 16% for boys aged 15 to 18 years (ns).

We have already shown that the amount of milk consumed, and in particular whole milk, declined as age increased (see *Chapter 4: Sections 4.2.1* and *4.3.3*); this is reflected in the proportion of energy obtained by young people from milk and milk products which tended to decline with age, ranging from 16% for girls aged 4 to 6 years, to 9% for girls aged 15 to 18 years (ns). Whole milk contributed 6% and 7% to energy intake for boys and girls aged 4 to 6 years, and 2% for both sexes aged 15 to 18 years (ns). Reduced fat milk, that is semi-skimmed and skimmed milk, contributed 3% to energy intake for boys and 2% for girls; this contribution was fairly constant across the age groups.

Sugar, preserves and confectionery provided 9% of the energy of the young people in the survey, of which more than half (5%) came from chocolate confectionery.

Overall young people obtained 6% of their energy from drinks, of which the majority, 4%, came from the consumption of soft drinks which were not low calorie. Alcoholic drinks contributed less than 0.5% to energy intake (see also *Chapter 6 Section 6.5.2* for further information on alcohol intakes). *(Table 5.14)*

Figures 5.1 to 5.4 show the contribution of the main food types to average daily energy intake for different subgroups in the sample of young people, that is by region, social class of head of household, whether the young person's 'parents' were in receipt of benefits, and gross weekly household income.

It has already been shown in Chapter 4 that there was some variation in the types and quantities of different foods eaten by young people living in different parts of Great Britain, for example, young people living in the Northern region were more likely to have eaten fried or coated white fish than young people living elsewhere, and young people in Scotland were more likely to have eaten confectionery. To some extent these variations are reflected in differences in the contribution of different foods to the average daily energy intake. However regional differences in the contribution of the main food types to average daily energy intake are generally less marked than the regional variation in dietary habits and none reached the level of statistical significance (p > 0.05). The data do suggest that both boys and girls living in London and the South East obtained a slightly higher proportion of their energy from cereals and cereal products (36% for boys and 35% for girls) than young people living elsewhere. The proportion of energy obtained from the consumption of sugar, preserves and confectionery was highest for boys living in Scotland (11%), while girls in Scotland appear to have obtained more of their energy from meat and meat products (14%) than other girls. The proportion of

energy from vegetables, potatoes and savoury snacks (17%) was somewhat higher for boys in the Northern region than for other boys. Girls in London and the South East obtained a somewhat lower proportion of their energy intake from vegetables, potatoes and savoury snacks, 17%, than girls in Scotland, 19%.

Differences in the percentage contribution of main food types to average daily energy intake of young people according to whether the head of household was in a non-manual or manual social class were also small and did not reach statistical significance (p > 0.05). The data do suggest that both boys and girls from a manual home background obtained a slightly higher proportion of their energy intake than did those from a non-manual background from the consumption of vegetables, which includes all forms of potatoes and savoury snacks (19% compared with 17%). Girls from a manual home background appear to have obtained less energy from cereals and cereal products (32%) than girls living in non-manual households (34%), and the same trend is apparent in the data for boys, but for both sexes the differences are not statistically significant (p > 0.05).

Boys living in households where one or both parents were currently receiving Income Support, Family Credit or Job Seeker's Allowance obtained a somewhat higher proportion of their average daily intake of energy from vegetables, potatoes and savoury snacks (19%) and a somewhat smaller proportion of energy from drinks (5%) compared with boys in households where these benefits were not being received (15% and 7%) (ns). Among girls there were similar, but smaller differences, 20% of energy came from vegetables, potatoes and savoury snacks and 5% from drinks for girls in households receiving benefits, compared with 17% and 6% for girls in households not receiving benefits (ns).

Although the differences did not reach the level of statistical significance (p > 0.05) the data suggest that there were a number of trends associated with gross weekly household income for both boys and girls in the percentage contribution to energy intake made by different food types.

For both sexes the percentage contribution to energy intake made by milk and milk products, and by drinks tended to increase with income group. For example, for those in the lowest gross weekly household income group, less than £160, drinks contributed about 5% to average daily energy intake for boys and girls. In the highest income group, £600 a week or more, drinks contributed 8% to average daily energy intake.

In contrast the contribution to average daily energy intake made by meat and meat products, and by vegetables, potatoes and savoury snacks, tended to decrease with increasing gross weekly household income. For example, girls in the lowest household income group obtained 20% of their average daily energy intake from vegetables, potatoes and savoury snacks, compared with 15% for girls in the highest income group. *(Figures 5.1 to 5.4)*

5.6 Comparisons with other studies

Table 5.15 compares data from this present survey of young people with equivalent data on energy intake from other national surveys, including the 1983 Department of Health study of the Diets of British Schoolchildren[4,15,16].

The youngest age group for which comparative data are available are for children aged 3½ to 4½ years, from the NDNS of pre-school children[4], carried out in 1992/3, compared with 4 to 6 year olds in this present survey. Not surprisingly, for both boys and girls the mean energy intake for the slightly older age group was greater than for the younger children, but the proportion of energy provided by protein, carbohydrate and total fat was broadly similar.

Comparative data for 10 to 11 year olds collected in 1983 shows a decrease over time in the mean energy intake for both boys and girls. For both boys and girls average energy intake has decreased by about 0.6MJ (143kcal) between 1983 and 1997. There also appears to have been a decline in the proportion of energy derived from total fat, for example, for boys from 37.4% in 1983 to 35.7% in 1997, and a corresponding increase in the proportion of energy derived from protein and carbohydrates. This is consistent with population trends seen in the National Food Survey (NFS)[17].

The same pattern is apparent for 14 to 15 year olds; mean daily energy intake has decreased over time, for example from 7.85MJ for girls in 1983 to 6.90MJ in 1997, and at the same time the contribution of total fat to energy intake has decreased.

Comparisons between the average energy intake of 16 to 24 year olds in 1986/7 Dietary and Nutritional Survey of British Adults and 15 to 18 year olds in this survey show a higher average energy intake in the older age group, but again suggest that the proportion of energy derived from total fat has fallen over time while the contribution from carbohydrates has increased. For example, for females aged 16 to 24 years, total fat contributed 39.8% to food energy intake in the 1986/7 survey, compared with 35.9% for females aged 15 to 18 years in this present survey, which is again consistent with data from the NFS[17].

Table 5.16 shows data on energy intakes and the contribution of macronutrients to energy intake taken from a variety of other published studies. It should be noted that these have mainly focussed on special population sub-groups or geographic areas and are generally not representative of the whole population of young people in the age group. Moreover, not all of the studies have used a weighed intake dietary methodology

and many had only a small sample size; these factors need to be taken into account when comparing with data from this present survey.

Nevertheless the other available data confirm the findings from this survey that generally intake of energy is below the Estimated Average Requirement for each age group and sex, that with increasing age the proportion of energy obtained from protein increases, from carbohydrate decreases, and from total fat shows little variation with age. *(Tables 5.15 and 5.16)*

References and endnotes

1 Department of Health. Report on Health and Social Subjects: 41. *Dietary Reference Values for Food Energy and Nutrients for the United Kingdom.* HMSO (London, 1991).

2 Tables showing the weighted base numbers by sex of the young person for key socio-demographic characteristics are given in Appendix R.

3 Calculated values quoted in the text are based on a conversion factor of 1kcal = 4.184 kJ. Table 5.2 shows average daily energy intake in kcals produced from analysis of the dataset. The small differences between these kcal values and equivalent values calculated using the conversion factor are due to rounding.

4 Gregory JR, Collins DL, Davies PSW, Hughes JM, Clarke PC. *National Diet and Nutrition Survey: children aged 1½ to 4½ years. Volume 1: Report of the diet and nutrition survey.* HMSO (London,1995).

5 Finch S, Doyle W, Lowe C, Bates CJ, Prentice A, Smithers G, Clarke PC. *National Diet and Nutrition Survey: people aged 65 years and over. Volume 1: Report of the diet and nutrition survey.* TSO (London, 1998).

6 Lowe S. *Feasibility study for the National Diet and Nutrition Survey: young people aged 4 to 18 years.* ONS *(In preparation).*

7 Smithers G, Gregory J, Coward WA, Wright A, Elsom R, Wenlock R. British National Diet and Nutrition Survey of young people aged 4 to 18 years: feasibility study of the dietary assessment methodology. Abstracts of the Third International conference on Dietary Assessment Methods. *Eur J Clin Nutr* 1998; **52**: S2. S76.

8 See Chapter 13: Section 13.5

9 Blading J. *Young people in 1994.* University of Exeter. Schools Health Education Unit. (Exeter,1995)

10 Hill AJ. Pre-adolescent dieting: implications for eating disorders. *Int Rev Psychiatry* 1993; **5**: 87-100.

11 Hill AJ. The socio-cultural context of children's eating. In *Making Sense of Food. Children in Focus.* Conference proceedings, October 1993. National Dairy Council. (London, 1993).

12 Bull NL. Dietary habits of 15 to 25 year olds. *Humn Nutr: Appl. Nutr* 1985; **35A**: Suppl. 1-68.

13 Chapter 3 includes information on the inter-relationships between the main socio-economic variables and gives tables of distributions for household type and gross weekly household income by sex and age group of young person – Tables 3.19 and 3.26.

14 See Appendix U 'Glossary' for information on the derivation of fieldwork wave for analysis purposes.

15 Gregory J, Foster K, Tyler H, Wiseman M. *The Dietary and Nutritional Survey of British Adults.* HMSO (London, 1990).

16 Department of Health. *The Diets of British Schoolchildren.* HMSO (London, 1989).

17 Ministry of Agriculture, Fisheries and Food. *National Food Survey 1998.* TSO (London, 1999).

Table 5.1 Average daily energy intake (MJ) by sex and age of young person

Energy intake (MJ)	Age (years)				All
	4–6	7–10	11–14	15–18	
	cum %	cum %	cum %	cum %	cum %
Males					
Less than 4.00	3	0	1	1	1
Less than 5.00	13	4	4	2	5
Less than 6.00	35	14	10	5	15
Less than 7.00	70	38	22	11	33
Less than 8.00	92	68	43	25	56
Less than 9.00	99	86	65	45	73
Less than 10.00	99	95	84	58	83
Less than 11.00	100	98	96	83	92
All		100	100	100	100
Base	*184*	*256*	*237*	*179*	*856*
Mean (average value)	6.39	7.47	8.28	9.60	8.01
Median	6.35	7.31	8.32	9.65	7.76
Lower 2.5 percentile	3.54	4.68	4.69	5.57	4.54
Upper 2.5 percentile	8.68	10.50	11.46	13.91	12.86
Standard deviation	1.27	1.49	1.83	2.36	2.13
	cum %	cum %	cum %	cum %	cum %
Females					
Less than 4.00	4	2	2	4	3
Less than 5.00	20	7	9	18	13
Less than 6.00	57	28	26	32	34
Less than 7.00	86	59	50	56	61
Less than 8.00	97	84	71	71	80
Less than 9.00	99	98	91	91	94
All	100	100	100	100	100
Base	*171*	*226*	*238*	*210*	*845*
Mean (average value)	5.87	6.72	7.03	6.82	6.65
Median	5.73	6.72	6.98	6.67	6.55
Lower 2.5 percentile	3.90	4.15	4.08	3.53	3.92
Upper 2.5 percentile	8.58	8.81	10.09	10.08	9.77
Standard deviation	1.15	1.18	1.56	1.75	1.50

Table 5.2 Average daily energy intake (kcal) by sex and age of young person

Energy intake (kcal)	Age (years) 4–6	7–10	11–14	15–18	All
	cum %	cum %	cum %	cum %	cum %
Males					
Less than 1000	5	0	1	0	1
Less than 1250	18	5	5	1	7
Less than 1500	47	20	14	6	20
Less than 1750	78	51	29	18	42
Less than 2000	97	76	53	33	63
Less than 2250	99	92	76	49	78
Less than 2500	100	98	91	65	88
Less than 2750		99	98	80	94
All		100	100	100	100
Base	*184*	*256*	*237*	*179*	*856*
Mean (average value)	1520	1777	1968	2285	1905
Median	1513	1739	1979	2296	1844
Lower 2.5 percentile	841	1113	1116	1331	1080
Upper 2.5 percentile	2072	2492	2738	3303	3056
Standard deviation	303	354	435	561	507
	cum %	cum %	cum %	cum %	cum %
Females					
Less than 1000	5	3	4	5	4
Less than 1250	30	10	13	19	17
Less than 1500	63	34	35	38	41
Less than 1750	92	72	59	63	70
Less than 2000	97	92	82	77	86
Less than 2250	99	99	94	95	97
All	100	100	100	100	100
Base	*171*	*226*	*138*	*210*	*845*
Mean (average value)	1397	1598	1672	1622	1582
Median	1368	1600	1660	1590	1561
Lower 2.5 percentile	927	987	972	841	932
Upper 2.5 percentile	2038	2104	2401	2399	2322
Standard deviation	275	281	371	417	357

Table 5.3 Average daily energy intake (MJ) as a percentage of the estimated average requirement (EAR) by sex and age of young person*

Sex and age of young person	Mean energy intake (MJ)	EAR (MJ)	Intake as % EAR**	*Base*
Males aged (years)				
4–6	6.39	7.16	89%	*184*
7–10	7.47	8.24	91%	*256*
11–14	8.28	9.27	89%	*237*
15–18	9.60	11.51	83%	*179*
Females aged (years)				
4–6	5.87	6.46	91%	*171*
7–10	6.72	7.28	92%	*226*
11–14	7.03	7.92	89%	*238*
15–18	6.82	8.83	77%	*210*

* Department of Health. Report on Health and Social Subjects: 41. *Dietary Reference Values for Food Energy and Nutrients for the United Kingdom.* HMSO (London, 1991).
** Energy intake as a percentage of EAR was calculated for each young person using the EAR appropriate for age and sex.

Table 5.4 Average daily energy intake (MJ) by reported smoking behaviour for girls aged 15 to 18 years

Girls aged 15 to 18 years – diary sample

Energy intake (MJ)	Whether ever smoked					All*
	Never smoked	Only tried once	Used to, but not now	Sometimes, but < 1 a week	Usually smokes	
Mean (average value)	7.12	6.86	6.48	7.04	6.61	6.82
Median	7.24	6.55	6.03	6.92	6.43	6.67
Lower 2.5 percentile	3.90	4.36	3.74	4.16	2.76	3.53
Upper 2.5 percentile	11.03	9.86	9.33	11.21	10.08	10.08
Standard deviation	1.60	1.65	1.95	1.69	1.82	1.75
Base	*65*	*38*	*27***	*17***	*60*	*210*

* Includes girls aged 15 to 18 not answering smoking behaviour questions.
** Small base numbers; results for this group should be treated with caution.

Table 5.5 Average daily energy intake (MJ) by whether currently dieting to lose weight for girls aged 15 to 18 years

Girls aged 15 to 18 years – diary sample

Energy intake (MJ)	Whether currently dieting to lose weight		All
	Dieting	Not dieting	
Mean (average value)	6.40	6.89	6.82
Median	6.43	6.67	6.67
Lower 2.5 percentile	2.76	3.53	3.53
Upper 2.5 percentile	10.39	9.90	10.08
Standard deviation	1.81	1.72	1.75
Base	*34*	*176*	*210*

Table 5.6 Average daily energy intake (MJ) by whether young person was reported as being unwell during the dietary recording period by sex

Energy intake (MJ)	Whether unwell during period			All
	Unwell and eating affected	Unwell and eating not affected	Not unwell	
	cum %	cum %	cum %	cum %
Males				
Less than 4.00	5	3	0	1
Less than 5.00	15	16	3	5
Less than 6.00	31	24	12	15
Less than 7.00	50	34	32	33
Less than 8.00	64	63	54	56
Less than 9.00	83	81	71	73
Less than 10.00	94	88	82	83
Less than 11.00	98	97	90	92
All	100	100	100	100
Base	*86*	*66*	*704*	*856*
Mean (average value)	7.10	7.55	8.16	8.01
Median	7.03	7.72	7.85	7.76
Lower 2.5 percentile	2.57	3.54	4.90	4.54
Upper 2.5 percentile	10.99	12.83	12.97	12.86
Standard deviation	2.05	2.09	2.11	2.13
	cum %	cum %	cum %	cum %
Females				
Less than 4.00	9	1	2	3
Less than 5.00	38	11	10	13
Less than 6.00	62	28	32	34
Less than 7.00	83	59	59	61
Less than 8.00	95	78	78	80
Less than 9.00	99	94	94	94
All	100	100	100	100
Base	*93*	*84*	*668*	*845*
Mean (average value)	5.63	6.71	6.78	6.65
Median	5.46	6.58	6.67	6.55
Lower 2.5 percentile	2.77	4.20	4.06	3.92
Upper 2.5 percentile	8.68	9.38	9.85	9.77
Standard deviation	1.42	1.38	1.47	1.50

Table 5.7 Macronutrient contribution to total and food energy intake by sex and age of young person

	Sex and age of young person									
	Males aged (years):				All	Females aged (years):				All
	4–6	7–10	11–14	15–18		4–6	7–10	11–14	15–18	
Average daily intake:										
Total energy MJ	6.39	7.47	8.28	9.60	8.01	5.87	6.72	7.03	6.82	6.65
Food energy MJ	6.39	7.47	8.27	9.37	7.95	5.87	6.72	7.02	6.69	6.61
Protein (g)	49.0	54.8	64.0	76.5	61.6	44.5	51.2	52.9	54.8	51.2
Carbohydrate (g)	209	248	271	301	260	191	218	228	214	214
Total fat (g)	60.1	69.8	77.2	89.0	74.7	55.9	63.8	67.2	64.0	63.1
Alcohol (g)	0.01	0.01	0.10	6.79	1.79	0.01	0.02	0.11	3.44	0.93
Percentage food energy from:										
Protein (%)	12.9	12.4	13.1	13.9	13.1	12.7	12.8	12.7	13.9	13.1
Carbohydrate (%)	51.6	52.4	51.7	50.5	51.6	51.4	51.3	51.2	50.6	51.1
Total fat (%)	35.5	35.2	35.2	35.9	35.4	35.9	35.9	36.1	35.9	35.9
Percentage total energy from:										
Protein (%)	12.9	12.4	13.1	13.6	13.0	12.7	12.8	12.7	13.6	13.0
Carbohydrate (%)	51.6	52.4	51.7	49.3	51.2	51.4	51.3	51.1	49.7	50.8
Total fat (%)	35.5	35.2	35.2	35.1	35.2	35.9	35.9	36.1	35.2	35.8
Alcohol (%)	<0.1	<0.1	<0.1	1.9	0.5	<0.1	<0.1	<0.1	1.4	0.4
Base	*184*	*256*	*237*	*179*	*856*	*171*	*226*	*238*	*210*	*845*

Table 5.8 Average daily energy intake (MJ) by region and sex of young person

Energy intake (MJ)	Region				All
	Scotland	Northern	Central, South West & Wales	London & the South East	
	cum %	cum %	cum %	cum %	cum %
Males					
Less than 4.00	–	1	0	2	1
Less than 5.00	4	6	4	6	5
Less than 6.00	15	15	12	18	15
Less than 7.00	37	34	31	35	33
Less than 8.00	63	55	53	58	56
Less than 9.00	75	72	74	72	73
Less than 10.00	84	82	84	84	83
Less than 11.00	90	92	94	89	92
All	100	100	100	100	100
Base	*68*	*243*	*300*	*245*	*856*
Mean (average value)	7.88	7.99	8.07	7.98	8.01
Median	7.26	7.86	7.88	7.59	7.76
Lower 2.5 percentile	4.91	4.47	4.81	4.17	4.54
Upper 2.5 percentile	13.91	12.33	12.44	12.85	12.86
Standard deviation	2.11	2.13	2.02	2.26	2.13
	cum %	cum %	cum %	cum %	cum %
Females					
Less than 4.00	5	2	2	4	3
Less than 5.00	15	9	13	17	13
Less than 6.00	39	32	35	35	34
Less than 7.00	71	57	60	64	61
Less than 8.00	84	79	78	82	80
Less than 9.00	95	95	93	96	94
All	100	100	100	100	100
Base	*69*	*217*	*306*	*253*	*845*
Mean (average value)	6.36	6.78	6.72	6.51	6.65
Median	6.39	6.73	6.62	6.43	6.55
Lower 2.5 percentile	3.36	4.35	4.00	3.65	3.92
Upper 2.5 percentile	9.54	9.68	9.93	9.38	9.77
Standard deviation	1.45	1.43	1.55	1.50	1.50

Table 5.9 Average daily energy intake (MJ) by fieldwork wave and sex of young person

Energy intake (MJ)	Fieldwork wave				All
	Wave 1 Jan–March	Wave 2 April–June	Wave 3 July–Sept	Wave 4 Oct–Dec	
	cum %	cum %	cum %	cum %	cum %
Males					
Less than 4.00	1	2	–	1	1
Less than 5.00	6	7	3	5	5
Less than 6.00	15	17	15	13	15
Less than 7.00	33	35	32	34	33
Less than 8.00	56	55	48	62	56
Less than 9.00	76	72	66	77	73
Less than 10.00	84	85	78	85	83
Less than 11.00	91	93	88	94	92
All	100	100	100	100	100
Base	*199*	*176*	*230*	*251*	*856*
Mean (average value)	7.94	7.94	8.33	7.89	8.01
Median	7.69	7.74	8.16	7.66	7.76
Lower 2.5 percentile	4.47	4.33	4.78	4.54	4.54
Upper 2.5 percentile	12.96	12.60	13.61	12.24	12.86
Standard deviation	2.09	2.14	2.21	2.08	2.13
	cum %	cum %	cum %	cum %	cum %
Females					
Less than 4.00	5	3	3	2	3
Less than 5.00	13	15	14	11	13
Less than 6.00	34	39	35	29	34
Less than 7.00	58	59	66	63	61
Less than 8.00	75	78	85	81	80
Less than 9.00	94	95	95	94	94
All	100	100	100	100	100
Base	*180*	*198*	*240*	*227*	*845*
Mean (average value)	6.69	6.62	6.58	6.71	6.65
Median	6.64	6.54	6.50	6.52	6.55
Lower 2.5 percentile	3.74	3.69	3.92	4.15	3.92
Upper 2.5 percentile	9.27	10.08	9.38	9.85	9.77
Standard deviation	1.53	1.58	1.45	1.43	1.50

Table 5.10 Average daily energy intake (MJ) by whether young person was living with both parents and sex of young person

Energy intake (MJ)	Whether living with both parents			All*
	Both parents and other children	Both parents and no other children	Single parent with/without other children	
	cum %	cum %	cum %	cum %
Males				
Less than 4.00	1	0	3	1
Less than 5.00	5	2	10	5
Less than 6.00	15	7	23	15
Less than 7.00	36	18	41	33
Less than 8.00	60	35	65	56
Less than 9.00	77	56	78	73
Less than 10.00	88	70	84	83
Less than 11.00	94	85	90	92
All	100	100	100	100
Base	*528*	*169*	*157*	*856*
Mean (average value)	7.77	8.98	7.72	8.01
Median	7.53	8.59	7.59	7.76
Lower 2.5 percentile	4.67	5.34	3.54	4.54
Upper 2.5 percentile	12.15	13.67	13.40	12.86
Standard deviation	1.83	2.36	2.46	2.13
	cum %	cum %	cum %	cum %
Females				
Less than 4.00	2	4	3	3
Less than 5.00	11	15	17	13
Less than 6.00	34	35	33	34
Less than 7.00	62	59	61	61
Less than 8.00	82	72	80	80
Less than 9.00	97	91	91	94
All	100	100	100	100
Base	*498*	*173*	*167*	*845*
Mean (average value)	6.62	6.76	6.66	6.65
Median	6.51	6.66	6.58	6.55
Lower 2.5 percentile	4.03	3.74	3.96	3.92
Upper 2.5 percentile	9.24	9.85	10.12	9.77
Standard deviation	1.37	1.70	1.63	1.50

* Includes nine young people (unweighted), two boys and seven girls, who were living with others, not parents.

Table 5.11 Average daily energy intake (MJ) by social class of head of household and sex of young person

Energy intake (MJ)	Social class of head of household		All*
	Non manual	Manual	
	cum %	cum %	cum %
Males			
Less than 4.00	1	1	1
Less than 5.00	3	5	5
Less than 6.00	12	15	15
Less than 7.00	30	35	33
Less than 8.00	52	57	56
Less than 9.00	71	73	73
Less than 10.00	82	83	83
Less than 11.00	91	91	92
All	100	100	100
Base	*414*	*385*	*856*
Mean (average value)	8.14	8.01	8.01
Median	7.89	7.71	7.76
Lower 2.5 percentile	4.58	4.71	4.54
Upper 2.5 percentile	12.60	13.32	12.86
Standard deviation	2.12	2.12	2.13
	cum %	cum %	cum %
Females			
Less than 4.00	3	2	3
Less than 5.00	13	11	13
Less than 6.00	29	39	34
Less than 7.00	58	65	61
Less than 8.00	79	80	80
Less than 9.00	95	94	94
All	100	100	100
Base	*401*	*361*	*845*
Mean (average value)	6.77	6.59	6.65
Median	6.74	6.38	6.55
Lower 2.5 percentile	3.92	4.10	3.92
Upper 2.5 percentile	9.72	9.71	9.77
Standard deviation	1.49	1.46	1.50

* Includes those for whom a social class could not be assigned.

Table 5.12 Average daily energy intake (MJ) by whether young person's 'parents' were receiving certain benefits and and sex of young person

Energy intake (MJ)	Whether receiving benefits		All
	Receiving benefits	Not receiving benefits	
	cum %	cum %	cum %
Males			
Less than 4.00	3	0	1
Less than 5.00	13	3	5
Less than 6.00	26	11	15
Less than 7.00	48	29	33
Less than 8.00	72	50	56
Less than 9.00	82	70	73
Less than 10.00	92	80	83
Less than 11.00	94	91	92
All	100	100	100
Base	*189*	*666*	*856*
Mean (average value)	7.22	8.27	8.01
Median	7.03	7.97	7.76
Lower 2.5 percentile	3.54	4.92	4.54
Upper 2.5 percentile	11.94	13.00	12.86
Standard deviation	2.04	2.10	2.13
	cum %	cum %	cum %
Females			
Less than 4.00	5	2	3
Less than 5.00	16	12	13
Less than 6.00	32	35	34
Less than 7.00	60	62	61
Less than 8.00	80	80	80
Less than 9.00	91	96	94
All	100	100	100
Base	*199*	*645*	*845*
Mean (average value)	6.64	6.66	6.65
Median	6.57	6.54	6.55
Lower 2.5 percentile	3.58	4.08	3.92
Upper 2.5 percentile	10.09	9.47	9.77
Standard deviation	1.62	1.45	1.50

Table 5.13 Average daily energy intake (MJ) by gross weekly household income and sex of young person

Energy intake (MJ)	Gross weekly household income					All*
	Less than £160	£160 to less than £280	£280 to less than £400	£400 to less than £600	£600 and over	
	cum %	cum %	cum %	cum %	cum %	cum %
Males						
Less than 4.00	4	2	–	–	–	1
Less than 5.00	12	13	2	0	1	5
Less than 6.00	25	22	13	6	11	15
Less than 7.00	47	40	32	23	29	33
Less than 8.00	72	65	52	47	48	56
Less than 9.00	80	82	68	67	70	73
Less than 10.00	89	90	79	80	82	83
Less than 11.00	92	95	92	89	91	92
All	100	100	100	100	100	100
Base	*133*	*159*	*157*	*173*	*208*	*856*
Mean (average value)	7.39	7.45	8.19	8.50	8.27	8.01
Median	7.08	7.38	7.82	8.18	8.17	7.76
Lower 2.5 percentile	3.54	4.17	5.04	5.30	5.33	4.54
Upper 2.5 percentile	13.06	11.94	12.42	13.41	12.15	12.86
Standard deviation	2.24	2.04	2.08	1.92	2.12	2.13
	cum %	cum %	cum %	cum %	cum %	cum %
Females						
Less than 4.00	5	2	1	3	3	3
Less than 5.00	19	14	8	13	11	13
Less than 6.00	39	33	36	34	29	34
Less than 7.00	62	63	60	61	59	61
Less than 8.00	80	82	79	79	79	80
Less than 9.00	90	93	93	97	96	94
All	100	100	100	100	100	100
Base	*131*	*146*	*145*	*192*	*196*	*845*
Mean (average value)	6.53	6.66	6.72	6.63	6.77	6.65
Median	6.35	6.57	6.47	6.57	6.79	6.55
Lower 2.5 percentile	3.53	4.15	4.21	3.97	3.85	3.92
Upper 2.5 percentile	10.37	9.90	9.66	9.24	9.27	9.77
Standard deviation	1.75	1.42	1.43	1.45	1.43	1.50

* Includes those not answering income question.

Table 5.14   Percentage contribution of food types–average daily energy intake (MJ) by sex and age of young person

Type of food	Males				All	Females				All
	4–6	7–10	11–14	15–18		4–6	7–10	11–14	15–18	
	%	%	%	%	%	%	%	%	%	%
Cereals & cereal products of which:	35	36	35	33	35	33	34	33	32	33
bread	*10*	*11*	*11*	*11*	*11*	*10*	*10*	*10*	*12*	*11*
breakfast cereals	*7*	*7*	*7*	*6*	*7*	*6*	*5*	*6*	*4*	*5*
biscuits, buns, cakes & pastries	*12*	*12*	*10*	*7*	*10*	*11*	*11*	*10*	*7*	*10*
Milk & milk products *of which:*	15	12	11	9	11	16	12	10	9	11
whole milk	*6*	*4*	*2*	*2*	*3*	*7*	*3*	*2*	*2*	*3*
reduced fat milk	*2*	*3*	*3*	*3*	*3*	*2*	*2*	*2*	*2*	*2*
cheese	*2*	*2*	*2*	*2*	*2*	*2*	*2*	*2*	*3*	*2*
Eggs & egg dishes	1	1	1	1	1	1	1	1	1	1
Fat spreads	3	4	3	3	3	4	3	3	3	3
Meat & meat products *of which:*	11	12	14	16	14	10	13	13	13	13
beef, veal dishes	*1*	*1*	*1*	*2*	*1*	*1*	*2*	*2*	*2*	*2*
coated chicken	*2*	*2*	*1*	*2*	*2*	*2*	*2*	*2*	*2*	*2*
chicken & turkey dishes	*1*	*2*	*2*	*2*	*2*	*2*	*2*	*2*	*2*	*2*
burgers & kebabs	*1*	*1*	*1*	*2*	*1*	*1*	*1*	*1*	*2*	*1*
sausages	*2*	*2*	*2*	*2*	*2*	*2*	*2*	*2*	*1*	*2*
meat pies & pastries	*2*	*2*	*2*	*3*	*2*	*2*	*2*	*2*	*2*	*2*
Fish & fish dishes	2	2	1	2	2	2	2	1	2	2
Vegetables, potatoes & savoury snacks *of which:*	16	16	17	16	16	15	17	20	18	18
potato chips	*5*	*5*	*6*	*7*	*6*	*4*	*5*	*7*	*7*	*6*
savoury snacks	*5*	*5*	*5*	*4*	*4*	*6*	*5*	*6*	*4*	*5*
Fruit & nuts	3	2	2	1	2	3	3	2	2	2
Sugar, preserves & confectionery *of which:*	7	9	10	8	9	9	8	9	8	9
chocolate confectionery	*4*	*5*	*5*	*5*	*5*	*5*	*5*	*6*	*5*	*5*
Drinks* *of which:*	5	5	6	9	6	5	5	6	8	6
fruit juice	*1*	*1*	*1*	*1*	*1*	*1*	*1*	*1*	*1*	*1*
soft drinks, not low calorie	*3*	*4*	*4*	*5*	*4*	*4*	*4*	*4*	*5*	*4*
alcoholic drinks	*0*	*0*	*0*	*0*	*0*	*0*	*0*	*0*	*0*	*0*
Miscellaneous**	1	1	1	2	2	1	2	2	3	2
Average daily intake (MJ)	6.39	7.47	8.28	9.60	8.01	5.87	6.72	7.03	6.82	6.65
Total number of young people	184	256	237	179	856	171	226	238	210	845

*Includes soft drinks, alcoholic drinks, tea, coffee & water.
**Includes powdered beverages (except tea & coffee), soup, sauces & condiments, & commercial toddlers' foods.

Table 5.15 Comparison of average daily energy intake and percentage contribution to energy intakes from macronutrients with other national surveys of young people

Sex and age of young person	Survey year	Av. daily energy intake (MJ)	Percentage food energy from:			Base = number of young people
			protein	carbohydrate	total fat	
Males aged (years)						
3½–4½	(1992/3)	5.36	12.4	52.3	35.3	250
4–6	(1997)	6.39	12.9	51.6	35.5	184
10–11	(1983)	8.67	12.0	50.5	37.4	902
10–11	(1997)	7.98	12.8	51.5	35.7	140
14–15	(1983)	10.40	12.3	49.8	37.9	513
14–15	(1997)	9.13	13.5	50.6	35.9	110
16–24	(1986/7)	10.29	13.7*	42.9*	40.2	214
15–18	(1997)	9.60	13.6*	49.3*	35.9	179
Females aged (years)						
3½–4½	(1992/3)	4.98	12.7	51.7	35.5	243
4–6	(1997)	5.87	12.7	51.4	35.9	171
10–11	(1983)	7.69	11.8	50.2	37.9	821
10–11	(1997)	7.04	12.7	51.2	36.6	118
14–15	(1983)	7.85	12.4	48.8	38.7	461
14–15	(1997)	6.90	13.2	50.8	36.1	113
16–24	(1986/7)	7.11	14.0*	44.9*	39.8	189
15–18	(1997)	6.82	13.6*	49.7*	35.9	210

1983 Department of Health. *The Diets of British Schoolchildren.* HMSO (London, 1989)
1986/7 Gregory JR et al. *The Dietary and Nutritional Survey of British Adults.* HMSO (London, 1990)
1992/3 Gregory JR et al. *National Diet and Nutrition Survey: children aged 1½ to 4½ years.* HMSO (London, 1995)
1997 National Diet and Nutrition Survey: young people aged 4 to 18 years.
* Macronutrient contribution to total energy, that is including alcohol.

Table 5.16 Comparison of average daily energy intake and percentage contribution to energy intakes from macronutrients with other surveys of young people

Reference (study date)	Age (years)	Sex	Sample size	Energy (MJ) intake/day	Percentage energy from:		
					fat	carbohydrate	protein
Ruxton (1991/2)	7–8	M	65	7.78	.37.4	50.8	11.8
		F	71	7.16	37.8	50.3	11.9
Nelson (1988)	7–10	M	25	7.59	36.6	n/a	n/a
		F	26	6.92	35.0	n/a	n/a
Hunt (1988, 1990)	8–11	M	111	7.61	37	51	n/a
		F	148	6.53	39	50	n/a
Nelson (1988)	11–12	M	76	7.74	37.5	n/a	n/a
		F	67	7.45	38.4	n/a	n/a
McNeill (1988/9)	12	M	18	8.96	n/a	n/a	n/a
		F	43	8.14	n/a	n/a	n/a
Strain (1990/1)	12	M	251	11.0	39	50	11
		F	258	9.2	38	50	11
Strain (1990/1)	15	M	252	13.1	39	50	11
		F	254	9.1	39	49	11
Bull (1982)	15–18	M	198	10.1	42	43	13
		F	184	7.8	43	43	13
Crawley (1986/7)	16–17	M	2006	11.4	41.4	44.2	12.5
		F	2754	8.8	41.6	43.9	12.5
Barker (1986/7)	16–29	M	105	10.7	39.2	43.5	13.0
		F	110	7.6	39.7	44.5	12.9

n/a not available

Ruxton (1991/2)   Ruxton CHS, Kirk TR and Belton NR. (1996) Energy and nutrient intakes in a sample of Edinburgh 7-8 year olds: a comparison with United Kingdom dietary reference values. *Br J Nutr* **75**: 151-160.
Nelson (1988)   Nelson M, Naismith DJ, Burley V et al. (1990) Nutrient intakes, vitamin-mineral supplementation, and intelligence in British schoolchildren. *Br J Nutr* **64**: 13-22.
Hunt (1988, 1990)   Hunt C and Rigley L. (1995) A study of the dietary habits, heights and weights of primary schoolchildren. *Nutr and Food Sci* **4**: 5-7.
McNeill (1988/9)   McNeill G, Davidson L, Morrison DC et al. (1991) Nutrient intake in schoolchildren: some practical considerations. *Proc Nutr Soc* **50**: 37-43.
Strain (1990/91)   Strain JJ, Robson PJ, Livingstone MBE et al. (1994) Estimates of food and macronutrient intake in a random sample of Northern Ireland adolescents. *Br J Nutr* **72**: 343-352.
Bull (1982)   Bull N. (1985) Dietary habits of 15-25 year olds. *Hum Nutr: Appl Nutr* **39A**: Suppl. 1, 1-68.
Crawley (1986/7)   Crawley HF. (1993) The energy, nutrient and food intakes of teenagers aged 16-17 years in Britain. *Br J Nutr*. **70**: 15-26
Barker (1986/7)   Barker ME, McClean SI, McKenna PG et al. *Diet, Lifestyle and Health in Northern Ireland*. Coleraine (Centre for Applied Health Studies, 1988).

Figure 5.1(a) Percentage contribution of food types to average daily energy intake by region – males

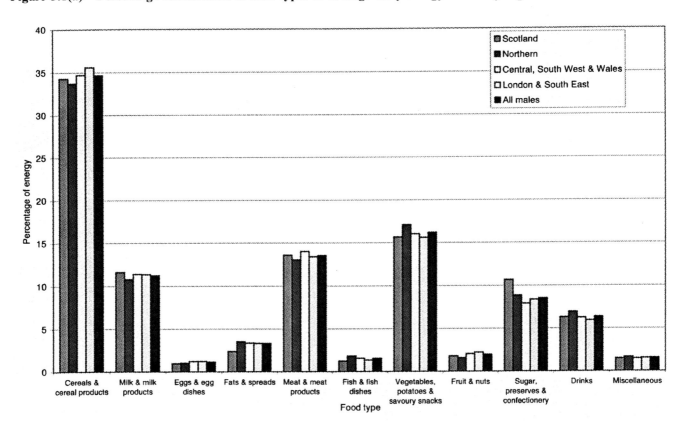

Figure 5.2(b) Percentage contribution of food types to average daily energy intake by region – females

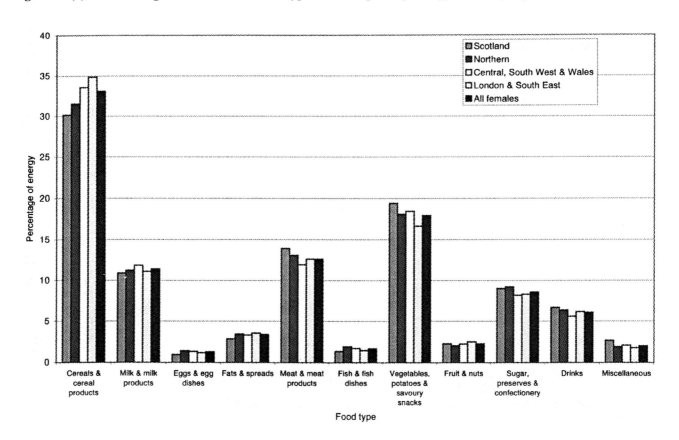

Figure 5.2(a) **Percentage contribution of food types to average daily intake of energy by social class of head of household – males**

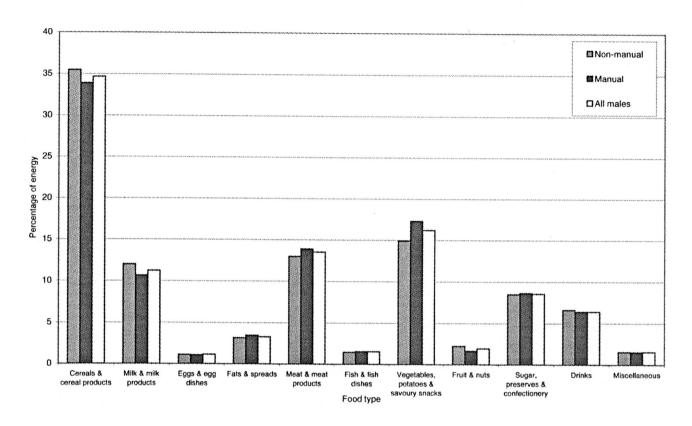

Figure 5.2(b) **Percentage contribution of food types to average daily energy intake by social class of head of household – females**

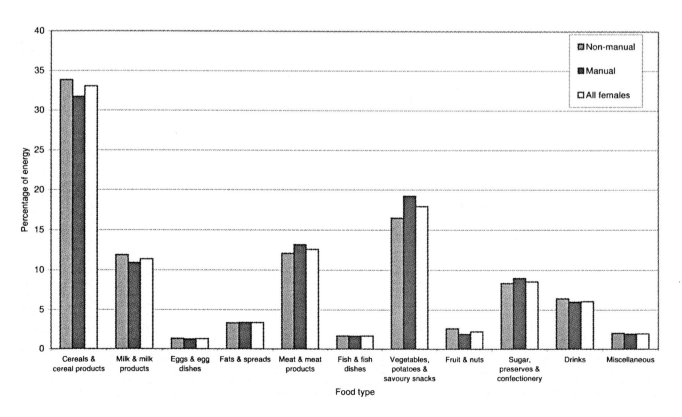

Figure 5.3(a)   Percentage contribution of food types to average daily energy intake by whether young person's 'parents' were receiving benefits – males

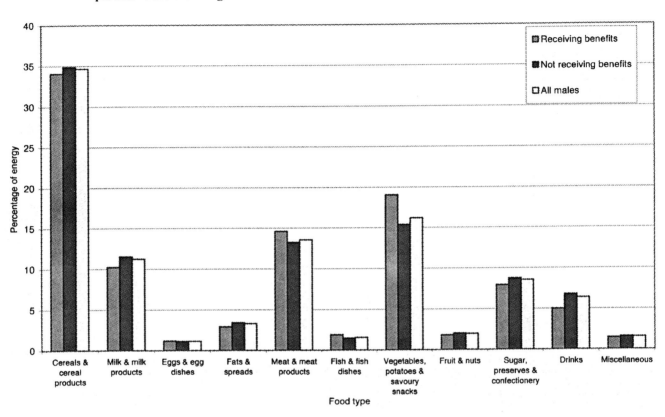

Figure 5.3(b)   Percentage contribution of food types to average daily energy intake by whether young person's 'parents' were receiving benefits – females

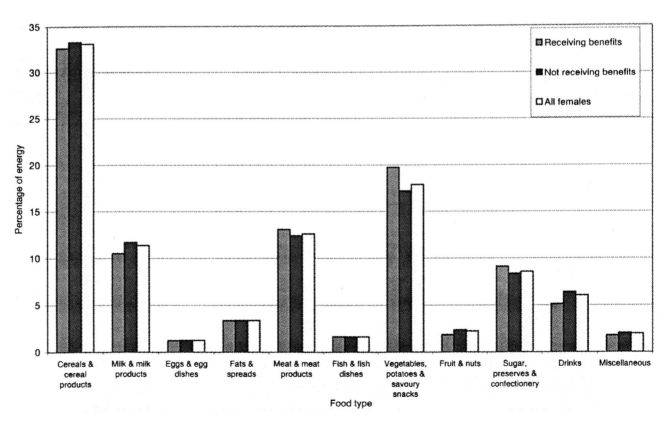

Figure 5.4(a)   Percentage contribution of food types to average daily energy intake by gross weekly household income – males

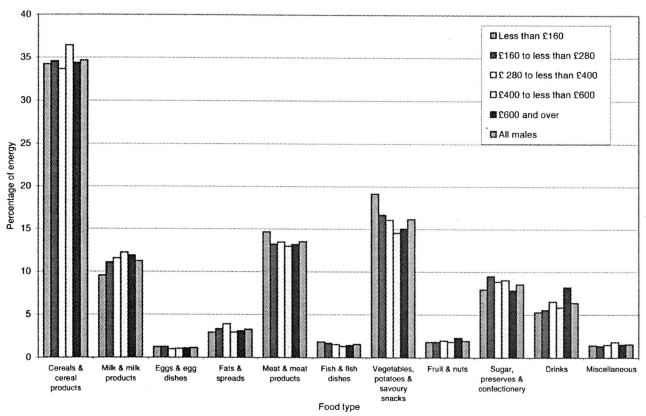

Figure 5.4(b)   Percentage contribution of food types to average daily energy intake by gross weekly household income – females

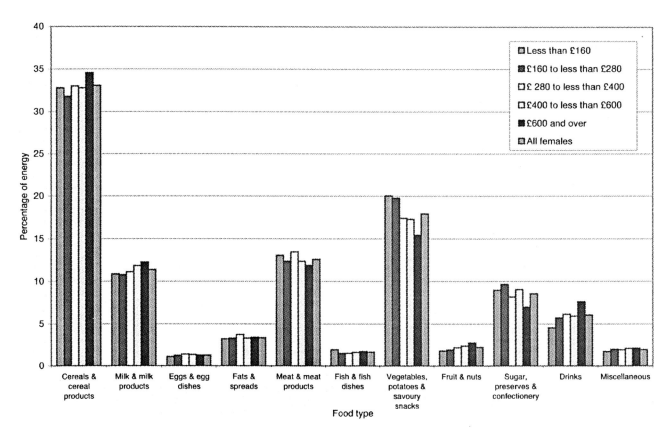

6 Protein, carbohydrate and alcohol intake

6.1 Introduction

In this and the following chapter, data are presented on intakes of protein, carbohydrate, alcohol, total fat and fatty acids, and on the percentage of food energy provided by each. Intakes are expressed as daily averages for the 1701 young people (unweighted) for whom a complete 7-day weighed intake record was obtained. Protein, carbohydrate and alcohol are considered in this chapter; for carbohydrate, information is shown separately for total carbohydrate, starch, total sugars, non-milk extrinsic sugars, intrinsic and milk sugars, intrinsic and milk sugars and starch, and non-starch polysaccharides ('fibre')[1]. Respondents were asked to keep a record of their bowel movements during the dietary recording period. These data are also presented in this chapter.

6.2 Protein

The current UK Reference Nutrient Intake (RNI) values for protein are shown in Table 6.1[2].

Mean daily protein intake for boys aged between 4 and 18 years was 61.6g (median 60.2g). Mean intake increased with age, being lowest for those aged 4 to 6 years, 49.0g, and highest for boys aged 15 to 18 years, 76.5g (differences between consecutive age groups all: $p < 0.01$). Mean daily protein intake for girls aged between 4 and 18 years was 51.2g (median 50.5g). Mean intake increased from 44.5g for girls aged 4 to 6 years to 54.8g for girls aged 15 to 18 years ($p < 0.01$), although the only significant difference between consecutive age groups was between girls aged 4 to 6 years and those aged 7 to 10 years ($p < 0.01$). *(Table 6.2)*

As Table 6.3 shows, average protein intakes were well in excess of the RNI, for example, mean protein intake for boys aged 4 to 6 years was 249% of the RNI. Although this percentage decreased with age, mean intake was still more than 120% of the RNI for both boys and girls aged 15 to 18 years.

As shown in Table 6.4, protein provided on average 13.1% of the food energy intake of the young people in the survey. Among boys, those aged 7 to 10 years derived the lowest proportion and those aged 15 to 18 years the highest proportion of their food energy from protein ($p < 0.01$). Girls aged 15 to 18 years obtained a higher proportion of their food energy from protein than younger girls ($p < 0.01$) but there was no significant increase with age for those aged under 14 years.

Table 6.5 shows that around three quarters of the protein consumed was derived from three main food types. Meat and meat products was the major source, providing on average 32% of daily intake for boys and 30% for girls. Cereals and cereal products provided 26% of the protein intake for girls and 27% for boys. Milk and milk products provided 18% of protein intake for both boys and girls. Compared with young people aged 15 to 18 years, the data suggest that the youngest children, aged 4 to 6 years, obtained a greater proportion of their protein from milk and milk products and somewhat less from meat and meat products although the differences did not reach the level of statistical significance ($p > 0.05$). There were only small differences between boys and girls in the proportion of their protein intake obtained from different food types. *(Tables 6.1 to 6.5)*

6.3 Total carbohydrate

The mean daily intake of total carbohydrate was 260g (median 252g) for boys and 214g (median 211g) for girls. Mean intake for boys was consistently higher than for girls for all age groups (all: $p < 0.01$). For boys, intake increased significantly with age, from a mean of 209g for boys aged 4 to 6 years to a mean of 301g for boys aged 15 to 18 years (differences between consecutive age groups all: $p < 0.01$). For girls, the data suggest that mean intakes increased with age up to the age of 11 to 14 years, although the only significant difference between consecutive age groups was between young people aged 4 to 6 years and those aged 7 to 10 years ($p < 0.01$). Mean intake then decreased to 214g for girls aged 15 to 18 years (girls 11 to 14 compared with girls 15 to 18 years: ns). The intake for girls at the lower 2.5 percentile of the distribution was lower for those aged 15 to 18 years than for those aged 4 to 6 years (107g compared with 124g).

Within each age and sex group the range of intakes was large; for example, for boys aged 15 to 18 years, 2.5% had an intake of 161g of total carbohydrate or less per day compared with 2.5% who had an intake of 506g or more a day.

Total carbohydrate provided on average 51.6% of food energy intake for boys and 51.1% for girls. There was no significant difference between boys and girls or between age groups in the proportion of food energy derived from total carbohydrate. At the lower 2.5

percentile, young people derived about 40% of their food energy from total carbohydrate. At the upper 2.5 percentile close to 60% of food energy was derived from this source, with little variation by age or sex.

The main sources of total carbohydrate did not vary significantly by age group or sex. Cereals and cereal products were the major source, contributing 45% of total carbohydrate intake for boys and 42% for girls, of which bread contributed 16% for both boys and girls and breakfast cereals contributed 11% for boys and 8% for girls. Vegetables, potatoes and savoury snacks contributed 16% of total carbohydrate for boys and 18% for girls, of which 7% came from roast or fried potatoes and chips. Drinks contributed 11% for both boys and girls, at least two thirds of which was from soft drinks (not low calorie). Sugars, preserves and confectionery also contributed 11% for both boys and girls, of which chocolate confectionery accounted for around half.   *(Tables 6.6 to 6.8)*

6.3.1 Sugars

As well as showing intakes of total sugars for the young people in the survey, information is also given on their intakes of *non-milk extrinsic sugars* and *intrinsic and milk sugars*. This distinction is made on the basis of cariogenicity. Relationships between the oral health of young people and their intakes of sugars are discussed in Section 6.2 of the Report of the Oral Health Survey[3].

Extrinsic sugars are any sugars which are not contained within the cellular structure of the food, whether natural and unprocessed or refined. Examples are the sugars in honey, table sugar and lactose in milk and milk products. Non-milk extrinsic sugars are therefore all extrinsic sugars *excluding* lactose in milk and milk products, which is seen to be a special case.

Intrinsic sugars are those contained within the cellular structure of the food; milk sugars include lactose in milk and milk products. The UK Dietary Reference Value[2] for non-milk extrinsic sugars is 10% of total dietary energy or 11% of food energy, expressed as a population average. It was recommended that starches and intrinsic and milk sugars should provide the balance of energy not provided by alcohol, protein, fat and non-milk extrinsic sugars, that is on average 37% of total dietary energy or 39% of food energy for the population. For comparative purposes, as well as being shown separately, information on intakes of intrinsic and milk sugars is also shown combined with information on intakes of starch.

Total sugars

Table 6.9 shows that the mean daily intake of total sugars was 117g (median 111g) for boys and 97g (median 95g) for girls (p < 0.01). For boys, mean intake for those aged 15 to 18 years was significantly higher than for those aged 4 to 6 years, 129g compared with

98g (p < 0.01). For girls, the highest mean intakes were for those in the 7 to 10 and the 11 to 14 year age groups (101g and 99g respectively). For all groups and particularly for older boys, the range of intakes was large; for example, for boys aged 15 to 18 years intakes ranged from 44g at the lower 2.5 percentile to 254g at the upper 2.5 percentile.

Table 6.10 shows that more than two thirds of the intake of total sugars came from three food types, drinks (24%), sugar, preserves and confectionery (23%) and cereals and cereal products (boys: 23%; girls: 22%). In the drinks group, soft drinks (not low calorie) accounted for 19% of the intake of total sugars for boys and 18% for girls.

In the sugar, preserves and confectionery group, chocolate confectionery accounted for 10% of total sugars intake for boys and girls and sugar confectionery 6% of intake for boys and 7% for girls.
                                    (Tables 6.9 and 6.10)

Non-milk extrinsic sugars

The mean daily intake of non-milk extrinsic sugars was 85g (median 78g) for boys and 69g (median 67g) for girls, representing about 72% of total sugars intake. For boys, intake increased significantly with age, from a mean of 66g for those aged 4 to 6 years to 97g for those aged 15 to 18 years (p < 0.01). For girls, there were no significant differences in mean intake by age. At the lower 2.5 percentile of the distribution, the intake for girls aged 15 to 18 years was below that for girls aged 4 to 6 years (17g compared with 19g).

The current UK recommendation is that the population average intake of non-milk extrinsic sugars should not exceed 10% of total dietary energy or 11% of food energy[2]. The mean percentage of food energy from non-milk extrinsic sugars was above the current recommendation for both boys (16.7%) and girls (16.4%) and for all age groups. Young people at the upper 2.5 percentile of the distribution were obtaining more than one quarter of their food energy from non-milk extrinsic sugars.

The main food sources of non-milk extrinsic sugars for both boys and girls were the drinks group and the sugar, preserves and confectionery group, each of which provided about one third of total intake. Chocolate confectionery provided 12% of intake for boys and girls. The proportion of non-milk extrinsic sugars provided by drinks increased with age, for example rising from 27% of intake for boys aged 4 to 6 years to 42% for boys aged 15 to 18 years (p < 0.05). Within the drinks group, carbonated soft drinks (not low calorie) were the main source of non-milk extrinsic sugars, providing 18% of intake for boys and 16% for girls and increasing with age.

The proportion of non-milk extrinsic sugars intake provided by sugar, preserves and confectionery did not vary significantly with age, although the data suggest that the contribution made by table sugar increased (ns) and the contribution made by sugar confectionery decreased with the age of the young person (both sexes: ns). It has already been shown (see *Chapter 4: Tables 4.12(a) and (b)*) that boys and girls aged 15 to 18 years were less likely to have consumed sugar confectionery than younger children, and that girls aged 15 to 18 years who consumed sugar confectionery ate smaller mean amounts than younger girls[4]. *(Tables 6.11 to 6.13)*

Intrinsic sugars and milk sugars
The mean daily intrinsic and milk sugars intake was 32g (median 30g) for boys and 28g (median 26g) for girls, representing about 27% and 29% respectively of total sugars intake. For boys, mean intake did not vary by age, although the intake of those at the upper 2.5 percentile of the distribution did increase with age, from 59g for boys aged 4 to 6 years to 67g for boys aged 15 to 18 years. For girls, mean daily intake was the same (29g) for those in the youngest two age groups, however the data suggest that intakes were lower for girls in the oldest two age groups (26g) (7 to 10 years compared with 11 to 14 years: p < 0.05; others ns).

As might be expected, the major source of intrinsic and milk sugars was milk and milk products, which accounted for 40% of intake for boys and 36% of intake for girls. The data suggest that the proportion of intrinsic and milk sugars obtained from milk and milk products decreased with age, from 44% for both boys and girls aged 4 to 6 years to 36% for boys and 30% for girls aged 15 to 18 years (ns). For both girls and boys, the proportion of intrinsic and milk sugars obtained from whole milk decreased significantly with age, for example from 22% for girls aged 4 to 6 years to 8% for girls aged 15 to 18 years (both: p < 0.01). This decrease reflects the fall in consumption of milk with age.

Fruit and nuts contributed a further 20% to the intake of intrinsic and milk sugars for boys and 24% for girls. Cereals and cereal products contributed 19% of intake for boys and 18% for girls, with bread accounting for about one third of this. *(Table 6.14 and 6.15)*

6.3.2 Starch
The mean daily starch intake was 143g (median 138g) for boys and 117g (median 114g) for girls, representing about 55% of total carbohydrate intake. For boys, starch intake increased with age, from a mean of 110g for boys aged 4 to 6 years to a mean of 172g for boys aged 15 to 18 years (p < 0.01). For girls, intakes increased from a mean of 96g for those aged 4 to 6 years to a mean of 129g for those aged 11 to 14 years (p < 0.01).

Overall, boys obtained 63% and girls 60% of their intake of starch from the consumption of cereals and cereal products, with bread contributing 28% and 27% and breakfast cereals 15% and 11% for boys and girls respectively. The only other food type contributing more than 10% to starch intake was vegetables, including potatoes and savoury snacks, which contributed 27% for boys and 29% for girls, of which 12% came from roast or fried potatoes and chips, and 6% for boys and 7% for girls from savoury snacks. There was little variation by age or sex in the contributions to starch intake made by different food types.
(Tables 6.16 and 6.17)

6.3.3 Intrinsic sugars, milk sugars and starch
This group includes starch and all sugars with the exception of non-milk extrinsic sugars as previously defined (see *Section 6.3.1* above); that is, total carbohydrate minus non-milk extrinsic sugars.

The COMA Panel on Dietary Reference Values recommended that starches and intrinsic and milk sugars should provide on average 39% of food energy for the population and that this should apply to children over 2 years old[2]. Table 6.18 shows that on average both boys and girls were obtaining around 35% of their food energy from this group of carbohydrates and that the proportion did not vary significantly by age or sex.
(Table 6.18)

6.3.4 Non-starch polysaccharides (NSP)
Adult dietary intakes of NSP in the UK are estimated to be between 11g/d and 13g/d, and the COMA Panel on Dietary Reference Values proposed that the diet of the adult population should contain on average 18g/d non-starch polysaccharides, with an individual range of 12g/d to 24g/d, from a variety of foods[2]. The Panel noted that there were no data on the physiological effects of NSP on children. However, they suggested that it is likely that any such effects are related to body size and therefore recommended that children should have proportionately lower intakes.

The mean daily intake of NSP was 11.2g (median 10.8g) for boys and significantly lower, 9.7g (median 9.3g), for girls (p < 0.01). For both boys and girls intakes increased with age, for example from a mean of 8.0g for girls aged 4 to 6 years to a mean of 10.6g for those aged 15 to 18 years (p < 0.01). Intakes at the upper 2.5 percentile were within the recommended range of intakes for adults for all age and sex groups.

The two main sources of non-starch polysaccharides were vegetables, potatoes and savoury snacks, which provided 40% of intake for boys and 42% for girls, and cereals and cereal products (40% for boys and 37% for girls). Vegetables, excluding potatoes, accounted for 15% to 21% of intake depending on the age and sex of the young person and roast or fried potatoes and chips another 9% to 13%. White bread and high fibre and whole grain breakfast cereals each accounted for around 10% of non-starch polysaccharides intake. There were no significant differences between boys and girls or between young people of different ages in the proportion of non-starch polysaccharides provided by different food types. *(Tables 6.19 and 6.20)*

6.4 Bowel movements

Over the seven days when the dietary record was being completed, young people were asked to keep a record of the number of bowel movements they had each day. A copy of the bowel movement diary is given in Appendix A.

The purpose of collecting this information was primarily to establish normative values for the population of young people aged between 4 and 18 years, which are not available from other sources, and to be able to relate the information on the number of bowel movements to other information collected, principally dietary data. In this section, information is presented on the average number of bowel movements per day and the mean NSP intake for young people according to their number of bowel movements.

Table 6.21 shows that, overall, almost two thirds of young people had at least one bowel movement a day, and 10% of boys and 13% of girls recorded at least two bowel movements a day. There was some evidence that both boys and girls in the older age groups were more likely to have recorded having at least two bowel movements a day than younger children. For example, 14% of girls and 17% of boys aged 15 to 18 years recorded at least two movements a day compared with 6% of boys and girls aged 4 to 6 years (boys: $p < 0.05$; girls: ns).

The data shown in Table 6.22 suggest a positive association between recorded number of bowel movements and mean daily intake of NSP, although the only significant difference was between young people who had fewer than one bowel movement a day and those who had between 1.0 and fewer than 1.5 bowel movements per day (10.0g compared with 10.7g: $p < 0.05$). Mean daily NSP intake was lower for young people who had 3.0 or more bowel movements per day than for those who had between 2.5 and fewer than 3.0 bowel movements per day, 10.2g compared with 11.2g, but the difference did not reach the level of statistical significance ($p > 0.05$). *(Tables 6.21 and 6.22)*

6.5 Alcohol

For adults, sustained excessive consumption of alcohol has the effect of increasing the risk of high blood pressure and stroke, as well as being a risk factor for other conditions, for example cancers and cirrhosis of the liver. Current recommendations for adults are that consistently drinking four or more units a day for men, or three or more units a day for women, is not advised as a sensible drinking level because of the progressive health risk it carries[5]. These conclusions apply particu-

larly to young adults (aged 16 to 24 years) as 'binge drinking' is a common and hazardous pattern of drinking in this age group. The Inter-Departmental Working Group also voiced its concern over young people aged under 16 years who may not have reached physical maturity who are drinking at or above the levels of sensible drinking recommended to adults.

Information on alcohol consumption was collected for young people aged 11 to 18 years in the self-completion section of the initial dietary interview and for young people aged 4 to 18 years in the 7-day dietary record (see *Chapter 4.3.2*). It should be noted that the data collected in the dietary interview relate to the consumption of alcoholic drinks only, while data from the dietary record may also include alcohol consumed as part of recipe dishes. Alcohol differed from nutrients measured in the survey in that for the majority of respondents estimated intake was zero. Intakes are therefore given for the total sample and for consumers only. The number of consumers aged 4 to 10 years identified from the dietary record was so small (17 young people aged 4 to 6 years and 29 young people aged 7 to 10 years) that intakes by age group are reported for young people aged 11 to 18 years only.

6.5.1 Data from the initial dietary interview

It was assumed that children aged 4 to 6 years would not report consuming alcoholic drinks and that a self-completion schedule would be too complex a task for them to complete. However, the feasibility study showed that 7 to 10 year olds were capable of completing the self-completion schedule and that a small number reported consuming alcohol[6]. At the main stage the questions were therefore asked of all young people aged 7 to 18 years.

Table 6.23 shows that about three quarters of both girls and boys aged 7 to 18 years reported not having consumed an alcoholic drink in the seven days prior to the interview. As would be expected, both the proportion of young people who reported having consumed alcohol in the previous seven days and the mean units of alcohol consumed increased significantly between the 11 to 14 year age group and the 15 to 18 year age group. For example, 18% of girls aged 11 to 14 years reported consuming alcohol compared with 59% of girls aged 15 to 18 years ($p < 0.01$).

Information was collected about the total consumption of alcoholic drinks in the seven days before the initial dietary interview. It is therefore not possible to identify those who consumed more than the recommended maximum number of units of alcohol for adults (or safe limit) on a daily basis. However, if a boy consumed more than 28 units of alcohol or a girl more than 21 units of alcohol in the seven days before the interview, then on average the boy will have consumed more than 4 units and the girl more than 3 units per day. Overall, 10% of all boys aged 15 to 18 years (18% of consumers) had consumed more than 28 units of alcohol in the seven-day period. For girls, 8% of those aged 15 to 18 years (14% of consumers) had consumed more than 21 units of alcohol in the seven-day period. No young people aged 7 to 14 years reported consuming more than the recommended maximum number of units of alcohol for adults.

Of those who reported consuming alcohol in the seven days before the interview 72% mentioned that they drank beer, lager or cider, 40% reported drinking spirits or liqueurs, 35% mentioned wine, 28% mentioned alcopops and 12% reported drinking shandy, Martini or sherry (table not shown).

The questions about alcohol consumption were taken from the drinking section of the survey 'Smoking among secondary school children in 1994'[7]. Table 6.24 is a comparison of data from the NDNS and equivalent data on reported alcohol consumption from the 1996 repeat of the 1994 survey, published as the Survey of Young Teenagers and Alcohol[8]. The proportion of young people aged 11 to 15 years who reported consuming alcohol in the seven days prior to the interview was similar for the two surveys. However, the mean units of alcohol consumed was lower for young people in the NDNS compared with those in the Survey of Young Teenagers and Alcohol, both overall and for consumers only.

The apparent under-reporting in this survey may be partly explained by differences in methodology between the two surveys. Although the questions and the way the number of units consumed was calculated were identical for the two surveys, in this NDNS of young people the questions were completed in the home, generally with the young person's parent present. In the Survey of Young Teenagers and Alcohol the self-completion questionnaire was completed in the classroom under the supervision of an interviewer but with no teacher present[9]. *(Tables 6.23 and 6.24)*

6.5.2 Data from the dietary record

Overall, 27% of boys and 23% of girls aged 11 to 18 years reported consuming items containing alcohol in the 7-day dietary record. For young people aged 11 to 18 years, the mean daily intake of alcohol was 3.4g for boys (12.9g for consumers only) and 1.8g for girls (7.6g for consumers only). There were too few consumers to allow reliable means to be calculated for young people aged 4 to 10 years.

For consumers, the data suggest that on average girls had lower alcohol intakes than boys, for example mean alcohol intake for girls aged 15 to 18 was 9.3g compared with 15.6g for boys, although perhaps due to the small numbers of consumers, the difference was not statistically significant ($p > 0.05$). Mean alcohol intakes were higher for both boys and girls aged 15 to 18 years than for those aged 11 to 14 years, for example 1.5g for girls

aged 11 to 14 years compared with 9.3g for girls aged 15 to 18 years ($p < 0.01$). As would be expected, the distribution of alcohol intake was positively skewed and median values both for the total sample and for consumers only were significantly lower than mean values.

The percentage of total energy derived from alcohol suggests a similar pattern to that of absolute intakes, for example for consumers, boys aged 11 to 18 years obtained a greater percentage of total energy from alcohol than girls (3.8% compared with 3.1%: ns). The percentage of total energy from alcohol increased for both male and female consumers between those aged 11 to 14 years and those aged 15 to 18 years (both: $p < 0.01$). *(Tables 6.25 to 6.26)*

6.5.3 Comparing data from the initial dietary interview with data from the dietary record

For young people aged 11 to 18 years, the mean alcohol intake estimated from information recorded in the dietary record was lower than the alcohol intake estimated from the dietary interview, both for the total sample (a mean of 2.6g compared with 3.2g) and for consumers only (a mean of 10.5g compared with 13.3g), although these differences did not reach the level of statistical significance (table not shown). All types of drinks, but alcoholic drinks in particular, are likely to be among the items most frequently under-recorded by respondents keeping a dietary record, especially in this age group. The fact that the dietary record may not have been kept confidential within the young person's household, unlike the self-completion questionnaire, may also account for this difference.

6.6 Variation in intake of protein, total carbohydrate and non-starch polysaccharides

Tables 6.27 to 6.32 show mean and median intakes of protein, total carbohydrate and non-starch polysaccharides for different groups of young people in the sample.

6.6.1 Young people reported as being unwell

It was shown in the previous chapter that young people who were reported as being unwell during the dietary recording period had lower average daily energy intakes than young people who were not unwell. Those whose eating was reported as being affected had the lowest mean energy intakes, but even for those whose eating was reported not to have been affected by being unwell, mean energy intakes were lower compared with young people not reported as being unwell (see *Chapter 5, Section 5.2.3*).

The mean intake for each nutrient shown in Table 6.27 was significantly lower for young people whose eating was reported to be affected by their being unwell than for young people who were not unwell (all: $p < 0.01$), with the exception of non-milk extrinsic sugars. Even for those who were reported as being unwell but whose eating was said not to have been affected, intakes of protein and non-starch polysaccharides were significantly lower than for young people who were not unwell (protein: $p < 0.05$; non-starch polysaccharides: $p < 0.01$). However, although absolute intakes were lower for young people who were unwell, the proportion of food energy derived from total carbohydrate was similar for all three groups of young people, suggesting that in respect of carbohydrates the reduced intake was due to the reduced energy intake and not to any selective avoidance of carbohydrates by young people who were reported as being unwell. *(Table 6.27)*

6.6.2 Region

In general, regional differences in average intakes of protein and total carbohydrate were small and did not reach the level of statistical significance.

The data suggest that young people in Scotland had the lowest mean intake of starch, although differences between regions did not reach the level of statistical significance. Mean intakes of non-starch polysaccharides were lowest in Scotland, 9.3g, significantly higher in the Northern region, 10.3g, and in London and the South East, 10.5g ($p < 0.05$) and highest in the Central and South West regions of England and Wales, 10.9g ($p < 0.01$). *(Table 6.28)*

6.6.3 Socio-economic status

As described in Chapter 3, a number of measures of the socio-economic status of the young person's household were derived from the interview data. It has also been noted that many of these measures are interrelated; for example, households receiving Family Credit, Income Support or Job Seeker's Allowance were more likely to be in the lower income groups and have a head of household from the manual, rather than the non-manual, social class group. Bearing such associations in mind, the data show a clear pattern of young people from households of lower economic status having lower mean intakes of protein, total carbohydrate, total sugars, non-milk extrinsic sugars and NSP than other young people.

Mean intakes of protein, total carbohydrate, total sugars, non-milk extrinsic sugars and NSP were significantly lower for young people from households in the lower income groups (gross weekly household income of less than £160 compared with £600 and over: total carbohydrate: $p < 0.05$; others: $p < 0.01$) and for those from households that were in receipt of benefits (NSP: $p < 0.05$; others: $p < 0.01$) than for other young people. The data suggest that young people from manual households had lower intakes of these nutrients than other young people, although the only significant difference was for total sugars ($p < 0.01$).

None of the indicators of lower economic status was associated with either significantly lower starch intakes or significantly lower percentages of food energy from total carbohydrate. Unlike children aged 1½ to 4½ years[10], there was no evidence that in young people from the lower economic status groups the mean daily intake of starch was higher. *(Tables 6.29 to 6.31)*

6.6.4 Household type

Comparisons for young people living in different household types may, as has already been noted, be affected by differences in the age composition of the different groups, particularly for boys where intakes vary markedly with age.

Table 6.32 shows that, compared with young people living with a single parent and those living with both parents and other children, those who were living with both parents and no other children had significantly higher mean daily intakes of protein (both: $p < 0.01$) and starch (both: $p < 0.05$). Those living with both parents and no other children also had a significantly higher mean daily intake of non-starch polysaccharides than those living with both parents and other children ($p < 0.05$), but the proportion of energy they derived from total carbohydrate was significantly lower ($p < 0.01$). *(Table 6.32)*

6.7 Variation in intake of alcohol

Tables 6.33 to 6.38 show mean alcohol intakes (from the dietary record data) for different groups of young people in the sample. Due to the large number of cases for whom estimated intake was zero, data are shown for young people aged 11 to 18 years only. In order to provide adequate numbers for analysis, some of the main classificatory variables have been combined. Data are presented for the total sample and, where the sizes of the groups allow, for consumers only.

6.7.1 Young people reported as being unwell

There was no significant difference in mean alcohol intake between young people who were reported to be unwell, either with or without their eating affected, and young people who were not unwell during the recording period. The proportion of young people who had consumed alcohol did not vary significantly according to whether they were reported as being unwell but there were too few consumers to allow reliable mean intakes to be calculated for consumers only. *(Table 6.33)*

6.7.2 Region

There were only small differences between mean alcohol intakes in different regions. The data suggest that mean daily intakes were highest for young people living in the Northern region, 3.3g, and London and the South East, 3.2g, lower for those living in the Central and South West regions of England and Wales, 1.9g, and lowest for those living in Scotland, 1.6g, although these differences did not reach the level of statistical significance ($p > 0.05$). The data suggest that both the proportions of consumers and the mean intakes for consumers followed the same pattern, indicating both that a greater proportion of young people in the Northern region consumed alcohol and that, for those who consumed alcohol, mean intakes were higher than for those living in other regions. *(Table 6.34)*

6.7.3 Socio-economic status

The data show a pattern of smaller proportions of young people from households with lower socio-economic status consuming alcohol. The data suggest that a smaller proportion of young people from manual households consumed alcohol compared with those from non-manual households (ns). A significantly smaller proportion of young people from households with the lowest gross weekly household income consumed alcohol compared with the highest income group (4% compared with 26%: p < 0.01). A smaller proportion of young people whose 'parents' were receiving benefits consumed alcohol compared with those whose 'parents' were not in receipt of benefits (p < 0.01).

There was no significant variation in mean alcohol intake by social class background for the total sample, although the data suggest that consumers from a manual background had higher mean intakes than those from a non-manual background (13.2g compared with 9.0g: ns).

For the total sample, mean daily alcohol intake increased with income, from a mean of 1.0g for young people from households with a gross weekly income of less than £160 to 5.6g for those from households with an income of £600 and over (p < 0.01). Young people from households that were in receipt of benefits had significantly lower mean alcohol intakes than other young people (p < 0.01). However, there were too few consumers for the lower income groups and for those receiving benefits to allow reliable mean intakes to be calculated for consumers. *(Tables 6.35 to 6.37)*

6.7.4 Household type

Young people aged 11 to 18 who were living with both parents and no other children had a significantly higher mean daily intake of alcohol and obtained a higher proportion of their energy from alcohol than young people living with both parents and other children (mean daily intake: p < 0.05; as % energy: p < 0.01). These differences are likely to be associated with there being a much higher proportion of young people aged 15 to 18 in the group living with both parents and no other children than in other household types.

Comparisons based on consumers only showed no significant differences associated with household type. *(Table 6.38)*

6.8 Comparisons with other studies

Table 6.39 compares data from this present NDNS of young people with equivalent data on the intake of protein and total carbohydrate from other national surveys, including the 1992/3 NDNS of pre-school children[11], the 1983 Department of Health study of the Diets of British Schoolchildren[12], and the 1986/87 Adults survey[13]. Comparisons of percentage energy from protein and total carbohydrate are given in *Chapter 5.6, Table 5.15.*

Table 5.15 showed that there was little difference in the percentage of food energy from either protein or total carbohydrate between the 1992/3 survey of pre-school children and this Survey for the youngest age groups for which comparable data are available.

Absolute intakes of protein and total carbohydrate were significantly higher for both boys and girls aged 4 to 6 years in 1997 compared with children aged 3½ to 4½ years in 1992/3, although this may be partly due to the age difference between the two groups (all: p < 0.01). Comparative data for boys and girls aged 10 to 11 years and 14 to 15 years collected in 1983 show no significant differences over time in the mean daily intake of protein. The data suggest that mean intakes of total carbohydrate have decreased over time for both boys and girls aged 10 to 11 years and 14 to 15 years, although the differences were only statistically significant for those aged 14 to 15 years, for example 324g for boys in 1983 compared with 294g for boys in 1997 (p < 0.05).

Table 5.15 showed that comparing young people aged 15 to 18 years in the current survey with those aged 16 to 24 years in the 1986/7 Adults survey, the percentage contribution to energy intakes from protein was similar. However, the percentage contribution to energy intakes from total carbohydrate was greater for young people in this present survey. For both boys and girls, there was no significant difference in mean protein intake for young people aged 15 to 18 years in 1997 compared to those aged 16 to 24 years in 1986/7. The data suggest that mean total carbohydrate intakes were higher in 1997 than in 1986/7, although the differences were not statistically significant. *(Table 6.39)*

References and endnotes

1. Non-starch polysaccharides refer to non–alpha–glucans as measured by the technique of Englyst and Cummings. Englyst HN, Cummings JH. Improved method for measurement of dietary fibre as non-starch polysaccharides in plant foods. *J Assoc Off Anal Chem* 1988: **71**: 808–814.
2. Department of Health. Report on Health and Social Subjects: 41. *Dietary Reference Values for Food Energy and Nutrients for the United Kingdom.* HMSO (London, 1991).
3. Walker A, Gregory J, Bradnock G, Nunn J, White D. *National Diet and Nutrition Survey: young people aged 4 to 18 years. Volume 2: Report of the Oral Health Survey.* TSO (London, 2000).

4   See Appendix J 'Under-reporting' for a discussion of possible selective under–reporting of non–milk extrinsic sugars.

5   Department of Health. *Sensible drinking – the report of an inter-departmental working group.* HMSO (London, 1996).

6   Lowe S. *Feasibility study for the National Diet and Nutrition Survey of young people aged 4 to 18 years.* ONS (*In preparation*). See also *Appendix C.*

7   Diamond A, Goddard E. *Smoking among secondary school children in 1994.* HMSO (London, 1995).

8   Goddard E. *Young Teenagers and Alcohol in 1996. Volume 1: England.* HMSO (London, 1997).

9   The under-reporting of the number of units of alcohol consumed in this present survey may be affected by a programming error which led to those who reported drinking a bottle or more of alcopops not being asked how much they drank. In the analysis, units were imputed as one unit of alcohol per consumer of alcopops. This was to allow valid comparisons with data from the Survey of Young Teenagers and Alcohol, where one bottle or can of alcopops was taken to contain 1.0 unit of alcohol. For consumers only, to impute 1.5 units rather than 1.0 units per consumer of alcopops increased the overall mean alcohol intake from 11.41 units to 11.49 units, while to impute 2.0 units increased the mean intake to 11.58.

10   Gregory JR, Collins DL, Davies PSW, Hughes JM, Clarke PC. *National Diet and Nutrition Survey: children aged 1½ to 4½ years. Volume 1: Report of the diet and nutrition survey.* HMSO (London, 1995).

11   Gregory JR et al (1995) p.76 and p.80. *(see ref 10)*

12   Department of Health. *The Diets of British Schoolchildren.* HMSO (London, 1989).

13   Gregory J, Foster K, Tyler H, Wiseman M. *The Dietary and Nutritional Survey of British Adults.* HMSO (London, 1990).

Table 6.1 Reference Nutrient Intakes (RNIs) for protein*

Sex and age (years) of young person	Protein
	g/d
Males	
4–6	19.7
7–10	28.3
11–14	42.1
15–18	55.2
Females	
4–6	19.7
7–10	28.3
11–14	41.2
15–18	45.4

*Source: Department of Health. *Report on Health and Social Subjects: 41. Dietary Reference Values for Food Energy and Nutrients for the United Kingdom.* HMSO (London, 1991).

Table 6.2 Average daily protein intake (g) by sex and age of young person

Average daily protein intake (g)	Age (years)				
	4–6	7–10	11–14	15–18	All
	cum %	cum %	cum %	cum %	cum %
Males					
Less than 19.7	1	0	0	-	0
Less than 28.3	3	1	1	-	1
Less than 42.1	29	13	7	2	12
Less than 55.2	75	53	25	14	40
Less than 65.0	91	78	51	28	61
Less than 75.0	96	96	76	49	79
Less than 85.0	99	98	92	68	89
All	100	100	100	100	100
Base	*184*	*256*	*237*	*179*	*856*
Mean (average value)	49.0	54.8	64.0	76.5	61.6
Median value	47.9	54.2	64.8	75.5	60.2
Lower 2.5 percentile	25.4	34.5	30.9	45.4	31.3
Upper 2.5 percentile	76.8	79.7	93.9	112.2	99.9
Standard deviation	13.52	12.25	15.36	19.61	18.55
	cum %	cum %	cum %	cum %	cum %
Females					
Less than 19.7	1	-	0	0	0
Less than 28.3	5	2	3	4	3
Less than 41.2	40	18	18	19	23
Less than 45.4	60	27	29	26	34
Less than 55.0	81	65	58	51	63
Less than 65.0	96	91	80	77	86
Less than 75.0	99	97	95	91	95
All	100	100	100	100	100
Base	*171*	*226*	*238*	*210*	*845*
Mean (average value)	44.5	51.2	52.9	54.8	51.2
Median value	42.7	50.7	51.7	53.9	50.5
Lower 2.5 percentile	26.3	29.5	26.9	26.4	26.8
Upper 2.5 percentile	66.8	75.2	78.4	87.4	78.4
Standard deviation	11.11	11.08	13.21	15.17	13.32

Table 6.3 Average daily protein intake as a percentage of Reference Nutrient Intake (RNI) by sex and age of young person

Sex and age (years) of young person	Average daily intake as % of RNI*			Base
	Mean	Median	sd	
Males				
4–6	249	243	69	184
7–10	194	192	43	256
11–14	152	154	36	237
15–18	139	137	36	179
All	180	171	62	856
Females				
4–6	226	217	56	171
7–10	181	179	39	226
11–14	128	126	32	238
15–18	121	119	33	210
All	161	154	58	845

*Protein intake as a percentage of RNI was calculated for each young person using the RNI appropriate for age and sex. The values were then pooled to give the mean, median and sd for each age and sex group.

Table 6.4 Percentage of food energy from protein by sex and age of young person

Percentage of food energy from protein	Age (years)				
	4–6	7–10	11–14	15–18	All
	cum %	cum %	cum %	cum %	cum %
Males					
10.0 or less	5	8	7	4	6
12.0 or less	32	42	32	20	32
14.0 or less	77	85	68	55	71
16.0 or less	96	96	90	82	91
18.0 or less	100	99	99	94	98
All	100	100	100	100	100
Base	184	256	237	179	856
Mean (average value)	12.9	12.4	13.1	13.9	13.1
Median value	12.9	12.4	13.0	13.6	12.9
Lower 2.5 percentile	9.6	9.0	8.9	9.4	9.3
Upper 2.5 percentile	16.3	17.1	17.6	19.6	17.8
Standard deviation	1.76	1.85	2.20	2.50	2.18
	cum %	cum %	cum %	cum %	cum %
Females					
10.0 or less	5	5	6	4	5
12.0 or less	34	34	42	20	33
14.0 or less	76	76	78	55	72
16.0 or less	94	94	93	82	90
18.0 or less	99	99	98	94	98
All	100	100	100	100	100
Base	171	226	238	210	845
Mean (average value)	12.7	12.8	12.7	13.9	13.1
Median value	12.6	12.8	12.5	13.7	13.0
Lower 2.5 percentile	9.4	9.5	9.2	9.9	9.5
Upper 2.5 percentile	17.1	16.7	17.9	18.9	17.8
Standard deviation	1.99	1.90	2.17	2.48	2.20

Table 6.5 Percentage contribution of food types–average daily protein intake by sex and age of young person

Type of food	Males aged (years)				All males	Females aged (years)				All females
	4–6	7–10	11–14	15–18		4–6	7–10	11–14	15–18	
	%	%	%	%	%	%	%	%	%	%
Cereals & cereal products	27	29	28	26	27	26	26	26	26	26
of which:										
bread	*11*	*12*	*11*	*12*	*12*	*11*	*11*	*11*	*12*	*11*
breakfast cereals	*5*	*5*	*4*	*4*	*4*	*4*	*3*	*3*	*2*	*3*
biscuits	*2*	*3*	*2*	*1*	*2*	*3*	*3*	*2*	*1*	*2*
buns, cakes & pastries	*3*	*3*	*2*	*2*	*2*	*2*	*2*	*2*	*2*	*2*
Milk & milk products	24	20	17	15	18	25	19	16	16	18
of which:										
whole milk	*10*	*6*	*3*	*3*	*5*	*10*	*5*	*3*	*3*	*5*
reduced fat milks	*6*	*7*	*8*	*6*	*7*	*5*	*6*	*6*	*5*	*5*
cheese	*3*	*3*	*3*	*4*	*4*	*5*	*4*	*4*	*5*	*5*
yogurt, fromage frais & other dairy desserts	*3*	*2*	*2*	*1*	*2*	*4*	*3*	*2*	*1*	*2*
Eggs & egg dishes	2	2	2	2	2	2	2	2	2	2
Fat spreads	0	0	0	0	0	0	0	0	0	0
Meat & meat products	27	28	32	37	32	26	30	32	32	30
of which:										
bacon & ham	*2*	*3*	*4*	*5*	*3*	*3*	*3*	*3*	*3*	*3*
beef, veal & dishes	*3*	*3*	*4*	*6*	*4*	*3*	*4*	*5*	*5*	*4*
chicken, turkey & dishes, including coated	*9*	*10*	*11*	*12*	*11*	*11*	*11*	*12*	*13*	*12*
sausages	*4*	*4*	*3*	*3*	*3*	*3*	*3*	*3*	*2*	*2*
Fish & fish dishes	5	4	4	4	4	5	5	4	5	5
Vegetables, potatoes & savoury snacks	11	10	10	11	10	10	11	12	12	12
of which:										
vegetables, excluding potatoes	*5*	*3*	*4*	*4*	*4*	*4*	*4*	*4*	*6*	*5*
roast or fried potatoes & chips	*3*	*3*	*3*	*4*	*3*	*3*	*3*	*4*	*3*	*3*
other potatoes	*2*	*2*	*2*	*2*	*2*	*2*	*2*	*2*	*2*	*2*
Fruit & nuts	1	1	1	1	1	1	1	1	1	1
Sugars, preserves & confectionery	2	3	3	2	2	2	2	3	2	3
Drinks*	1	1	0	1	1	1	1	1	1	1
Miscellaneous**	1	1	1	1	1	1	1	1	2	1
Average daily intake (g)	**49.0**	**54.8**	**64.0**	**76.5**	**61.6**	**44.5**	**51.2**	**52.9**	**54.8**	**51.2**
Total number of young people	**184**	**256**	**237**	**179**	**856**	**171**	**226**	**238**	**210**	**845**

*Includes soft drinks, alcoholic drinks, tea, coffee & water.
**Includes powdered beverages (except tea and coffee), soups, sauces and condiments and commercial toddlers' foods.

Table 6.6 Average daily total carbohydrate intake (g) by sex and age of young person

Average daily carbohydrate intake (g)	Age (years)				
	4–6	7–10	11–14	15–18	All
	cum %	cum %	cum %	cum %	cum %
Males					
Less than 150	8	2	1	2	3
Less than 200	40	16	12	7	18
Less than 250	80	53	38	30	49
Less than 300	99	87	70	55	77
Less than 350	100	97	90	76	90
Less than 400		99	98	88	96
All		100	100	100	100
Base	*184*	*256*	*237*	*179*	*856*
Mean (average value)	209	248	271	301	260
Median value	209	248	270	290	252
Lower 2.5 percentile	126	156	161	161	143
Upper 2.5 percentile	284	355	391	506	422
Standard deviation	42	51	64	84	71
	cum %	cum %	cum %	cum %	cum %
Females					
Less than 150	13	7	7	14	10
Less than 200	62	33	32	42	41
Less than 250	96	73	65	74	76
Less than 300	99	98	90	93	95
Less than 350	100	100	99	99	99
All			100	100	100
Base	*171*	*226*	*238*	*210*	*845*
Mean (average value)	191	218	228	214	214
Median value	190	218	226	213	211
Lower 2.5 percentile	124	124	130	107	124
Upper 2.5 percentile	259	299	342	329	323
Standard deviation	40	42	56	58	51

Table 6.7 Percentage of food energy from total carbohydrate by sex and age of young person

Percentage of food energy from carbohydrate	Age (years)				
	4–6	7–10	11–14	15–18	All
	cum %	cum %	cum %	cum %	cum %
Males					
40.0 or less	1	-	2	3	1
45.0 or less	7	5	7	13	8
50.0 or less	36	26	34	49	36
55.0 or less	75	77	78	79	77
60.0 or less	98	97	99	95	97
All	100	100	100	100	100
Base	*184*	*256*	*237*	*179*	*856*
Mean (average value)	51.6	52.4	51.7	50.5	51.6
Median value	51.6	52.4	51.8	50.1	51.6
Lower 2.5 percentile	43.0	44.2	42.5	39.9	42.5
Upper 2.5 percentile	59.4	60.5	59.8	60.7	60.5
Standard deviation	4.33	4.10	4.57	5.41	4.68
	cum %	cum %	cum %	cum %	cum %
Females					
40.0 or less	1	-	2	3	1
45.0 or less	10	8	8	15	10
50.0 or less	38	40	45	47	43
55.0 or less	78	81	79	83	80
60.0 or less	95	98	95	94	96
All	100	100	100	100	100
Base	*171*	*226*	*238*	*210*	*845*
Mean (average value)	51.4	51.3	51.2	50.6	51.1
Median value	51.7	50.8	50.7	50.3	50.8
Lower 2.5 percentile	42.1	42.6	42.2	39.9	41.1
Upper 2.5 percentile	60.5	59.9	62.8	64.0	61.3
Standard deviation	5.01	4.32	5.24	5.62	5.07

Table 6.8 Percentage contribution of food types–average daily total carbohydrate intake by age and sex of young person

Type of food	Males aged (years)				All males	Females aged (years)				All females
	4–6	7–10	11–14	15–18		4–6	7–10	11–14	15–18	
	%	%	%	%	%	%	%	%	%	%
Cereals & cereal products	45	47	44	44	45	43	43	42	41	42
of which:										
bread	*14*	*16*	*16*	*17*	*16*	*14*	*15*	*15*	*18*	*16*
breakfast cereals	*12*	*12*	*11*	*10*	*11*	*10*	*9*	*9*	*6*	*8*
biscuits	*6*	*6*	*5*	*4*	*5*	*7*	*6*	*5*	*3*	*5*
buns, cakes & pastries	*6*	*6*	*5*	*4*	*5*	*5*	*5*	*5*	*4*	*5*
puddings	*3*	*2*	*1*	*1*	*2*	*2*	*2*	*1*	*1*	*2*
Milk & milk products	10	8	7	5	7	10	8	6	5	7
of which:										
milk (whole, semi-skimmed, skimmed)	*5*	*4*	*4*	*3*	*4*	*5*	*3*	*3*	*3*	*3*
Eggs & egg dishes	0	0	0	0	0	0	0	0	0	0
Fat spreads	0	0	0	0	0	0	0	0	0	0
Meat & meat products	4	3	4	5	4	3	4	4	5	4
Fish & fish dishes	1	1	1	1	1	1	1	1	1	1
Vegetables, potatoes & savoury snacks	16	15	16	17	16	15	17	19	19	18
of which:										
vegetables, excluding potatoes	*3*	*2*	*3*	*3*	*3*	*3*	*3*	*3*	*4*	*3*
roast or fried potatoes & chips	*6*	*6*	*7*	*8*	*7*	*5*	*6*	*8*	*8*	*7*
other potatoes	*3*	*3*	*3*	*4*	*3*	*3*	*4*	*4*	*4*	*4*
savoury snacks	*4*	*4*	*4*	*3*	*3*	*4*	*4*	*5*	*3*	*4*
Fruit & nuts	4	3	2	2	3	5	4	3	3	3
Sugars, preserves & confectionery	10	11	12	11	11	12	11	11	10	11
of which:										
table sugar	*2*	*2*	*2*	*3*	*2*	*2*	*2*	*2*	*4*	*2*
sugar confectionery	*3*	*4*	*4*	*2*	*3*	*4*	*4*	*3*	*1*	*3*
chocolate confectionery	*4*	*5*	*5*	*5*	*5*	*4*	*4*	*5*	*5*	*5*
Drinks*	9	10	10	13	11	10	10	10	13	11
of which:										
fruit juice	*2*	*2*	*2*	*2*	*2*	*2*	*2*	*2*	*3*	*2*
soft drinks, not low calorie	*6*	*8*	*8*	*11*	*9*	*7*	*7*	*8*	*9*	*8*
alcoholic drinks	*0*	*0*	*0*	*1*	*0*	*0*	*0*	*0*	*1*	*0*
Miscellaneous**	1	1	1	2	2	1	2	2	2	2
Average daily intake (g)	209	248	271	301	260	191	218	228	214	214
Total number of young people	184	256	237	179	856	171	226	238	210	845

*Includes soft drinks, alcoholic drinks, tea, coffee & water.
**Includes powdered beverages (except tea and coffee), soups, sauces and condiments and commercial toddlers' foods.

144

Table 6.9 Average daily total sugars intake (g) by sex and age of young person

Average daily total sugars intake (g)	Age (years)				
	4–6	7–10	11–14	15–18	All
	cum %	cum %	cum %	cum %	cum %
Males					
Less than 60	9	6	7	6	7
Less than 90	39	22	29	24	28
Less than 120	79	58	51	50	59
Less than 150	97	84	76	70	81
Less than 180	100	94	89	83	91
Less than 210		99	97	92	97
All		100	100	100	100
Base	*184*	*256*	*237*	*179*	*856*
Mean (average value)	98	115	122	129	117
Median value	96	111	118	120	111
Lower 2.5 percentile	46	52	47	44	47
Upper 2.5 percentile	155	185	215	254	215
Standard deviation	28.5	36.0	44.8	55.3	44.2
	cum %	cum %	cum %	cum %	cum %
Females					
Less than 60	11	9	15	20	14
Less than 90	43	40	42	52	44
Less than 120	82	75	74	81	78
Less than 150	98	93	92	92	93
Less than 180	100	100	97	98	99
All			100	100	100
Base	*171*	*226*	*238*	*210*	*845*
Mean (average value)	95	101	99	92	97
Median value	95	101	98	90	95
Lower 2.5 percentile	40	40	39	29	37
Upper 2.5 percentile	146	166	181	179	166
Standard deviation	28.3	30.7	36.8	36.5	33.6

Table 6.10 Percentage contribution of food types to average daily total sugars intake by sex and age of young person

Type of food	Males aged (years)				All males	Females aged (years)				All females
	4–6	7–10	11–14	15–18		4–6	7–10	11–14	15–18	
	%	%	%	%	%	%	%	%	%	%
Cereals & cereal products	26	26	22	20	23	22	24	23	17	22
of which:										
high fibre & whole grain breakfast cereals	*2*	*2*	*2*	*2*	*2*	*2*	*2*	*2*	*1*	*2*
other breakfast cereals	*5*	*5*	*5*	*4*	*5*	*4*	*4*	*4*	*2*	*4*
biscuits	*6*	*6*	*5*	*4*	*5*	*6*	*6*	*5*	*3*	*5*
buns, cakes & pastries	*7*	*7*	*6*	*4*	*6*	*6*	*6*	*7*	*5*	*6*
puddings	*4*	*2*	*2*	*1*	*2*	*2*	*3*	*2*	*2*	*2*
Milk & milk products	20	17	15	12	16	20	16	14	12	15
of which:										
milk (whole, semi-skimmed, skimmed)	*11*	*8*	*8*	*7*	*8*	*10*	*7*	*6*	*7*	*7*
yogurt, fromage frais & other dairy desserts	*5*	*4*	*3*	*2*	*3*	*6*	*4*	*4*	*3*	*4*
Eggs & egg dishes	0	0	0	0	0	0	0	0	0	0
Fat spreads	0	0	0	0	0	0	0	0	0	0
Meat & meat products	1	1	2	2	2	1	1	2	2	2
Fish & fish dishes	0	0	0	0	0	0	0	0	0	0
Vegetables, potatoes & savoury snacks	4	3	4	4	4	3	4	4	5	4
of which:										
vegetables, excluding potatoes	*3*	*2*	*2*	*3*	*3*	*2*	*3*	*3*	*4*	*3*
Fruit & nuts	9	7	4	4	6	9	8	6	7	7
Sugars, preserves & confectionery	20	23	26	24	23	22	22	25	23	23
of which:										
table sugar	*4*	*4*	*5*	*8*	*6*	*3*	*4*	*5*	*8*	*5*
preserves & sweet spreads	*2*	*2*	*2*	*2*	*2*	*2*	*2*	*1*	*1*	*2*
sugar confectionery	*6*	*8*	*9*	*3*	*6*	*9*	*8*	*7*	*3*	*7*
chocolate confectionery	*7*	*10*	*10*	*11*	*10*	*8*	*9*	*11*	*10*	*10*
Drinks*	18	21	23	31	24	20	21	24	29	24
of which:										
fruit juice	*4*	*4*	*4*	*4*	*4*	*5*	*5*	*5*	*6*	*5*
soft drinks, not low calorie	*13*	*16*	*19*	*25*	*19*	*15*	*16*	*19*	*21*	*18*
alcoholic drinks	*0*	*0*	*0*	*2*	*0*	*0*	*0*	*0*	*2*	*0*
Miscellaneous**	2	2	2	2	2	2	2	2	3	2
Average daily intake (g)	**98**	**115**	**122**	**129**	**117**	**95**	**101**	**99**	**92**	**97**
Total number of young people	**184**	**256**	**237**	**179**	**856**	**171**	**226**	**238**	**210**	**845**

*Includes soft drinks, alcoholic drinks, tea, coffee & water.
**Includes powdered beverages (except tea and coffee), soups, sauces and condiments and commercial toddlers' foods.

146

Table 6.11 Average daily non-milk extrinsic sugars intake (g) by sex and age of young person

Average daily non-milk extrinsic sugars intake (g)	Age (years)				
	4–6	7–10	11–14	15–18	All
	cum %	cum %	cum %	cum %	cum %
Males					
Less than 40	14	8	8	9	9
Less than 60	41	21	23	24	27
Less than 80	75	50	43	42	51
Less than 100	91	75	64	61	72
Less than 120	100	87	81	75	85
Less than 140		94	89	83	91
Less than 160		99	95	87	95
All		100	100	100	100
Base	*184*	*256*	*237*	*179*	*856*
Mean (average value)	66	83	90	97	85
Median value	64	80	87	89	78
Lower 2.5 percentile	26	32	33	24	28
Upper 2.5 percentile	115	147	177	224	177
Standard deviation	23.1	30.8	38.6	49.1	38.7
	cum %	cum %	cum %	cum %	cum %
Females					
Less than 40	15	10	15	22	15
Less than 60	42	37	35	46	40
Less than 80	71	62	62	70	66
Less than 100	92	86	83	87	87
Less than 120	99	96	92	94	95
Less than 140	100	100	97	97	98
All			100	100	100
Base	*171*	*226*	*238*	*210*	*845*
Mean (average value)	66	72	73	66	69
Median value	65	70	72	63	67
Lower 2.5 percentile	19	29	23	17	20
Upper 2.5 percentile	116	133	151	144	133
Standard deviation	24.2	26.3	31.5	31.7	29.0

Table 6.12 Percentage of food energy from non-milk extrinsic sugars by sex and age of young person

Percentage of food energy from non-milk extrinsic sugars	Age (years)				
	4–6	7–10	11–14	15–18	All
	cum %	cum %	cum %	cum %	cum %
Males					
11.0 or less*	15	11	12	21	15
15.0 or less	39	33	39	49	40
20.0 or less	78	70	75	78	75
25.0 or less	95	91	94	90	92
All	100	100	100	100	100
Base	*184*	*256*	*237*	*179*	*856*
Mean (average value)	16.2	17.5	16.9	15.8	16.7
Median value	16.2	17.0	16.2	15.1	16.2
Lower 2.5 percentile	7.0	6.9	7.1	5.8	6.9
Upper 2.5 percentile	26.1	28.8	31.4	29.9	28.7
Standard deviation	4.80	5.51	5.42	6.02	5.52
	cum %	cum %	cum %	cum %	cum %
Females					
11.0 or less*	12	15	17	22	17
15.0 or less	35	36	41	48	40
20.0 or less	68	75	77	83	76
25.0 or less	90	94	95	94	93
All	100	100	100	100	100
Base	*171*	*226*	*238*	*210*	*845*
Mean (average value)	17.6	16.7	16.2	15.3	16.4
Median value	17.2	16.7	16.3	15.0	16.4
Lower 2.5 percentile	7.2	7.4	6.8	5.1	6.7
Upper 2.5 percentile	28.9	26.8	27.1	27.8	27.9
Standard deviation	5.63	4.95	5.45	5.77	5.50

*The current recommendation is that intake of non-milk extrinsic sugars should not exceed 11% of food energy.

Table 6.13 Percentage contribution of food types to average daily non-milk extrinsic sugars intake by sex and age of young person

Type of food	Males aged (years)				All males	Females aged (years)				All females
	4–6	7–10	11–14	15–18		4–6	7–10	11–14	15–18	
	%	%	%	%	%	%	%	%	%	%
Cereals & cereal products	30	28	23	19	25	26	26	24	17	23
of which:										
high fibre & whole grain breakfast cereals	2	2	2	2	2	2	2	2	1	2
other breakfast cereals	6	7	5	5	6	6	5	5	3	5
biscuits	8	8	6	6	7	8	8	7	4	7
buns, cakes & pastries	9	8	7	5	7	7	7	8	6	7
puddings	4	2	2	1	2	2	3	1	2	2
Milk & milk products	9	7	7	4	6	9	8	6	5	7
Eggs & egg dishes	0	0	0	0	0	0	0	0	0	0
Fat spreads	0	-	0	0	0	0	0	0	0	0
Meat & meat products	0	0	0	1	0	0	0	0	1	0
Fish & fish dishes	0	0	0	0	0	0	0	0	0	0
Vegetables, potatoes & savoury snacks	1	1	1	2	1	1	1	1	1	1
Fruit & nuts	1	1	0	0	1	1	1	1	0	1
Sugars, preserves & confectionery	28	31	33	30	31	31	30	32	31	31
of which:										
table sugar	6	6	7	11	8	5	5	7	12	7
preserves & sweet spreads	3	2	2	2	2	3	3	2	2	2
sugar confectionery	9	11	11	4	9	13	11	10	4	9
chocolate confectionery	9	12	12	12	12	10	11	14	13	12
Drinks*	27	29	31	42	33	29	30	32	41	33
of which:										
fruit juice	6	6	5	6	6	7	7	6	8	7
carbonated soft drinks not low calorie	9	13	19	28	18	11	12	19	23	16
concentrated soft drinks not low calorie	6	7	4	4	5	6	6	4	4	5
ready to drink soft drinks not low calorie	4	4	2	1	3	4	4	2	2	3
alcoholic drinks	0	0	0	2	1	0	0	0	2	1
Miscellaneous**	3	2	3	2	2	3	3	2	3	3
Average daily intake (g)	**66**	**83**	**90**	**97**	**85**	**66**	**72**	**73**	**66**	**69**
Total number of young people	**184**	**256**	**237**	**179**	**856**	**171**	**226**	**238**	**210**	**845**

*Includes soft drinks, alcoholic drinks, tea, coffee & water.
**Includes powdered beverages (except tea and coffee), soups, sauces and condiments and commercial toddlers' foods.

149

Table 6.14   Average daily intrinsic and milk sugars intake (g) by sex and age of young person

Average daily intrinsic and milk sugars intake (g)	Age (years)				
	4–6	7–10	11–14	15–18	All
	cum %	cum %	cum %	cum %	cum %
Males					
Less than 15	6	4	7	7	6
Less than 30	50	46	54	53	51
Less than 45	86	88	83	83	85
Less than 60	98	98	96	96	97
All	100	100	100	100	100
Base	*184*	*256*	*237*	*179*	*856*
Mean (average value)	32	32	31	32	32
Median value	30	31	29	29	30
Lower 2.5 percentile	12	13	11	11	12
Upper 2.5 percentile	59	60	65	67	63
Standard deviation	12.4	11.5	13.3	15.1	13.2
	cum %	cum %	cum %	cum %	cum %
Females					
Less than 15	7	7	14	19	12
Less than 30	59	61	68	68	64
Less than 45	91	94	94	93	93
Less than 60	99	98	99	99	99
All	100	100	100	100	100
Base	*171*	*226*	*238*	*210*	*845*
Mean (average value)	29	29	26	26	28
Median value	29	28	23	24	26
Lower 2.5 percentile	11	11	11	9	11
Upper 2.5 percentile	53	57	53	53	53
Standard deviation	10.6	10.7	11.1	13.4	11.6

Table 6.15 Percentage contribution of food types to average daily intrinsic and milk sugars intake by sex and age of young person

Type of food	Males aged (years)				All males	Females aged (years)				All females
	4–6	7–10	11–14	15–18		4–6	7–10	11–14	15–18	
	%	%	%	%	%	%	%	%	%	%
Cereals & cereal products	16	19	20	21	19	15	18	19	18	18
of which:										
bread	*5*	*7*	*8*	*9*	*7*	*5*	*6*	*7*	*8*	*7*
breakfast cereals	*3*	*4*	*4*	*4*	*4*	*3*	*3*	*3*	*2*	*3*
buns, cakes & pastries	*2*	*3*	*3*	*2*	*2*	*2*	*2*	*3*	*2*	*2*
puddings	*3*	*2*	*2*	*1*	*2*	*2*	*3*	*2*	*2*	*2*
Milk & milk products	44	41	41	36	40	44	36	34	30	36
of which:										
whole milk	*21*	*14*	*9*	*9*	*13*	*22*	*11*	*8*	*8*	*12*
reduced fat milks	*12*	*16*	*21*	*20*	*17*	*10*	*14*	*16*	*15*	*14*
yogurt, fromage frais										
& other dairy										
desserts	*7*	*6*	*5*	*3*	*5*	*7*	*7*	*6*	*4*	*6*
Eggs & egg dishes	0	0	0	0	0	0	0	0	0	0
Fat spreads	0	0	0	0	0	0	0	0	0	0
Meat & meat products	3	3	5	7	5	3	4	5	5	4
Fish & fish dishes	0	0	0	0	0	0	0	0	0	0
Vegetables, potatoes & savoury snacks	8	8	10	12	10	8	10	13	15	12
Fruit & nuts	24	23	16	16	20	26	26	20	23	24
Sugars, preserves & confectionery	3	4	5	5	4	3	4	5	4	4
Drinks*	0	0	0	0	0	0	0	0	0	0
Miscellaneous**	1	1	1	2	1	1	1	1	2	1
Average daily intake (g)	**32**	**32**	**31**	**32**	**32**	**29**	**29**	**26**	**26**	**28**
Total number of young people	**184**	**256**	**237**	**179**	**856**	**171**	**226**	**238**	**210**	**845**

*Includes soft drinks, alcoholic drinks, tea, coffee & water.
**Includes powdered beverages (except tea and coffee), soups, sauces and condiments and commercial toddlers' foods.

151

Table 6.16 Average daily starch intake (g) by sex and age of young person

Average daily starch intake (g)	Age (years)				
	4–6	7–10	11–14	15–18	All
	cum %	cum %	cum %	cum %	cum %
Males					
Less than 90	19	4	3	2	6
Less than 120	70	34	15	8	30
Less than 150	93	73	54	33	62
Less than 180	99	95	83	63	84
Less than 210	100	98	95	81	93
All		100	100	100	100
Base	*184*	*256*	*237*	*179*	*856*
Mean (average value)	110	133	149	172	143
Median value	109	130	147	168	138
Lower 2.5 percentile	61	86	88	95	77
Upper 2.5 percentile	163	200	224	272	236
Standard deviation	25.4	31.4	34.0	44.2	41.2
	cum %	cum %	cum %	cum %	cum %
Females					
Less than 60	3	-	-	2	1
Less than 90	45	12	10	17	20
Less than 120	86	57	43	46	56
Less than 150	97	90	74	82	85
Less than 180	99	99	95	95	97
All	100	100	100	100	100
Base	*171*	*226*	*238*	*210*	*845*
Mean (average value)	96	117	129	122	117
Median value	95	116	127	122	114
Lower 2.5 percentile	57	73	74	62	64
Upper 2.5 percentile	162	173	195	185	182
Standard deviation	23.2	24.2	31.2	32.7	30.6

Table 6.17 **Percentage contribution of food types to average daily starch intake by age and sex of young person**

Type of food	Males aged (years)				All males	Females aged (years)				All females
	4–6	7–10	11–14	15–18		4–6	7–10	11–14	15–18	
	%	%	%	%	%	%	%	%	%	%
Cereals & cereal products	63	65	62	62	63	63	60	58	59	60
of which:										
bread	26	28	27	29	28	27	26	25	31	27
breakfast cereals	17	15	14	13	15	15	11	11	8	11
biscuits	6	6	4	3	5	7	6	4	3	5
buns, cakes & pastries	5	5	4	3	4	5	4	4	4	4
Milk & milk products	0	0	0	0	0	0	0	0	0	0
Eggs & egg dishes	0	0	0	0	0	0	0	0	0	0
Fat spreads	-	0	-	-	0	-	-	-	-	-
Meat & meat products	6	5	7	8	7	5	6	6	7	6
Fish & fish dishes	2	1	1	1	1	2	1	1	1	1
Vegetables, potatoes & savoury snacks	27	26	27	27	27	27	29	31	29	29
of which:										
vegetables, excluding potatoes	3	2	3	3	3	3	3	3	4	3
roast or fried potatoes & chips	10	11	12	13	12	10	11	13	13	12
other potatoes	6	6	5	6	6	6	7	6	7	7
savoury snacks	7	7	6	5	6	8	8	8	6	7
Fruit & nuts	0	0	0	0	0	0	0	0	0	0
Sugars, preserves & confectionery	1	1	1	1	1	1	1	1	1	1
Drinks*	0	0	0	0	0	0	0	0	0	0
Miscellaneous**	1	1	1	1	1	1	1	1	2	1
Average daily intake (g)	110	133	149	172	143	96	117	129	122	117
Total number of young people	184	256	237	179	856	171	226	238	210	845

*Includes soft drinks, alcoholic drinks, tea, coffee & water.
**Includes powdered beverages (except tea and coffee), soups, sauces and condiments and commercial toddlers' foods.

Table 6.18 Percentage of food energy from intrinsic and milk sugars and starch by sex and age of young person

Percentage of food energy from intrinsic and milk sugars and starch	Age (years)				
	4–6	7–10	11–14	15–18	All
	cum %	cum %	cum %	cum %	cum %
Males					
25.0 or less	–	1	3	3	2
30.0 or less	9	11	16	20	14
35.0 or less	54	53	52	53	53
39.0 or less	78	82	84	83	82
40.0 or less	83	89	86	87	86
45.0 or less	97	99	98	96	98
All	100	100	100	100	100
Base	*184*	*256*	*237*	*179*	*856*
Mean (average value)	35.4	34.9	34.8	34.7	34.9
Median value	34.4	34.7	34.9	34.5	34.6
Lower 2.5 percentile	26.5	27.2	24.3	24.6	25.7
Upper 2.5 percentile	45.1	42.6	44.1	45.7	44.8
Standard deviation	4.54	4.40	4.89	5.15	4.76
	cum %	cum %	cum %	cum %	cum %
Females					
25.0 or less	1	1	1	0	1
30.0 or less	18	15	16	18	17
35.0 or less	66	61	53	53	58
39.0 or less	92	85	82	76	83
40.0 or less	94	89	88	81	88
45.0 or less	98	97	97	95	97
All	100	100	100	100	100
Base	*171*	*226*	*238*	*210*	*845*
Mean (average value)	33.8	34.5	35.0	35.3	34.7
Median value	33.6	34.1	34.9	34.5	34.3
Lower 2.5 percentile	26.5	26.5	25.8	26.5	26.3
Upper 2.5 percentile	43.4	45.8	45.6	47.2	46.3
Standard deviation	4.46	4.66	5.27	5.70	5.09

Table 6.19 Average daily non-starch polysaccharides intake (g) by sex and age of young person

Average daily non-starch polysaccharides intake (g)	Age (years)				
	4–6	7–10	11–14	15–18	All
	cum %	cum %	cum %	cum %	cum %
Males					
Less than 6.0	13	4	4	2	5
Less than 8.0	37	22	13	7	19
Less than 10.0	67	51	33	22	42
Less than 12.0	83	72	59	42	63
Less than 14.0	94	87	78	61	79
Less than 16.0	97	96	89	78	90
Less than 18.0	99	99	95	89	95
Less than 20.0	100	100	98	93	98
All			100	100	100
Base	*184*	*256*	*237*	*179*	*856*
Mean (average value)	9.1	10.3	11.6	13.3	11.2
Median value	8.8	9.9	11.5	12.5	10.8
Lower 2.5 percentile	4.0	5.7	4.9	7.0	5.0
Upper 2.5 percentile	16.3	16.5	19.8	23.4	19.8
Standard deviation	2.96	2.99	3.44	4.42	3.83
	cum %	cum %	cum %	cum %	cum %
Females					
Less than 6.0	24	8	5	8	11
Less than 8.0	54	29	27	23	32
Less than 10.0	79	57	54	50	59
Less than 12.0	94	78	74	72	79
Less than 14.0	97	93	86	84	90
Less than 16.0	98	97	96	91	96
Less than 18.0	99	99	98	96	98
All	100	100	100	100	100
Base	*171*	*226*	*238*	*210*	*845*
Mean (average value)	8.0	9.8	10.2	10.6	9.7
Median value	7.5	9.6	9.6	10.0	9.3
Lower 2.5 percentile	4.1	5.3	5.2	4.1	4.5
Upper 2.5 percentile	15.1	16.5	17.0	19.8	17.5
Standard deviation	2.82	2.82	3.21	4.21	3.46

Table 6.20 Percentage contribution of food types to average daily non-starch polysaccharides intake by sex and age of young person

Type of food	Males aged (years)				All males	Females aged (years)				All females
	4–6	7–10	11–14	15–18		4–6	7–10	11–14	15–18	
	%	%	%	%	%	%	%	%	%	%
Cereals & cereal products	40	43	41	39	40	39	37	35	36	37
of which:										
white bread	*8*	*10*	*10*	*11*	*10*	*9*	*9*	*9*	*9*	*9*
wholemeal bread	*4*	*4*	*3*	*3*	*3*	*4*	*4*	*3*	*4*	*4*
high fibre & whole grain breakfast cereals	*11*	*11*	*10*	*9*	*10*	*10*	*8*	*7*	*6*	*8*
other breakfast cereals	*2*	*2*	*2*	*2*	*2*	*2*	*2*	*1*	*1*	*1*
biscuits	*4*	*4*	*3*	*2*	*3*	*4*	*4*	*3*	*2*	*3*
buns, cakes & pastries	*3*	*3*	*3*	*2*	*3*	*3*	*3*	*3*	*2*	*3*
Milk & milk products	1	1	1	0	1	1	1	1	0	1
Eggs & egg dishes	0	0	0	0	0	0	0	0	0	0
Fat spreads	-	-	-	-	-	-	-	-	-	-
Meat & meat products	5	5	6	8	6	5	6	6	6	6
Fish & fish dishes	1	1	1	1	1	1	1	1	1	1
Vegetables, potatoes & savoury snacks	39	38	39	42	40	39	41	44	43	42
of which:										
vegetables, excluding potatoes	*18*	*15*	*16*	*18*	*17*	*18*	*17*	*17*	*21*	*18*
roast or fried potatoes & chips	*9*	*10*	*12*	*13*	*11*	*9*	*10*	*13*	*11*	*11*
other potatoes	*5*	*6*	*6*	*6*	*6*	*5*	*7*	*7*	*6*	*6*
savoury snacks	*7*	*7*	*6*	*5*	*6*	*7*	*7*	*8*	*5*	*7*
Fruit & nuts	10	9	6	5	7	11	10	7	7	9
Sugars, preserves & confectionery	2	3	3	3	3	2	2	3	2	2
Drinks*	0	0	0	0	0	0	0	0	0	0
Miscellaneous**	1	1	1	2	1	1	1	2	3	2
Average daily intake (g)	**9.1**	**10.3**	**11.6**	**13.3**	**11.2**	**8.0**	**9.8**	**10.2**	**10.6**	**9.7**
Total number of young people	**184**	**256**	**237**	**179**	**856**	**171**	**226**	**238**	**210**	**845**

*Includes soft drinks, alcoholic drinks, tea, coffee & water.
**Includes powdered beverages (except tea and coffee), soups, sauces and condiments and commercial toddlers' foods.

Table 6.21　Average number of bowel movements per day during dietary recording period by sex and age of young person

Those completing a 7-day bowel movement record

Average number of bowel movements per day	Males aged (years)				All males	Females aged (years)				All females
	4–6	7–10	11–14	15–18		4–6	7–10	11–14	15–18	
	%	%	%	%	%	%	%	%	%	%
Fewer than 1.0 per day	33	43	36	31	36	34	40	41	37	38
1.0 to fewer than 1.5 per day	53	44	43	43	45	50	42	33	40	41
1.5 to fewer than 2.0 per day	9	8	10	10	9	10	10	4	9	8
2.0 to fewer than 2.5 per day	4	4	6	8	5	4	5	9	4	6
2.5 to fewer than 3.0 per day	1	1	2	4	2	2	1	3	4	3
3.0 or more per day	1	0	4	5	3	0	2	9	6	4
Mean number of bowel movements	1.1	1.0	1.2	1.4	1.2	1.1	1.1	1.3	1.3	1.2
Base	*200*	*267*	*254*	*203*	*924*	*190*	*244*	*256*	*236*	*926*

Table 6.22　Average number of bowel movements per day during dietary recording period by average daily intake of non-starch polysaccharides (g)

Those completing a 7-day bowel movement record

Average number of bowel movements per day	Average daily intake of non-starch polysaccharides (g)			*Base*
	Mean	Median	sd	
Fewer than 1.0	10.0	9.6	3.62	*620*
1.0 to fewer than 1.5	10.7	10.3	3.58	*705*
1.5 to fewer than 2.0	10.8	10.2	3.60	*145*
2.0 to fewer than 2.5	11.0	10.0	4.35	*93*
2.5 to fewer than 3.0	11.2	9.3	5.37	*33*
3.0 or more	10.2	10.0	3.23	*59*
All young people	10.5	10.0	3.70	*1659*

Table 6.23   Alcohol consumption in the last seven days as reported in the initial dietary interview by sex and age of young person

Responding sample – young people aged 7 to 18 years

Reported alcohol consumption (units)	Males aged (years) 7–10	11–14	15–18	All males	Females aged (years) 7–10	11–14	15–18	All females
a) Total sample	%	%	%	%	%	%	%	%
None	94	86	43	75	90	82	41	71
Less than 1.00	1	4	4	3	–	5	7	4
1.00 – 1.75	0	3	4	3	1	6	4	4
2.00 – 3.75	–	2	7	3	–	2	6	3
4.00 – 5.75	–	0	6	2	0	0	7	3
6.00 – 9.75	–	2	5	2	–	0	12	4
10.00 – 14.75	–	1	8	3	–	1	9	3
15.00–20.75	–	1	6	2	–	1	3	1
21.00–27.75	–	–	6	2	–	–	3	1
28.00 or more	–	–	10	3	–	–	5	2
Not answered	5	2	1	3	9	2	2	4
Mean number of units consumed in 7 days	0.0	0.5	9.1	3.2	0.0	0.5	6.7	2.4
Base	*304*	*290*	*258*	*852*	*277*	*280*	*264*	*821*
b) Consumers only*	No.	%	%	%	No.	%	%	%
Less than 1.00	[2]	35	7	13	–	31	12	16
1.00 – 1.75	[1]	24	8	11	[3]	37	8	15
2.00 – 3.75	–	13	13	13	–	12	11	11
4.00 – 5.75	–	3	11	9	[1]	3	13	11
6.00 – 9.75	–	14	9	10	–	2	21	17
10.00 – 14.75	–	6	14	12	–	7	16	14
15.00–20.75	–	5	10	9	–	8	5	5
21.00–27.75	–	–	10	8	–	–	6	5
28.00 or more	–	–	18	14	–	–	8	7
Mean number of units consumed in 7 days	**	3.6	16.1	13.7	**	3.4	11.4	9.5
Base	*3*	*39*	*146*	*188*	*4*	*44*	*132*	*152*

*[ ] indicates number (unweighted) not percentage.
** Base numbers are too small to allow reliable means to be calculated.

Table 6.24   Alcohol consumption in the last seven days as reported in the initial dietary interview compared with data from the 1996 Survey of Young Teenagers and Alcohol

Total reported alcohol consumption in 7 days (units)	NDNS responding sample – young people aged 11–15 years: England only Total sample	Consumers only	1996 Survey of Young Teenagers and Alcohol: England* All pupils	Consumers only
	%	%	%	%
None	79	–	78	-
Less than 1.00	5	26	2	8
1.00 – 1.75	5	24	3	12
2.00 – 3.75	3	17	5	21
4.00 – 5.75	2	10	3	14
6.00 – 9.75	2	10	4	18
10.00 – 14.75	1	7	2	10
15.00 or more	1	6	4	17
Not answered	1	–	–	–
Mean number of units consumed in 7 days	0.7	3.9	1.8	8.4
Base	*545*	*105*	*2676*	*585*

*Goddard E. *Young teenagers and alcohol in 1996 Volume 1: England.* HMSO (London, 1997).

Table 6.25 Average daily alcohol intake (g) by sex and age of young person

Diary sample

Average daily alcohol intake (g)	Males aged (years)				Females aged (years)			
	11–14	15–18	11–18	4–18*	11–14	15–18	11–18	4–18*
a) Total sample	cum %	cum %	cum %	cum %	cum %	cum %	cum %	cum %
Zero	90	56	73	84	90	63	77	85
Less than 1.0	96	60	79	89	97	67	82	91
Less than 2.0	98	63	81	90	98	70	84	92
Less than 5.0	100	74	87	93	99	76	88	94
Less than 10.0		80	90	95	100	89	94	97
Less than 20.0		89	95	97		96	98	99
Less than 30.0		94	97	98		98	99	100
All		100	100	100		100	100	100
Base	*237*	*179*	*416*	*856*	*238*	*210*	*448*	*845*
Mean (average value)	0.1	6.8	3.4	1.8	0.1	3.4	1.8	0.9
Median value	0.0	0.0	0.0	0.0	0.0	0.0	0.0	0.0
Upper 2.5 percentile	1.8	48.1	0.0	23.7	1.6	23.8	0.0	12.2
Standard deviation	0.5	18.1	13.2	9.7	1.0	7.6	5.6	4.2
b) Consumers only								
Mean (average value)	1.1	15.6	12.9	11.0	1.5	9.3	7.6	6.3
Median value	0.4	7.4	4.7	3.4	0.4	6.2	5.2	3.1
Upper 2.5 percentile	4.7	51.0	51.0	49.5	12.3	41.8	31.8	31.8
Standard deviation	1.42	24.75	23.09	21.71	2.78	10.02	9.53	9.07
Base	*22***	*81*	*103*	*127*	*25***	*86*	*111*	*133*

*17 young people aged 4–6 years, and 29 young people aged 7 to 10 years reported consuming foods or drinks containing alcohol during the 7-day recording period. Some alcohol may have been consumed as part of recipe dishes.
** Small base number; results for this group should therefore be treated with caution.

Table 6.26 **Percentage of energy from alcohol by sex and age of young person**

Diary sample

Percentage of energy from alcohol	Males aged (years)				Females aged (years)			
	11–14	15–18	11–18	4–18*	11–14	15–18	11–18	4–18*
a) Total sample	cum %	cum %	cum %	cum %	cum %	cum %	cum %	cum %
Zero	90	56	73	84	90	63	77	85
Less than 1.0%	96	60	79	89	97	67	82	91
Less than 2.0%	98	63	81	90	98	70	84	92
Less than 5.0%	100	74	87	93	99	76	88	94
Less than 10.0%		80	90	95	100	89	94	97
All		100	100	100		100	100	100
Base	*237*	*179*	*416*	*856*	*238*	*210*	*448*	*845*
Mean	0.0	1.9	1.0	0.5	0.1	1.4	0.7	0.4
Median value	0.0	0.0	0.0	0.0	0.0	0.0	0.0	0.0
Upper 2.5 percentile	0.6	14.0	10.1	6.7	0.6	8.4	6.9	4.8
Standard deviation	0.18	4.53	3.33	2.45	0.39	3.02	2.25	1.66
b) Consumers only								
Mean	0.4	4.5	3.8	3.2	0.6	3.8	3.1	2.6
Median value	0.2	2.3	1.3	1.0	0.2	2.7	2.3	1.5
Upper 2.5 percentile	1.6	18.1	17.7	17.3	4.5	14.8	14.6	9.4
Standard deviation	0.47	6.03	5.70	5.42	1.09	3.95	3.77	3.61
Base	*22***	*81*	*103*	*127*	*25***	*86*	*111*	*133*

*17 young people aged 4 to 6 years, and 29 young people aged 7 to 10 years reported consuming foods or drinks containing alcohol during the 7-day recording period. Some alcohol may have been consumed as part of recipe dishes.
** Small base number; results for this group should therefore be treated with caution.

Table 6.27 Average daily intake of protein, carbohydrates and non-starch polysaccharides (g) by whether young person was reported as being unwell during the dietary recording period

Nutrient	Whether young person was unwell during dietary recording period								
	Unwell and eating affected			Unwell and eating not affected			Not unwell		
	Mean	Median	sd	Mean	Median	sd	Mean	Median	sd
Protein (g)	48.6	47.0	17.09	53.8	51.3	15.79	57.8	55.6	16.86
Total carbohydrate (g)	205	199	63.5	231	228	60.3	242	235	66.2
Total carbohydrate as % food energy	51.5	51.9	5.65	51.5	51.6	4.62	51.3	51.2	4.80
Total sugars (g)	94	89	40.4	103	104	37.2	109	106	40.7
Non-milk extrinsic sugars (g)	70	64	36.7	76	77	31.9	78	74	35.2
Starch (g)	111	107	35.1	128	124	33.0	133	127	38.9
Non-starch polysaccharides (g)	8.7	8.3	3.44	9.8	9.3	2.92	10.8	10.2	3.77
Base	*179*			*150*			*1372*		

Table 6.28 Average daily intake of protein, carbohydrates and non-starch polysaccharides (g) by region

Nutrient	Region											
	Scotland			Northern			Central, South West and Wales			London and the South East		
	Mean	Median	sd	Mean	Median	sd	Mean	Median	sd	Mean	Median	sd
Protein (g)	54.8	51.5	16.65	56.1	55.0	15.63	57.8	56.1	17.51	55.9	52.6	17.75
Total carbohydrate (g)	229	216	71.7	238	232	66.3	241	235	64.1	235	230	67.4
Total carbohydrate as % food energy	50.6	50.7	4.98	51.1	51.2	4.77	51.6	51.5	4.69	51.5	51.4	5.15
Total sugars (g)	106	97	44.0	108	105	40.0	108	105	39.9	106	102	41.1
Non-milk extrinsic sugars (g)	77	71	37.8	79	75	35.4	78	74	34.7	76	71	34.9
Starch (g)	124	123	38.3	130	125	39.6	132	127	36.6	129	125	39.8
Non-starch polysaccharides (g)	9.3	9.1	3.19	10.3	9.9	3.39	10.9	10.5	3.62	10.5	9.6	4.18
Base	*137*			*460*			*606*			*498*		

Table 6.29 Average daily intake of protein, carbohydrates and non-starch polysaccharides (g) by social class of head of household

| Nutrient | Social class of head of household | | | | | | | | |
| | Non-manual | | | Manual | | | Unclassified* | | |
	Mean	Median	sd	Mean	Median	sd	Mean	Median	sd
Protein (g)	58.1	56.1	17.50	55.9	53.7	16.37	52.1	50.3	16.78
Total carbohydrate (g)	242	237	67.8	237	229	64.6	218	218	63.8
Total carbohydrate as % food energy	51.4	51.4	4.89	51.2	51.1	4.70	51.4	50.9	5.59
Total sugars (g)	113	110	40.9	104	99	38.7	92	89	41.8
Non-milk extrinsic sugars (g)	81	77	35.6	76	72	34.4	66	61	33.9
Starch (g)	129	125	38.6	132	127	39.5	126	124	33.7
Non-starch polysaccharides (g)	10.8	10.2	3.84	10.3	9.8	3.61	9.9	9.6	3.54
Base		*815*			*746*			*140*	

*Includes those for whom social class could not be assigned.

Table 6.30 Average daily intake of protein, carbohydrates and non-starch polysaccharides (g) by gross weekly household income

Nutrient	Gross weekly household income														
	Less than £160			£160 to less than £280			£280 to less than £400			£400 to less than £600			£600 and over		
	Mean	Median	sd	Mean	Median	sd	Mean	Median	sd	Mean	Median	sd	Mean	Median	sd
Protein (g)	53.2	51.7	16.42	52.6	51.2	15.66	56.8	55.1	15.90	58.8	56.8	17.08	59.7	57.4	17.07
Total carbohydrate (g)	226	220	69.9	231	228	60.2	240	229	65.8	245	244	68.9	243	233	65.7
Total carbohydrate as % food energy	51.2	51.3	4.81	51.9	51.7	5.06	50.8	50.9	4.72	51.5	51.5	4.52	51.4	51.3	4.99
Total sugars (g)	96	92	40.8	102	96	38.2	108	103	39.8	114	111	41.1	115	111	40.7
Non-milk extrinsic sugars (g)	69	63	35.0	74	69	32.9	79	72	35.9	82	77	35.6	82	78	35.5
Starch (g)	130	124	42.4	129	127	35.6	132	125	38.7	131	128	39.4	128	123	36.4
Non-starch polysaccharides (g)	10.0	9.6	3.53	10.0	9.6	3.33	10.4	9.9	3.66	10.7	10.3	3.69	10.9	10.3	3.87
Base	375			144			522			268			321		

Table 6.31 Average daily intake of protein, carbohydrates and non-starch polysaccharides (g) by whether young person's 'parents' were receiving certain benefits

Nutrient	Whether 'parents' receiving benefits					
	Receiving benefits			Not receiving benefits		
	Mean	Median	sd	Mean	Median	sd
Protein (g)	52.3	51.1	15.43	58.0	55.7	17.27
Total carbohydrate (g)	224	223	63.0	242	236	66.9
Total carbohydrate as % food energy	51.2	51.1	4.95	51.4	51.3	4.85
Total sugars (g)	96	92	39.3	111	108	40.3
Non-milk extrinsic sugars (g)	69	63	33.1	80	76	35.4
Starch (g)	129	125	38.4	131	126	38.6
Non-starch polysaccharides (g)	10.0	9.5	3.67	10.7	10.1	3.73
Base		*388*			*1311*	

Table 6.32 Average daily intake of protein, carbohydrates and non-starch polysaccharides (g) by whether the young person was living with both parents

Nutrient	Young person living with*:								
	Both parents and other children			Both parents and no other children			Single parent with/out other children		
	Mean	Median	sd	Mean	Median	sd	Mean	Median	sd
Protein (g)	54.9	52.8	15.13	63.4	61.5	19.60	55.0	53.2	18.16
Carbohydrate (g)	236	230	59.0	249	244	80.2	231	225	69.7
Total carbohydrate as % food energy	51.7	51.5	4.78	50.4	50.2	4.99	51.3	51.4	4.89
Total sugars (g)	108	105	38.0	111	106	47.8	103	98	42.0
Non-milk extrinsic sugars (g)	78	74	32.6	81	73	40.9	74	70	36.3
Starch (g)	128	125	35.4	138	136	43.9	128	124	40.9
Non-starch polysaccharides (g)	10.3	9.8	3.49	11.2	10.9	4.23	10.4	9.9	3.82
Base		*1026*			*342*			*324*	

*Excludes 9 young people who were living with others, not parents.

Table 6.33 Average daily intake of alcohol (g) by whether young person was reported as being unwell during dietary recording period

Young people aged 11 to 18 years

Nutrient	Whether young person reported as unwell during dietary recording period								
	Unwell and eating affected			Unwell and eating not affected			Not unwell		
	Mean	Median	sd	Mean	Median	sd	Mean	Median	sd
(a) Total sample									
Alcohol (g)	2.7	0.0	8.66	1.6	0.0	5.79	2.8	0.0	10.85
Alcohol as % total energy	0.9	0.0	2.73	0.6	0.0	2.25	0.9	0.0	2.94
Base = all aged 11 to 18 years		*95*			*86*			*683*	
(b) Consumers only*									
Percentage consumers		22%			19%			26%	
Base = all consumers		*21*			*16*			*180*	

* Base numbers are too small to allow reliable means to be calculated.

Table 6.34 Average daily intake of alcohol (g) by region

Young people aged 11 to 18 years

Nutrient	Region														
	Scotland			Northern			Central, South West and Wales			London and the South East		
	Mean	Median	sd	Mean	Median	sd	Mean	Median	sd	Mean	Median	sd
(a) Total sample												
Alcohol (g)	1.6	0.0	6.37	3.3	0.0	9.59	1.9	0.0	5.78	3.2	0.0	15.03
Alcohol as % total energy	0.6	0.0	2.12	1.1	0.0	2.90	0.7	0.0	2.05	1.0	0.0	3.72
Base = all aged 11 to 18 years		*63*			*229*			*312*			*260*	
(b) Consumers only												
Alcohol (g)	*	*		12.0	6.5	15.14	8.9	5.3	9.76	10.7	3.7	25.98
Alcohol as % total energy	*	*		3.9	2.4	4.42	3.1	1.5	3.52	3.2	1.4	6.26
Percentage consumers	19%			29%			21%			28%		
Base = all consumers		*12*			*67*			*64*			*74*	

* Base numbers are too small to allow reliable means to be calculated.

Table 6.35 Average daily intake of alcohol (g) by social class of head of household

Young people aged 11 to 18 years

Nutrient	Social class of head of household								
	Non-manual			Manual			All*		
	Mean	Median	sd	Mean	Median	sd	Mean	Median	sd
a) Total sample									
Alcohol (g)	2.8	0.0	8.21	3.0	0.0	12.86	0.4	0.0	2.11
Alcohol as % total energy	0.9	0.0	2.74	0.9	0.0	3.23	0.2	0.0	0.83
Base = all aged 11 to 18 years		402			386			864	
b) Consumers only									
Alcohol (g)	9.0	4.4	12.72	13.2	6.5	24.49	4.5	2.0	5.38
Alcohol as % total energy	3.0	1.5	4.23	4.1	2.5	5.78	1.8	0.7	2.12
Percentage consumers		29%			22%			25%	
Base = all consumers		118			87			214	

*Includes those for whom social class could not be assigned.

Table 6.36 Average daily intake of alcohol by gross weekly household income

Young people aged 11 to 18 years

Nutrient	Gross weekly household income														
	Less than £160			£160 to less than £280			£280 to less than £400			£400 to less than £600			£600 and over		
	Mean	Median	sd	Mean	Median	sd	Mean	Median	sd	Mean	Median	sd	Mean	Median	sd
(a) Total sample															
Alcohol (g)	1.0	0.0	5.44	1.7	0.0	6.11	2.8	0.0	7.91	1.3	0.0	4.15	5.6	0.0	17.76
Alcohol as % total energy	0.3	0.0	1.51	0.6	0.0	2.13	0.9	0.0	2.59	0.5	0.0	1.52	1.7	0.0	4.57
Base = all aged 11 to 18 years		*375*			*144*			*522*			*268*			*321*	
(b) Consumers only															
Alcohol (g)		*			*		10.2	4.8	12.43	5.7	2.9	7.02	13.7	6.7	25.79
Alcohol as % total energy		*			*		3.4	1.6	4.04	2.1	1.1	2.55	4.3	2.3	6.37
Percentage consumers		4%			17%			7%			18%			26%	
Base = all consumers		*16*			*24*			*37*			*48*			*85*	

* Base numbers are too small to allow reliable means to be calculated.

Table 6.37 Average daily intake of alcohol (g) by whether young person's 'parents' were receiving certain benefits

Young people aged 11 to 18 years

| Nutrient | Whether 'parents' receiving benefits | | | | | |
| | Receiving benefits | | | Not receiving benefits | | |
	Mean	Median	sd	Mean	Median	sd
Total sample						
Alcohol (g)	0.8	0.0	4.51	3.1	0.0	11.34
Alcohol as % total energy	0.3	0.0	1.43	1.0	0.0	3.13
Base = all aged 11 to 18 years		168			694	
(b) Consumers only*						
Percentage consumers		11%			29%	
Base = all consumers		19			198	

* Base numbers are too small to allow reliable means to be calculated.

Table 6.38 Average daily intake of alcohol (g) by whether the young person was living with both parents

Young people aged 11 to 18 years

| Nutrient | Young person living with*: | | | | | | | | |
| | Both parents and other children | | | Both parents and no other children | | | Single parent with/out other children | | |
	Mean	Median	sd	Mean	Median	sd	Mean	Median	sd
(a) Total sample									
Alcohol (g)	1.3	0.0	5.25	5.2	0.0	16.57	2.3	0.0	7.13
Alcohol as % total energy	0.4	0.0	1.82	1.7	0.0	4.26	0.7	0.0	2.25
Base = all aged 11 to 18 years		430			260			165	
(b) Consumers only									
Alcohol (g)	7.0	3.4	10.60	14.3	6.7	25.00	9.1	3.5	11.92
Alcohol as % total energy	2.4	1.3	3.69	4.5	2.6	6.08	2.9	1.1	3.76
Percentage consumers		19%			35%			25%	
Base = all consumers aged 11 to 18 years		80			90			42	

*Excludes 9 young people (5 consumers) who were living with others, not parents.

Table 6.39 Average daily intake from protein and total carbohydrate compared with data from other surveys of young people

Sex and age of young person	Survey year	Average daily intake (g)						Base*
		protein			total carbohydrate			
		Mean	se	sd	Mean	se	sd	
Males aged (years)								
3½–4½	(1992/3)	39.4	0.66		177	2.60		250
4–6	(1997)	49.0		13.5	209		42	184
10–11	(1983)	61.0		12.0	274		52	902
10–11	(1997)	60.4		12.5	261		54	140
14–15	(1983)	74.6		17.5	324		75	513
14–15	(1997)	71.9		16.9	294		78	110
16–24	(1986/7)	81.6	1.48		282	6.00		214
15–18	(1997)	76.5		19.6	301		84	179
Females aged (years)								
3½–4½	(1992/3)	37.7	0.67		162	2.10		243
4–6	(1997)	44.5		11.1	191		40	172
10–11	(1983)	53.2		11.8	241		58	821
10–11	(1997)	52.9		11.6	229		45	118
14–15	(1983)	56.2		12.6	240		59	461
14–15	(1997)	53.7		14.1	221		58	113
16–24	(1986/7)	58.5	1.09		204	4.30		189
15–18	(1997)	54.8		15.2	214		58	210

*Bases for 1983 are weighted.

1983 Department of Health. *The Diets of British Schoolchildren.* HMSO (London, 1989).
1986/7 Gregory JR et al. *The Dietary and Nutritional Survey of British Adults.* HMSO (London, 1990).
1992/3 Gregory JR et al. *The National Diet and Nutrition Survey: Children aged 1½ to 4½ years.* HMSO (London, 1995).
1997 *National Diet and Nutrition Survey: young people aged 4 to 18 years.*

7 Fat and fatty acids intake

7.1 Introduction

This chapter presents data on the intakes of fat and fatty acids for young people in the survey who kept a 7-day weighed intake dietary record. Data are shown separately for intakes of total fat, saturated, *trans* unsaturated, and *cis* monounsaturated and *cis* polyunsaturated fatty acids (n-3 and n-6) and for cholesterol[1]. Figure 7.1 shows the intakes of fat and fatty acids by age and sex. *(Figure 7.1)*

7.1.1 Current recommendations on fat intakes for adults and children

Dietary Reference Values (DRVs) for fat and fatty acids have been formulated for adults[2] and are expressed as population averages. Current recommendations are that total fat intake should contribute a population average of no more than 35% of daily food energy intake, that is excluding alcohol (33% of daily total energy intake, including alcohol). Saturated fatty acids should contribute an average of no more than 11%, *cis* polyunsaturated fatty acids an average of 6.5%, *cis* monounsaturated fatty acids 13%, and *trans* fatty acids an average of no more than 2% of food energy intake for the population. *(Table 7.1)*

In this chapter the proportion of energy derived from fat and fatty acids for young people in the survey is compared with the DRVs for adults. DRVs for fat and fatty acids have not been formulated separately for children, since the relationship between dietary fat intake in children and plasma cholesterol concentrations and the significance of any long-term effects are less well established for children than for adults. However it is recommended that the dietary patterns of fat intake recommended for adults should be appropriate for children from the age of five years. Up to the age of five years it is expected that the proportion of energy derived from dietary fat will fall from about 50%, as supplied by breast feeding or infant formula, to the levels recommended for adults, but that moderating dietary fat intake should not generally begin below the age of two years[3].

7.2 Total fat

The mean daily total fat intake for boys was 74.7g and for girls 63.1g (medians 72.1g and 62.7g respectively) and for each age group mean intake was higher for boys than for girls (p < 0.01). Mean intakes increased with age for boys, the increase being particularly marked between the two oldest age cohorts (p < 0.01). Among girls mean intakes increased with age except for the oldest age group where mean intake was 64g, very close to that for girls aged 7 to 10 years, (age 4 to 6 years compared with age 11 to 14 years: p < 0.01; 11 to 14 compared with 15 to 18 years: ns).

Among boys, intakes at the lower 2.5 percentile were about half the median amount while at the upper 2.5 percentile intakes ranged from 95.0g for boys aged 4 to 6 years to 134.3g for those aged 15 to 18 years. Among girls intakes at the lower 2.5 percentile showed much less variation by age than for boys, ranging between 26.7g for girls aged 15 to 18 years to 36.3g for girls aged 7 to 10 years. The variation in intake at the upper 2.5 percentile was also less than for boys, but, as for boys, increased steadily with age, from 83.5g for girls aged 4 to 6 years to 102.6g for girls aged 15 to 18 years.

Boys derived a mean of 35.4% and girls 35.9% of their food energy intake from fat. Although absolute intakes of total fat increased with age for boys and for girls up to the age of 14 years, there was no increase in the mean proportion of food energy derived from total fat intake associated with age. Among boys values at the lower 2.5 percentile also showed very little variation with age, ranging from 26.0% for those aged 11 to 14 years, to 28.8% for those aged 7 to 10 years. At the upper 2.5 percentile the percentage of food energy derived from total fat ranged from 42.5% for boys aged 4 to 6 years to 45.3% for boys aged 15 to 18 years. Among girls the proportion of food energy derived from fat by those at the lower 2.5 percentile was lower for the older girls (23.3% and 22.7% for those in the two oldest age groups) than for the younger girls (26.2% for those aged 4 to 6 years). Values at the upper 2.5 percentile of the distribution were very close to those for boys and showed no clear association with age.

As noted above the DRV for the population average percentage contribution to food energy intake from total fat for adults is 35%. The average percentage of food energy from fat was close to the DRV for each age and sex group. *(Figure 7.1; Tables 7.2 and 7.3)*

7.3 Saturated fatty acids

Tables 7.4 and 7.5 show the average daily intake of saturated fatty acids for young people in the survey, and the contribution made by saturated fatty acids to their food energy intake.

Overall boys in the survey had a mean daily intake of saturated fatty acids of 29.8g; the mean intake for girls was 25.2g (p < 0.01). Median intakes were close to the mean values, 28.7g and 25.1g for boys and girls respectively.

Among boys mean intake increased steadily with age, rising from 25.1g for boys aged 4 to 6 years to 34.7g for boys aged 15 to 18 years (p < 0.01).

Among girls mean intake increased with age through the first three age cohorts, rising from 23.8g for girls aged 4 to 6 years to 26.2g for girls aged 11 to 14 years (p < 0.05). However mean intake for the oldest group of girls, 24.7g, was not significantly different from the mean intake for the youngest age group or for girls aged 11 to 14 years.

Intakes at the lower 2.5 percentile were generally about half the median value, except for girls aged 15 to 18 years, where the intake for the lower 2.5 percentile was only 9.4g saturated fatty acids per day.

At the upper end of the distribution, intakes for boys at the top 2.5 percentile ranged from 40.6g for those aged 4 to 6 years, to 53.8g for those aged 15 to 18 years. Among girls the variation in intake by age at the upper 2.5 percentile was smaller than for boys, ranging from 35.1g for girls aged 4 to 6 years, to 41.8g for girls aged 11 to 14 years.

For adults the DRV for the population average percentage contribution to food energy intake from saturated fatty acids is 11%. In this survey the mean percentage of food energy derived from saturated fatty acids was 14.2% for boys and 14.3% for girls and for both sexes declined with age, for example from 14.8% for boys aged 4 to 6 years to 13.9% for boys aged 15 to 18 years (both sexes: p < 0.01).

At the lower 2.5 percentile values were below 11% for each age/sex group, but at the upper 2.5 percentile values ranged from 21.2% for girls aged 4 to 6 years to 17.6% for boys aged 15 to 18 years. *(Tables 7.4 and 7.5)*

7.4 *Trans* unsaturated fatty acids (*trans* fatty acids)

Mean intake of *trans* fatty acids was 2.87g per day for boys and 2.36g for girls (p < 0.01). Median intakes were close to mean values for both sexes, 2.69g for boys and 2.30g for girls. Mean intake of *trans* fatty acids for boys increased steadily with age from 2.26g for boys aged 4 to 6 years, to 3.45g for boys aged 15 to 18 years (p < 0.01). Among girls mean daily intake rose from 2.09g for girls aged 4 to 6 years to 2.48g for girls aged 7 to 10 years (p < 0.01). There was then no further significant change in mean intake either for girls aged 11 to 14 years, 2.48g, or for girls aged 15 to 18 years, 2.34g.

At the upper 2.5 percentile intakes for boys increased consistently with age, ranging from 3.91g for boys aged 4 to 6 years to 6.33g for boys aged 15 to 18 years. As found for intakes of total fat and saturated fatty acids, intakes of *trans* fatty acids for girls at the upper 2.5 percentile of the distribution showed less variation by age than for boys and only increased with age across the first three age cohorts.

The DRV set for adults for the population average percentage contribution to food energy intake from *trans* fatty acids is no more than 2%. In this survey the mean percentage of food energy from *trans* fatty acids was 1.4% for boys and 1.3% for girls. At the upper 2.5 percentile of the distribution *trans* fatty acids provided 2.1% of the food energy intake for both boys and girls.
(Tables 7.6 and 7.7)

7.5 *Cis* monounsaturated fatty acids

Mean daily intakes of *cis* monounsaturated fatty acids were 24.6g and 20.6g for boys and girls respectively (p < 0.01). Median intakes for both sexes were close to the mean values, 23.6g and 20.4g respectively.

As for other fatty acids, mean intake of *cis* monounsaturated fatty acids for boys increased steadily with age, from 19.4g for boys aged 4 to 6 years to 29.6g for boys aged 15 to 18 years (p < 0.01). The pattern of intake associated with age for girls was as found for other fatty acids with an increase in mean intake from 17.8g for the 4 to 6 year olds to 22.4g for the 11 to 14 year group (p < 0.01); mean intake for 15 to 18 year-old girls, 20.9g, was not significantly different from that for 11 to 14 year olds and was the same as for 7 to 10 year olds.

The DRV for adults in respect of *cis* monounsaturated fatty acids is that they should provide 13% of food energy as a population average. Table 7.9 shows that the mean values for both boys and girls were below this level, 11.7% and 11.8% respectively.
(Tables 7.8 and 7.9)

7.6 Polyunsaturated fatty acids

Cis polyunsaturated fatty acids can be divided into two main groups, *cis* n-3 and *cis* n-6 polyunsaturated fatty acids; each group has different biological functions and is found in different foods.

Fish oils are the richest source of *cis* n-3 polyunsaturated fatty acids, but they are also found in seed oils and margarines. *Cis* n-6 polyunsaturated fatty acids are mainly found in plant oils, including soya, corn and sunflower oils and margarines derived from these oils.

7.6.1 Total cis polyunsaturated fatty acids

The mean daily intake of total *cis* polyunsaturated fatty acids for boys in the survey was 12.5g; median intake was 11.7g. Mean and median intakes and intakes at the upper 2.5 percentile of the distribution increased for boys throughout the age range. For example, for boys aged 4 to 6 years and 15 to 18 years mean intakes were 9.3g and 15.5g respectively (p < 0.01) and intakes at the upper 2.5 percentile of the distribution were 15.0g and 28.8g.

Intakes for boys at the lower 2.5 percentile of the distribution increased with age in the first three cohorts from 4.3g for those aged 4 to 6 years to 7.4g for those aged 11 to 14 years. The comparable intake for boys aged 15 to 18 years was 7.2g.

Girls had a mean daily intake of total *cis* polyunsaturated fatty acids of 10.7g (median 10.1g) significantly lower than for boys (p < 0.01). Mean and median intakes for girls at the upper and lower 2.5 percentiles of the distribution increased with age up to ages 11 to 14 years. Comparable intakes for girls aged 15 to 18 years were not significantly different from the intakes for girls aged 11 to 14 years. *(Table 7.10)*

7.6.2 Cis n-3 polyunsaturated fatty acids

Overall boys had a significantly higher mean daily intake of *cis* n-3 polyunsaturated fatty acids than girls, 1.77g compared with 1.48g (p < 0.01). Median intakes were about 10% below mean intakes, 1.59g for boys and 1.36g for girls.

Mean daily intake for boys increased with age from 1.29g for boys aged 4 to 6 years to 2.19g for boys aged 15 to 18 years (p < 0.01).

For girls mean daily intake of *cis* n-3 polyunsaturated fatty acids increased with age from 1.15g for those aged 4 to 6 years to 1.65g for those aged 11 to 14 years. There was then a slight fall in mean intake to 1.61g for girls aged 15 to 18 years (ns). *(Table 7.11)*

7.6.3 Cis n-6 polyunsaturated fatty acids

The mean daily intakes of *cis* n-6 polyunsaturated fatty acids for boys and girls in the survey were 10.7g and 9.3g respectively (p < 0.01). Median intakes for both boys and girls were close to the mean values, 10.0g and 8.7g respectively. For boys mean daily intake increased consistently with age, from 8.0g for boys aged 4 to 6 years to 13.3g for boys aged 15 to 18 years (p < 0.01). Mean intake for girls increased from 7.2g for girls aged 4 to 6 years, up to 10.2g for girls aged 11 to 14 and 15 to 18 years (p < 0.01). *(Table 7.12)*

7.6.4 Percentage energy from cis polyunsaturated fatty acids

COMA recommended that the population average intake of *cis* polyunsaturated fatty acids should be 6.5% of food energy intake. Moreover individual intakes should not contribute more than 10% of total energy. For infants, children and adults COMA

recommended that linoleic acid (*cis* n-6) should provide at least 1% of total energy and α-linolenic acid (*cis* n-3) at least 0.2% of total energy[2]. Subsequently, in the Report on Nutritional Aspects of Cardiovascular Disease, COMA recommended that in respect of *cis* n-6 polyunsaturated fatty acids there should be no further increase in average intakes and that the proportion of the population with intakes providing more than 10% of their energy should not increase. In respect of average daily intakes of long chain *cis* n-3 polyunsaturated fatty acids COMA recommended an increase from about 0.1g to 0.2g[4].

The mean percentage contribution to food energy intakes from total *cis* polyunsaturated fatty acids (*cis* n-3 and *cis* n-6) was 5.9% for boys and 6.1% for girls, close to the DRV of 6.5%.

The mean percentage of food energy from *cis* n-3 polyunsaturated fatty acids was 0.8% for boys and girls and from *cis* n-6 polyunsaturated fatty acids 5.1% for boys and 5.3% for girls and for both sexes increased significantly (boys: p < 0.5; girls: p < 0.01). For both boys and girls the percentage of energy from *cis* n-6 polyunsaturated fatty acids increased with age from 4.8% and 4.6% for boys and girls respectively aged 4 to 6 years to 5.3% and 5.7% for boys and girls aged 15 to 18 years (boys: p < 0.05; girls: p < 0.01).

The DRV for α-linolenic acid, part of the *cis* n-3 group, is at least 0.2% of total energy for individuals, and for linoleic acid, part of the *cis* n-6 group, at least 1% of total energy for individuals. This survey did not collect information on intakes of individual fatty acids. However intakes of total *cis* n-3 and total *cis* n-6 polyunsaturated fatty acids as a percentage of food energy at the lower 2.5 percentile of the distribution were well above the DRVs set for individual fatty acids, indicating that the percentage of young people who failed to meet the DRVs was likely to be low. *(Tables 7.13 to 7.15)*

7.7 Cholesterol

Dietary cholesterol has a relatively small and variable effect on serum and plasma cholesterol levels and for that reason COMA set no DRV for cholesterol. However, in its Report on Nutritional Aspects of Cardiovascular Disease COMA recommended that average daily population intakes should not rise above the 1992 level of 245mg[4]. The FAO/WHO expert committee on Fats and Oils in Human Nutrition advised 'reasonable restriction' on dietary cholesterol at below 300mg a day; whether this applies to individuals or is a population average is not made clear.[5]

The mean daily intake of cholesterol was 198g for boys and 169g for girls (p < 0.01). Among boys intakes increased significantly with age, rising from 158mg for boys aged 4 to 6 years to 243mg for boys aged 15 to 18 years (p < 0.01). Among girls mean intakes increased between the youngest two age groups, from 156mg to 170mg, and then rose slightly to a maximum of 177mg for girls aged 15 to 18 years; however none of these differences reached the level of statistical significance.

Median intakes were close to mean values, 186mg for boys and 160mg for girls. Among boys intakes at the lower and upper 2.5 percentiles, like mean values, increased sharply with age. For example, at the upper 2.5 percentile, from 330mg for boys aged 4 to 6 years to 428mg for boys aged 15 to 18 years. Just over a quarter, 27%, of the oldest group of boys had daily intakes of cholesterol at or above 300mg a day.

For girls, daily intakes at the upper 2.5 percentile tended to increase with age ranging from 282mg for the youngest group to 346mg for the oldest girls. Seven per cent of the oldest girls had cholesterol intakes at or above 300mg per day.   *(Table 7.16)*

7.8 Sources of fat in the diet

7.8.1 *Total fat, saturated, trans unsaturated and cis monounsaturated fatty acids*

Tables 7.17 to 7.20 show the percentage contribution of food types to the average daily intake of total fat (Table 7.17), saturated (Table 7.18), *trans* unsaturated (Table 7.19) and *cis* monounsaturated fatty acids (Table 7.20) for young people in the survey, by sex and age.

The four main sources of total fat, saturated, *trans* and *cis* monounsaturated fatty acids in the diets of young people were cereals and cereal products, milk and milk products, meat and meat products, and vegetables, potatoes and savoury snacks.

Overall *cereals and cereal products* accounted for just over a fifth of the intake of total fat, a similar proportion of saturated fatty acids, and a slightly smaller proportion of *cis* monounsaturated fatty acids intake. The contribution made by this food type to the daily intake of *trans* fatty acids was higher, with about a third of the intake coming from cereals and cereal products.

Apart from *trans* fatty acids there was very little variation by age in the contribution of cereals and cereal products to the intake of fat and these fatty acids. For *trans* fatty acids, although the differences were not statistically significant, there was a consistent pattern for the contribution made by cereals and cereal products to intake to fall with age, for example, from 33% of intake for boys aged 4 to 6 years to 25% for those aged 15 to 18 years. Among girls the comparable proportions were 32% and 27%.

Within the cereals and cereal products food group the main sources of fat, saturated, *trans* and *cis* monounsaturated fatty acids were biscuits, and buns, cakes and pastries. The contribution of these sub-groups decreased with increasing age for both boys and girls.

The contribution made to the intake of total fat and saturated, *trans* and *cis* monounsaturated fatty acids by *milk and milk products,* although not statistically significant, declined steadily as the age of the young person increased. For example, for boys aged 4 to 6 years milk and milk products contributed 20% to the intake of total fat, and 30% to the intake of saturated fatty acids. By age 15 to 18 years, milk and milk products provided only 13% and 20% of the intake for boys of total fat and saturated fatty acids. The same pattern is seen in the data for girls and reflects the fall in milk consumption with age, particularly of whole milk.

Meat and meat products contributed 21% to the intake of total fat for boys and 18% for girls, 19% to the intake of saturated fatty acids for boys and 16% for girls, in a similar range for *trans* fatty acids, 15% for both boys and girls, but slightly higher for *cis* monounsaturated fatty acids, 25% and 22% respectively.

Among boys the contribution made by meat and meat products to intakes of total fat, saturated, *trans* and *cis* monounsaturated fatty acids generally increased steadily with increasing age. Among girls the percentage contribution increased between the youngest two age groups, but then stayed at about the same level, with no further increase up to age 15 to 18 years. For example, meat and meat products contributed 15% to the intake of total fat for girls aged 4 to 6 years; at age 7 to 10 years this had increased to 19%, but then remained at this level in the two older age groups.

Within the meat and meat products food group, the principal sources of total fat, and saturated, *trans* and *cis* monounsaturated fatty acids for both boys and girls and all age groups were sausages, and meat pies and pastries. These two groups together provided 8% of total fat intake for boys and 6% for girls. Burgers and kebabs provided 4% of the intake of saturated fatty acids for boys aged 15 to 18 years.

The consumption of *vegetables, potatoes and savoury snacks* also accounted for a substantial proportion of the intake of total fat for young people, 18% for boys and 20% for girls. This food group contributed 13% and 15% to the intake of saturated fatty acids for boys and girls respectively and 21% and 23% to the intake of *cis* monounsaturated fatty acids. In each case there was very little variation by age in the contribution made by this food group, except for girls aged 11 to 14 years. Although not statistically significant, the contribution made by vegetables, potatoes and savoury snacks to intakes of total fat and saturated and *cis* monounsaturated fatty acids was consistently higher for this age group than for any other age/sex group.

Within the vegetables, potatoes and savoury snacks group the main contributors to intakes of fat, saturated and *cis* monounsaturated fatty acids were roast and fried potatoes and chips, and savoury snacks. For example, the consumption of roast and fried potatoes, and chips by boys aged 15 to 18 years accounted for 10% of their total fat intake, 5% of their intake of saturated fatty acids and 12% of their *cis* monounsaturated fatty acids intake. The contribution of savoury snacks to the intake of total fat, saturated and *cis* monounsaturated fatty acids tended to decrease with age.

Fat spreads contributed 9% to the intake of total fat for both boys and girls, 8% to the intake of both saturated and *cis* monounsaturated fatty acids, again for both boys and girls. The contribution made by this food type to intakes of *trans* fatty acids was slightly higher, 13% for both sexes. The contributions made by fat spreads to intakes of total fat, saturated, *trans* unsaturated, and *cis* monounsaturated fatty acids varied very little by age.

Chocolate confectionery provided 6% of both total fat and *cis* monounsaturated fatty acids intake for boys and girls, 9% of saturated fatty acid intake for both boys and girls, and for *trans* fatty acids 9% for boys and 8% for girls. *(Tables 7.17 to 7.20)*

7.8.2 Cis n-3 and n-6 polyunsaturated fatty acids

The main sources of *cis n-3 polyunsaturated fatty acids* were vegetables, potatoes and savoury snacks, cereals and cereal products, and meat and meat products. Vegetables, potatoes and savoury snacks provided over a third of intake (34% for boys and 38% for girls) mainly from roast and fried potatoes and chips. There was no clear pattern associated with age group for either sex, but the contribution provided by this food group ranged from 32% for boys aged 7 to 10 years, to 42% for girls aged 11 to 14 years (ns).

Cereals and cereal products contributed 18% to intakes of *cis* n-3 polyunsaturated fatty acids for boys and 16% for girls, with very little variation for either sex by age group.

Meat and meat products provided 17% of the intake of *cis* n-3 polyunsaturated fatty acids for boys, and 16% for girls. For both boys and girls, coated chicken and chicken and turkey dishes were major sources within this food group.

Nuts and seeds contributed 8% to *cis* n-3 polyunsaturated fatty acids intake for boys and 4% for girls. The contribution declined markedly in the oldest group of both boys and girls.

Milk and milk products provided 5% of *cis* n-3 polyunsaturated fatty acids intake for both boys and girls, with the contribution reducing as age increased.

Overall fish and fish dishes provided 5% of *cis* n-3 polyunsaturated fatty acids intake for boys and 6% for girls, mainly in the form of coated and fried white fish. Oily fish, which is a rich source of *cis* n-3 polyunsaturated fatty acids, provided 2% of intake for both boys and girls. *(Table 7.21)*

The main sources of *cis n-6 polyunsaturated fatty acids* in the diets of young people in the survey were vegetables, potatoes and savoury snacks, (27% of intake for boys and 29% for girls) cereals and cereal products (23% for boys and 21% for girls), fat spreads (16% for both boys and girls), and meat and meat products (18% for boys and 16% for girls).

There was very little variation for either sex by age group in the contribution to intake of *cis* n-6 polyunsaturated fatty acids from vegetables, potatoes and savoury snacks. For both boys and girls, roasted and fried potatoes and chips were major sources, contributing 14% to intake for both sexes. Savoury snacks contributed a further 7% for boys and 8% for girls.

The contribution to *cis* n-6 polyunsaturated fatty acids intake from cereals and cereal products varied very little by age. Within this food group the main sources were white bread (4% for both boys and girls) and buns, cakes and pastries (5% for boys and 4% for girls).

The contribution to intake from fat spreads tended to fall steadily with age for both boys and girls, although the differences were not statistically significant, and within this food group the main contributor was polyunsaturated reduced fat spreads, contributing 9% to intake for boys and 10% for girls.

For boys the contribution to intake from meat and meat products increased steadily, but not significantly with age. Within the food group the main contributors to intake were coated chicken, chicken and turkey dishes, and sausages. *(Table 7.22)*

7.9 Variation in intake of fat

Young people reported as being unwell
It has already been shown that the mean energy intake for young people who reported being unwell and whose eating was affected during the 7-day dietary recording period was significantly lower than for other young people in the survey (see *Table 5.5*). As Table 7.23 shows, young people who reported being unwell also had lower mean daily intakes of total fat and all fatty acids than other young people; this generally applied whether or not their eating was reported to have been affected by their being unwell, although differences between these groups were generally not statistically significant. For example, the mean daily intake of total fat for boys whose eating was affected was 65.6g

compared with 70.9g for those whose eating was not affected (ns) and 76.1g for boys who were not reported as being unwell (not unwell compared with unwell, eating affected: p < 0.01). However when intakes of fat and fatty acids were expressed as percentage of food energy intake, there were no significant differences between the well and unwell groups. This indicates that the lower fat and fatty acids intakes in the unwell group were due to the overall lower energy intakes and not a selective fall in fat and fatty acids intakes. *(Table 7.23)*

Region
There were no significant regional differences in average daily intakes of fat or fatty acids for boys or girls. However the data show a consistent pattern for girls living in the Northern region having higher mean intakes of total fat, saturated fatty acids, and *cis* monounsaturated fatty acids than girls living elsewhere, although the differences did not reach statistical significance.

When energy intake was taken into account there were no significant regional differences for boys in the percentage of food energy derived from total fat and fatty acids intake. For girls there were no significant differences in the percentage of food energy derived from total fat, saturated, *trans* or polyunsaturated fatty acids intakes. However girls living in Scotland and the Northern region derived significantly more food energy from *cis* monounsaturated fatty acids than girls in the Central and South West regions of England and Wales. Therefore the fatty acid density of the diets of girls in these regions differed from other girls and was not purely the result of differences in their food energy intake. *(Table 7.24)*

Socio-economic characteristics
Tables 7.25 to 7.27 show mean intakes of total fat and fatty acids, and the percentage of food energy they provided for boys and girls according to whether they were living in a household receiving benefits, by the social class of the head of their household and by gross weekly household income.

Table 7.25 clearly shows that boys living in *households receiving benefits* had significantly lower mean intakes of total fat and nearly all fatty acids (except *cis* n-3 polyunsaturated fatty acids) compared with boys living in households not receiving benefits (total fat, saturated and *trans* fatty acids: p < 0.01; other fatty acids: p < 0.05). This reflects the lower energy intakes for boys in households receiving benefits (see *Table 5.12)*.

In contrast the data for girls show no significant differences in mean intakes. This is at least partially explained by differences in the age composition of the benefit and non-benefit sub groups in the sample and the real difference in intakes between girls aged 15 to 18 years and boys in the same age group. As shown previously (see *Table 3.29)* young people aged 15 to 18

were less likely to live in benefit households than those in younger groups. The relatively high proportion of girls aged 15 to 18 years living in households not receiving benefits therefore affects the data on intakes of fat and fatty acids, since the oldest group of girls, as has been shown earlier in this chapter, had much lower mean intakes of total fat and most fatty acids than boys in the same age group.

When intakes were expressed as a percentage of food energy intake, there were no significant differences in the fatty acids composition of the diets of young people from households receiving and not receiving benefits.

For boys, mean daily intakes of total fat, saturated, *trans* and *cis* n-6 polyunsaturated fatty acids and cholesterol were lowest in the two lowest income groups, that is for boys living in households where the *gross weekly household income* was less than £280. Mean daily intake of total fat was highest for boys in the middle household income group, £280 to less than £400 (p < 0.05). For saturated and *trans* fatty acids and cholesterol mean intakes were highest for boys living in households where the gross weekly household income was between £400 and £600, reflecting higher energy intakes in the higher income groups (saturated fatty acids: p < 0.01; *trans* fatty acids: p < 0.05; cholesterol: ns) (see *Table 5.13)*. When intakes were expressed as a percentage of food energy boys in households where the gross weekly household income was between £400 and £600 had significantly lower percentage energy from total *cis* and *cis* n-6 polyunsaturated fatty acids than boys in the lowest household income group and boys in households where the gross weekly income was between £280 and £400 (for *cis* n-6 polyunsaturated fatty acids compared with the lowest income group: p < 0.05; others: p < 0.01).

For girls mean intakes of total fat and saturated fatty acids were lowest for those living in households in the lowest income group, less than £160 a week, but there were no statistically significant differences in fat and fatty acids intake associated with household income level. When intakes were expressed as a percentage of energy intake the only marked difference was the relatively low proportion of food energy derived from *cis* monounsaturated fatty acids for girls in the highest household income group (£600 a week or more). This group derived an average of 11.4% food energy from *cis* monounsaturated fatty acids compared with 12.1% for girls in the lowest household income group (p < 0.05).

There were no significant differences associated with the social class of the head of household for either boys or girls in absolute intakes of fat or fatty acids (Table 7.27).

When fat and fatty acids intake was expressed as a percentage of food energy intake the data show that the diets of boys from a manual home background were richer in *cis* monounsaturated, total *cis* polyunsaturated and *cis* n-6 polyunsaturated fatty acids. The proportion of food energy they derived from these fatty acids was significantly higher than for other boys (*cis* monounsaturated and total polyunsaturated: $p < 0.01$; *cis* n-6 polyunsaturated: $p < 0.05$).

For girls, there were no significant differences in the percentage of food energy from total fat and fatty acids between the two groups. *(Tables 7.25 to 7.27)*

Household type

An analysis of fat and fatty acid intake by *household type* (Table 7.28) showed that for boys living with both parents and no other children intakes of total fat and each fatty acid were consistently higher than mean intakes for boys living with both parents and other children or in one-parent households, reflecting higher energy intake in this group. For example, boys living with both parents but no other children had a mean daily total fat intake of 83.5g, compared with 72.3g for boys in two-parent, other children households, and 72.8g for boys in one-parent households (all: $p < 0.01$). However it should be noted that young people living with both parents and no other children were significantly more likely to be in the oldest age group. Therefore these differences for boys in absolute intakes of fat and fatty acids are likely to be, at least partly, explained by differences in the age structure of the groups.

Indeed, when intakes were expressed as a percentage of food energy intakes most of these differences were no longer apparent. However boys living with both parents and no other children, and living in one-parent households, both derived a higher proportion of their food energy from *cis* monounsaturated fatty acids, than did boys living with both their parents and other children ($p < 0.05$).

For girls the only significant difference in absolute intake was for total *cis* polyunsaturated fatty acids; girls living with both parents and no other children had a higher mean intake than girls living with both parents and other children ($p < 0.05$). This group also derived a higher proportion of food energy from total *cis* polyunsaturated fatty acids, and from *cis* n-6 polyunsaturated fatty acids than girls living with both parents and other children (both: $p < 0.05$).
(Table 7.28)

7.10 Comparisons with other studies

Table 7.29 and 7.30 compare data from this present survey of young people with equivalent data on fat and fatty acids intake from other national surveys, including the 1983 Department of Health study of the Diets of British Schoolchildren, the 1986/7 survey of adults and the 1992/3 survey of pre-school children[6,7,8].

Table 7.29 compares data on the intake of fat and fatty acids and the percentage of food energy from fat and fatty acids for children aged 3½ to 4½ years, from the NDNS of pre-school children, with data for young people aged 4 to 6 years from this present survey[9].

Allowing for the differences in the age groupings, which will largely account for differences in average daily intakes, the data suggest that since the pre-school children's survey in 1992/3, the diets of very young children, and particularly boys, are becoming less rich in saturated fatty acids, as suggested by the fall in the mean proportion of energy obtained from saturated fatty acids over the period. Similarly there appears to be a reduction in the *trans* fatty acid density of the diet, with the percentage of energy derived from this source falling from 1.7% for the 1992/3 cohort to 1.3% for the present survey cohort. The data also suggest that the present cohort of young children are consuming a diet richer in *cis* monounsaturated fatty acids and in *cis* n-6 polyunsaturated acids, as indicated by the increase between the two surveys in the mean proportion of energy derived from these fatty acids.

Table 7.29 also gives similar data for the oldest age group in the present survey, young people aged 15 to 18 years, and compares these with data for young people aged 16 to 24 years, taken from the 1986/7 survey of British adults. The two age groups are less well matched than for the previous comparison and the interval between the two surveys is much greater, but bearing these points in mind the data suggest that the overall percentage of food energy derived from fat for young people has declined, possibly by up to 10%, over the period since 1986/7. This is in line with the trend seen in the National Food Survey for a decline in the percentage of energy from fat[10]. Thus in 1986/7 16 to 24 year-old males obtained 40.2% of food energy from fat, whereas in 1997 15 to 18 year-old males obtained 35.9% of food energy from fat. Similarly there appears to have been a marked reduction in the proportion of food energy obtained for both boys and girls from saturated and *trans* fatty acids and, to a somewhat smaller extent, from *cis* monounsaturated fatty acids, and an increase in the proportion of energy derived from *cis* n-3 polyunsaturated fatty acids.

Table 7.30 compares the mean daily intake of total fat and the percentage of food energy derived from fat for boys and girls aged 10 to 11 years and 14 to 15 years from the 1983 survey of the diets of British school-children with equivalent data from the present survey.

Although the age groups have been matched for comparison, differences in the sample design and dietary methodologies of the two surveys need to be borne in mind when considering differences in the data[11].

For both sexes and both age groups mean daily intakes

of total fat and the percentage of food energy derived from total fat intake were higher in the 1983 than the 1997 survey. In the present survey mean daily fat intakes were about 14% lower for the younger group, and about 20% lower for those aged 14 to 15 years. The 1983 survey reported that for both age groups and sexes about 4% of total fat intake came from milk, that chips contributed 3% for the younger children and 4% for the older group, and butter contributed about 2%, except for the older group of boys where it contributed 3% to total fat intake (*Table not shown*). The present survey found that whole milk now contributed about 3% to total fat intake, butter about 2% and chips about 8%.

Despite the quite substantial proportional reductions in absolute fat intake, reductions in the proportion of food energy derived from fat are much smaller, about 5% for the younger age group and 7% for those aged 14 to 15 years. It was noted earlier (see *Chapter 5: Section 5.6*) that over this period there has been a reduction in the energy intake of these age groups and this present comparison confirms that the reduction in mean daily fat intake is largely associated with the reduction in energy intake. Nevertheless the diets of the present cohort of young people are less rich in total fat that the equivalent group of young people in 1983.

(Table 7.29 and 7.30)

References and endnotes

1   Fat is a mixture of triglycerides (1 unit glycerol with 3 fatty acids), phospholipids, sterols and related compounds. Total fat includes all these components.

2   Department of Health. Report on Health and Social Subjects: 41. *Dietary Reference Values for Food Energy and Nutrients for the United Kingdom*. HMSO (London, 1991).

3   Department of Health. Report on Health and Social Subjects: 45. *Weaning and the Weaning Diet*. HMSO (London, 1994).

4   Department of Health. Report on Health and Social Subjects: 46 *Nutritional Aspects of Cardiovascular Disease*. HMSO (London, 1994).

5   Food and Agriculture Organisation. Food and Nutrition Paper: 57 *Fats and Oils in Human Nutrition*. FAO (Rome, 1994).

6   Gregory JR, Collins DL, Davies PSW, Hughes JM, Clarke PC. *National Diet and Nutrition Survey: children aged 1½ to 4 ½ years. Volume 1: Report of the diet and nutrition survey*. HMSO (London, 1995).

7   Gregory J, Foster K, Tyler H, Wiseman M. *The Dietary and Nutritional Survey of British Adults*. HMSO (London, 1990).

8   Department of Health. Report on Health and Social Subjects: 36 The *Diets of British Schoolchildren*. HMSO (London, 1989).

9   The different age groupings in the different surveys should be taken into account when making comparisons between surveys.

10 Ministry of Agriculture, Fisheries and Food. *National Food Survey 1998*. TSO (London 1999).

11 See *Appendix W* for an account of the 1983 survey methodology and sample design.

Table 7.1 **Dietary reference values for adults for fat as a percentage of daily total energy intake* (percentage of food energy)****

Fat and fatty acids	Individual minimum	Population average	Individual maximum
Saturated fatty acids		10 (11)	
Cis polyunsaturated fatty acids		6 (6.5)	10
	n-3 0.2		
	n-6 1		
Cis monounsaturated fatty acids		12 (13)	
Trans fatty acids		2 (2)	
Total fatty acids		30 (32.5)	
Total fat		33 (35)	

* Total energy includes energy from alcohol.
** Department of Health. Report on Health and Social Subjects: 41. *Dietary Reference Values for Food Energy and Nutrients for the United Kingdom*. HMSO (London, 1991).

Table 7.2 Average daily total fat intake (g) by sex and age of young person

Total fat intake (g)	Age (years)				All
	4–6	7–10	11–14	15–18	
Males	cum %	cum %	cum %	cum %	cum %
Less than 40	7	3	2	1	3
Less than 60	51	27	16	10	25
Less than 70	80	53	35	23	46
Less than 80	92	73	59	39	65
Less than 100	99	96	91	68	88
Less than 120	100	99	98	93	97
All		100	100	100	100
Base	*184*	*256*	*237*	*179*	*856*
Mean (average value)	60.1	69.8	77.2	89.0	74.7
Median	59.8	68.4	76.7	89.9	72.1
Lower 2.5 percentile	30.9	39.1	41.5	42.8	38.3
Upper 2.5 percentile	95.0	104.8	120.9	134.3	125.3
Standard deviation	14.47	16.95	20.85	24.16	22.15
Females	cum %	cum %	cum %	cum %	cum %
Less than 40	10	5	8	12	9
Less than 60	64	39	35	41	44
Less than 70	86	66	55	64	67
Less than 80	95	86	76	79	83
Less than 100	99	99	99	95	98
All	100	100	100	100	100
Base	*171*	*226*	*238*	*210*	*845*
Mean (average value)	55.9	63.8	67.2	64.0	63.1
Median	54.2	63.4	67.7	64.7	62.7
Lower 2.5 percentile	30.6	36.3	33.4	26.7	33.4
Upper 2.5 percentile	83.5	90.0	99.3	102.6	98.3
Standard deviation	13.76	13.84	17.56	20.14	17.09

Table 7.3 Percentage food energy intake from total fat by sex and age of young person

Percentage food energy intake from total fat	Age (years)				All
	4–6	7–10	11–14	15–18	
	cum %	cum %	cum %	cum %	cum %
Males					
30 or less	6	8	11	12	10
33 or less	26	27	28	24	26
35 or less	43	47	49	38	44
38 or less	76	80	76	66	74
40 or less	90	90	88	83	88
45 or less	99	100	99	97	99
All	100		100	100	100
Base	*184*	*256*	*237*	*179*	*856*
Mean (average value)	35.5	35.2	35.2	35.9	35.4
Median	35.9	35.2	35.1	36.3	35.5
Lower 2.5 percentile	27.9	28.8	26.0	26.3	26.6
Upper 2.5 percentile	42.5	42.9	43.6	45.3	43.6
Standard deviation	3.90	3.69	4.27	4.68	4.17
	cum %	cum %	cum %	cum %	cum %
Females					
30 or less	8	7	8	14	10
33 or less	22	21	23	28	23
35 or less	39	41	40	39	40
38 or less	71	67	67	67	68
40 or less	87	87	80	79	83
45 or less	98	98	96	97	97
	100	100	100	100	100
Base	*171*	*226*	*238*	*210*	*845*
Mean (average value)	35.9	35.9	36.1	35.9	35.9
Median	36.0	36.0	36.0	36.6	36.2
Lower 2.5 percentile	26.2	26.6	23.3	22.7	26.2
Upper 2.5 percentile	44.8	44.2	45.2	45.6	45.0
Standard deviation	4.42	4.14	4.98	5.37	4.76

Table 7.4 Average daily intake of saturated fatty acids (g) by sex and age of young person

Intake of saturated fatty acids (g)	Age (years)				All
	4–6	7–10	11–14	15–18	
	cum %	cum %	cum %	cum %	cum %
Males					
Less than 20	20	11	11	7	12
Less than 25	55	35	24	18	32
Less than 30	82	61	50	33	55
Less than 35	92	82	77	52	75
Less than 40	97	95	90	69	87
Less than 45	100	98	96	84	94
All		100	100	100	100
Base	*184*	*256*	*237*	*179*	*856*
Mean (average value)	25.1	28.3	30.3	34.7	29.8
Median	24.0	27.7	30.1	34.4	28.7
Lower 2.5 percentile	13.4	15.5	13.8	16.5	14.5
Upper 2.5 percentile	40.6	42.7	51.0	53.8	50.4
Standard deviation	6.98	7.47	9.04	10.41	9.28
	cum %	cum %	cum %	cum %	cum %
Females					
Less than 15	5	4	8	17	9
Less than 20	27	19	23	32	25
Less than 25	61	46	43	51	50
Less than 30	85	74	70	70	74
Less than 35	97	92	85	88	90
Less than 40	99	99	96	96	97
All	100	100	100	100	100
Base	*171*	*226*	*238*	*210*	*845*
Mean (average value)	23.8	25.7	26.2	24.7	25.2
Median	22.7	25.9	26.2	24.5	25.1
Lower 2.5 percentile	11.2	13.5	11.6	9.4	11.3
Upper 2.5 percentile	35.1	38.3	41.8	41.3	40.1
Standard deviation	6.42	6.27	7.83	8.59	7.42

Table 7.5 Percentage food energy intake from saturated fatty acids by sex and age of young person

Percentage food energy intake from saturated fatty acids	Age (years)				All
	4–6	7–10	11–14	15–18	
	cum %	cum %	cum %	cum %	cum %
Males					
11 or less	5	4	11	7	7
13 or less	22	27	34	32	29
15 or less	53	64	77	70	67
17 or less	85	92	92	93	91
19 or less	94	97	99	99	97
All	100	100	100	100	100
Base	*184*	*256*	*237*	*179*	*856*
Mean (average value)	14.8	14.3	13.8	13.9	14.2
Median	14.9	14.2	13.8	13.9	14.2
Lower 2.5 percentile	10.6	10.5	9.8	9.4	9.9
Upper 2.5 percentile	19.7	19.3	18.6	17.6	19.0
Standard deviation	2.36	2.11	2.19	2.07	2.21
	cum %	cum %	cum %	cum %	cum %
Females					
11 or less	4	7	11	10	8
13 or less	19	26	35	34	29
15 or less	47	61	67	72	63
17 or less	78	88	89	91	87
19 or less	92	97	99	97	96
All	100	100	100	100	100
Base	*171*	*226*	*238*	*210*	*845*
Mean (average value)	15.3	14.5	14.0	13.8	14.3
Median	15.2	14.4	13.9	13.9	14.3
Lower 2.5 percentile	10.4	9.2	9.3	8.8	9.2
Upper 2.5 percentile	21.2	19.2	18.7	19.3	19.3
Standard deviation	2.52	2.29	2.50	2.52	2.51

Table 7.6 Average daily intake of *trans* fatty acids (g) by sex and age of young person

Intake of *trans* fatty acids (g)	Age (years)				All
	4–6	7–10	11–14	15–18	
	cum %	cum %	cum %	cum %	cum %
Males					
Less than 1.5	14	9	7	5	8
Less than 2.0	37	20	16	11	20
Less than 2.5	63	45	35	26	41
Less than 3.0	90	66	56	42	62
Less than 3.5	94	80	78	55	76
Less than 4.0	98	90	87	69	85
Less than 4.5	100	97	93	78	92
All		100	100	100	100
Base	*184*	*256*	*237*	*179*	*856*
Mean (average value)	2.26	2.74	2.92	3.45	2.87
Median	2.25	2.63	2.87	3.29	2.69
Lower 2.5 percentile	1.03	1.15	1.21	1.30	1.20
Upper 2.5 percentile	3.91	4.61	5.36	6.33	5.77
Standard deviation	0.696	0.960	1.065	1.346	1.134
	cum %	cum %	cum %	cum %	cum %
Females					
Less than 1.5	18	10	15	21	16
Less than 2.0	51	29	31	39	36
Less than 2.5	75	54	50	60	59
Less than 3.0	93	77	75	74	79
Less than 3.5	96	90	90	90	91
Less than 4.0	97	95	95	96	96
Less than 4.5	98	99	97	99	99
All	100	100	100	100	100
Base	*171*	*226*	*238*	*210*	*845*
Mean (average value)	2.09	2.48	2.48	2.34	2.36
Median	1.99	2.40	2.49	2.30	2.30
Lower 2.5 percentile	0.99	1.20	0.98	0.85	0.96
Upper 2.5 percentile	4.10	4.26	4.77	4.37	4.29
Standard deviation	0.705	0.778	0.954	0.905	0.860

Table 7.7 Percentage food energy intake from *trans* fatty acids by sex and age of young person

Percentage food energy intake from *trans* fatty acids	Age (years)				All
	4–6	7–10	11–14	15–18	
	cum %	cum %	cum %	cum %	cum %
Males					
1.0 or less	12	13	16	12	13
1.2 or less	35	33	38	36	36
1.4 or less	64	59	65	59	61
1.6 or less	82	77	80	77	79
1.8 or less	93	88	93	88	90
2.0 or less	98	96	97	93	96
All	100	100	100	100	100
Base	*184*	*256*	*237*	*179*	*856*
Mean (average value)	1.3	1.4	1.3	1.4	1.4
Median	1.3	1.3	1.3	1.3	1.3
Lower 2.5 percentile	0.8	0.8	0.7	0.7	0.8
Upper 2.5 percentile	2.0	2.2	2.0	2.1	2.1
Standard deviation	0.29	0.34	0.33	0.37	0.34
	cum %	cum %	cum %	cum %	cum %
Females					
1.0 or less	11	11	19	20	16
1.2 or less	32	30	40	40	35
1.4 or less	65	56	61	62	61
1.6 or less	84	76	80	81	80
1.8 or less	92	88	91	90	90
2.0 or less	97	96	95	95	96
All	100	100	100	100	100
Base	*171*	*226*	*238*	*210*	*845*
Mean (average value)	1.3	1.4	1.3	1.3	1.3
Median	1.3	1.3	1.3	1.3	1.3
Lower 2.5 percentile	0.8	0.8	0.7	0.7	0.7
Upper 2.5 percentile	2.0	2.2	2.2	2.2	2.1
Standard deviation	0.30	0.33	0.38	0.37	0.35

Table 7.8 Average daily intake of *cis* monounsaturated fatty acids (g) by sex and age

Intake of *cis* monounsaturated fatty acids (g)	Age (years)				All
	4–6	7–10	11–14	15–18	
	cum %	cum %	cum %	cum %	cum %
Males					
Less than 16	19	11	6	4	10
Less than 20	61	31	19	11	29
Less than 24	83	60	43	26	52
Less than 28	95	83	66	45	71
Less than 32	98	96	86	64	85
Less than 36	100	97	94	80	92
All		100	100	100	100
Base	*184*	*256*	*237*	*179*	*856*
Mean (average value)	19.4	22.8	25.6	29.6	24.6
Median	18.8	22.3	24.7	29.0	23.6
Lower 2.5 percentile	10.3	13.2	13.6	15.0	12.7
Upper 2.5 percentile	29.7	36.7	42.1	46.4	41.7
Standard deviation	4.87	6.08	7:21	8.35	7.72
	cum %	cum %	cum %	cum %	cum %
Females					
Less than 12	9	3	4	10	7
Less than 16	35	16	16	27	23
Less than 20	72	45	34	45	48
Less than 24	90	74	56	70	72
Less than 28	99	93	85	84	90
Less than 32	100	98	95	94	96
All		100	100	100	100
Base	*171*	*226*	*238*	*210*	*845*
Mean (average value)	17.8	20.9	22.4	20.9	20.6
Median	17.6	20.6	22.3	20.8	20.4
Lower 2.5 percentile	10.4	11.8	9.7	7.5	9.7
Upper 2.5 percentile	26.6	30.7	34.6	35.2	33.8
Standard deviation	4.38	4.89	6.10	6.87	5.90

Table 7.9 Percentage food energy intake from *cis* monounsaturated fatty acids by sex and age of young person

Intake of *cis* monounsaturated fatty acids (g)	Age (years)				All
	4–6	7–10	11–14	15–18	
	cum %	cum %	cum %	cum %	cum %
Males					
9 or less	5	3	7	7	5
10 or less	16	18	18	19	18
11 or less	42	38	37	31	37
12 or less	68	69	55	49	60
13 or less	83	84	79	71	79
14 or less	93	93	90	86	90
All	100	100	100	100	100
Base	*184*	*256*	*237*	*179*	*856*
Mean (average value)	11.5	11.5	11.7	12.0	11.7
Median	11.3	11.4	11.9	12.1	11.6
Lower 2.5 percentile	8.5	8.9	8.4	8.2	8.4
Upper 2.5 percentile	15.0	14.8	15.2	16.2	15.6
Standard deviation	1.57	1.55	1.77	. 2.10	1.78
	cum %	cum %	cum %	cum %	cum %
Females					
9 or less	7	7	6	10	7
10 or less	16	12	16	22	16
11 or less	35	32	29	35	33
12 or less	64	57	50	52	55
13 or less	83	79	71	73	76
14 or less	96	91	85	85	89
All	100	100	100	100	100
Base	*171*	*226*	*238*	*210*	*845*
Mean (average value)	11.5	11.8	12.0	11.7	11.8
Median	11.5	11.8	12.0	11.8	11.7
Lower 2.5 percentile	8.2	8.3	8.0	6.6	8.0
Upper 2.5 percentile	15.1	15.4	17.1	15.6	15.9
Standard deviation	1.69	1.75	2.16	2.19	1.98

Table 7.10 Average daily intake of total *cis* polyunsaturated fatty acids (g) (*cis* n-3 + *cis* n-6) by sex and age of young person

Intake of *cis* monounsaturated fatty acids (g)	Age (years)				All
	4–6	7–10	11–14	15–18	
	cum %	cum %	cum %	cum %	cum %
Males					
Less than 7	20	9	2	2	8
Less than 10	64	39	22	10	32
Less than 13	90	73	56	38	63
Less than 16	98	90	79	60	81
Less than 19	100	96	88	77	90
All		100	100	100	100
Base	*184*	*256*	*237*	*179*	*856*
Mean (average value)	9.3	11.3	13.3	15.5	12.5
Median	9.2	10.7	12.5	14.6	11.7
Lower 2.5 percentile	4.3	5.4	7.4	7.2	5.5
Upper 2.5 percentile	15.0	21.5	22.7	28.8	23.8
Standard deviation	2.91	3.64	4.31	5.21	4.72
	cum %	cum %	cum %	cum %	cum %
Females					
Less than 7	41	14	9	14	18
Less than 10	75	51	35	39	49
Less than 13	93	82	63	63	74
Less than 16	98	93	87	84	90
Less than 19	99	99	96	95	97
All	100	100	100	100	100
Base	*171*	*226*	*238*	*210*	*845*
Mean (average value)	8.4	10.5	11.8	11.8	10.7
Median	7.9	9.9	11.6	11.2	10.1
Lower 2.5 percentile	4.1	5.6	5.4	4.9	5.1
Upper 2.5 percentile	15.2	18.1	20.1	21.3	19.5
Standard deviation	3.01	3.31	3.85	4.40	3.94

Table 7.11 Average daily intake of *cis* n-3 polyunsaturated fatty acids (g) by sex and age of young person

Intake of *cis* n-3 polyunsaturated fatty acids (g)	Age (years)				All
	4–6	7–10	11–14	15–18	
	cum %	cum %	cum %	cum %	cum %
Males					
Less than 0.7	9	4	2	0	4
Less than 1.0	33	15	7	3	14
Less than 1.5	74	53	35	19	44
Less than 2.0	90	82	66	49	71
Less than 2.5	95	91	80	73	84
All	100	100	100	100	100
Base	*184*	*256*	*237*	*179*	*856*
Mean (average value)	1.29	1.58	1.95	2.19	1.77
Median	1.18	1.42	1.67	2.01	1.59
Lower 2.5 percentile	0.52	0.65	0.83	0.95	0.64
Upper 2.5 percentile	2.92	3.48	4.08	4.60	3.77
Standard deviation	0.570	0.692	1.239	0.862	0.949
	cum %	cum %	cum %	cum %	cum %
Females					
Less than 0.7	16	4	3	4	6
Less than 1.0	45	18	16	16	23
Less than 1.5	80	66	47	50	60
Less than 2.0	96	85	76	76	83
Less than 2.5	98	95	91	92	94
All	100	100	100	100	100
Base	*171*	*226*	*238*	*210*	*845*
Mean (average value)	1.15	1.44	1.65	1.61	1.48
Median	1.07	1.36	1.59	1.50	1.36
Lower 2.5 percentile	0.51	0.67	0.67	0.65	0.58
Upper 2.5 percentile	2.32	3.04	3.42	3.12	3.17
Standard deviation	0.499	0.548	0.716	0.640	0.639

Table 7.12 Average daily intake of *cis* n-6 polyunsaturated fatty acids (g) by sex and age of young person

Intake of *cis* n-6 polyunsaturated fatty acids (g)	Age (years)				All
	4–6	7–10	11–14	15–18	
	cum %	cum %	cum %	cum %	cum %
Males					
Less than 6	21	10	2	2	8
Less than 8	50	31	17	6	25
Less than 10	79	61	39	25	50
Less than 12	93	78	63	44	68
Less than 14	99	91	79	61	82
Less than 16	100	96	88	75	89
All		100	100	100	100
Base	*184*	*256*	*237*	*179*	*856*
Mean (average value)	8.0	9.7	11.4	13.3	10.7
Median	7.9	9.2	10.6	12.5	10.0
Lower 2.5 percentile	3.6	4.7	6.2	6.1	4.7
Upper 2.5 percentile	13.4	18.8	19.3	24.8	20.5
Standard deviation	2.56	3.27	3.68	4.56	4.10
	cum %	cum %	cum %	cum %	cum %
Females					
Less than 6	39	13	9	15	18
Less than 8	68	42	28	33	41
Less than 10	88	66	51	55	64
Less than 12	95	86	72	68	80
Less than 14	98	94	87	84	90
Less than 16	98	97	94	92	95
All	100	100	100	100	100
Base	*171*	*226*	*238*	*210*	*845*
Mean (average value)	7.2	9.0	10.2	10.2	9.3
Median	6.7	8.5	9.8	9.5	8.7
Lower 2.5 percentile	3.6	4.7	4.9	4.1	4.2
Upper 2.5 percentile	13.5	16.7	17.8	18.9	17.6
Standard deviation	2.72	3.00	3.37	3.98	3.51

Table 7.13 Percentage food energy intake from total *cis* polyunsaturated fatty acids (*cis* n-3 + *cis* n-6) by sex and age of young person

Percentage food energy intake from *cis* n-3 + *cis* n-6 polyunsaturated fatty acids	Age (years)				All
	4–6	7–10	11–14	15–18	
Males	cum %	cum %	cum %	cum %	cum %
4.5 or less	23	19	10	12	16
5.5 or less	51	49	36	36	42
6.5 or less	82	77	67	59	71
7.5 or less	91	88	86	77	85
8.5 or less	97	96	93	89	94
10.0 or less	100	99	98	99	99
All		100	100	100	100
Base	*184*	*256*	*237*	*179*	*856*
Mean (average value)	5.5	5.7	6.1	6.3	5.9
Median	5.5	5.5	5.9	6.1	5.7
Lower 2.5 percentile	3.1	3.5	3.8	3.7	3.6
Upper 2.5 percentile	8.5	9.4	9.5	9.4	9.3
Standard deviation	1.34	1.49	1.43	1.60	1.50
Females	cum %	cum %	cum %	cum %	cum %
4.5 or less	28	20	11	12	17
5.5 or less	60	42	35	26	40
6.5 or less	79	70	54	48	62
7.5 or less	91	82	74	72	79
8.5 or less	98	94	89	85	91
10.0 or less	100	99	97	95	98
All		100	100	100	100
Base	*171*	*226*	*238*	*210*	*845*
Mean (average value)	5.4	5.9	6.4	6.7	6.1
Median	5.2	5.7	6.3	6.6	5.9
Lower 2.5 percentile	3.2	3.4	3.8	3.7	3.4
Upper 2.5 percentile	8.4	9.4	10.2	10.6	9.9
Standard deviation	1.35	1.53	1.68	1.87	1.70

Table 7.14 Percentage food energy from *cis* n-3 polyunsaturated fatty acids by sex and age of young person

Percentage food energy intake from *cis* n-3 polyunsaturated fatty acids	Age (years)				All
	4–6	7–10	11–14	15–18	
	cum %	cum %	cum %	cum %	cum %
Males					
0.5 or less	12	11	11	6	10
0.6 or less	31	26	19	17	23
0.7 or less	55	46	36	28	40
0.8 or less	67	62	51	48	57
0.9 or less	76	74	66	56	68
1.0 or less	87	81	73	71	78
1.5 or less	96	96	94	93	95
All	100	100	100	100	100
Base	*184*	*256*	*237*	*179*	*856*
Mean (average value)	0.8	0.8	0.9	0.9	0.8
Median	0.7	0.7	0.8	0.9	0.8
Lower 2.5 percentile	0.4	0.4	0.4	0.5	0.4
Upper 2.5 percentile	1.8	1.7	1.9	1.6	1.7
Standard deviation	0.30	0.33	0.45	0.30	0.36
	cum %	cum %	cum %	cum %	cum %
Females					
0.5 or less	17	10	9	4	9
0.6 or less	34	21	20	13	21
0.7 or less	51	37	34	30	37
0.8 or less	69	58	49	45	55
0.9 or less	77	73	60	53	65
1.0 or less	87	80	68	63	74
1.5 or less	98	97	94	95	96
All	100	100	100	100	100
Base	*171*	*226*	*238*	*210*	*845*
Mean (average value)	0.7	0.8	0.9	0.9	0.8
Median	0.7	0.8	0.8	0.9	0.8
Lower 2.5 percentile	0.4	0.4	0.4	0.5	0.4
Upper 2.5 percentile	1.3	1.5	2.0	1.6	1.6
Standard deviation	0.27	0.29	0.36	0.31	0.32

Table 7.15 Percentage food energy intake from *cis* n-6 polyunsaturated fatty acids by sex and age of young person

Percentage food energy intake from *cis* n-6 polyunsaturated fatty acids	Age (years)				All
	4–6	7–10	11–14	15–18	
	cum %	cum %	cum %	cum %	cum %
Males					
3 or less	5	2	1	2	2
4 or less	29	24	15	17	21
5 or less	61	61	48	50	55
6 or less	88	83	80	72	80
7 or less	93	93	91	86	91
8 or less	99	97	97	98	98
All	100	100	100	100	100
Base	*184*	*256*	*237*	*179*	*856*
Mean (average value)	4.8	4.9	5.2	5.3	5.1
Median	4.7	4.7	5.1	5.0	4.9
Lower 2.5 percentile	2.7	3.0	3.3	3.0	3.0
Upper 2.5 percentile	7.4	8.4	8.4	7.9	7.9
Standard deviation	1.20	1.37	1.23	1.40	1.33
	cum %	cum %	cum %	cum %	cum %
Females					
3 or less	5	3	1	2	3
4 or less	32	24	16	18	22
5 or less	68	51	40	37	48
6 or less	85	77	66	63	72
7 or less	94	91	84	79	87
8 or less	100	95	95	91	95
All		100	100	100	100
Base	*171*	*226*	*238*	*210*	*845*
Mean (average value)	4.6	5.1	5.5	5.7	5.3
Median	4.5	4.9	5.4	5.6	5.1
Lower 2.5 percentile	2.7	2.9	3.2	3.1	2.9
Upper 2.5 percentile	7.6	8.5	8.6	9.4	8.7
Standard deviation	1.24	1.41	1.46	1.68	1.52

Table 7.16 Average daily intake of cholesterol (mg) by sex and age of young person

Intake of cholesterol (mg)	Age (years)				All
	4–6	7–10	11–14	15–18	
	cum %	cum %	cum %	cum %	cum %
Males					
Less than 100	15	9	7	3	8
Less than 150	57	35	27	15	32
Less than 200	78	67	52	37	58
Less than 250	91	85	79	57	77
Less than 300	96	95	90	73	88
All	100	100	100	100	100
Base	*184*	*256*	*237*	*179*	*856*
Mean (average value)	158	181	201	243	198
Median	143	174	195	239	186
Lower 2.5 percentile	64	67	78	97	75
Upper 2.5 percentile	330	335	401	428	390
Standard deviation	71.4	66.9	80.3	95.4	85.1
	cum %	cum %	cum %	cum %	cum %
Females					
Less than 100	15	11	15	14	14
Less than 150	48	44	42	40	43
Less than 200	77	73	72	68	72
Less than 250	93	88	89	84	88
Less than 300	98	94	94	93	95
All	100	100	100	100	100
Base	*171*	*226*	*238*	*210*	*845*
Mean (average value)	156	170	169	177	169
Median	151	160	160	170	160
Lower 2.5 percentile	62	61	54	53	60
Upper 2.5 percentile	282	329	345	346	329
Standard deviation	59.6	67.0	72.2	80.4	71.0

Table 7.17 Percentage contribution of food types to average daily intake of total fat by sex and age of young person

Type of food	Males aged (years)				All males	Females aged (years)				All females
	4–6	7–10	11–14	15–18		4–6	7–10	11–14	15–18	
	%	%	%	%	%	%	%	%	%	%
Cereals & cereal products	22	24	23	21	22	21	23	21	21	21
of which:										
pizza	2	3	4	4	3	2	2	2	3	2
white bread	2	2	2	2	2	2	2	2	2	2
biscuits	7	7	6	5	6	7	7	5	3	6
buns, cakes & pastries	6	6	5	4	5	5	5	5	5	5
Milk & milk products	20	16	14	13	15	21	16	13	13	15
of which:										
whole milk	10	5	3	3	5	10	5	3	3	4
semi-skimmed milk	2	3	3	2	2	2	2	2	2	2
cheese (incl. cottage cheese)	3	3	3	5	4	5	4	5	6	5
ice cream	2	2	2	1	2	2	2	2	1	2
Eggs & egg dishes	2	2	2	2	2	3	3	2	3	2
Fat spreads	9	10	9	9	9	11	9	9	10	9
of which:										
butter	2	2	2	2	2	3	2	1	2	2
reduced fat spreads	5	6	5	4	5	5	4	4	5	4
Meat & meat products	17	18	20	25	21	15	19	19	19	18
of which:										
bacon & ham	1	1	2	2	2	1	1	1	1	1
beef, veal & dishes	1	2	2	3	2	1	2	2	2	2
lamb & dishes	1	1	1	1	1	1	1	1	1	1
pork & dishes	1	1	1	1	1	1	1	1	1	1
coated chicken	2	2	2	2	2	3	3	3	3	3
chicken & turkey dishes	1	2	2	3	2	2	2	2	3	2
burgers & kebabs	1	1	2	3	2	1	1	2	2	2
sausages	5	4	3	4	4	3	4	3	2	3
meat pies & pastries	3	3	4	4	4	3	3	4	3	3
other meat products	1	1	1	1	1	1	1	0	0	1
Fish & fish dishes	2	2	2	2	2	2	2	2	2	2
of which:										
coated & fried white fish	2	1	1	1	1	2	1	1	1	1
Vegetables, potatoes & savoury snacks	19	18	19	18	18	17	19	23	20	20
of which:										
roast & fried potatoes, & chips	7	7	9	10	8	6	8	10	9	8
savoury snacks	8	8	7	6	7	9	8	9	6	8
Fruit & nuts	1	1	1	1	1	1	1	1	1	1
Sugar, preserves & confectionery	6	8	8	7	7	7	7	8	7	7
of which:										
chocolate confectionery	5	7	7	6	6	6	6	7	6	6
Drinks*	0	0	0	0	0	0	0	0	0	0
Miscellaneous**	1	2	2	2	2	1	2	2	4	4
Average daily intake (g)	**60.1**	**69.8**	**77.2**	**89.0**	**74.7**	**55.9**	**63.8**	**67.2**	**64.0**	**63.1**
Number of young people	**184**	**256**	**237**	**179**	**856**	**171**	**226**	**238**	**210**	**845**

* Includes soft drinks, alcoholic drinks, tea, coffee and water.
** Includes powdered beverages (except tea and coffee), soups, sauces and condiments and commercial toddlers' foods.

Table 7.18 Percentage contribution of food types to average daily intake of saturated fatty acids by sex and age of young person

Type of food	Males aged (years) 4–6	7–10	11–14	15–18	All males	Females aged (years) 4–6	7–10	11–14	15–18	All females
	%	%	%	%	%	%	%	%	%	%
Cereals & cereal products	22	24	23	20	22	21	23	22	21	22
of which:										
pizza	2	3	4	4	3	2	2	3	3	3
white bread	1	1	2	2	2	1	1	1	2	1
biscuits	8	8	7	6	7	9	9	7	4	7
buns, cakes & pastries	5	6	5	4	5	4	5	5	4	5
Milk & milk products	30	24	22	20	23	31	24	20	21	23
of which:										
whole milk	15	8	5	5	8	15	7	4	5	7
semi-skimmed milk	3	4	5	4	4	3	3	3	3	3
cheese (incl. cottage cheese)	5	5	6	8	6	7	7	7	10	8
ice cream	2	3	3	2	2	3	3	2	1	2
Eggs & egg dishes	1	2	2	2	2	2	2	2	2	2
Fat spreads	7	9	7	8	8	9	7	7	9	8
of which:										
butter	2	4	3	3	3	4	3	2	4	3
reduced fat spreads	3	3	3	3	3	3	3	3	3	3
Meat & meat products	15	16	19	24	19	13	17	18	18	16
of which:										
bacon & ham	1	1	2	2	1	1	1	1	1	1
beef, veal and dishes	1	1	2	3	2	1	2	2	3	2
lamb & dishes	1	1	1	2	1	1	1	1	1	1
pork & dishes	1	1	1	1	1	0	1	1	1	1
coated chicken	1	1	1	1	1	1	1	2	2	2
chicken & turkey dishes	1	1	2	2	2	1	1	2	2	2
burgers & kebabs	1	1	2	4	2	1	2	2	3	2
sausages	4	4	3	4	4	3	3	3	2	3
meat pies & pastries	3	3	4	4	4	3	3	4	3	3
other meat products	1	1	1	1	1	0	1	0	0	1
Fish & fish dishes	1	1	1	1	1	1	1	1	1	1
of which:										
coated & fried white fish	1	1	1	1	1	1	1	1	1	1
Vegetables, potatoes & savoury snacks	14	13	14	13	13	13	14	17	15	15
of which:										
roasted & fried potatoes, & chips	4	4	5	5	4	3	4	5	5	4
savoury snacks	8	8	7	6	7	8	8	9	6	8
Fruit & nuts	1	1	1	0	1	0	1	1	0	0
Sugar, preserves & confectionery	8	10	10	9	9	9	9	11	9	9
of which:										
chocolate confectionery	7	9	10	9	9	8	8	10	9	9
Drinks*	0	0	0	0	0	0	0	0	0	0
Miscellaneous**	1	1	1	2	2	1	2	2	3	3
Average daily intake (g)	**25.1**	**28.3**	**30.3**	**34.7**	**29.8**	**23.8**	**25.7**	**26.2**	**24.7**	**25.2**
Number of young people	**184**	**256**	**237**	**179**	**856**	**171**	**226**	**238**	**210**	**845**

* Includes soft drinks, alcoholic drinks, tea, coffee and water.
** Includes powdered beverages (except tea and coffee), soups, sauces and condiments and commercial toddlers' foods.

Table 7.19 Percentage contribution of food types to average daily intake of *trans* fatty acids by sex and age of young person

Type of food	Males aged (years)				All males	Females aged (years)				All females
	4–6	7–10	11–14	15–18		4–6	7–10	11–14	15–18	
	%	%	%	%	%	%	%	%	%	%
Cereals & cereal products	33	33	29	25	30	32	32	29	27	30
of which:										
pizza	*2*	*2*	*3*	*3*	*3*	*2*	*2*	*2*	*3*	*2*
white bread	*1*	*1*	*2*	*2*	*1*	*1*	*1*	*1*	*1*	*1*
biscuits	*14*	*13*	*11*	*10*	*12*	*15*	*14*	*12*	*7*	*12*
buns, cakes & pastries	*11*	*11*	*9*	*7*	*9*	*9*	*10*	*9*	*9*	*9*
Milk & milk products	21	16	15	14	17	23	17	15	16	17
of which:										
whole milk	*9*	*5*	*3*	*3*	*4*	*10*	*5*	*3*	*3*	*4*
semi-skimmed milk	*3*	*3*	*4*	*3*	*2*	*2*	*2*	*2*	*3*	*2*
cheese (incl. cottage cheese)	*4*	*4*	*4*	*6*	*6*	*6*	*5*	*6*	*8*	*6*
ice cream	*2*	*2*	*2*	*1*	*2*	*2*	*3*	*2*	*1*	*2*
Eggs & egg dishes	1	1	1	2	2	2	2	1	2	2
Fat spreads	11	13	12	13	13	14	12	12	14	13
of which:										
butter	*2*	*2*	*2*	*2*	*2*	*3*	*2*	*2*	*3*	*2*
soft margarine, not polyunsaturated	*3*	*3*	*4*	*4*	*4*	*4*	*4*	*4*	*5*	*4*
polyunsaturated reduced fat spread	*2*	*2*	*1*	*1*	*2*	*2*	*2*	*1*	*1*	*2*
other reduced fat spread	*3*	*3*	*3*	*3*	*3*	*3*	*2*	*2*	*3*	*3*
Meat & meat products	14	14	16	22	15	12	16	16	17	15
of which:										
beef, veal & dishes	*2*	*2*	*2*	*3*	*2*	*1*	*2*	*2*	*3*	*2*
lamb & dishes	*2*	*2*	*2*	*3*	*2*	*1*	*2*	*2*	*2*	*2*
coated chicken	*2*	*1*	*1*	*1*	*2*	*2*	*2*	*2*	*2*	*2*
chicken & turkey dishes	*1*	*1*	*1*	*1*	*1*	*1*	*1*	*1*	*1*	*1*
burgers & kebabs	*1*	*1*	*2*	*4*	*2*	*1*	*1*	*2*	*2*	*2*
sausages	*1*	*1*	*1*	*1*	*1*	*1*	*1*	*1*	*1*	*1*
meat pies & pastries	*5*	*5*	*6*	*8*	*6*	*4*	*6*	*6*	*6*	*5*
other meat products	*0*	*0*	*1*	*1*	*1*	*0*	*1*	*0*	*0*	*0*
Fish & fish dishes	2	2	2	1	2	2	2	1	2	2
of which:										
coated & fried white fish	*2*	*1*	*1*	*1*	*1*	*2*	*1*	*1*	*1*	*1*
Vegetables, potatoes & savoury snacks	9	10	11	11	10	7	9	12	12	10
of which:										
roast & fried potatoes, & chips	*4*	*4*	*6*	*7*	*6*	*4*	*5*	*7*	*7*	*6*
savoury snacks	*2*	*3*	*3*	*2*	*3*	*1*	*2*	*3*	*2*	*2*
Fruit & nuts	0	0	-	-	0	0	0	-	-	0
Sugar, preserves & confectionery	7	11	12	10	10	8	9	11	9	9
of which:										
chocolate confectionery	*6*	*9*	*10*	*10*	*9*	*6*	*8*	*10*	*8*	*8*
Drinks*	-	-	-	0	0	-	-	-	-	0
Miscellaneous**	1	1	1	1	1	1	1	1	2	2
Average daily intake (g)	**2.26**	**2.74**	**2.92**	**3.45**	**2.87**	**2.09**	**2.48**	**2.48**	**2.34**	**2.36**
Number of young people	**184**	**256**	**237**	**179**	**856**	**171**	**226**	**238**	**210**	**845**

* Includes soft drinks, alcoholic drinks, tea, coffee and water.
** Includes powdered beverages (except tea and coffee), soups, sauces and condiments and commercial toddlers' foods.

Table 7.20 Percentage contribution of food types to average daily intake of *cis* monounsaturated fatty acids by sex and age of young person

Type of food	Males aged (years)				All males	Females aged (years)				All females
	4–6	7–10	11–14	15–18		4–6	7–10	11–14	15–18	
	%	%	%	%	%	%	%	%	%	%
Cereals & cereal products	19	20	20	18	19	20	21	21	23	20
of which:										
pizza	2	2	4	4	3	2	3	4	5	2
white bread	1	1	2	2	2	1	1	2	2	1
biscuits	6	6	5	4	5	6	6	5	5	5
buns, cakes & pastries	6	6	5	4	5	7	6	5	5	5
Milk & milk products	13	13	11	10	11	18	14	11	12	11
of which:										
whole milk	7	4	2	2	3	8	4	3	3	3
semi-skimmed milk	2	2	2	2	2	2	2	2	2	1
cheese(incl. cottage cheese)	3	2	2	4	3	3	2	3	5	4
ice cream	2	2	2	1	1	2	2	1	1	2
Eggs & egg dishes	2	2	3	3	3	2	2	3	3	3
Fat spreads	8	9	8	8	8	9	8	7	8	8
of which:										
butter	1	2	1	1	1	1	2	1	1	1
soft margarine, not polyunsaturated	1	1	2	2	1	2	2	1	2	2
polyunsaturated reduced fat spread	2	2	2	2	2	2	2	2	2	2
other reduced fat spread	3	4	2	2	3	3	2	2	2	2
Meat & meat products	22	22	24	29	25	19	22	21	20	22
of which:										
bacon & ham	1	1	2	3	2	1	1	1	1	1
beef, veal and dishes	2	2	2	3	2	1	2	2	3	2
lamb & dishes	1	1	1	1	1	1	1	1	1	1
pork & dishes	1	1	1	1	1	1	1	1	1	1
coated chicken	3	3	2	3	3	3	3	3	3	3
chicken & turkey dishes	2	2	3	3	3	2	2	2	3	3
burgers & kebabs	2	2	2	4	3	2	2	2	2	2
sausages	6	6	4	5	5	5	4	4	3	4
meat pies & pastries	4	4	5	5	4	3	4	4	3	4
other meat products	1	1	1	1	1	1	1	1	0	1
Fish & fish dishes	3	2	2	2	2	3	2	1	2	2
of which:										
coated & fried white fish	2	2	1	1	2	2	2	1	1	2
Vegetables, potatoes & savoury snacks	22	21	21	21	21	20	22	25	21	23
of which:										
roast & fried potatoes, & chips	9	9	11	12	10	7	9	12	10	10
savoury snacks	10	9	8	7	8	11	10	10	7	10
Fruit & nuts	1	2	2	1	1	1	1	1	1	1
Sugar, preserves & confectionery	5	7	7	6	7	6	6	7	6	7
of which:										
chocolate confectionery	5	6	6	5	6	5	5	6	5	6
Drinks*	0	0	0	0	0	0	0	0	0	0
Miscellaneous**	1	2	2	2	2	1	2	2	3	3
Average daily intake (g)	**19.4**	**22.8**	**25.6**	**29.6**	**24.6**	**17.8**	**20.9**	**22.4**	**20.9**	**20.6**
Number of young people	**184**	**256**	**237**	**179**	**856**	**171**	**226**	**238**	**210**	**845**

* Includes soft drinks, alcoholic drinks, tea, coffee and water.

Table 7.21 Percentage contribution of food types to average daily intake of *cis* n-3 polyunsaturated fatty acids by sex and age of young person

Type of food	Males aged (years)				All males	Females aged (years)				All females
	4–6	7–10	11–14	15–18		4–6	7–10	11–14	15–18	
	%	%	%	%	%	%	%	%	%	%
Cereals & cereal products	16	18	18	18	18	15	17	15	17	16
of which:										
pizza	3	4	5	5	4	3	3	3	4	3
white bread	2	2	2	2	2	2	2	2	2	2
biscuits	2	2	1	1	1	2	2	1	1	1
buns, cakes & pastries	4	4	3	2	3	3	3	3	2	3
Milk & milk products	6	5	4	4	5	7	5	4	4	5
of which:										
whole milk	2	1	1	1	1	2	1	1	1	1
cheese (incl. cottage cheese)	2	1	1	2	2	2	2	2	2	2
Eggs & egg dishes	1	1	2	1	1	2	2	1	1	1
Fat spreads	6	8	6	6	6	8	6	6	6	6
of which:										
butter	1	1	1	1	1	1	1	1	1	1
soft margarine, not polyunsaturated	1	1	2	2	2	2	2	2	2	2
polyunsaturated reduced fat spread	1	1	1	1	1	1	1	1	1	1
other reduced fat spread	3	4	2	2	3	4	2	2	2	2
Meat & meat products	15	16	16	19	17	15	16	15	16	16
of which:										
coated chicken	5	5	3	4	4	6	5	4	5	5
chicken & turkey dishes	2	3	3	4	3	3	3	3	4	3
sausages	3	2	2	2	2	2	2	2	1	2
meat pies & pastries	1	1	2	2	2	1	1	1	1	1
Fish & fish dishes	6	5	5	5	5	8	6	4	6	6
of which:										
coated & fried white fish	4	3	2	3	3	4	3	2	3	3
oily fish	2	2	2	2	2	3	2	1	3	2
Vegetables, potatoes & savoury snacks	34	32	34	36	34	33	37	42	39	38
of which:										
roast & fried potatoes, & chips	21	22	25	26	24	20	25	29	23	25
savoury snacks	5	4	3	2	3	5	5	4	3	4
Fruit & nuts	11	11	10	4	9	7	6	6	2	5
of which:										
nuts & seeds	10	10	10	4	8	5	5	5	2	4
Sugar, preserves & confectionery	2	2	2	2	2	2	1	2	2	2
Drinks*	0	0	0	0	0	0	0	0	0	0
Miscellaneous**	2	2	2	3	3	2	3	4	4	4
Average daily intake (g)	**1.29**	**1.58**	**1.95**	**2.19**	**1.77**	**1.15**	**1.44**	**1.65**	**1.61**	**1.48**
Number of young people	**184**	**256**	**237**	**179**	**856**	**171**	**226**	**238**	**210**	**845**

* Includes soft drinks, alcoholic drinks, tea, coffee and water.
** Includes powdered beverages (except tea and coffee), soups, sauces and condiments and commercial toddlers' foods.

199

Table 7.22 Percentage contribution of food types to average daily intake of *cis* n-6 polyunsaturated fatty acids by sex and age of young person

Type of food	Sex and age of young person									
	Males aged (years)				All males	Females aged (years)				All females
	4–6	7–10	11–14	15–18		4–6	7–10	11–14	15–18	
	%	%	%	%	%	%	%	%	%	%
Cereals & cereal products	23	24	23	22	23	22	22	21	21	21
of which:										
pizza	*2*	*2*	*4*	*3*	*3*	*2*	*2*	*2*	*2*	*2*
white bread	*4*	*4*	*4*	*4*	*4*	*4*	*4*	*4*	*4*	*4*
whole grain and high fibre b'fast cereals	*2*	*2*	*2*	*1*	*2*	*2*	*1*	*1*	*1*	*1*
biscuits	*4*	*4*	*3*	*2*	*3*	*4*	*4*	*3*	*2*	*3*
buns, cakes & pastries	*6*	*6*	*5*	*4*	*5*	*5*	*5*	*5*	*3*	*4*
Milk & milk products	4	3	3	2	3	4	3	2	2	2
Eggs & egg dishes	2	2	3	3	2	3	3	2	2	2
Fat spreads	18	18	16	15	16	19	17	15	15	16
of which:										
polyunsaturated margarine	*1*	*1*	*1*	*1*	*1*	*1*	*1*	*1*	*1*	*1*
polyunsaturated low fat spread	*1*	*3*	*2*	*1*	*2*	*1*	*1*	*2*	*2*	*2*
polyunsaturated reduced fat spread	*11*	*10*	*9*	*8*	*9*	*11*	*10*	*9*	*8*	*10*
other reduced fat spread	*2*	*3*	*2*	*2*	*2*	*3*	*2*	*1*	*2*	*2*
Meat & meat products	16	16	17	20	18	15	17	16	16	16
of which:										
coated chicken	*4*	*4*	*3*	*4*	*4*	*5*	*4*	*4*	*5*	*1*
chicken & turkey dishes	*2*	*2*	*3*	*3*	*3*	*2*	*2*	*3*	*3*	*2*
sausages	*5*	*4*	*3*	*3*	*4*	*3*	*3*	*3*	*2*	*3*
meat pies & pastries	*2*	*2*	*3*	*3*	*2*	*2*	*2*	*2*	*2*	*2*
Fish & fish dishes	3	3	2	3	3	4	3	2	3	3
of which:										
coated & fried white fish	*3*	*2*	*2*	*2*	*2*	*3*	*2*	*2*	*2*	*2*
Vegetables, potatoes & savoury snacks	27	26	28	27	27	26	28	33	29	29
of which:										
roasted & fried potatoes, & chips	*12*	*12*	*15*	*16*	*14*	*11*	*13*	*17*	*13*	*14*
savoury snacks	*9*	*9*	*7*	*6*	*7*	*10*	*9*	*9*	*6*	*8*
Fruit & nuts	1	1	1	1	1	1	2	1	1	1
of which:										
nuts & seeds	*1*	*1*	*1*	*1*	*1*	*1*	*1*	*1*	*1*	*1*
Sugar, preserves & confectionery	2	3	4	3	3	2	2	3	3	3
Drinks*	0	0	0	0	0	0	0	0	0	0
Miscellaneous**	3	3	3	5	4	3	4	4	9	6
Average daily intake (g)	**8.0**	**9.7**	**11.4**	**13.3**	**10.7**	**7.2**	**9.0**	**10.2**	**10.2**	**9.3**
Number of young people	**184**	**256**	**237**	**179**	**856**	**171**	**226**	**238**	**210**	**845**

* Includes soft drinks, alcoholic drinks, tea, coffee and water.
** Includes powdered beverages (except tea and coffee), soups, sauces and condiments and commercial toddlers' foods.

Table 7.23 Total fat, fatty acids and cholesterol intake by sex of young person and whether young person was reported as being unwell during dietary recording period: average daily intake and percentage contribution to food energy intake

Fatty acids	Whether unwell during period								
	Unwell and eating affected			Unwell and eating not affected			Not unwell		
	Mean	Median	SD	Mean	Median	SD	Mean	Median	SD
Males									
Total fat (g)	65.6	65.4	20.22	70.9	69.6	21.15	76.1	72.8	22.18
Saturated fatty acids (g)	26.4	25.9	9.03	28.4	27.2	8.50	30.3	29.2	9.28
Trans fatty acids (g)	2.52	2.39	1.038	2.70	2.67	1.017	2.93	2.72	1.146
Cis monounsaturated fatty acids (g)	21.5	21.3	6.82	23.4	22.7	7.39	25.1	24.0	7.76
Total *cis* polyunsaturated fatty acids (g)	10.9	10.4	3.79	11.8	10.6	4.53	12.8	11.8	4.79
Cis n-3 polyunsaturated fatty acids (g)	1.57	1.42	0.740	1.76	1.52	0.929	1.80	1.63	0.970
Cis n-6 polyunsaturated fatty acids (g)	9.3	8.6	3.31	10.1	9.0	3.91	11.0	10.2	4.17
Cholesterol (mg)	182	175	82.2	188	174	85.8	200	188	85.2
Females									
Total fat (g)	54.1	54.4	16.46	63.3	63.6	17.01	64.2	63.7	16.83
Saturated fatty acids (g)	21.6	21.7	7.09	25.0	24.0	7.83	25.7	25.7	7.27
Trans fatty acids (g)	1.99	1.89	0.772	2.31	2.28	0.869	2.42	2.34	0.857
Cis monounsaturated fatty acids (g)	17.7	17.8	5.71	20.8	20.8	5.75	21.0	20.6	5.84
Total *cis* polyunsaturated fatty acids (g)	9.4	8.5	3.69	11.2	10.3	4.24	10.9	10.2	3.89
Cis n-3 polyunsaturated fatty acids (g)	1.31	1.28	0.690	1.52	1.33	0.744	1.50	1.38	0.614
Cis n-6 polyunsaturated fatty acids (g)	8.1	7.3	3.19	9.6	8.9	3.68	9.4	8.8	3.50
Cholesterol (mg)	144	139	71.9	163	153	67.6	173	164	70.6
Percentage food energy from:									
Males									
Total fat	35.1	35.1	4.24	35.6	35.7	2.97	35.5	35.5	4.26
Saturated fatty acids	14.1	14.2	2.35	14.3	14.2	1.92	14.1	14.1	2.22
Trans fatty acids	1.3	1.3	0.32	1.3	1.3	0.28	1.4	1.3	0.34
Cis monounsaturated fatty acids	11.5	11.6	1.74	11.7	11.6	1.35	11.7	11.6	1.82
Total *cis* polyunsaturated fatty acids	5.9	5.8	1.37	5.9	5.5	1.21	5.9	5.7	1.54
Cis n-3 polyunsaturated fatty acids	0.8	0.8	0.33	0.9	0.8	0.35	0.8	0.8	0.36
Cis n-6 polyunsaturated fatty acids	5.0	5.0	1.22	5.0	4.7	1.06	5.1	4.9	1.36
Females									
Total fat	36.3	35.9	5.55	35.7	36.3	4.90	35.9	36.2	4.63
Saturated fatty acids	14.4	14.5	2.80	14.0	14.0	2.69	14.4	14.3	2.45
Trans fatty acids	1.3	1.3	0.35	1.3	1.3	0.37	1.3	1.3	0.35
Cis monounsaturated fatty acids	11.9	11.6	2.31	11.8	12.0	2.00	11.7	11.7	1.93
Total *cis* polyunsaturated fatty acids	6.3	6.1	1.76	6.3	6.0	1.89	6.1	5.9	1.67
Cis n-3 polyunsaturated fatty acids	0.9	0.8	0.38	0.9	0.8	0.35	0.8	0.8	0.30
Cis n-6 polyunsaturated fatty acids	5.4	5.2	1.61	5.4	5.2	1.65	5.2	5.0	1.48
Total number of males	86			66			704		
Total number of females	93			84			668		

Table 7.24 Total fat, fatty acids and cholesterol intake by sex and region: average daily intake and percentage contribution to food energy intake

Fatty acids	Region											
	Scotland			Northern			Central, South West and Wales			London and the South East		
	Mean	Median	SD	Mean	Median	SD	Mean	Median	SD	Mean	Median	SD
Males												
Total fat (g)	73.9	70.5	20.01	74.9	72.2	21.49	75.0	73.3	22.00	74.2	71.4	23.51
Saturated fatty acids (g)	29.9	27.3	9.32	29.7	28.4	9.02	29.9	29.4	9.24	29.7	28.7	9.57
Trans fatty acids (g)	2.81	2.63	1.210	2.88	2.70	1.108	2.91	2.71	1.111	2.85	2.65	1.163
Cis monounsaturated fatty acids (g)	24.6	23.2	6.97	24.6	24.0	7.34	24.8	24.2	7.82	24.2	22.8	8.16
Total *cis* polyunsaturated fatty acids (g)	12.0	11.7	3.64	12.9	11.9	4.99	12.4	11.4	4.53	12.4	11.8	4.91
Cis n-3 polyunsaturated fatty acids (g)	1.73	1.60	0.935	1.74	1.56	0.792	1.76	1.63	0.922	1.83	1.68	1.110
Cis n-6 polyunsaturated fatty acids (g)	10.3	10.4	3.14	11.1	10.2	4.46	10.6	9.7	3.92	10.6	10.0	4.18
Cholesterol (mg)	183	181	74.2	194	184	79.5	201	187	82.7	202	187	95.0
Females												
Total fat (g)	61.9	61.1	16.31	65.0	65.4	15.51	63.0	61.5	17.30	61.6	62.3	18.28
Saturated fatty acids (g)	24.1	23.7	6.92	26.0	26.1	6.63	25.4	25.8	7.57	24.5	23.6	7.96
Trans fatty acids (g)	2.24	2.12	0.858	2.45	2.35	0.809	2.37	2.31	0.869	2.30	2.25	0.889
Cis monounsaturated fatty acids (g)	20.7	20.4	5.83	21.4	21.3	5.38	20.4	19.9	5.99	20.2	20.0	6.23
Total *cis* polyunsaturated fatty acids (g)	11.0	10.9	3.99	11.0	10.2	4.12	10.7	10.1	3.72	10.4	9.8	3.98
Cis n-3 polyunsaturated fatty acids (g)	1.48	1.35	0.586	1.53	1.39	0.691	1.45	1.34	0.606	1.47	1.35	0.637
Cis n-6 polyunsaturated fatty acids (g)	9.5	9.2	3.58	9.5	8.9	3.67	9.2	8.7	3.34	9.0	8.2	3.53
Cholesterol (mg)	154	137	62.5	177	168	72.4	169	159	76.3	164	158	63.9
Percentage food energy from:												
Males												
Total fat	35.8	36.2	4.02	35.8	35.7	4.01	35.2	35.3	4.17	35.3	35.4	4.33
Saturated fatty acids	14.4	14.2	2.17	14.2	14.2	2.17	14.0	13.9	2.20	14.2	14.3	2.26
Trans fatty acids	1.3	1.3	0.31	1.4	1.3	0.34	1.4	1.3	0.34	1.3	1.3	0.34
Cis monounsaturated fatty acids	12.0	11.9	1.90	11.8	11.7	1.76	11.6	11.6	1.74	11.5	11.4	1.80
Total *cis* polyunsaturated fatty acids	5.9	5.8	1.50	6.1	5.9	1.57	5.8	5.6	1.45	5.9	5.8	1.49
Cis n-3 polyunsaturated fatty acids	0.8	0.7	0.39	0.8	0.8	0.32	0.8	0.8	0.33	0.9	0.8	0.41
Cis n-6 polyunsaturated fatty acids	5.0	4.8	1.37	5.2	5.1	1.39	5.0	4.8	1.28	5.0	4.9	1.29
Females												
Total fat	37.0	37.5	4.59	36.5	36.6	4.36	35.4	35.7	4.57	35.7	36.2	5.28
Saturated fatty acids	14.4	14.6	2.32	14.6	14.4	2.27	14.3	14.2	2.53	14.2	14.0	2.74
Trans fatty acids	1.3	1.3	0.39	1.4	1.4	0.33	1.3	1.3	0.34	1.3	1.3	0.37
Cis monounsaturated fatty acids	12.4	12.2	2.06	12.0	12.0	1.93	11.5	11.6	1.89	11.7	11.9	2.04
Total *cis* polyunsaturated fatty acids	6.6	6.6	1.88	6.2	5.9	1.76	6.0	5.8	1.57	6.1	5.8	1.73
Cis n-3 polyunsaturated fatty acids	0.9	0.9	0.30	0.9	0.8	0.34	0.8	0.8	0.27	0.9	0.8	0.34
Cis n-6 polyunsaturated fatty acids	5.7	5.4	1.70	5.3	5.1	1.51	5.2	5.0	1.44	5.2	5.0	1.54
Total number of males	*68*			*243*			*300*			*245*		
Total number of females	*69*			*217*			*306*			*253*		

Table 7.25 Total fat, fatty acids and cholesterol intake by sex of young person and whether young person's 'parents' were receiving certain benefits: average daily intake and percentage contribution to food energy intake

Fatty acids	Whether receiving benefits					
	Receiving benefits			Not receiving benefits		
	Mean	Median	SD	Mean	Median	SD
Males						
Total fat (g)	68.3	64.7	22.75	76.7	73.9	21.58
Saturated fatty acids (g)	26.6	25.4	9.82	30.8	30.1	8.86
Trans fatty acids (g)	2.55	2.40	1.219	2.98	2.81	1.085
Cis monounsaturated fatty acids (g)	23.0	22.2	7.87	25.1	24.3	7.61
Total *cis* polyunsaturated fatty acids (g)	11.7	11.1	4.33	12.8	11.8	4.81
Cis n-3 polyunsaturated fatty acids (g)	1.80	1.58	1.118	1.77	1.59	0.888
Cis n-6 polyunsaturated fatty acids (g)	9.9	9.4	3.56	11.0	10.2	4.23
Cholesterol (mg)	184	167	77.3	202	190	87.1
Females						
Total fat (g)	63.7	64.3	17.80	62.9	61.8	16.78
Saturated fatty acids (g)	25.2	25.5	7.73	25.2	25.1	7.28
Trans fatty acids (g)	2.49	2.34	1.006	2.32	2.26	0.795
Cis monounsaturated fatty acids (g)	21.1	21.2	6.06	20.5	20.0	5.83
Total *cis* polyunsaturated fatty acids (g)	10.9	10.5	4.04	10.7	10.1	3.90
Cis n-3 polyunsaturated fatty acids (g)	1.51	1.37	0.691	1.47	1.36	0.619
Cis n-6 polyunsaturated fatty acids (g)	9.4	8.8	3.54	9.2	8.6	3.51
Cholesterol (mg)	167	156	71.5	170	161	70.6
Percentage food energy from:						
Males						
Total fat	35.7	36.1	4.54	35.4	35.4	4.04
Saturated fatty acids	13.9	14.0	2.31	14.3	14.2	2.17
Trans fatty acids	1.3	1.3	0.36	1.4	1.3	0.33
Cis monounsaturated fatty acids	12.0	11.9	2.00	11.6	11.5	1.69
Total *cis* polyunsaturated fatty acids	6.2	5.9	1.51	5.9	5.6	1.49
Cis n-3 polyunsaturated fatty acids	0.9	0.9	0.41	0.8	0.8	0.33
Cis n-6 polyunsaturated fatty acids	5.2	5.0	1.29	5.0	4.8	1.33
Females						
Total fat	36.3	36.4	4.74	35.8	36.2	4.77
Saturated fatty acids	14.3	14.3	2.54	14.4	14.3	2.50
Trans fatty acids	1.4	1.4	0.39	1.3	1.3	0.33
Cis monounsaturated fatty acids	12.0	12.1	1.96	11.7	11.6	1.98
Total *cis* polyunsaturated fatty acids	6.2	6.1	1.63	6.1	5.9	1.72
Cis n-3 polyunsaturated fatty acids	0.9	0.8	0.34	0.8	0.8	0.31
Cis n-6 polyunsaturated fatty acids	5.3	5.2	1.43	5.2	5.0	1.54
Total number of males		189			666	
Total number of females		199			645	

Table 7.26 Total fat, fatty acids and cholesterol intake by sex of young person and gross weekly household income: average daily intake and percentage contribution to food energy intake

Fatty acids	Gross weekly household income														
	Less than £160			£160 to less than £280			£280 to less than £400			£400 to less than £600			£600 and over		
	Mean	Median	SD	Mean	Median	SD	Mean	Median	SD	Mean	Median	SD	Mean	Median	SD
Males															
Total fat (g)	69.6	64.7	23.77	70.0	67.5	22.59	78.3	77.6	21.16	77.5	73.4	19.78	75.5	74.1	21.22
Saturated fatty acids (g)	26.8	24.8	9.37	27.9	27.3	9.62	30.6	29.5	8.14	31.9	30.7	8.59	30.6	29.8	9.01
Trans fatty acids (g)	2.62	2.37	1.281	2.63	2.55	1.073	3.01	2.87	1.079	3.09	3.00	1.056	2.92	2.67	1.070
Cis monounsaturated fatty acids (g)	23.4	22.2	8.36	23.2	22.6	7.82	25.9	24.8	7.85	25.2	24.2	6.89	24.5	24.0	7.29
Total cis polyunsaturated fatty acids (g)	12.3	11.2	5.20	11.6	10.9	4.32	13.6	12.8	5.12	12.3	11.6	4.07	12.4	11.6	4.59
Cis n-3 polyunsaturated fatty acids (g)	1.86	1.66	1.232	1.69	1.55	0.841	1.84	1.62	0.929	1.69	1.57	0.794	1.76	1.54	0.963
Cis n-6 polyunsaturated fatty acids (g)	10.4	9.5	4.41	9.9	9.4	3.69	11.8	11.2	4.48	10.6	9.8	3.63	10.6	9.9	3.99
Cholesterol (mg)	189	166	80.4	183	164	89.4	190	185	69.2	208	199	79.8	205	192	85.5
Females															
Total fat (g)	62.4	62.8	18.51	63.1	62.1	16.43	64.5	64.9	16.72	62.9	61.9	16.01	63.6	63.4	17.44
Saturated fatty acids (g)	24.6	23.6	8.25	25.0	25.7	6.81	25.8	25.2	7.41	25.5	25.4	7.17	25.6	25.5	7.36
Trans fatty acids (g)	2.45	2.26	1.063	2.34	2.21	0.865	2.43	2.40	0.805	2.30	2.23	0.770	2.38	2.36	0.805
Cis monounsaturated fatty acids (g)	20.7	20.6	6.22	20.8	20.7	5.96	21.2	21.3	5.72	20.5	20.1	5.45	20.4	20.0	6.04
Total cis polyunsaturated fatty acids (g)	10.6	10.2	3.64	10.8	10.3	4.15	10.9	10.0	4.39	10.5	10.1	3.57	10.9	10.2	3.94
Cis n-3 polyunsaturated fatty acids (g)	1.50	1.36	0.646	1.51	1.42	0.752	1.41	1.33	0.545	1.45	1.33	0.597	1.52	1.40	0.616
Cis n-6 polyunsaturated fatty acids (g)	9.1	8.8	3.20	9.3	8.6	3.65	9.5	8.5	4.00	9.1	8.7	3.19	9.4	8.8	3.55
Cholesterol (mg)	170	158	71.8	153	138	69.4	173	165	62.4	170	156	81.9	180	177	65.1
Percentage food energy from:															
Males															
Total fat	35.6	36.1	4.37	35.5	35.7	4.46	36.3	36.0	3.59	34.6	34.7	4.01	35.0	35.1	4.07
Saturated fatty acids	13.7	13.7	2.28	14.1	14.2	2.16	14.3	14.2	2.05	14.2	14.4	2.16	14.2	14.2	2.27
Trans fatty acids	1.3	1.3	0.36	1.3	1.3	0.34	1.4	1.3	0.34	1.4	1.3	0.30	1.4	1.3	0.34
Cis monounsaturated fatty acids	11.9	11.9	1.89	11.8	11.9	1.87	12.0	11.8	1.73	11.3	11.0	1.65	11.4	11.3	1.59
Total cis polyunsaturated fatty acids	6.2	6.0	1.44	5.9	5.6	1.43	6.3	6.1	1.67	5.5	5.3	1.27	5.7	5.6	1.47
Cis n-3 polyunsaturated fatty acids	0.9	0.9	0.42	0.9	0.8	0.34	0.8	0.8	0.34	0.8	0.7	0.31	0.8	0.7	0.36
Cis n-6 polyunsaturated fatty acids	5.3	5.1	1.25	5.0	4.8	1.21	5.4	5.3	1.53	4.7	4.5	1.15	4.8	4.7	1.28
Females															
Total fat	36.2	35.8	4.84	35.8	36.1	4.73	36.5	37.1	4.92	36.0	35.9	4.16	35.6	35.9	4.79
Saturated fatty acids	14.2	14.2	2.56	14.2	14.3	2.41	14.6	14.5	2.66	14.5	14.3	2.25	14.3	14.2	2.57
Trans fatty acids	1.4	1.4	0.38	1.3	1.3	0.39	1.4	1.3	0.36	1.3	1.3	0.31	1.3	1.3	0.30
Cis monounsaturated fatty acids	12.1	12.0	2.04	11.8	11.8	2.10	12.0	12.1	2.04	11.7	11.6	1.75	11.4	11.6	1.87
Total cis polyunsaturated fatty acids	6.2	5.9	1.43	6.1	5.9	1.79	6.1	5.8	1.84	6.1	5.9	1.68	6.1	6.0	1.69
Cis n-3 polyunsaturated fatty acids	0.9	0.8	0.33	0.9	0.8	0.37	0.8	0.8	0.26	0.8	0.8	0.32	0.9	0.8	0.29
Cis n-6 polyunsaturated fatty acids	5.3	5.1	1.24	5.3	4.9	1.60	5.3	5.0	1.61	5.2	5.1	1.51	5.2	5.1	1.55
Total number of males	*133*			*159*			*157*			*173*			*208*		
Total number of females	*131*			*146*			*145*			*192*			*196*		

Table 7.27   Total fat, fatty acids and cholesterol intake by sex of young person and social class of head of household: average daily intake and percentage contribution to food energy intake

Fatty acids	Social class of head of household					
	Non-manual			Manual		
	Mean	*Median*	*SD*	*Mean*	*Median*	*SD*
Males						
Total fat (g)	75.3	73.0	21.51	75.3	71.0	22.89
Saturated fatty acids (g)	30.6	29.4	8.94	29.7	28.4	9.54
Trans fatty acids (g)	2.98	2.83	1.162	2.84	2.63	1.121
Cis monounsaturated fatty acids (g)	24.5	23.8	7.53	25.1	23.8	7.93
Total *cis* polyunsaturated fatty acids (g)	12.3	11.6	4.58	12.8	11.7	4.91
Cis n-3 polyunsaturated fatty acids (g)	1.7	1.5	0.920	1.8	1.7	0.995
Cis n-6 polyunsaturated fatty acids (g)	10.6	10.0	3.98	11.0	10.1	4.27
Cholesterol (mg)	202	191	87.7	192	179	80.5
Females						
Total fat (g)	64.1	64.1	17.13	62.7	61.1	16.23
Saturated fatty acids (g)	25.9	25.8	7.43	24.8	24.5	7.00
Trans fatty acids (g)	2.40	2.33	0.820	2.32	2.26	0.861
Cis monounsaturated fatty acids (g)	20.8	20.5	5.92	20.7	20.3	5.67
Total *cis* polyunsaturated fatty acids (g)	10.7	10.1	3.78	10.8	10.3	4.06
Cis n-3 polyunsaturated fatty acids (g)	1.49	1.36	0.609	1.48	1.37	0.676
Cis n-6 polyunsaturated fatty acids (g)	9.3	8.7	3.39	9.3	8.8	3.59
Cholesterol (mg)	178	173	74.1	161	152	65.9
Percentage food energy from:						
Males						
Total fat	35.2	35.1	4.16	35.7	36.1	4.09
Saturated fatty acids	14.3	14.3	2.22	14.1	14.1	2.17
Trans fatty acids	1.4	1.3	0.36	1.3	1.3	0.32
Cis monounsaturated fatty acids	11.4	11.3	1.70	11.9	11.9	1.75
Total *cis* polyunsaturated fatty acids	5.7	5.6	1.48	6.1	5.8	1.46
Cis n-3 polyunsaturated fatty acids	0.8	0.7	0.34	0.9	0.8	0.37
Cis n-6 polyunsaturated fatty acids	4.9	4.7	1.31	5.2	5.0	1.28
Females						
Total fat	35.9	36.0	4.61	36.1	36.5	4.68
Saturated fatty acids	14.5	14.4	2.42	14.3	14.2	2.51
Trans fatty acids	1.3	1.3	0.33	1.3	1.3	0.36
Cis monounsaturated fatty acids	11.6	11.5	1.93	11.9	12.0	1.97
Total *cis* polyunsaturated fatty acids	6.0	5.9	1.64	6.2	6.1	1.76
Cis n-3 polyunsaturated fatty acids	0.8	0.8	0.30	0.9	0.8	0.33
Cis n-6 polyunsaturated fatty acids	5.2	4.9	1.49	5.3	5.2	1.54
Total number of males		*414*			*385*	
Total number of females		*401*			*361*	

Table 7.28 Total fat, fatty acids and cholesterol intake by sex of young person and whether living with both parents: average daily intake and percentage contribution to food energy intake

Fatty acids	Young person living with:								
	Both parents & other children			Both parents & no other children			Single parent with/out other children		
	Mean	*Median*	*SD*	*Mean*	*Median*	*SD*	*Mean*	*Median*	*SD*
Males									
Total fat (g)	72.3	69.4	19.67	83.5	81.0	22.99	72.8	69.6	26.27
Saturated fatty acids (g)	29.0	28.0	8.31	33.0	32.0	9.62	28.9	26.4	11.16
Trans fatty acids (g)	2.81	2.63	1.041	3.21	3.07	1.273	2.72	2.58	1.215
Cis monounsaturated fatty acids (g)	23.7	22.6	6.97	27.6	26.5	8.00	24.2	23.2	8.85
Total *cis* polyunsaturated fatty acids (g)	12.0	11.4	4.26	14.2	13.4	5.19	12.2	11.5	5.06
Cis n-3 polyunsaturated fatty acids (g)	1.68	1.54	0.878	2.06	1.78	1.172	1.79	1.63	0.831
Cis n-6 polyunsaturated fatty acids (g)	10.3	9.8	3.71	12.1	11.5	4.47	10.4	9.7	4.46
Cholesterol (mg)	185	174	76.7	233	223	86.9	204	186	98.0
Females									
Total fat (g)	62.9	62.4	16.33	64.3	62.8	19.05	62.8	63.0	17.44
Saturated fatty acids (g)	25.4	25.5	7.17	25.1	25.1	8.15	25.0	24.9	7.44
Trans fatty acids (g)	2.36	2.32	0.844	2.30	2.24	0.827	2.41	2.29	0.935
Cis monounsaturated fatty acids (g)	20.5	20.1	5.60	21.1	20.1	6.62	20.7	21.2	6.09
Total *cis* polyunsaturated fatty acids (g)	10.5	9.9	3.90	11.6	11.1	4.37	10.6	10.3	3.54
Cis n-3 polyunsaturated fatty acids (g)	1.45	1.33	0.654	1.54	1.47	0.573	1.48	1.36	0.633
Cis n-6 polyunsaturated fatty acids (g)	9.1	8.4	3.46	10.0	9.3	4.01	9.2	8.6	3.11
Cholesterol (mg)	167	156	67.2	181	168	84.2	165	161	68.7
Percentage food energy from:									
Males									
Total fat	35.2	35.3	4.02	35.9	36.1	4.31	35.8	36.0	4.46
Saturated fatty acids	14.1	14.1	2.19	14.2	14.2	2.14	14.2	14.2	2.34
Trans fatty acids	1.4	1.3	0.33	1.4	1.4	0.36	1.3	1.3	0.33
Cis monounsaturated fatty acids	11.5	11.4	1.72	11.9	11.8	1.89	11.9	11.8	1.83
Total *cis* polyunsaturated fatty acids	5.9	5.6	1.45	6.1	5.9	1.71	6.0	5.9	1.40
Cis n-3 polyunsaturated fatty acids	0.8	0.8	0.35	0.9	0.8	0.43	0.9	0.8	0.30
Cis n-6 polyunsaturated fatty acids	5.0	4.9	1.30	5.1	4.9	1.46	5.1	4.8	1.26
Females									
Total fat	35.9	36.2	4.88	36.4	36.5	4.66	35.6	35.7	4.44
Saturated fatty acids	14.5	14.4	2.62	14.1	14.1	2.45	14.1	14.2	2.24
Trans fatty acids	1.3	1.3	0.35	1.3	1.3	0.31	1.4	1.3	0.35
Cis monounsaturated fatty acids	11.7	11.6	1.99	11.9	12.1	1.85	11.8	11.8	1.93
Total *cis* polyunsaturated fatty acids	6.0	5.8	1.66	6.6	6.5	1.97	6.1	5.8	1.47
Cis n-3 polyunsaturated fatty acids	0.8	0.8	0.32	0.9	0.8	0.29	0.8	0.8	0.31
Cis n-6 polyunsaturated fatty acids	5.1	5.0	1.48	5.6	5.6	1.78	5.2	4.9	1.31
Total number of males		528			169			157	
Total number of females		498			173			167	

Table 7.29 Comparison of fat and fatty acids intake and percentage food energy from fat and fatty acids by young people in three surveys: 1992/3 NDNS: children aged 1½ to 4½ years; 1986/7 British Adults; 1997 NDNS young people aged 4 to 18 years (present survey).

	Age and sex of young person							
	1992/3: 3½–4½*		1997: 4–6		1986/7: 16–24**		1997: 15–18	
	Males	Females	Males	Females	Males	Females	Males	Females
Fat (g)	50.1	47.2	60.1	55.9	103.5	73.6	89.0	64.0
% food energy from fat	35.3	35.5	35.5	35.9	40.2	39.8	35.9	35.9
Saturated fatty acids (g)	21.9	20.6	25.1	23.8	41.6	30.4	34.7	24.7
% food energy from saturated fatty acids	15.4	15.5	14.8	15.3	16.1	16.4	13.9	13.8
Trans fatty acids (g)	2.4	2.3	2.3	2.1	5.9	4.0	3.5	2.3
% food energy from *trans* fatty acids	1.7	1.7	1.3	1.3	2.3	2.2	1.4	1.3
Cis monounsaturated fatty acids (g)	15.7	14.8	19.4	17.8	32.4	22.7	29.6	20.9
% food energy from *cis* monounsaturated fatty acids	11.1	11.1	11.5	11.5	12.6	12.3	12.0	11.7
Cis n-3 polyunsaturated fatty acids	1.0	1.0	1.3	1.2	2.0	1.4	2.2	1.6
% food energy from *cis* n-3 polyunsaturated fatty acids (g)	0.7	0.7	0.8	0.7	0.8	0.8	0.9	0.9
Cis n-6 polyunsaturated fatty acids (g)	5.8	5.5	8.0	7.2	14.2	9.9	13.3	10.2
% food energy from *cis* n-6 polyunsaturated fatty acids	4.1	4.1	4.8	4.6	5.5	5.3	5.3	5.7
Base – number of young people	*250*	*243*	*184*	*171*	*214*	*189*	*179*	*210*

*Gregory JR et al. *National Diet and Nutrition Survey: children aged 1½ to 4½ years.* HMSO (London, 1995).
** Gregory J et al. *The Dietary and Nutritional Survey of British Adults* HMSO (London, 1990).

Table 7.30 Comparison of fat intake and percentage energy from fat by young people aged between 10 and 15 years in two surveys: 1983 The Diets of British Schoolchildren; 1997 NDNS young people aged 4 to 18 years (present survey).

	Sex and age of young person (years)n							
	1983*		1997		1983*		1997	
	10–11		10–11		14–15		14–15	
	Males	Females	Males	Females	Males	Females	Males	Females
Fat (g)/day	87.6	78.9	75.8	67.2	106.3	82.2	86.5	65.9
% food energy from fat	37.4	37.9	35.7	36.0	37.9	38.7	35.9	36.1
No. of children	*902*	*821*	*140*	*118*	*513*	*461*	*110*	*113*

* Department of Health. Report on Health and Social Subjects: 36. *The Diets of British Schoolchildren* HMSO (London, 1989).

Figure 7.1   Average daily intake of total fat and fatty acids (g) by sex and age of young person*

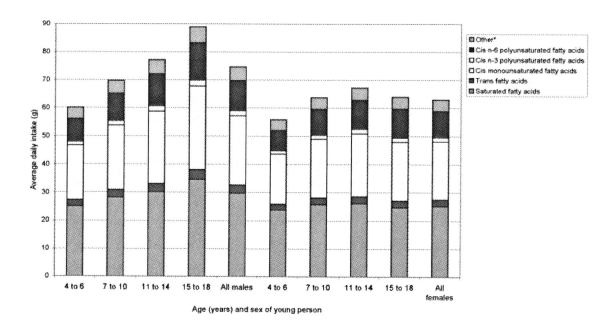

* Total fat consists of a mixture of triglycerides (each triglyceride is made up of three fatty acids with one unit of glycerol) and phospholipids, sterols and other related compounds. Other refers to the non fatty acid component of total fat, estimated as the difference between total fat and the sum of fatty acids.

8 Vitamins

8.1 Introduction

Vitamins are organic compounds, which are required in small amounts for growth and metabolism. They are essential substances which, with the exception of vitamin D, cannot be synthesised in the body and are therefore required in the diet.

This chapter presents data on the daily intakes of vitamins and some precursors, for example carotene, which were derived from the quantities of food being consumed and from the intake of dietary supplements.

Dietary supplements may have a marked impact on the intakes of some vitamins; 20% of the boys and 19% of the girls completing seven-day dietary records recorded intakes of supplements. In this chapter data are therefore presented for intakes for the 1701 (unweighted) young people who completed a seven-day dietary record including any dietary supplements, referred to as intakes from *all sources*, and excluding dietary supplements, referred to as intakes from *food sources*.

For those vitamins where UK Reference Nutrient Intake values (RNI) have been published for the appropriate sex and age group[1], the proportion of young people with intakes below the Lower Reference Nutrient Intake (LRNI) for each vitamin are shown, and average daily intakes are compared with the RNIs, which are shown in Table 8.1.   *(Table 8.1)*

Average daily intakes of vitamins from food sources per megajoule (MJ) energy intake are also presented, providing a measure of nutrient density commonly used to assess the quality of the diet.

8.1.1 Reference Nutrient Intake (RNI)

The RNI for a vitamin or mineral is an amount of that nutrient that is sufficient, or more than sufficient, for about 97% of the people in that group. If the average intake of the group is at the RNI, then the risk of deficiency in the group is judged to be very small. However, if the average intake is lower than the RNI then it is possible that some of the group will have an intake below their requirement. This is even more likely if a proportion of the group have an intake below the Lower Reference Nutrient Intake (LRNI). The LRNI for a vitamin or mineral is the amount of that nutrient that is enough for only the few people in a group who

have low needs. For further definitions of the RNI and LRNI see Department of Health (1991)[1,2].

8.2 Vitamin A (retinol and carotene)

Vitamin A as pre-formed retinol is only available from animal products, especially liver, kidneys, oily fish and dairy products[3]. However a number of carotenoids can be converted to retinol in the body, and these are primarily found in the yellow and orange pigments of vegetables; carrots and dark green vegetables are rich sources. Carotene is also added to margarine and fat spreads.

8.2.1 Pre-formed retinol

Table 8.2 shows the average daily intake of pre-formed retinol from food sources and all sources, for boys and girls in different age groups.

Mean daily intake from food sources was 302μg for boys and 262μg for girls (medians 256μg and 218μg). Intake increased significantly with age for boys and, apart from for the youngest age group, was somewhat higher for boys than girls in each age group, the difference increasing with age. For example, for boys mean daily intake of pre-formed retinol ranged from 250μg for those aged 4 to 6 years, to 333μg for those aged 15 to 18 years (p < 0.01). For girls the comparable intakes were 253μg and 272μg.

The range of intakes within age and sex group was wide and the distributions skewed, reflecting the limited distribution of pre-formed retinol in foods. Median intakes were about 10% to 20% lower than mean intakes. At the lower 2.5 percentile intakes were about one third of the median intakes and at the upper 2.5 percentile intakes were about 2½ to three times the median intakes. For example, for 15 to 18 year old boys intakes at the lower 2.5 and upper 2.5 percentiles were 87μg and 889μg respectively.

Dietary supplements providing pre-formed retinol increased the mean intake from that from food sources alone for boys by 13%, from 302μg to 340μg, and for girls by 11%, from 262μg to 290μg. For both sexes, the effect of supplements on mean intake decreased with age, reflecting the fact that retinol-containing supplements were more likely to be taken by the younger children. For example, for boys aged 4 to 6 years mean intake of pre-formed retinol from all sources was nearly one third higher than mean intake from food sources alone, 327µg compared with 250µg, while for the oldest group of boys, supplements only increased mean intake by about 5%, from 333µg to 348µg.

The effect of dietary supplements on intakes of pre-formed retinol was particularly marked at the upper 2.5 percentile. Thus for boys dietary supplements increased intakes at the upper 2.5 percentile by between 12% and 73%, depending on age. For girls the effect was even greater; dietary supplements increased intakes at the upper 2.5 percentile by between 36%, for girls aged 11 to 14 years, and 94% for girls aged 7 to 10 years.

Table 8.3 shows intakes of vitamins from food sources after allowing for variation in total energy intake, that is expressed per MJ total energy intake. Any variation in average daily intake of vitamins, after allowing for differences in total energy intake, indicates variation in the nutrient density of the diet, in respect of that vitamin. If there are no differences in average daily vitamin intake expressed per unit energy, then the inference is that the differences are explained by differences in energy intake.

Intakes for boys of pre-formed retinol from food sources, expressed per MJ total energy intake, showed very little variation for the three youngest age groups and were slightly, but not significantly lower for boys aged 15 to 18 years. For girls, there was no clear pattern associated with age. *(Tables 8.2 and 8.3)*

8.2.2 Total carotene (ß-carotene equivalents)

Total carotene is expressed as ß-carotene equivalents, that is the sum of ß-carotene and half the amount of α-carotene and ß-cryptoxanthin.

As the dietary supplements taken by young people in this survey did not provide any carotene the intakes presented are from food sources.

Mean daily total carotene intake for boys in the survey was 1411µg, and for girls was 1354µg. The distribution of intakes was skewed; median intakes were about one fifth lower than mean intakes, 1111µg for boys and 1112µg for girls.

Mean daily intake of total carotene increased significantly with age for both boys and girls, for example from 1248µg for boys aged 4 to 6 years, to 1680µg for boys aged 15 to 18 years (p < 0.05). The comparable intakes for girls in these two age groups were 1175µg and 1637µg (p < 0.05).

There was a wide range of intakes of total carotene within each age and sex group with median intakes being about 4½ times greater than intakes at the lower 2.5 percentile. At the upper 2.5 percentile intakes were between 2½ times and 5½ times greater than the median.

The differences between age groups in mean daily intake of total carotene are largely associated with differences in energy intake between the age groups. As Table 8.3 shows, the average daily intake of total carotene per MJ total energy did not vary significantly with age except for the oldest group of girls where average intake was significantly higher than for girls aged 11 to 14 years (p < 0.05). It has already been shown that girls aged 15 to 18 years were more likely to report being vegetarian than younger girls (see *Table 4.10*) and since, as is shown below, vegetables are the main source of total carotene, it is not surprising to find that the oldest group of girls were eating a diet richer in total carotene than other, younger girls.

Boys and girls in the survey obtained over half (56% and 57% respectively) their total carotene intake from vegetables, potatoes and savoury snacks. Cooked carrots were the largest single provider accounting for 32% of intake for boys and 30% for girls; raw carrots provided 9% of intake for both boys and girls.

Meat and meat products provided a further 12% of the carotene intake for boys and 11% for girls, mainly from vegetables added to meat dishes. Drinks provided a further 6% for both sexes, nearly all of which came from the consumption of soft drinks; ß-carotene is often used as a colour in orange-coloured drinks.

(Tables 8.4 and 8.5)

8.2.3 ß-carotene, α-carotene and ß-cryptoxanthin

ß-carotene, α-carotene and ß-cryptoxanthin are all carotenoids with vitamin A activity. Only a few of the more than 100 carotenoids have structures that enable them to serve as precursors of vitamin A; ß-carotene is the most important of these. α-carotene and ß-cryptoxanthin have approximately half the pro-vitamin A activity of ß-carotene on a weight-for-weight basis.

Mean daily intake of ß-carotene from food sources was 1271µg for boys and 1220µg for girls (medians 1011µg and 1016µg). Mean intakes increased steadily with age for both boys and girls, for example from 1120µg and 1060µg for boys and girls aged 4 to 6 years, to 1512µg and 1470µg for boys and girls aged 15 to 18 years (p < 0.05).

Mean daily intake of α-carotene was 244µg for boys and 232µg for girls (medians 139µg and 163µg) and for ß-cryptoxanthin, 35µg and 34µg respectively (medians 23µg and 24µg). Intakes of ß-cryptoxanthin increased markedly with age for both boys and girls (comparing youngest and oldest age groups: p < 0.01) but the slight increases in mean intakes of α-carotene with age were not statistically significant.

For all three carotenoids there was a wide range of intakes within age and sex groups, and some young people had zero intakes of some carotenoids during the

7-day dietary recording period. Overall 2% of both boys and girls had zero intake of α-carotene, and the same proportions had zero intake of ß-cryptoxanthin. Intakes of ß-carotene for boys aged 15 to 18 years at the lower 2.5 percentile, 270µg, were only about one quarter of the median intake, 1153µg, while intakes for this age group at the upper 2.5 percentile, 5903µg, were five times the median intake.

None of the dietary supplements taken by young people in the survey provided any of these three carotenoids.

(Tables 8.6 to 8.8)

8.2.4 Vitamin A (retinol equivalents)

The total vitamin A content of the diet is usually expressed as retinol equivalents using the conversion factor, of 6µg ß-carotene being equivalent to 1µg retinol.

The mean daily intake of vitamin A from food sources by young people in the survey was 537µg (boys) and 487µg (girls). The distribution of intakes was skewed, with median intakes being about 13% lower than mean intakes, 465µg for boys and 424µg for girls.

Mean intakes of vitamin A from food sources appeared to increase with age for both sexes, for example from 458µg for boys and 449µg for girls aged 4 to 6 years, to 613µg and 545µg for boys and girls aged 15 to 18 years (boys: p < 0.01; girls: ns).

The range of intakes of vitamin A from food sources, like those for pre-formed retinol, α- and ß- carotene and ß-cryptoxanthin, was very large. Mean intakes were between two and 3½ times greater than intakes at the lower 2.5 percentile, depending on age and sex, and intakes at the upper 2.5 percentile were about 2½ times greater than mean intakes, again depending on age and sex.

Table 8.1 shows the current UK RNI and LRNI values for vitamin A for young people in each of four age groups.

The mean daily intake of vitamin A from food sources was 98% of the RNI for boys and 93% of the RNI for girls and tended to decrease as age increased[4] (see *Table 8.10*). For example, for boys aged 4 to 6 years intake was 114% of the RNI compared with 88% for boys aged 15 to 18 years.

For boys, between 8% and 13% had a vitamin A intake from food sources which was below the LRNI. For girls, the proportions with intakes below the LRNI were 6% and 10% for those aged 4 to 6 years and 7 to 10 years. In the top two age groups, 20% and 12% of girls had average daily intakes of vitamin A below the LRNI.

After allowing for differences in energy intake there were no significant age differences in the average daily

intake of vitamin A from food sources for boys or girls (see *Table 8.3*).

Dietary supplements containing pre-formed retinol increased the mean intakes of vitamin A from food sources alone by 7% for boys and by 6% for girls. However the effect of supplements on mean intakes was more marked for the youngest children, where mean intakes from food sources were increased by supplement taking by 17% for boys and 12% for girls aged 4 to 6 years. For the oldest group of boys and girls supplement taking only increased mean vitamin A intakes by about 3%.

The effect of supplements on intakes was marked at the upper 2.5 percentile of the distribution, where overall, for boys, the intake from food sources increased by 9% from 1288µg to 1402µg with the addition of supplements; for girls the intake from food sources increased by 12% from 1158µg to 1296µg with supplements. Again, this effect was most noticeable for the younger children. For example, intakes at the upper 2.5 percentile of the distribution for girls aged 4 to 6 years were 955µg from food sources and 1265µg from all sources, an increase of about one third.

The main food groups contributing to average daily intake of vitamin A were vegetables, potatoes and savoury snacks (contributing about 27% to average intake, mainly from vegetables); milk and milk products (contributing about 20%); meat and meat products, (about 15%, of which about half came from liver and liver products) and fat spreads and cereals and cereal products, (each contributing about 13% to average daily intake).

Overall there was almost no difference between boys and girls in the main sources of vitamin A in their diets, and only the contribution made by milk and milk products varied with age, decreasing as age increased. This was due to the decrease in the consumption of milk, particularly whole milk, for boys and girls, as age increased. Thus milk and milk products contributed 24% of intake of vitamin A for boys aged 4 to 6 years and 26% of intake for girls in the same age group, of which 11% and 10% of intake respectively came from the consumption of whole milk. For boys and girls aged 15 to 18 years, milk and milk products provided 19% and 16% of vitamin A intake, of which 4% and 3% came from whole milk (whole milk, both sexes, comparing youngest and oldest age groups: ns).

(Tables 8.9 to 8.11)

8.3 B vitamins

8.3.1 Thiamin (vitamin B₁)

Mean daily intake of thiamin from food sources for all boys was 1.59mg and for girls 1.31mg (p < 0.01) (medians 1.45mg and 1.20mg). For boys mean intake increased steadily with age from 1.27mg for boys aged 4 to 6 years to 1.90mg for boys aged 15 to 18 years (p < 0.01). Mean intake for girls increased from 1.14mg for girls aged 4 to 6 years up to 1.40mg for girls aged 11 to 14 years (p < 0.01); intake by the oldest girls was close to that of the 11 to 14 year olds (1.38mg).

At the lower 2.5 percentile intakes of thiamin from food sources were about half the median values, and at the upper 2.5 percentile about twice the median values.

Table 8.13 shows that the average daily intakes of thiamin from food sources were well above the RNIs for boys and girls in each age group. Overall, mean intakes from food sources were 187% and 180% of the RNI for boys and girls respectively[4].

Intakes of thiamin from food sources at the lower 2.5 percentile were above the LRNI for each age/sex group. There were no boys aged between 4 and 10 or 15 and 18 years of age with intakes below the LRNI, and less than 0.5% of 11 to 14 year-old boys had intakes below the LRNI. For girls, 1% of 11 to 14 year olds and 2% of those aged 15 to 18 years had intakes below the LRNI.

Table 8.3 shows that average daily intakes of thiamin per MJ total energy did not vary with the sex and age of the young person. The variations in intake associated with age described above are therefore accounted for by differences between the various sex and age groups in their energy intake.

Dietary supplements provided very little thiamin and mean daily intakes from all sources were very close to intakes from food sources.

Most breakfast cereals are fortified with thiamin and cereals and cereal products were the main dietary source of thiamin for young people in the survey, providing 43% of the intake for boys and 38% for girls, of which just over one fifth came from breakfast cereals and just under 10% from white bread. Vegetables, potatoes and savoury snacks provided about one fifth of the thiamin intake for boys and just over one quarter of the intake for girls. The consumption of meat and meat products, mainly as bacon and ham, and chicken and turkey, provided just under a further one fifth of intake.

(Tables 8.12 to 8.14)

8.3.2 Riboflavin (vitamin B₂)

The mean daily intakes of riboflavin from food sources were 1.71mg and 1.34mg for boys and girls respectively (p < 0.01) (medians 1.58mg and 1.30mg).

For boys, but not girls, mean intake from food sources increased steadily with age, from 1.56mg for boys aged 4 to 6 years, to 1.92mg for boys aged 15 to 18 years (p < 0.01). At the lower 2.5 percentile, intakes were about 40% of median intakes for boys and about 35%

of median intakes for girls. At the upper 2.5 percentile, intakes from food sources were about twice median intakes. For example, for boys 15 to 18 years, daily intakes of riboflavin from food sources at the lower 2.5, 50th and upper 2.5 percentiles were 0.68mg, 1.82mg and 3.88mg respectively.

Mean riboflavin intake from food sources was above the RNI for all age/sex groups. Mean intake was 160% of the RNI for boys and 136% for girls and decreased with age (see *Table 8.16*). Six per cent of boys in the top two age groups had intakes below the LRNI as did 22% of girls aged 11 to 14 years and 21% of girls aged 15 to 18 years.

There were no significant differences in riboflavin intakes from food sources per MJ energy intake for boys or girls.

Dietary supplements made a negligible contribution to mean riboflavin intakes. At the upper 2.5 percentile supplements providing riboflavin increased intakes from food sources alone by no more than 5%.

One third of the mean daily intake of riboflavin by young people in the survey came from cereals and cereal products, mainly from breakfast cereals, many of which are fortified with riboflavin. A further third of intake came from milk and milk products. It has already been clearly shown in Chapter 4 (see, for example, *Table 4.3*) that the consumption of milk, and in particular whole milk, declined with increasing age for both boys and girls, and it is therefore not surprising to find that the importance of whole milk as a source of riboflavin in the diets of these young people reduced as age increased. For example, young people aged 4 to 6 years obtained nearly one quarter of their daily mean intake of riboflavin from whole milk while for 15 to 18 year olds whole milk contributed less than one tenth to their riboflavin intake (both sexes, comparing youngest and oldest age groups: p < 0.01). The only other food group contributing more than 10% to average daily riboflavin intake was meat and meat products, providing 11% of intake for both boys and girls, and 14% of intake for the oldest group of boys. *(Tables 8.15 to 8.17)*

8.3.3 Niacin equivalents

Niacin is a B vitamin, which can be obtained pre-formed from the diet or can be made in the body from the amino acid, tryptophan. Niacin intake is expressed as niacin equivalents, defined as the total amount of niacin plus one sixtieth of the weight, in mg, of tryptophan.

The mean daily intake of niacin from food sources was 29.1mg for boys and significantly lower for girls, 23.6mg (p < 0.01) (medians 27.9mg and 22.8mg). For boys intakes increased throughout the age range, from 22.8mg for boys aged 4 to 6 years, to 36.6mg for boys aged 15 to 18 years (p < 0.01). For girls, mean daily intake increased from 20.4mg for girls aged 4 to 6 years, to 25.2mg for girls aged 15 to 18 years (p < 0.01).

Median intakes were close to mean values, and at the lower 2.5 percentile intakes were about half of median intakes. Intakes at the upper 2.5 percentile were about 55% to 70% higher than median intakes depending on the age and sex of the young person.

Mean daily intake of niacin from food sources was about 200% of the RNI for boys and girls in each age group[4] (see *Table 8.19*). Intakes were above the LRNI for young people in all age groups except girls aged 15 to 18 years, 1% of whom had intakes below the LRNI.

As described above, the average daily intake of niacin from food sources varied according to the sex and age of the young person. After allowing for differences between the groups in their average daily intake of total energy (see *Table 8.3*) the oldest boys and girls still had niacin intakes which were higher than those for the youngest age group, although the differences were only statistically significant for boys (p < 0.01; girls: ns). This suggests that the oldest group of boys in the survey were consuming diets richer in niacin than the youngest group of children.

Supplements provided very little niacin and thus mean and median intakes from all sources were close to intakes of niacin from food sources alone. At the upper 2.5 percentile supplements providing niacin increased daily intakes by up to 7% for boys and up to 6% for girls, depending on age.

Boys and girls in the survey derived 38% and 34% respectively of their average daily intake of niacin from cereals and cereal products, about half of which came from breakfast cereals, which are often fortified with niacin. For boys a further 30%, and for girls 29% of intake came from their consumption of meat and meat products, mainly in the form of chicken, turkey and dishes.

The contribution to niacin intake made by meat and meat products tended to increase with age for both boys and girls, for example, providing 25% of the niacin intake of boys aged 4 to 6 years and 34% of that of 15 to 18 year olds, although the differences are not statistically significant (p > 0.05).

Vegetables, potatoes and savoury snacks provided a further 11% to 12% of intake.

Milk and milk products contributed a further 10% to average niacin intake, the contribution tending to reduce as milk consumption decreased with increasing age. *(Tables 8.18 to 8.20)*

8.3.4 Vitamin B₆

The mean daily intake of vitamin B_6 from food sources for boys was 2.2mg, significantly higher than the mean intake for girls, 1.8mg, (p < 0.01) (medians 2.0mg and 1.7mg). Mean intake for boys increased with age from 1.7mg for boys aged 4 to 6 years, to 2.7mg for boys aged 15 to 18 years (p < 0.01) and in each age group boys had a significantly higher intake compared with girls of the same age (p < 0.01). Mean intake of vitamin B_6 from food sources for girls increased from 1.5mg for those aged 4 to 6 years to 1.9mg for those aged 11 to 14 years (p < 0.01); mean intake then fell slightly to 1.8mg for the oldest group of girls (ns).

Overall, median intakes of vitamin B_6 from food sources were only slightly below mean intakes for both boys and girls. Intakes at the lower 2.5 percentile were about half the median intake for both boys and girls. At the upper 2.5 percentile, intakes for boys were higher than the median intake by between about 60% and 120%. For girls intakes at the upper 2.5 percentile were between about 80% and 95% higher than median intakes.

Table 8.22 shows that the mean daily intake of vitamin B_6 from food sources was at least 150% of the RNI for each sex/age group. One per cent of boys aged 11 to 14 years had an average daily intake which was below the LRNI, as did 1% of girls aged 7 to 10 and 11 to 14 years. For 5% of girls in the top age group, average daily intake of vitamin B_6 was below the LRNI.

As described above mean intakes of vitamin B_6 from food sources were strongly associated with the sex and age of the young person; however these differences were largely accounted for by differences in the average daily energy intake of the different groups. As Table 8.3 shows, after allowing for variation in total energy intake, there were almost no differences between boys and girls or between different age groups in the average daily intake per MJ of this vitamin from food sources.

The contribution of dietary supplements to vitamin B_6 intakes was very small, except for the oldest group of girls, where supplements providing vitamin B_6 increased mean intake from that from food sources by about 11% from 1.8mg to 2.0mg.

The two main sources of vitamin B_6 in the diets of young people were cereals and cereal products and vegetables, potatoes and savoury snacks, each providing nearly 30% of the average intake. About two thirds of the contribution made by cereals and cereal products came from breakfast cereals, many of which are fortified with vitamin B_6. The contribution from vegetables, potatoes and savoury snacks came mainly from potatoes.

Meat and meat products contributed 15% to average daily vitamin B_6 intake, the contribution increasing slightly with age.

About one eighth (12%) of average intake came from milk and milk products, the contribution made by whole milk reducing as age increased.

(Tables 8.21 to 8.23)

8.3.5 Vitamin B_{12}

Mean daily intake of vitamin B_{12} from food sources for boys in the survey was 4.4μg; for girls mean intake was significantly lower, 3.4μg, (p < 0.01) (medians 4.0μg and 3.2μg). For boys, mean intake appeared to increase slightly with age, from 3.9μg for boys aged 7 to 10 years, to 4.5μg for 11 to 14 year olds (p < 0.05) and to 5.0μg for the oldest boys (ns). For girls variation in mean intake was not clearly associated with age; the highest intake was by the youngest age group, 3.6μg and the lowest for girls aged 11 to 14 years, 3.2μg (ns).

Intakes at the lower 2.5 percentile were about 40% of median intakes for both boys and girls and at the upper 2.5 percentile were at least twice the median intake.

Mean daily intakes of vitamin B_{12} from food sources were well in excess of the RNI, 394% of the RNI for boys and 316% of the RNI for girls (see *Table 8.25*). One per cent of girls aged 7 to 14 years and 2% aged 15 to 18 years had intakes below the LRNI.

Although mean daily intakes of vitamin B_{12} varied very little by age group, the quality of the diet, in relation to the vitamin B_{12} content, varied significantly by age for both boys and girls. The data show that, after allowing for differences between the age groups in their average daily energy intake, there were significant differences in average vitamin B_{12} intake per MJ energy (see *Table 8.3*). For both boys and girls, mean intake per MJ total energy reduced as age increased, for example from 0.62μg/MJ and 0.61μg/MJ for boys and girls aged 4 to 6 years, to 0.52μg/MJ and 0.50μg/MJ for boys and girls aged 15 to 18 years (both sexes: p < 0.01). This is probably associated with the decline in the consumption of milk, particularly whole milk, as age increased, since, as will be shown below, milk and milk products were a major contributor to intakes of this vitamin by young people in the survey.

Dietary supplements taken by young people in the survey provided very little vitamin B_{12}, and the contribution to mean intakes was negligible.

Vitamin B_{12} is found only in animal products. The main contributors to vitamin B_{12} intake for young people in the survey were milk and milk products, providing about 47% of average daily intake, mainly from whole and semi-skimmed milk, and meat and meat products, providing a further 23%. The only other major contribution to vitamin B_{12} intake came from the consumption of cereals and cereal products, which accounted for 12% of average daily intake.

(Tables 8.24 to 8.26)

8.3.6 Folate

Overall boys in the survey had a significantly higher mean daily intake of folate from food sources than girls, 240μg and 194μg respectively (p < 0.01) (medians 221μg and 187μg).

For boys, mean folate intake from food sources increased steadily with age by nearly 60% from 191μg for boys aged 4 to 6 years, to 305μg for 15 to 18 year-old boys (p < 0.01). Mean intake for girls also increased steadily with age, but by a proportionately much smaller amount, about 25%, from 169μg for the youngest age group, to 210μg for the oldest group (p < 0.01).

Intakes from food sources at the lower 2.5 percentile of the distribution were about half median intakes for both boys and girls in each age group, and at the upper 2.5 percentile intakes were between about 70% and 120% higher than median intakes, depending on age and sex.

As can be seen from Table 8.28 mean daily intakes of folate from food sources were above the appropriate RNI for each sex and age group, providing 149% and 123% of the RNI for boys and girls respectively[4]. However, for girls in the top two age groups, median intakes were slightly below the RNI, providing 99% and 98% of the RNI respectively.

One per cent of boys aged 11 to 14 years had intakes below the LRNI. There were no intakes below the LRNI for boys in the other age groups. For girls, 2% of those aged 7 to 10 years, 3% of those aged 11 to 14 years and 4% of 15 to 18 year olds had an average daily folate intake below the LRNI.

Table 8.3 shows that after allowing for differences in intake of energy there remained some variation in folate intake associated with age for girls. For girls mean intake per MJ ranged from 28μg/MJ for girls aged 7 to 10 years to 31μg/MJ for girls aged 15 to 18 years (p < 0.05). This indicates that the diets of the oldest group of girls were more folate dense than the diets of the younger age group.

The effect of supplements providing folate was only apparent for girls aged between 7 and 18 years and at the upper 2.5 percentile of the distribution. At the upper 2.5 percentile and in the 11 to 14 year-old group of girls supplements providing folate increased intakes from food sources alone by 13%; in the 7 to 10 year and 15 to 18 year age groups, the increase in intakes was smaller, 7% and 5% respectively.

Table 8.29 shows the percentage contribution of food types to average daily intake of folate for boys and girls in the survey. The two main sources of folate in the diets of these young people were cereals and cereal products and vegetables, potatoes and savoury snacks. Cereals and cereal products contributed 44% and 37% respectively to the intake of folate for boys and girls, of which 25% and 20% respectively came from breakfast cereals, many of which are fortified with folate. For both sexes the contribution made by breakfast cereals tended to fall slightly with age.

Vegetables, potatoes and savoury snacks contributed 24% and 28% to the average daily intake of folate for boys and girls respectively, of which about half came from potatoes in some form.

Milk and milk products contributed 12% to average daily folate intake for both boys and girls, the proportion tending to fall as age increased. For example for girls aged 4 to 6 years, milk and milk products contributed 17% to daily intake of folate, but only 10% to intake for girls aged 15 to 18 years (ns).

Drinks contributed 11% and 9% to the average daily folate intake of the oldest group of boys and girls respectively; this included 6% for boys and 3% for girls contributed by beers and lagers. *(Tables 8.27 to 8.29)*

8.3.7 Biotin and pantothenic acid

Mean daily intake of *biotin* from food sources for boys in the survey was 25µg, and for girls, significantly lower, 20µg (p < 0.01) (medians 23µg and 20µg). Mean daily intake for boys increased steadily and significantly with age from 22µg for boys aged 4 to 6 years, to 29µg for 15 to 18 year olds (p < 0.01). There was no significant increase in mean intake for girls associated with age.

Median intakes were up to 9% below mean intake for each sex and age group; intakes at the lower and upper 2.5 percentiles were about half and twice the median intakes respectively.

Dietary supplements taken by the young people in the survey provided very little biotin and the contribution of supplements to average intakes was negligible.

The mean daily intake of *pantothenic acid* from food sources for boys, 5.1mg, was significantly higher than the mean intake for girls, 4.1mg (p < 0.01) (medians 4.8mg and 4.0mg). For boys there was a steady and marked increase in mean intake associated with age, intakes rising from 4.4mg for 4 to 6 year olds, to 5.8mg for 15 to 18 year-old boys (p < 0.01). There was no difference in mean intake associated with age for girls in the survey.

Dietary supplements taken by young people in the survey provided very little pantothenic acid, and the contribution of supplements to average intakes was negligible.

For boys, but not girls, median intakes were, for each age group, up to 7% lower than mean intakes. Intakes at the lower and upper 2.5 percentiles were about half

and twice the median intakes respectively.

There are no DRVs set for either pantothenic acid or biotin. However intakes for biotin within the range 10mg to 200mg are considered safe and adequate as are intakes for pantothenic acid in the range of 3mg to 7mg[1]. Mean intakes of both biotin and pantothenic acid were within these ranges. Three per cent of boys and 5% of girls had intakes of biotin below 10mg. For pantothenic acid, 8% of boys had intakes below 3mg and 10% had intakes at or above 7.5mg. For girls the proportion with intakes below 3mg was much larger, 20%, but only 2% of girls had intakes at or above 7.5mg. *(Tables 8.30 and 8.31)*

8.4 Vitamin C

The mean daily intakes of vitamin C from food sources for boys and girls in the survey were similar, 75.2mg and 71.2mg respectively (medians 60.9mg and 60.6mg). For both sexes there were no significant differences by age. However the data show that mean intake for boys increased steadily with age, from 67.0mg for those aged 4 to 6 years, to 83.3mg for boys aged 15 to 18 years. For girls, intake increased slightly at the lower end of the age range, from 65.2mg for girls aged 4 to 6 years, to 73.5mg for 7 to 10 year olds but mean intake then remained at about this level in the two upper age groups.

The distribution of intakes was skewed with median intakes between 11% and 20% lower than mean intakes depending on sex and age. For both sexes this skewness increased with age.

The range of intakes was large, with intakes at the lower 2.5 percentile about one third of median intakes and at the upper 2.5 percentile between about 2½ and 4½ times larger than median intakes, depending on age and sex. The oldest group of boys had particularly high intakes; at the upper 2.5 percentile intake of vitamin C from food sources was 292.3mg, over seven times the RNI (40mg/d).

Mean intakes of vitamin C from food sources were above the RNI for each sex and age group, and as Table 8.33 shows, provided 223% of the RNI for boys and 213% of the RNI for girls[4]. No more than 1% of any sex/age group had an intake below the appropriate LRNI.

Although the differences are not statistically significant the data suggest that for boys, the quality of their diets, in relation to vitamin C content, varied by age group, as there were age differences in the average daily intake of vitamin C from food sources per MJ total energy (Table 8.3). While absolute intakes of vitamin C for boys increased steadily with age, intakes of vitamin C per MJ total energy intake tended to *decrease* as age increased. Thus as boys get older their diets become less rich in vitamin C. Average daily intakes of vitamin C from food sources per MJ total energy for boys ranged from

10.5mg/MJ for boys aged 4 to 6 years to 8.8mg/MJ for boys aged 15 to 18 years. For girls, the data suggest that the vitamin C density of the diet is similar across the age groups; intakes for girls ranged from 10.1mg/MJ for 11 to 14 year olds to 11.2mg/MJ for 4 to 6 year-old girls (ns).

Dietary supplements providing vitamin C taken by young people in the survey increased mean intake from that from food sources alone by 5% for boys and 7% for girls. For boys the effect of supplements on mean intake was most marked for the youngest age group, where intake of vitamin C from all sources was 11% higher than from food sources alone; for the oldest boys supplements increased mean intake by 4%. The data for girls show no variation with age.

Nearly half the average daily intake of vitamin C in the diets of young people in the survey came from fruit juice and from soft drinks, which may be fortified with vitamins, including vitamin C. For example, for boys, drinks contributed 47% overall to daily intake of vitamin C, of which 22% came from fruit juice and 25% from soft drinks. The proportions were very similar for girls, and for both sexes the contribution made by fruit juice tended to increase with increasing age, while the contribution from soft drinks decreased with age.

Vegetables, potatoes and savoury snacks contributed 27% and 28% to the average intake of vitamin C for boys and girls respectively, the contribution increasing slightly as age increased. Over half of this came from potatoes in some form.

Fruit and nuts contributed 10% to the vitamin C intake for boys and 13% for girls. *(Tables 8.32 to 8.34)*

8.5   Vitamin D

Most of the body's requirement for vitamin D can be synthesised by the skin in the presence of sufficient sunlight of the appropriate wavelength, that is between April and October in England. Adequate summer exposure provides sufficient vitamin D stores throughout winter. Food sources are therefore particularly important for those who do not receive adequate sunlight. No RNIs have been set for vitamin D for this age group. Vitamin D is found naturally in some animal products, including oily fish. Some foods, such as margarine and fat spreads, some yogurts and breakfast cereals, are fortified with vitamin D.

Mean daily intake of vitamin D from food sources for boys in the survey was 2.6µg, significantly higher than that for girls, 2.1µg (p < 0.01) (medians 2.4µg and 1.9µg).

As for most other vitamins, mean intake of vitamin D from food sources for boys increased steadily and significantly with age from 2.1µg for the youngest boys

to 3.2µg for boys aged 15 to 18 years (p < 0.01). For girls mean intake increased slightly with age, from 1.8µg for the youngest group to 2.2µg for 11 to 14 year olds (p < 0.01), and then remained at about the same level for the oldest group of girls (2.1µg).

The distribution of intakes of vitamin D for both boys and girls was skewed, with median intakes being between 4% and 14% lower than mean intakes depending on sex and age. Intakes of vitamin D from food sources at the lower 2.5 percentile were between about 25% and 35% of median intakes, and at the upper 2.5 percentile were two to three times higher than median intakes depending on age and sex.

Although there were some differences in average daily intake of vitamin D associated with the sex and age of the young person, these were largely accounted for by differences in energy intake between the various sex/age groups. Thus, as Table 8.3 shows, after allowing for differences in total energy intake, average daily intake of vitamin D per MJ showed little variation by age or sex.

Supplements providing vitamin D increased mean intakes from that from food sources by 8% for boys and by 5% for girls. However supplements providing vitamin D were predominantly being taken by younger children in the survey; in the 4 to 6 year age group supplements increased mean intakes by 19% for boys and 22% for girls.

The largest contribution to average intake of vitamin D for both boys and girls was made by cereals and cereal products, accounting for 37% of intake for boys and 35% of intake for girls. Many breakfast cereals are fortified with vitamin D, and breakfast cereals alone contributed one quarter of the intake of vitamin D for boys and one fifth of the intake for girls.

Fat spreads and meat and meat products each contributed about 20% to average daily intake of vitamin D for both boys and girls[5]. About half the contribution made by fat spreads came from reduced fat spreads. For boys, 7% of vitamin D intake came from eating oily fish, which is a rich source of vitamin D. For girls, oily fish contributed 9% to vitamin D intake.
 (Tables 8.35 and 8.36)

8.6   Vitamin E

The mean daily intakes of vitamin E from food sources for boys and girls in the survey were 8.6mg and 7.6mg respectively (p < 0.01) (medians 8.1mg and 7.0mg). For boys, mean intake increased across the four age groups from 6.6mg to 10.3mg (p < 0.01). For girls, mean intake rose from 6.3mg for 4 to 6 year olds, to 8.1mg for the top two age groups, that is from 11 to 18 years (p < 0.01). Median intakes of vitamin E from food sources were between 5% and 10% below mean intakes depending on sex and age. The range of intakes was wide with intake at the lower 2.5 percentile being about half the median intake, and at the upper 2.5 percentile about twice median intake.

Average daily intakes of vitamin E from food sources per MJ total energy ranged between 1.0mg/MJ and 1.2mg/MJ (ns) (see *Table 8.3*). Thus the differences in absolute intake associated with age and sex described above, were largely attributable to differences between the sexes and age groups in energy intake.

Supplements providing vitamin E being taken by young people in the survey had little effect on mean intakes, increasing intakes from food sources alone by 2% overall for boys and 3% for girls. However for the youngest group, intakes from all sources were 9% higher for boys and 5% higher for girls than intakes of vitamin E from food sources alone. For girls aged 15 to 18 years supplements increased vitamin E intake from food sources by 6%.

There are no DRVs set for vitamin E. However intakes above 4mg/d for adult men and above 3mg/d for adult women are considered safe[1]. Mean intakes for both boys and girls in each age group were above these levels. Overall, 4% of boys had an average daily intake of vitamin E below 4mg, the proportion decreasing with age, from 12% of 4 to 6 year olds, to 1% of 15 to 18 year olds. Overall, 1% of girls, and no more than 2% in any age group had an intake of less than 3mg.

Just under one third of the average daily intake of vitamin E by young people in the survey came from vegetables, potatoes and savoury snacks. Within this food group, potatoes, mainly as roast or fried potatoes or chips, and savoury snacks were the main contributors, where the vitamin E was provided by the oil used in cooking and frying.

Fat spreads contributed 23% and 22% to the vitamin E intake of boys and girls respectively, including 13% from polyunsaturated reduced fat spreads.

Cereals and cereal products provided 17% of vitamin E intake for boys and 15% for girls, about half of which came from biscuits, buns, cakes and pastries.

(Tables 8.37 and 8.38)

8.7 Vitamin intakes for young people who were reported to be taking dietary supplements

Table 8.39 shows average daily intakes of vitamins for young people who reported, as part of the initial dietary interview, taking dietary supplements; their intakes are shown from all sources and from food sources. Also shown are intakes from food sources for those young people who said that they were not currently taking any dietary supplements.

For young people who were taking dietary supplements, mean daily intakes from *food sources* alone of vitamin A, thiamin, riboflavin, niacin (girls only), vitamin B_6 (boys only), vitamins B_{12} and C, folate, biotin and pantothenic acid were higher than intakes from *food sources* by young people who were not taking dietary supplements. The relatively small number of young people taking dietary supplements may account for none of the differences for boys and girls separately reaching the level of statistical significance ($p > 0.05$). However when the data for boys and girls were combined, differences in respect of intakes of vitamins B_{12} and C, and pantothenic acid were significant (all: $p < 0.05$). Other national dietary surveys of pre-school children, elderly persons, and adults[6,7,8] have also found that those taking dietary supplements have higher average daily intakes of many vitamins from food sources alone than those who are not taking any supplements.

(Table 8.39)

8.8 Variations in vitamin intake

In this section variation in the average daily intake of vitamins from *food sources* in relation to the main characteristics of the sample is considered. Since mean daily vitamin intake may be related to energy intake, the quality of the diet, in respect of vitamins, is compared by looking at vitamin intakes from *food sources* for boys and girls in the survey per MJ *total energy*.

Young people reported as being unwell
Compared with young people who reported not being unwell during the 7-day dietary recording period those who said they were unwell and their eating was affected had lower average daily intakes of all vitamins from food sources. Girls whose eating was affected by being unwell had significantly lower average daily intakes from food sources than girls who were not unwell of pre-formed retinol, vitamin A, riboflavin, niacin, vitamins B_6 and B_{12}, folate and pantothenic acid (all: $p < 0.01$) and of total carotene, biotin and vitamin C (all: $p < 0.05$). Boys who reported being unwell and whose eating was affected had significantly lower average daily intakes from food sources of pantothenic acid and vitamin E ($p < 0.01$) and of riboflavin and vitamin B_6 (all: $p < 0.05$).

When differences in energy intake were taken into account, very few of the differences in vitamin intake between those who were unwell and whose eating was affected and those who were not unwell remained. This suggests that in respect of intakes of most vitamins the quality of the diet did not change when the young person was unwell, they simply had a lower total energy intake. However, for boys, those who were unwell and whose eating was affected had a significantly lower intake of pantothenic acid per MJ energy than boys who were not unwell ($p < 0.01$). For girls there remained differences between the unwell and eating affected group and those who were not unwell in intakes per

MJ energy for biotin and pantothenic acid (both: p < 0.01). *(Tables 8.40 and 8.41)*

Region
Boys living in Scotland had lower absolute intakes than boys living elsewhere for all vitamins except vitamins B_6 and B_{12}, although for most vitamins the differences did not reach statistical significance. Boys living in the Central and South West regions of England, and in Wales had the highest absolute intakes of pre-formed retinol, vitamin A, thiamin, riboflavin, niacin, folate and vitamins B_{12} and D. Differences between intakes for boys living in Scotland and boys in the Central and South West regions of England and in Wales were statistically significant only for vitamin D (p < 0.05). Intakes of vitamin E were highest for boys living in the Northern region but not significantly different from intakes of vitamin E for boys in Scotland. Intakes of total carotene, biotin, pantothenic acid and vitamin C were highest for boys living in London and the South East, but not significantly different from those for boys living in Scotland.

Girls living in Scotland had the lowest absolute intakes of all vitamins except vitamin C, which was lowest for girls living in the Northern region, and vitamin E, lowest for girls living in London and the South East. Girls living in the Central and South West regions of England and in Wales had the highest absolute intakes of all vitamins except total carotene and vitamin E, which were highest for girls in the Northern region, and vitamin C, which was highest for girls in London and the South East. Differences between intakes for girls in Scotland and in the Central and South West and Wales were statistically significant for folate and pantothenic acid (all: p < 0.05). Differences between girls in regions with the highest and lowest intakes were not statistically significant for any of the other vitamins.

When differences in energy intake were taken into account, the variation in absolute intakes of many vitamins for boys living in different regions was no longer apparent. The only significant difference that remained, indicating a difference in the quality of the diet was for vitamin D, between boys in Scotland who had the lowest intake per MJ energy, and boys living in the Central and South West regions of England and Wales (p < 0.05).

For girls, after allowing for differences in energy intake, those in Scotland had significantly lower intakes per MJ of energy for thiamin, folate and pantothenic acid than girls who lived in the Central and South West regions and Wales (all: p < 0.05). *(Tables 8.42 and 8.43)*

Socio-economic factors
Tables 8.44 to 8.49 show mean intakes of vitamins from food for boys and girls according to whether they were living in a household receiving benefits, by the social class of the head of their household and by gross weekly household income. Intakes are expressed both on an absolute basis and also per MJ energy intake as a measure of the nutrient density of the diet.

Absolute mean daily intakes of nearly all vitamins were lower for boys in *households receiving benefits* than in households not receiving benefits (Family Credit, Income Support or Job Seeker's Allowance). The largest differences for boys were for intakes from food sources of thiamin, riboflavin, niacin, vitamin B_6, folate, biotin and pantothenic acid, vitamin C and vitamin E (all: p < 0.01).

There was much less variation in the intakes of vitamins for girls living in benefit and non-benefit households. Only for vitamin C (p < 0.01) and biotin (p < 0.05) were average intakes significantly lower for girls in benefit households.

After allowing for differences in energy intake between the two groups many of the differences were no longer evident. However both boys and girls living in benefit households had significantly lower average daily intakes of vitamin C from food sources per MJ total energy than young people in non-benefit households (boys: p < 0.05; girls: p < 0.01). Boys in benefit households also had significantly lower intakes per MJ of energy of biotin and pantothenic acid (both: p < 0.01). For girls, but not boys, intakes per MJ of both riboflavin and niacin were also lower for those living in benefit households (both: p < 0.05). *(Tables 8.44 and 8.45)*

Generally, and before allowing for differences in total energy intake, average daily intakes from food sources of most vitamins increased significantly as *gross weekly household income* increased.

For boys, intakes were lowest in the lowest household income group, except for total carotene and vitamins C and E, all of which were lowest for boys in households with a gross weekly income of between £160 and £280. There was no clear association with household income for boys for vitamin D. Intakes were highest for boys in the top two household income groups, except for intakes of vitamin E, which were highest for boys in households with a gross weekly income of between £280 and £400.

The most marked differences between highest and lowest intakes associated with household income for boys were for riboflavin, niacin, folate, biotin, pantothenic acid, and vitamin C (all: p < 0.01). There were also significant differences between the highest and lowest intakes for boys for total carotene, thiamin and vitamins B_6, B_{12} and E (p < 0.05)[9].

For girls, intakes of all vitamins were lowest for those in the lowest household income group, except for intakes of pre-formed retinol and vitamin E, which were lowest for girls in households with an income of between £400 and £600 a week, and for vitamins B_6 and D, which showed almost no variation by household income group. Intakes of all vitamins, except B_6, D and E were highest for girls in households in the highest income group. For vitamin E intakes were highest for girls in households with a gross weekly income of between £280 and £400.

The most marked differences between highest and lowest intakes associated with household income for girls were for biotin and vitamin C (both: $p < 0.01$). There were also significant differences between the highest and lowest intakes for girls for total carotene, niacin and folate $(p < 0.05)$[9].

After allowing for differences in total energy intake, the only significant differences associated with household income for boys were for biotin and pantothenic acid $(p < 0.01)$ where the boys in the lowest income households had significantly lower average daily intakes per MJ than boys in the highest income households. Intakes of vitamin C per MJ energy were significantly lower for boys in households with a gross weekly income of between £280 and £400 than for boys in the highest household income group $(p < 0.05)$. Intakes of vitamin D per MJ were significantly lower for boys in households with a gross weekly income of between £400 and £600 than for boys in households with a gross weekly income of up to £280 $(p < 0.05)$.

For girls, intakes of vitamin C, total carotene and niacin were still significantly lower for the lowest income group compared with the highest income group, after allowing for differences in energy intake (vitamin C: $p < 0.01$; others $p < 0.05$). *(Tables 8.46 and 8.47)*

Although there was a general pattern for young people from manual *social class* backgrounds to have lower average daily intakes from food sources of most vitamins than young people from non-manual home backgrounds, there were very few statistically significant differences in mean intake. For both boys and girls mean intakes of vitamin C were markedly lower for those from a manual social class background (both sexes: $p < 0.01$). For boys from a manual background intake of pantothenic acid was lower and for girls from a manual background mean intake of biotin was lower (boys – pantothenic acid: $p < 0.05$; girls – biotin: $p < 0.01$).

As can be seen from Table 8.49 many of these differences were associated with differences in total energy intake. Thus after allowing for differences in energy intake, mean intake of vitamin C from food sources varied significantly by social class for both boys and girls $(p < 0.01)$. For boys there also remained a significant difference in intake per MJ energy for pantothenic acid $(p < 0.05)$ and for girls for intake per MJ energy for biotin $(p < 0.01)$.
(Tables 8.48 and 8.49)

Household type
It has already been noted that a much higher proportion of young people who were living with both parents and no other children were aged 15 to 18 years compared with other household types. This difference in the age distribution may account for differences in nutrient intake associated with household type, including intakes of vitamins.

Table 8.50 shows that for boys, those living in households with both parents and no other children had the highest average daily intake of all vitamins. Intakes for boys living with both parents and other children and boys in single-parent households, with or without other children had average intakes which were very similar to each other.

Comparing average daily intakes for boys in two-parent, no other children households and boys in single-parent households, there were significant differences in the average daily intakes of niacin $(p < 0.01)$ and of vitamins B_{12} and B_{12}, folate, biotin and vitamin E (all: $p < 0.05$). In each case boys from single-parent households had a significantly lower average daily intake from food sources of the vitamin.

For girls the differences in intakes between those living in different household types were not as marked as for boys, and the pattern was less clear. None of the differences between intakes for girls living in different household types reached the level of statistical significance $(p > 0.05)$.

After allowing for differences in total energy intake between boys living in different household types, intakes per MJ total energy were still generally highest for boys in two-parent, no other children households, although the differences between the three groups were much less. Indeed the only difference to reach the level of statistical significance was between average daily intake of niacin per MJ for boys living in two-parent households with other children, 3.6mg/MJ, and for boys living in two-parent households with no other children, 3.9mg/MJ $(p < 0.01)$. *(Tables 8.50 and 8.51)*

8.9 Comparisons with other studies
Tables 8.52 and 8.53 compare data from this present survey of young people with equivalent data on average daily intakes of vitamins from food sources from other national surveys, including the 1983 Department of Health study of the Diets of British Schoolchildren[10].

Table 8.52 compares the average daily intake of vitamins for boys and girls aged 10 to 11 years and 14 to 15 years from the 1983 survey of the diets of British schoolchildren with equivalent data from the present survey.

For both sexes and both age groups there were significant differences in average daily intakes for the majority of the vitamins. For thiamin, vitamin C, vitamin D and vitamin B_6, young people in the present survey had markedly higher intakes (vitamins C, D and B_6, both age groups, both sexes: $p < 0.01$; thiamin, girls aged 14 to 15: $p < 0.05$; thiamin, others: $p < 0.01$). For example, for boys aged 14 to 15 years, mean daily intake of vitamin C was more than 50% and vitamin D more than 80% higher than intakes in 1983; for vitamin C, 76.0mg compared with 49.3mg, and for vitamin D, 3.00 µg compared with1.63µg.

However, compared with 1983, average daily intakes of retinol and retinol equivalents by young people in the present survey, and for boys, ß-carotene, were markedly lower (retinol and retinol equivalents, both age groups, both sexes: $p < 0.01$; ß-carotene, boys aged 10 to 11 years: $p < 0.01$; ß-carotene, others: ns).

The extent to which these differences represent changes in the diets of young people over the period is not clear. Many factors contribute to any differences, including changes in nutrient composition data due to both actual changes in nutrient composition and, as noted previously, new analytical methods[3,5], increase in fortification practices and changes in food consumption patterns. However, given that, as was shown in Chapter 5, average daily intakes of total energy have decreased over the period between these surveys (see *Table 5.15*) it is likely that at least part of the increase in average daily intakes of thiamin and vitamins C and B_6 is attributable to changes in the quality of the diet, with the diets of young people being richer in these vitamins than previously. Given the reduction in average daily energy intake and the revision of retinol values in milk, the decline in intakes of retinol, retinol equivalents, and for younger boys of ß-carotene may be mainly attributable to these factors and not to changes in the quality of the diet in respect of these vitamins.

A comparison of intakes of vitamins by boys and girls aged 3½ to 4½ years in the 1992/3 survey of pre-school children[6] with intakes by 4 to 6 year olds in the present NDNS shows that intakes of all vitamins from food sources, except vitamin A, and, for boys, total carotene, were significantly higher in the present survey (girls, total carotene: $p < 0.05$; all other vitamins for boys and girls: $p < 0.01$). As noted above, retinol values in milk have been revised downwards since the earlier survey, and this may account for the apparent decline in intakes between the surveys. Comparing 16 to 24 year olds in

the 1986/7 survey[8] with intakes for 15 to 18 year olds in the present survey shows, for boys, a general pattern of lower intakes in the present survey, probably associated with age differences between the two cohorts. However boys in the present survey had higher intakes of thiamin, vitamin B_6, folate, and vitamins C, D and E. Of these the differences were statistically significant only for vitamin C ($p < 0.05$). Boys aged 15 to 18 years in the present survey had significantly lower intakes of vitamin A, probably associated with the revised values for retinol in milk, and of vitamin B_{12} (vitamin A: $p < 0.01$; vitamin B_{12}: $p < 0.05$). Girls aged 15 to 18 years in the present NDNS had significantly higher intakes of vitamin E ($p < 0.01$) and significantly lower intakes of vitamin A ($p < 0.01$) and B_{12} ($p < 0.05$).

(Tables 8.52 and 8.53)

References and endnotes

1   Department of Health. Report on Health and Social Subjects: 41. *Dietary Reference Values for Food Energy and Nutrients for the United Kingdom*. HMSO (London, 1991).

2   Department of Health. *Dietary Reference Values. A Guide*. HMSO (London, 1991).

3   New analytical values for retinol in pasteurised milk became available in 1996 and have resulted in lower assessed intakes of retinol for this survey.

4   Intakes as a percentage of RNI were calculated for each young person, taking the appropriate RNI for each sex/age group. The values for all young people in each age group were then pooled to give a mean, median and standard deviation.

5   Measurable amounts of vitamin D and its metabolites have now been found in meats as a result of new analytical methods. New data for poultry and meat products became available for this survey resulting in higher assessed intakes of vitamin D compared with previous surveys.

6   Gregory JR, Collins DL, Davies PSW, Hughes JM, Clarke PC. *National Diet and Nutrition Survey: children aged 1½ to 4½ years. Volume 1: Report of the diet and nutrition survey*. HMSO (London, 1995).

7   Finch S, Doyle W, Lowe C, Bates CJ, Prentice A, Smithers G, Clarke PC. *National Diet and Nutrition Survey: people aged 65 years and over. Volume 1: Report of the diet and nutrition survey*. TSO (London, 1998).

8   Gregory J, Foster K, Tyler H, Wiseman M. *The Dietary and Nutritional Survey of British Adults*. HMSO (London, 1990).

9   p values are based on comparisons between young people in household income groups with the lowest and highest vitamin intakes.

10 Department of Health. Report on Health and Social Subjects: 36. *The Diets of British Schoolchildren*. HMSO (London, 1989).

Table 8.1 Reference Nutrient Intakes (RNIs) and Lower Reference Nutrient Intakes (LRNIs) for vitamins*

RNI and LRNI by age (years) and sex		Vitamins							
		Vitamin A	Thiamin***	Riboflavin	Niacin***	Vitamin B_6**	Vitamin B_{12}	Folate	Vitamin C
Males		μg/d	mg/d	mg/d	mg/d	mg/d	μg/d	μg/d	mg/d
4–6	RNI	400	0.7	0.8	11.0	0.9	0.8	100	30.0
	LRNI	200	0.4	0.4	8.0	0.7	0.5	50	8.0
7–10	RNI	500	0.7	1.0	12.0	1.0	1.0	150	30.0
	LRNI	250	0.5	0.5	9.0	0.8	0.6	75	8.0
11–14	RNI	600	0.9	1.2	15.0	1.2	1.2	200	35.0
	LRNI	250	0.5	0.8	10.0	0.9	0.8	100	9.0
15–18	RNI	700	1.1	1.3	18.0	1.5	1.5	200	40.0
	LRNI	300	0.6	0.8	12.0	1.1	1.0	100	10.0
Females		μg/d	mg/d	mg/d	mg/d	mg/d	μg/d	μg/d	mg/d
4–6	RNI	400	0.7	0.8	11.0	0.9	0.8	100	30.0
	LRNI	200	0.4	0.4	7.0	0.6	0.5	50	8.0
7–10	RNI	500	0.7	1.0	12.0	1.0	1.0	150	30.0
	LRNI	250	0.4	0.5	8.0	0.7	0.6	75	8.0
11–14	RNI	600	0.7	1.1	12.0	1.0	1.2	200	35.0
	LRNI	250	0.4	0.8	8.0	0.7	0.8	100	9.0
15–18	RNI	600	0.8	1.1	14.0	1.2	1.5	200	40.0
	LRNI	250	0.5	0.8	9.0	0.9	1.0	100	10.0

*Source: Department of Health. Report on Health and Social Subjects: 41. *Dietary Reference Values for Food Energy and Nutrients for the United Kingdom.* HMSO (London, 1991).
**Based on protein providing 14.7% of the Estimated Average Requirement (EAR) for energy. Calculated values from quoted LRNIs μg/g protein
***Calculated values based on EARs for energy; calculated values from quoted LRNIs mg/1000 kcal.

Table 8.2 Average daily intake of pre-formed retinol (µg) by sex and age of young person

Pre-formed retinol (µg)	Males aged (years)				All males	Females aged (years)				All females
	4–6	7–10	11–14	15–18		4–6	7–10	11–14	15–18	
	cum %	cum %	cum %	cum %	cum %	cum %	cum %	cum %	cum %	cum %
(a) Intakes from *all* sources										
Less than 100	6	4	5	4	5	5	5	10	8	7
Less than 150	20	10	14	10	13	16	14	26	24	20
Less than 200	38	28	27	23	28	34	37	47	46	41
Less than 300	66	63	64	51	61	67	70	73	70	70
Less than 400	78	81	81	72	78	81	87	89	86	86
Less than 600	86	88	94	91	90	91	94	95	95	94
All	100	100	100	100	100	100	100	100	100	100
Base	*184*	*256*	*237*	*179*	*856*	*171*	*226*	*238*	*210*	*845*
Mean (average value)	327	339	344	348	340	307	298	271	289	290
Median value	238	259	270	293	267	251	235	214	232	233
Lower 2.5 percentile	81	88	74	89	78	81	85	59	60	68
Upper 2.5 percentile	1040	1162	990	996	1069	1015	1004	895	940	959
Standard deviation of the mean	248	285	530	246	352	218	288	367	347	314
	cum %	cum %	cum %	cum %	cum %	cum %	cum %	cum %	cum %	cum %
(b) Intakes from *food* sources										
Less than 100	6	4	6	4	5	5	6	10	8	7
Less than 150	22	11	15	10	14	18	16	27	24	21
Less than 200	42	30	28	23	30	39	41	48	47	44
Less than 300	78	68	67	54	66	80	76	75	72	76
Less than 400	91	89	85	75	85	91	92	91	88	90
Less than 600	97	96	96	94	96	97	98	97	97	98
All	100	100	100	100	100	100	100	100	100	100
Base	*184*	*256*	*237*	*179*	*856*	*171*	*226*	*238*	*210*	*845*
Mean (average value)	250	289	325	333	302	253	264	256	272	262
Median value	217	248	261	283	256	229	219	205	214	218
Lower 2.5 percentile	81	88	74	87	76	79	83	59	60	68
Upper 2.5 percentile	821	671	786	889	730	604	517	658	637	598
Standard deviation of the mean	149	216	525	234	323	159	258	355	334	292

Table 8.3   Average daily intake of vitamins from food sources per MJ total energy by sex and age of young person

Vitamins	Age of young person (years)											
	4–6			7–10			11–14			15–18		
	Mean	Median	sd	Mean	Median	sd	Mean	Median	sd	Mean	Median	sd
Males												
Pre-formed retinol (µg)	39	36	21	39	35	34	40	31	34	34	31	21
Total carotene (β-carotene equivalents) (µg)	192	146	158	175	144	158	168	139	136	181	139	162
Vitamin A (retinol equivalents) (µg)	71	63	33.7	68	61	39.8	68	56	39.8	64	56	34.1
Thiamin (mg)	0.20	0.19	0.067	0.19	0.19	0.067	0.21	0.19	0.043	0.20	0.19	0.069
Riboflavin (mg)	0.24	0.24	0.068	0.22	0.21	0.068	0.21	0.20	0.064	0.20	0.19	0.079
Niacin equivalents (mg)	3.6	3.5	0.59	3.5	3.4	0.59	3.7	3.6	0.57	3.9	3.8	0.85
Vitamin B$_6$ (mg)	0.27	0.26	0.051	0.26	0.26	0.051	0.27	0.26	0.060	0.28	0.27	0.094
Vitamin B$_{12}$ (µg)	0.62	0.62	0.201	0.53	0.51	0.201	0.54	0.49	0.190	0.52	0.51	0.184
Folate (µg)	30	29	6.7	29	28	6.7	30	29	6.3	32	31	10.6
Vitamin C (mg)	10.5	9.0	5.46	9.9	7.9	5.46	9.2	7.5	6.36	8.8	7.2	7.17
Vitamin D (µg)	0.33	0.30	0.152	0.32	0.30	0.152	0.32	0.30	0.139	0.34	0.31	0.172
Vitamin E (α-tocopherol equivalents) (mg)	1.0	1.0	0.30	1.1	1.0	0.30	1.1	1.0	0.37	1.1	1.0	0.32
Base	*184*			*256*			*237*			*179*		
Females												
Pre-formed retinol (µg)	42	40	24	39	34	24	36	30	38	40	33	55
Total carotene (β-carotene equivalents) (µg)	199	174	120	195	180	120	181	141	113	247	195	271
Vitamin A (retinol equivalents) (µg)	76	70	32.8	72	66	32.8	66	58	43.7	81	64	72.0
Thiamin (mg)	0.19	0.19	0.081	0.19	0.18	0.081	0.20	0.19	0.050	0.20	0.18	0.110
Riboflavin (mg)	0.24	0.23	0.060	0.20	0.20	0.060	0.19	0.19	0.067	0.19	0.17	0.083
Niacin equivalents (mg)	3.5	3.4	0.69	3.5	3.5	0.69	3.5	3.4	0.66	3.7	3.7	0.84
Vitamin B$_6$ (mg)	0.26	0.25	0.066	0.26	0.25	0.066	0.27	0.27	0.065	0.27	0.26	0.071
Vitamin B$_{12}$ (µg)	0.61	0.59	0.207	0.51	0.49	0.207	0.46	0.43	0.197	0.50	0.45	0.301
Folate (µg)	29	27	7.0	28	28	7.0	29	28	6.9	31	30	10.3
Vitamin C (mg)	11.2	10.1	5.34	10.8	9.7	5.34	10.1	8.7	5.45	11.1	9.3	7.24
Vitamin D (µg)	0.31	0.29	0.143	0.31	0.29	0.143	0.31	0.28	0.141	0.32	0.29	0.166
Vitamin E (α-tocopherol equivalents) (mg)	1.1	1.0	0.29	1.1	1.1	0.29	1.2	1.1	0.35	1.2	1.1	0.38
Base	*171*			*226*			*238*			*210*		

223

Table 8.4 Average daily intake of total carotene (β-carotene equivalents) (μg) by sex and age of young person

Total carotene (β-carotene equivalents) (μg)	Males aged (years)				All males	Females aged (years)				All females
	4–6	7–10	11–14	15–18		4–6	7–10	11–14	15–18	
	cum %	cum %	cum %	cum %	cum %	cum %	cum %	cum %	cum %	cum %
Intakes from *food sources**										
Less than 300	8	5	6	3	5	7	5	8	2	5
Less than 600	31	26	22	17	24	23	17	28	18	22
Less than 900	50	39	39	32	40	44	37	46	32	40
Less than 1200	62	56	54	47	55	56	51	62	47	54
Less than 1500	72	71	63	59	66	73	68	71	60	68
Less than 2100	85	86	78	73	80	87	83	86	74	82
All	100	100	100	100	100	100	100	100	100	100
Base	*184*	*256*	*237*	*179*	*856*	*171*	*226*	*238*	*210*	*845*
Mean (average value)	1248	1295	1396	1680	1411	1175	1304	1268	1637	1354
Median value	903	1046	1112	1269	1111	1035	1169	967	1241	1112
Lower 2.5 percentile	194	239	242	293	246	233	262	226	300	236
Upper 2.5 percentile	3955	3943	3852	6837	4255	2840	3045	3991	4327	3776
Standard deviation of the mean	1100	1045	980	1343	1137	726	792	1005	1774	1177

*None of the dietary supplements taken by young people in this survey provided any carotene.

Table 8.5   **Percentage contribution of food types to average daily intake of total carotene (β-carotene equivalents) by sex and age of young person**

Type of food	Males aged (years)				All males	Females aged (years)				All females
	4–6	7–10	11–14	15–18		4–6	7–10	11–14	15–18	
	%	%	%	%	%	%	%	%	%	%
Cereals & cereal products	5	6	6	7	6	5	5	6	5	5
Milk & milk products	4	4	4	4	4	5	4	3	3	3
of which: *milk (whole, semi-skimmed, skimmed)*	*3*	*2*	*2*	*2*	*2*	*3*	*2*	*1*	*1*	*2*
Eggs & egg dishes	0	0	0	0	0	0	0	0	0	0
Fat spreads	4	5	4	4	4	4	4	4	3	4
Meat & meat products	10	10	13	15	12	9	12	11	11	11
Fish & fish dishes	0	0	1	0	0	0	0	0	0	0
Vegetables, potatoes & savoury snacks	61	56	54	56	56	58	56	57	57	57
of which: *raw carrots*	*15*	*10*	*4*	*10*	*9*	*10*	*9*	*6*	*11*	*9*
cooked carrots	*34*	*31*	*35*	*31*	*32*	*34*	*31*	*32*	*26*	*30*
other cooked vegetables, excluding potatoes	*9*	*9*	*10*	*9*	*9*	*11*	*10*	*13*	*13*	*12*
Fruit & nuts	5	6	4	4	4	5	6	3	5	5
Sugars, preserves & confectionery	2	2	2	2	2	2	2	2	1	2
Drinks*	6	7	6	4	6	7	6	6	4	6
of which: *soft drinks, including low calorie*	*6*	*7*	*6*	*4*	*6*	*7*	*6*	*6*	*4*	*6*
Miscellaneous**	2	4	4	5	4	4	4	4	5	5
Average daily intake (µg)	1248	1295	1396	1680	1411	1175	1304	1268	1637	1354
Total number of young people	184	256	237	179	856	171	226	238	210	845

*Includes soft drinks, alcoholic drinks, tea, coffee & water.
** Includes powdered beverages (except tea and coffee), soups, sauces and condiments and commercial toddlers' foods.

Table 8.6 Average daily intake of β-carotene (µg) by sex and age of young person

β-carotene (µg)	Males aged (years)				All males	Females aged (years)				All females
	4–6	7–10	11–14	15–18		4–6	7–10	11–14	15–18	
	cum %	cum %	cum %	cum %	cum %	cum %	cum %	cum %	cum %	cum %
Intakes from *food sources***										
Less than 200	3	1	2	1	1	2	1	2	1	1
Less than 400	15	13	11	7	11	14	10	14	8	11
Less than 600	32	28	25	17	25	26	21	29	20	24
Less than 800	48	37	37	29	37	44	34	42	30	37
Less than 1600	79	80	68	63	72	80	78	77	68	76
Less than 2400	91	92	89	85	90	97	94	90	86	92
All	100	100	100	100	100	100	100	100	100	100
Base	*184*	*256*	*237*	*179*	*856*	*171*	*226*	*238*	*210*	*845*
Mean (average value)	1120	1167	1261	1512	1271	1060	1176	1148	1470	1220
Median value	832	974	1011	1153	1011	951	1064	892	1142	1016
Lower 2.5 percentile	190	235	229	270	235	232	245	212	300	233
Upper 2.5 percentile	3437	3318	3459	5903	3655	2539	2665	3486	3839	3343
Standard deviation of the mean	949	898	851	1159	982	634	685	884	1580	1040

*None of the dietary supplements taken by young people in this survey provided any β-carotene.

Table 8.7 Average daily intake of α-carotene (µg) by sex and age of young person

α-carotene (µg)	Males aged (years)				All males	Females aged (years)				All females
	4–6	7–10	11–14	15–18		4–6	7–10	11–14	15–18	
	cum %	cum %	cum %	cum %	cum %	cum %	cum %	cum %	cum %	cum %
Intakes from *food sources***										
Zero	1	2	3	2	2	1	0	3	2	2
Less than 10	22	21	27	18	22	18	16	25	14	18
Less than 25	26	25	30	27	27	25	22	32	19	24
Less than 75	38	38	39	34	38	34	32	40	28	34
Less than 150	53	52	50	49	51	50	48	54	40	48
Less than 300	72	75	67	66	70	71	72	72	66	70
Less than 600	91	93	89	86	90	96	93	92	88	92
All	100	100	100	100	100	100	100	100	100	100
Base	*184*	*256*	*237*	*179*	*856*	*171*	*226*	*238*	*210*	*845*
Mean (average value)	230	223	236	288	244	204	224	209	286	232
Median value	132	134	152	160	139	152	170	130	195	163
Lower 2.5 percentile	0	0	0	0	0	0	0	0	0	0
Upper 2.5 percentile	949	1018	952	1547	1095	624	778	982	1072	937
Standard deviation of the mean	302	310	266	372	317	195	225	261	387	281

*None of the dietary supplements taken by young people in this survey provided any α-carotene.

Table 8.8 Average daily intake of β-cryptoxanthin (μg) by sex and age of young person

β-cryptoxanthin (μg)	Males aged (years)				All males	Females aged (years)				All females
	4–6	7–10	11–14	15–18		4–6	7–10	11–14	15–18	
	cum %	cum %	cum %	cum %	cum %	cum %	cum %	cum %	cum %	cum %
Intakes from *food sources*										
Zero	1	1	2	5	2	1	2	3	2	2
Less than 2	4	5	6	11	7	7	6	6	3	6
Less than 5	16	16	12	16	15	15	15	14	9	13
Less than 10	29	24	24	27	26	29	26	25	20	25
Less than 15	44	37	36	34	37	43	36	40	28	36
Less than 30	69	63	62	48	60	75	60	65	48	61
Less than 60	92	87	84	75	84	91	87	87	72	84
All	100	100	100	100	100	100	100	100	100	100
Base	*184*	*256*	*237*	*179*	*856*	*171*	*226*	*238*	*210*	*845*
Mean (average value)	26	32	33	48	35	26	31	30	47	34
Median value	18	24	23	32	23	19	25	21	33	24
Lower 2.5 percentile	1	1	0	0	0	1	1	0	0	0
Upper 2.5 percentile	97	137	158	201	141	103	130	106	177	130
Standard deviation of the mean	24.7	32.0	36.5	68.6	45.1	28.7	31.0	28.7	50.7	37.1

*None of the dietary supplements taken by young people in this survey provided any β-cryptoxanthin.

227

Table 8.9 Average daily intake of vitamin A (retinol equivalents) (µg) by sex and age of young person

Vitamin A (retinol equivalents) (µg)	Males aged (years)				All males	Females aged (years)				All females
	4–6	7–10	11–14	15–18		4–6	7–10	11–14	15–18	
	cum %	cum %	cum %	cum %	cum %	cum %	cum %	cum %	cum %	cum %
(a) Intakes from *all* sources										
Less than 200	8	3	6	4	5	6	4	12	5	7
Less than 250	13	9	12	6	10	11	9	20	12	13
Less than 300	23	14	19	12	17	20	18	29	20	22
Less than 400	42	35	35	30	35	42	43	52	40	44
Less than 500	57	57	51	42	52	60	59	63	55	59
Less than 600	71	72	65	52	65	74	76	74	70	73
Less than 700	78	78	77	69	75	83	84	84	76	82
All	100	100	100	100	100	100	100	100	100	100
Base	*184*	*256*	*237*	*179*	*856*	*171*	*226*	*238*	*210*	*845*
Mean (average value)	535	555	577	628	575	502	515	482	562	516
Median value	432	460	485	584	485	437	460	380	475	439
Lower 2.5 percentile	131	196	145	188	157	166	174	126	156	145
Upper 2.5 percentile	1314	1451	1277	1579	1402	1265	1331	1296	1413	1296
Standard deviation of the mean	320	341	563	355	411	269	333	419	464	384
	cum %	cum %	cum %	cum %	cum %	cum %	cum %	cum %	cum %	cum %
(b) Intakes from *food* sources										
Less than 200	8	3	6	4	5	6	5	12	5	7
Less than 250	16	9	13	6	11	13	10	20	12	14
Less than 300	27	15	20	12	18	23	19	29	20	23
Less than 400	48	39	37	31	38	47	45	54	40	46
Less than 500	66	62	54	43	56	69	64	65	56	63
Less than 600	83	78	67	54	70	81	81	76	71	77
Less than 700	88	84	79	70	80	90	88	86	78	86
All	100	100	100	100	100	100	100	100	100	100
Base	*184*	*256*	*237*	*179*	*856*	*171*	*226*	*238*	*210*	*845*
Mean (average value)	458	505	558	613	537	449	481	467	545	487
Median value	407	443	476	549	465	414	448	377	472	424
Lower 2.5 percentile	131	196	147	188	157	166	174	126	156	145
Upper 2.5 percentile	1176	1279	1218	1579	1288	955	937	1234	1281	1158
Standard deviation of the mean	251	276	556	347	386	220	302	410	452	364

Table 8.10 Average daily intake of vitamin A (retinol equivalents) as a percentage of Reference Nutrient Intake (RNI) by sex and age of young person

Sex and age (years) of young person	Average daily intake as % of RNI*							
	(a) All sources			Base	(b) Food sources			Base
	Mean	Median	sd		Mean	Median	sd	
Males								
4–6	134	108	80.0	184	114	102	62.8	184
7–10	111	92	68.2	256	101	89	55.3	256
11–14	96	81	93.8	237	93	79	92.7	237
15–18	90	83	50.7	179	88	78	49.6	179
All	103	92	76.2	856	98	87	68.0	856
Females								
4–6	126	109	67.1	171	112	103	55.1	171
7–10	103	92	66.7	226	96	90	60.4	226
11–14	80	63	69.9	238	78	63	68.2	238
15–18	94	79	77.3	210	91	79	75.3	210
All	99	86	72.2	845	93	83	66.6	845

*Intake as a percentage of RNI was calculated for each young person. The values for all young people in each age group were then pooled to give a mean, median and sd.

Table 8.11 Percentage contribution of food types to average daily intake of vitamin A (retinol equivalents) by sex and age of young person

Type of food	Males aged (years)				All males	Females aged (years)				All females
	4–6	7–10	11–14	15–18		4–6	7–10	11–14	15–18	
	%	%	%	%	%	%	%	%	%	%
Cereals & cereal products	12	14	13	12	13	11	13	13	12	12
of which:										
buns, cakes & pastries	5	6	4	3	5	4	5	5	4	4
pizza	2	3	4	4	4	2	2	3	3	3
Milk & milk products	24	21	19	19	20	26	20	18	16	19
of which:										
whole milk	11	6	4	4	6	10	5	3	3	5
reduced fat milks	4	5	6	5	5	3	4	4	3	4
cheese	5	5	5	8	6	7	6	7	8	7
Eggs & egg dishes	3	4	4	4	4	4	4	4	3	4
Fat spreads	11	14	12	13	13	13	12	12	12	12
of which:										
polyunsaturated reduced fat spreads	4	3	3	3	3	4	4	3	3	3
butter	2	4	2	3	3	4	3	2	3	3
Meat & meat products	11	13	19	16	15	10	15	15	15	14
of which:										
liver & liver dishes	5	6	10	5	7	5	8	8	8	7
Fish & fish dishes	1	0	1	1	1	0	1	1	1	1
Vegetables, potatoes & savoury snacks	29	25	25	27	26	27	27	29	30	28
of which:										
vegetables, excluding potatoes	28	23	23	26	25	25	25	26	29	27
Fruit & nuts	1	1	1	0	1	1	1	1	1	1
Sugars, preserves & confectionery	1	1	1	1	1	1	1	1	1	1
Drinks*	5	5	4	4	4	5	5	4	3	4
Miscellaneous**	1	2	2	3	2	2	2	2	3	3
Average daily intake (µg)	**458**	**505**	**558**	**613**	**537**	**449**	**481**	**467**	**545**	**487**
Total number of young people	**184**	**256**	**237**	**179**	**856**	**171**	**226**	**238**	**210**	**845**

*Includes soft drinks, alcoholic drinks, tea, coffee & water.
** Includes powdered beverages (except tea and coffee), soups, sauces and condiments and commercial toddlers' foods.

Table 8.12 Average daily intake of thiamin (mg) by sex and age of young person

Thiamin (mg)	Males aged (years)				All males	Females aged (years)				All females
	4–6	7–10	11–14	15–18		4–6	7–10	11–14	15–18	
	cum %	cum %	cum %	cum %	cum %	cum %	cum %	cum %	cum %	cum %
(a) Intakes from *all* sources										
Less than 0.40	–	–	0	–	0	–	–	1	1	0
Less than 0.50	2	–	0	–	0	1	2	1	2	1
Less than 0.60	3	1	0	–	1	4	2	1	3	2
Less than 0.70	6	1	2	–	2	8	2	3	6	4
Less than 0.80	11	4	5	1	5	15	7	7	13	10
Less than 0.90	19	7	6	2	8	28	14	14	19	18
Less than 1.10	37	22	13	7	19	53	35	31	36	38
Less than 1.50	77	63	45	30	52	84	78	66	68	74
Less than 2.10	96	94	81	64	83	96	96	92	90	93
All	100	100	100	100	100	100	100	100	100	100
Base	*184*	*256*	*237*	*179*	*856*	*171*	*226*	*238*	*210*	*845*
Mean (average value)	1.28	1.43	1.71	1.93	1.60	1.17	1.29	1.42	1.41	1.33
Median value	1.23	1.37	1.55	1.83	1.46	1.07	1.23	1.30	1.24	1.21
Lower 2.5 percentile	0.51	0.77	0.72	0.84	0.72	0.57	0.70	0.68	0.53	0.60
Upper 2.5 percentile	2.60	2.38	2.97	3.86	3.09	2.38	2.31	2.51	2.77	2.58
Standard deviation of the mean	0.516	0.427	1.278	0.733	0.854	0.494	0.423	0.789	0.857	0.678
	cum %	cum %	cum %	cum %	cum %	cum %	cum %	cum %	cum %	cum %
(b) Intakes from *food* sources										
Less than 0.40	–	–	0	–	0	–	–	1	1	0
Less than 0.50	2	–	0	–	0	1	2	1	2	1
Less than 0.60	3	1	0	–	1	4	2	1	3	2
Less than 0.70	6	1	2	–	2	8	2	3	6	4
Less than 0.80	11	4	5	1	5	15	7	8	13	10
Less than 0.90	19	7	6	2	8	30	14	14	19	19
Less than 1.10	37	22	13	7	19	56	35	32	36	39
Less than 1.50	78	64	46	30	53	88	79	68	70	76
Less than 2.10	96	95	82	64	84	97	97	93	92	95
All	100	100	100	100	100	100	100	100	100	100
Base	*184*	*256*	*237*	*179*	*856*	*171*	*226*	*238*	*210*	*845*
Mean (average value)	1.27	1.42	1.70	1.90	1.59	1.14	1.27	1.40	1.38	1.31
Median value	1.22	1.37	1.54	1.81	1.45	1.05	1.23	1.29	1.21	1.20
Lower 2.5 percentile	0.51	0.77	0.72	0.84	0.72	0.56	0.70	0.68	0.53	0.60
Upper 2.5 percentile	2.60	2.29	2.97	3.70	3.06	2.33	2.17	2.45	2.78	2.46
Standard deviation of the mean	0.504	0.396	1.278	0.682	0.837	0.479	0.404	0.783	0.841	0.666

Table 8.13 Average daily intake of thiamin as a percentage of Reference Nutrient Intake (RNI) by sex and age of young person

Sex and age (years) of young person	Average daily intake as % of RNI*							
	(a) All sources			*Base*	(b) Food sources			*Base*
	Mean	Median	sd		Mean	Median	sd	
Males								
4–6	183	175	73.7	*184*	181	174	72.1	*184*
7–10	205	195	61.0	*256*	202	195	56.6	*256*
11–14	190	172	142.0	*237*	189	172	142.0	*237*
15–18	175	166	66.6	*179*	173	165	62.0	*179*
All	189	180	93.1	*856*	187	179	91.3	*856*
Females								
4–6	167	153	70.6	*171*	163	150	68.4	*171*
7–10	184	176	60.4	*226*	182	176	57.7	*226*
11–14	202	186	112.7	*238*	200	184	111.8	*238*
15–18	176	155	107.1	*210*	172	151	105.1	*210*
All	183	170	91.9	*845*	180	168	90.3	*845*

*Intake as a percentage of RNI was calculated for each young person. The values for all young people in each age group were then pooled to give a mean, median and sd.

Table 8.14 Percentage contribution of food types to average daily intake of thiamin by sex and age of young person

Type of food	Males aged (years)				All males	Females aged (years)				All females
	4–6	7–10	11–14	15–18		4–6	7–10	11–14	15–18	
	%	%	%	%	%	%	%	%	%	%
Cereals & cereal products	44	48	42	42	43	43	40	38	33	38
of which:										
white bread	8	10	9	10	9	8	9	9	9	9
high fibre & whole grain breakfast cereals	10	10	8	7	9	9	7	7	4	7
other breakfast cereals	15	17	14	14	15	14	12	12	8	12
Milk & milk products	8	7	5	4	6	8	6	5	5	6
of which:										
milk (whole, semi-skimmed, skimmed)	5	4	4	3	4	5	4	3	3	4
Eggs & egg dishes	0	0	0	1	1	1	1	0	1	1
Fat spreads	0	0	0	0	0	0	0	0	0	0
Meat & meat products	15	17	19	23	19	16	20	18	19	18
of which:										
bacon & ham	3	4	5	7	5	4	5	4	4	4
chicken, turkey & dishes including coated	5	6	6	7	6	6	7	7	7	7
pork & dishes	2	2	2	2	2	2	2	2	3	2
Fish & fish dishes	1	1	1	1	1	1	1	1	1	1
Vegetables, potatoes & savoury snacks	23	19	24	22	22	23	23	28	31	27
of which:										
vegetables, excluding potatoes	9	4	9	7	7	9	6	10	15	10
roast or fried potatoes & chips	7	7	8	9	8	6	8	10	8	8
other potatoes	4	5	5	5	5	4	6	6	6	6
savoury snacks	3	3	2	2	2	3	3	3	2	3
Fruit & nuts	2	2	1	1	1	2	3	2	2	2
Sugars, preserves & confectionery	1	1	1	1	1	1	1	1	1	1
Drinks*	2	2	2	2	2	3	3	3	3	3
Miscellaneous**	3	3	2	3	3	3	3	3	3	3
Average daily intake (mg)	1.27	1.42	1.70	1.90	1.59	1.14	1.27	1.40	1.38	1.31
Total number of young people	184	256	237	179	856	171	226	238	210	845

*Includes soft drinks, alcoholic drinks, tea, coffee & water.
** Includes powdered beverages (except tea and coffee), soups, sauces and condiments and commercial toddlers' foods.

233

Table 8.15 Average daily intake of riboflavin (mg) by sex and age of young person

Riboflavin (mg)	Males aged (years)				All males	Females aged (years)				All females
	4–6	7–10	11–14	15–18		4–6	7–10	11–14	15–18	
	cum %	cum %	cum %	cum %	cum %	cum %	cum %	cum %	cum %	cum %
(a) Intakes from *all* sources										
Less than 0.40	–	–	1	–	0	–	1	1	3	1
Less than 0.50	–	1	1	1	1	–	1	4	6	3
Less than 0.80	10	3	6	6	6	7	9	22	21	15
Less than 1.00	14	12	14	11	13	18	21	34	35	27
Less than 1.10	18	16	20	17	18	25	30	40	40	34
Less than 1.20	23	23	25	24	24	32	37	46	47	41
Less than 1.30	31	32	31	28	30	44	47	49	55	49
Less than 1.60	56	54	48	42	50	67	72	70	74	71
Less than 2.00	81	76	64	59	69	88	89	88	84	87
Less than 2.40	93	90	85	72	85	97	94	94	91	94
All	100	100	100	100	100	100	100	100	100	100
Base	*184*	*256*	*237*	*179*	*856*	*171*	*226*	*238*	*210*	*845*
Mean (average value)	1.57	1.64	1.74	1.95	1.73	1.43	1.38	1.35	1.34	1.37
Median value	1.50	1.52	1.65	0.86	1.60	1.39	1.35	1.31	1.25	1.31
Lower 2.5 percentile	0.58	0.80	0.63	0.68	0.63	0.62	0.57	0.45	0.39	0.48
Upper 2.5 percentile	3.05	2.92	3.49	3.88	3.56	2.55	2.62	2.79	3.00	2.72
Standard deviation of the mean	0.591	0.594	0.706	0.911	0.730	0.467	0.498	0.622	0.669	0.575
	cum %	cum %	cum %	cum %	cum %	cum %	cum %	cum %	cum %	cum %
(b) Intakes from *food* sources										
Less than 0.40	–	–	1	–	0	–	1	1	3	1
Less than 0.50	–	1	1	1	1	–	1	4	6	3
Less than 0.80	10	3	6	6	6	7	9	22	21	15
Less than 1.00	14	12	14	11	13	18	21	35	35	28
Less than 1.10	18	17	20	17	18	26	30	41	42	35
Less than 1.20	23	23	25	24	24	34	37	47	48	42
Less than 1.30	31	32	31	28	31	46	47	50	58	50
Less than 1.60	57	54	48	44	50	72	72	72	76	73
Less than 2.00	82	77	65	60	70	89	90	89	86	89
Less than 2.40	94	91	85	74	86	98	96	95	93	95
All	100	100	100	100	100	100	100	100	100	100
Base	*184*	*256*	*237*	*179*	*856*	*171*	*226*	*238*	*210*	*845*
Mean (average value)	1.56	1.62	1.73	1.92	1.71	1.40	1.37	1.32	1.30	1.34
Median value	1.49	1.52	1.62	1.82	1.58	1.35	1.34	1.30	1.22	1.30
Lower 2.5 percentile	0.58	0.80	0.63	0.68	0.63	0.62	0.57	0.45	0.39	0.48
Upper 2.5 percentile	2.96	2.83	3.49	3.88	3.47	2.44	2.58	2.69	3.00	2.68
Standard deviation of the mean	0.576	0.556	0.705	0.893	0.713	0.449	0.475	0.578	0.631	0.543

Table 8.16 Average daily intake of riboflavin as a percentage of Reference Nutrient Intake (RNI) by sex and age of young person

Sex and age (years) of young person	Average daily intake as % of RNI*							
	(a) All sources			*Base*	(b) Food sources			*Base*
	Mean	Median	sd		Mean	Median	sd	
Males								
4–6	197	187	73.9	*184*	194	186	72.0	*184*
7–10	163	152	59.4	*256*	162	152	55.6	*256*
11–14	145	137	58.8	*237*	144	135	58.8	*237*
15–18	150	143	70.0	*179*	148	140	68.7	*179*
All	162	154	68.0	*856*	160	154	66.2	*856*
Females								
4–6	179	174	58.4	*171*	175	168	56.1	*171*
7–10	138	135	49.8	*226*	137	134	47.5	*226*
11–14	123	119	56.5	*238*	120	118	52.6	*238*
15–18	122	114	60.8	*210*	118	110	57.4	*210*
All	138	132	60.4	*845*	136	130	57.4	*845*

*Intake as a percentage of RNI was calculated for each young person. The values for all young people in each age group were then pooled to give a mean, median and sd.

Table 8.17 **Percentage contribution of food types to average daily intake of riboflavin by sex and age of young person**

Type of food	Males aged (years)				All males	Females aged (years)				All females
	4–6	7–10	11–14	15–18		4–6	7–10	11–14	15–18	
	%	%	%	%	%	%	%	%	%	%
Cereals & cereal products	32	36	35	34	34	31	32	34	27	31
of which:										
high fibre & whole grain breakfast cereals	9	10	9	8	9	8	8	8	5	7
other breakfast cereals	14	16	15	16	15	13	13	14	10	12
Milk & milk products	42	37	34	30	36	43	36	31	31	35
of which:										
whole milk	22	13	9	7	12	23	12	7	8	12
semi-skimmed milk	11	15	18	16	16	10	13	14	14	13
yogurt, fromage frais & other dairy desserts	6	5	4	2	4	7	6	4	3	5
Eggs & egg dishes	2	2	2	2	2	2	3	2	3	2
Fat spreads	0	0	0	0	0	0	0	0	0	0
Meat & meat products	9	9	11	14	11	8	11	11	13	11
of which:										
chicken, turkey & dishes including coated	2	2	3	3	3	2	3	3	4	3
Fish & fish dishes	1	1	1	1	1	1	1	1	1	1
Vegetables, potatoes & savoury snacks	5	4	4	5	4	4	4	6	8	5
Fruit & nuts	1	1	1	1	1	1	1	1	1	1
Sugars, preserves & confectionery	5	6	6	5	5	6	6	7	6	6
Drinks*	0	0	1	5	2	0	1	1	3	1
Miscellaneous**	4	4	4	3	4	4	4	4	5	4
Average daily intake (mg)	**1.56**	**1.62**	**1.73**	**1.92**	**1.71**	**1.40**	**1.37**	**1.32**	**1.30**	**1.34**
Total number of young people	**184**	**256**	**237**	**179**	**856**	**171**	**226**	**238**	**210**	**845**

*Includes soft drinks, alcoholic drinks, tea, coffee & water.
** Includes powdered beverages (except tea and coffee), soups, sauces and condiments and commercial toddlers' foods.

Table 8.18 Average daily intake of niacin equivalents (mg) by sex and age of young person

Niacin equivalents (mg)	Males aged (years)				All males	Females aged (years)				All females
	4–6	7–10	11–14	15–18		4–6	7–10	11–14	15–18	
	cum %	cum %	cum %	cum %	cum %	cum %	cum %	cum %	cum %	cum %
(a) Intakes from *all* sources										
Less than 7.0	–	0	0	–	0	–	–	–	0	0
Less than 8.0	–	0	0	–	0	–	–	–	1	0
Less than 9.0	–	0	0	–	0	1	1	1	1	1
Less than 10.0	2	0	0	–	1	2	1	1	2	1
Less than 11.0	2	0	0	–	1	2	1	1	2	1
Less than 12.0	3	0	1	–	1	3	2	2	2	2
Less than 14.0	3	0	4	–	2	9	3	4	5	5
Less than 15.0	7	1	4	–	3	15	6	6	10	9
Less than 18.0	21	7	6	–	8	30	16	14	17	19
Less than 25.0	69	46	28	12	37	81	63	57	49	62
Less than 35.0	97	92	77	50	78	98	97	91	89	94
All	100	100	100	100	100	100	100	100	100	100
Base	*184*	*256*	*237*	*179*	*856*	*171*	*226*	*238*	*210*	*845*
Mean (average value)	22.9	26.1	30.0	36.8	29.2	20.7	23.6	24.8	25.6	23.8
Median value	22.0	25.6	29.8	35.0	27.9	20.2	23.0	24.0	25.0	23.0
Lower 2.5 percentile	11.6	16.1	13.6	19.4	14.6	11.6	13.7	13.7	12.8	12.3
Upper 2.5 percentile	38.3	42.2	47.0	60.9	51.9	33.3	35.8	40.7	44.9	40.7
Standard deviation of the mean	7.01	6.22	8.33	10.65	9.70	5.67	6.21	6.93	8.06	7.04
	cum %	cum %	cum %	cum %	cum %	cum %	cum %	cum %	cum %	cum %
(b) Intakes from *food* sources										
Less than 7.0	–	0	0	–	0	–	–	–	0	0
Less than 8.0	–	0	0	–	0	–	–	–	1	0
Less than 9.0	–	0	0	–	0	1	1	1	1	1
Less than 10.0	2	0	0	–	1	2	1	1	2	1
Less than 11.0	2	0	0	–	1	2	1	1	2	1
Less than 12.0	3	0	1	–	1	3	2	2	2	2
Less than 14.0	3	0	4	–	2	9	3	4	5	5
Less than 15.0	7	1	4	–	3	15	6	7	10	9
Less than 18.0	21	7	6	–	8	33	16	14	17	19
Less than 25.0	70	46	28	12	37	83	63	57	50	62
Less than 35.0	97	93	77	50	79	99	97	92	90	94
All	100	100	100	100	100	100	100	100	100	100
Base	*184*	*256*	*237*	*179*	*856*	*171*	*226*	*238*	*210*	*845*
Mean (average value)	22.8	26.0	30.0	36.6	29.1	20.4	23.4	24.6	25.2	23.6
Median value	22.0	25.6	29.8	35.0	27.9	19.9	23.0	23.8	25.0	22.8
Lower 2.5 percentile	11.6	16.1	13.6	19.4	14.6	11.6	13.7	13.7	12.8	12.3
Upper 2.5 percentile	35.9	40.5	47.0	57.5	51.6	33.3	35.3	40.5	42.4	39.6
Standard deviation of the mean	6.83	5.89	8.33	10.45	9.55	5.30	5.91	6.79	7.62	6.74

Table 8.19 Average daily intake of niacin equivalents as a percentage of Reference Nutrient Intake (RNI) by sex and age of young person

Sex and age (years) of young person	Average daily intake as % of RNI*							
	(a) All sources			*Base*	(b) Food sources			*Base*
	Mean	Median	sd		Mean	Median	sd	
Males								
4–6	208	200	63.7	*184*	207	200	62.1	*184*
7–10	218	214	51.8	*256*	216	214	49.1	*256*
11–14	200	198	55.5	*237*	200	198	55.6	*237*
15–18	204	194	59.2	*179*	203	194	58.0	*179*
All	208	204	57.7	*856*	207	204	56.3	*856*
Females								
4–6	188	183	51.5	*171*	186	181	48.1	*171*
7–10	196	192	51.8	*226*	195	192	49.2	*226*
11–14	207	200	57.7	*238*	205	199	56.6	*238*
15–18	183	179	57.5	*210*	180	179	54.4	*210*
All	194	189	55.6	*845*	192	188	53.2	*845*

*Intake as a percentage of RNI was calculated for each young person. The values for all young people in each age group were then pooled to give a mean, median and sd.

Table 8.20 Percentage contribution of food types to average daily intake of niacin equivalents by sex and age of young person

Type of food	Males aged (years)				All males	Females aged (years)				All females
	4–6	7–10	11–14	15–18		4–6	7–10	11–14	15–18	
	%	%	%	%	%	%	%	%	%	%
Cereals & cereal products	38	41	37	34	38	38	36	34	31	34
of which:										
white bread	8	9	8	8	9	8	8	8	9	8
high fibre & whole grain breakfast cereals	8	8	7	5	7	7	6	6	4	5
other breakfast cereals	12	12	11	10	11	11	9	9	6	9
Milk & milk products	13	11	9	8	10	14	10	8	9	10
of which:										
milk (whole, semi-skimmed, skimmed)	8	6	5	4	6	8	5	4	4	5
Eggs & egg dishes	1	1	1	1	1	2	2	1	1	1
Fat spreads	0	0	0	0	0	0	0	0	0	0
Meat & meat products	25	26	30	34	30	26	30	30	32	29
of which:										
bacon & ham	2	3	4	4	3	3	3	3	3	3
beef, veal & dishes	3	3	3	5	3	2	4	4	4	4
chicken, turkey & dishes including coated	11	11	12	13	12	12	13	14	15	13
Fish & fish dishes	4	4	4	3	4	4	4	4	5	4
Vegetables, potatoes & savoury snacks	11	11	11	11	11	11	12	13	13	12
of which:										
vegetables, excluding potatoes	3	3	3	3	3	3	3	3	5	4
roast or fried potatoes and chips	3	3	4	4	4	3	4	4	4	4
Fruit & nuts	2	2	2	1	2	2	2	2	1	2
Sugars, preserves & confectionery	1	2	2	1	1	1	2	2	1	2
Drinks*	2	2	2	5	3	2	2	2	3	2
Miscellaneous**	2	2	1	1	1	1	2	1	2	2
Average daily intake (mg)	22.8	26.0	30.0	36.6	29.1	20.4	23.4	24.6	25.2	23.6
Total number of young people	184	256	237	179	856	171	226	238	210	845

*Includes soft drinks, alcoholic drinks, tea, coffee & water.
** Includes powdered beverages (except tea and coffee), soups, sauces and condiments and commercial toddlers' foods.

239

Table 8.21 Average daily intake of vitamin B₆ (mg) by sex and age of young person

Vitamin B₆ (mg)	Males aged (years)				All males	Females aged (years)				All females
	4–6	7–10	11–14	15–18		4–6	7–10	11–14	15–18	
	cum %	cum %	cum %	cum %	cum %	cum %	cum %	cum %	cum %	cum %
(a) Intakes from *all* sources										
Less than 0.6	–	–	1	–	0	–	0	0	–	0
Less than 0.7	–	–	1	–	0	1	0	1	1	1
Less than 0.8	1	–	1	–	0	3	0	1	2	2
Less than 0.9	3	0	3	–	1	5	1	2	5	4
Less than 1.0	4	1	4	0	2	11	1	3	9	6
Less than 1.1	9	2	6	0	3	16	1	7	12	10
Less than 1.2	15	4	11	1	5	25	3	11	18	16
Less than 1.5	36	24	31	5	19	53	15	29	33	35
Less than 2.0	78	59	74	26	50	89	43	64	71	74
Less than 3.0	99	95	97	69	87	99	88	94	96	96
All	100	100	100	100	100	100	100	100	100	100
Base	*184*	*256*	*237*	*179*	*856*	*171*	*226*	*238*	*210*	*845*
Mean (average value)	1.7	2.0	2.2	2.7	2.2	1.6	1.8	1.9	2.0	1.8
Median value	1.7	1.9	2.1	2.4	2.0	1.5	1.7	1.9	1.7	1.7
Lower 2.5 percentile	0.9	1.2	1.2	1.4	1.1	0.8	0.9	0.9	0.8	0.9
Upper 2.5 percentile	2.8	3.4	4.1	5.2	4.3	2.9	3.6	3.5	3.8	3.4
Standard deviation of the mean	0.52	0.57	0.72	1.08	0.85	0.49	0.75	0.68	2.39	1.35
	cum %	cum %	cum %	cum %	cum %	cum %	cum %	cum %	cum %	cum %
(b) Intakes from *food* sources										
Less than 0.6	–	–	0	–	0	–	1	0	–	0
Less than 0.7	–	–	0	–	0	1	1	1	1	1
Less than 0.8	1	–	0	–	0	3	1	1	2	2
Less than 0.9	3	0	1	–	1	5	3	2	5	4
Less than 1.0	4	1	1	0	2	11	4	3	9	6
Less than 1.1	9	2	1	0	3	16	6	7	12	10
Less than 1.2	15	4	3	1	5	25	11	11	18	16
Less than 1.5	36	24	15	5	19	53	31	29	33	35
Less than 2.0	78	59	43	26	50	89	74	64	71	74
Less than 3.0	99	95	88	69	87	99	97	94	96	96
All	100	100	100	100	100	100	100	100	100	100
Base	*184*	*256*	*237*	*179*	*856*	*171*	*226*	*238*	*210*	*845*
Mean (average value)	1.7	1.9	2.2	2.7	2.2	1.5	1.7	1.9	1.8	1.8
Median value	1.7	1.9	2.1	2.4	2.0	1.5	1.7	1.9	1.7	1.7
Lower 2.5 percentile	0.9	1.2	1.2	1.4	1.1	0.8	0.9	0.9	0.8	0.9
Upper 2.5 percentile	2.8	3.4	4.1	5.2	4.3	2.8	3.1	3.4	3.3	3.3
Standard deviation of the mean	0.50	0.55	0.71	1.03	0.82	0.46	0.53	0.65	0.63	0.59

Table 8.22   Average daily intake of vitamin B$_6$ as a percentage of Reference Nutrient Intake (RNI) by sex and age of young person

Sex and age (years) of young person	Average daily intake as % of RNI*							
	(a) All sources			Base	(b) Food sources			Base
	Mean	Median	sd		Mean	Median	sd	
Males								
4–6	191	188	57.5	184	189	188	55.1	184
7–10	196	190	56.9	256	194	190	54.5	256
11–14	183	172	59.9	237	182	172	59.2	237
15–18	182	163	72.3	179	180	163	68.5	179
All	188	180	62.4	856	186	179	60.0	856
Females								
4–6	173	165	54.8	171	169	164	51.4	171
7–10	180	169	74.8	226	174	169	52.6	226
11–14	194	186	67.7	238	190	185	64.8	238
15–18	170	145	199.4	210	150	144	52.1	210
All	179	165	117.1	845	171	164	57.6	845

*Intake as a percentage of RNI was calculated for each young person. The values for all young people in each age group were then pooled to give a mean, median and sd.

Table 8.23 Percentage contribution of food types to average daily intake of vitamin B_6 by sex and age of young person

Type of food	Males aged (years)				All males	Females aged (years)				All females
	4–6	7–10	11–14	15–18		4–6	7–10	11–14	15–18	
	%	%	%	%	%	%	%	%	%	%
Cereals & cereal products	31	32	30	27	30	29	27	27	22	26
of which:										
white bread	2	3	3	3	3	2	3	2	3	3
high fibre & whole grain breakfast cereals	5	6	5	4	5	5	4	5	3	4
other breakfast cereals	16	17	15	14	16	15	13	13	9	12
Milk & milk products	17	14	12	9	12	17	13	10	10	12
of which:										
whole milk	9	5	3	2	4	9	4	2	2	4
semi-skimmed milk	5	5	6	5	5	4	4	4	4	4
Eggs & egg dishes	0	0	1	1	1	1	1	0	1	1
Fat spreads	0	0	0	0	0	0	0	0	0	0
Meat & meat products	12	13	16	18	15	12	15	16	17	15
of which:										
beef, veal & dishes	2	2	2	3	3	2	3	3	3	3
chicken, turkey & dishes including coated	4	5	5	6	5	5	6	7	7	7
Fish & fish dishes	2	2	2	2	2	2	2	2	2	2
Vegetables, potatoes & savoury snacks	27	28	30	29	29	27	31	35	34	32
of which:										
vegetables, excluding potatoes	4	3	4	4	3	4	4	4	6	5
roast or fried potatoes & chips	12	13	15	15	14	12	14	17	15	15
other potatoes	6	7	6	7	7	6	8	8	8	7
savoury snacks	6	5	5	4	5	6	6	6	5	6
Fruit & nuts	5	5	3	2	4	6	5	3	4	4
Sugars, preserves & confectionery	0	1	1	0	0	0	0	0	0	0
Drinks*	4	4	4	11	6	4	5	4	6	5
of which:										
beers & lagers	0	0	0	6	2	0	0	0	3	1
Miscellaneous**	1	1	1	1	1	1	1	1	2	1
Average daily intake (mg)	1.7	1.9	2.2	2.7	2.2	1.5	1.7	1.9	1.8	1.8
Total number of young people	184	256	237	179	856	171	226	238	210	845

*Includes soft drinks, alcoholic drinks, tea, coffee & water.
** Includes powdered beverages (except tea and coffee), soups, sauces and condiments and commercial toddlers' foods.

242

Vitamin B$_{12}$ (µg)	Males aged (years)				All males	Females aged (years)				All females
	4–6	7–10	11–14	15–18		4–6	7–10	11–14	15–18	
	cum %	cum %	cum %	cum %	cum %	cum %	cum %	cum %	cum %	cum %
(a) Intakes from *all* sources										
Less than 0.5	–	–	–	–	–	–	0	–	0	0
Less than 0.6	–	–	0	–	0	–	1	–	1	0
Less than 0.8	–	–	0	–	0	0	1	1	1	1
Less than 1.0	–	0	1	–	0	0	2	2	2	2
Less than 1.2	1	1	1	–	1	1	3	3	4	3
Less than 1.5	1	2	3	1	2	2	6	9	10	7
Less than 3.0	26	29	22	17	24	39	40	50	48	45
Less than 4.5	71	68	62	48	62	76	79	80	77	79
Less than 6.0	90	91	84	72	84	92	96	94	94	94
All	100	100	100	100	100	100	100	100	100	100
Base	*184*	*256*	*237*	*179*	*856*	*171*	*226*	*238*	*210*	*845*
Mean (average value)	4.0	4.0	4.5	5.0	4.4	3.6	3.5	3.3	3.4	3.4
Median value	3.8	3.8	4.0	4.6	4.0	3.4	3.4	3.0	3.1	3.2
Lower 2.5 percentile	1.6	1.6	1.4	2.1	1.6	1.6	1.2	1.1	1.1	1.2
Upper 2.5 percentile	8.5	7.8	9.3	10.0	9.0	7.6	6.9	7.2	7.6	7.3
Standard deviation of the mean	1.66	1.54	2.72	2.10	2.11	1.46	1.50	1.62	1.99	1.67
	cum %	cum %	cum %	cum %	cum %	cum %	cum %	cum %	cum %	cum %
(b) Intakes from *food* sources										
Less than 0.5	–	–	–	–	–	–	0	–	0	0
Less than 0.6	–	–	0	–	0	–	1	–	1	0
Less than 0.8	–	–	0	–	0	0	1	1	1	1
Less than 1.0	–	0	1	–	0	0	2	2	2	2
Less than 1.2	1	1	1	–	1	1	3	4	4	3
Less than 1.5	1	2	3	1	2	2	6	10	10	7
Less than 3.0	26	29	22	17	24	40	41	51	50	46
Less than 4.5	71	68	62	48	62	78	80	81	78	79
Less than 6.0	90	92	94	72	84	93	96	95	94	95
All	100	100	100	100	100	100	100	100	100	100
Base	*184*	*256*	*237*	*179*	*856*	*171*	*226*	*238*	*210*	*845*
Mean (average value)	4.0	3.9	4.5	5.0	4.4	3.6	3.5	3.2	3.4	3.4
Median value	3.8	3.7	4.0	4.6	4.0	3.4	3.4	3.0	3.0	3.2
Lower 2.5 percentile	1.6	1.6	1.4	2.1	1.6	1.6	1.2	1.1	1.1	1.2
Upper 2.5 percentile	8.3	7.8	9.3	9.5	8.6	7.6	6.9	7.1	7.3	7.2
Standard deviation of the mean	1.62	1.52	2.72	2.04	2.09	1.44	1.49	1.59	1.95	1.64

243

Table 8.25   Average daily intake of vitamin B$_{12}$ as a percentage of Reference Nutrient Intake (RNI) by sex and age of young person

Sex and age (years) of young person	Average daily intake as % of RNI*							
	(a) All sources			*Base*	(b) Food sources			*Base*
	Mean	Median	sd		Mean	Median	sd	
Males								
4–6	502	474	206.9	*184*	499	474	202.2	*184*
7–10	397	376	154.0	*256*	395	375	151.8	*256*
11–14	373	331	226.8	*237*	372	329	227.0	*237*
15–18	333	306	139.7	*179*	330	306	136.3	*179*
All	396	364	193.0	*856*	394	363	190.9	*856*
Females								
4–6	453	423	182.2	*171*	446	422	180.5	*171*
7–10	349	339	149.7	*226*	347	338	149.4	*226*
11–14	273	250	135.4	*238*	270	248	132.5	*238*
15–18	229	207	132.6	*210*	225	203	130.0	*210*
All	320	292	170.1	*845*	316	289	168.2	*845*

*Intake as a percentage of RNI was calculated for each young person. The values for all young people in each age group were then pooled to give a mean, median and sd.

Table 8.26   Percentage contribution of food types to average daily intake of vitamin B$_{12}$ by sex and age of young person

Type of food	Males aged (years)				All males	Females aged (years)				All females
	4–6	7–10	11–14	15–18		4–6	7–10	11–14	15–18	
	%	%	%	%	%	%	%	%	%	%
Cereals & cereal products	12	14	12	12	12	11	12	14	11	12
Milk & milk products	57	52	45	39	47	58	46	41	38	46
of which:										
whole milk	*33*	*21*	*13*	*11*	*18*	*34*	*18*	*12*	*11*	*19*
semi-skimmed milk	*16*	*23*	*26*	*22*	*22*	*14*	*18*	*21*	*19*	*18*
Eggs & egg dishes	3	4	5	5	4	4	5	4	5	4
Fat spreads	0	0	0	0	0	0	0	0	0	0
Meat & meat products	17	20	26	28	23	16	23	27	26	23
of which:										
liver & liver dishes	*1*	*1*	*5*	*1*	*2*	*2*	*2*	*2*	*4*	*2*
beef, veal & dishes	*4*	*4*	*4*	*7*	*5*	*3*	*6*	*7*	*7*	*6*
burgers & kebabs	*2*	*3*	*4*	*6*	*4*	*2*	*3*	*5*	*4*	*4*
Fish & fish dishes	6	7	7	8	7	7	9	8	12	9
of which:										
oily fish	*3*	*3*	*4*	*4*	*3*	*3*	*4*	*4*	*7*	*5*
Vegetables, potatoes & savoury snacks	2	1	1	1	1	1	1	1	2	1
Fruit & nuts	0	0	0	0	0	0	0	0	0	0
Sugars, preserves & confectionery	1	1	1	1	1	1	1	1	1	1
Drinks*	1	2	1	5	3	1	2	2	2	2
Miscellaneous**	1	1	1	1	1	1	1	1	1	1
Average daily intake (µg)	**4.0**	**3.9**	**4.5**	**5.0**	**4.4**	**3.6**	**3.5**	**3.2**	**3.4**	**3.4**
Total number of young people	184	256	237	179	856	171	226	238	210	845

*Includes soft drinks, alcoholic drinks, tea, coffee & water.
** Includes powdered beverages (except tea and coffee), soups, sauces and condiments and commercial toddlers' foods.

Table 8.27   Average daily intake of folate (µg) by sex and age of young person

Folate (µg)	Males aged (years)				All males	Females aged (years)				All females
	4–6	7–10	11–14	15–18		4–6	7–10	11–14	15–18	
	cum %	cum %	cum %	cum %	cum %	cum %	cum %	cum %	cum %	cum %
(a) Intakes from *all* sources										
Less than 50	–	–	–	–	–	–	–	1	–	0
Less than 75	1	–	0	–	0	1	2	1	1	1
Less than 100	4	1	1	–	1	5	4	3	4	4
Less than 150	21	13	9	5	12	41	22	23	22	26
Less than 200	60	48	33	18	39	78	60	50	52	59
Less than 250	84	76	57	37	63	94	88	74	72	82
Less than 300	94	92	74	54	78	97	96	89	85	91
Less than 400	100	99	97	78	93	99	100	98	97	98
All		100	100	100	100	100		100	100	100
Base	*184*	*256*	*237*	*179*	*856*	*171*	*226*	*238*	*210*	*845*
Mean (average value)	192	213	247	309	242	171	190	210	215	197
Median value	185	203	234	284	222	162	187	200	197	188
Lower 2.5 percentile	93	123	114	130	109	89	93	90	88	90
Upper 2.5 percentile	350	373	405	615	480	317	341	398	402	370
Standard deviation of the mean	61.0	61.1	81.0	123.5	96.6	55.6	57.0	83.5	81.9	73.0
	cum %	cum %	cum %	cum %	cum %	cum %	cum %	cum %	cum %	cum %
(b) Intakes from *food* sources										
Less than 50	–	–	–	–	–	–	–	1	–	0
Less than 75	1	–	0	–	0	1	2	1	1	1
Less than 100	4	1	1	–	1	6	4	3	4	4
Less than 150	21	13	9	5	12	42	23	23	22	27
Less than 200	61	48	33	18	39	79	61	51	53	60
Less than 250	85	77	58	37	64	94	89	75	74	83
Less than 300	94	93	75	55	79	97	96	90	87	93
Less than 400	100	100	97	79	94	99	100	100	98	99
All			100	100	100	100		100	100	100
Base	*184*	*256*	*237*	*179*	*856*	*171*	*226*	*238*	*210*	*845*
Mean (average value)	191	212	245	305	240	169	188	205	210	194
Median value	184	203	234	283	221	159	186	198	197	187
Lower 2.5 percentile	93	123	114	130	109	89	93	90	88	90
Upper 2.5 percentile	350	348	405	615	478	317	320	353	383	349
Standard deviation of the mean	60.7	58.4	80.8	118.7	94.0	54.9	54.2	73.1	76.9	67.7

Table 8.28   Average daily intake of folate as a percentage of Reference Nutrient Intake (RNI) by sex and age of young person

Sex and age (years) of young person	Average daily intake as % of RNI*							
	(a) All sources			*Base*	(b) Food sources			*Base*
	Mean	Median	sd		Mean	Median	sd	
Males								
4–6	192	185	61	*184*	191	184	61	*184*
7–10	142	136	41	*256*	141	135	39	*256*
11–14	123	117	40	*237*	123	117	40	*237*
15–18	154	142	62	*179*	152	142	59	*179*
All	151	142	57	*856*	149	141	55	*856*
Females								
4–6	171	162	56	*171*	169	159	55	*171*
7–10	127	125	38	*226*	126	124	36	*226*
11–14	105	100	42	*238*	102	99	36	*238*
15–18	107	98	41	*210*	105	98	38	*210*
All	125	119	50	*845*	123	117	48	*845*

*Intake as a percentage of RNI was calculated for each young person. The values for all young people in each age group were then pooled—give a mean, median and sd.

245

Table 8.29 Percentage contribution of food types to average daily intake of folate by sex and age of young person

Type of food	Males aged (years)				All males	Females aged (years)				All females
	4–6	7–10	11–14	15–18		4–6	7–10	11–14	15–18	
	%	%	%	%	%	%	%	%	%	%
Cereals & cereal products	44	45	45	41	44	40	38	38	34	37
of which:										
white bread	5	6	6	6	6	5	6	6	6	6
wholemeal & other bread	3	2	3	3	3	3	3	2	4	3
high fibre & whole grain breakfast cereals	8	8	8	6	7	8	7	6	4	6
other breakfast cereals	20	20	18	17	18	17	15	15	10	14
Milk & milk products	15	13	12	9	12	17	13	10	10	12
of which:										
whole milk	7	4	2	2	3	7	3	2	2	3
semi-skimmed milk	4	5	6	5	5	4	4	4	4	4
Eggs & egg dishes	1	1	1	1	1	2	2	1	1	2
Fat spreads	0	0	0	0	0	0	0	0	0	0
Meat & meat products	5	5	6	7	6	5	6	6	6	6
Fish & fish dishes	1	1	1	1	1	1	1	1	1	1
Vegetables, potatoes & savoury snacks	23	24	24	25	24	24	28	30	30	28
of which:										
vegetables, excluding potatoes	9	9	9	10	9	11	11	12	15	12
roast or fried potatoes & chips	7	7	8	9	8	6	8	10	8	8
other potatoes	4	5	4	5	4	4	6	5	5	5
savoury snacks	3	3	2	2	2	3	3	3	2	3
Fruit & nuts	3	3	2	2	2	3	4	2	3	3
Sugars, preserves & confectionery	1	1	1	1	1	1	1	1	1	1
Drinks*	4	4	4	11	6	5	5	5	9	6
of which:										
fruit juice	3	3	3	3	3	4	4	4	4	4
beers & lagers	0	0	0	6	2	0	0	0	3	1
Miscellaneous**	2	3	2	2	2	2	3	3	4	3
Average daily intake (µg)	191	212	245	305	240	169	188	205	210	194
Total number of young people	184	256	237	179	856	171	226	238	210	845

*Includes soft drinks, alcoholic drinks, tea, coffee & water.
** Includes powdered beverages (except tea and coffee), soups, sauces and condiments and commercial toddlers' foods.

246

Table 8.30   Average daily intake of biotin (µg) by sex and age of young person

Biotin (µg)	Males aged (years)				All males	Females aged (years)				All females
	4–6	7–10	11–14	15–18		4–6	7–10	11–14	15–18	
	cum %	cum %	cum %	cum %	cum %	cum %	cum %	cum %	cum %	cum %
(a) Intakes from *all* sources										
Less than 10	5	2	3	2	3	4	3	6	6	5
Less than 15	20	11	13	8	13	27	20	32	22	25
Less than 20	48	40	30	22	35	58	52	51	45	51
Less than 25	74	62	55	44	58	82	81	76	73	78
Less than 30	84	79	74	59	73	94	91	90	86	90
Less than 40	97	96	94	86	93	99	98	96	98	98
All	100	100	100	100	100	100	100	100	100	100
Base	*184*	*256*	*237*	*179*	*856*	*171*	*226*	*238*	*210*	*845*
Mean (average value)	22	24	25	29	25	19	21	21	21	21
Median value	20	22	24	27	23	18	20	20	21	20
Lower 2.5 percentile	8	11	9	12	10	8	7	9	9	9
Upper 2.5 percentile	43	50	51	57	52	32	40	44	40	40
Standard deviation of the mean	8.3	10.9	10.9	11.7	10.9	6.6	12.5	12.7	8.4	10.6
	cum %	cum %	cum %	cum %	cum %	cum %	cum %	cum %	cum %	cum %
(b) Intakes from *food* sources										
Less than 10	5	2	3	2	3	4	3	6	6	5
Less than 15	20	11	13	8	13	27	21	32	22	25
Less than 20	48	40	30	22	35	58	52	51	45	51
Less than 25	74	62	55	44	58	82	82	76	74	78
Less than 30	84	79	74	59	73	94	92	90	86	90
Less than 40	97	96	94	86	93	99	98	97	98	98
All	100	100	100	100	100	100	100	100	100	100
Base	*184*	*256*	*237*	*179*	*856*	*171*	*226*	*238*	*210*	*845*
Mean (average value)	22	24	25	29	25	19	20	20	21	20
Median value	20	22	24	27	23	18	19	20	21	20
Lower 2.5 percentile	8	11	9	12	10	8	7	9	9	8
Upper 2.5 percentile	43	41	51	57	51	32	39	42	40	40
Standard deviation of the mean	8.3	8.3	10.9	11.6	10.2	6.6	7.0	8.4	8.4	7.7

Table 8.31 Average daily intake of pantothenic acid (mg) by sex and age of young person

Pantothenic acid (mg)	Males aged (years)				All males	Females aged (years)				All females
	4–6	7–10	11–14	15–18		4–6	7–10	11–14	15–18	
	cum %	cum %	cum %	cum %	cum %	cum %	cum %	cum %	cum %	cum %
(a) Intakes from _all_ sources										
Less than 2.5	6	1	5	0	3	8	6	9	10	8
Less than 3.0	16	5	9	3	8	23	13	21	23	20
Less than 3.5	28	18	15	8	17	37	30	37	37	35
Less than 4.5	60	48	39	31	44	69	64	63	66	65
Less than 5.5	81	75	60	52	66	84	88	85	87	86
Less than 7.5	97	95	89	79	90	99	99	97	96	98
All	100	100	100	100	100	100	100	100	100	100
Base	_184_	_256_	_237_	_179_	_856_	_171_	_226_	_238_	_210_	_845_
Mean (average value)	4.4	4.8	5.2	5.8	5.1	4.1	4.2	4.2	4.1	4.1
Median value	4.2	4.6	4.9	5.5	4.8	3.9	4.0	4.0	4.0	4.0
Lower 2.5 percentile	2.1	2.8	2.1	2.7	2.4	2.1	2.3	1.8	1.6	1.9
Upper 2.5 percentile	8.0	7.7	9.2	10.8	9.3	7.4	7.0	7.6	8.9	7.4
Standard deviation of the mean	1.55	1.36	1.76	2.06	1.78	1.39	1.18	1.51	1.60	1.43
	cum %	cum %	cum %	cum %	cum %	cum %	cum %	cum %	cum %	cum %
(b) Intakes from _food_ sources										
Less than 2.5	6	1	5	0	3	8	7	9	10	9
Less than 3.0	16	5	9	3	8	24	13	21	23	20
Less than 3.5	28	18	15	8	17	37	31	38	38	36
Less than 4.5	60	48	39	31	44	70	64	63	67	66
Less than 5.5	81	75	60	52	66	85	89	85	89	87
Less than 7.5	98	96	89	79	90	100	100	97	97	98
All	100	100	100	100	100			100	100	100
Base	_184_	_256_	_237_	_179_	_856_	_171_	_226_	_238_	_210_	_845_
Mean (average value)	4.4	4.7	5.2	5.8	5.1	4.0	4.1	4.2	4.0	4.1
Median value	4.2	4.6	4.9	5.4	4.8	3.9	4.0	4.0	4.0	4.0
Lower 2.5 percentile	2.1	2.8	2.1	2.7	2.4	2.1	2.3	1.8	1.6	1.9
Upper 2.5 percentile	7.5	7.6	9.2	10.8	9.2	6.9	6.7	7.6	7.7	7.1
Standard deviation of the mean	1.41	1.33	1.76	2.06	1.76	1.28	1.12	1.50	1.42	1.34

Table 8.32 Average daily intake of vitamin C (mg) by sex and age of young person

Vitamin C (mg)	Males aged (years)				All males	Females aged (years)				All females
	4–6	7–10	11–14	15–18		4–6	7–10	11–14	15–18	
	cum %	cum %	cum %	cum %	cum %	cum %	cum %	cum %	cum %	cum %
(a) Intakes from *all* sources										
Less than 8.0	–	–	–	–	–	0	–	–	0	0
Less than 9.0	–	–	–	–	–	0	–	1	0	0
Less than 10.0	–	–	–	–	–	0	–	1	0	0
Less than 30.0	8	8	11	9	9	9	9	10	12	10
Less than 35.0	16	13	14	17	15	14	13	20	20	17
Less than 40.0	22	19	22	20	21	18	18	26	26	22
Less than 60.0	47	46	46	46	46	49	43	51	46	47
Less than 80.0	66	67	67	60	65	67	64	67	65	66
Less than 100.0	82	78	78	73	78	84	76	81	76	79
All	100	100	100	100	100	100	100	100	100	100
Base	*184*	*256*	*237*	*179*	*856*	*171*	*226*	*238*	*210*	*845*
Mean (average value)	74.2	77.1	78.4	86.5	79.3	69.1	78.9	73.7	81.2	76.1
Median value	63.8	64.9	63.0	66.9	64.6	60.6	68.5	59.4	65.0	63.1
Lower 2.5 percentile	19.3	23.9	24.2	21.0	20.8	19.7	19.3	17.4	20.2	19.6
Upper 2.5 percentile	195.9	235.0	215.4	292.3	258.1	163.9	216.2	230.6	207.5	202.8
Standard deviation of the mean	53.66	51.60	52.90	68.72	57.38	34.82	56.41	56.07	74.72	58.32
	cum %	cum %	cum %	cum %	cum %	cum %	cum %	cum %	cum %	cum %
(b) Intakes from *food* sources										
Less than 8.0	–	–	–	–	–	0	–	–	0	0
Less than 9.0	–	–	–	–	–	0	–	1	0	0
Less than 10.0	–	–	–	–	–	0	–	1	0	0
Less than 30.0	8	9	11	9	10	9	10	10	13	10
Less than 35.0	16	15	14	17	16	14	13	20	20	17
Less than 40.0	24	21	22	20	22	18	19	26	26	22
Less than 60.0	52	50	48	47	49	53	45	52	47	49
Less than 80.0	72	72	70	61	68	77	67	68	66	69
Less than 100.0	85	80	79	76	80	89	78	84	78	82
All	100	100	100	100	100	100	100	100	100	100
Base	*184*	*256*	*237*	*179*	*856*	*171*	*226*	*238*	*210*	*845*
Mean (average value)	67.0	72.8	76.3	83.3	75.2	65.2	73.5	70.8	74.0	71.2
Median value	59.3	59.8	60.6	65.8	60.9	57.8	65.1	59.2	62.3	60.6
Lower 2.5 percentile	19.3	23.9	24.2	21.0	20.7	19.7	19.3	17.4	20.2	19.3
Upper 2.5 percentile	159.6	206.2	215.4	292.3	219.3	161.6	180.7	198.5	206.3	188.7
Standard deviation of the mean	38.35	45.67	51.27	65.03	51.82	32.52	41.31	46.28	49.68	43.48

Table 8.33 Average daily intake of vitamin C as a percentage of Reference Nutrient Intake (RNI) by sex and age of young person

Sex and age (years) of young person	Average daily intake as % of RNI*							
	(a) All sources			*Base*	(b) Food sources			*Base*
	Mean	Median	sd		Mean	Median	sd	
Males								
4–6	247	212	178.9	*184*	223	198	127.8	*184*
7–10	257	216	172.0	*256*	243	199	152.2	*256*
11–14	224	180	151.1	*237*	218	173	146.5	*237*
15–18	216	167	171.8	*179*	208	165	162.6	*179*
All	236	190	169.0	*856*	223	184	149.4	*856*
Females								
4–6	230	202	116.1	*171*	217	193	108.4	*171*
7–10	263	228	188.0	*226*	245	217	137.7	*226*
11–14	210	170	160.2	*238*	202	169	132.2	*238*
15–18	203	163	186.8	*210*	185	156	124.2	*210*
All	227	190	169.5	*845*	213	184	129.1	*845*

*Intake as a percentage of RNI was calculated for each young person. The values for all young people in each age group were then pooled to give a mean, median and sd.

Table 8.34 Percentage contribution of food types to average daily intake of vitamin C by sex and age of young person

Type of food	Males aged (years)				All males	Females aged (years)				All females
	4–6	7–10	11–14	15–18		4–6	7–10	11–14	15–18	
	%	%	%	%	%	%	%	%	%	%
Cereals & cereal products	3	4	4	4	4	3	3	4	4	4
Milk & milk products	8	7	7	5	7	7	5	5	4	5
of which:										
milk (whole, semi-skimmed, skimmed)	*7*	*6*	*6*	*5*	*6*	*6*	*4*	*4*	*3*	*4*
Eggs & egg dishes	0	0	0	0	0	0	0	0	0	0
Fat spreads	0	0	0	0	0	0	0	0	0	0
Meat & meat products	3	3	4	5	4	2	3	3	3	3
Fish & fish dishes	0	0	0	0	0	0	0	0	0	0
Vegetables, potatoes & savoury snacks	23	24	27	32	27	23	25	31	32	28
of which:										
vegetables, excluding potatoes	*7*	*8*	*8*	*11*	*9*	*9*	*9*	*10*	*15*	*11*
roast or fried potatoes & chips	*9*	*10*	*13*	*14*	*12*	*8*	*10*	*13*	*11*	*11*
other potatoes	*5*	*5*	*6*	*6*	*5*	*5*	*6*	*6*	*6*	*6*
savoury snacks	*1*	*1*	*1*	*1*	*1*	*1*	*1*	*1*	*1*	*1*
Fruit & nuts	12	13	8	8	10	14	15	11	13	13
Sugars, preserves & confectionery	0	0	0	0	0	0	0	0	0	0
Drinks*	50	48	48	44	47	50	48	45	41	46
of which:										
fruit juice	*18*	*19*	*22*	*26*	*22*	*20*	*19*	*23*	*26*	*22*
soft drinks, including low calorie	*32*	*29*	*26*	*17*	*25*	*30*	*29*	*22*	*15*	*24*
Miscellaneous**	0	0	0	0	0	0	0	0	1	0
Average daily intake (mg)	**67.0**	**72.8**	**76.3**	**83.3**	**75.2**	**65.2**	**73.5**	**70.8**	**74.0**	**71.2**
Total number of young people	**184**	**256**	**237**	**179**	**856**	**171**	**226**	**238**	**210**	**845**

*Includes soft drinks, alcoholic drinks, tea, coffee & water.
** Includes powdered beverages (except tea and coffee), soups, sauces and condiments and commercial toddlers' foods.

250

Table 8.35　Average daily intake of vitamin D (µg) by sex and age of young person

Vitamin D (µg)	Males aged (years)				All males	Females aged (years)				All females
	4–6	7–10	11–14	15–18		4–6	7–10	11–14	15–18	
	cum %	cum %	cum %	cum %	cum %	cum %	cum %	cum %	cum %	cum %
(a) Intakes from *all* sources										
Less than 0.5	1	2	1	-	1	1	2	2	1	2
Less than 1.0	10	5	6	2	6	17	9	13	13	13
Less than 1.5	27	17	16	12	17	36	31	29	34	32
Less than 2.0	47	39	32	22	34	55	51	49	52	52
Less than 3.0	74	71	66	53	66	80	78	81	79	80
Less than 5.0	94	93	93	84	91	97	97	97	96	97
All	100	100	100	100	100	100	100	100	100	100
Base	*184*	*256*	*237*	*179*	*856*	*171*	*226*	*238*	*210*	*845*
Mean (average value)	2.5	2.7	2.7	3.3	2.8	2.2	2.3	2.3	2.2	2.2
Median value	2.1	2.5	2.5	2.9	2.5	1.8	2.0	2.0	1.9	2.0
Lower 2.5 percentile	0.7	0.8	0.8	1.0	0.8	0.5	0.5	0.6	0.5	0.6
Upper 2.5 percentile	5.9	7.5	5.7	7.6	6.7	5.7	5.8	5.8	6.2	5.8
Standard deviation of the mean	1.67	1.54	1.31	1.74	1.59	1.28	1.39	1.32	1.33	1.33
	cum %	cum %	cum %	cum %	cum %	cum %	cum %	cum %	cum %	cum %
(b) Intakes from *food* sources										
Less than 0.5	1	2	1	-	1	2	2	2	1	2
Less than 1.0	12	7	6	3	7	20	10	15	13	14
Less than 1.5	31	20	17	12	20	42	32	31	34	34
Less than 2.0	54	43	34	23	38	64	55	50	53	55
Less than 3.0	87	77	70	54	71	90	84	83	81	84
Less than 5.0	97	97	94	85	93	100	99	98	97	98
All	100	100	100	100	100		100	100	100	100
Base	*184*	*256*	*237*	*179*	*856*	*171*	*226*	*238*	*210*	*845*
Mean (average value)	2.1	2.4	2.6	3.2	2.6	1.8	2.1	2.2	2.1	2.1
Median value	1.9	2.3	2.4	2.9	2.4	1.7	1.9	2.0	1.9	1.9
Lower 2.5 percentile	0.7	0.7	0.8	1.0	0.8	0.5	0.5	0.6	0.5	0.5
Upper 2.5 percentile	5.3	5.0	5.7	7.6	5.8	3.7	4.3	4.7	5.4	4.5
Standard deviation of the mean	1.24	1.14	1.27	1.68	1.41	0.91	1.16	1.16	1.16	1.12

Table 8.36 Percentage contribution of food types to average daily intake of vitamin D by sex and age of young person

Type of food	Males aged (years)				All males	Females aged (years)				All females
	4–6	7–10	11–14	15–18		4–6	7–10	11–14	15–18	
	%	%	%	%	%	%	%	%	%	%
Cereals & cereal products	40	42	35	34	37	38	34	37	30	35
of which:										
breakfast cereals	*25*	*26*	*22*	*25*	*24*	*23*	*19*	*23*	*17*	*20*
buns, cakes & pastries	*10*	*11*	*8*	*6*	*8*	*10*	*9*	*10*	*7*	*9*
Milk & milk products	3	2	2	3	2	3	2	2	3	2
Eggs & egg dishes	5	6	7	7	7	8	7	6	7	7
Fat spreads	20	23	21	19	21	23	21	22	22	22
of which:										
soft margarine, not poly- unsaturated	*3*	*3*	*4*	*4*	*3*	*4*	*4*	*4*	*5*	*4*
low fat spreads	*3*	*5*	*5*	*3*	*4*	*3*	*4*	*6*	*4*	*4*
reduced fat spreads	*12*	*13*	*11*	*10*	*12*	*14*	*11*	*11*	*11*	*11*
Meat & meat products	19	19	22	26	22	18	21	21	21	20
of which:										
sausages	*6*	*5*	*4*	*4*	*5*	*4*	*4*	*4*	*3*	*4*
meat pies & pastries	*3*	*2*	*3*	*3*	*3*	*2*	*3*	*3*	*2*	*3*
chicken, turkey & dishes including coated	*4*	*4*	*4*	*5*	*4*	*4*	*4*	*4*	*5*	*4*
Fish & fish dishes	8	6	9	9	8	8	11	7	13	10
of which:										
oily fish	*7*	*5*	*9*	*8*	*7*	*7*	*11*	*7*	*12*	*9*
Vegetables, potatoes & savoury snacks	2	2	1	2	2	1	2	2	2	2
Fruit & nuts	0	0	0	0	0	0	0	0	0	0
Sugars, preserves & confectionery	0	0	0	0	0	0	0	0	0	0
Drinks*	0	0	0	0	0	0	0	0	0	0
Miscellaneous**	3	0	1	1	1	0	1	1	1	1
Average daily intake (µg)	**2.1**	**2.4**	**2.6**	**3.2**	**2.6**	**1.8**	**2.1**	**2.2**	**2.1**	**2.1**
Total number of young people	**184**	**256**	**237**	**179**	**856**	**171**	**226**	**238**	**210**	**845**

*Includes soft drinks, alcoholic drinks, tea, coffee & water.
** Includes powdered beverages (except tea and coffee), soups, sauces and condiments and commercial toddlers' foods.

Table 8.37 Average daily intake of vitamin E (α-tocopherol equivalents) (mg) by sex and age of young person

Vitamin E (α-tocopherol equivalents) (mg)	Males aged (years)				All males	Females aged (years)				All females
	4–6	7–10	11–14	15–18		4–6	7–10	11–14	15–18	
	cum %	cum %	cum %	cum %	cum %	cum %	cum %	cum %	cum %	cum %
(a) Intakes from *all* sources										
Less than 3.0	0	0	1	–	1	2	1	1	2	1
Less than 4.0	12	3	3	1	4	10	4	4	9	6
Less than 5.0	21	11	6	5	10	26	14	13	16	17
Less than 6.0	43	23	13	9	21	50	30	24	30	33
Less than 7.0	60	42	28	18	36	67	47	39	45	48
Less than 8.0	71	53	41	30	48	80	60	56	56	62
Less than 10.0	91	77	68	56	72	91	82	76	71	80
Less than 15.0	98	96	95	88	94	97	96	98	97	97
All	100	100	100	100	100	100	100	100	100	100
Base	*184*	*256*	*237*	*179*	*856*	*171*	*226*	*238*	*210*	*845*
Mean (average value)	7.2	8.3	9.1	10.3	8.8	6.6	7.8	8.2	8.6	7.8
Median value	6.3	7.5	8.6	9.3	8.2	6.0	7.2	7.6	7.5	7.1
Lower 2.5 percentile	3.3	4.0	3.5	4.4	3.5	3.2	3.8	3.8	3.3	3.4
Upper 2.5 percentile	14.7	18.3	16.5	19.6	18.5	16.3	15.7	15.5	16.1	15.7
Standard deviation of the mean	5.05	3.32	3.32	4.09	4.09	2.80	3.04	3.08	7.21	4.53
	cum %	cum %	cum %	cum %	cum %	cum %	cum %	cum %	cum %	cum %
(b) Intakes from *food* sources										
Less than 3.0	0	0	1	1	1	2	1	1	2	1
Less than 4.0	12	3	3	1	4	10	5	4	9	7
Less than 5.0	21	11	6	5	10	29	15	13	16	18
Less than 6.0	44	24	13	10	22	54	31	24	31	34
Less than 7.0	62	43	28	18	36	72	48	40	47	50
Less than 8.0	73	54	41	31	48	84	61	57	57	64
Less than 10.0	94	78	68	56	73	95	84	78	73	82
Less than 15.0	100	97	95	88	95	100	97	98	97	97
All		100	100	100	100		100	100	100	100
Base	*184*	*256*	*237*	*179*	*856*	*171*	*226*	*238*	*210*	*845*
Mean (average value)	6.6	8.1	9.1	10.3	8.6	6.3	7.6	8.1	8.1	7.6
Median value	6.2	7.5	8.6	9.3	8.1	5.7	7.1	7.5	7.2	7.0
Lower 2.5 percentile	3.3	4.0	3.5	4.4	3.4	3.2	3.8	3.8	3.3	3.4
Upper 2.5 percentile	12.4	15.8	16.5	19.6	17.8	11.2	15.3	15.0	16.1	15.3
Standard deviation of the mean	2.26	2.97	3.32	4.09	3.51	2.47	2.82	2.97	3.39	3.04

253

Table 8.38   Percentage contribution of food types to average daily intake of vitamin E by sex and age of young person

Type of food	Males aged (years)				All males	Females aged (years)				All females
	4–6	7–10	11–14	15–18		4–6	7–10	11–14	15–18	
	%	%	%	%	%	%	%	%	%	%
Cereals & cereal products	17	18	17	17	17	17	16	15	14	15
of which:										
breakfast cereals	*4*	*4*	*3*	*4*	*4*	*3*	*2*	*2*	*2*	*2*
biscuits	*5*	*5*	*4*	*3*	*4*	*5*	*5*	*4*	*2*	*4*
buns, cakes & pastries	*5*	*5*	*4*	*3*	*4*	*4*	*4*	*4*	*3*	*4*
Milk & milk products	5	4	4	3	4	5	4	3	3	4
Eggs & egg dishes	2	2	2	3	2	2	2	2	2	2
Fat spreads	23	24	22	21	23	23	22	22	21	22
of which:										
polyunsaturated low fat spreads	*3*	*6*	*4*	*2*	*4*	*3*	*3*	*4*	*4*	*3*
polyunsaturated reduced fat spreads	*15*	*13*	*12*	*11*	*13*	*14*	*14*	*12*	*12*	*13*
Meat & meat products	9	9	10	12	10	8	9	9	10	9
of which:										
chicken, turkey & dishes including coated	*4*	*4*	*4*	*5*	*4*	*4*	*4*	*4*	*5*	*4*
Fish & fish dishes	2	2	2	3	2	3	2	2	3	2
Vegetables, potatoes & savoury snacks	30	28	29	28	29	30	30	34	30	31
of which:										
vegetables, excluding potatoes	*6*	*5*	*5*	*7*	*6*	*6*	*6*	*7*	*11*	*8*
roast or fried potatoes & chips	*9*	*9*	*12*	*12*	*11*	*9*	*10*	*12*	*9*	*10*
other potatoes	*2*	*2*	*2*	*2*	*2*	*2*	*2*	*2*	*2*	*2*
savoury snacks	*13*	*11*	*10*	*8*	*10*	*13*	*12*	*13*	*8*	*11*
Fruit & nuts	4	4	3	2	3	4	4	3	3	3
Sugars, preserves & confectionery	4	6	7	6	6	4	4	6	5	5
Drinks*	1	1	1	1	1	1	1	1	1	1
Miscellaneous**	3	3	3	4	3	3	3	4	7	4
Average daily intake (mg)	**6.6**	**8.1**	**9.1**	**10.3**	**8.6**	**6.3**	**7.6**	**8.1**	**8.1**	**7.6**
Total number of young people	**184**	**256**	**237**	**179**	**856**	**171**	**226**	**238**	**210**	**845**

*Includes soft drinks, alcoholic drinks, tea, coffee & water.
** Includes powdered beverages (except tea and coffee), soups, sauces and condiments and commercial toddlers' foods.

Table 8.39 Average daily intake of vitamins by whether young person reported taking dietary supplements during the dietary recording period

Vitamins	Whether young person reported taking any dietary supplements								
	(a) Not taking supplements			(b) Taking supplements					
	Intake from food sources			Intake from all sources			Intake from food sources		
	Mean	Median	sd	Mean	Median	sd	Mean	Median	sd
Males									
Pre-formed retinol (µg)	303	252	344.7	501	410	337.9	303	272	210.8
Total carotene (β-carotene equivalents) (µg)	1400	1109	1100	1458	1132	1284	1458	1132	1284
Vitamin A (retinol equivalents) (µg)	536	460	402.5	744	654	406.5	546	474	310.7
Thiamin (mg)	1.56	1.45	0.581	1.80	1.50	1.535	1.72	1.47	1.494
Riboflavin (mg)	1.70	1.55	0.710	1.88	1.75	0.794	1.79	1.69	0.722
Niacin equivalents (mg)	29.1	28.0	9.64	29.8	27.4	9.94	29.1	27.2	9.18
Vitamin B_6 (mg)	2.1	2.0	0.80	2.3	2.0	1.00	2.2	2.0	0.87
Vitamin B_{12} (µg)	4.3	3.9	2.10	4.7	4.2	2.15	4.6	4.2	2.04
Folate (µg)	240	221	92.2	253	231	113.0	242	226	101.4
Biotin (µg)	25	23	10.2	27	24	13.2	26	24	10.2
Pantothenic acid (mg)	5.0	4.7	1.72	5.4	5.1	2.00	5.3	5.1	1.89
Vitamin C (mg)	72.9	59.3	49.3	106.5	83.1	77.8	86.9	66.2	65.3
Vitamin D (µg)	2.6	2.4	1.43	3.6	3.1	2.00	2.5	2.2	1.40
Vitamin E (α-tocopherol equivalents) (mg)	8.7	8.1	3.54	9.4	8.3	5.86	8.4	8.0	3.43
Base		689			167			167	
Females									
Pre-formed retinol (µg)	263	216	313.1	411	315	290.1	259	225	173.9
Total carotene (β-carotene equivalents) (µg)	1298	1051	943	1602	1305	1871	1602	1305	1871
Vitamin A (retinol equivalents) (µg)	479	411	368.2	678	597	409.8	525	471	344.7
Thiamin (mg)	1.28	1.20	0.536	1.52	1.30	1.086	1.40	1.20	1.060
Riboflavin (mg)	1.33	1.29	0.542	1.55	1.44	0.672	1.39	1.32	0.543
Niacin equivalents (mg)	23.5	22.7	6.77	25.3	23.8	7.94	23.9	23.2	6.59
Vitamin B_6 (mg)	1.8	1.7	0.60	2.2	1.9	2.85	1.7	1.7	0.54
Vitamin B_{12} (µg)	3.4	3.2	1.68	3.7	3.6	1.58	3.5	3.4	1.46
Folate (µg)	193	187	66.8	217	190	93.5	200	186	71.1
Biotin (µg)	20	19	7.8	23	22	18.1	21	21	7.1
Pantothenic acid (mg)	4.1	3.9	1.35	4.4	4.2	1.69	4.2	4.1	1.26
Vitamin C (mg)	70.1	58.9	43.56	102.4	79.3	95.82	76.3	67.9	43.15
Vitamin D (µg)	2.1	1.9	1.12	2.9	2.4	1.90	2.0	1.8	1.13
Vitamin E (α-tocopherol equivalents) (mg)	7.7	7.0	3.15	8.6	7.3	8.17	7.2	7.0	2.55
Base		683			162			162	

Table 8.40 Average daily intake of vitamins from food sources by whether young person was reported as being unwell during dietary recording period

| Vitamins | Whether unwell during period | | | | | | | | |
| | Unwell and eating affected | | | Unwell and eating not affected | | | Not unwell | | |
	Mean	Median	sd	Mean	Median	sd	Mean	Median	sd
Males									
Pre-formed retinol (µg)	288	243	242	258	241	145	308	259	343
Total carotene (β-carotene equivalents) (µg)	1168	896	1079	1267	1086	1046	1454	1141	1148
Vitamin A (retinol equivalents) (µg)	483	415	296	469	412	249	550	479	405
Thiamin (mg)	1.39	1.26	0.707	1.41	1.37	0.521	1.63	1.49	0.870
Riboflavin (mg)	1.52	1.36	0.670	1.53	1.40	0.698	1.75	1.62	0.712
Niacin equivalents (mg)	26.6	25.9	9.18	26.8	25.0	9.79	29.6	28.2	9.49
Vitamin B_6 (mg)	1.9	1.7	0.77	2.0	1.8	0.77	2.2	2.0	0.82
Vitamin B_{12} (µg)	4.0	4.0	1.80	3.8	3.4	1.68	4.5	4.0	2.14
Folate (µg)	219	192	100.1	222	208	88.9	244	226	93.2
Biotin (µg)	23	21	9.5	22	23	9.9	25	23	10.3
Pantothenic acid (mg)	4.5	4.5	1.53	4.5	4.2	1.64	5.2	4.9	1.77
Vitamin C (mg)	70.2	56.7	42.28	76.6	60.6	63.29	75.7	61.7	51.60
Vitamin D (µg)	2.2	2.0	1.18	2.6	2.1	1.72	2.6	2.4	1.39
Vitamin E (α-tocopherol equivalents) (mg)	7.0	6.7	2.64	8.1	7.3	3.30	8.9	8.3	3.57
Base		86			66			704	
Females									
Pre-formed retinol (µg)	196	172	101	281	191	326	268	229	303
Total carotene (β-carotene equivalents) (µg)	1069	897	707	1428	1101	1143	1383	1152	1226
Vitamin A (retinol equivalents) (µg)	374	351	167	519	412	389	498	436	377
Thiamin (mg)	1.19	0.98	1.227	1.30	1.24	0.406	1.32	1.22	0.579
Riboflavin (mg)	1.05	0.96	0.430	1.24	1.21	0.556	1.40	1.34	0.540
Niacin equivalents (mg)	19.2	18.6	5.75	23.5	22.9	5.91	24.2	23.3	6.74
Vitamin B_6 (mg)	1.4	1.3	0.50	1.7	1.7	0.52	1.8	1.7	0.59
Vitamin B_{12} (µg)	2.7	2.5	1.26	3.1	3.0	1.47	3.5	3.3	1.68
Folate (µg)	155	146	52.7	186	179	55.7	201	191	69.0
Biotin (µg)	18	15	7.5	18	18	5.7	21	20	7.8
Pantothenic acid (mg)	3.3	3.1	1.11	4.0	3.8	1.32	4.2	4.1	1.33
Vitamin C (mg)	58.1	50.7	37.84	70.5	59.2	41.85	73.0	62.3	44.09
Vitamin D (µg)	1.8	1.6	0.93	1.9	1.7	0.89	2.1	1.9	1.16
Vitamin E (α-tocopherol equivalents) (mg)	6.9	6.2	2.88	7.8	7.3	3.06	7.6	7.0	3.04
Base		93			84			668	

Table 8.41 Average daily intake of vitamins from food sources per MJ total energy by whether young person was reported as being unwell during dietary recording period

Vitamins	Whether unwell during period								
	Unwell and eating affected			Unwell and eating not affected			Not unwell		
	Mean	Median	sd	Mean	Median	sd	Mean	Median	sd
Males									
Pre-formed retinol (µg)	38	33	45.7	34	31	15.3	38	33	45.7
Total carotene (β-carotene equivalents) (µg)	163	126	136	173	146	151	180	143	144
Vitamin A (retinol equivalents) (µg)	70	58	52.1	62	57	31.0	68	59	51.7
Thiamin (mg)	0.20	0.18	0.080	0.18	0.18	0.044	0.20	0.19	0.099
Riboflavin (mg)	0.22	0.20	0.078	0.20	0.19	0.067	0.22	0.21	0.073
Niacin equivalents (mg)	3.8	3.6	0.82	3.5	3.4	0.72	3.6	3.6	0.73
Vitamin B_6 (mg)	0.27	0.27	0.080	0.26	0.25	0.070	0.27	0.26	0.072
Vitamin B_{12} (µg)	0.57	0.55	0.230	0.51	0.48	0.181	0.55	0.52	0.253
Folate (µg)	31	28	10.9	29	29	7.5	30	29	8.1
Biotin (µg)	23	21	9.5	22	23	9.9	25	23	10.3
Pantothenic acid (mg)	4.5	4.5	1.53	4.5	4.2	1.64	5.2	4.9	1.77
Vitamin C (mg)	10.2	8.2	6.11	9.8	7.8	6.90	9.5	7.7	6.26
Vitamin D (µg)	0.32	0.29	0.171	0.34	0.30	0.188	0.33	0.31	0.145
Vitamin E (α-tocopherol equivalents) (mg)	1.0	1.0	0.32	1.1	1.0	0.29	1.1	1.0	0.33
Base		86			66			704	
Females									
Pre-formed retinol (µg)	34	33	12.8	41	29	47.1	40	34	46.5
Total carotene (β-carotene equivalents) (µg)	191	170	127	210	164	154	207	173	186
Vitamin A (retinol equivalents) (µg)	66	65	24.7	74	66	56.9	74	66	56.9
Thiamin (mg)	0.22	0.18	0.252	0.20	0.18	0.073	0.20	0.18	0.073
Riboflavin (mg)	0.19	0.17	0.083	0.21	0.20	0.071	0.21	0.20	0.071
Niacin equivalents (mg)	3.5	3.3	0.88	3.6	3.5	0.73	3.6	3.5	0.73
Vitamin B_6 (mg)	0.25	0.23	0.087	0.27	0.26	0.069	0.27	0.26	0.069
Vitamin B_{12} (µg)	0.50	0.45	0.235	0.52	0.50	0.237	0.52	0.50	0.237
Folate (µg)	28	26	8.1	30	29	8.7	30	29	8.7
Biotin (µg)	17.6	14.9	7.5	18.4	18.3	5.7	20.9	20.2	7.8
Pantothenic acid (mg)	3.3	3.1	1.11	4.0	3.8	1.32	4.2	4.1	1.33
Vitamin C (mg)	10	10	6.20	11	9	6.21	11	9	6.21
Vitamin D (µg)	0.32	0.27	0.170	0.31	0.29	0.153	0.31	0.29	0.153
Vitamin E (α-tocopherol equivalents) (mg)	1.2	1.1	0.41	1.1	1.1	0.34	1.1	1.1	0.34
Base		93			84			668	

Table 8.42 Average daily intake of vitamins from food sources by region

Vitamins	Region											
	Scotland			Northern			Central, South West and Wales			London and the South East		
	Mean	Median	sd	Mean	Median	sd	Mean	Median	sd	Mean	Median	sd
Males												
Pre-formed retinol (µg)	238	235	111	291	257	215	324	254	470	304	266	205
Total carotene (β-carotene equivalents) (µg)	1267	850	1390	1241	976	1015	1495	1180	1191	1513	1269	1080
Vitamin A (retinol equivalents) (µg)	449	383	241	497	443	287	573	471	518	556	514	295
Thiamin (mg)	1.42	1.37	0.469	1.57	1.46	0.607	1.62	1.53	0.602	1.61	1.37	1.248
Riboflavin (mg)	1.60	1.43	0.657	1.67	1.61	0.647	1.76	1.59	0.720	1.72	1.59	0.772
Niacin equivalents (mg)	28.1	26.8	9.25	28.4	27.5	8.74	29.8	28.6	9.45	29.3	27.5	10.40
Vitamin B_6 (mg)	2.1	1.8	0.84	2.1	2.0	0.82	2.2	2.0	0.79	2.1	1.9	0.84
Vitamin B_{12} (µg)	4.3	3.8	1.97	4.2	3.9	1.68	4.5	4.0	2.51	4.4	4.0	1.88
Folate (µg)	216	197	82.8	236	225	87.1	249	231	90.4	240	215	105.6
Biotin (µg)	23	21	8.8	24	22	8.9	25	23	10.3	26	24	11.5
Pantothenic acid (mg)	4.7	4.3	1.48	5.0	4.8	1.65	5.1	4.8	1.65	5.2	4.9	2.01
Vitamin C (mg)	63.8	54.4	43.04	70.3	60.1	42.77	77.8	61.7	56.52	80.0	64.6	55.10
Vitamin D (µg)	2.2	1.9	1.17	2.6	2.3	1.40	2.7	2.4	1.41	2.6	2.4	1.47
Vitamin E (α-tocopherol equivalents) (mg)	7.8	7.2	2.66	8.9	8.4	3.82	8.6	8.1	3.41	8.7	7.9	3.49
Base	*68*			*243*			*300*			*245*		
Females												
Pre-formed retinol (µg)	216	187	132	257	232	200	287	222	420	249	212	190
Total carotene (β-carotene equivalents) (µg)	1129	860	837	1393	1132	1049	1377	1162	967	1351	1108	1546
Vitamin A (retinol equivalents) (µg)	404	346	224	489	439	270	516	439	468	474	416	323
Thiamin (mg)	1.13	1.06	0.425	1.31	1.21	0.627	1.37	1.26	0.636	1.27	1.16	0.773
Riboflavin (mg)	1.21	1.10	0.600	1.34	1.31	0.526	1.43	1.36	0.558	1.29	1.24	0.508
Niacin equivalents (mg)	22.5	21.9	6.55	23.4	23.0	6.41	24.3	23.2	7.09	23.1	22.6	6.59
Vitamin B_6 (mg)	1.7	1.6	0.64	1.8	1.7	0.54	1.8	1.7	0.64	1.7	1.6	0.54
Vitamin B_{12} (µg)	3.2	2.9	1.52	3.5	3.3	1.43	3.6	3.4	1.92	3.2	3.0	1.46
Folate (µg)	174	157	67.7	189	186	60.2	204	191	67.7	194	187	72.6
Biotin (µg)	19	16	8.0	21	20	7.2	21	20	7.7	20	19	8.0
Pantothenic acid (mg)	3.7	3.4	1.29	4.1	4.0	1.33	4.3	4.2	1.33	4.0	3.7	1.34
Vitamin C (mg)	67.2	53.8	41.38	66.5	59.6	36.07	72.8	61.3	43.36	74.9	62.9	49.83
Vitamin D (µg)	1.8	1.6	1.06	2.1	1.9	1.05	2.2	2.0	1.24	1.9	1.7	1.01
Vitamin E (α-tocopherol equivalents) (mg)	7.6	7.1	3.05	7.8	7.2	3.08	7.6	6.9	3.08	7.3	6.6	2.91
Base	*69*			*217*			*306*			*253*		

Table 8.43 Average daily intake of vitamins from food sources per MJ total energy by region

Vitamins	Region											
	Scotland			Northern			Central, South West and Wales			London and the South East		
	Mean	Median	sd	Mean	Median	sd	Mean	Median	sd	Mean	Median	sd
Males												
Pre-formed retinol (µg)	30	29	12.5	37	32	34.5	40	33	64.7	38	33	22.6
Total carotene (β-carotene equivalents) (µg)	160	107	193	158	128	127	187	151	148	191	155	134
Vitamin A (retinol equivalents) (µg)	57	51	30.0	64	55	40.9	72	59	69.5	70	64	31.4
Thiamin (mg)	0.18	0.18	0.051	0.20	0.19	0.069	0.20	0.20	0.062	0.20	0.19	0.143
Riboflavin (mg)	0.20	0.20	0.067	0.21	0.21	0.072	0.22	0.22	0.074	0.22	0.21	0.075
Niacin equivalents (mg)	3.6	3.5	0.78	3.6	3.5	0.75	3.7	3.6	0.74	3.7	3.6	0.69
Vitamin B_6 (mg)	0.26	0.25	0.079	0.27	0.26	0.072	0.28	0.27	0.078	0.27	0.26	0.063
Vitamin B_{12} (µg)	0.55	0.51	0.182	0.53	0.51	0.200	0.56	0.53	0.317	0.56	0.53	0.197
Folate (µg)	28	26	8.31	30	29	8.55	31	30	8.42	30	29	7.91
Biotin (µg)	23	21	8.8	24	22	8.9	25	23	10.3	26	24	11.5
Pantothenic acid (mg)	4.7	4.3	1.48	5.0	4.8	1.65	5.1	4.8	1.65	5.2	4.9	2.01
Vitamin C (mg)	8.2	7.2	4.7	9.1	7.4	5.8	9.8	8.2	6.7	10.1	8.0	6.6
Vitamin D (µg)	0.29	0.27	0.131	0.32	0.29	0.153	0.34	0.31	0.157	0.32	0.30	0.145
Vitamin E (α-tocopherol equivalents) (mg)	1.0	0.9	0.30	1.1	1.1	0.35	1.1	1.0	0.33	1.1	1.0	0.31
Base		*68*			*243*			*300*			*245*	
Females												
Pre-formed retinol (µg)	34	31	15.6	37	34	27.3	43	33	65.3	38	34	27.9
Total carotene (β-carotene equivalents) (µg)	179	143	120	205	170	145	211	175	159	207	176	233
Vitamin A (retinol equivalents) (µg)	63	57	27.6	72	66	35.6	78	66	73.0	73	65	47.0
Thiamin (mg)	0.18	0.17	0.053	0.19	0.18	0.082	0.21	0.19	0.082	0.20	0.18	0.152
Riboflavin (mg)	0.19	0.18	0.078	0.20	0.20	0.068	0.21	0.21	0.078	0.20	0.20	0.070
Niacin equivalents (mg)	3.6	3.6	0.75	3.5	3.3	0.69	3.6	3.5	0.78	3.6	3.5	0.75
Vitamin B_6 (mg)	0.27	0.26	0.077	0.26	0.26	0.059	0.27	0.26	0.077	0.26	0.25	0.069
Vitamin B_{12} (µg)	0.50	0.46	0.209	0.52	0.47	0.195	0.54	0.51	0.282	0.50	0.47	0.212
Folate (µg)	27	26	7.8	28	27	7.1	31	29	9.3	30	29	8.5
Biotin (µg)	19	16	8.0	21	20	7.2	21	20	7.7	20	19	8.0
Pantothenic acid (mg)	3.7	3.4	1.29	4.1	4.0	1.33	4.3	4.2	1.33	4.0	3.7	1.34
Vitamin C (mg)	10.7	9.0	6.57	9.9	9.1	4.89	10.9	9.5	6.18	11.4	10.4	6.90
Vitamin D (µg)	0.28	0.26	0.132	0.31	0.29	0.149	0.33	0.30	0.164	0.30	0.27	0.144
Vitamin E (α-tocopherol equivalents) (mg)	1.2	1.2	0.40	1.1	1.1	0.32	1.1	1.1	0.35	1.1	1.1	0.35
Base		*69*			*217*			*306*			*253*	

Table 8.44 Average daily intake of vitamins from food sources by whether young person's parents were receiving benefits

Vitamin	Whether receiving benefits					
	Receiving benefits			Not receiving benefits		
	Mean	Median	sd	Mean	Median	sd
Males						
Pre-formed retinol (μg)	291	210	531	306	270	216
Total carotene (β-carotene equivalents) (μg)	1243	961	1178	1468	1173	1118
Vitamin A (retinol equivalents) (μg)	498	395	568	550	482	303
Thiamin (mg)	1.40	1.34	0.509	1.65	1.50	0.911
Riboflavin (mg)	1.47	1.37	0.615	1.79	1.68	0.724
Niacin equivalents (mg)	25.5	24.6	7.88	30.3	29.0	9.77
Vitamin B_6 (mg)	1.9	1.9	0.60	2.2	2.0	0.87
Vitamin B_{12} (μg)	4.0	3.6	2.63	4.5	4.1	1.86
Folate (μg)	213	195	84.5	249	231	95.3
Biotin (μg)	21	20	10.0	26	24	10.0
Pantothenic acid (mg)	4.5	4.1	1.46	5.2	4.9	1.80
Vitamin C (mg)	57.7	53.9	31.24	80.9	65.6	55.81
Vitamin D (μg)	2.5	2.3	1.39	2.6	2.4	1.41
Vitamin E (α-tocopherol equivalents) (mg)	7.8	7.4	2.96	8.9	8.4	3.63
Base	*189*			*666*		
Females						
Pre-formed retinol (μg)	251	219	313	266	218	284
Total carotene (β-carotene equivalents) (μg)	1353	1033	1682	1357	1136	933
Vitamin A (retinol equivalents) (μg)	476	399	434	492	437	335
Thiamin (mg)	1.24	1.15	0.473	1.33	1.23	0.721
Riboflavin (mg)	1.29	1.24	0.560	1.37	1.32	0.534
Niacin equivalents (mg)	22.5	21.4	7.12	24.0	23.3	6.53
Vitamin B_6 (mg)	1.7	1.6	0.60	1.8	1.7	0.59
Vitamin B_{12} (μg)	3.4	3.1	1.86	3.4	3.3	1.56
Folate (μg)	189	186	70.1	197	188	66.7
Biotin (μg)	19	18	7.6	21	20	7.7
Pantothenic acid (mg)	4.0	3.9	1.47	4.1	4.0	1.28
Vitamin C (mg)	60.4	49.2	39.91	75.2	66.5	44.07
Vitamin D (μg)	2.2	1.9	1.22	2.0	1.8	1.08
Vitamin E (α-tocopherol equivalents) (mg)	7.8	7.2	3.22	7.5	6.9	2.97
Base	*199*			*645*		

Table 8.45 Average daily intake of vitamins from food sources per MJ total energy by whether young person's parents were receiving benefits

Vitamin	Whether receiving benefits					
	Receiving benefits			Not receiving benefits		
	Mean	Median	sd	Mean	Median	sd
Males						
Pre-formed retinol (µg)	41	30	79.7	37	33	23.4
Total carotene (β-carotene equivalents) (µg)	172	127	161	180	144	137
Vitamin A (retinol equivalents) (µg)	70	56	83.8	67	61	32.9
Thiamin (mg)	0.20	0.19	0.055	0.20	0.19	0.103
Riboflavin (mg)	0.21	0.20	0.072	0.22	0.21	0.073
Niacin equivalents (mg)	3.6	3.5	0.77	3.7	3.6	0.72
Vitamin B_6 (mg)	0.27	0.27	0.060	0.27	0.26	0.077
Vitamin B_{12} (µg)	0.56	0.51	0.355	0.55	0.52	0.199
Folate (µg)	30	29	9.3	30	29	8.0
Biotin (µg)	21	20	10.0	26	24	10.0
Pantothenic acid (mg)	4.5	4.1	1.46	5.2	4.9	1.80
Vitamin C (mg)	8.3	7.2	4.97	10.0	8.1	6.63
Vitamin D (µg)	0.35	0.33	0.160	0.32	0.29	0.148
Vitamin E (α-tocopherol equivalents) (mg)	1.1	1.0	0.31	1.1	1.0	0.34
Base		*189*			*666*	
Females						
Pre-formed retinol (µg)	38	34	53.1	40	34	40.6
Total carotene (β-carotene equivalents) (µg)	208	167	261	205	175	136
Vitamin A (retinol equivalents) (µg)	73	61	70.2	74	66	47.2
Thiamin (mg)	0.19	0.18	0.072	0.20	0.19	0.116
Riboflavin (mg)	0.19	0.19	0.070	0.21	0.20	0.074
Niacin equivalents (mg)	3.4	3.3	0.76	3.6	3.5	0.74
Vitamin B_6 (mg)	0.26	0.25	0.067	0.27	0.25	0.072
Vitamin B_{12} (µg)	0.51	0.48	0.278	0.52	0.49	0.218
Folate (µg)	29	27	8.8	30	29	8.3
Biotin (µg)	19	18	7.6	21	20	7.7
Pantothenic acid (mg)	4.0	3.9	1.47	4.1	4.0	1.28
Vitamin C (mg)	9.2	7.5	5.97	11.3	10.0	6.10
Vitamin D (µg)	0.32	0.29	0.164	0.31	0.29	0.147
Vitamin E (α-tocopherol equivalents) (mg)	1.2	1.1	0.34	1.1	1.1	0.35
Base		*199*			*645*	

Table 8.46 Average daily intake of vitamins from food sources by gross weekly household income

Vitamins	Gross weekly household income														
	Less than £160			£160 to less than £280			£280 to less than £400			£400 to less than £600			£600 and over		
	Mean	Median	sd	Mean	Median	sd	Mean	Median	sd	Mean	Median	sd	Mean	Median	sd
Males															
Pre-formed retinol (µg)	258	213	206	315	224	591	292	248	216	310	287	189	313	273	210
Total carotene (β-carotene equivalents) (µg)	1346	987	1339	1196	948	882	1388	1130	985	1560	1298	1179	1538	1181	1227
Vitamin A (retinol equivalents) (µg)	482	412	300	514	411	618	523	459	306	571	527	275	570	510	306
Thiamin (mg)	1.42	1.38	0.536	1.52	1.35	1.372	1.64	1.55	0.607	1.64	1.55	0.643	1.65	1.49	0.687
Riboflavin (mg)	1.46	1.37	0.585	1.63	1.48	0.703	1.73	1.74	0.621	1.86	1.82	0.691	1.81	1.67	0.781
Niacin equivalents (mg)	26.1	24.8	8.46	26.9	25.4	8.81	29.3	28.4	8.95	31.5	30.3	9.02	30.8	28.7	10.41
Vitamin B_6 (mg)	2.0	1.9	0.82	2.0	1.9	0.69	2.1	2.0	0.68	2.3	2.1	0.80	2.3	2.1	0.97
Vitamin B_{12} (µg)	4.0	3.7	1.72	4.1	3.6	2.87	4.2	4.0	1.58	4.7	4.5	1.77	4.6	4.2	2.00
Folate (µg)	213	196	87.4	229	209	96.7	240	218	91.4	248	237	77.0	258	238	104.9
Biotin (µg)	21	20	9.4	22	20	10.3	25	23	9.8	27	26	8.3	28	25	11.0
Pantothenic acid (mg)	4.6	4.3	1.54	4.6	4.3	1.66	5.1	4.9	1.48	5.5	5.3	1.64	5.4	5.0	2.01
Vitamin C (mg)	60.6	55.4	39.14	60.0	53.0	33.94	76.5	58.6	56.64	79.2	65.8	50.54	93.7	76.5	62.46
Vitamin D (µg)	2.6	2.3	1.42	2.6	2.5	1.20	2.7	2.4	1.36	2.5	2.3	1.35	2.6	2.3	1.49
Vitamin E (α-tocopherol equivalents) (mg)	8.1	7.6	3.69	8.0	7.6	3.04	9.4	8.7	3.85	8.8	8.0	3.30	8.6	8.2	3.52
Base		*133*			*159*			*157*			*173*			*208*	
Females															
Pre-formed retinol (µg)	258	206	381	266	208	416	260	214	236	249	214	177	286	256	228
Total carotene (β-carotene equivalents) (µg)	1194	922	922	1230	1047	863	1483	1046	2023	1361	1222	784	1553	1279	1043
Vitamin A (retinol equivalents) (µg)	457	363	449	471	380	445	507	421	394	476	455	239	544	496	301
Thiamin (mg)	1.21	1.15	0.436	1.35	1.24	0.831	1.30	1.21	0.541	1.26	1.20	0.448	1.41	1.20	0.899
Riboflavin (mg)	1.28	1.25	0.578	1.35	1.29	0.525	1.30	1.21	0.527	1.36	1.33	0.540	1.42	1.37	0.531
Niacin equivalents (mg)	22.6	21.4	7.51	22.6	21.7	6.57	23.7	23.0	6.59	23.6	23.4	6.63	25.3	24.4	5.85
Vitamin B_6 (mg)	1.7	1.6	0.60	1.8	1.7	0.61	1.7	1.6	0.61	1.7	1.7	0.54	1.8	1.7	0.55
Vitamin B_{12} (µg)	3.3	2.9	2.09	3.4	3.3	1.43	3.4	3.1	1.48	3.4	3.2	1.41	3.7	3.4	1.79
Folate (µg)	186	185	71.2	193	186	61.5	186	178	65.4	195	190	73.1	210	197	62.4
Biotin (µg)	18	18	7.2	20	19	7.8	19	18	5.9	21	21	8.1	23	21	8.0
Pantothenic acid (mg)	4.0	3.9	1.56	4.0	3.9	1.35	4.0	3.9	1.15	4.2	4.1	1.35	4.2	4.2	1.24
Vitamin C (mg)	58.6	46.9	40.36	62.0	56.8	30.01	69.4	55.4	47.38	72.1	66.7	41.24	91.1	83.3	46.13
Vitamin D (µg)	2.1	1.9	1.32	2.0	1.9	1.09	2.3	2.1	1.23	2.0	1.8	0.93	2.0	1.8	1.03
Vitamin E (α-tocopherol equivalents) (mg)	7.6	7.2	3.10	7.7	7.0	3.15	7.8	7.0	3.50	7.2	6.9	2.54	7.7	7.0	2.98
Base		*131*			*146*			*145*			*192*			*196*	

262

Table 8.47 Average daily intake of vitamins from food sources per MJ total energy by gross weekly household income

Vitamins	Gross weekly household income														
	Less than £160			£160 to less than £280			£280 to less than £400			£400 to less than £600			£600 and over		
	Mean	Median	sd	Mean	Median	sd	Mean	Median	sd	Mean	Median	sd	Mean	Median	sd
Males															
Pre-formed retinol (µg)	36	31	38.0	43	31	84.6	35	31	19.6	37	35	20.2	38	33	23.3
Total carotene (β-carotene equivalents) (µg)	183	139	183	162	121	115	172	144	126	188	152	148	188	141	147
Vitamin A (retinol equivalents) (µg)	67	57	46.5	70	56	87.4	64	57	30.1	68	64	31.2	69	63	33.3
Thiamin (mg)	0.19	0.18	0.058	0.21	0.19	0.165	0.20	0.20	0.061	0.19	0.19	0.072	0.20	0.19	0.067
Riboflavin (mg)	0.20	0.19	0.071	0.22	0.22	0.075	0.22	0.21	0.069	0.22	0.22	0.072	0.22	0.21	0.074
Niacin equivalents (mg)	3.6	3.5	0.72	3.6	3.6	0.82	3.6	3.5	0.68	3.7	3.6	0.75	3.7	3.6	0.70
Vitamin B$_6$ (mg)	0.27	0.27	0.060	0.27	0.27	0.074	0.26	0.26	0.062	0.27	0.26	0.075	0.28	0.26	0.086
Vitamin B$_{12}$ (µg)	0.55	0.51	0.204	0.55	0.51	0.377	0.53	0.52	0.195	0.56	0.54	0.187	0.56	0.52	0.215
Folate (µg)	29	29	8.6	31	30	9.9	29	30	7.5	29	29	7.4	31	30	8.1
Biotin (µg)	21	20	9.4	22	20	10.3	25	23	9.8	27	26	8.3	28	25	11.0
Pantothenic acid (mg)	4.6	4.3	1.54	4.6	4.3	1.66	5.1	4.9	1.48	5.5	5.3	1.64	5.4	5.0	2.01
Vitamin C (mg)	8.4	7.1	4.80	8.3	7.4	4.96	9.4	7.5	6.07	9.5	7.8	6.15	11.7	9.5	8.04
Vitamin D (µg)	0.35	0.33	0.163	0.35	0.33	0.149	0.33	0.30	0.143	0.29	0.28	0.136	0.31	0.27	0.153
Vitamin E (α-tocopherol equivalents) (mg)	1.1	1.1	0.30	1.1	1.0	0.30	1.2	1.1	0.39	1.0	0.9	0.31	1.0	1.0	0.33
Base	*133*			*159*			*157*			*173*			*208*		
Females															
Pre-formed retinol (µg)	40	34	65.1	40	32	60.7	38	33	32.7	38	33	25.9	42	37	31.3
Total carotene (β-carotene equivalents) (µg)	180	153	128	191	170	140	220	163	303	211	189	128	232	196	157
Vitamin A (retinol equivalents) (µg)	70	59	73.2	72	61	65.5	75	66	56.8	73	66	35.7	80	73	40.8
Thiamin (mg)	0.19	0.18	0.052	0.21	0.19	0.174	0.19	0.18	0.087	0.19	0.18	0.052	0.21	0.19	0.116
Riboflavin (mg)	0.20	0.20	0.074	0.20	0.20	0.069	0.20	0.18	0.075	0.21	0.20	0.070	0.21	0.20	0.073
Niacin equivalents (mg)	3.5	3.4	0.77	3.4	3.3	0.69	3.5	3.5	0.74	3.6	3.5	0.74	3.8	3.7	0.71
Vitamin B$_6$ (mg)	0.27	0.26	0.064	0.27	0.25	0.074	0.26	0.26	0.068	0.26	0.25	0.067	0.27	0.25	0.069
Vitamin B$_{12}$ (µg)	0.51	0.47	0.327	0.50	0.49	0.181	0.50	0.46	0.209	0.52	0.48	0.206	0.54	0.51	0.245
Folate (µg)	29	27	8.5	29	28	9.6	28	27	8.1	29	28	8.4	31	31	7.4
Biotin (µg)	18	18	7.2	20	19	7.8	19	18	5.9	21	21	8.1	23	21	8.0
Pantothenic acid (mg)	4.0	3.9	1.56	4.0	3.9	1.35	4.0	3.9	1.15	4.2	4.1	1.35	4.2	4.2	1.24
Vitamin C (mg)	9.0	7.3	5.89	9.6	8.4	5.18	10.3	9.0	6.29	10.9	10.2	5.38	13.6	12.2	6.61
Vitamin D (µg)	0.33	0.28	0.182	0.31	0.28	0.155	0.34	0.33	0.154	0.30	0.29	0.125	0.30	0.27	0.137
Vitamin E (α-tocopherol equivalents) (mg)	1.2	1.1	0.30	1.1	1.0	0.38	1.1	1.1	0.37	1.1	1.0	0.33	1.1	1.1	0.35
Base	*131*			*146*			*145*			*192*			*196*		

263

Table 8.48 Average daily intake of vitamins from food sources by social class of head of household

Vitamins	Social class of head of household								
	Non-manual			Manual			All*		
	Mean	Median	sd	Mean	Median	sd	Mean	Median	sd
Males									
Pre-formed retinol (μg)	303	266	197	294	247	235	302	256	323
Total carotene (β-carotene equivalents) (μg)	1451	1180	1082	1391	1051	1172	1411	1111	1137
Vitamin A (retinol equivalents) (μg)	545	484	290	525	446	311	537	465	386
Thiamin (mg)	1.66	1.48	1.085	1.55	1.48	0.514	1.59	1.45	0.837
Riboflavin (mg)	1.80	1.69	0.734	1.67	1.54	0.659	1.71	1.59	0.713
Niacin equivalents (mg)	30.0	28.7	9.83	28.8	27.5	9.18	29.1	27.9	9.55
Vitamin B_6 (mg)	2.2	2.0	0.88	2.1	2.0	0.77	2.2	2.0	0.82
Vitamin B_{12} (μg)	4.5	4.2	1.87	4.2	3.9	1.75	4.4	4.0	2.09
Folate (μg)	250	231	97.7	235	213	90.7	240	221	94.0
Biotin (μg)	26	25	10.1	24	22	9.9	25	23	10.2
Pantothenic acid (mg)	5.3	4.9	1.87	4.9	4.7	1.59	5.1	4.8	1.76
Vitamin C (mg)	84.6	67.1	57.44	67.4	57.2	45.54	75.2	60.9	51.82
Vitamin D (μg)	2.6	2.3	1.38	2.6	2.5	1.39	2.6	2.3	1.41
Vitamin E (α-tocopherol equivalents) (mg)	8.6	8.1	3.42	8.7	8.2	3.64	8.6	8.1	3.51
Base		*414*			*385*			*856*	
Females									
Pre-formed retinol (μg)	274	241	214	257	203	382	262	218	292
Total carotene (β-carotene equivalents) (μg)	1407	1224	944	1327	1031	1440	1354	1111	1177
Vitamin A (retinol equivalents) (μg)	508	460	281	478	386	458	487	424	364
Thiamin (mg)	1.39	1.23	0.871	1.25	1.20	0.417	1.30	1.20	0.666
Riboflavin (mg)	1.41	1.34	0.545	1.31	1.26	0.532	1.35	1.30	0.543
Niacin equivalents (mg)	24.4	23.8	6.67	23.1	22.6	6.52	23.6	22.8	6.74
Vitamin B_6 (mg)	1.8	1.7	0.61	1.7	1.7	0.55	1.8	1.7	0.59
Vitamin B_{12} (μg)	3.5	3.4	1.64	3.3	3.1	1.67	3.4	3.2	1.64
Folate (μg)	200	191	67.7	188	184	64.7	194	187	67.7
Biotin (μg)	22	21	7.7	19	19	7.5	20	20	7.7
Pantothenic acid (mg)	4.2	4.1	1.30	4.0	3.9	1.33	4.1	4.0	1.34
Vitamin C (mg)	80.0	72.0	45.91	64.3	55.4	40.34	71.2	60.6	43.48
Vitamin D (μg)	2.1	1.8	1.15	2.0	1.9	1.05	2.1	1.9	1.12
Vitamin E (α-tocopherol equivalents) (mg)	7.5	7.0	2.85	7.7	7.1	3.11	7.6	7.0	3.03
Base		*401*			*361*			*845*	

*Includes those for whom social class could not be assigned.

Table 8.49 Average daily intake of vitamins from food sources per MJ total energy by social class of head of household head of household

| Vitamins | Social class of head of household | | | | | | | | |
| | Non-manual | | | Manual | | | All* | | |
	Mean	Median	sd	Mean	Median	sd	Mean	Median	sd
Males									
Pre-formed retinol (µg)	37	34	20.2	37	31	33.1	38	32	44.4
Total carotene (β-carotene equivalents) (µg)	180	146	131	177	138	153	178	141	143
Vitamin A (retinol equivalents) (µg)	67	62	30.4	67	58	40.8	68	59	50.4
Thiamin (mg)	0.20	0.19	0.125	0.20	0.19	0.052	0.20	0.19	0.094
Riboflavin (mg)	0.22	0.22	0.071	0.21	0.21	0.074	0.22	0.21	0.073
Niacin equivalents (mg)	3.7	3.6	0.70	3.6	3.6	0.73	3.6	3.6	0.74
Vitamin B_6 (mg)	0.27	0.26	0.078	0.27	0.26	0.070	0.27	0.26	0.073
Vitamin B_{12} (µg)	0.56	0.54	0.198	0.53	0.51	0.191	0.55	0.52	0.246
Folate (µg)	31	30	7.9	30	29	8.7	30	29	8.4
Biotin (µg)	26	25	10.1	24	22	9.9	25	23	10.2
Pantothenic acid (mg)	5.3	4.9	1.87	4.9	4.7	1.59	5.1	4.8	1.76
Vitamin C (mg)	10.6	8.7	7.03	8.6	7.4	5.52	9.6	7.8	6.30
Vitamin D (µg)	0.32	0.29	0.147	0.33	0.31	0.143	0.33	0.30	0.151
Vitamin E (α-tocopherol equivalents) (mg)	1.1	1.0	0.33	1.1	1.0	0.32	1.1	1.0	0.33
Base		*414*			*385*			*856*	
Females									
Pre-formed retinol (µg)	40	36	29.6	39	32	60.0	39	34	44.2
Total carotene (β-carotene equivalents) (µg)	211	180	142	202	163	216	206	172	178
Vitamin A (retinol equivalents) (µg)	75	69	38.8	73	61	70.8	73	65	54.2
Thiamin (mg)	0.21	0.19	0.146	0.19	0.18	0.051	0.20	0.18	0.106
Riboflavin (mg)	0.21	0.20	0.073	0.20	0.20	0.072	0.20	0.20	0.073
Niacin equivalents (mg)	3.6	3.5	0.77	3.5	3.5	0.69	3.6	3.5	0.75
Vitamin B_6 (mg)	0.27	0.25	0.074	0.26	0.26	0.064	0.27	0.25	0.071
Vitamin B_{12} (µg)	0.52	0.49	0.225	0.51	0.47	0.255	0.52	0.48	0.235
Folate (µg)	30	29	8.0	29	27	7.8	29	28	8.5
Biotin (µg)	22	21	7.7	19	19	7.5	20	20	7.7
Pantothenic acid (mg)	4.2	4.1	1.30	4.0	3.9	1.33	4.1	4.0	1.34
Vitamin C (mg)	11.9	10.6	6.47	9.8	8.6	5.60	10.8	9.5	6.14
Vitamin D (µg)	0.31	0.28	0.149	0.31	0.29	0.152	0.31	0.29	0.152
Vitamin E (α-tocopherol equivalents) (mg)	1.1	1.0	0.33	1.2	1.1	0.35	1.1	1.1	0.35
Base		*401*			*361*			*845*	

*Includes those for whom social class could not be assigned.

Table 8.50 Average daily intake of vitamins from food sources by whether the young person was living with both parents

Vitamins	Young person living with:								
	Both parents and other children			Both parents and no other children			Single parent with/out other children		
	Mean	Median	sd	Mean	Median	sd	Mean	Median	sd
Males									
Pre-formed retinol (µg)	278	245	182	395	289	616	285	252	208
Total carotene (β-carotene equivalents) (µg)	1384	1045	1174	1578	1266	1137	1333	1117	984
Vitamin A (retinol equivalents) (µg)	509	438	284	658	552	649	507	446	274
Thiamin (mg)	1.52	1.39	0.562	1.83	1.65	1.421	1.56	1.48	0.728
Riboflavin (mg)	1.68	1.54	0.672	1.86	1.69	0.798	1.65	1.49	0.733
Niacin equivalents (mg)	27.7	26.5	8.44	34.2	33.0	10.24	28.4	27.4	10.30
Vitamin B$_6$ (mg)	2.0	1.9	0.69	2.5	2.3	1.00	2.1	2.0	0.88
Vitamin B$_{12}$ (µg)	4.1	3.8	1.73	5.2	4.6	3.00	4.3	4.0	1.77
Folate (µg)	229	213	80.9	278	267	111.9	236	213	102.3
Biotin (µg)	24	22	9.5	28	26	11.1	24	23	10.8
Pantothenic acid (mg)	4.9	4.6	1.66	5.6	5.3	1.78	5.0	4.6	1.91
Vitamin C (mg)	73.2	60.4	48.64	86.2	70.3	62.12	69.1	57.2	45.15
Vitamin D (µg)	2.5	2.2	1.32	2.9	2.7	1.44	2.7	2.4	1.61
Vitamin E (α-tocopherol equivalents) (mg)	8.4	8.0	3.19	9.6	8.9	3.90	8.1	7.2	3.80
Base		*528*			*169*			*157*	
Females									
Pre-formed retinol (µg)	253	219	198	287	219	433	265	218	359
Total carotene (β-carotene equivalents) (µg)	1377	1132	1312	1410	1198	1020	1250	1033	874
Vitamin A (retinol equivalents) (µg)	482	427	305	522	443	472	473	399	409
Thiamin (mg)	1.30	1.20	0.645	1.30	1.20	0.513	1.33	1.19	0.828
Riboflavin (mg)	1.38	1.35	0.532	1.25	1.17	0.535	1.35	1.27	0.573
Niacin equivalents (mg)	23.3	22.6	6.46	24.7	24.9	7.09	23.5	22.6	7.16
Vitamin B$_6$ (mg)	1.7	1.7	0.57	1.8	1.7	0.61	1.8	1.7	0.63
Vitamin B$_{12}$ (µg)	3.5	3.3	1.59	3.2	3.1	1.51	3.3	3.0	1.88
Folate (µg)	194	187	66.7	196	190	67.3	194	183	70.7
Biotin (µg)	21	20	7.5	21	20	9.0	19	18	7.0
Pantothenic acid (mg)	4.1	4.1	1.26	4.0	3.9	1.35	4.1	3.8	1.53
Vitamin C (mg)	73.9	61.0	44.84	71.1	66.7	43.26	64.5	52.7	39.05
Vitamin D (µg)	2.1	1.9	1.11	2.0	1.8	0.97	2.1	1.9	1.22
Vitamin E (α-tocopherol equivalents) (mg)	7.6	7.0	3.04	7.9	7.2	3.31	7.5	7.0	2.73
Base		*498*			*173*			*167*	

*Excludes 9 young people who were living with others, not parents.

Table 8.51 Average daily intake of vitamins from food sources per MJ total energy by whether the young person was living with both parents*

Vitamins	Young person living with:								
	Both parents and other children			Both parents and no other children			Single parent with/out other children		
	Mean	Median	sd	Mean	Median	sd	Mean	Median	sd
Males									
Pre-formed retinol (µg)	36	32	20.6	46	34	86.1	39	32	37.8
Total carotene (β-carotene equivalents) (µg)	179	137	149	180	143	138	175	148	129
Vitamin A (retinol equivalents) (µg)	65	58	32.0	76	59	89.4	68	60	43.1
Thiamin (mg)	0.20	0.19	0.059	0.21	0.19	0.171	0.20	0.19	0.072
Riboflavin (mg)	0.22	0.21	0.072	0.21	0.20	0.078	0.22	0.21	0.071
Niacin equivalents (mg)	3.6	3.5	0.68	3.9	3.8	0.88	3.7	3.6	0.71
Vitamin B_6 (mg)	0.27	0.26	0.065	0.28	0.27	0.098	0.27	0.27	0.063
Vitamin B_{12} (µg)	0.54	0.51	0.195	0.59	0.53	0.395	0.56	0.55	0.183
Folate (µg)	30	29	7.7	31	30	9.5	31	29	9.0
Biotin (µg)	24	22	9.5	28	26	11.1	24	23	10.8
Pantothenic acid (mg)	4.9	4.6	1.66	5.6	5.3	1.78	5.0	4.6	1.91
Vitamin C (mg)	9.5	8.0	5.93	9.9	7.7	7.50	9.3	7.6	6.07
Vitamin D (µg)	0.32	0.30	0.145	0.32	0.29	0.153	0.36	0.35	0.169
Vitamin E (α-tocopherol equivalents) (mg)	1.1	1.0	0.33	1.1	1.0	0.34	1.0	1.0	0.29
Base		528			169			157	
Females									
Pre-formed retinol (µg)	38	34	28.3	42	32	62	40	34	60.6
Total carotene (β-carotene equivalents) (µg)	209	173	197	211	180	152	192	163	141
Vitamin A (retinol equivalents) (µg)	73	66	43.7	77	64	66.6	72	62	68.2
Thiamin (mg)	0.20	0.18	0.087	0.19	0.18	0.063	0.21	0.19	0.167
Riboflavin (mg)	0.21	0.21	0.072	0.19	0.17	0.075	0.20	0.20	0.076
Niacin equivalents (mg)	3.5	3.4	0.70	3.7	3.7	0.83	3.6	3.4	0.79
Vitamin B_6 (mg)	0.26	0.25	0.070	0.27	0.25	0.074	0.27	0.26	0.071
Vitamin B_{12} (µg)	0.53	0.49	0.219	0.49	0.47	0.206	0.51	0.48	0.294
Folate (µg)	29	28	8.0	29	29	7.7	30	27	10.2
Biotin (µg)	21	20	7.5	21	20	9.0	19	18	7.0
Pantothenic acid (mg)	4.1	4.1	1.26	4.0	3.9	1.35	4.1	3.8	1.53
Vitamin C (mg)	11.2	10.0	6.22	10.6	9.2	5.73	10.0	8.0	6.19
Vitamin D (µg)	0.31	0.29	0.151	0.29	0.27	0.136	0.32	0.29	0.156
Vitamin E (α-tocopherol equivalents) (mg)	1.1	1.1	0.35	1.2	1.1	0.38	1.1	1.1	0.30
Base		498			173			167	

* Excludes 9 young people who were living with others, not parents.

Table 8.52 Comparison of vitamin intake from food sources by young people aged between 10 and 15 years in two surveys: 1983 The Diets of British Schoolchildren; 1997 NDNS young people aged 4 to 18 years (present survey)

Vitamin	Sex and age of young person							
	1983*		1997		1983*		1997	
	10–11		10–11		14–15		14–15	
	Males	Females	Males	Females	Males	Females	Males	Females
Thiamin (mg)								
mean	1.21	1.03	1.52	1.29	1.47	1.04	1.85	1.42
median	1.17	0.99	1.48	1.26	1.39	1.00	1.76	1.22
sd	0.35	0.31	0.43	0.38	0.49	0.31	0.81	1.08
Riboflavin (mg)								
mean	1.70	1.40	1.69	1.34	1.89	1.32	1.81	1.29
median	1.63	1.35	1.59	1.31	1.84	1.24	1.66	1.20
sd	0.59	0.47	0.61	0.50	0.72	0.50	0.82	0.56
Vitamin C (mg)								
mean	49.3	49.0	74.9	73.4	49.3	48.0	76.0	73.1
median	39.4	38.3	64.2	61.8	41.4	41.5	60.3	58.0
sd	32.9	37.5	49.3	45.7	29.4	27.7	47.8	50.6
Retinol (μg)								
mean	589	460	299	275	696	558	387	294
median	309	259	263	227	348	271	288	220
sd	902	590	263	280	1004	803	665	431
β-carotene (μg)								
mean	1553	1386	1183	1252	1644	1454	1360	1307
median	1228	1087	941	1051	1355	1144	1162	999
sd	1261	1157	963	818	1353	1267	934	961
Vitamin A (retinol equivalents) (μg)								
mean	854	691	518	507	969	801	638	534
median	565	482	433	452	653	496	571	420
sd	466	638	329	328	1050	870	690	486
Vitamin D (μg)								
mean	1.48	1.32	2.44	2.31	1.63	1.24	3.00	2.11
median	1.22	1.10	2.27	2.10	1.28	1.05	2.64	1.92
sd	1.09	0.98	1.10	1.11	1.30	0.89	1.48	1.16
Vitamin B_6 (mg)**								
mean	1.17	1.03	2.06	1.81	1.35	1.06	2.35	1.81
median	1.14	1.00	1.98	1.72	1.28	1.04	2.22	1.68
sd	0.31	0.27	0.56	0.57	0.37	0.29	0.84	0.57
Base	*902*	*821*	*140*	*118*	*513*	*461*	*110*	*113*

* Department of Health. Report on Health and Social Subjects: 36. *The Diets of British Schoolchildren* HMSO (London, 1989)
** Reported as pyridoxine in 1983 survey

Table 8.53 Comparison of vitamin intake from food sources by young people in three surveys: 1992/3 NDNS: children aged 1½–4½ years; 1986/7 British Adults; 1997 NDNS young people aged 4–18 years (present survey)

Vitamin	Age and sex of young person							
	1992/3: 3½–4½*		1997: 4–6		1986/7: 16–24**		1997: 15–18	
	Males	Females	Males	Females	Males	Females	Males	Females
Total carotene (μg)								
mean	1029	884	1248	1175	1893	1576	1680	1637
median	700	6212	903	1035	1229	1179	1269	1241
se/sd***	66	52	1100	726	118.2	101.5	1343	1774
Vitamin A (retinol equivalents) (μg)								
mean	484	462	458	449	1164	1051	613	545
median	411	360	407	414	786	633	549	472
se/sd***	23.8	42.0	251	220	85.8	98.7	347	452
Thiamin (mg)								
mean	0.9	0.8	1.27	1.14	1.72	1.26	1.90	1.38
median	0.9	0.8	1.22	1.05	1.68	1.23	1.81	1.21
se/sd***	0.02	0.02	0.504	0.479	0.04	0.03	0.682	0.841
Riboflavin (mg)								
mean	1.2	1.1	1.56	1.40	1.96	1.45	1.92	1.30
median	1.2	1.1	1.49	1.35	1.91	1.33	1.82	1.22
se/sd***	0.02	0.02	0.576	0.449	0.05	0.04	0.893	0.631
Niacin equivalents (mg)								
mean	17.9	17.1	22.8	20.4	39.0	27.3	36.6	25.2
median	17.9	16.5	22.0	19.9	38.3	27.1	35.0	25.0
se/sd***	0.3	0.3	6.83	5.30	0.77	0.54	10.45	7.62
Vitamin B_6 (mg)								
mean	1.3	1.3	1.7	1.5	2.57	1.63	2.7	1.8
median	1.3	1.2	1.7	1.5	2.47	1.63	2.4	1.7
se/sd***	0.03	0.03	0.50	0.46	0.07	0.04	1.03	0.63
Vitamin B_{12} (μg)								
mean	2.8	2.8	4.0	3.6	6.2	4.4	5.0	3.4
median	2.6	2.4	3.8	3.4	5.1	3.4	4.6	3.0
se/sd***	0.09	0.10	1.62	1.44	0.29	0.28	2.04	1.95
Folate (μg)								
mean	143	138	191	169	302	198	305	210
median	138	134	184	159	285	194	283	197
se/sd***	3.0	2.9	60.7	54.9	7.6	4.7	118.7	76.9
Vitamin C (mg)								
mean	50.8	45.9	67.0	65.2	64.9	60.4	83.3	74.0
median	38.4	38.7	59.3	57.0	52.6	48.8	65.8	62.3
se/sd***	2.6	2.0	38.35	32.52	3.26	3.27	65.03	49.68
Vitamin D (μg)								
mean	1.4	1.3	2.1	1.8	2.81	2.10	3.2	2.1
median	1.1	1.1	1.9	1.7	2.39	1.86	2.9	1.9
se/sd***	0.07	0.05	1.24	0.91	0.14	0.09	1.68	1.16
Vitamin E (α-tocopherol equivalents) (mg)								
mean	5.0	4.5	6.6	6.3	9.7	6.8	10.3	8.1
median	4.5	4.1	6.2	5.7	9.2	6.1	9.3	7.2
se/sd***	0.13	0.12	2.26	2.47	0.26	0.22	4.09	3.39
Base – number of young people	*250*	*243*	*184*	*171*	*214*	*189*	*179*	*210*

* Gregory JR et al. *National Diet and Nutrition Survey: children aged 1½–4½ years.* HMSO (London, 1995).
** Gregory J et al. *The Dietary and Nutritional Survey of British Adults* HMSO (London, 1990).
*** 1992/3 and 1986/7 surveys reported standard errors; present survey reports standard deviations.

9 Minerals

9.1 Introduction

Minerals are inorganic elements. Some minerals are required for the body's normal function and these essential minerals are derived from the diet; they include iron, calcium, phosphorus, potassium, magnesium, sodium and chloride. Trace elements are required in minute amounts, and include zinc, copper, iodine and manganese.

Data are presented in this chapter for average daily intakes of the above minerals, which were derived from the records of the 1701 (unweighted) young people in the survey who completed a full seven-day dietary record.

Correlations between dietary intakes of sodium and potassium and blood pressure measurements are reported in *Chapter 11, Blood pressure*, and correlations between dietary intakes of sodium and potassium and urinary sodium and potassium are presented in this chapter.

This chapter also presents results for urinary sodium and urinary potassium, which are also presented as ratios to urinary creatinine. The results are based on first void on rising urine samples (see *Section 9.11*).

Iron and zinc were the only minerals for which dietary supplements made a noticeable contribution to intake and so iron and zinc intakes are presented from *all sources*, including dietary supplements, and from *food sources* alone. For the remaining minerals, intakes are only presented from food sources alone.

For those minerals where UK Reference Nutrient Intake values (RNIs) and Lower Reference Nutrient Intake values (LRNIs) have been published for young people in the appropriate sex and age groups, the proportion of young people with intakes below the LRNIs are shown, and average daily intakes are compared with current RNIs, which are shown in Table 9.1[1]. A further explanation of RNIs and LRNIs can be found in Chapter 8, Section 8.1.1. Intakes are also shown per megajoule (MJ) of daily energy intake, providing a measure of nutrient density commonly used to assess the quality of diets.   *(Table 9.1)*

9.2 Total iron, haem and non-haem iron

Dietary iron occurs in two forms. About 90% of iron in the average British diet is in the form of iron salts and is referred to as *non-haem iron*[2]. The extent to which this type of iron is absorbed is highly variable and depends both on the individual's iron status and on other components of the diet. The other 10% of dietary iron is in the form of *haem iron* and comes mainly from the haemoglobin and myoglobin of meat. Haem iron is well absorbed, and its absorption is less strongly influenced by the individual's iron stores or other constituents of the diet.

Ascorbic acid (vitamin C) enhances the absorption of non-haem iron, as do meat, fish and poultry. Bran, polyphenols, oxalates, phytates, the tannins in tea, and phosphates inhibit absorption. Haem iron itself promotes the absorption of non-haem iron. As an example of how these factors interact in the diet, beverages can improve or inhibit the absorption of iron depending on their type; orange juice or soft drinks fortified with vitamin C can double the absorption of non-haem iron from an entire meal, while tea decreases it[3]. Data presented in Table 4.11 shows that 45% of boys and 48% of girls in the survey consumed tea over the seven-day recording period and the average amount consumed (by consumers) was between 499g and 1966g a day, depending on sex and age.

The mean daily intake of *total iron* from food sources was 10.4mg for boys and, significantly lower, 8.3mg for girls (medians 9.8mg and 7.9mg) (p < 0.01). Haem iron contributed a mean of 0.4mg and 0.3mg (medians 0.4mg and 0.3mg) towards total iron intake for boys and girls, while non-haem iron from food sources contributed 10.0mg and 8.0mg respectively (medians 9.3mg and 7.5mg) (differences between sexes for haem and non-haem iron: p < 0.01).

For boys, and for girls except the oldest age group, mean intake of total iron from food sources increased with age, for example from 8.2mg and 7.3mg for boys and girls aged 4 to 6 years to 12.5mg for boys aged 15 to 18 years, and 8.8mg for girls aged 11 to 14 years (p < 0.01). Mean daily intake of haem iron and non-haem iron also increased significantly with age (p < 0.01), except for intake of non-haem iron for girls aged 15 to 18 years where mean daily intake from food sources was slightly lower than for girls aged 11 to 14 years (ns).

Intakes of total iron at the lower 2.5 percentile were about half median intakes and at the upper 2.5 percentile increased with age, being less than twice the median intake in each group, except for girls aged 15 to 18 years.

As Table 9.5 shows, for boys the mean intake of total iron from food sources was 112% of the RNI and was above the RNI in each age group except for those aged 11 to 14 years (95% of RNI).

For girls, mean intake from food sources was 82% of the RNI overall and fell markedly with age. Only for the youngest girls was mean intake of total iron from food sources above the RNI, but for all other age groups was below the RNI and for 15 to 18 year-old girls mean intake was only just above half the RNI, 58%.

No more than 3% of boys in any age group or girls in the two younger age groups had an average daily intake of total iron from food sources below the LRNI. However, the proportion of older girls with intakes below the LRNI was much higher, 45% of 11 to 14 year olds and 50% of 15 to 18 year olds. The inclusion of iron supplements had little effect on these proportions.

As Table 9.2 shows, dietary supplements providing iron made almost no difference to mean daily intakes of total iron, or to intakes at the lower 2.5 percentile. At the upper 2.5 percentile, supplements increased intakes of total iron for boys aged 4 to 6 years by 7% from 13.5mg to 14.4mg, and overall for girls, by just over 10% from 14.9mg to 16.5mg. For girls there were marked differences in the contribution of supplements between the age groups; intakes of total iron at the upper 2.5 percentile were increased by supplement taking by about 7% for the youngest and oldest groups of girls, but for 7 to 10 year olds and 11 to 14 year olds supplements providing iron increased intake at the upper 2.5 percentile by 13% and 20% respectively.

Table 9.6 shows the average daily intake of minerals from food sources for boys and girls in the survey, adjusted for variation in energy intake, that is intake of minerals per megajoule energy intake.

As this table shows, the variation in average daily intake of both haem and non-haem iron associated with sex and age largely disappeared when the variation in energy intake was taken into account. This indicates that the differences reported above are largely associated with differences in the intakes of energy between the sex and age groups.   (Tables 9.2 to 9.6)

Food sources of total iron, haem and non-haem iron
Some foods are fortified with iron, for example white flour and many breakfast cereals. Thus food groups such as cereals and cereal products were found to be major sources of iron for young people in this survey. Indeed as Table 9.7 shows, young people in the survey

obtained about half their average daily intake of total iron from cereals and cereal products. Within this group the major sources were breakfast cereals, providing 29% of total iron for boys and 23% for girls, and white bread, contributing 11% for both boys and girls. Although the contribution made by cereals and cereal products to total iron intake appeared to fall as age increased, from 57% for boys and girls aged 4 to 6 years, to 52% for boys and 47% for girls aged 15 to 18 years, this difference was not statistically significant.

The two other main sources of iron in the diets of young people in the survey were vegetables, potatoes and savoury snacks, and meat and meat products. Vegetables, potatoes and savoury snacks provided 16% and 18% respectively of intake for boys and girls, about half of which came from potatoes. Meat and meat products contributed 14% to total iron intake for boys and 13% for girls, of which about 3% came from beef, veal and dishes, 3% from chicken and turkey and dishes, and a further 3% from burgers, kebabs and sausages. On average, liver, liver products and liver dishes contributed less than 0.5% to total iron intake for any sex or age group.

Tables 9.8 and 9.9 show the food sources of haem and non-haem iron in the diets of the young people in the survey. Haem iron is found mainly in the haemoglobin and myoglobin of meat and over 90% of haem iron in the diets of the young people in the survey came from meat and meat products, principally beef, veal, chicken, turkey and dishes made from these and from burgers and kebabs. In contrast, meat and meat products contributed only 10% to average daily intake of non-haem iron. Over half of intake of non-haem iron came from cereals and cereal products, and a further 17% and 19% for boys and girls respectively from vegetables, potatoes and savoury snacks.   (Tables 9.7 to 9.9)

9.3   Calcium
Calcium is the most abundant mineral in the body. Of the 1000g or so in the human adult body, about 99% is in the bones and teeth where its primary role is structural.

Boys in the survey had a significantly higher mean daily intake of calcium from food sources (784mg) than girls (652mg) (medians 748mg and 644mg) (p < 0.01). Intakes increased significantly with age for boys (p < 0.01) but not for girls, and in the oldest group intake for boys was a third higher than for girls (p < 0.01).

For both boys and girls the range of intakes was wide. For both boys and girls, intakes at the lower 2.5 percentile were between a third and a half of median intakes depending on age group, and intakes at the upper 2.5 percentile were 60% to 95% higher than median intakes.

Overall, mean intake of calcium was 113% and 105% of the RNI for boys and girls respectively. Average intakes were above the RNI for the two younger groups but were below the RNI for both boys and girls aged 11 to 14 and 15 to 18 years.

One in eight boys and one in four girls in the 11 to 14 age group had a daily intake below the LRNI. For 15 to 18 year olds 9% of boys and 19% of girls had an intake below the LRNI.

After adjusting for differences between boys and girls in different age groups in intake of energy there were still significant differences between the groups in average daily calcium intake (see *Table 9.6*). For both boys and girls, those aged 4 to 6 years had a significantly higher average daily intake of calcium from food sources per MJ energy than young people in each of the older age groups (p < 0.01). This is probably accounted for by the higher milk consumption by the younger age groups.

The contribution of calcium-containing supplements to intakes was negligible.   *(Tables 9.10 and 9.11)*

Food sources of calcium [4]

The main source of calcium for young people in the survey was milk and milk products, contributing 48% to average intake for boys and 47% for girls. Within this group, whole milk, semi-skimmed milk and cheese were the main contributors. The contribution made by milk, particularly whole milk, to average daily calcium intake, was, not surprisingly, strongly associated with age, since, as has been noted previously, the consumption of whole milk decreased with increasing age (see *Table 4.3*). Thus whole milk contributed 25% to average calcium intake for children aged 4 to 6 years, but only 8% to intake for those aged 15 to 18 years (p < 0.01).

White flour is fortified with calcium, and cereals and cereal products were therefore another main source of calcium in the diets of the young people, contributing 27% to average intake. Within this group, 10% came from bread, mainly as white bread, about 5% from pizzas and a further 5% from biscuits, cakes, buns and pastries. The data suggest that cereals and cereal products were a slightly more important source of calcium for older children, but the differences by age were not statistically significant (p > 0.05).

(Table 9.12)

9.4   Phosphorus

Phosphorus is the second most abundant mineral in the body and has a variety of functions.

Mean daily intake of phosphorus from food sources for boys increased with age from 919mg for boys aged 4 to 6 years to 1330mg for those aged 15 to 18 years (p < 0.01). For girls, intakes were lower than for boys in each age group, ranging from 848mg for the youngest group of girls to 959mg for girls aged 15 to 18 years (p < 0.01). The overall mean intake for girls, 917mg, was significantly lower than the mean intake for boys, 1105mg (p < 0.01).

Median intakes were slightly below mean intakes (1066mg and 896mg for boys and girls respectively). Intakes at the lower 2.5 percentile were between about 45% and 65% of median intakes, depending on the sex and age of the young person, and at the upper 2.5 percentile were between about 40% and 70% higher than median intakes, again depending on sex and age of the young person.

Mean intakes were 198% and 184% of the RNI for boys and girls respectively and were above the RNI for each age group.

As Table 9.6 shows, after adjusting for variation in energy intake, boys and girls aged 4 to 6 years had a higher average intake of phosphorus from food sources per MJ energy than young people aged 7 to 10 years (both sexes: p < 0.05) and for girls, compared with girls aged 11 to 14 years (p < 0.01), suggesting that the youngest children in the survey were having a diet richer in this mineral than these older groups of boys and girls.

None of the dietary supplements taken by young people in the survey provided any phosphorus.

(Tables 9.13 and 9.14)

Food sources of phosphorus

The two main sources of phosphorus in the diets of young people in the survey were cereals and cereal products, and milk and milk products, each contributing about one quarter of the average intake. The contribution made by cereals and cereal products did not vary significantly with age, and included contributions from white and wholemeal bead (7%), breakfast cereals (about 5%) and biscuits, buns, cakes and pastries (5%).

Reduced fat milks contributed 10% and 8% respectively to the average intake of phosphorus for boys and girls, and whole milk a further 8% for boys and 7% for girls. As for other minerals and some vitamins, the percentage contribution from whole milk decreased significantly with age, from 15% for both boys and girls aged 4 to 6 years, to 4% for those aged 15 to 18 years (both sexes combined: p < 0.01).

Meat and meat products contributed just under one fifth to average intake of phosphorus, coming mainly from the consumption of chicken, turkey and dishes, and from burgers, kebabs and sausages.

Boys obtained 12% and girls 13% of their average intake of phosphorus from vegetables, potatoes and savoury snacks.   *(Table 9.15)*

9.5 Magnesium

The mean daily intake of magnesium from food sources for boys, 212mg, was about one fifth higher than that for girls, 178mg ($p < 0.01$). For both sexes intake increased significantly with age, from 172mg and 155mg for boys and girls aged 4 to 6 years to 256mg and 191mg for boys and girls aged 15 to 18 years ($p < 0.01$).

Median intakes were close to mean intakes, and were 204mg and 175mg for boys and girls respectively. Overall, intakes at the lower 2.5 percentile were about 50% of median intake for both boys and girls, but for boys there was quite wide variation between age groups. For example, for boys aged 4 to 6 years, intake of magnesium at the lower 2.5 percentile was only 67mg, about 40% of the median intake, while for those aged 7 to 10 years, intake at the lower 2.5 percentile was 117mg, about 63% of median intake. Intakes at the upper 2.5 percentile were between about 45% and 70% higher than median intakes depending on the sex and age of the young person, and ranged between 264mg and 390mg for boys and between 244mg and 314mg for girls.

Overall, mean intakes of magnesium for boys and girls in the survey were, respectively, 98% and 85% of the RNI and were above the RNI only for 4 to 6 year-old boys and girls. For the 11 to 14 year age group mean intakes were 78% and 65% of the RNI for boys and girls respectively, and for the 15 to 18 year age group, 85% and 64%. For boys in the top two age groups 28% and 18% respectively had intakes below the LRNI. Half the girls in the top two age groups had a daily intake of magnesium below the LRNI, 51% of 11 to 14 year olds and 53% of 15 to 18 year olds.

The differences in average daily intake of magnesium for boys and girls of different ages that are described above are largely associated with differences in energy intake between the groups, since after adjusting for this variation, there were no significant differences in intake of magnesium per MJ energy associated with sex or age (see *Table 9.6*).

None of the dietary supplements taken by young people in the survey provided any magnesium.

(Tables 9.16 and 9.17)

Food sources of magnesium
Just under one third (32% for boys and 30% for girls) of the average intake of magnesium for young people in the survey came from their consumption of cereals and cereal products, including 7% from white bread, about 8% from breakfast cereals and 5% from biscuits, buns, cakes and pastries. The data indicate that the contribution made by cereals and cereal products reduced slightly as age increased, but the differences between the age groups were not statistically significant ($p > 0.05$).

The other main source of magnesium in the diets of the young people was vegetables, potatoes and savoury snacks, contributing 21% to average intake of magnesium for boys and 23% for girls. Over half of this (12% for both sexes) came from the consumption of potatoes.

Milk and milk products contributed a further 16% to intake for boys and 15% for girls, mainly from whole and semi-skimmed milk. As found previously, the contribution made by whole milk was highest for the youngest children, and reduced significantly with age. For example, 4 to 6 year-old boys and girls derived on average 10% of their intake of magnesium from whole milk, compared with 3% for 15 to 18 year olds (both sexes combined: $p < 0.01$).

Meat and meat products contributed 11% overall to average magnesium intake, with about one third of this coming from the consumption of chicken, turkey and dishes.

Beers and lagers contributed 4% to magnesium intake for boys aged 15 to 18 years and 2% to intake for girls in the same age group. *(Table 9.18)*

9.6 Sodium and chloride
Sodium and chloride are the principal cation and anion respectively in extracellular fluid in the body. Both sodium and chloride are required in small amounts in the diet and their concentrations are maintained by a variety of regulatory mechanisms.

Sodium and chloride are not generally found in high concentrations in unprocessed foods, but tend to be added to many foods during processing as well as in the home during cooking or at the table. Although the average sodium and chloride content of foods was assessed, it was not possible to measure the amount of salt added to the young person's food during cooking or at the table. Thus intakes of both sodium and chloride are based on average values attributed to foods eaten and do not allow for additions in cooking and at the table. The results are therefore underestimates of total sodium and chloride intake.

Questions on the habitual use of salt in cooking the young person's food and on the addition of salt at the table were asked in the initial interview. These questions did not ask how much salt was used, only about frequency of use.

It was reported that about two thirds of the young people usually had salt added to their food in cooking[5] and that salt was added to food at the table, either usually or occasionally, by about half of the young people (see *Table 9.19*). There was no difference between boys and girls in the likelihood of salt being used in cooking or at the table, but salt was more likely to be used as age increased. For example, it was reported that salt was usually added in cooking for 54%

of boys and 56% of girls aged 4 to 6 years; however 70% of boys and 69% of girls aged 15 to 18 years had salt added to their food in cooking (p < 0.05). Similarly the use of salt at the table increased with age; 10% of boys and 13% of girls aged 4 to 6 years usually had salt added to their food at the table. In the 15 to 18 year age group, 33% of boys and 30% of girls were usually adding salt to their food at the table (both sexes: p < 0.01).

The use of salt in cooking and the addition of salt to food at the table are to some extent related. Table 9.20 shows that for 23% of boys and 24% of girls salt was usually added to their food in cooking and at the table, and for 53% and 54% salt was not added in cooking *and* rarely or never used at the table.

(Tables 9.19 and 9.20)

The mean daily intakes of *sodium* from food sources, excluding additions in cooking or at the table, for boys and girls in the survey were 2630mg and 2156mg respectively (p < 0.01). For both sexes intake increased significantly with age from 2069mg and 1857mg for boys and girls aged 4 to 6 years to 3265mg and 2281mg for those aged 15 to 18 years (p < 0.01).

Median intakes were close to mean values, 2542mg for boys and 2119mg for girls. Intakes at the upper 2.5 percentile were between about 50% and 70% higher than median intakes and ranged from 3361mg and 2905mg for boys and girls aged 4 to 6 years, to 5031mg and 3603mg for those aged 15 to 18 years.

Mean intake of sodium was well above the RNI for each age and sex group, and overall was over twice the RNI for boys, 212%, and 178% of the RNI for girls. Less than 0.5% of both boys and girls had an intake below the LRNI. Intakes at the upper 2.5 percentile for boys were between 2½ and nearly five times the RNI, depending on age, and for girls between two and four times the RNI.

None of the dietary supplements taken by young people in the survey provided any sodium.

(Tables 9.21 and 9.22)

The average daily *chloride* intake was, like intake of sodium, several grams per day. Mean daily intakes for boys and girls were 3954mg and 3241mg respectively (p < 0.01), representing 206% and 173% of the RNI. Chloride intake increased significantly with age (p < 0.01), particularly for boys, and median intakes were close to mean values, 3821mg for boys and 3190mg for girls. Intakes at the upper 2.5 percentile were between about 45% and 65% higher than median intakes and between two and 4½ times greater than the RNI for boys and girls, depending on age.

None of the dietary supplements taken by young people in the survey provided any chloride.

(Tables 9.23 and 9.24)

The data suggest that the oldest group of boys and girls were consuming a diet richer in both sodium and chloride than younger children in the survey, since, even after allowing for variation in intake of energy, there remained differences in average intakes of sodium and chloride per MJ energy associated with age group. As Table 9.6 shows, young people, and particularly boys, aged 15 to 18 years, had an average intake of sodium per MJ energy significantly higher than those aged 4 to 6 years (both sexes: p < 0.05). Similarly, average intake of chloride per MJ energy was significantly higher for boys and girls aged 15 to 18 years, than for those aged 4 to 6 years (boys: p < 0.05; girls: p < 0.01). These differences in intake per MJ energy between the oldest and youngest groups are, as has already been shown, compounded by the greater use of salt in cooking and at the table by the oldest age group.

Food sources of sodium and chloride[6]
The main food sources of sodium and chloride in the diets of young people were very similar, since these two minerals are generally found together in foods in the form of salt; only the food sources of sodium are discussed here, but Table 9.26 shows the percentage contribution made by food types to average daily intake of chloride.

Nearly two fifths (40% for boys and 38% for girls) of the average intake of sodium came from cereals and cereal products, with white bread alone providing about 15% of average daily intake, about 8% from breakfast cereals, 5% from biscuits, cakes, buns and pastries, and about a further 4% from pizza. The contribution made by cereals and cereal products varied very little with age.

Meat and meat products contributed 24% to the average intake of sodium for boys and 21% for girls; there was no significant difference in the percentage contribution associated with age. Bacon and ham, chicken and turkey and dishes, and sausages each contributed about 5%.

Vegetables, potatoes and savoury snacks provided about 15% of intake, of which savoury snacks contributed 6% for boys and 7% for girls, and vegetables, excluding potatoes, a further 6% and 7% respectively, mainly from vegetable dishes.

(Tables 9.25 and 9.26)

9.7 Potassium

The mean daily intake of potassium from food sources for boys in the survey was 2343mg and for girls, significantly lower, 2026mg (p < 0.01). For both sexes, mean intakes increased significantly with age, for example, from 1944mg and 1774mg for boys and girls aged 4 to 6 years, to 2833mg and 2162mg for 15 to 18 year olds (p < 0.01). Median intakes were close to mean intakes, 2267mg for boys and 2010mg for girls.

Intakes at the lower 2.5 percentile were about half median intakes and intakes at the upper 2.5 percentile were between 50% and 60% higher than median intakes for boys, and about 40% to 65% higher for girls, depending on age group.

Mean intake of potassium from food sources for boys in the survey provided 107% of the RNI, and 95% of the RNI for girls. Mean intakes as a percentage of the RNI decreased markedly with age and were above the RNI for the two younger age groups, but below the RNI for the older age groups. For example, for the youngest boys mean intake of potassium provided 177% of the RNI, but only 81% for 15 to 18 year-old boys. The pattern was similar for girls, with the mean intake providing 161% of the RNI for 4 to 6 year olds, but only 62% for the oldest girls.

When intakes are compared with LRNIs the data show no more than 1% of boys and girls aged 4 to 10 years had intakes below the LRNI. These proportions then increased with age so that one in ten boys and one in five girls aged 11 to 14 years had an intake of potassium below the LRNI. For the oldest group nearly one in seven boys and more than one in three girls had intakes below the LRNI.

After allowing for variation in intake of energy, average intake of potassium per MJ energy for boys was significantly higher for those aged 4 to 6 years compared with boys aged 7 to 10 years ($p < 0.05$) (see *Table 9.6*). For girls, differences associated with age in average intake of potassium per MJ were also evident, but, in contrast to boys, the oldest group of girls had a significantly higher intake per MJ than younger girls ($p < 0.05$).

None of the dietary supplements taken by young people in the survey provided any potassium.

(Tables 9.27 and 9.28)

Food sources of potassium
Boys obtained 34% and girls 36% of their average intake of potassium from the consumption of vegetables, potatoes and savoury snacks. Within this group, the main contributor was potatoes, which provided 22%. The data suggest that the percentage contribution made by this group increased with age, but the differences between the age groups did not reach the level of statistical significance ($p > 0.05$).

Milk and milk products contributed 18% for boys and 16% for girls to average intake of potassium. In the youngest age group, whole milk alone contributed 12% to intake, but this declined with age, so that by age 15 to 18 years, whole milk only contributed 3% to average potassium intake (both sexes combined: $p < 0.01$). Semi-skimmed milk contributed 8% for boys and 6% for girls and unlike whole milk there was little variation in the percentage contribution made by semi-skimmed milk associated with age.

Cereals and cereal products contributed about 15% to average intake of potassium, with almost no variation between age groups. This was principally in the form of white bread (3%), biscuits, buns, cakes and pastries (3%) and high fibre or wholegrain breakfast cereals (2%).

Meat and meat products contributed about 13% to average potassium intake, and for boys, the contribution increased with age from 10% for boys aged 4 to 6 years to 16% for boys aged 15 to 18 years (ns).

9.8 Trace elements

9.8.1 Zinc
The mean daily intake of zinc from food sources for boys in the survey was 6.9mg and for girls significantly lower, 5.7mg ($p < 0.01$). For both sexes, mean intakes increased with age, for example, from 5.5mg for boys aged 4 to 6 years, to 8.7mg for boys aged 15 to 18 years ($p < 0.01$).

Median intakes, 6.5mg for boys and 5.5mg for girls were only slightly lower than mean intakes. At the lower 2.5 percentile intakes were about half the median, and at the upper 2.5 percentile about 60% to 80% higher than median intakes, depending on the sex and age of the young person.

Mean daily intake of zinc from food sources was 86% of the RNI for boys and 77% of the RNI for girls and was below the RNI for all age groups.

When the intake of zinc from food sources is compared with LRNIs, the proportions with intakes below the LRNIs ranged from one in twenty boys aged 7 to 10 years to about one in seven boys aged 11 to 14 years and one in eight boys in the youngest age group. For girls aged 7 to 10 years and 15 to 18 years, one in ten had a daily intake of zinc from food sources below the LRNI, rising to one in four girls aged 4 to 6 years, and more than one in three for the 11 to 14 year olds.

Supplements providing zinc made very little contribution to intakes. As Table 9.30 shows the only noticeable difference was in intakes at the upper 2.5 percentile for boys aged 4 to 10 years and girls aged 4 to 6 years. Supplements providing zinc had no effect on the proportions in each age/sex group with intakes below the LRNI.

After allowing for differences in energy intake, both boys and girls aged 15 to 18 years still had significantly higher intakes of zinc from food sources than boys and girls in the youngest age group ($p < 0.05$) (see *Table 9.6*). This suggests that the oldest children were consuming diets richer in zinc than those in the youngest age group.

(Tables 9.30 and 9.31)

Food sources of zinc
Just under one third of the average intake of zinc came from the consumption of meat and meat products (31% for boys and 30% for girls). For both sexes this included about 7% contributed by beef and veal and dishes and about 6% each from chicken, turkey and dishes, and burgers, kebabs and sausages.

One quarter of zinc intake came from cereals and cereal products, chiefly in the form of white bread (6%), and breakfast cereals, mainly of the wholegrain or high fibre type (about 5%).

There were no significant differences associated with sex or age in the contribution made by either meat and meat products or cereals and cereal products to average zinc intake, but milk and milk products, which contributed about one fifth overall to average intake, were a more important source of this trace element for younger children in the survey. In the youngest age group whole milk contributed 12% to average intake of zinc for boys and 13% for girls, compared with only 3% for 15 to 18 year olds (both sexes combined: p < 0.01).

Vegetables, potatoes and savoury snacks was the only other food group contributing more than 10% to average intake of zinc.   *(Table 9.32)*

9.8.2 Copper

The mean daily intake of copper from food sources was 0.88mg for boys in the survey, and for girls was significantly lower, 0.75mg (p < 0.01). Mean daily intake increased with age for boys from 0.70mg for 4 to 6 year olds, to 1.06mg for 15 to 18 year olds (p < 0.01). For girls, there was a similar increase with age with mean daily intake rising from 0.64mg to 0.80mg (p < 0.01).

Median intakes were slightly below mean intakes, 0.83mg for boys and 0.71mg for girls.

At the lower 2.5 percentile average daily intakes of copper for boys were about 50% to 60% lower than mean intake, ranging from 0.33mg for 4 to 6 year olds, to 0.58mg for 15 to 18 year-old boys. For girls, intakes at the lower 2.5 percentile were also about 50% to 60% below mean intakes but there was no clear association with age.

Intakes at the upper 2.5 percentile ranged between 1.33mg and 1.68mg for boys, and 1.22mg and 1.39mg for girls, depending on age.

Overall for boys, mean intake of copper exceeded the RNI, providing 113% of the reference value, and was above the RNI for all age groups. However, the mean intake for girls was 97% of the RNI, and mean intakes for the 11 to 14 and 15 to 18 year age groups were below the RNI at 98% and 80% of the RNI respectively.

There are no LRNIs for copper.

The differences in average daily intake of copper associated with age above are largely accounted for by differences in energy intake between the age groups. As Table 9.6 shows, after allowing for differences in energy intake, intake of copper per MJ energy did not vary significantly between the age groups for either boys or girls in the survey.

Dietary supplements taken by young people in the survey provided only negligible amounts of copper.
                                        (Tables 9.33 and 9.34)

Food sources of copper
For boys, 41% and for girls, 38% of average intake of copper came from the consumption of cereals and cereal products, including about 13% from bread. There was no significant variation associated with age (p > 0.05).

Vegetables, potatoes and savoury snacks contributed between 18% and 23% of the average copper intake for boys and girls, depending on age, the contribution increasing slightly with age. Potatoes were the major contributor from this group.

Meat and meat products contributed 14% to average copper intake for boys and 13% for girls; for boys, the percentage contribution increased with age from 12% for 4 to 6 year-old boys to 17% for 15 to 18 year olds (ns).   *(Table 9.35)*

9.8.3 Iodine

The mean daily intake of iodine from food sources for boys in the survey was 163µg; mean intake for girls was significantly lower, 134µg (p < 0.01). For boys, mean daily intake increased with age, from 156µg for 4 to 6 year olds to 181µg for 15 to 18 year olds (p < 0.05); there was no association between mean iodine intakes and age for girls.

Median intakes were slightly below mean intakes, 150µg for boys and 125µg for girls.

For boys, intake at the lower 2.5 percentile was between about 40% and 45% of median intake, and for girls, between about 35% and 40% of median intake. At the upper 2.5 percentile the intake for both boys and girls was at least twice the median intake. For example, for young people aged 15 to 18 years, intakes at the lower 2.5, 50th and upper 2.5 percentiles were 78µg, 168µg and 348µg for boys, and 41µg, 126µg and 279µg for girls.

As Table 9.37 shows, mean intakes of iodine were in excess of the RNI for both boys and girls, providing 139% and 111% of the reference value respectively. However, mean daily intakes for girls in the top two age groups were slightly below the reference value, providing 92% and 96% of the RNIs.

No more than 3% of boys in any age group had an intake of iodine below the LRNI. The proportion of girls with intakes below the LRNI was greater than for boys, and ranged from 2% in the youngest group to 13% for girls aged 11 to 14 years (p < 0.01).

The data suggest that the youngest children in the survey, those aged 4 to 6 years, were consuming a diet richer in iodine than that of older boys and girls (see *Table 9.6*). After allowing for differences between the age groups in their average daily intake of energy, boys and girls aged 4 to 6 years had a higher average intake of iodine per MJ energy than older boys and girls (p < 0.05). This is at least partly due to the higher consumption of milk by younger children.

Dietary supplements taken by young people in the survey provided only negligible amounts of iodine.

(Tables 9.36 and 9.37)

Food sources of iodine

Milk and milk products were clearly the most important source of iodine in the diets of young people in the survey. About half (51% for boys and 48% for girls) of the average daily intake of iodine came from milk and milk products, mainly in the form of either whole milk (17%) or semi-skimmed milk (22% for boys and 17% for girls). As has previously been noted, whole milk as a provider of minerals and vitamins, made a greater contribution to average intake in the younger age groups, while the contribution made by semi-skimmed milk tended to increase with age. Thus 4 to 6 year-old boys and girls in the survey obtained nearly one third (31%) of their average intake of iodine from whole milk, while for the 15 to 18 year olds, this source contributed just 11% (both sexes combined: p < 0.01).

The other major source of iodine was cereals and cereal products, contributing 16% to average intake for both boys and girls, and tending to increase slightly with increasing age. This includes about 4% from bread, and 5% from biscuits, buns, cakes and pastries.

Fish and fish dishes, which are a rich source of iodine, contributed 8% to intake for both boys and girls.

(Table 9.38)

9.8.4 Manganese

The mean daily intake of manganese for boys in the survey was 2.20mg, and significantly lower for girls, 1.87mg (p < 0.01) (medians 2.03mg and 1.73mg). For both sexes mean intakes increased with age from 1.78mg and 1.56mg for boys and girls aged 4 to 6 years to 2.62mg and 2.04mg for boys and girls aged 15 to 18 years (both sexes: p < 0.01).

The range of intakes of manganese was wide, with intakes at the lower 2.5 percentile being between 40% and 60% of median daily intake, and at the upper 2.5 percentile between two and 2½ times greater than median intakes.

There are no RNIs for manganese but safe intakes are believed to lie above 1.4mg/d for adults and above 16µg/kg/d for infants and children[1]. Mean intakes were above the adult safe level for each age and sex group and at the lower 2.5 percentile were above the safe level for infants and children.

The differences in average daily intake of manganese for boys associated with age are largely accounted for by differences between the groups in average daily energy intake. However, for girls, even after allowing for variation in energy intake, those aged 15 to 18 years had a significantly higher average intake of manganese than girls aged 4 to 6 years (p < 0.05) (see *Table 9.6*).

The contribution of manganese-containing supplements to intakes was negligible. *(Table 9.39)*

Food sources of manganese

The principal source of manganese for both boys and girls in the survey was cereals and cereal products, contributing respectively 59% and 56% of average intake. This included 20% from bread, mainly white, and a similar proportion from breakfast cereals, mainly high fibre and wholegrain. Biscuits alone contributed 5% to average intake for both boys and girls.

The only other main source of manganese in the diets of the young people was vegetables, potatoes and savoury snacks, which contributed 17% to average intake for boys and 19% for girls.

Tea, which is a rich source of manganese, contributed 3% to intake overall for boys and girls; but almost twice this for the oldest age group, 5% for boys and 6% for girls (all differences: ns). *(Table 9.40)*

9.9 Variations in intakes

In this section, the variation in the average daily intake of minerals from *food sources* in relation to the main characteristics of the sample is considered. Since, as has been shown above, absolute intakes are related to energy intake, the quality of diets in respect of minerals, is compared by looking at mineral intakes from *food sources* for boys and girls in the survey per MJ energy intake.

Young people reported as being unwell

Compared with young people who reported not being unwell during the 7-day dietary recording period, those who said they were unwell and their eating was affected had lower average daily intakes of all minerals from food sources. Differences were particularly marked for girls, with intakes of all minerals, except haem iron, being markedly lower for those whose eating was affected by being unwell (all: p < 0.01). For boys average daily intakes of phosphorus, magnesium and potassium were most affected by being unwell (p < 0.01), although average daily intakes of non-haem iron, sodium, chloride, zinc, copper and iron, were also significantly lower for the unwell group of boys ($p < 0.05$).

When differences in average daily intake of energy were taken into account, none of the differences between those who were unwell and whose eating was affected and those who were not unwell remained. This suggests that the quality of the diet did not change when the young person was unwell, but they simply had a lower energy intake.   *(Tables 9.41 and 9.42)*

Region
Table 9.43 shows the average daily intake of minerals from food sources for boys and girls in the sample living in different regions.

The data suggest that compared with boys living elsewhere those living in Scotland tended to have lower average daily intakes from food sources of most minerals. However, the power to detect differences is limited by the relatively small size of the Scottish sample, so that very few differences reached the level of statistical significance. However there were significant differences between boys in Scotland and boys in London and the South East for intakes of copper and magnesium ($p < 0.05$).

Girls living in Scotland had the lowest absolute intakes of total and non-haem iron, calcium, magnesium, zinc, copper, iodine and manganese. Highest intakes of all these minerals, except iodine, were for girls living in the Central and South West regions of England and Wales. Intake of iodine was highest for girls in the Northern region. Of these, only differences in intake of total and non-haem iron and magnesium were statistically significant ($p < 0.05$). Intakes of sodium and chloride were highest for girls in the Northern region and lowest for those in London and the South East (both: $p < 0.05$).

When differences in energy intake were taken into account the variation that was seen in absolute intake of many minerals for young people living in different regions was no longer apparent. However, a few differences remained, indicating differences in the quality of the diets. For boys, there were significant differences for total and non-haem iron between boys living in Scotland, who had the lowest intake per MJ, and boys living in the Central and South West regions of England and Wales, who had the highest intake per MJ (both: $p < 0.05$). Boys in Scotland also had a lower intake per MJ of manganese compared with boys living in London and the South East ($p < 0.05$). Intake of zinc per MJ energy for boys living in the Northern region was significantly lower than for all other boys except those living in Scotland ($p < 0.05$).

Compared with girls living in the Northern region, girls living in the Central and South West regions of England and Wales had significantly higher intakes per MJ of total and non-haem iron and manganese (all: $p < 0.05$).

Girls in the Central and South West regions of England and Wales also had a higher intake of potassium per MJ than girls in London and the South East ($p < 0.05$). Compared with girls in London and the South East the diets of girls in Scotland were richer in sodium, since the intake, after allowing for variation in energy intake, was significantly higher ($p < 0.05$).   *(Tables 9.43 and 9.44)*

Socio-economic characteristics
Tables 9.45 to 9.50 show average daily intakes of minerals before and after allowing for differences in energy intake, for boys and girls according to whether they were living in households where one or both parents were receiving state benefits, by gross weekly household income and by the social class of the head of the household.

Average daily intakes of all minerals, except haem iron, were significantly lower for boys living in *benefit households*, than for those in households where neither parent was receiving Family Credit, Income Support or Job Seeker's Allowance (copper: $p < 0.05$; all others: $p < 0.01$).

In contrast there were no significant differences in average daily intake of minerals between girls living in benefit and non-benefit households.

Most of the differences in mineral intake for boys were accounted for by differences between the two groups in energy intake. Only for calcium was the average daily intake significantly lower for boys in benefit households when calculated per MJ energy (calcium: $p < 0.01$). For girls, those living in households where neither parent was receiving benefits had diets richer in calcium, phosphorus and iodine, than girls in benefit households, since the average intake per MJ energy for these minerals was significantly higher for the non-benefit group (iodine: $p < 0.05$; others: $p < 0.01$).

Before allowing for differences in energy intake, average daily intakes from food sources of most minerals increased for boys as *gross weekly household income* increased up to a gross weekly household income of between £400 and £600. Thereafter there was no significant difference in absolute intake for any of the minerals. Comparing intakes for boys in the lowest household income group with those for boys in households with an income of between £400 and £600 a week, there were statistically significant differences for all minerals except intake of haem iron and copper (manganese: $p < 0.05$; others: $p < 0.01$). For girls, average daily intakes of all minerals, except sodium and chloride, also increased as gross weekly household income increased, being highest in the top household income group but the differences in intake between the bottom and top income groups only reached the level of statistical significance for calcium, phosphorus and magnesium (magnesium: $p < 0.01$; others $p < 0.05$).

There were no significant differences in intake of sodium or chloride associated with household income level for girls.

After allowing for differences in average energy intake the only difference remaining for boys was for calcium, with boys in households with a weekly income of between £400 and £600 consuming a diet richer in calcium than those in the lowest income group ($p < 0.01$). For girls, average daily intakes of calcium, phosphorus and magnesium were still significantly higher in the highest income group than in the lowest income group when calculated per MJ energy (calcium: $p < 0.05$; others: $p < 0.01$).

Although there was a general pattern for young people from a manual *social class* background to have lower average intakes of most minerals than those from non-manual home backgrounds, there were few statistically significant differences. For boys intakes of calcium, and for girls intakes of phosphorus, and for both sexes intakes of iodine, were lower for those from a manual background (calcium for boys: $p < 0.01$; others: $p < 0.05$). Additionally girls from a manual social class home background had a lower average intake of magnesium and manganese than girls from a non-manual background (both: $p < 0.05$).

Most of these differences are likely to reflect differences in the quality of the diet in respect of these minerals, since after allowing for differences in energy intake, boys from a manual background had a lower average intake of calcium, phosphorus, magnesium and iodine, than boys from a non-manual background (calcium and phosphorus: $p < 0.01$; others: $p < 0.05$). For girls, intakes of phosphorus, magnesium, iodine and manganese per MJ energy were lower for the manual group, while adjusted intakes of sodium were higher for this same group of girls ($p < 0.05$). *(Table 9.45 to 9.50)*

Household type
It has already been noted that the age distribution of the different household types varied significantly, with a much higher proportion of older boys and girls living with both parents and no other children. This difference needs to be borne in mind when considering apparent differences between the groups in mineral and other nutrient intakes, particularly in the data for boys whose intakes are more strongly associated with age than for girls.

Table 9.51 shows that for boys, those living in households with both parents and no other children had the highest average daily intake of all minerals, including sodium and chloride. Comparing boys in two-parent households with and without other children, differences in average intakes of all minerals were statistically significant (total and non-haem iron: $p < 0.05$; others: $p < 0.01$).

For girls, the differences associated with household type were very small; comparing girls living in two-parent households with and without other children, none of the differences in average intake of any of the minerals reached the level of statistical significance ($p > 0.05$).

Intakes for boys and girls living with both parents and other children and boys and girls in single-parent households with or without other children were very similar to each other.

After allowing for differences in average energy intake between boys living in different household types, average intakes of minerals per MJ energy were still generally highest for boys living in two-parent households with no other children, although the differences between the three household types were much less than for the unadjusted intakes. The only differences to reach the level of statistical significance were for average intakes of phosphorus, potassium and zinc per MJ for boys in two-parent, no other children households, compared with boys in two-parent other children households (phosphorus and zinc: $p < 0.01$; potassium: $p < 0.05$). There were no significant differences for girls after allowing for differences in average energy intake ($p > 0.05$). *(Tables 9.51 and 9.52)*

9.10 Comparisons with other studies
Tables 9.53 and 9.54 compare data from this present survey of young people with data on average daily intakes of minerals from other national surveys; the 1983 Department of Health study of the Diets of British Schoolchildren, the 1992/93 survey of pre-school children and the 1986/87 survey of adults[7,8,9].

Table 9.53 compares the average daily intake of total iron and calcium from food sources for boys and girls aged 10 to 11 years and 14 to 15 years from the 1983 survey of the diets of British schoolchildren[7] with equivalent data from the present survey.

There are no significant differences in the average daily intake of total iron from food sources between the two surveys for boys in either of the two age groups, or for girls aged between 10 and 11 years. The data suggest that average daily intake of total iron for girls aged between 14 and 15 years may have declined over the period. In 1983, average daily intake for this sub-group was 9.3mg and in 1997, 8.6mg, but this difference was not statistically significant ($p > 0.05$).

For both sexes and both age groups there were no significant differences between the two sets of survey data for average daily intake of calcium from food sources, although the general trend was for intakes to be somewhat lower in the present survey.

As noted in Chapter 8 (see *Section 8.9)* the extent to which differences represent changes in the diets of young people over the period is difficult to assess. Many factors may contribute to any differences, including changes in nutrient composition data due to both actual changes in nutrient composition and new analytical methods, changes in fortification practices, and changes in food consumption patterns.

The 1983 survey data were not reported per unit energy intake. However, it has already been shown (see *Table 5.15*) that average daily intakes of energy are lower in the present survey than in 1983. It is therefore likely that the small decreases in average intake of both total iron and calcium are at least partly accounted for by changes in average energy intake, and probably do not represent a decline in the quality of young people's diets in respect of these minerals.

Table 9.54 compares mineral intake from food sources for boys and girls from the 1992/3 NDNS of children aged 1½ to 4½ years[8] and from the 1986/7 Dietary and Nutritional Survey of British Adults[9]. It should be noted that absolute intakes are shown, that is they do not take into account differences in energy intake, and that the age groups are not exactly matched.

Comparing mineral intakes for 3½ to 4½ year old boys and girls with those for 4 to 6 year olds clearly shows higher intakes for the generally older cohort from the present survey. For both boys and girls intakes of all minerals were significantly higher, except for calcium intakes by girls aged 4 to 6 years (boys: calcium $p < 0.05$; other minerals $p < 0.01$; girls: calcium ns; other minerals $p < 0.01$). The higher intakes are probably due, at least in part, to higher energy intake by the slightly older cohort. The decline in the consumption of milk, and in particular of whole milk as age increases, probably accounts for there being less difference between the cohorts in calcium intake.

For the older cohorts, there are fewer significant differences, and the data are less easy to interpret given the age groups are less well matched. However the data from the current survey suggest that for both boys and girls there has been a decline in the intake of magnesium, and of the trace elements, zinc, copper and iodine (boys: all $p < 0.01$; girls: magnesium and iodine $p < 0.05$; zinc and copper $p < 0.01$). Additionally for girls intake of total iron is significantly lower in the present survey than for the 16 to 24 year-old group of women in 1986/7 ($p < 0.05$).   *(Tables 9.53 and 9.54)*

9.11 Urine analytes

The following section presents data based on the analysis of the spot urine samples provided by young people in the survey. As described in Chapter 2 (see *Section 2.10*) the main reason for collecting spot urine samples from young people was to provide an indirect estimate of sodium intake, since it is not possible to measure intake directly as the amount of salt added to food in cooking or at the table cannot be accurately assessed. Chapter 2 also describes the procedure for obtaining a spot urine sample; the response rate for the urine sample is given in Chapter 3. Appendix S describes the processing of the urine samples and quality control procedures.

9.11.1 Results used in the analysis

A total of 1851 young people (unweighted) provided a spot urine sample and 1829 samples were analysed; 22 samples were received in an unsuitable condition for analysis and have been excluded from the urine analysis results.

The samples were analysed for concentrations of urinary sodium, urinary potassium and urinary creatinine. As was noted in Chapter 2 the rates of excretion of urinary sodium and urinary potassium vary with dietary intake, and their concentration in the urine may also vary with the volume of liquid recently consumed. In an attempt to reduce the intra-subject variation young people were asked to collect the sample of their urine from the first void on rising. Although those providing a sample were asked to confirm that it was from the first void on rising, which the majority did, (97%) there was no practical way of checking this information and it is possible that some samples were obtained from subsequent voidings. Other than for the 22 samples that were not suitable for analysis, the results for *all* the remaining 1829 samples are presented in the tables in this section. Hence some analytical values are likely to have been more affected than others by recent dietary intakes and by the volume of liquid consumed prior to collecting the sample.

By measuring urinary creatinine in the samples comparisons can be made between groups based on the ratios of urinary sodium to urinary creatinine and urinary potassium to urinary creatinine, which adjust for differences in urinary dilution.

9.11.2 Urinary sodium to urinary creatinine ratio

In adults, creatinine excretion is generally higher for men than women; this is associated with the higher proportion of lean body tissue in men. Urinary concentrations of sodium and potassium relative to urinary concentrations of creatinine are therefore generally lower for men than women. This general pattern for adults was reflected only in the results for the oldest age group of young people in this survey, those aged 15 to 18 years. For this age group the mean concentration of urinary creatinine was higher for boys than girls, 17.4mmol/l and 14.1mmol/l, ($p < 0.01$) while the mean urinary sodium to (urinary) creatinine ratio was lower for boys than girls, 9.2mol/mol and 11.4mol/mol ($p < 0.05$).

In the age group covered by this survey, it would be expected that urinary sodium and potassium concentrations relative to urinary creatinine concentration would decrease as the proportion of lean body mass increased, that is with increasing age, particularly for boys. Mean urinary sodium to creatinine ratio was lowest for the oldest group of boys and girls, those aged 15 to 18 years compared with those aged 4 to 6 years (both sexes p < 0.01). In the younger age groups there were no significant differences between boys and girls in either the mean concentration of creatinine or the mean ratio of urinary sodium to creatinine.

For both sexes the mean concentration of urinary sodium was lowest for the oldest age group, 134.4mmol/l and 138.5mmol/l respectively for boys and girls aged 15 to 18 years compared with 149.7mmol/l and 144.4mmol/l for boys and girls aged 4 to 6 years, but the differences did not reach the level of statistical significance.

As Table 9.56 shows, the distribution of values for the ratio of urinary sodium to creatinine was skewed and the range of values wide. Median values were below mean values by about 10%. At the lower 2.5 percentile values were between about one quarter and one third of median values and at the upper 2.5 percentile values were 2½ to 3½ times the median value, depending on the sex and age of the young person. For example, for boys aged 15 to 18 years the ratios at the lower 2.5, 50th and upper 2.5 percentiles were 2.1mol/mol, 7.6mol/mol and 25.7mol/mol respectively. *(Tables 9.55 and 9.56)*

9.11.3 Urinary potassium to urinary creatinine ratio

For both sexes the mean ratio of urinary potassium to urinary creatinine decreased as age increased, from 7.1mol/mol for both boys and girls aged 4 to 6 years, to 3.0mol/mol and 3.7mol/mol respectively for those aged 15 to 18 years (both sexes: p < 0.01). There were no significant differences by age group between boys and girls in mean ratio of urinary potassium to (urinary) creatinine.

For both boys and girls in the three youngest age groups the mean urinary concentration of potassium tended to decrease as age increased, from 55.0mmol/l for boys and 52.1mmol/l for girls aged 4 to 6 years, to 47.3mmol/l for boys and 43.4mmol/l for girls aged 11 to 14 years, however these differences did not reach the level of statistical significance. The mean urinary concentrations of potassium for boys and girls aged 15 to 18 years were slightly higher than the concentrations for those aged 11 to 14 years, but the differences were not significant (p > 0.05).

For both boys and girls the median urinary potassium to creatinine ratios were lower than the mean value, median values being about three-quarters the mean value. The range of ratios was also large with values at the lower 2.5 percentile being between about one third of median values and values at the upper 2.5 percentile

being between 3 and 5 times greater than median values, depending on the sex and age group. For example, for girls aged 15 to 18 years the ratios at the lower 2.5, 50th and upper 2.5 percentiles were 1.0mol/mol, 2.8mol/mol and 12.6mol/mol respectively. *(Tables 9.55 and 9.57)*

9.11.4 Urinary sodium to urinary potassium ratio

The mean urinary sodium to (urinary) potassium ratio for both boys and girls was 3.9mol/mol. As Table 9.58 shows, values increased very slightly across the youngest three age groups for boys, from 3.7mol/mol for boys aged 4 to 6 years to 4.1mol/mol for boys aged 11 to 14 years (ns) and for girls, from 3.7mol/mol for those in the youngest age group to 4.3mol/mol for girls aged 11 to 14 years (ns).

Median values were about 12% lower than mean values for both boys and girls, but there was considerable variation by age, particularly for girls, where median values were between about 10% and 20% lower than mean values, depending on age. Ratios at the lower 2.5 percentile were between a fifth and quarter of median values, ranging from 0.6mol/mol (boys aged 4 to 6 years) to 0.9mol/mol (boys aged 11 to 14 years). At the upper 2.5 percentile, values were 2½ to 3 times median values and ranged from 9.2mol/mol (boys aged 11 to 14 years) to 11.9mol/mol (girls aged 11 to 14 years). *(Tables 9.55 and 9.58)*

9.11.5 Correlations with dietary intakes

Tables 9.59 to 9.61 show correlation coefficients for urinary analyte ratios with estimated dietary intakes, for the eight age and sex groups of young people[10]. The tables are thus based on young people who provided both a spot urine sample and completed a seven-day weighed intake dietary record. The tables indicate those coefficients that are statistically significant, but it should be noted in relation to non-significant coefficients that the spot urine samples were not always collected during or immediately after the dietary recording period. It should also be noted that since these are bivariate correlations, causal relationships between the dietary and urinary variables cannot be assumed; there may be other associations, which might affect the size of the coefficient.

Urinary sodium to urinary creatinine ratio with dietary intake of sodium[11]
Within age group correlations between dietary intake of sodium and the urinary sodium to creatinine ratio were generally weak and positive in direction. Only the coefficients for all boys (-0.10), for boys aged 7 to 10 years (+0.28) and for girls aged 4 to 6 years (+0.20) were statistically significant (all: p < 0.01).

Urinary potassium to urinary creatinine ratio with dietary intake of potassium
Correlations between dietary intakes of potassium and the urinary potassium to creatinine ratio were strongest

for boys and girls in the younger age groups. The coefficients were statistically significant for boys aged 4 to 6 years ($+0.16$: $p < 0.05$) and 7 to 10 years ($+0.23$: $p < 0.01$) and for girls aged 4 to 6 years ($+0.22$: $p < 0.01$).

Urinary sodium to urinary potassium ratio with sodium to potassium ratio for dietary intakes[11]
There was generally a strong positive correlation between the ratio of urinary sodium to urinary potassium and the ratio of the dietary intake of these minerals for both boys and girls within age group, and overall for both sexes ($p < 0.01$, except for girls aged 11 to 14 years, where $p < 0.05$). The only exception was for boys aged 15 to 18 years, where the correlation was not statistically significant ($p > 0.05$).

(Tables 9.59 to 9.61)

9.11.6 Correlations with body mass index[12]

As in the previous surveys of pre-school children[8] and older people[13] correlations between urinary analyte ratios and body mass index (BMI) are reported (Tables 9.62 to 9.64).

Since urinary creatinine concentration is related to lean body mass, and urinary sodium and potassium concentrations relative to urinary creatinine concentration are lower for those with a higher proportion of lean body mass, it would be expected that the urinary analyte ratios relative to urinary creatinine would be inversely correlated with body mass index. As Tables 9.62 and 9.63 show, generally within age groups, the correlations were negative, and did not reach the level of statistical significance. However for girls aged 15 to 18 years there were significant positive correlations between BMI and the urinary sodium to creatinine ratio and BMI and the urinary sodium to potassium ratio (both: $p < 0.01$).

(Tables 9.62 to 9.64)

9.11.7 Variation in urinary analyte levels

Tables 9.65 to 9.70 show the mean concentration of the three urinary analytes measured and the urinary analyte ratios for boys and girls according to the main socio-demographic characteristics of the sample, and whether the young person was unwell during the dietary recording period.

There were very few clear patterns in the data or significant differences between sub-groups, including between those who were well and those who were unwell during the dietary recording period.

There were no differences in the urinary sodium to urinary creatinine ratios associated with social class for both boys and girls or with whether the young person's parents were in receipt of benefits. Again, although the differences were not significant ($p > 0.05$), for boys there was a general pattern for urinary analyte ratios to decrease as gross weekly household income increased.

For girls the highest urinary analyte ratios were for those in the second lowest household gross income band, £160 to less than £280 a week, but thereafter, as for boys, the urinary analyte ratios decreased with increasing income level.

For boys and girls living with both parents and no other children ratios of urinary sodium to creatinine and urinary potassium to creatinine were significantly lower than for those living in other household types ($p < 0.01$). However, as has been pointed out in other chapters, any differences associated with household type are likely to be a reflection, at least in part, of the significantly different age composition and BMI of the different household types (see, for example, *Chapter 11, Section 11.3*).

(Tables 9.65 to 9.70)

References and endnotes

1   Department of Health. Report on Health and Social Subjects: 41. *Dietary Reference Values for Food Energy and Nutrients for the United Kingdom.* HMSO (London, 1991).
2   Bull NI, Buss DH. Haem and Non-haem Iron in British Diets. *J Hum Nutr* 1980; **34:** 141–145
3   Oski FA. Iron deficiency in infancy and childhood. *N Engl J Med* 1993; **329**(3): 190–193
4   Hard water typically provides 200mg calcium daily, while in soft water areas it provides none. Due to regional differences it was not possible to ascertain the contribution of water to calcium intake. In addition, it was not possible to distinguish whether tap water consumed had been filtered, which could reduce the levels of calcium, chloride and heavy metals, for example, found in tap water.
5   Includes the use of a salt alternative in cooking.
6   Excludes salt added in cooking or at the table.
7   Department of Health. Report on Health and Social Subjects: 36. *The Diets of British Schoolchildren.* HMSO (London, 1989).
8   Gregory JR, Collins DL, Davies PSW, Hughes JM, Clarke PC. *National Diet and Nutrition Survey: children aged 1½ to 4½ years. Volume 1: Report of the diet and nutrition survey.* HMSO (London, 1995).
9   Gregory J, Foster K, Tyler H, Wiseman M. *The Dietary and Nutritional Survey of British Adults.* HMSO (London, 1990).
10 Pearson correlation coefficients were calculated in SPSS. Weighting factors, for non-response and sampling probability, were scaled (normalised) to approximate to the original, unweighted, sample size before running the SPSS procedure on weighted data. Pearson correlation coefficients are robust to departures from normally distributed data, that is skewed data, provided the value of the population coefficient is low, which it is for these data. *See:*
    Gayen AK. The distribution of Student's t in random samples of any size drawn from non-normal universes. *Biometrica.* 1949; **36:** 353
    Gayen AK. The distribution of the variance ratio in random samples of any size drawn for non-normal universes. Significance of difference between the means of two non-random samples. *Biometrica.* 1950: **37:** 236, 399
    Gayen AK. The frequency distribution of the product-moment correlation coefficient in random samples of any size drawn for non-normal universes. *Biometrica.* 1951: **38:** 219

[11] Intake of sodium from food sources only; excludes further additions of salt in cooking or at the table.

[12] See Chapter 10 for results and information on the derivation and interpretation of body mass index for young people in the survey.

[13] Finch S, Doyle W, Lowe C, Bates CJ, Prentice A, Smithers G, Clarke PC. *National Diet and Nutrition Survey: people aged 65 years and over. Volume 1: Report of the diet and nutrition survey.* TSO (London, 1998).

Table 9.1 Reference Nutrient Intakes (RNIs) and Lower Reference Nutrient Intakes (LRNIs) for minerals*

RNI and LRNI by age (years) and sex		Minerals									
		Iron	Calcium	Phosphorus**	Magnesium	Sodium	Chloride***	Potassium	Zinc	Copper	Iodine
		mg/d	mg/d	mg/d	mg/d	mg/d	mg/d	mg/d	mg/d	mg/d	µg/d
Males											
4–6	RNI	6.1	450	350	120	700	1100	1100	6.5	0.60	100
	LRNI	3.3	275	215	70	280	430	600	4.0	n/a	50
7–10	RNI	8.7	550	450	200	1200	1800	2000	7.0	0.70	110
	LRNI	4.7	325	250	115	350	530	950	4.0	n/a	55
11–14	RNI	11.3	1000	775	280	1600	2500	3100	9.0	0.80	130
	LRNI	6.1	480	370	180	460	710	1600	5.3	n/a	65
15–18	RNI	11.3	1000	775	300	1600	2500	3500	9.5	1.00	140
	LRNI	6.1	480	370	190	575	890	2000	5.5	n/a	70
Females		mg/d	mg/d	mg/d	mg/d	mg/d	mg/d	mg/d	mg/d	mg/d	µg/d
4–6	RNI	6.1	450	350	120	700	1100	1100	6.5	0.60	100
	LRNI	3.3	275	215	70	280	430	600	4.0	n/a	50
7–10	RNI	8.7	550	450	200	1200	1800	2000	7.0	0.70	110
	LRNI	4.7	325	250	115	350	530	950	4.0	n/a	55
11–14	RNI	14.8	800	625	280	1600	2500	3100	9.0	0.80	130
	LRNI	8.0	450	350	180	460	710	1600	5.3	n/a	65
15–18	RNI	14.8	800	625	300	1600	2500	3500	7.0	1.00	140
	LRNI	8.0	450	350	190	575	890	2000	4.0	n/a	70

*Source: Department of Health. Report on Health and Social Subjects: 41. *Dietary Reference Values for Food Energy and Nutrients for the United Kingdom*. HMSO (London, 1991).
** RNIs and LRNIs for phosphorus are set equal to the RNI for calcium in molar terms.
*** RNIs and LRNIs for chloride correspond to those for sodium in molar terms.
n/a no reference value set

Table 9.2 Average daily intake of total iron (mg) by sex and age of young person

Total iron (mg)	Males aged (years)				All males	Females aged (years)				All females
	4–6	7–10	11–14	15–18		4–6	7–10	11–14	15–18	
	cum %	cum %	cum %	cum %	cum %	cum %	cum %	cum %	cum %	cum %
(a) Intakes from *all* sources										
Less than 3.3	–	0	0	–	0	1	–	–	0	0
Less than 4.7	4	1	1	–	1	6	3	2	6	4
Less than 6.1	14	5	3	2	5	28	14	16	18	19
Less than 8.0	49	26	16	10	24	68	47	44	48	51
Less than 8.7	64	39	24	15	34	77	59	52	57	60
Less than 11.3	91	75	60	43	66	97	92	80	81	87
Less than 14.8	98	96	91	74	90	99	97	96	93	96
All	100	100	100	100	100	100	100	100	100	100
Base	*184*	*256*	*237*	*179*	*856*	*171*	*226*	*238*	*210*	*845*
Mean (average value)	8.3	9.8	10.8	12.6	10.5	7.4	8.5	9.1	8.9	8.5
Median value	8.0	9.3	10.4	11.7	9.9	7.1	8.2	8.6	8.2	8.0
Lower 2.5 percentile	4.4	5.7	5.8	6.9	5.1	3.9	4.7	4.8	3.9	4.2
Upper 2.5 percentile	14.4	15.8	17.6	22.3	19.0	11.8	15.0	17.4	17.6	16.5
Standard deviation of the mean	2.55	2.74	3.15	4.07	3.55	2.20	2.42	3.20	3.56	2.99
	cum %	cum %	cum %	cum %	cum %	cum %	cum %	cum %	cum %	cum %
(b) Intakes from *food* sources										
Less than 3.3	–	0	0	–	0	1	–	–	0	0
Less than 4.7	4	1	1	–	1	6	3	2	6	4
Less than 6.1	14	5	3	2	6	28	14	17	19	19
Less than 8.0	51	26	16	11	25	71	47	45	50	52
Less than 8.7	65	40	24	15	35	80	59	53	59	62
Less than 11.3	92	76	61	44	67	98	92	82	82	88
Less than 14.8	99	97	92	74	90	99	98	98	94	97
All	100	100	100	100	100	100	100	100	100	100
Base	*184*	*256*	*237*	*179*	*856*	*171*	*226*	*238*	*210*	*845*
Mean (average value)	8.2	9.7	10.8	12.5	10.4	7.3	8.4	8.8	8.7	8.3
Median value	7.9	9.3	10.4	11.6	9.8	7.1	8.2	8.4	8.0	7.9
Lower 2.5 percentile	4.4	5.7	5.8	6.6	5.1	3.9	4.7	4.8	3.9	4.2
Upper 2.5 percentile	13.5	15.7	17.6	22.3	19.0	10.9	13.3	14.5	16.6	14.9
Standard deviation of the mean	2.47	2.54	3.11	4.09	3.49	2.08	2.28	2.74	3.21	2.69

Table 9.3   Average daily intake of haem iron (mg) by sex and age of young person

Haem iron (mg)	Males aged (years)				All males	Females aged (years)				All females
	4–6	7–10	11–14	15–18		4–6	7–10	11–14	15–18	
	cum %	cum %	cum %	cum %	cum %	cum %	cum %	cum %	cum %	cum %
Intakes from *food sources*										
Less than 0.1	14	9	6	2	7	16	7	10	15	12
Less than 0.2	36	28	16	7	21	49	30	26	27	32
Less than 0.3	66	55	33	15	42	77	54	50	43	55
Less than 0.4	84	78	58	30	62	91	72	64	63	72
Less than 0.5	96	88	75	50	77	99	87	82	80	87
Less than 0.6	98	95	87	64	86	100	96	94	88	94
Less than 0.8	99	98	91	73	90		97	96	91	96
All	100	100	100	100	100		100	100	100	100
Base	*184*	*256*	*237*	*179*	*856*	*171*	*226*	*238*	*210*	*845*
Mean (average value)	0.3	0.3	0.4	0.6	0.4	0.2	0.3	0.4	0.4	0.3
Median value	0.2	0.3	0.4	0.5	0.4	0.2	0.3	0.3	0.3	0.3
Lower 2.5 percentile	0.0	0.0	0.1	0.1	0.0	0.0	0.0	0.0	0.0	0.0
Upper 2.5 percentile	0.7	0.7	1.1	1.4	1.1	0.5	0.8	0.9	1.1	0.9
Standard deviation of the mean	0.18	0.18	0.26	0.32	0.28	0.11	0.19	0.23	0.26	0.22

*None of the dietary supplements taken by young people in this survey provided any haem iron.

Table 9.4 Average daily intake of non-haem iron (mg) by sex and age of young person

Non-haem iron (mg)	Males aged (years)				All males	Females aged (years)				All females
	4–6	7–10	11–14	15–18		4–6	7–10	11–14	15–18	
	cum %	cum %	cum %	cum %	cum %	cum %	cum %	cum %	cum %	cum %
(a) Intakes from *all* sources										
Less than 4.0	2	0	0	–	1	3	2	1	4	2
Less than 6.0	17	6	5	2	7	29	16	21	21	21
Less than 8.0	57	31	21	13	29	70	52	50	54	56
Less than 10.0	83	65	49	35	57	93	83	67	79	80
Less than 12.0	95	83	73	58	76	98	95	86	89	92
Less than 14.0	97	94	89	71	88	99	97	96	93	96
All	100	100	100	100	100	100	100	100	100	100
Base	*184*	*256*	*237*	*179*	*856*	*171*	*226*	*238*	*210*	*845*
Mean (average value)	8.0	9.5	10.4	12.0	10.0	7.2	8.1	8.7	8.5	8.2
Median value	7.8	9.0	10.1	11.1	9.4	6.9	7.9	8.1	7.8	7.7
Lower 2.5 percentile	4.2	5.5	5.5	6.4	4.9	3.8	4.4	4.5	3.9	4.0
Upper 2.5 percentile	14.1	15.6	17.4	21.5	18.4	11.4	14.6	17.3	17.6	16.0
Standard deviation of the mean	2.49	2.71	3.12	4.04	3.46	2.17	2.39	3.20	3.54	2.96
	cum %	cum %	cum %	cum %	cum %	cum %	cum %	cum %	cum %	cum %
(b) Intakes from *food* sources										
Less than 4.0	2	0	0	–	1	3	2	1	4	2
Less than 6.0	17	6	5	2	7	29	17	21	22	22
Less than 8.0	58	32	21	14	30	73	53	51	56	57
Less than 10.0	85	66	51	35	58	93	83	69	80	81
Less than 12.0	96	84	74	58	77	98	96	89	89	93
Less than 14.0	98	95	90	72	88	99	98	98	94	97
All	100	100	100	100	100	100	100	100	100	100
Base	*184*	*256*	*237*	*179*	*856*	*171*	*226*	*238*	*210*	*845*
Mean (average value)	7.9	9.4	10.3	11.9	10.0	7.1	8.0	8.5	8.3	8.0
Median value	7.7	8.9	9.8	11.1	9.3	6.8	7.8	8.0	7.6	7.5
Lower 2.5 percentile	4.2	5.5	5.5	6.1	4.9	3.8	4.4	4.5	3.9	4.0
Upper 2.5 percentile	13.4	15.5	17.4	21.5	18.1	10.8	12.8	14.3	16.4	14.5
Standard deviation of the mean	2.41	2.51	3.08	4.04	3.41	2.05	2.25	2.72	3.18	2.65

Table 9.5 Average daily intake of total iron as a percentage of Reference Nutrient Intake (RNI) by sex and age of young person

Sex and age (years) of young person	Average daily intake as % of RNI*							
	(a) All sources			*Base*	(b) Food sources			*Base*
	Mean	Median	sd		Mean	Median	sd	
Males								
4–6	136	132	41.8	*184*	134	130	40.4	*184*
7–10	112	107	31.5	*256*	111	107	29.2	*256*
11–14	96	92	27.9	*237*	95	92	27.5	*237*
15–18	111	103	36.0	*179*	111	103	36.2	*179*
All	113	107	36.8	*856*	112	106	35.8	*856*
Females								
4–6	121	116	36.1	*171*	119	116	34.1	*171*
7–10	97	94	27.9	*226*	96	94	26.2	*226*
11–14	61	58	21.6	*238*	60	57	18.5	*238*
15–18	60	55	24.0	*210*	58	54	21.7	*210*
All	83	77	37.1	*845*	82	77	35.5	*845*

*Intake as a percentage of RNI was calculated for each young person. The values for all young people in each age group were then pooled to give a mean, median and sd.

288

Table 9.6 Average daily intake of minerals from food sources per MJ total energy intake by sex and age of young person

Minerals	Age of young person (years)											
	4–6			7–10			11–14			15–18		
	Mean	Median	sd	Mean	Median	sd	Mean	Median	sd	Mean	Median	sd
Males												
Total iron (mg)	1.3	1.3	0.25	1.3	1.3	0.26	1.3	1.3	0.31	1.3	1.3	0.36
Haem iron (mg)	0.04	0.04	0.026	0.04	0.04	0.025	0.05	0.05	0.036	0.07	0.06	0.038
Non-haem iron (mg)	1.2	1.2	0.25	1.3	1.2	0.26	1.3	1.2	0.30	1.3	1.2	0.36
Calcium (mg)	110	107	29.4	99	95	24.1	96	94	26.4	91	91	21.4
Phosphorus (mg)	143	142	22.3	135	135	21.3	137	136	21.9	140	139	22.2
Magnesium (mg)	27	26	4.3	26	26	4.3	26	26	4.7	27	26	5.0
Sodium (mg)*	325	316	55.2	322	320	53.3	325	321	62.9	348	338	84.7
Chloride (mg)*	487	480	82.0	483	475	81.3	489	482	93.7	525	515	126.0
Potassium (mg)	304	303	44.4	288	289	44.0	291	285	48.2	298	295	58.7
Zinc (mg)	0.86	0.86	0.164	0.82	0.81	0.158	0.87	0.85	0.198	0.93	0.89	0.257
Copper (mg)	0.11	0.10	0.029	0.11	0.10	0.030	0.11	0.11	0.023	0.11	0.11	0.023
Iodine (µg)	24	23	9.5	21	19	7.0	19	19	7.1	19	18	6.2
Manganese (mg)	0.28	0.26	0.082	0.28	0.26	0.091	0.28	0.26	0.089	0.28	0.26	0.085
Base	184			256			237			179		
Females												
Total iron (mg)	1.2	1.2	0.27	1.2	1.2	0.27	1.3	1.2	0.31	1.3	1.2	0.36
Haem iron (mg)	0.04	0.04	0.019	0.05	0.04	0.027	0.05	0.05	0.034	0.06	0.05	0.040
Non-haem iron (mg)	1.2	1.2	0.27	1.2	1.1	0.27	1.2	1.2	0.31	1.2	1.1	0.36
Calcium (mg)	111	109	27.5	97	97	23.4	91	90	24.9	96	94	30.3
Phosphorus (mg)	144	143	21.7	136	135	20.1	133	131	21.7	141	139	23.5
Magnesium (mg)	26	26	4.2	26	26	4.6	26	25	3.9	28	27	5.5
Sodium (mg)*	318	314	59.2	322	319	56.4	325	323	64.1	339	332	66.7
Chloride (mg)*	477	465	87.9	482	476	82.4	488	486	92.6	515	505	99.6
Potassium (mg)	302	299	49.6	302	297	45.6	301	297	53.4	321	316	61.9
Zinc (mg)	0.83	0.82	0.146	0.85	0.83	0.159	0.85	0.82	0.178	0.90	0.87	0.212
Copper (mg)	0.11	0.10	0.029	0.11	0.10	0.024	0.11	0.11	0.024	0.12	0.11	0.028
Iodine (µg)	24	23	9.1	20	18	6.9	18	17	8.3	20	19	8.9
Manganese (mg)	0.27	0.25	0.078	0.28	0.25	0.092	0.28	0.26	0.090	0.30	0.28	0.106
Base	171			226			238			210		

* Data in this table include intakes from food only and do not include further additions of salt in cooking or at the table

Table 9.7   Percentage contribution of food types to average daily intake of total iron by age and sex of young person

Type of food	Males aged (years)				All males	Females aged (years)				All females
	4–6	7–10	11–14	15–18		4–6	7–10	11–14	15–18	
	%	%	%	%	%	%	%	%	%	%
Cereals & cereal products	57	59	54	52	55	57	52	50	47	51
of which:										
white bread	*10*	*11*	*11*	*12*	*11*	*10*	*11*	*11*	*12*	*11*
wholemeal bread	*2*	*2*	*2*	*2*	*2*	*2*	*2*	*2*	*2*	*2*
high fibre & whole grain breakfast cereals	*13*	*13*	*12*	*10*	*12*	*12*	*10*	*9*	*7*	*9*
other breakfast cereals	*18*	*19*	*16*	*16*	*17*	*18*	*14*	*14*	*11*	*14*
biscuits	*4*	*4*	*3*	*2*	*3*	*4*	*4*	*3*	*2*	*4*
buns, cakes & pastries	*4*	*4*	*3*	*3*	*3*	*4*	*4*	*4*	*3*	*4*
Milk & milk products	3	3	3	2	3	4	3	3	3	3
Eggs & egg dishes	1	2	2	2	2	2	2	2	2	2
Fat spreads	0	0	0	0	0	0	0	0	0	0
Meat & meat products	11	11	14	17	14	10	13	14	14	13
of which:										
beef, veal & dishes	*2*	*2*	*2*	*4*	*3*	*2*	*3*	*3*	*4*	*3*
chicken, turkey & dishes, including coated	*2*	*2*	*3*	*3*	*3*	*2*	*3*	*3*	*4*	*3*
burgers, kebabs & sausages	*3*	*3*	*3*	*4*	*3*	*3*	*3*	*3*	*2*	*3*
liver, liver products & dishes	*0*	*0*	*0*	*0*	*0*	*0*	*0*	*0*	*0*	*0*
Fish & fish dishes	2	1	1	1	1	2	2	1	2	2
Vegetables, potatoes & savoury snacks	17	15	16	17	16	16	18	19	20	18
of which:										
vegetables, excluding potatoes	*8*	*6*	*7*	*7*	*7*	*8*	*8*	*8*	*10*	*8*
all potatoes	*6*	*6*	*7*	*8*	*7*	*6*	*7*	*8*	*8*	*7*
Fruit & nuts	2	2	1	1	1	2	2	1	1	2
Sugars, preserves & confectionery	3	4	4	4	4	3	3	4	4	4
Drinks*	1	1	1	2	1	2	2	1	3	2
Miscellaneous**	3	2	2	2	2	2	2	2	3	2
Average daily intake (mg)	**8.2**	**9.7**	**10.8**	**12.5**	**10.4**	**7.3**	**8.4**	**8.8**	**8.7**	**8.3**
Total number of young people	**184**	**256**	**237**	**179**	**856**	**171**	**226**	**238**	**210**	**845**

*Includes soft drinks, alcoholic drinks, tea, coffee & water.
**Includes powdered beverages (except tea and coffee), soups, sauces and condiments and commercial toddlers' foods.

Table 9.8 Percentage contribution of food types to average daily intake of haem iron by age and sex of young person*

Type of food	Males aged (years)				All males	Females aged (years)				All females
	4–6	7–10	11–14	15–18		4–6	7–10	11–14	15–18	
	%	%	%	%	%	%	%	%	%	%
Meat & meat products	90	91	92	93	92	91	92	92	87	91
of which:										
bacon & ham	6	7	7	7	7	8	7	5	5	6
liver, liver products & dishes	3	3	4	2	3	3	3	3	3	3
beef, veal & dishes	18	18	16	23	19	16	22	22	24	22
chicken, turkey & dishes, including coated	16	17	16	15	16	20	17	19	19	18
lamb & lamb dishes	9	11	10	8	9	8	10	9	7	8
pork & pork dishes	5	5	5	4	4	5	5	5	6	5
burgers & kebabs	10	10	11	16	13	11	9	12	11	11
sausages	13	11	8	7	9	11	9	7	4	7
meat pies & pastries	4	4	6	4	5	5	4	6	4	5
Fish & fish dishes	5	4	4	4	4	5	5	4	8	6
of which:										
oily fish	3	4	3	2	3	4	4	3	6	4
Average daily intake (mg)	**0.3**	**0.3**	**0.4**	**0.6**	**0.4**	**0.2**	**0.3**	**0.4**	**0.4**	**0.3**
Total number of young people	**184**	**256**	**237**	**179**	**856**	**171**	**226**	**238**	**210**	**845**

* Other food groups made a very small contribution to intakes of haem iron.

Table 9.9 Percentage contribution of food types to average daily intake of non-haem iron by age and sex of young person

Type of food	Males aged (years)				All males	Females aged (years)				All females
	4–6	7–10	11–14	15–18		4–6	7–10	11–14	15–18	
	%	%	%	%	%	%	%	%	%	%
Cereals & cereal products	59	61	56	55	57	58	54	52	49	53
of which:										
white bread	*10*	*11*	*11*	*12*	*11*	*10*	*11*	*11*	*12*	*11*
wholemeal bread	*2*	*2*	*2*	*2*	*2*	*2*	*2*	*2*	*2*	*2*
high fibre & whole grain										
breakfast cereals	*14*	*13*	*12*	*10*	*12*	*12*	*10*	*10*	*7*	*10*
other breakfast cereals	*18*	*19*	*16*	*17*	*18*	*18*	*15*	*15*	*11*	*15*
biscuits	*4*	*4*	*3*	*2*	*3*	*5*	*5*	*3*	*2*	*4*
buns, cakes & pastries	*4*	*4*	*3*	*3*	*4*	*4*	*4*	*4*	*3*	*4*
Milk & milk products	3	4	3	2	3	4	4	3	3	3
Eggs & egg dishes	2	2	2	2	2	2	2	2	2	2
Fat spreads	0	0	0	0	0	0	0	0	0	0
Meat & meat products	8	9	11	13	10	8	10	11	11	10
of which:										
beef, veal & dishes	*1*	*2*	*2*	*3*	*2*	*1*	*2*	*2*	*3*	*2*
chicken, turkey & dishes,										
including coated	*2*	*2*	*2*	*3*	*2*	*2*	*2*	*2*	*3*	*2*
Fish & fish dishes	1	1	1	1	1	2	1	1	2	1
Vegetables, potatoes & savoury snacks	17	15	16	18	17	16	18	20	21	19
of which:										
vegetables, excluding										
potatoes	*8*	*6*	*7*	*8*	*7*	*8*	*8*	*8*	*11*	*9*
all potatoes	*6*	*6*	*7*	*8*	*7*	*6*	*7*	*9*	*8*	*8*
Fruit & nuts	2	2	1	1	1	2	2	1	1	2
Sugars, preserves & confectionery	3	4	4	4	4	4	4	4	4	4
Drinks*	1	1	1	2	1	2	2	2	3	2
Miscellaneous**	3	2	2	3	2	2	2	2	3	2
Average daily intake (mg)	**7.9**	**9.4**	**10.3**	**11.9**	**10.0**	**7.1**	**8.0**	**8.5**	**8.3**	**8.0**
Total number of young people	**184**	**256**	**237**	**179**	**856**	**171**	**226**	**238**	**210**	**845**

*Includes soft drinks, alcoholic drinks, tea, coffee & water.
**Includes powdered beverages (except tea and coffee), soups, sauces and condiments and commercial toddlers' foods.

Table 9.10 Average daily intake of calcium (mg) from food sources by sex and age of young person

Calcium (mg)	Males aged (years)				All males	Females aged (years)				All females
	4–6	7–10	11–14	15–18		4–6	7–10	11–14	15–18	
	cum %	cum %	cum %	cum %	cum %	cum %	cum %	cum %	cum %	cum %
Intakes from *food sources*										
Less than 275	3	1	2	0	2	2	2	3	3	3
Less than 325	5	2	4	1	3	4	5	7	7	6
Less than 450	10	9	10	6	8	15	13	24	19	18
Less than 480	13	11	12	9	11	20	15	28	22	22
Less than 550	26	19	20	14	19	33	29	38	30	33
Less than 600	36	31	25	17	27	43	38	45	44	42
Less than 800	73	65	54	41	57	79	78	79	76	78
Less than 1000	89	85	79	68	80	92	95	93	90	93
All	100	100	100	100	100	100	100	100	100	100
Base	*184*	*256*	*237*	*179*	*856*	*171*	*226*	*238*	*210*	*845*
Mean (average value)	706	741	799	878	784	657	656	641	653	652
Median value	666	700	781	850	748	635	664	630	631	644
Lower 2.5 percentile	249	349	299	384	307	280	279	254	258	270
Upper 2.5 percentile	1303	1251	1499	1474	1413	1243	1058	1200	1162	1151
Standard deviation of the mean	256.8	234.6	288.4	298.2	278.3	219.9	194.2	235.7	242.4	223.6

* Dietary supplements taken by young people in this survey provided only negligible amounts of calcium.

Table 9.11 Average daily intake of calcium from food sources as a percentage of Reference Nutrient Intake (RNI) by sex and age of young person

Sex and age (years) of young person	Average daily intake as % of RNI*			*Base*
	Mean	Median	sd	
Males				
4–6	157	148	57.1	*184*
7–10	135	127	42.7	*256*
11–14	80	78	28.8	*237*
15–18	88	85	29.8	*179*
All	113	105	50.9	*856*
Females				
4–6	146	141	48.9	*171*
7–10	119	121	35.3	*226*
11–14	80	79	29.5	*238*
15–18	82	79	30.3	*210*
All	105	98	44.8	*845*

* Intake as a percentage of RNI was calculated for each young person. The values for all young people in each age group were then pooled to give a mean, median and sd.

Table 9.12 Percentage contribution of food types to average daily intake of calcium by age and sex of young person

Type of food	Males aged (years)				All males	Females aged (years)				All females
	4–6	7–10	11–14	15–18		4–6	7–10	11–14	15–18	
	%	%	%	%	%	%	%	%	%	%
Cereals & cereal products	24	28	28	28	27	23	27	28	27	27
of which:										
white & wholemeal bread	*8*	*10*	*10*	*11*	*10*	*8*	*9*	*10*	*11*	*10*
breakfast cereals	*3*	*2*	*2*	*2*	*2*	*3*	*2*	*2*	*1*	*2*
pizza	*2*	*4*	*6*	*6*	*5*	*3*	*4*	*4*	*5*	*4*
biscuits, buns, cakes &										
pastries	*5*	*6*	*5*	*4*	*5*	*5*	*6*	*5*	*4*	*5*
puddings	*3*	*2*	*2*	*1*	*2*	*2*	*3*	*2*	*2*	*2*
Milk & milk products	55	49	47	44	48	56	48	44	44	47
of which:										
whole milk	*25*	*15*	*10*	*8*	*14*	*25*	*13*	*8*	*8*	*13*
semi-skimmed milk	*13*	*17*	*21*	*18*	*18*	*11*	*14*	*15*	*15*	*14*
cheese	*6*	*7*	*7*	*11*	*8*	*9*	*9*	*10*	*13*	*10*
yogurt, fromage frais &										
other dairy desserts	*6*	*5*	*4*	*3*	*4*	*7*	*6*	*5*	*3*	*5*
Eggs & egg dishes	1	1	1	1	1	1	1	1	1	1
Fat spreads	0	0	0	0	0	0	0	0	0	0
Meat & meat products	5	6	6	8	6	4	6	7	6	6
Fish & fish dishes	2	2	2	2	2	2	2	1	2	2
Vegetables, potatoes & savoury snacks	5	5	6	6	6	5	6	7	8	7
Fruit & nuts	1	1	1	1	1	1	1	1	1	1
Sugars, preserves & confectionery	3	5	5	4	4	4	4	5	4	5
Drinks*	2	3	3	4	3	3	3	3	4	3
Miscellaneous**	1	1	1	1	1	1	1	2	2	2
Average daily intake (mg)	**706**	**741**	**799**	**878**	**784**	**657**	**656**	**641**	**653**	**652**
Total number of young people	**184**	**256**	**237**	**179**	**856**	**171**	**226**	**238**	**210**	**845**

*Includes soft drinks, alcoholic drinks, tea, coffee & water.
**Includes powdered beverages (except tea and coffee), soups, sauces and condiments and commercial toddlers' foods.

Table 9.13 Average daily intake of phosphorus (mg) from food sources by sex and age of young person

Phosphorus (mg)	Males aged (years)				All males	Females aged (years)				All females
	4–6	7–10	11–14	15–18		4–6	7–10	11–14	15–18	
	cum %	cum %	cum %	cum %	cum %	cum %	cum %	cum %	cum %	cum %
Intakes from *food sources*										
Less than 350	1	0	-	-	0	1	-	0	1	0
Less than 450	4	0	2	-	1	2	2	2	3	2
Less than 625	8	5	4	1	4	14	7	10	9	9
Less than 775	28	18	10	5	14	40	23	25	26	28
Less than 900	49	38	22	9	28	65	47	51	43	51
Less than 1100	81	66	44	26	53	88	85	74	74	80
Less than 1300	94	88	71	49	75	98	98	93	90	95
Less than 1500	99	97	90	70	89	99	99	98	96	98
Less than 1700	100	98	98	85	95	100	100	99	99	100
All		100	100	100	100			100	100	
Base	*184*	*256*	*237*	*179*	*856*	*171*	*226*	*238*	*210*	*845*
Mean (average value)	919	1008	1132	1330	1105	848	915	932	959	917
Median value	901	991	1140	1310	1066	829	910	898	955	896
Lower 2.5 percentile	412	595	513	759	570	452	484	477	413	452
Upper 2.5 percentile	1453	1632	1678	1913	1851	1297	1296	1413	1623	1459
Standard deviation of the mean	250.8	242.8	291.4	345.1	324.1	215.3	198.5	251.1	273.4	239.9

*None of the dietary supplements taken by young people in this survey provided any phosphorus.

Table 9.14 Average daily intake of phosphorus from food sources as a percentage of Reference Nutrient Intake (RNI) by sex and age of young person

Sex and age (years) of young person	Average daily intake as % of RNI*			Base
	Mean	Median	sd	
Males				
4–6	263	257	71.7	*184*
7–10	224	220	54.0	*256*
11–14	146	147	37.6	*237*
15–18	172	169	44.5	*179*
All	198	191	68.3	*856*
Females				
4–6	242	237	61.5	*171*
7–10	203	202	44.1	*226*
11–14	149	144	40.2	*238*
15–18	153	153	43.7	*210*
All	184	180	60.0	*845*

*Intake as a percentage of RNI was calculated for each young person. The values for all young people in each age group were then pooled to give a mean, median and sd.

Table 9.15 Percentage contribution of food types to average daily intake of phosphorus by age and sex of young person

Type of food	Males aged (years)				All males	Females aged (years)				All females
	4–6	7–10	11–14	15–18		4–6	7–10	11–14	15–18	
	%	%	%	%	%	%	%	%	%	%
Cereals & cereal products	25	28	26	24	26	24	26	26	25	25
of which:										
white & wholemeal bread	*6*	*7*	*7*	*7*	*7*	*6*	*7*	*7*	*7*	*7*
breakfast cereals	*6*	*6*	*5*	*5*	*5*	*5*	*4*	*4*	*3*	*4*
biscuits, buns, cakes &										
pastries	*6*	*6*	*5*	*4*	*5*	*6*	*6*	*6*	*4*	*5*
pizza	*1*	*2*	*3*	*4*	*3*	*2*	*2*	*2*	*3*	*2*
Milk & milk products	35	30	26	23	28	36	28	24	23	27
of which:										
whole milk	*15*	*9*	*5*	*4*	*8*	*15*	*8*	*4*	*4*	*7*
reduced fat milks	*8*	*10*	*12*	*10*	*10*	*7*	*9*	*9*	*9*	*8*
Eggs & egg dishes	1	2	2	2	2	2	2	2	2	2
Fat spreads	0	0	0	0	0	0	0	0	0	0
Meat & meat products	16	17	19	22	19	15	18	19	19	18
of which:										
chicken, turkey & dishes,										
including coated	*5*	*5*	*6*	*7*	*6*	*6*	*6*	*7*	*7*	*7*
burgers, kebabs &										
sausages	*4*	*4*	*4*	*5*	*5*	*3*	*4*	*4*	*3*	*4*
Fish & fish dishes	3	3	3	3	3	3	3	3	3	3
Vegetables, potatoes & savoury snacks	12	12	12	13	12	11	13	14	15	13
of which:										
vegetables, excluding										
potatoes	*5*	*4*	*4*	*5*	*4*	*4*	*5*	*5*	*7*	*5*
roast or fried potatoes &										
chips	*3*	*4*	*4*	*5*	*4*	*3*	*4*	*5*	*4*	*4*
Fruit & nuts	2	2	1	1	1	2	2	1	1	1
Sugars, preserves & confectionery	3	4	4	3	3	3	3	4	3	3
Drinks*	3	3	5	8	5	3	3	4	7	4
of which:										
soft drinks, including low										
calorie	*2*	*3*	*4*	*5*	*4*	*2*	*3*	*4*	*4*	*3*
beers & lagers	*0*	*0*	*0*	*2*	*1*	*0*	*0*	*0*	*1*	*0*
Miscellaneous**	1	1	1	1	1	1	1	2	2	2
Average daily intake (mg)	**919**	**1008**	**1132**	**1330**	**1105**	**848**	**915**	**932**	**959**	**917**
Total number of young people	**184**	**256**	**237**	**179**	**856**	**171**	**226**	**238**	**210**	**845**

*Includes soft drinks, alcoholic drinks, tea, coffee & water.
**Includes powdered beverages (except tea and coffee), soups, sauces and condiments and commercial toddlers' foods.

Table 9.16 Average daily intake of magnesium (mg) from food sources by sex and age of young person

Magnesium (mg)	Males aged (years)				All males	Females aged (years)				All females
	4–6	7–10	11–14	15–18		4–6	7–10	11–14	15–18	
	cum %	cum %	cum %	cum %	cum %	cum %	cum %	cum %	cum %	cum %
Intakes from *food sources**										
Less than 70	3	-	-	-	1	1	-	0	1	1
Less than 115	9	2	4	1	4	10	5	7	6	7
Less than 120	11	3	4	1	5	13	6	8	7	8
Less than 150	31	15	10	5	14	55	24	26	21	30
Less than 180	61	44	28	13	35	73	55	51	41	54
Less than 190	70	51	35	18	42	83	63	59	53	64
Less than 200	76	56	39	23	47	89	75	69	63	74
Less than 240	93	84	66	43	71	97	93	89	83	90
Less than 280	99	95	86	66	86	99	99	97	93	97
Less than 300	100	97	90	75	90	99	99	98	97	98
All		100	100	100	100	100	100	100	100	100
Base	184	256	237	179	856	171	226	238	210	845
Mean (average value)	172	194	218	256	212	155	177	182	191	178
Median value	170	187	214	254	204	145	176	176	189	175
Lower 2.5 percentile	67	117	97	145	107	92	98	102	84	94
Upper 2.5 percentile	264	302	351	390	358	244	261	290	314	285
Standard deviation of the mean	46.0	46.1	59.8	72.2	65.1	39.9	41.0	48.1	57.5	49.0

*None of the dietary supplements taken by young people in this survey provided any magnesium.

Table 9.17 Average daily intake of magnesium from food sources as a percentage of Reference Nutrient Intake (RNI) by sex and age of young person

Sex and age (years) of young person	Average daily intake as % of RNI*			*Base*
	Mean	Median	sd	
Males				
4–6	143	141	38.4	184
7–10	97	94	23.0	256
11–14	78	76	21.3	237
15–18	85	85	24.1	179
All	98	91	35.8	856
Females				
4–6	129	121	33.3	171
7–10	89	88	20.5	226
11–14	65	63	17.2	238
15–18	64	63	19.2	210
All	85	78	33.9	845

*Intake as a percentage of RNI was calculated for each young person. The values for all young people in each age group were then pooled to give a mean, median and sd.

Table 9.18 Percentage contribution of food types to average daily intake of magnesium by age and sex of young person

Type of food	Males aged (years)				All males	Females aged (years)				All females
	4–6	7–10	11–14	15–18		4–6	7–10	11–14	15–18	
	%	%	%	%	%	%	%	%	%	%
Cereals & cereal products	32	34	32	29	32	31	31	30	29	30
of which:										
white bread	*6*	*8*	*8*	*8*	*7*	*7*	*7*	*7*	*7*	*7*
breakfast cereals	*10*	*10*	*9*	*8*	*9*	*9*	*8*	*7*	*5*	*7*
biscuits, buns, cakes &										
pastries	*6*	*6*	*5*	*4*	*5*	*6*	*6*	*6*	*4*	*5*
Milk & milk products	20	17	15	12	16	21	16	13	12	15
of which:										
whole milk	*10*	*5*	*3*	*3*	*5*	*10*	*5*	*3*	*3*	*4*
semi-skimmed milk	*5*	*6*	*7*	*6*	*6*	*4*	*5*	*5*	*5*	*5*
Eggs & egg dishes	1	1	1	1	1	1	1	1	1	1
Fat spreads	0	0	0	0	0	0	0	0	0	0
Meat & meat products	9	10	12	14	11	9	11	11	11	11
of which:										
chicken, turkey & dishes,										
including coated	*3*	*3*	*4*	*5*	*4*	*4*	*4*	*4*	*5*	*4*
Fish & fish dishes	2	2	2	2	2	2	2	2	2	2
Vegetables, potatoes & savoury snacks	20	20	22	22	21	19	22	25	24	23
of which:										
vegetables, excluding										
potatoes	*7*	*6*	*7*	*7*	*7*	*7*	*7*	*7*	*9*	*8*
all potatoes	*10*	*11*	*12*	*13*	*12*	*9*	*12*	*14*	*12*	*12*
Fruit & nuts	6	5	4	3	4	6	5	4	4	5
Sugars, preserves & confectionery	4	5	5	4	5	5	5	6	4	5
Drinks*	4	5	6	10	7	5	5	6	9	6
of which:										
fruit juice	*2*	*2*	*2*	*2*	*2*	*2*	*2*	*2*	*2*	*2*
beers & lagers	*0*	*0*	*0*	*4*	*1*	*0*	*0*	*0*	*2*	*1*
Miscellaneous**	2	2	2	2	2	2	2	2	3	2
Average daily intake (mg)	**172**	**194**	**218**	**256**	**212**	**155**	**177**	**182**	**191**	**178**
Total number of young people	**184**	**256**	**237**	**179**	**856**	**171**	**226**	**238**	**210**	**845**

*Includes soft drinks, alcoholic drinks, tea, coffee & water.
**Includes powdered beverages (except tea and coffee), soups, sauces and condiments and commercial toddlers' foods.

Table 9.19 Use of salt in cooking and at the table by sex and age of young person*

Responding sample

Use of salt in cooking and at the table	Males aged (years)				All males	Females aged (years)				All females
	4–6	7–10	11–14	15–18		4–6	7–10	11–14	15–18	
	%	%	%	%	%	%	%	%	%	%
Salt added to cooking:										
usually added	54	62	62	70	62	56	60	66	69	63
uses salt alternative	3	3	6	4	4	2	0	6	6	4
not usually added	43	36	32	27	34	42	39	28	25	33
Salt added at table:										
usually	10	19	27	33	23	13	15	27	30	22
occasionally	23	29	25	29	27	27	39	30	28	31
rarely	23	26	24	13	22	22	24	21	17	21
never	45	26	24	25	29	38	22	22	26	26
Base	*230*	*304*	*290*	*258*	*1082*	*224*	*277*	*280*	*264*	*1045*

*As reported in the dietary interview.

Table 9.20 Use of salt in cooking and at the table by age and sex of young person*

Responding sample

Sex of young person and use of salt at the table	Use of salt in cooking and age of young person (years)															All
	Salt added**					No salt added					All					
	4-6	7-10	11-14	15-18	All	4-6	7-10	11-14	15-18	All	4-6	7-10	11-14	15-18	All	
	%	%	%	%	%	%	%	%	%	%	%	%	%	%	%	%
Males																
Use salt at the table:																
Usually	12	18	27	32	23	8	20	27	33	21	10	19	27	33	23	23
Occasionally	24	30	24	30	27	21	29	27	26	26	23	29	25	29	27	27
Rarely or never	64	53	49	37	49	71	51	46	42	53	67	52	48	38	51	51
Base	*127*	*193*	*195*	*185*	*700*	*103*	*111*	*95*	*73*	*382*	*230*	*304*	*290*	*258*	*1082*	*1082*
Females																
Use salt at the table:																
Usually	13	18	30	31	24	13	11	20	25	16	13	15	27	30	22	22
Occasionally	30	43	28	29	32	23	33	36	25	30	27	39	30	28	31	31
Rarely or never	57	40	42	40	44	63	56	44	49	54	60	46	42	42	47	47
Base	*126*	*166*	*198*	*198*	*688*	*98*	*111*	*82*	*66*	*357*	*224*	*277*	*280*	*264*	*1045*	*1045*

* As reported in the dietary interview.
** Includes cases where salt alternative used

Table 9.21 Average daily intake of sodium (mg) from food sources by sex and age of young person*

Sodium (mg)	Males aged (years)				All males	Females aged (years)				All females
	4–6	7–10	11–14	15–18		4–6	7–10	11–14	15–18	
	cum %	cum %	cum %	cum %	cum %	cum %	cum %	cum %	cum %	cum %
Intakes from *food sources*										
Less than 280	–	–	–	–	–	–	–	–	–	–
Less than 350	–	–	–	–	–	–	–	0	–	0
Less than 460	–	–	0	–	0	–	–	0	–	0
Less than 575	–	–	0	–	0	–	–	0	0	0
Less than 700	–	0	1	–	0	–	–	0	0	0
Less than 1200	3	1	4	–	2	5	2	3	3	3
Less than 1600	16	7	6	1	7	27	12	12	14	16
Less than 2000	50	25	13	6	22	70	40	32	32	42
Less than 2500	82	59	38	18	48	93	77	69	67	42
Less than 3000	95	86	69	43	72	99	94	87	86	76
Less than 3500	100	94	89	66	87	100	99	98	97	91
Less than 4000		99	96	77	93		100	100	99	100
Less than 4500		100	99	92	97				100	
All			100	100	100					
Base	*184*	*256*	*237*	*179*	*856*	*171*	*226*	*238*	*210*	*845*
Mean (average value)	2069	2402	2683	3265	2630	1857	2155	2272	2281	2156
Median value	2000	2346	2688	3171	2542	1831	2080	2270	2276	2119
Lower 2.5 percentile	1128	1306	1138	1765	1229	889	1255	1121	1060	1093
Upper 2.5 percentile	3361	3732	4058	5031	4509	2905	3285	3473	3603	3389
Standard deviation of the mean	536.4	592.5	727.2	895.7	827.6	454.3	496.3	605.7	632.3	578.7

* Data in this table are for intakes from food only and do not include further additions of salt in cooking or at the table.
** None of the dietary supplements taken by young people in this survey provided any sodium.

Table 9.22 Average daily intake of sodium from food sources as a percentage of Reference Nutrient Intake (RNI) by sex and age of young person*

Sex and age (years) of young person	Average daily intake as % of RNI**			*Base*
	Mean	Median	sd	
Males				
4–6	296	286	76.6	*184*
7–10	200	195	49.4	*256*
11–14	168	168	45.4	*237*
15–18	204	198	56.0	*179*
All	212	198	72.3	*856*
Females				
4–6	265	262	64.9	*171*
7–10	180	173	41.4	*226*
11–14	142	142	37.9	*238*
15–18	143	142	39.5	*210*
All	178	165	66.0	*845*

* Data in this table are for intakes from food only and do not include further additions of salt in cooking or at the table.
** Intake as a percentage of RNI was calculated for each young person. The values for all young people in each age group were then pooled to give a mean, median and sd.

Table 9.23 Average daily intake of chloride (mg) from food sources by sex and age of young person*

Chloride (mg)	Males aged (years)				All males	Females aged (years)				All females
	4–6	7–10	11–14	15–18		4–6	7–10	11–14	15–18	
	cum %	cum %	cum %	cum %	cum %	cum %	cum %	cum %	cum %	cum %
Intakes from *food sources*										
Less than 1100	–	0	1	–	0	–	–	0	0	0
Less than 1800	4	1	4	–	2	7	2	2	3	3
Less than 2500	20	7	7	1	8	32	15	16	13	18
Less than 3000	52	26	13	6	23	64	41	33	31	41
Less than 4000	86	72	49	24	56	94	87	75	73	82
Less than 5000	98	94	86	57	83	99	98	95	94	97
Less than 6000	100	99	98	83	94	100	100	100	100	100
All		100	100	100	100					
Base	*184*	*256*	*237*	*179*	*856*	*171*	*226*	*238*	*210*	*845*
Mean (average value)	3105	3594	4030	4938	3954	2785	3222	3403	3465	3241
Median value	2971	3575	4020	4725	3821	2749	3196	3357	3508	3190
Lower 2.5 percentile	1613	2012	1678	2539	1953	1366	1870	1880	1574	1751
Upper 2.5 percentile	4828	5581	6244	7860	6808	4353	4663	5296	5303	5180
Standard deviation of the mean	798.5	887.1	1071.4	1372.5	1252.6	676.5	726.8	884.8	939.6	856.7

* Data in this table are for intakes from food only and do not include further additions of salt in cooking or at the table.
** None of the dietary supplements taken by young people in this survey provided any chloride.

Table 9.24 Average daily intake of chloride from food sources as a percentage of Reference Nutrient Intake (RNI) by sex and age of young person*

Sex and age (years) of young person	Average daily intake as % of RNI**			*Base*
	Mean	Median	sd	
Males				
4–6	282	270	72.6	*184*
7–10	200	199	49.3	*256*
11–14	161	161	42.9	*237*
15–18	198	189	54.9	*179*
All	206	195	69.0	*856*
Females				
4–6	253	250	61.5	*171*
7–10	179	178	40.4	*226*
11–14	136	134	35.4	*238*
15–18	139	140	37.6	*210*
All	173	162	62.6	*845*

* Data in this table are for intakes from food only and do not include further additions of salt in cooking or at the table.
** Intake as a percentage of RNI was calculated for each young person. The values for all young people in each age group were then pooled to give a mean, median and sd.

Table 9.25 Percentage contribution of food types to average daily intake of sodium by age and sex of young person*

Type of food	Males aged (years)				All males	Females aged (years)				All females
	4–6	7–10	11–14	15–18		4–6	7–10	11–14	15–18	
	%	%	%	%	%	%	%	%	%	%
Cereals & cereal products	40	42	40	38	40	39	38	38	37	38
of which:										
white bread	*13*	*15*	*15*	*15*	*15*	*13*	*14*	*14*	*15*	*14*
breakfast cereals	*9*	*10*	*9*	*8*	*9*	*9*	*7*	*7*	*5*	*7*
biscuits, buns, cakes &										
pastries	*6*	*6*	*5*	*3*	*5*	*6*	*6*	*5*	*4*	*5*
pizza	*2*	*3*	*4*	*4*	*4*	*2*	*3*	*3*	*3*	*3*
Milk & milk products	9	8	7	7	7	10	8	7	7	8
of which:										
milk	*5*	*4*	*4*	*3*	*4*	*5*	*3*	*3*	*3*	*3*
cheese	*3*	*3*	*2*	*3*	*3*	*4*	*3*	*3*	*4*	*4*
Eggs & egg dishes	1	1	1	1	1	1	1	1	2	1
Fat spreads	2	3	3	2	3	3	3	3	3	3
Meat & meat products	20	21	24	28	24	19	22	22	21	21
of which:										
bacon & ham	*3*	*4*	*6*	*7*	*5*	*4*	*5*	*4*	*4*	*4*
chicken, turkey & dishes,										
including coated	*4*	*4*	*4*	*5*	*4*	*4*	*4*	*5*	*6*	*5*
sausages	*6*	*6*	*4*	*5*	*5*	*5*	*5*	*4*	*3*	*4*
Fish & fish dishes	3	2	2	2	2	3	3	2	3	3
Vegetables, potatoes & savoury snacks	17	14	15	13	14	16	17	16	15	16
of which:										
vegetables, excluding										
potatoes	*8*	*5*	*6*	*7*	*6*	*6*	*7*	*6*	*8*	*7*
savoury snacks	*7*	*7*	*6*	*4*	*6*	*8*	*8*	*8*	*5*	*7*
Fruit & nuts	0	0	0	0	0	0	0	0	0	0
Sugars, preserves & confectionery	1	2	2	1	1	1	1	2	1	1
Drinks**	2	1	1	2	1	2	1	1	2	1
Miscellaneous***	4	5	5	6	5	5	5	7	9	7
Average daily intake (mg)	**2069**	**2402**	**2683**	**3265**	**2630**	**1857**	**2155**	**2272**	**2281**	**2156**
Total number of young people	**184**	**256**	**237**	**179**	**856**	**171**	**226**	**238**	**210**	**845**

* Data in this table are for intakes from food only and do not include additions of salt at the table or in cooking.
** Includes soft drinks, alcoholic drinks, tea, coffee & water.
***Includes powdered beverages (except tea and coffee), soups, sauces and condiments and commercial toddlers' foods.

Table 9.26 Percentage contribution of food types to average daily intake of chloride by age and sex of young person*

Type of food	Males aged (years)				All males	Females aged (years)				All females
	4–6	7–10	11–14	15–18		4–6	7–10	11–14	15–18	
	%	%	%	%	%	%	%	%	%	%
Cereals & cereal products	39	42	40	38	40	38	37	38	37	38
of which:										
white bread	*14*	*16*	*15*	*16*	*15*	*14*	*14*	*15*	*15*	*15*
breakfast cereals	*9*	*10*	*8*	*8*	*9*	*9*	*7*	*7*	*5*	*7*
biscuits, buns, cakes &										
pastries	*5*	*5*	*4*	*3*	*4*	*5*	*5*	*4*	*3*	*4*
pizza	*2*	*3*	*4*	*5*	*4*	*2*	*3*	*3*	*3*	*3*
Milk & milk products	11	9	8	7	9	12	9	8	8	9
of which:										
milk	*7*	*5*	*5*	*4*	*5*	*7*	*5*	*4*	*4*	*4*
cheese	*2*	*2*	*2*	*3*	*2*	*3*	*3*	*3*	*4*	*3*
Eggs & egg dishes	1	1	1	1	1	1	1	1	1	1
Fat spreads	2	3	3	2	3	3	3	3	3	3
Meat & meat products	19	20	22	26	22	18	21	21	19	20
of which:										
bacon & ham	*3*	*4*	*5*	*6*	*5*	*4*	*5*	*4*	*4*	*4*
chicken, turkey & dishes,										
including coated	*3*	*3*	*4*	*4*	*4*	*4*	*4*	*4*	*5*	*4*
sausages	*6*	*5*	*4*	*4*	*5*	*4*	*4*	*4*	*2*	*4*
Fish & fish dishes	3	2	2	2	2	3	3	2	3	3
Vegetables, potatoes & savoury snacks	18	16	16	14	16	17	18	18	17	18
of which:										
vegetables, excluding										
potatoes	*8*	*5*	*6*	*7*	*6*	*6*	*7*	*6*	*8*	*7*
savoury snacks	*8*	*7*	*6*	*5*	*6*	*8*	*8*	*8*	*5*	*7*
Fruit & nuts	1	1	0	0	0	1	1	0	0	0
Sugars, preserves & confectionery	1	2	2	1	1	1	1	2	1	1
Drinks**	0	0	0	1	0	0	0	0	1	0
Miscellaneous***	4	5	5	6	5	4	5	6	8	6
Average daily intake (mg)	**3105**	**3594**	**4030**	**4938**	**3954**	**2785**	**3222**	**3403**	**3465**	**3241**
Total number of young people	**184**	**256**	**237**	**179**	**856**	**171**	**226**	**238**	**210**	**845**

* Data in this table are for intakes from food only and do not include further additions of salt in cooking or at the table.
** Includes soft drinks, alcoholic drinks, tea, coffee & water.
***Includes powdered beverages (except tea and coffee), soups, sauces and condiments and commercial toddlers' foods.

Table 9.27 Average daily intake of potassium (mg) from food sources by sex and age of young person

Potassium (mg)	Males aged (years)				All males	Females aged (years)				All females
	4–6	7–10	11–14	15–18		4–6	7–10	11–14	15–18	
	cum %	cum %	cum %	cum %	cum %	cum %	cum %	cum %	cum %	cum %
Intakes from *food sources*										
Less than 600	–	–	–	–	–	–	–	–	0	0
Less than 950	2	–	1	–	1	1	1	1	1	1
Less than 1100	5	–	1	1	2	5	3	2	3	3
Less than 1600	20	13	10	2	11	47	15	19	17	23
Less than 2000	58	43	27	15	35	69	46	46	38	49
Less than 2400	84	71	54	29	58	91	84	72	67	78
Less than 2800	97	91	74	53	78	99	97	88	85	92
Less than 3100	98	97	88	67	87	99	99	97	95	97
Less than 3500	99	99	96	85	95	99	100	99	99	99
All	100	100	100	100	100	100		100	100	100
Base	*184*	*256*	*237*	*179*	*856*	*171*	*226*	*238*	*210*	*845*
Mean (average value)	1944	2136	2392	2833	2343	1774	2019	2100	2162	2026
Median value	1889	2086	2344	2775	2267	1661	2029	2025	2148	2010
Lower 2.5 percentile	1045	1280	1201	1636	1209	1016	1098	1176	1063	1074
Upper 2.5 percentile	3019	3110	3653	4416	4009	2721	2827	3159	3334	3110
Standard deviation of the mean	502.9	488.2	608.2	820.2	703.6	458.9	420.2	549.5	592.7	529.7

*None of the dietary supplements taken by young people in this survey provided any potassium.

Table 9.28 Average daily intake of potassium from food sources as a percentage of Reference Nutrient Intake (RNI) by sex and age of young person

Sex and age (years) of young person	Average daily intake as % of RNI*			*Base*
	Mean	Median	sd	
Males				
4–6	177	172	45.7	*184*
7–10	107	104	24.4	*256*
11–14	77	76	19.6	*237*
15–18	81	79	23.4	*179*
All	107	95	47.4	*856*
Females				
4–6	161	151	41.7	*171*
7–10	101	101	21.0	*226*
11–14	68	65	17.7	*238*
15–18	62	61	16.9	*210*
All	95	84	45.1	*845*

*Intake as a percentage of RNI was calculated for each young person. The values for all young people in each age group were then pooled to give a mean, median and sd.

Table 9.29 Percentage contribution of food types to average daily intake of potassium by age and sex of young person

Type of food	Males aged (years)				All males	Females aged (years)				All females
	4–6	7–10	11–14	15–18		4–6	7–10	11–14	15–18	
	%	%	%	%	%	%	%	%	%	%
Cereals & cereal products	15	17	16	15	15	14	15	14	14	14
of which:										
white bread	3	3	3	3	3	3	3	3	3	3
high fibre & whole grain breakfast cereals	2	3	2	2	2	2	2	2	1	2
biscuits, buns, cakes & pastries	3	4	3	2	3	3	4	3	2	3
Milk & milk products	24	20	18	14	18	24	17	14	13	16
of which:										
whole milk	12	7	4	3	6	12	6	3	3	6
semi-skimmed milk	6	8	9	7	8	5	6	6	6	6
Eggs & egg dishes	1	1	1	1	1	1	1	1	1	1
Fat spreads	0	0	0	0	0	0	0	0	0	0
Meat & meat products	10	11	14	16	13	10	12	13	13	12
of which:										
beef, veal & dishes	2	2	2	3	2	2	2	2	3	2
chicken, turkey & dishes, including coated	3	4	4	5	4	4	4	5	5	4
Fish & fish dishes	2	2	2	2	2	2	2	2	2	2
Vegetables, potatoes & savoury snacks	31	32	35	36	34	30	35	40	38	36
of which:										
vegetables, excluding potatoes	7	6	7	8	7	7	7	7	10	8
all potatoes	18	20	23	24	22	17	21	26	23	22
savoury snacks	6	6	5	4	5	6	6	7	4	6
Fruit & nuts	7	6	4	3	5	8	7	4	5	6
Sugars, preserves & confectionery	2	3	3	3	3	3	3	3	3	3
Drinks*	5	6	6	9	7	6	6	6	9	7
of which:										
fruit juice	3	3	3	3	3	4	4	4	4	4
Miscellaneous**	2	2	2	2	2	2	2	2	3	2
Average daily intake (mg)	**1944**	**2136**	**2392**	**2833**	**2343**	**1774**	**2019**	**2100**	**2162**	**2026**
Total number of young people	**184**	**256**	**237**	**179**	**856**	**171**	**226**	**238**	**210**	**845**

*Includes soft drinks, alcoholic drinks, tea, coffee & water.
**Includes powdered beverages (except tea and coffee), soups, sauces and condiments and commercial toddlers' foods.

Table 9.30 Average daily intake of zinc (mg) by sex and age of young person

Zinc (mg)	Males aged (years)				All males	Females aged (years)				All females
	4–6	7–10	11–14	15–18		4–6	7–10	11–14	15–18	
	cum %	cum %	cum %	cum %	cum %	cum %	cum %	cum %	cum %	cum %
(a) Intakes from *all* sources										
Less than 4.0	12	5	5	1	6	26	10	12	10	14
Less than 5.3	48	30	14	7	24	62	39	37	39	43
Less than 5.5	56	34	17	9	27	67	48	43	42	49
Less than 6.5	79	63	38	19	49	89	73	66	61	71
Less than 7.0	85	73	49	24	56	92	83	76	72	80
Less than 8.0	92	90	71	41	73	98	95	87	86	91
Less than 9.0	97	95	84	61	84	99	97	96	93	96
Less than 9.5	97	97	88	68	87	99	99	98	95	98
All	100	100	100	100	100	100	100	100	100	100
Base	*184*	*256*	*237*	*179*	*856*	*171*	*226*	*238*	*210*	*845*
Mean (average value)	5.6	6.1	7.2	8.7	7.0	5.0	5.7	5.9	6.1	5.7
Median value	5.4	6.0	7.0	8.5	6.6	4.8	5.6	5.8	6.0	5.5
Lower 2.5 percentile	2.5	3.4	3.6	4.6	3.3	2.6	3.1	2.6	2.6	2.8
Upper 2.5 percentile	10.3	10.3	11.3	15.5	12.4	7.9	9.2	9.4	10.7	9.3
Standard deviation of the mean	1.80	1.60	1.97	2.66	2.37	1.39	1.37	1.73	2.02	1.71
	cum %	cum %	cum %	cum %	cum %	cum %	cum %	cum %	cum %	cum %
(b) Intakes from *food* sources										
Less than 4.0	12	5	5	1	6	26	10	12	10	14
Less than 5.3	49	30	14	8	24	65	39	37	40	44
Less than 5.5	57	34	17	9	28	69	48	43	43	50
Less than 6.5	80	63	38	20	49	91	73	66	61	72
Less than 7.0	86	73	49	24	57	93	83	77	73	81
Less than 8.0	93	90	71	41	73	98	95	88	86	92
Less than 9.0	98	95	84	62	84	99	97	97	93	96
Less than 9.5	98	97	88	69	88	99	100	98	95	98
All	100	100	100	100	100	100	100	100	100	100
Base	*184*	*256*	*237*	*179*	*856*	*171*	*226*	*238*	*210*	*845*
Mean (average value)	5.5	6.1	7.1	8.7	6.9	4.9	5.7	5.9	6.1	5.7
Median value	5.3	6.0	7.0	8.5	6.5	4.8	5.6	5.8	5.9	5.5
Lower 2.5 percentile	2.5	3.4	3.6	4.6	3.3	2.6	3.1	2.6	2.6	2.8
Upper 2.5 percentile	9.0	10.0	11.2	15.5	12.4	7.6	9.1	9.3	10.7	9.3
Standard deviation of the mean	1.70	1.58	1.94	2.67	2.35	1.32	1.35	1.64	2.02	1.67

Table 9.31 Average daily intake of zinc as a percentage of Reference Nutrient Intake (RNI) by sex and age of young person

Sex and age (years) of young person	Average daily intake as % of RNI*							
	(a) All sources			*Base*	(b) Food sources			*Base*
	Mean	Median	sd		Mean	Median	sd	
Males								
4–6	86	82	27.6	*184*	85	82	26.2	*184*
7–10	88	86	22.8	*256*	88	86	22.6	*256*
11–14	79	78	21.9	*237*	79	78	21.5	*237*
15–18	92	89	28.0	*179*	92	89	28.1	*179*
All	86	84	25.5	*856*	86	84	25.0	*856*
Females								
4–6	77	74	21.3	*171*	75	74	20.2	*171*
7–10	81	79	19.5	*226*	81	79	19.3	*226*
11–14	66	64	19.2	*238*	66	64	18.3	*238*
15–18	87	85	28.9	*210*	87	85	28.9	*210*
All	78	76	23.9	*845*	77	75	23.5	*845*

*Intake as a percentage of RNI was calculated for each young person. The values for all young people in each age group were then pooled to give a mean, median and sd.

Table 9.32 Percentage contribution of food types to average daily intake of zinc by age and sex of young person

Type of food	Males aged (years)				All males	Females aged (years)				All females
	4–6	7–10	11–14	15–18		4–6	7–10	11–14	15–18	
	%	%	%	%	%	%	%	%	%	%
Cereals & cereal products	26	29	27	26	27	26	27	26	26	26
of which:										
white bread	5	6	6	6	6	5	6	6	6	6
wholemeal bread	2	2	2	1	2	2	2	2	2	2
high fibre & whole grain										
breakfast cereals	5	5	5	5	5	4	4	4	3	4
other breakfast cereals	2	2	2	1	2	2	2	1	1	1
pizza	1	2	3	3	2	2	2	2	2	2
biscuits, buns, cakes &										
pastries	5	5	4	3	4	5	5	5	3	4
Milk & milk products	26	22	19	16	20	28	20	17	17	20
of which:										
whole milk	12	7	4	3	6	13	6	3	3	6
semi-skimmed milk	6	8	9	7	7	6	6	6	6	6
Eggs & egg dishes	2	2	2	2	2	2	2	2	2	2
Fat spreads	0	0	0	0	0	0	0	0	0	0
Meat & meat products	26	27	32	37	31	24	30	32	31	30
of which:										
beef, veal & dishes	6	6	7	10	7	5	8	8	9	8
chicken, turkey & dishes,										
including coated	5	5	5	6	5	5	5	6	6	6
burgers, kebabs &										
sausages	6	6	7	9	7	5	5	6	6	6
Fish & fish dishes	2	1	1	2	1	2	2	1	2	2
Vegetables, potatoes & savoury snacks	12	11	12	12	12	11	13	14	14	13
Fruit & nuts	2	2	1	1	2	2	2	2	1	2
Sugars, preserves & confectionery	2	3	3	2	2	3	3	3	2	3
Drinks*	0	0	0	1	0	0	0	0	1	0
Miscellaneous**	1	1	1	1	1	2	1	1	2	2
Average daily intake (mg)	**5.5**	**6.1**	**7.1**	**8.7**	**6.9**	**4.9**	**5.7**	**5.9**	**6.1**	**5.7**
Total number of young people	**184**	**256**	**237**	**179**	**856**	**171**	**226**	**238**	**210**	**845**

*Includes soft drinks, alcoholic drinks, tea, coffee & water.
**Includes powdered beverages (except tea and coffee), soups, sauces and condiments and commercial toddlers' foods.

Table 9.33 Average daily intake of copper (mg) from food sources by sex and age of young person

Copper (mg)	Males aged (years)				All males	Females aged (years)				All females
	4–6	7–10	11–14	15–18		4–6	7–10	11–14	15–18	
	cum %	cum %	cum %	cum %	cum %	cum %	cum %	cum %	cum %	cum %
Intakes from *food sources*										
Less than 0.30	2	0	0	–	1	1	–	–	1	1
Less than 0.40	5	2	2	–	2	6	4	1	4	3
Less than 0.50	14	5	5	1	6	29	9	7	10	13
Less than 0.60	38	15	11	3	15	52	23	21	25	29
Less than 0.70	59	33	18	7	27	70	49	41	39	49
Less than 0.80	73	53	35	20	44	82	68	60	56	66
Less than 1.00	89	83	69	50	72	93	91	84	78	86
Less than 1.20	96	93	89	70	87	97	96	93	92	94
All	100	100	100	100	100	100	100	100	100	100
Base	*184*	*256*	*237*	*179*	*856*	*171*	*226*	*238*	*210*	*845*
Mean (average value)	0.70	0.81	0.90	1.06	0.88	0.64	0.74	0.79	0.80	0.75
Median value	0.66	0.79	0.87	1.00	0.83	0.60	0.70	0.75	0.75	0.71
Lower 2.5 percentile	0.33	0.44	0.44	0.58	0.41	0.34	0.37	0.43	0.36	0.37
Upper 2.5 percentile	1.45	1.33	1.50	1.68	1.55	1.22	1.25	1.35	1.39	1.35
Standard deviation of the mean	0.238	0.234	0.261	0.334	0.299	0.213	0.207	0.250	0.282	0.248

* Dietary supplements taken by young people in the survey provided negligible amounts of copper.

Table 9.34 Average daily intake of copper from food sources as a percentage of Reference Nutrient Intake (RNI) by sex and age of young person

Sex and age (years) of young person	Average daily intake as % of RNI*			*Base*
	Mean	Median	sd	
Males				
4–6	117	110	39.6	*184*
7–10	116	113	33.4	*256*
11–14	112	108	32.6	*237*
15–18	106	100	33.4	*179*
All	113	108	34.8	*856*
Females				
4–6	106	99	35.5	*171*
7–10	105	101	29.5	*226*
11–14	98	94	31.3	*238*
15–18	80	75	28.2	*210*
All	97	93	32.7	*845*

*Intake as a percentage of RNI was calculated for each young person. The values for all young people in each age group were then pooled to give a mean, median and sd.

Table 9.35 Percentage contribution of food types to average daily intake of copper by age and sex of young person

Type of food	Males aged (years)				All males	Females aged (years)				All females
	4–6	7–10	11–14	15–18		4–6	7–10	11–14	15–18	
	%	%	%	%	%	%	%	%	%	%
Cereals & cereal products	42	44	42	39	41	40	40	38	37	38
of which:										
white & wholemeal bread	*12*	*14*	*13*	*13*	*13*	*12*	*13*	*12*	*13*	*12*
breakfast cereals	*9*	*8*	*8*	*6*	*8*	*8*	*6*	*6*	*4*	*6*
pasta	*3*	*3*	*3*	*3*	*3*	*3*	*3*	*3*	*4*	*3*
pizza	*1*	*2*	*3*	*4*	*3*	*2*	*2*	*2*	*3*	*2*
biscuits, buns, cakes &										
pastries	*11*	*11*	*9*	*7*	*9*	*10*	*10*	*9*	*6*	*9*
Milk & milk products	3	3	2	2	2	4	2	2	2	2
Eggs & egg dishes	1	1	1	1	1	1	1	1	1	1
Fat spreads	0	0	0	0	0	0	0	0	0	0
Meat & meat products	12	12	14	17	14	12	13	13	13	13
of which:										
chicken, turkey & dishes										
including coated	*3*	*3*	*3*	*4*	*3*	*3*	*3*	*4*	*4*	*4*
Fish & fish dishes	1	1	1	2	1	1	1	1	2	1
Vegetables, potatoes & savoury snacks	18	19	20	22	20	19	21	23	23	22
of which:										
vegetables, excluding potatoes	*4*	*3*	*4*	*5*	*4*	*4*	*4*	*5*	*6*	*5*
all potatoes	*11*	*13*	*14*	*15*	*14*	*12*	*13*	*15*	*14*	*14*
Fruit & nuts	11	9	5	5	7	10	10	6	5	8
of which:										
fruit	*10*	*7*	*4*	*4*	*6*	*9*	*9*	*5*	*5*	*7*
Sugars, preserves & confectionery	5	7	8	7	7	6	6	8	7	7
Drinks*	1	1	1	2	1	1	1	1	3	2
Miscellaneous**	4	4	4	4	4	6	4	4	6	5
Average daily intake (mg)	**0.70**	**0.81**	**0.90**	**1.06**	**0.88**	**0.64**	**0.74**	**0.79**	**0.80**	**0.75**
Total number of young people	**184**	**256**	**237**	**179**	**856**	**171**	**226**	**238**	**210**	**845**

*Includes soft drinks, alcoholic drinks, tea, coffee & water.
**Includes powdered beverages (except tea and coffee), soups, sauces and condiments and commercial toddlers' foods.

Table 9.36 Average daily intake of iodine (µg) from food sources by sex and age of young person

Iodine (µg)	Males aged (years)				All males	Females aged (years)				All females
	4–6	7–10	11–14	15–18		4–6	7–10	11–14	15–18	
	cum %	cum %	cum %	cum %	cum %	cum %	cum %	cum %	cum %	cum %
Intakes from *food sources*										
Less than 50	2	–	1	–	1	2	2	4	5	3
Less than 55	2	1	2	0	1	3	3	4	5	4
Less than 65	3	3	3	1	2	5	5	13	9	8
Less than 70	6	3	5	1	4	9	8	17	10	11
Less than 100	19	15	20	10	16	27	28	37	32	31
Less than 110	26	24	27	13	22	34	39	44	39	39
Less than 130	37	40	37	29	36	45	56	61	53	54
Less than 140	47	47	42	33	42	53	65	65	61	62
Less than 170	64	70	59	51	61	73	82	80	76	78
Less than 200	81	82	73	66	75	87	90	88	90	89
Less than 250	91	91	90	82	88	94	97	96	95	96
All	100	100	100	100	100	100	100	100	100	100
Base	*184*	*256*	*237*	*179*	*856*	*171*	*226*	*238*	*210*	*845*
Mean (average value)	156	154	162	181	163	143	131	129	135	134
Median value	144	142	153	168	150	133	123	119	126	125
Lower 2.5 percentile	61	65	59	78	65	54	51	48	41	48
Upper 2.5 percentile	336	309	341	348	332	318	258	268	279	268
Standard deviation of the mean	72.9	61.6	69.2	73.6	70.0	66.3	52.4	64.9	71.4	64.0

* Dietary supplements taken by young people in the survey provided only negligible amounts of iodine.

Table 9.37 Average daily intake of iodine from food sources as a percentage of Reference Nutrient Intake (RNI) by sex and age of young person

Sex and age (years) of young person	Average daily intake as % of RNI*			*Base*
	Mean	Median	sd	
Males				
4–6	156	144	72.9	*184*
7–10	140	129	56.0	*256*
11–14	124	118	53.2	*237*
15–18	139	130	56.6	*179*
All	139	130	60.3	*856*
Females				
4–6	143	133	66.3	*171*
7–10	119	112	47.6	*226*
11–14	92	85	46.3	*238*
15–18	96	90	51.0	*210*
All	111	102	56.1	*845*

*Intake as a percentage of RNI was calculated for each young person. The values for all young people in each age group were then pooled to give a mean, median and sd.

Table 9.38 Percentage contribution of food types to average daily intake of iodine by age and sex of young person

Type of food	Males aged (years)				All males	Females aged (years)				All females
	4–6	7–10	11–14	15–18		4–6	7–10	11–14	15–18	
	%	%	%	%	%	%	%	%	%	%
Cereals & cereal products	14	18	17	17	16	14	17	18	16	16
of which:										
bread	3	4	4	5	4	3	4	4	5	4
biscuits, buns, cakes &										
pastries	4	6	5	3	5	4	5	5	3	5
Milk & milk products	58	54	50	43	51	58	49	43	41	48
of which:										
whole milk	31	20	12	11	17	31	16	10	11	17
semi-skimmed milk	16	22	26	22	22	14	18	18	18	17
yogurt, fromage frais &										
other dairy desserts	7	7	6	4	6	8	9	8	5	7
Eggs & egg dishes	2	3	3	3	3	3	4	3	3	3
Fat spreads	2	2	2	2	2	2	2	2	2	2
Meat & meat products	4	5	6	8	6	4	6	7	7	6
Fish & fish dishes	8	8	8	8	8	8	10	8	8	8
of which:										
coated & fried white fish	7	6	5	6	6	6	7	6	5	6
Vegetables, potatoes &										
savoury snacks	4	4	5	5	5	4	5	6	6	5
Fruit & nuts	1	1	1	1	1	1	1	1	1	1
Sugars, preserves &										
confectionery	2	3	3	2	2	2	3	3	3	3
Drinks*	1	1	1	9	3	1	1	1	6	2
of which:										
beers & lagers	0	0	0	7	2	0	0	0	3	1
Miscellaneous**	3	1	1	2	2	3	2	5	6	4
Average daily intake (μg)	**156**	**154**	**162**	**181**	**163**	**143**	**131**	**129**	**135**	**134**
Total number of young people	**184**	**256**	**237**	**179**	**856**	**171**	**226**	**238**	**210**	**845**

*Includes soft drinks, alcoholic drinks, tea, coffee & water.
**Includes powdered beverages (except tea and coffee), soups, sauces and condiments and commercial toddlers' foods.

Table 9.39 Average daily intake of manganese (mg) from food sources by sex and age of young person

Manganese (mg)	Males aged (years)				All males	Females aged (years)				All females
	4–6	7–10	11–14	15–18		4–6	7–10	11–14	15–18	
	cum %	cum %	cum %	cum %	cum %	cum %	cum %	cum %	cum %	cum %
Intakes from *food sources*										
Less than 0.80	3	1	1	1	1	2	2	1	3	2
Less than 1.20	15	7	5	2	7	28	12	15	12	16
Less than 1.40	30	14	12	4	14	45	28	25	20	29
Less than 1.60	44	28	18	8	23	62	43	38	30	42
Less than 2.00	71	56	43	26	48	82	67	62	55	66
Less than 2.40	83	77	65	50	68	95	82	77	73	81
Less than 2.80	92	87	78	66	80	97	94	88	87	91
Less than 3.20	98	93	88	77	88	98	96	94	91	94
All	100	100	100	100	100	100	100	100	100	100
Base	*184*	*256*	*237*	*179*	*856*	*171*	*226*	*238*	*210*	*845*
Mean (average value)	1.78	2.05	2.28	2.62	2.20	1.56	1.85	1.96	2.04	1.87
Median value	1.68	1.92	2.10	2.40	2.03	1.44	1.70	1.81	1.92	1.73
Lower 2.5 percentile	0.67	1.08	1.01	1.21	1.00	0.82	0.86	0.89	0.74	0.83
Upper 2.5 percentile	3.17	4.22	4.79	4.98	4.36	2.92	4.19	4.21	4.19	3.91
Standard deviation of the mean	0.623	0.728	0.860	0.955	0.862	0.599	0.694	0.769	0.869	0.765

*None of the dietary supplements taken by young people in this survey provided any manganese.

Table 9.40 Percentage contribution of food types to average daily intake of manganese by age and sex of young person

Type of food	Males aged (years)				All males	Females aged (years)				All females
	4–6	7–10	11–14	15–18		4–6	7–10	11–14	15–18	
	%	%	%	%	%	%	%	%	%	%
Cereals & cereal products	60	62	59	55	59	60	57	56	52	56
of which:										
white bread	*12*	*14*	*14*	*16*	*14*	*13*	*14*	*13*	*14*	*14*
wholemeal bread	*7*	*6*	*5*	*5*	*6*	*6*	*7*	*5*	*6*	*6*
high fibre & whole grain										
breakfast cereals	*15*	*14*	*12*	*10*	*13*	*14*	*10*	*11*	*6*	*10*
other breakfast cereals	*6*	*6*	*5*	*4*	*5*	*6*	*5*	*4*	*3*	*4*
biscuits	*6*	*6*	*5*	*4*	*5*	*6*	*6*	*5*	*3*	*5*
Milk & milk products	1	1	1	1	1	2	1	1	1	1
Eggs & egg dishes	0	0	0	0	0	0	0	0	0	0
Fat spreads	0	0	0	0	0	0	0	0	0	0
Meat & meat products	5	6	7	9	7	5	6	6	6	6
Fish & fish dishes	1	1	1	1	1	1	1	1	1	1
Vegetables, potatoes & savoury snacks	17	15	18	18	17	17	18	20	20	19
of which:										
vegetables, excluding potatoes	*8*	*6*	*8*	*8*	*8*	*8*	*8*	*9*	*11*	*9*
all potatoes	*6*	*7*	*7*	*8*	*7*	*6*	*7*	*8*	*8*	*8*
Fruit & nuts	7	6	4	3	5	7	6	4	4	5
of which:										
fruit	*6*	*5*	*3*	*3*	*4*	*6*	*5*	*3*	*4*	*4*
Sugars, preserves & confectionery	3	4	4	4	4	3	3	4	4	4
Drinks*	4	4	4	7	5	3	4	6	9	6
of which:										
fruit juice	*3*	*2*	*2*	*2*	*2*	*2*	*2*	*3*	*2*	*2*
tea	*1*	*2*	*2*	*5*	*3*	*1*	*2*	*3*	*6*	*3*
Miscellaneous**	1	1	1	2	1	1	2	2	2	2
Average daily intake (mg)	**1.78**	**2.05**	**2.28**	**2.62**	**2.20**	**1.56**	**1.85**	**1.96**	**2.04**	**1.87**
Total number of young people	**184**	**256**	**237**	**179**	**856**	**171**	**226**	**238**	**210**	**845**

*Includes soft drinks, alcoholic drinks, tea, coffee & water.
**Includes powdered beverages (except tea and coffee), soups, sauces and condiments and commercial toddlers' foods.

Table 9.41 Average daily intake of minerals from food sources by whether young person was reported as being unwell during dietary recording period

| Minerals | Whether unwell during period | | | | | | | | |
| | Unwell and eating affected | | | Unwell and eating not affected | | | Not unwell | | |
	Mean	Median	sd	Mean	Median	sd	Mean	Median	sd
Males									
Total iron (mg)	9.4	8.6	3.53	9.6	9.1	3.17	10.6	10.0	3.49
Haem iron (mg)	0.4	0.3	0.30	0.3	0.3	0.23	0.4	0.4	0.28
Non-haem iron (mg)	8.9	8.0	3.44	9.2	8.7	3.14	10.2	9.5	3.40
Calcium (mg)	691	689	278.1	719	690	274.5	802	763	275.6
Phosphorus (mg)	985	1021	316.9	1026	1013	337.3	1127	1091	319.4
Magnesium (mg)	188	187	63.1	192	190	65.5	216	206	64.3
Sodium (mg)*	2365	2273	738.1	2508	2520	810.8	2673	2569	832.4
Chloride (mg)*	3566	3559	1112.9	3777	3703	1247.2	4017	3860	1259.1
Potassium (mg)	2033	1995	606.5	2131	2137	680.8	2400	2292	703.0
Zinc (mg)	6.2	6.2	2.28	6.3	6.3	2.23	7.1	6.7	2.34
Copper (mg)	0.78	0.77	0.293	0.79	0.79	0.265	0.90	0.84	0.299
Iodine (µg)	143	134	68.2	147	136	59.6	167	152	70.5
Manganese (mg)	1.94	1.85	0.887	1.98	1.90	0.822	2.25	2.08	0.854
Base		*86*			*66*			*704*	
Females									
Total iron (mg)	6.8	6.6	2.10	8.2	7.6	2.30	8.6	8.1	2.74
Haem iron (mg)	0.3	0.2	0.20	0.4	0.3	0.23	0.3	0.3	0.21
Non-haem iron (mg)	6.6	6.3	2.08	7.8	7.3	2.27	8.2	7.8	2.70
Calcium (mg)	544	543	206.8	587	580	205.5	674	661	222.3
Phosphorus (mg)	758	752	215.4	870	866	211.7	944	919	237.3
Magnesium (mg)	147	144	41.9	172	170	37.8	182	179	49.6
Sodium (mg)*	1816	1754	567.5	2170	2126	590.6	2199	2165	563.7
Chloride (mg)*	2727	2637	835.4	3247	3100	858.5	3308	3249	836.2
Potassium (mg)	1663	1633	482.6	2008	2000	443.1	2077	2044	526.6
Zinc (mg)	4.7	4.6	1.46	5.6	5.3	1.59	5.8	5.6	1.67
Copper (mg)	0.65	0.64	0.215	0.77	0.72	0.263	0.76	0.71	0.248
Iodine (µg)	113	103	55.8	121	112	50.5	138	129	65.8
Manganese (mg)	1.54	1.45	0.594	1.76	1.72	0.508	1.92	1.77	0.798
Base		*93*			*84*			*668*	

* Includes intakes from food only; excludes further additions of salt in cooking or at the table.

Table 9.42   Average daily intake of minerals from food sources per MJ total energy by whether young person was reported as being unwell during dietary recording period

| Minerals | Whether unwell during period | | | | | | | | |
| | Unwell and eating affected | | | Unwell and eating not affected | | | Not unwell | | |
	Mean	Median	sd	Mean	Median	sd	Mean	Median	sd
Males									
Total iron (mg)	1.34	1.27	0.401	1.27	1.25	0.252	1.31	1.28	0.290
Haem iron (mg)	0.06	0.04	0.044	0.05	0.05	0.028	0.05	0.04	0.032
Non-haem iron (mg)	1.28	1.22	0.392	1.22	1.20	0.255	1.25	1.23	0.289
Calcium (mg)	96	99	24.8	94	90	24.9	99	96	26.3
Phosphorus (mg)	139	139	21.3	135	132	22.7	139	138	22.1
Magnesium (mg)	26	26	4.7	25	25	4.4	27	26	4.6
Sodium (mg)*	338	333	87.9	332	327	56.8	329	325	64.2
Chloride (mg)*	509	490	127.7	499	483	86.0	494	485	96.7
Potassium (mg)	290	283	50.0	282	281	43.8	296	296	50.0
Zinc (mg)	0.88	0.87	0.207	0.84	0.82	0.195	0.87	0.85	0.203
Copper (mg)	0.11	0.10	0.037	0.10	0.10	0.019	0.11	0.11	0.025
Iodine (µg)	20	18	7.5	20	19	6.6	21	20	7.8
Manganese (mg)	0.27	0.25	0.097	0.26	0.25	0.086	0.28	0.26	0.086
Base		86			66			704	
Females									
Total iron (mg)	1.24	1.18	0.357	1.23	1.23	0.272	1.27	1.21	0.303
Haem iron (mg)	0.05	0.04	0.037	0.06	0.05	0.036	0.05	0.04	0.031
Non-haem iron (mg)	1.19	1.11	0.362	1.17	1.16	0.270	1.22	1.16	0.302
Calcium (mg)	98	97	32.9	88	89	25.6	100	98	26.6
Phosphorus (mg)	136	131	26.2	131	129	22.6	140	138	21.3
Magnesium (mg)	26	25	4.9	26	25	4.8	27	26	4.6
Sodium (mg)*	323	309	69.2	324	323	61.4	327	324	61.3
Chloride (mg)*	486	466	104.4	485	474	90.7	492	486	90.4
Potassium (mg)	297	293	59.8	303	302	52.3	308	302	52.9
Zinc (mg)	0.85	0.82	0.202	0.84	0.81	0.196	0.86	0.84	0.172
Copper (mg)	0.12	0.11	0.027	0.12	0.11	0.030	0.11	0.11	0.026
Iodine (µg)	21	18	10.8	18	18	7.2	20	19	8.3
Manganese (mg)	0.28	0.25	0.092	0.27	0.26	0.082	0.28	0.26	0.095
Base		93			84			668	

* Includes intakes from food only; excludes further additions of salt in cooking or at the table.

Table 9.43 Average daily intake of minerals from food sources by region

Minerals	Region Scotland			Northern			Central, South West and Wales			London and the South East		
	Mean	Median	sd	Mean	Median	sd	Mean	Median	sd	Mean	Median	sd
Males												
Total iron (mg)	9.6	8.8	3.41	10.1	9.8	3.22	10.7	10.0	3.25	10.5	9.8	3.97
Haem iron (mg)	0.4	0.4	0.24	0.4	0.3	0.24	0.4	0.4	0.29	0.4	0.4	0.29
Non-haem iron (mg)	9.1	8.5	3.29	9.8	9.3	3.17	10.2	9.5	3.16	10.1	9.3	3.87
Calcium (mg)	784	775	297.9	779	755	264.9	800	745	278.5	770	741	284.4
Phosphorus (mg)	1085	1059	325.5	1087	1076	303.9	1122	1075	328.5	1107	1063	336.1
Magnesium (mg)	196	184	65.0	209	201	63.0	214	209	61.3	215	205	70.6
Sodium (mg)*	2691	2620	841.3	2637	2606	767.6	2673	2548	784.5	2553	2417	921.0
Chloride (mg)*	4057	3896	1336.3	3975	3906	1146.3	4013	3871	1182.7	3834	3598	1394.5
Potassium (mg)	2189	1990	688.0	2332	2267	678.8	2393	2317	694.2	2337	2202	735.6
Zinc (mg)	6.7	6.2	2.20	6.6	6.3	2.02	7.2	6.7	2.53	7.1	6.7	2.40
Copper (mg)	0.80	0.76	0.241	0.85	0.82	0.269	0.89	0.86	0.304	0.91	0.84	0.329
Iodine (µg)	152	141	66.4	164	156	65.3	166	150	73.1	164	150	71.2
Manganese (mg)	1.94	1.83	0.679	2.12	1.96	0.843	2.25	2.11	0.825	2.30	2.15	0.944
Base	*68*			*243*			*300*			*245*		
Females												
Total iron (mg)	7.6	7.2	2.42	8.2	7.9	2.43	8.7	8.3	2.70	8.2	7.6	2.92
Haem iron (mg)	0.3	0.3	0.24	0.3	0.3	0.21	0.3	0.3	0.24	0.3	0.3	0.18
Non-haem iron (mg)	7.3	7.0	2.35	7.9	7.4	2.39	8.4	8.0	2.65	7.9	7.3	2.91
Calcium (mg)	604	573	233.2	661	660	209.5	674	648	224.4	629	630	229.1
Phosphorus (mg)	901	869	255.6	920	917	227.6	942	933	246.9	887	877	235.0
Magnesium (mg)	165	155	47.0	178	178	44.0	184	181	49.3	174	168	52.8
Sodium (mg)*	2172	2119	547.4	2219	2161	601.6	2189	2146	562.2	2051	2028	571.3
Chloride (mg)*	3241	3061	786.5	3347	3282	887.7	3286	3218	840.4	3085	3016	844.0
Potassium (mg)	1943	1892	544.6	2066	2070	493.1	2097	2041	544.5	1926	1895	523.4
Zinc (mg)	5.5	5.0	1.88	5.7	5.6	1.54	5.8	5.6	1.72	5.6	5.4	1.66
Copper (mg)	0.69	0.65	0.266	0.73	0.72	0.220	0.77	0.74	0.252	0.74	0.70	0.260
Iodine (µg)	119	108	57.0	140	132	56.5	136	128	56.2	130	119	79.0
Manganese (mg)	1.71	1.50	0.799	1.78	1.74	0.623	1.94	1.79	0.741	1.91	1.70	0.884
Base	*69*			*217*			*306*			*253*		

* Includes intakes from food only; excludes further additions of salt in cooking or at the table.

Table 9.44 Average daily intake of minerals from food sources per MJ total energy by region

Minerals	Region											
	Scotland			Northern			Central, South West and Wales			London and the South East		
	Mean	Median	sd	Mean	Median	sd	Mean	Median	sd	Mean	Median	sd
Males												
Total iron (mg)	1.21	1.21	0.276	1.29	1.20	0.340	1.33	1.30	0.265	1.32	1.30	0.301
Haem iron (mg)	0.05	0.05	0.028	0.05	0.04	0.033	0.05	0.05	0.034	0.05	0.05	0.033
Non-haem iron (mg)	1.16	1.18	0.272	1.24	1.16	0.333	1.28	1.25	0.265	1.26	1.25	0.302
Calcium (mg)	99	92	25.8	98	95	26.6	99	98	24.8	97	95	27.0
Phosphorus (mg)	138	137	20.4	137	138	22.5	139	137	21.5	139	138	22.7
Magnesium (mg)	25	25	4.1	26	26	4.5	27	26	4.1	27	26	5.3
Sodium (mg)*	345	332	66.7	333	328	68.5	332	328	59.1	320	314	71.0
Chloride (mg)*	519	510	105.8	502	494	99.5	499	489	89.7	480	474	106.5
Potassium (mg)	279	278	48.6	294	290	50.4	298	299	50.7	294	293	47.3
Zinc (mg)	0.84	0.85	0.166	0.83	0.81	0.187	0.89	0.86	0.216	0.89	0.87	0.204
Copper (mg)	0.10	0.10	0.016	0.11	0.10	0.027	0.11	0.11	0.024	0.11	0.11	0.030
Iodine (µg)	19	19	6.4	21	19	7.2	21	19	8.2	21	19	7.8
Manganese (mg)	0.25	0.24	0.059	0.27	0.25	0.085	0.28	0.27	0.078	0.29	0.27	0.101
Base	*68*			*243*			*300*			*245*		
Females												
Total iron (mg)	1.21	1.15	0.284	1.21	1.17	0.254	1.30	1.24	0.314	1.27	1.21	0.338
Haem iron (mg)	0.05	0.05	0.041	0.05	0.04	0.030	0.05	0.04	0.034	0.05	0.04	0.028
Non-haem iron (mg)	1.15	1.11	0.281	1.16	1.12	0.253	1.26	1.19	0.314	1.22	1.16	0.339
Calcium (mg)	95	94	27.4	97	96	25.3	101	99	26.6	97	95	30.2
Phosphorus (mg)	142	142	22.1	136	135	20.8	141	139	22.9	137	134	22.1
Magnesium (mg)	26	25	4.7	26	26	4.0	27	26	4.9	27	26	4.9
Sodium (mg)*	347	346	65.5	327	325	58.7	329	321	60.1	317	315	65.4
Chloride (mg)*	517	521	91.6	494	491	85.7	493	483	88.9	478	476	99.4
Potassium (mg)	307	305	54.0	306	302	48.3	314	307	55.6	298	296	55.0
Zinc (mg)	0.86	0.82	0.225	0.84	0.83	0.165	0.87	0.85	0.177	0.86	0.84	0.176
Copper (mg)	0.11	0.10	0.030	0.11	0.10	0.023	0.11	0.11	0.026	0.11	0.11	0.027
Iodine (µg)	19	17	7.3	21	20	7.2	20	19	8.0	20	18	10.5
Manganese (mg)	0.27	0.24	0.097	0.26	0.25	0.076	0.29	0.27	0.095	0.29	0.27	0.103
Base	*69*			*217*			*306*			*253*		

* Includes intakes from food only; excludes further additions of salt in cooking or at the table.

Table 9.45 Average daily intake of minerals from food sources by whether young person's 'parents' were receiving certain benefits

Minerals	Whether receiving benefits					
	Receiving benefits			Not receiving benefits		
	Mean	Median	sd	Mean	Median	sd
Males						
Total iron (mg)	9.3	8.8	2.87	10.7	10.1	3.61
Haem iron (mg)	0.4	0.3	0.27	0.4	0.4	0.28
Non-haem iron (mg)	8.9	8.4	2.82	10.3	9.6	3.51
Calcium (mg)	656	628	255.7	826	790	272.7
Phosphorus (mg)	969	936	296.5	1150	1109	320.6
Magnesium (mg)	187	176	60.0	220	210	64.6
Sodium (mg)*	2362	2237	851.8	2716	2635	801.2
Chloride (mg)*	3565	3397	1272.9	4080	3944	1220.5
Potassium (mg)	2143	2058	618.9	2408	2311	717.6
Zinc (mg)	6.3	6.0	2.12	7.1	6.7	2.37
Copper (mg)	0.81	0.77	0.306	0.90	0.86	0.294
Iodine (μg)	143	133	60.4	170	157	71.6
Manganese (mg)	1.99	1.83	0.888	2.27	2.10	0.843
Base		189			666	
Females						
Total iron (mg)	8.3	7.8	2.80	8.4	7.9	2.65
Haem iron (mg)	0.3	0.3	0.20	0.3	0.3	0.22
Non-haem iron (mg)	7.9	7.5	2.75	8.0	7.5	2.62
Calcium (mg)	614	599	219.6	666	656	222.4
Phosphorus (mg)	882	877	248.1	931	905	234.0
Magnesium (mg)	171	172	49.0	180	176	48.6
Sodium (mg)*	2142	2159	614.4	2164	2119	563.2
Chloride (mg)*	3219	3203	921.6	3253	3190	830.1
Potassium (mg)	1980	1961	551.5	2045	2025	519.8
Zinc (mg)	5.6	5.5	1.63	5.7	5.5	1.68
Copper (mg)	0.73	0.69	0.256	0.75	0.72	0.245
Iodine (μg)	129	119	59.1	136	127	65.4
Manganese (mg)	1.83	1.68	0.738	1.88	1.75	0.773
Base		199			645	

* Includes intakes from food only; excludes further additions of salt in cooking or at the table.

Table 9.46 Average daily intake of minerals from food sources per MJ total energy by whether young person's 'parents' were receiving certain benefits

Minerals	Whether receiving benefits					
	Receiving benefits			Not receiving benefits		
	Mean	Median	sd	Mean	Median	sd
Males						
Total iron (mg)	1.31	1.27	0.301	1.30	1.28	0.301
Haem iron (mg)	0.06	0.05	0.040	0.05	0.04	0.030
Non-haem iron (mg)	1.25	1.22	0.297	1.25	1.23	0.299
Calcium (mg)	91	87	24.9	101	98	26.0
Phosphorus (mg)	135	134	23.7	140	139	21.4
Magnesium (mg)	26	25	5.1	27	26	4.5
Sodium (mg)*	329	327	80.8	330	325	60.9
Chloride (mg)*	497	484	120.3	496	485	91.6
Potassium (mg)	300	301	48.5	292	290	50.0
Zinc (mg)	0.88	0.86	0.214	0.86	0.85	0.196
Copper (mg)	0.11	0.11	0.033	0.11	0.11	0.024
Iodine (µg)	20	19	6.8	21	19	7.9
Manganese (mg)	0.28	0.26	0.096	0.28	0.26	0.084
Base		*189*			*666*	
Females						
Total iron (mg)	1.25	1.20	0.315	1.26	1.21	0.304
Haem iron (mg)	0.05	0.04	0.030	0.05	0.04	0.033
Non-haem iron (mg)	1.20	1.15	0.311	1.21	1.16	0.305
Calcium (mg)	92	93	23.1	101	99	28.5
Phosphorus (mg)	133	134	20.4	140	139	22.3
Magnesium (mg)	26	25	4.5	27	27	4.7
Sodium (mg)*	325	323	62.7	327	323	62.0
Chloride (mg)*	488	484	94.5	492	485	91.2
Potassium (mg)	300	297	51.2	309	303	54.5
Zinc (mg)	0.85	0.83	0.160	0.86	0.84	0.184
Copper (mg)	0.11	0.10	0.029	0.11	0.11	0.025
Iodine (µg)	19	19	7.5	21	19	8.8
Manganese (mg)	0.28	0.25	0.094	0.28	0.26	0.094
Base		*199*			*645*	

* Includes intakes from food only; excludes further additions of salt in cooking or at the table.

319

Table 9.47 Average daily intake of minerals from food sources by gross weekly household income

Minerals	Gross weekly household income														
	Less than £160			£160 to less than £280			£280 to less than £400			£400 to less than £600			£600 and over		
	Mean	Median	sd	Mean	Median	sd	Mean	Median	sd	Mean	Median	sd	Mean	Median	sd
Males															
Total iron (mg)	9.5	9.2	2.98	9.8	9.5	3.32	10.4	9.8	3.29	11.1	10.8	3.38	10.8	9.7	3.96
Haem iron (mg)	0.4	0.4	0.27	0.4	0.3	0.26	0.4	0.3	0.28	0.4	0.4	0.27	0.4	0.4	0.28
Non-haem iron (mg)	9.1	8.7	2.90	9.5	8.9	3.22	10.0	9.4	3.20	10.7	10.2	3.30	10.4	9.3	3.87
Calcium (mg)	658	649	241.0	713	670	281.2	797	783	256.6	888	858	272.5	837	807	270.9
Phosphorus (mg)	987	945	302.8	1004	983	308.6	1115	1103	295.7	1206	1182	292.3	1173	1105	338.4
Magnesium (mg)	190	176	62.0	192	181	60.3	214	202	61.9	227	225	57.0	227	217	70.2
Sodium (mg)*	2425	2331	904.6	2485	2345	835.8	2672	2699	722.9	2851	2779	795.3	2628	2546	759.7
Chloride (mg)*	3665	3482	1369.7	3747	3575	1257.8	4003	3991	1091.3	4280	4189	1186.2	3936	3771	1167.2
Potassium (mg)	2180	2118	666.9	2130	2026	660.0	2332	2218	650.9	2472	2445	618.4	2507	2405	768.1
Zinc (mg)	6.5	6.0	2.27	6.3	6.1	2.11	6.8	6.6	2.09	7.5	7.4	2.18	7.3	6.7	2.61
Copper (mg)	0.84	0.80	0.324	0.80	0.81	0.259	0.87	0.82	0.295	0.92	0.90	0.258	0.92	0.89	0.332
Iodine (µg)	144	133	60.6	148	137	66.1	159	151	55.2	180	174	67.8	178	164	82.0
Manganese (mg)	2.07	1.88	0.923	2.03	1.92	0.799	2.19	1.99	0.821	2.38	2.22	0.892	2.30	2.20	0.852
Base	*133*			*159*			*157*			*173*			*208*		
Females															
Total iron (mg)	8.3	7.8	3.00	8.3	7.8	2.49	8.3	8.1	2.41	8.4	7.8	2.93	7.9	7.9	2.51
Haem iron (mg)	0.3	0.3	0.22	0.3	0.3	0.21	0.3	0.3	0.22	0.3	0.3	0.20	0.3	0.3	0.22
Non-haem iron (mg)	7.9	7.5	2.96	8.0	7.5	2.43	7.9	7.7	2.35	8.1	7.5	2.90	8.1	7.5	2.49
Calcium (mg)	611	585	243.6	636	635	204.2	644	616	194.2	664	662	222.3	707	674	231.8
Phosphorus (mg)	876	850	268.8	882	877	217.7	908	879	199.2	928	905	232.8	985	966	247.6
Magnesium (mg)	168	166	50.9	174	175	44.7	173	170	39.6	179	176	48.1	191	185	52.6
Sodium (mg)*	2097	2049	609.4	2198	2180	575.7	2243	2214	587.5	2178	2102	580.8	2134	2069	516.6
Chloride (mg)*	3149	3063	896.0	3320	3301	873.0	3354	3391	890.2	3270	3228	844.0	3205	3086	756.3
Potassium (mg)	1966	1961	566.1	2021	2015	511.5	1981	1974	480.9	2037	2014	531.4	2127	2064	520.2
Zinc (mg)	5.5	5.4	1.67	5.5	5.3	1.53	5.6	5.4	1.53	5.8	5.7	1.69	6.0	5.8	1.80
Copper (mg)	0.71	0.66	0.246	0.75	0.72	0.263	0.73	0.70	0.209	0.75	0.72	0.236	0.77	0.72	0.269
Iodine (µg)	131	119	62.7	130	127	45.9	129	118	56.9	139	124	69.4	142	131	77.1
Manganese (mg)	1.79	1.68	0.716	1.80	1.68	0.635	1.76	1.73	0.595	1.87	1.69	0.786	2.03	1.81	0.926
Base	*131*			*146*			*145*			*192*			*196*		

* Includes intakes from food only; excludes further additions of salt in cooking or at the table.

Table 9.48 Average daily intake of minerals from food sources per MJ total energy by gross weekly household income

Minerals	Gross weekly household income														
	Less than £160			£160 to less than £280			£280 to less than £400			£400 to less than £600			£600 and over		
	Mean	Median	sd	Mean	Median	sd	Mean	Median	sd	Mean	Median	sd	Mean	Median	sd
Males															
Total iron (mg)	1.31	1.29	0.297	1.34	1.30	0.355	1.27	1.26	0.247	1.31	1.27	0.279	1.30	1.27	0.302
Haem iron (mg)	0.06	0.05	0.033	0.05	0.04	0.037	0.05	0.04	0.032	0.05	0.04	0.031	0.05	0.04	0.032
Non-haem iron (mg)	1.25	1.24	0.296	1.29	1.24	0.346	1.22	1.19	0.246	1.26	1.22	0.279	1.25	1.22	0.300
Calcium (mg)	90	87	24.4	95	93	23.6	99	94	26.6	105	104	26.2	102	100	26.5
Phosphorus (mg)	135	132	24.4	135	136	20.5	137	137	20.5	143	140	22.4	142	141	21.4
Magnesium (mg)	26	25	5.5	26	26	4.3	26	26	4.2	27	26	4.8	27	27	4.4
Sodium (mg)*	329	327	70.6	335	329	75.1	329	325	55.9	337	329	68.7	320	316	56.5
Chloride (mg)*	498	492	107.0	504	484	112.5	493	491	84.0	506	497	102.5	478	471	83.5
Potassium (mg)	298	298	47.6	288	284	49.9	287	283	47.4	293	289	51.5	303	301	50.0
Zinc (mg)	0.89	0.84	0.223	0.85	0.85	0.185	0.84	0.82	0.187	0.88	0.85	0.184	0.89	0.87	0.221
Copper (mg)	0.11	0.11	0.036	0.11	0.11	0.023	0.11	0.10	0.025	0.11	0.10	0.023	0.11	0.11	0.025
Iodine (µg)	20	19	7.3	20	18	6.9	20	19	6.3	21	20	7.8	22	20	9.2
Manganese (mg)	0.28	0.25	0.105	0.27	0.26	0.080	0.27	0.25	0.072	0.28	0.26	0.094	0.28	0.26	0.084
Base	133			159			157			173			208		
Females															
Total iron (mg)	1.27	1.21	0.336	1.25	1.20	0.286	1.24	1.19	0.284	1.26	1.21	0.300	1.25	1.19	0.289
Haem iron (mg)	0.05	0.04	0.038	0.04	0.04	0.030	0.05	0.04	0.032	0.05	0.04	0.028	0.05	0.05	0.032
Non-haem iron (mg)	1.22	1.17	0.332	1.20	1.15	0.287	1.19	1.14	0.280	1.21	1.15	0.303	1.20	1.14	0.289
Calcium (mg)	93	95	25.6	96	94	29.0	97	93	25.2	101	97	27.4	104	100	27.5
Phosphorus (mg)	135	135	21.2	133	132	19.7	136	134	21.3	141	138	21.5	146	144	23.1
Magnesium (mg)	26	25	4.1	26	25	4.8	26	26	4.1	27	26	4.4	28	27	4.9
Sodium (mg)*	325	324	63.3	332	325	64.6	335	331	62.4	330	326	60.2	318	311	55.1
Chloride (mg)*	488	485	92.8	501	483	98.8	500	496	94.3	496	488	86.2	477	475	80.7
Potassium (mg)	303	298	45.7	305	300	56.1	297	297	52.8	309	302	53.2	316	312	57.2
Zinc (mg)	0.85	0.82	0.173	0.83	0.81	0.156	0.84	0.83	0.192	0.87	0.84	0.163	0.90	0.87	0.197
Copper (mg)	0.11	0.10	0.025	0.11	0.11	0.030	0.11	0.11	0.024	0.11	0.11	0.024	0.11	0.11	0.027
Iodine (µg)	20	19	7.5	20	19	6.1	19	18	7.9	21	19	8.9	21	19	10.2
Manganese (mg)	0.28	0.27	0.090	0.27	0.25	0.089	0.26	0.25	0.079	0.28	0.26	0.091	0.30	0.28	0.106
Base	131			146			145			192			196		

* Includes intakes from food only; excludes further additions of salt in cooking or at the table.

Table 9.49 Average daily intake of minerals from food sources by social class of head of household

Minerals	Social class of head of household								
	Non-manual			Manual			All*		
	Mean	Median	sd	Mean	Median	sd	Mean	Median	sd
Males									
Total iron (mg)	10.7	10.1	3.85	10.3	9.8	3.14	10.4	9.8	3.49
Haem iron (mg)	0.4	0.3	0.27	0.4	0.4	0.27	0.4	0.4	0.28
Non-haem iron (mg)	10.3	9.6	3.75	9.8	9.3	3.05	10.0	9.3	3.41
Calcium (mg)	834	807	270.0	760	726	265.9	784	748	278.3
Phosphorus (mg)	1149	1106	327.6	1084	1046	302.5	1105	1067	324.1
Magnesium (mg)	220	210	67.8	208	200	58.8	212	204	65.1
Sodium (mg)**	2650	2580	823.8	2650	2542	834.5	2630	2542	827.6
Chloride (mg)**	3985	3843	1260.8	3983	3860	1254.8	3954	3821	1252.6
Potassium (mg)	2411	2308	752.5	2315	2201	646.7	2343	2267	703.4
Zinc (mg)	7.1	6.7	2.51	6.8	6.5	2.13	6.9	6.5	2.35
Copper (mg)	0.91	0.86	0.321	0.86	0.83	0.265	0.88	0.83	0.299
Iodine (µg)	173	163	73.6	157	145	64.9	163	150	70.0
Manganese (mg)	2.28	2.08	0.905	2.15	2.00	0.772	2.20	2.03	0.862
Base		*414*			*385*			*856*	
Females									
Total iron (mg)	8.5	7.9	2.81	8.2	7.8	2.55	8.3	7.9	2.69
Haem iron (mg)	0.3	0.3	0.22	0.3	0.3	0.22	0.3	0.3	0.22
Non-haem iron (mg)	8.2	7.7	2.78	7.8	7.5	2.52	8.0	7.5	2.65
Calcium (mg)	680	664	226.2	633	614	216.3	652	644	223.6
Phosphorus (mg)	951	931	241.9	894	872	229.6	917	896	239.9
Magnesium (mg)	185	181	50.0	172	170	47.3	178	175	49.0
Sodium (mg)**	2151	2089	567.5	2181	2143	583.3	2156	2119	578.7
Chloride (mg)**	3230	3164	839.5	3278	3192	866.6	3241	3190	856.7
Potassium (mg)	2069	2041	532.3	2005	2002	522.0	2026	2010	529.7
Zinc (mg)	5.8	5.6	1.75	5.6	5.5	1.56	5.7	5.5	1.67
Copper (mg)	0.77	0.72	0.265	0.73	0.70	0.232	0.75	0.71	0.248
Iodine (µg)	141	130	72.5	127	121	53.4	134	125	64.0
Manganese (mg)	1.96	1.78	0.831	1.76	1.64	0.690	1.87	1.73	0.765
Base		*401*			*361*			*845*	

*Includes those for whom social class could not be assigned.
**Includes intakes from food only; excludes further additions of salt in cooking or at the table.

Table 9.50 Average daily intake of minerals from food sources per MJ total energy by social class of head of household

Minerals	Social class of head of household								
	Non-manual			Manual			All*		
	Mean	Median	sd	Mean	Median	sd	Mean	Median	sd
Males									
Total iron (mg)	1.30	1.27	0.288	1.30	1.27	0.316	1.31	1.28	0.300
Haem iron (mg)	0.05	0.04	0.029	0.05	0.05	0.032	0.05	0.04	0.033
Non-haem iron (mg)	1.26	1.22	0.288	1.25	1.22	0.313	1.25	1.22	0.298
Calcium (mg)	103	100	26.1	96	92	24.6	98	96	26.1
Phosphorus (mg)	142	140	21.9	136	136	21.1	139	137	22.1
Magnesium (mg)	27	26	4.6	26	26	4.5	26	26	4.6
Sodium (mg)**	326	322	58.2	333	328	68.1	330	326	66.3
Chloride (mg)**	489	482	88.8	500	492	101.4	496	485	99.4
Potassium (mg)	297	296	52.4	292	289	47.8	294	292	49.7
Zinc (mg)	0.88	0.85	0.205	0.86	0.85	0.193	0.87	0.85	0.203
Copper (mg)	0.11	0.11	0.026	0.11	0.10	0.026	0.11	0.11	0.026
Iodine (μg)	22	20	8.3	20	19	7.0	21	19	7.7
Manganese (mg)	0.28	0.26	0.087	0.27	0.26	0.084	0.28	0.26	0.087
Base		*414*			*385*			*856*	
Females									
Total iron (mg)	1.27	1.21	0.317	1.24	1.20	0.278	1.26	1.21	0.306
Haem iron (mg)	0.05	0.04	0.031	0.05	0.05	0.033	0.05	0.04	0.032
Non-haem iron (mg)	1.22	1.16	0.317	1.19	1.15	0.278	1.21	1.15	0.307
Calcium (mg)	101	100	27.6	96	95	27.6	98	97	27.5
Phosphorus (mg)	141	139	23.3	136	135	20.9	138	137	22.2
Magnesium (mg)	27	26	4.9	26	26	4.1	27	26	4.7
Sodium (mg)**	320	313	59.8	333	328	62.0	326	323	62.2
Chloride (mg)**	481	476	88.5	500	491	91.8	491	484	92.0
Potassium (mg)	308	303	55.2	305	299	53.1	307	301	53.7
Zinc (mg)	0.87	0.83	0.188	0.85	0.84	0.170	0.86	0.84	0.178
Copper (mg)	0.11	0.11	0.028	0.11	0.11	0.025	0.11	0.11	0.026
Iodine (μg)	21	19	9.4	19	18	7.3	20	19	8.5
Manganese (mg)	0.29	0.27	0.099	0.27	0.25	0.083	0.28	0.26	0.094
Base		*401*			*361*			*845*	

*Includes those for whom social class could not be assigned.
**Includes intakes from food only; excludes further additions of salt in cooking or at the table.

Table 9.51 Average daily intake of minerals from food sources by whether living with both parents

Minerals	Household type*								
	Young person living with:								
	Both parents and other children			Both parents and no other children			Single parent with/out other children		
	Mean	Median	sd	Mean	Median	sd	Mean	Median	sd
Males									
Total iron (mg)	10.2	9.7	3.26	11.3	10.5	3.67	10.1	9.5	3.88
Haem iron (mg)	0.4	0.3	0.24	0.5	0.5	0.3	0.4	0.3	0.27
Non-haem iron (mg)	9.8	9.2	3.18	10.8	10.0	3.59	9.6	9.2	3.80
Calcium (mg)	768	728	271.5	880	890	286.7	738	706	270.8
Phosphorus (mg)	1058	1029	292.6	1279	1230	339.8	1077	1036	345.0
Magnesium (mg)	203	198	58.4	242	235	69.0	207	192	71.8
Sodium (mg)**	2526	2426	733.5	2998	2996	866.8	2575	2479	952.8
Chloride (mg)**	3796	3680	1098.0	4506	4517	1334.4	3877	3706	1449.9
Potassium (mg)	2241	2154	618.4	2700	2603	773.7	2300	2187	761.8
Zinc (mg)	6.5	6.2	1.99	8.3	7.9	2.66	6.8	6.5	2.57
Copper (mg)	0.84	0.81	0.261	1.00	0.97	0.345	0.87	0.81	0.334
Iodine (µg)	159	145	68.3	185	175	75.2	157	144	65.7
Manganese (mg)	2.13	2.00	0.772	2.45	2.25	0.980	2.18	1.95	0.974
Base		*528*			*169*			*157*	
Females									
Total iron (mg)	8.3	7.9	2.56	8.3	7.8	2.75	8.5	7.9	3.01
Haem iron (mg)	0.3	0.3	0.19	0.4	0.3	0.27	0.3	0.3	0.22
Non-haem iron (mg)	8.0	7.5	2.53	7.9	7.5	2.67	8.2	7.6	2.99
Calcium (mg)	660	653	225.0	649	647	240.2	635	618	201.3
Phosphorus (mg)	910	897	226.8	945	912	276.1	912	886	241.8
Magnesium (mg)	176	173	45.4	184	181	58.7	177	175	49.1
Sodium (mg)**	2125	2090	542.7	2237	2174	652.9	2179	2160	601.5
Chloride (mg)**	3194	3166	801.8	3373	3303	962.8	3266	3207	894.7
Potassium (mg)	2012	2001	502.8	2087	2056	600.8	2018	1984	530.1
Zinc (mg)	5.6	5.5	1.55	5.9	5.6	2.09	5.6	5.5	1.59
Copper (mg)	0.73	0.69	0.240	0.77	0.73	0.260	0.76	0.71	0.259
Iodine (µg)	137	128	64.1	130	122	73.5	129	119	54.3
Manganese (mg)	1.85	1.70	0.731	1.94	1.79	0.935	1.85	1.72	0.684
Base		*498*			*173*			*167*	

* Excludes nine young people who were living with others, not parents.
** Includes intakes from food only; excludes further additions of salt in cooking and at the table.

Table 9.52 Average daily intake of minerals from food sources per MJ total energy by whether living with both parents

Minerals	Household type*								
	Young person living with:								
	Both parents and other children			Both parents and no other children			Single parent with/out other children		
	Mean	Median	sd	Mean	Median	sd	Mean	Median	sd
Males									
Total iron (mg)	1.31	1.29	0.278	1.28	1.24	0.343	1.32	1.27	0.327
Haem iron (mg)	0.05	0.04	0.029	0.06	0.05	0.043	0.05	0.05	0.032
Non-haem iron (mg)	1.26	1.24	0.275	1.22	1.17	0.336	1.26	1.22	0.330
Calcium (mg)	99	96	26.9	99	98	24.5	97	93	24.5
Phosphorus (mg)	136	135	21.3	144	141	21.1	141	139	24.6
Magnesium (mg)	26	26	4.5	27	27	4.4	27	26	5.1
Sodium (mg)**	326	321	65.5	338	332	70.0	335	332	64.5
Chloride (mg)**	491	480	97.6	507	499	103.8	504	503	99.8
Potassium (mg)	289	287	47.0	304	301	53.9	301	299	51.8
Zinc (mg)	0.84	0.83	0.171	0.94	0.90	0.257	0.89	0.86	0.218
Copper (mg)	0.11	0.10	0.025	0.11	0.11	0.026	0.11	0.11	0.031
Iodine (μg)	21	19	7.9	21	19	7.6	21	19	7.0
Manganese (mg)	0.28	0.26	0.085	0.28	0.26	0.088	0.28	0.26	0.092
Base		528			169			157	
Females									
Total iron (mg)	1.25	1.21	0.298	1.24	1.20	0.288	1.29	1.20	0.346
Haem iron (mg)	0.05	0.04	0.027	0.05	0.05	0.036	0.05	0.04	0.035
Non-haem iron (mg)	1.21	1.16	0.299	1.18	1.14	0.285	1.24	1.15	0.347
Calcium (mg)	100	98	28.0	96	91	31.4	96	96	21.7
Phosphorus (mg)	138	136	22.6	140	139	23.2	138	137	19.5
Magnesium (mg)	27	26	4.5	27	27	4.9	27	26	5.0
Sodium (mg)**	322	319	58.1	333	330	65.1	331	328	69.3
Chloride (mg)**	484	477	84.9	502	504	97.6	497	488	103.5
Potassium (mg)	305	299	54.7	310	306	50.9	306	306	52.8
Zinc (mg)	0.85	0.83	0.164	0.88	0.86	0.203	0.85	0.82	0.175
Copper (mg)	0.11	0.10	0.026	0.11	0.11	0.024	0.12	0.11	0.030
Iodine (μg)	21	19	9.0	19	17	8.7	20	19	6.7
Manganese (mg)	0.28	0.26	0.090	0.29	0.27	0.102	0.28	0.26	0.094
Base		498			173			167	

*Excludes nine young people who were living with others, not parents.
**Includes intakes from food only; excludes further additions of salt in cooking or at the table.

Table 9.53 Comparison of average daily intake of total iron and calcium from food sources by young people aged between 10 and 15 years in two surveys: 1983 The Diets of British Schoolchildren; 1997 NDNS young people aged 4 to 18 years (present survey)

Mineral	Sex and age of young person							
	1983*		1997		1983*		1997	
	10–11		10–11		14–15		14–15	
	Males	Females	Males	Females	Males	Females	Males	Females
Total iron (mg)								
mean	10.0	8.6	10.3	8.5	12.2	9.3	12.0	8.6
median	9.7	8.4	10.3	8.2	11.8	9.0	11.5	8.0
sd	2.3	1.9	2.7	2.2	3.3	2.5	3.9	2.9
Calcium (mg)								
mean	833	702	790	659	925	692	869	645
median	803	672	773	649	884	671	835	656
sd	253	217	270	214	303	223	306	219
Base	902	821	140	118	513	461	110	113

* Department of Health. Report on Health and Social Subjects: 36. *The Diets of British Schoolchildren*. HMSO (London, 1989)

Table 9.54 Comparison of mineral intakes from food sources by young people in three surveys: 1992/3 NDNS: children aged 1½ to 4½ years; 1986/7 British Adults*; 1997 NDNS young people aged 4 to 18 years (present survey)

Mineral	Age and sex of young person							
	1992/3: 3½–4½**		1997: 4–6		1986/7: 16–24***		1997: 15–18	
	Males	Females	Males	Females	Males	Females	Males	Females
Total iron (mg)								
mean	6.1	5.6	8.2	7.3	12.6	9.8	12.5	8.7
median	5.9	5.5	7.9	7.1	12.4	9.1	11.6	8.0
se/sd****	0.11	0.10	2.47	2.08	0.29	0.28	4.09	3.21
Calcium (mg)								
mean	625	595	706	657	894	675	878	653
median	598	584	666	635	858	656	850	631
se/sd****	14.3	13.6	256.8	219.9	23.1	19.4	298.2	242.4
Phosphorus (mg)								
mean	767	736	919	848	1382	986	1330	959
median	750	711	901	829	1360	943	1310	955
se/sd****	13.4	13.3	250.8	215.3	28.2	21.5	345.1	273.4
Magnesium (mg)								
mean	146	137	172	155	304	215	256	191
median	141	134	170	145	298	208	254	189
se/sd****	2.4	2.3	46.0	39.9	6.8	5.2	72.2	57.5
Sodium (mg)*****								
mean	1658	1632	2069	1857	3432	2334	3265	2281
median	1645	1508	2000	1831	3430	2291	3171	2276
se/sd****	28.6	31.9	536.4	454.3	78.2	49.1	895.7	632.3
Chloride (mg)*****								
mean	2464	2436	3105	2787	5245	3572	4938	3465
median	2444	2287	2971	2749	5252	3497	4725	3508
se/sd****	42.8	47.0	798.5	676.5	115.4	74.0	1372.5	939.6
Potassium (mg)								
mean	1573	1501	1944	1774	3018	2259	2833.0	2162
median	1531	1459	1889	1661	3006	2228	2775	2148
se/sd****	26.6	25.3	502.9	458.9	60	45	820	592
Zinc(mg)								
mean	4.7	4.4	5.5	4.9	10.7	7.6	8.7	6.1
median	4.6	4.2	5.3	4.8	10.4	7.5	8.5	5.9
se/sd****	0.09	0.09	1.70	1.32	0.24	0.16	2.67	2.02
Copper(mg)								
mean	0.5	0.5	0.70	0.64	1.40	1.09	1.06	0.80
median	0.5	0.5	0.66	0.60	1.37	1.01	1.00	0.75
se/sd****	0.01	0.01	0.238	0.213	0.03	0.04	0.344	0.282
Iodine (µg)								
mean	121	113	156	143	225	158	181	135
median	111	102	144	133	217	144	168	126
se/sd****	3.6	3.6	72.9	66.3	6.6	4.6	73.6	71.4
Manganese (mg)								
mean	1.4	1.3	1.78	1.56	n/a	n/a	2.62	2.04
median	1.3	1.1	1.68	1.44	n/a	n/a	2.40	1.92
se/sd****	0.03	0.03	0.623	0.599	n/a	n/a	0.955	0.869
Base — number of young people	250	243	184	171	214	189	179	210

* Intakes of phosphorus, magnesium, sodium, chloride, potassium and zinc reported for 1986/87 survey as average daily intakes from *all* sources.
** Gregory JR et al. *National Diet and Nutrition Survey: children aged 1½ to 4½ years.* HMSO (London, 1995)
*** Gregory J et al. *The Dietary and Nutritional Survey of British Adults* HMSO (London, 1990)
**** 1992/3 and 1986/7 surveys reported standard errors; present survey reports standard deviations
*****Intakes from food only; excludes further additions of salt in cooking or at the table.
n/a not available

Table 9.55 Mean concentration of urine analytes by sex and age of young person

Sex of young person and urine analytes	Age of young person (years)																			
	4–6				7–10				11–14				15–18				All			
	Mean	Median	Std Dev	Base	Mean	Median	Std Dev	Base	Mean	Median	Std Dev	Base	Mean	Median	Std Dev	Base	Mean	Median	Std Dev	Base
Males																				
Urinary sodium (mmol/l)	149.7	149.1	59.92	199	149.7	150.9	56.93	271	154.6	156.5	63.45	259	134.4	133.7	54.11	202	147.1	147.7	59.12	931
Urinary potassium (mmol/l)	55.0	47.9	32.54	199	50.8	41.5	31.57	271	47.3	41.4	27.36	259	48.2	37.0	33.63	202	50.1	41.5	31.40	931
Urinary creatinine (mmol/l)	9.5	8.5	4.61	199	10.9	10.1	4.25	271	13.1	12.8	5.07	259	17.4	15.9	7.67	202	12.8	11.7	6.31	931
Urinary sodium: creatinine ratio (mol/mol)	18.9	16.7	12.92	199	15.3	14.1	7.55	271	13.5	12.1	8.67	259	9.2	7.7	5.70	202	14.0	12.2	9.48	931
Urinary potassium: urinary creatinine ratio (mol/mol)	7.1	5.4	5.75	199	5.3	4.1	4.02	271	4.1	3.2	3.19	259	3.0	2.3	2.23	202	4.8	3.5	4.16	931
Urinary sodium: urinary potassium ratio (mol/mol)	3.7	3.1	2.49	199	4.0	3.3	2.59	271	4.1	3.6	2.35	259	4.0	3.4	2.64	202	4.0	3.4	2.53	931
Females																				
Urinary sodium (mmol/l)	144.4	142.6	57.77	181	147.6	149.0	57.94	243	144.9	139.3	56.61	245	138.5	135.7	58.01	229	143.9	141.5	57.66	898
Urinary potassium (mmol/l)	52.1	43.7	33.17	181	49.6	42.9	30.68	243	43.4	38.5	26.46	245	45.8	36.5	29.47	229	47.5	39.9	30.03	898
Urinary creatinine (mmol/l)	8.8	8.2	3.71	181	10.9	10.6	4.69	243	13.1	12.7	5.41	245	14.1	13.2	5.99	229	11.9	10.9	5.45	898
Urinary sodium: creatinine ratio (mol/mol)	19.1	17.1	10.89	181	15.6	13.7	8.13	243	12.4	11.4	5.90	245	11.4	10.5	6.36	229	14.4	12.8	8.38	898
Urinary potassium: urinary creatinine ratio (mol/mol)	7.1	5.4	6.27	181	5.2	4.0	3.55	243	3.5	3.0	2.22	245	3.7	2.8	2.79	229	4.8	3.5	4.09	898
Urinary sodium: urinary potassium ratio (mol/mol)	3.7	3.1	2.36	181	3.8	3.5	2.15	243	4.3	3.7	2.67	245	3.8	3.5	2.27	229	3.9	3.4	2.38	898

327

Table 9.56　Percentage distribution of urinary sodium: urinary creatinine ratio by sex and age of young person

Urinary sodium: urinary creatinine ratio (mol/mol)	Males aged (years)					Females aged (years)				
	4–6	7–10	11–14	15–18	All males	4–6	7–10	11–14	15–18	All females
	cum %	cum %	cum %	cum %	cum %	cum %	cum %	cum %	cum %	cum %
Less than 5.0	3	3	8	20	9	4	6	4	13	7
Less than 7.5	10	13	19	48	23	11	13	22	31	20
Less than 10.0	18	22	34	70	37	18	26	40	48	34
Less than 12.5	30	41	54	80	52	31	39	55	65	48
Less than 15.0	43	55	70	87	65	42	55	70	77	62
Less than 20.0	65	78	86	93	81	61	79	92	90	81
All	100	100	100	100	100	100	100	100	100	100
Base	*199*	*271*	*259*	*202*	*931*	*181*	*243*	*245*	*229*	*898*
Mean	18.9	15.3	13.5	9.2	14.0	19.1	15.6	12.4	11.4	14.4
Median	16.7	14.1	12.1	7.6	12.2	17.1	13.7	11.4	10.5	12.8
Lower 2.5 percentile	4.4	4.5	3.3	2.1	3.0	4.5	4.4	3.7	3.1	3.6
Upper 2.5 percentile	44.6	38.3	30.9	25.7	37.2	50.6	36.9	26.8	28.7	37.6
Standard deviation	12.92	7.55	8.67	5.70	9.48	10.89	8.13	5.90	6.36	8.38

Table 9.57　Percentage distribution of urinary potassium: urinary creatinine ratio by sex and age of young person

Urinary potassium: urinary creatinine ratio (mol/mol)	Males aged (years)					Females aged (years)				
	4–6	7–10	11–14	15–18	All males	4–6	7–10	11–14	15–18	All females
	cum %	cum %	cum %	cum %	cum %	cum %	cum %	cum %	cum %	cum %
Less than 2.0	6	11	18	41	20	6	12	22	21	16
Less than 3.0	21	32	45	67	42	20	29	50	56	40
Less than 4.0	34	48	66	77	57	31	50	68	72	57
Less than 5.0	46	64	78	87	70	47	61	82	81	69
Less than 8.0	71	84	91	95	86	77	84	97	93	88
All	100	100	100	100	100	100	100	100	100	100
Base	*199*	*271*	*259*	*202*	*931*	*181*	*243*	*245*	*229*	*898*
Mean	7.1	5.3	4.1	3.0	4.8	7.1	5.2	3.5	3.7	4.8
Median	5.4	4.1	3.2	2.3	3.5	5.4	4.0	3.0	2.8	3.5
Lower 2.5 percentile	1.4	1.5	1.2	0.8	1.1	1.8	1.4	1.4	1.0	1.3
Upper 2.5 percentile	25.4	16.2	13.5	10.5	16.6	26.7	15.1	9.4	12.6	17.1
Standard deviation	5.75	4.02	3.19	2.23	4.16	6.27	3.55	2.22	2.79	4.09

Table 9.58　Percentage distribution of urinary sodium: urinary potassium ratio by sex and age of young person

Urinary sodium: urinary potassium ratio (mol/mol)	Males aged (years)					Females aged (years)				
	4–6	7–10	11–14	15–18	All males	4–6	7–10	11–14	15–18	All females
	cum %	cum %	cum %	cum %	cum %	cum %	cum %	cum %	cum %	cum %
Less than 1.0	9	5	3	9	6	7	5	2	5	5
Less than 2.0	29	23	16	22	22	23	20	14	21	19
Less than 3.0	48	44	37	41	42	47	41	34	42	41
Less than 4.0	62	59	58	62	60	63	59	56	62	60
Less than 6.0	84	82	83	83	83	84	86	80	84	84
All	100	100	100	100	100	100	100	100	100	100
Base	*199*	*271*	*259*	*202*	*931*	*181*	*243*	*245*	*229*	*898*
Mean	3.7	4.0	4.1	4.0	3.9	3.7	3.8	4.3	3.8	3.9
Median	3.1	3.3	3.6	3.4	3.4	3.1	3.5	3.7	3.5	3.4
Lower 2.5 percentile	0.6	0.8	0.9	0.6	0.7	0.7	0.7	0.9	0.9	0.8
Upper 2.5 percentile	9.4	9.9	9.2	10.9	10.1	9.6	9.4	11.9	9.4	9.9
Standard deviation	2.49	2.59	2.35	2.64	2.53	2.36	2.15	2.67	2.27	2.38

Table 9.59 Correlation coefficients between urinary sodium to urinary creatinine ratio and dietary intake of sodium†

Sex and age of young person	Correlation coefficient	Number of young people
Males aged (years)		
4–6	0.14	180
7–10	0.28**	249
11–14	−0.01	232
15–18	0.02	168
All males	−0.10**	829
Females aged (years)		
4–6	0.20**	161
7–10	0.12	219
11–14	0.09	221
15–18	0.11	207
All females	0.01	808

† Dietary intake of sodium excludes additions of salt in cooking or at the table.
** p < 0.01

Table 9.60 Correlation coefficients between urinary potassium to urinary creatinine ratio and dietary intake of potassium

Sex and age of young person	Correlation coefficient	Number of young people
Males aged (years)		
4–6	0.16*	180
7–10	0.23**	249
11–14	0.04	232
15–18	−0.01	168
All males	−0.07	829
Females aged (years)		
4–6	0.22**	161
7–10	0.10	219
11–14	0.07	221
15–18	0.01	207
All females	0.00	808

** p < 0.01
* p < 0.05

Table 9.61 Correlation coefficients between urinary sodium to urinary potassium ratio and sodium to potassium ratio for dietary intakes†

Sex and age of young person	Correlation coefficient	Number of young people
Males aged (years)		
4–6	0.40**	180
7–10	0.46**	249
11–14	0.24**	232
15–18	0.09	168
All males	0.28**	829
Females aged (years)		
4–6	0.28**	161
7–10	0.18**	219
11–14	0.15*	221
15–18	0.21**	207
All females	0.20**	808

† Dietary intake of sodium excludes additions of salt in cooking or at the table.
* p < 0.05
** p < 0.01

Table 9.62 Correlation coefficients between urinary sodium to urinary creatinine ratio and body mass index

Sex and age of young person	Correlation coefficient	Number of young people
Males aged (years)		
4–6	−0.08	199
7–10	−0.04	269
11–14	−0.09	258
15–18	0.08	201
All males	−0.22**	927
Females aged (years)		
4–6	−0.07	180
7–10	−0.08	241
11–14	0.02	243
15–18	0.18**	227
All females	−0.18**	891

** p < 0.01

Table 9.63 Correlation coefficients between urinary potassium to urinary creatinine ratio and body mass index

Sex and age of young person	Correlation coefficient	Number of young people
Males aged (years)		
4–6	−0.03	199
7–10	−0.05	269
11–14	−0.03	258
15–18	−0.05	201
All males	−0.22**	927
Females aged (years)		
4–6	0.03	180
7–10	−0.03	241
11–14	−0.12	243
15–18	0.00	227
All females	−0.19**	891

** p < 0.01

Table 9.64 Correlation coefficients between urinary sodium to urinary potassium ratio and body mass index

Sex and age of young person	Correlation coefficient	Number of young people
Males aged (years)		
4–6	−0.02	199
7–10	0.04	269
11–14	−0.06	258
15–18	0.10	201
All males	0.04	927
Females aged (years)		
4–6	−0.07	180
7–10	−0.01	241
11–14	0.08	243
15–18	0.23**	227
All females	0.09**	891

** p < 0.01

Table 9.65 Mean concentration of urine analytes by sex of young person and whether unwell during the dietary recording period

Sex of young person and urine analytes	Whether unwell during period												All			
	Unwell and eating affected				Unwell and eating not affected				Not unwell							
	Mean	Median	Std Dev	Base	Mean	Median	Std Dev	Base	Mean	Median	Std Dev	Base	Mean	Median	Std Dev	Base
Males																
Urinary sodium (mmol/l)	141.4	139.8	56.31	87	157.0	158.3	60.97	113	146.2	147.4	59.01	742	147.1	147.7	59.12	942
Urinary potassium (mmol/l)	49.7	40.9	33.07	87	53.0	45.4	32.49	113	49.7	41.4	31.03	742	50.1	41.5	31.40	942
Urinary creatinine (mmol/l)	12.3	11.6	6.22	87	13.2	12.3	5.60	113	12.8	11.8	6.41	742	12.8	11.7	6.31	942
Urinary sodium: creatinine ratio (mol/mol)	14.7	13.0	11.44	87	13.8	13.5	7.17	113	14.0	12.0	9.54	742	14.0	12.2	9.48	942
Urinary potassium: urinary creatinine ratio (mol/mol)	4.8	3.7	4.00	87	4.6	3.4	3.44	113	4.8	3.5	4.28	742	4.8	3.5	4.16	942
Urinary sodium: urinary potassium ratio (mol/mol)	3.9	3.3	2.39	87	4.1	3.4	2.77	113	3.9	3.4	2.50	742	3.9	3.4	2.53	942
Females																
Urinary sodium (mmol/l)	138.5	139.5	62.82	96	142.3	140.9	58.68	119	144.8	142.1	56.74	694	143.9	141.5	57.66	909
Urinary potassium (mmol/l)	50.8	43.9	31.31	96	45.0	37.4	27.43	119	47.5	39.9	30.25	694	47.5	39.9	30.03	909
Urinary creatinine (mmol/l)	12.7	11.7	6.10	96	12.2	11.5	5.08	119	11.7	10.8	5.40	694	11.9	10.9	5.45	909
Urinary sodium: creatinine ratio (mol/mol)	13.6	12.0	9.47	96	13.5	12.4	7.34	119	14.7	13.0	8.37	694	14.4	12.8	8.38	909
Urinary potassium: urinary creatinine ratio (mol/mol)	4.9	3.5	3.98	96	4.3	3.2	3.56	119	4.8	3.7	4.18	694	4.8	3.5	4.09	909
Urinary sodium: urinary potassium ratio (mol/mol)	3.4	3.0	2.09	96	4.1	3.3	2.64	119	4.0	3.5	2.36	694	3.9	3.4	2.38	909

Table 9.66 Mean concentration of urine analytes by sex of young person and region

Sex of young person and urine analytes	Region Scotland Mean	Median	Std Dev	Base	Northern Mean	Median	Std Dev	Base	Central, South West & Wales Mean	Median	Std Dev	Base	London & South East Mean	Median	Std Dev	Base	All Mean	Median	Std Dev	Base
Males																				
Urinary sodium (mmol/l)	160.7	165.3	60.33	74	148.6	147.4	55.44	256	145.6	147.9	59.64	329	143.7	139.5	61.03	283	147.1	147.7	59.12	942
Urinary potassium (mmol/l)	52.1	43.6	33.70	74	49.0	41.0	30.92	256	48.7	42.7	27.28	329	52.4	40.8	35.55	283	50.1	41.5	31.40	942
Urinary creatinine (mmol/l)	12.0	11.1	6.34	74	13.2	12.5	6.00	256	13.1	11.7	6.73	329	12.4	11.5	6.01	283	12.8	11.7	6.31	942
Urinary sodium: creatinine ratio (mol/mol)	18.1*	14.5	17.20	74	13.4	12.2	7.66	256	13.7	11.9	8.25	329	13.9	12.4	9.19	283	14.0	12.2	9.48	942
Urinary potassium: urinary creatinine ratio (mol/mol)	6.0	3.6	5.56	74	4.4	3.1	4.00	256	4.4	3.5	2.93	329	5.2	3.7	4.97	283	4.8	3.5	4.16	942
Urinary sodium: urinary potassium ratio (mol/mol)	4.4	3.6	3.16	74	4.2	3.6	2.64	256	3.9	3.4	2.45	329	3.7	3.3	2.27	283	3.9	3.4	2.53	942
Females																				
Urinary sodium (mmol/l)	151.9	158.9	64.03	72	133.8	125.5	56.99	239	150.4	149.0	59.36	328	143.0	144.0	52.76	270	143.9	141.5	57.66	909
Urinary potassium (mmol/l)	44.1	37.8	25.51	72	49.1	39.9	34.69	239	47.2	41.2	27.64	328	47.3	38.8	29.25	270	47.5	39.9	30.03	909
Urinary creatinine (mmol/l)	14.0	12.7	6.78	72	11.8	11.2	5.59	239	11.4	10.5	4.98	328	11.8	11.0	5.31	270	11.9	10.9	5.45	909
Urinary sodium: creatinine ratio (mol/mol)	12.9	10.6	7.42	72	13.9	12.2	8.74	239	15.1	13.6	8.44	328	14.4	12.5	8.12	270	14.4	12.8	8.38	909
Urinary potassium: urinary creatinine ratio (mol/mol)	3.6	3.0	2.03	72	4.9	3.5	4.14	239	4.9	3.8	4.67	328	4.7	3.6	3.65	270	4.8	3.5	4.09	909
Urinary sodium: urinary potassium ratio (mol/mol)	4.3	3.6	2.42	72	3.8	3.2	2.74	239	4.1	3.7	2.38	328	3.7	3.4	1.95	270	3.9	3.4	2.38	909

331

Table 9.67 Mean concentration of urine analytes by sex of young person and social class of head of household

Sex of young person and urine analytes	Social class of head of household											
	Non-manual				Manual				All*			
	Mean	Median	Std Dev	Base	Mean	Median	Std Dev	Base	Mean	Median	Std Dev	Base
Males												
Urinary sodium (mmol/l)	138.6	134.1	58.55	440	153.8	154.7	59.39	431	147.1	147.7	59.12	942
Urinary potassium (mmol/l)	48.8	41.0	31.45	440	51.8	42.1	31.74	431	50.1	41.5	31.40	942
Urinary creatinine (mmol/l)	12.6	11.6	5.84	440	13.1	12.0	6.53	431	12.8	11.7	6.31	942
Urinary sodium: creatinine ratio (mol/mol)	13.5	11.4	10.52	440	14.3	12.6	8.20	431	14.0	12.2	9.48	942
Urinary potassium: urinary creatinine ratio (mol/mol)	4.7	3.4	4.28	440	4.8	3.6	4.14	431	4.8	3.5	4.16	942
Urinary sodium: urinary potassium ratio (mol/mol)	3.9	3.2	2.68	440	3.9	3.5	2.36	431	3.9	3.4	2.53	942
Females												
Urinary sodium (mmol/l)	139.7	138.2	55.72	418	146.0	143.8	58.97	398	143.9	141.5	57.66	909
Urinary potassium (mmol/l)	48.0	39.8	30.14	418	45.8	40.0	27.65	398	47.5	39.9	30.03	909
Urinary creatinine (mmol/l)	11.5	10.5	5.33	418	11.9	11.1	5.43	398	11.9	10.9	5.45	909
Urinary sodium: creatinine ratio (mol/mol)	14.4	12.8	8.60	418	14.4	13.0	7.95	398	14.4	12.8	8.38	909
Urinary potassium: urinary creatinine ratio (mol/mol)	5.0	3.6	4.45	418	4.5	3.5	3.79	398	4.8	3.5	4.09	909
Urinary sodium: urinary potassium ratio (mol/mol)	3.7	3.4	2.15	418	4.1	3.5	2.52	398	3.9	3.4	2.38	909

* Includes those for whom a social class could not be assigned.

Table 9.68 Mean concentration of urine analytes by sex of young person and whether 'parents' were receiving certain benefits

Sex of young person and urine analytes	Whether 'parents' were receiving benefits											
	Receiving benefits				Not receiving benefits				All			
	Mean	Median	Std Dev	Base	Mean	Median	Std Dev	Base	Mean	Median	Std Dev	Base
Males												
Urinary sodium (mmol/l)	157.0	163.2	61.25	220	143.5	140.4	58.01	721	147.1	147.7	59.12	942
Urinary potassium (mmol/l)	52.8	47.0	30.50	220	49.2	40.8	31.69	721	50.1	41.5	31.40	942
Urinary creatinine (mmol/l)	12.7	11.5	6.69	220	12.9	11.9	6.17	721	12.8	11.7	6.31	942
Urinary sodium: creatinine ratio (mol/mol)	15.6	13.7	9.69	220	13.5	12.0	9.35	721	14.0	12.2	9.48	942
Urinary potassium: urinary creatinine ratio (mol/mol)	5.3	3.9	4.58	220	4.6	3.3	3.99	721	4.8	3.5	4.16	942
Urinary sodium: urinary potassium ratio (mol/mol)	4.0	3.4	2.72	220	3.9	3.4	2.46	721	3.9	3.4	2.53	942
Females												
Urinary sodium (mmol/l)	147.0	149.0	56.09	225	142.4	139.0	58.13	683	143.9	141.5	57.66	909
Urinary potassium (mmol/l)	48.0	38.6	33.30	225	47.3	40.3	28.75	683	47.5	39.9	30.03	909
Urinary creatinine (mmol/l)	11.6	11.3	5.63	225	12.0	10.8	5.38	683	11.9	10.9	5.45	909
Urinary sodium: creatinine ratio (mol/mol)	15.8	14.1	9.60	225	13.9	12.3	7.81	683	14.4	12.8	8.38	909
Urinary potassium: urinary creatinine ratio (mol/mol)	5.2	3.7	5.44	225	4.6	3.5	3.44	683	4.8	3.5	4.09	909
Urinary sodium: urinary potassium ratio (mol/mol)	4.1	3.6	2.56	225	3.8	3.4	2.31	683	3.9	3.4	2.38	909

Table 9.69 Mean concentration of urine analytes by sex of young person and gross weekly household income

Sex of young person and urine analytes	Gross weekly household income																								All*			
	Less than £160				£160 to less than £280				£280 to less than £400				£400 to less than £600				£600 and over											
	Mean	Median	Std Dev	Base	Mean	Median	Std Dev	Base	Mean	Median	Std Dev	Base	Mean	Median	Std Dev	Base	Mean	Median	Std Dev	Base	Mean	Median	Std Dev	Base	Mean	Median	Std Dev	Base
Males																												
Urinary sodium (mmol/l)	157.0	164.1	58.45	148	154.7	151.1	65.24	171	146.0	149.3	55.27	178	145.6	143.3	59.54	185	133.2	128.2	53.27	226	147.1	147.7	59.12	942				
Urinary potassium (mmol/l)	51.7	48.1	26.86	148	49.0	41.2	28.94	171	51.0	41.1	32.25	178	49.0	40.8	31.47	185	50.4	40.2	35.39	226	50.1	41.5	31.40	942				
Urinary creatinine (mmol/l)	12.2	10.7	6.37	148	13.4	12.0	7.59	171	12.3	11.3	5.72	178	12.8	12.1	5.47	185	13.0	11.7	6.07	226	12.8	11.7	6.31	942				
Urinary sodium: creatinine ratio (mol/mol)	16.5	14.4	10.36	148	14.6	12.9	8.89	171	13.9	12.4	7.27	178	13.5	11.1	11.72	185	12.7	11.3	8.90	226	14.0	12.2	9.48	942				
Urinary potassium: urinary creatinine ratio (mol/mol)	5.4	4.1	4.78	148	4.5	3.6	3.81	171	4.9	3.6	3.81	178	4.5	3.5	3.72	185	4.8	3.1	4.67	226	4.8	3.5	4.16	942				
Urinary sodium: urinary potassium ratio (mol/mol)	3.9	3.4	2.45	148	4.1	3.6	2.67	171	3.9	3.4	2.59	178	4.0	3.6	2.42	185	3.7	3.2	2.41	226	3.9	3.4	2.53	942				
Females																												
Urinary sodium (mmol/l)	146.2	145.9	57.93	149	151.6	157.5	59.92	160	151.3	150.3	56.10	151	141.3	137.5	58.28	208	131.1	130.5	53.61	203	143.9	141.5	57.66	909				
Urinary potassium (mmol/l)	49.7	38.0	34.86	149	46.6	40.2	27.74	160	49.2	40.8	33.33	151	47.0	39.3	29.39	208	46.1	40.7	25.44	203	47.5	39.9	30.03	909				
Urinary creatinine (mmol/l)	11.9	11.7	5.23	149	11.5	10.6	5.81	160	11.6	10.9	4.89	151	11.7	10.5	5.35	208	12.5	11.1	5.82	203	11.9	10.9	5.45	909				
Urinary sodium: creatinine ratio (mol/mol)	14.6	12.9	8.81	149	16.2	14.0	10.04	160	14.6	13.6	6.67	151	14.1	12.1	8.29	208	12.6	11.2	7.34	203	14.4	12.8	8.38	909				
Urinary potassium: urinary creatinine ratio (mol/mol)	4.8	3.8	4.35	149	5.4	3.5	5.56	160	4.7	3.7	3.55	151	4.8	3.3	3.86	208	4.3	3.5	2.89	203	4.8	3.5	4.09	909				
Urinary sodium: urinary potassium ratio (mol/mol)	4.0	3.5	2.37	149	4.3	3.6	2.85	160	4.1	3.8	2.45	151	3.8	3.3	2.18	208	3.5	3.2	1.99	203	3.9	3.4	2.38	909				

* Includes those not answering income question.

Table 9.70 Mean concentration of urine analytes by sex of young person and whether living with both parents

Sex of young person and urine analytes	Living with: both parents and other children				no other children				single parent with/out other children				All*			
	Mean	Median	Std Dev	Base	Mean	Median	Std Dev	Base	Mean	Median	Std Dev	Base	Mean	Median	Std Dev	Base
Males																
Urinary sodium (mmol/l)	148.9	149.6	58.88	574	138.0	138.6	58.86	181	150.9	150.5	59.46	183	147.1	147.7	59.12	942
Urinary potassium (mmol/l)	51.0	41.8	31.89	574	49.2	40.4	32.47	181	48.4	43.1	28.74	183	50.1	41.5	31.40	942
Urinary creatinine (mmol/l)	12.3	11.5	5.89	574	14.7	13.0	6.94	181	12.7	11.4	6.59	183	12.8	11.7	6.31	942
Urinary sodium: creatinine ratio (mol/mol)	14.7	13.0	10.10	574	11.1	9.7	6.47	181	15.0	12.4	9.33	183	14.0	12.2	9.48	942
Urinary potassium: urinary creatinine ratio (mol/mol)	5.1	3.7	4.52	574	3.7	2.9	2.60	181	4.8	3.4	4.04	183	4.8	3.5	4.16	942
Urinary sodium: urinary potassium ratio (mol/mol)	3.9	3.5	2.59	574	3.7	3.3	2.20	181	4.1	3.7	2.63	183	3.9	3.4	2.53	942
Females																
Urinary sodium (mmol/l)	142.9	139.6	55.37	532	139.4	131.4	61.16	179	150.8	158.9	60.02	189	143.9	141.5	57.66	909
Urinary potassium (mmol/l)	48.3	41.1	30.80	532	44.3	38.4	27.05	179	47.9	38.7	30.06	189	47.5	39.9	30.03	909
Urinary creatinine (mmol/l)	11.3	10.5	5.06	532	13.2	11.7	5.97	179	12.3	11.9	5.78	189	11.9	10.9	5.45	909
Urinary sodium: creatinine ratio (mol/mol)	14.8	13.1	8.23	532	12.2	10.9	6.80	179	15.1	13.4	9.66	189	14.4	12.8	8.38	909
Urinary potassium: urinary creatinine ratio (mol/mol)	5.0	3.7	3.86	532	3.7	3.1	2.54	179	5.1	3.4	5.44	189	4.8	3.5	4.09	909
Urinary sodium: urinary potassium ratio (mol/mol)	3.9	3.3	2.42	532	3.9	3.5	2.28	179	4.0	3.7	2.32	189	3.9	2.4	3.04	909

* Includes 13 young people (unweighted). four boys and nine girls, who were living with others, not parents.

10 Anthropometry

10.1 Introduction

This chapter presents anthropometric data on the height, weight and mid upper-arm circumference (MUAC) of young people aged 4 to 18 years and on the waist and hip circumferences of young people aged 11 to 18 years. Data are also presented on the derived measures of body mass index (BMI) and waist to hip ratio. Descriptive statistics are presented for boys and girls separately by age group and individual year of age. Both bivariate and multivariate analyses are presented showing the relationship between variations in the anthropometric measurements and various socio-demographic, behavioural and dietary factors.

Data from the 1995-97 Health Survey for England[1] and the 1994 National Study of Health and Growth (NSHG)[2] are presented for comparison. Data from the Health Survey are available on height, weight and BMI for young people aged 4 to 18 years and on mid upper-arm circumference for young people aged 4 to 15 years. Data from the NSHG are available on height, weight and BMI for young people aged 5 to 10 years.

The rationale for each of the anthropometric measurements and the equipment and methodologies used are described in Chapter 3 together with the response rate for each measurement. Further information, including the protocol for each measurement, is given in Appendix L.

Not all of the young people co-operated with every measurement. The bases shown in the tables of results for this chapter therefore vary between measurements. The number of cases for which individual measurements were missing was small enough that it was possible to use a single set of non-response weights for all of the measurements[3].

Data are presented for young people by individual year of age and by age group. For the purpose of these analyses age was calculated by subtracting the young person's date of birth from the date when each measurement was made. There was no requirement for all of the anthropometric measurements to be made at the same visit. Some young people may therefore be classified in different age groups for different measurements as well as being classified in different age groups for the measurements than for other stages of the survey.

The interviewers were asked to attempt each measurement twice. In the analysis, the mean of the two measurements was taken. Not all participants co-operated with both measurements. In the small number of cases where only one measurement was recorded, this measurement was used in the analysis.

The interviewers were asked to record any special circumstances encountered when taking the measurement, for example if the young person was unco-operative or would not stand still while the measurement was made. In addition, consistency checks were made within the data for each measurement. Where a measurement lay at either extreme of the distribution, all of the anthropometric measurements for the individual were scrutinised for inconsistency. Measurements that were considered unreliable were excluded from the analysis.

10.2 Anthropometric measurements for young people in the UK

Anthropometric data are widely used to estimate the nutritional status of children. The height and weight of a child are useful indices of development, reflecting the various influences on growth, including nutrition. Indeed, the monitoring of a child's increase in height and weight by age using growth charts is widely used to identify failure to thrive. The UK reference curves of stature, weight and BMI for children from birth to 20 years were revised in 1995 using data collected between 1978 and 1990[4,5].

10.2.1 The relationship between age and anthropometric measurements in young people

A particular problem in presenting and interpreting data on anthropometric measurements in young people is that, being at a developmental stage of relatively rapid growth, they vary with age. When considering variations in anthropometric measurements the effect of age must therefore be considered.

Descriptive data are presented for boys and girls separately by age group and individual year of age. Correlation coefficients are presented by sex and age group as well as for all boys and all girls aged 4 to 18 years. Multiple regression methods allow for the effect of age to be controlled, independent of other effects and associations. However, in interpreting the tables that show variations in measurements for all boys and all girls aged 4 to 18 years, where no standardisation has been applied, the correlation between age and each measurement should be remembered.

10.2.2 The relationship between stage of sexual development and anthropometric measurements in young people

This section describes how the information on stage of sexual development was collected. Tables 10.1 to 10.3 show descriptive statistics for stage of sexual development for boys and girls.

Although young people grow rapidly, the onset of puberty means that there is a close association between stage of sexual development and body shape and size, with both sexes undergoing an adolescent growth spurt and accompanying changes in body dimensions. Previous studies have shown that growth is steady for young people from the age of 2 years to the onset of puberty, at which time there is an increase in growth velocity. For boys, the onset of this growth spurt begins when they are on average two years older than girls and results in a greater achieved height[4,6].

As part of the self-completion section, girls aged 10 to 18 years were asked whether they had started menstruating and, if they had, the age at which they started menstruating. For boys aged 10 to 16 years plasma testosterone concentration was measured to establish whether they were pre- or post-pubertal.

Table 10.1 shows that mean plasma testosterone concentration increased significantly with age for boys aged 10 to 16 years (differences between boys aged 10 years and those aged 12 to 16 years all: $p < 0.01$)[7]. Table 10.2 shows tertiles of plasma testosterone concentration by individual year of age for boys aged 10 to 16 years[8] and shows that, as would be expected, a greater proportion of boys at younger individual years of age had a plasma testosterone concentration in the bottom tertile compared with older boys, and that a greater proportion of boys at older individual years of age had a plasma testosterone concentration in the top tertile compared with younger boys. For example 85% of those in the bottom tertile were aged 10 or 11 years and 71% of those in the top tertile were aged 14 to 16 years.

Table 10.3 shows that menarché was reported to have occurred for 4% of girls aged 10 years, 62% of girls aged 13 years and all girls aged 18 years. Among girls aged 18 years the median age at menarché was 13.0 years.

In girls, puberty is defined as precocious if the onset is before the age of 8 years and is regarded as delayed if there are no signs of puberty by the age of 13 years or menarché has not occurred by the age of 16½ years[6]. In this present Survey only girls aged 10 to 18 years were asked if menarché had occurred, none of whom reported their age at menarché being less than 8 years. However, 3% of girls aged 16½ years and over reported that menarché had not occurred (unweighted this represents 4 girls out of a total of 152 aged 16½ years and over; table not shown).

Indicators of stage of sexual development were included in the analysis looking at variation in the anthropometric measurements. For girls, the indicator was whether menarché had occurred and for boys age-specific tertiles for plasma testosterone concentration were used. The small numbers of younger girls who had reached menarché and older girls who had not did not allow for a full analysis of the relationship between the anthropometric measurements and menarché by individual year of age. However, it was possible to look at this relationship for girls aged 12 years and 13 years where there were more than 20 individuals who had started and more than 20 who had not started menstruating (see *Section 10.10.1*).

(Tables 10.1 to 10.3)

10.3 Height

All 2127 young people in the survey were eligible to have height measured. Height measurements were achieved for a total of 1949 young people; for three young people the measurements were excluded from the analyses as likely to be unreliable. These measurements were excluded due to inconsistency with other anthropometric measurements; the remaining measurements for these individuals were retained if they were consistent with each other. There were two young people for whom only one measurement of height was made.

Acceptable measures of height were obtained for 990 boys and 956 girls (unweighted). Tables 10.4 and 10.5 give descriptive statistics for height for boys and girls separately by age group and individual year of age.

The distribution of height was close to normal with the median values close to mean values. The data showed very little change in variability around the mean as age increased (see *Figures 10.1a and 10.1b*).

Mean height increased with grouped age (all: $p < 0.01$) and individual year of age for both boys and girls.

There was no significant difference in mean height between boys and girls for the three youngest age groups. However, boys aged 15 to 18 years were on average significantly taller than girls of the same age group, 175cm compared with 162cm ($p < 0.01$). Table 10.5 shows that boys were significantly taller than girls from the age of 14 years (all: $p < 0.01$).

(Tables 10.4 and 10.5; Figures 10.1a and 10.1b)

10.4 Weight

There are a number of difficulties associated with the measurement of weight, not least that it can vary for the same individual at different times of the same day. It is not easy to control for this variation within the constraints imposed by a general population household-based survey. In the context of an already onerous survey programme, it would have been unacceptable to impose a standard time of day at which the measurements should be taken.

In addition, there are problems associated with the interpretation of weight measurements, in that for adults and children they are highly correlated with height. Moreover, weight alone is not a measure of body fat, since it also includes the weight of non-fat tissue and body fluids. For further discussion of the interpretation of height and weight measurements see *Section 10.5.*

All young people who took part in the survey were eligible to be weighed. Measurements were achieved for 1946 young people, none of which was excluded. There were no cases where only one measurement was recorded. Results were available for 991 boys and 955 girls (unweighted).

Tables 10.6 and 10.7 give descriptive statistics for weight for boys and girls separately by age group and individual year of age.

The distribution of weight was positively skewed for boys and girls in all age groups. Median values were up to 7% (average 3%) lower than mean values depending on sex and individual year of age. For both boys and girls the variability of weight around the mean increased with age (see *Figures 10.2a* and *10.2b*).

Mean weight increased with both grouped age (all: $p < 0.01$) and individual year of age for both boys and girls.

The data suggest that in the youngest age group boys were heavier than girls, and that in the 7 to 14 year age group girls were heavier than boys, although neither of these differences reached the level of statistical significance. Boys aged 15 to 18 years were on average significantly heavier than girls of the same age, 68kg compared with 60kg ($p < 0.01$). Table 10.7 suggests that girls were on average heavier than boys at the ages of 7 to 9 years and 12 to 13 years, although the differences did not reach the level of statistical significance ($p > 0.05$). Boys were significantly heavier than girls from the age of 16 years (16 years and 17 years: $p < 0.05$; 18 years: $p < 0.01$).

(Tables 10.6 and 10.7; Figures 10.2a and 10.2b)

10.5 Body mass index (BMI)

Body weight and height, if considered independently, each reflect a child's size (large compared with small) at least as much as their body shape (fat compared with thin). Weight can be adjusted for height to give an indicator of body shape that is independent of height and this is used as a measure of 'fatness'. Of the various indices that standardise weight by height, the most widely used is the Quetelet or Body Mass Index (BMI). BMI is strongly correlated with the percentage of weight attributable to fat, yet much less so with height. The index is calculated as weight (kg)/height (m^2).

In adults the relationship between different levels of BMI and all cause mortality is used to define categories which identify individuals as underweight, average, overweight and obese; the category of obese is divided into classes I, II and III[9]. No data are available on the relationship between mortality risks and different levels of BMI for children. Age-independent categories can be used for adults because BMI increases fairly slowly with age whereas child BMI varies substantially with age and therefore needs to be assessed using age-specific categories.

Given the limitations of using the adult BMI classification for child BMI data and the lack of a recognised standard child BMI classification, for the purpose of presenting variations in BMI in this Report the data have been divided into age-sex specific quintiles.

Measurements of weight and height that were excluded for reasons described above were also excluded from the calculation of BMI. BMI was therefore calculated for a total of 989 boys and 953 girls (unweighted).

Tables 10.8 and 10.9 give descriptive statistics for BMI for boys and girls separately by age group and individual year of age.

The distribution of BMI was positively skewed for both boys and girls in all age groups. Median values were up to 10% (average 3%) lower than mean values depending on sex and individual year of age. The variability of BMI around the mean increased with age for both boys and girls (see *Figures 10.3a* and *10.3b*).

For both boys and girls, mean BMI increased significantly with grouped age ($p < 0.01$). Data for single-year age groups show that mean BMI was the same (16) for boys from the age of 4 to 8 years and girls from the age of 4 to 7 years. The data suggest that overall, mean BMI then increased steadily with individual year of age; however, BMI rose significantly for boys between the ages of 8 and 9, 9 and 10, and 13 and 14 years, and for girls between the ages of 11 and 12 years (all: $p < 0.05$; differences between all other consecutive individual years of age: ns).

Mean BMI was the same (16) for boys and girls in the youngest age group. The data suggest that mean BMI was lower for boys aged 7 to 18 years than for girls in the same age groups although the differences did not reach the level of statistical significance. Table 10.9 shows that mean BMI was the same for boys and girls at most individual years of age, however the data suggest that girls had a higher mean BMI than boys at the ages of 8, 9, 12, 13 and 15 to 17 years (ns).

(Tables 10.8 and 10.9; Figures 10.3a and 10.3b)

10.6 Mid upper-arm circumference

The measurement of mid upper-arm circumference (MUAC) is used as an indicator of body size and in conjunction with other measures can be used to estimate body fat as a percentage of weight.

The interviewers attempted to measure the mid upper-arm circumference of all young people who took part in the survey. Mid upper-arm circumference measurements were achieved for a total of 1944 young people; the measurements for one young person were excluded as there was a difference of more than 15% between the first and second measurement. There were two cases where only one measurement was taken. Reliable results were obtained for 985 boys and 958 girls (unweighted).

Tables 10.10 and 10.11 give descriptive statistics for MUAC for boys and girls separately by age group and individual year of age.

Mean MUAC was positively skewed for both boys and girls in all age groups and strongly so for young people aged 7 to 10 years. Median values were up to 5% (average 1%) lower than mean values depending on sex and individual year of age. The variability of MUAC around the mean increased with age for girls, while for boys, variability increased with age until 13 years, after which it decreased with age (see *Figures 10.4a and 10.4b*).

For both boys and girls mean MUAC increased significantly with grouped age between those aged 4 to 6 years and those aged 15 to 18 years (both sexes: p < 0.01). The data suggest a steady increase in mean MUAC with individual year of age for boys aged 4 to 16 years and girls aged 6 to 16 years. Differences were significant for boys between ages 4, 5 and 6, 7 and 8, 9 and 10, 11 and 12, 13 and 14, and 15 and 16 (all: p < 0.05). For girls differences were significant between ages 9 and 10 (p < 0.05) and 11 and 12 years (p < 0.01).

Boys aged 7 to 10 years and 15 to 18 years had a significantly greater MUAC than girls in the same age groups (7 to 10 years: p < 0.05; 15 to 18 years: p < 0.01).

(Tables 10.10 and 10.11; Figures 10.4a and 10.4b)

10.7 Waist and hip circumferences

The distribution as well as the amount of body fat in adults is a risk factor in the development of heart disease. The risk of developing heart disease is greater for those whose body fat is distributed to a greater extent centrally rather than peripherally compared with those whose body fat is distributed to a greater extent peripherally than centrally[10,11]. The waist to hip ratio (waist circumference (cm)/hip circumference (cm)) is an indicator for the distribution of body fat. The higher the value of the waist to hip ratio, the greater the extent to which body fat is deposited on the waist rather than the hips. For example, a waist circumference of 60cm and a hip circumference of 90cm gives a waist to hip ratio of 0.67; a waist circumference of 120cm and a hip circumference of 90cm gives a waist to hip ratio of 1.33. Since the relevance of waist to hip ratio for pre-pubescent young people is unknown, waist and hip circumferences were not measured for those aged 4 to 10 years.

All young people aged 11 to 18 years who took part in the survey were ask to agree to having their waist and hip circumferences measured by the interviewer. Waist and hip circumference measurements were achieved for 987 young people. After checking the data, all of the measurements were included in the analysis. There were two cases where only one of each measurement was recorded. Results were available for 490 boys and 497 girls aged 11 to 18 years (unweighted).

Tables 10.12 to 10.17 give descriptive statistics for waist and hip circumference and for waist to hip ratio for boys and girls separately by age group and individual year of age.

The distribution of waist circumference was strongly positively skewed for boys and girls in both age groups. The distribution of hip circumference was positively skewed for boys and girls in both age groups but less strongly so. The distribution of waist to hip ratio was positively skewed for young people in both age groups but only strongly so for girls aged 15 to 18 years. For waist circumference, median values were up to 4% (average 2%) lower than mean values, for hip circumference median values were up to 3% (average 1%) lower than mean values and for waist to hip ratio median values were up to 1% (average 1%) lower than mean values depending on sex and individual year of age.

For boys, the variability around the mean for both waist circumference and waist to hip ratio did not change with age, while the variability of hip circumference decreased slightly with age. For girls, the variability around the mean for both waist and hip circumference increased with age to 13 years, then decreased slightly with age. For waist to hip ratio there was an overall pattern for girls of increasing variability with age, although this decreased between the ages of 13 years and 14 years.

(Figures 10.5a to 10.7b)

Mean waist circumference increased significantly with grouped age (all: p < 0.01). Table 10.13 suggests a steady increase in waist circumference with age for boys (ns). Mean waist circumference for girls was significantly smaller for those aged 11 years than for those aged 12 years, 65cm compared with 70cm (p < 0.01). Although there were no further significant differences between girls at consecutive individual years of age, the data suggest a steady increase from 12 years to 16 years, after which mean waist circumference did not change (ns).

Table 10.12 shows that mean waist circumference was significantly greater for boys than for girls in both age groups (p < 0.01). Mean waist circumference was greater for boys than girls at each individual year of age but only significantly so at ages of 14, 16, 17 and 18 years (14, 16 and 17 years: p < 0.05; 18 years: p < 0.01).

Mean hip circumference increased significantly with grouped age (all: p < 0.01), but between individual year of age only increased significantly for girls between ages 11 and 12 (p < 0.01).

Mean hip circumference was significantly greater for girls aged 11 to 14 years than for boys of the same age (89cm compared with 86cm; p < 0.05), while there was no significant difference by sex for young people aged 15 to 18 years, 97cm for boys compared with 98cm for girls (ns). The data suggest that mean hip circumference was greater for girls aged 12 to 15 years than for boys of the same age, although the difference was only significant for those aged 13 years, 92cm compared with 87cm (p < 0.05).

Waist to hip ratio did not vary by grouped age or individual year of age for boys. Girls aged 15 to 18 years had a significantly lower mean waist to hip ratio than girls aged 11 to 14 years, 0.75 compared with 0.77 (p < 0.01). Table 10.17 suggests that waist to hip ratio decreased with age from the age of 12 years, although the only significant difference was for girls between the ages of 12 and 13 years (p < 0.05). This indicates that, at least partly as a result of their stage of sexual development, the body fat of older girls was deposited to a greater extent on their hips rather than on their waists when compared with younger girls.

Tables 10.16 and 10.17 show that mean waist to hip ratio was significantly greater for boys than girls in both age groups and at each individual year of age (all: p < 0.01). *(Tables 10.12 to 10.17; Figures 10.5a to 10.7b)*

10.8 Correlations between measurements

Table 10.18 gives a correlation coefficient matrix for the relationships between various anthropometric measurements. Each individual measurement was highly correlated with age; *partial correlation coefficients* have therefore been calculated which allow for the effect of

age to be controlled. Coefficients are given both for the whole sample and for the four age groups separately, each controlling for age.

With the exception of the relationships between height and BMI and height and waist to hip ratio, each pair of measurements were significantly correlated at the p < 0.01 level and the relationships between each pair of measurements were in the same direction and of a similar magnitude for boys and girls both overall and within age group. For boys, the value of the coefficients for the relationship between height and BMI was similar overall and for each age group (all: p < 0.01) while for girls, the value of the coefficients decreased with age, falling below the level of statistical significance (p > 0.05) for girls in the top two age groups and being statistically significant only at the p < 0.05 level overall. Height and waist to hip ratio were significantly negatively correlated for all girls aged 11 to 18 years, girls in both age groups and for boys aged 11 to 14 years (girls 11 to 14 years: p < 0.05; boys aged 11 to 18: p < 0.05; others: p < 0.01), while for boys aged 15 to 18 years, the correlation was positive without reaching the level of statistical significance. *(Table 10.18)*

10.9 Correlations with dietary intake

Partial correlation coefficients were calculated for the relationships between those measurements used to indicate body shape or 'fatness' (BMI, MUAC and waist to hip ratio) and those aspects of dietary intake which might be related to body shape or 'fatness' (average daily energy intake and percentage of energy from total fat, total carbohydrate and total sugars). As discussed above, the calculation controlled for the effect of age (see *Section 10.8*).

The positive associations between average daily energy intake and both MUAC and BMI were most marked for boys and girls in the first two age groups. There was no significant relationship between average daily energy intake and waist to hip ratio.

Percentage energy from total fat was significantly negatively correlated with MUAC for girls aged 11 to 14 years (p < 0.01) and with BMI for boys aged 7 to 10 years and girls aged 11 to 14 years (p < 0.05 and p < 0.01 respectively). Percentage energy from total carbohydrate was significantly positively correlated with MUAC for boys aged 4 to 6 years (p < 0.05). Percentage energy from total sugars was strongly negatively correlated with BMI for all boys aged 4 to 18 years and for girls aged 11 to 14 years, with MUAC for boys aged 11 to 14 years and with waist to hip ratio for all girls aged 11 to 16 years (all: p < 0.05). *(Table 10.19)*

10.10 Variations in measurements

In this section, variation in the average measurements in

relation to the main characteristics of the sample is considered.

Tables 10.20 to 10.25 show the relationships between mean measurements and key socio-demographic characteristics, including, for girls, whether menarché had occurred, and for boys, plasma testosterone concentration. The means for each measurement were strongly related to age. It should therefore be remembered when looking at these tables that socio-demographic characteristics that appear to explain variations in measurements might not be found to be significant when the effects of factors such as age are controlled (see *Section 10.11*).

Tables 10.26 to 10.31 show variations in age-sex specific BMI quintile. This method of presenting the results controls the effects of age. Quintiles were defined separately for boys and girls at each individual year of age; the values were then pooled to give quintiles for boys and girls aged 4 to 18 years.

For further analysis of the relationship between the anthropometric measurements and the socio-demographic characteristics, see *Section 10.11* where the technique of multiple regression was used to produce standardised regression coefficients for a number of characteristics associated with variation in the measurements used to indicate body shape or 'fatness' (BMI and waist to hip ratio).

10.10.1 Findings

Variation in height
There was no variation in height according to the region in which the young person lived or their social class background.

For boys height increased significantly as gross weekly household income increased (all: $p < 0.05$). For girls, the only significant difference was between those from households with an income of less than £160 per week and those from households with an income of £600 or more per week ($p < 0.05$). There were no significant differences in the mean height of either boys or girls according to household receipt of benefits.

Table 10.25 suggests that girls aged 12 and 13 years for whom menarché had occurred were on average taller than girls of the same age who had not reached menarché, although the differences did not reach the level of statistical significance.

(Tables 10.20 to 10.25)

Variation in weight
There was no variation in weight according to the region in which the young person lived or their social class background.

For both sexes mean weight increased as income increased (comparing lowest and highest income groups – boys: $p < 0.01$; girls: $p < 0.05$). For boys weight increased significantly between each income group. The data suggest that mean weight was lower for young people from households that were in receipt of benefits than for those from households that were not receiving benefits, although the difference was only significant for girls ($p < 0.05$).

Table 10.24 shows that there was no statistically significant variation in mean weight according to tertile of plasma testosterone concentration ($p > 0.05$). Table 10.25 shows that for girls aged 12 and 13 years, those who reached menarché were on average significantly heavier than girls who had not (both ages: $p < 0.05$).

(Tables 10.20 to 10.25)

Variation in BMI
There was no variation in BMI according to the region in which the young person lived or their social class background.

Among boys, the data suggest that mean BMI was higher for young people from households with higher incomes, although the only significant difference was between boys from households with a gross weekly household income of less than £160 per week and those from households with a gross income of £600 or more per week, BMI of 18 compared with BMI of 19 ($p < 0.05$). There was no significant variation in mean BMI with gross weekly household income for girls. There was no significant variation in mean BMI for either boys or girls by household receipt of benefits.

Tables 10.26 to 10.31 show variations in age-specific BMI quintile according to key socio-demographic characteristics, including for girls whether menarché had occurred, and for boys, plasma testosterone concentration. The proportion of young people in each BMI quintile did not vary significantly by region, social class background, household income group or household receipt of benefits.

Table 10.24 shows that there was no statistically significant variation in mean BMI according to tertile of plasma testosterone concentration. The onset of menstruation was related to BMI for girls. The proportion of girls aged 10 to 18 years for whom menarché had occurred increased with each BMI quintile, although the only significant difference was between the proportions in the bottom and top two quintiles, 49% compared with 70% and 74% ($p < 0.05$ and $p < 0.01$ respectively).

The data suggest that the proportion of young people who reported that they were dieting to lose weight increased with BMI quintile, although the only significant difference was between the top and bottom quintiles for girls (14% compared with 1%: $p < 0.01$).

Table 10.31 shows that 9% of boys and 14% of girls in the top BMI quintile were dieting to lose weight. One percent of girls in the bottom quintile and small proportions of boys and girls in the second quintile (1% of boys and 3% of girls) reported dieting to lose weight.

For further analysis of the relationship between BMI and the socio-demographic characteristics, see *Section 10.11* where the technique of multiple regression was used to produce standardised regression coefficients for a number of characteristics associated with variation in BMI. *(Tables 10.20 to 10.31)*

Variation in mid upper-arm circumference
There was no variation in mid upper-arm circumference (MUAC) according to the region in which the young person lived or their social class background.

For boys, mean MUAC varied with gross weekly household income. Boys from households with a gross income of less than £160 per week had on average a significantly lower MUAC than those from households with an income of £600 or more per week (all: $p < 0.01$). Boys in households receiving benefits also had a lower MUAC than boys in households not receiving benefits ($p < 0.05$). There was no significant variation in mean MUAC by income or according to household receipt of benefits for girls.

Table 10.24 shows that there was no statistically significant variation in mean MUAC according to tertile of plasma testosterone concentration. *(Tables 10.20 to 10.25)*

Variation in waist and hip circumferences
Table 10.20 shows that there was no significant difference in mean waist circumference or hip circumference between boys living in different regions. Waist to hip ratio was highest for boys living in the Northern region, 0.84, and lowest for boys in Scotland and London and the South East, 0.81 (Northern compared with Scotland: $p < 0.05$; Northern compared with London and the South East: $p < 0.01$).

For girls, mean waist circumference varied by region. Girls living in the Central and South West regions of England and Wales had the greatest mean waist circumference (73cm) and those living in Scotland and London and the South East of England had the smallest mean waist circumferences (70cm), although the only significant difference was between the Central and South West regions and Wales and London and the South East ($p < 0.05$). Although there were no significant variations in either hip circumference or waist to hip ratio by region, the data suggest that both were highest for girls from the Central and South West regions of England and Wales (ns).

For girls, mean waist circumference did not vary by social class, however girls from a non-manual social class background had a significantly greater hip circumference and hence a significantly smaller waist to hip ratio than girls from a manual background (hip circumference: $p < 0.05$; waist to hip ratio: $p < 0.01$).

For boys, both waist and hip circumference varied with gross weekly household income although waist to hip ratio did not. Boys from households with a gross weekly income of less than £160 had significantly smaller mean waist and hip circumferences than those from households with an income of £600 or more per week (waist circumference: $p < 0.05$; hip circumference: $p < 0.01$).

For girls, waist circumference did not show any clear pattern of variation with gross weekly household income. The data suggest an increase in hip circumference with increasing income and a significant decrease in waist to hip ratio between girls from households with an income of less than £160 per week and those from households with an income of £600 or more per week ($p < 0.01$).

There was no significant variation in mean waist or hip circumference or in mean waist to hip ratio for boys by household receipt of benefits. For girls, mean waist circumference did not vary by receipt of benefits, although the data suggest that girls from households in receipt of benefits had a smaller mean hip circumference and a greater mean waist to hip ratio than girls from households not in receipt of benefits (hip circumference: ns; waist to hip ratio: $p < 0.05$).

Tables 10.24 and 10.25 show that there was no statistically significant variation in mean waist circumference, hip circumference or waist to hip ratio for boys according to tertile of plasma testosterone concentration or for girls by whether menarché had occurred. *(Tables 10.20 to 10.25)*

10.11 Characteristics found to be independently associated with the anthropometric measurements

Tables 10.33 and 10.34 give standardised regression coefficients for a number of characteristics, the independent variables, associated with variation in the anthropometric measurements, the dependent variable, produced using the technique of multiple regression. Multiple regression analyses have been carried out for BMI and waist to hip ratio.

Various socio-demographic characteristics have been shown to be associated with variations in body size (see *Section 10.10*), but some of these factors are known to be inter-related. This section considers the combined effects of these variables on BMI for young people aged 7 to 18 years and waist to hip ratio for young people aged 11 to 18 years. The characteristics are analysed using the multiple regression technique to identify those with the strongest relationships with the anthropometric measurements. The tables of results identify those characteristics where the regression coefficients were significantly related to the measurements after controlling the effects of the other characteristics included in the analysis ($p < 0.05$, $p < 0.01$ or $p < 0.001$). Further information on the statistical method and interpretation of output from multiple regression analysis is given in Appendix E.

As noted above, for young people there is a strong association between age and measures of 'body size'. To control for this effect, age was included in each multiple regression analysis; thus differences in the measurements have been tested for significance after taking account of any age variation between groups. There is also a strong association between sex and the measurements; each multiple regression analysis is therefore presented separately for boys and girls. Both BMI and waist to hip ratio were significantly skewed[12] and they were therefore log transformed (natural log, ln) before being included in the analysis.

The technique of multiple regression calculates coefficients based on the number of cases for which there are valid values for all the variables included in the analysis. Among the variables of interest was physical activity level, as indicated by the calculated activity level score. However this was only derived for young people aged 7 to 18 years who completed a full 7-day physical activity diary, a total of 711 boys and 713 girls; young people aged 4 to 6 years did not keep physical activity diaries (see *Chapter 13*). Additionally for boys, the effect of blood testosterone level on BMI and waist to hip ratio was of interest. Blood testosterone concentration was only measured for boys aged 10 to 16 years who provided a blood sample, a total of 260 boys (see *Chapter 12*). Including physical activity score and, in the analysis for boys, blood testosterone level, in a single regression would therefore markedly reduce the number of cases available for analysis. It was therefore decided that a number of separate analyses should be run:

for BMI:
- all aged 4 to 18 years, *excluding* physical activity score and, for boys, blood testosterone level – Tables 10.33(a) and (d);
- all aged 7 to 18 years, *including* physical activity score, but, for boys, *excluding* blood testosterone level – Tables 10.33(b) and (e);
- all boys aged 10 to 16 years, *including* physical activity score and blood testosterone level – Table 10.33(c);

for waist to hip ratio:
- all aged 11 to 18 years, *including* physical activity score but, for boys, *excluding* blood testosterone level – Tables 10.34(a) and (c);
- all boys aged 11 to 16 years, *including* physical activity score and blood testosterone level – Table 10.34(b).

Except for those analyses that included blood testosterone level the regression analyses were carried out after weighting for differential sampling probabilities and differential non-response. The analyses for boys that included blood testosterone level were not weighted (see *Chapter 12; Section 12.1.2*)[13].

Parents' reported height
The association between the height of parents and the achieved height of their children is widely reported[14,15]. Where available, the heights of both the young person's mother and father were included in the multivariate analysis for BMI and waist to hip ratio. The section below describes how the information was collected and Table 10.32 gives descriptive statistics for these measurements.

After all the measurements of the young person had been made or attempted, the interviewer asked the young person or their mother figure the height of the young person's mother and father. These measurements were recorded for biological or 'birth' parents only and were self or proxy-reported; interviewers were not asked to take measurements of the parents. Although there is evidence to show that self-reported heights are often inaccurate[16], it would not have been possible in the context of an already onerous survey programme to collect measurements of both parents. In cases where one or both birth parents were not living in the household, proxy information was collected where possible about the absent parent's height.

The measurement was recorded in either imperial or metric units; imperial measurements were converted to metric units for the analysis.

The height of the young person's mother was collected for 1920 young people and the height of the young person's father was collected for 1867 young people (unweighted). Table 10.32 shows that mean reported height for fathers was 177cm and mean reported height for mothers was 162cm. *(Table 10.32)*

10.11.1 Findings

Characteristics independently associated with BMI
After controlling for the effects of the other characteristics entered into the model, BMI remained significantly positively associated with age for both boys and girls (both: $p < 0.001$).

Characteristics that were positively associated with BMI for both boys and girls aged 4 to 18 years were systolic blood pressure (both sexes: $p < 0.001$), average daily total energy intake (boys: $p < 0.001$; girls: $p < 0.01$) and whether the young person reported currently dieting to lose weight (both sexes: $p < 0.001$).

In addition, for boys aged 4 to 18 years BMI was

significantly associated with region, percentage energy from total fat ($p < 0.05$) and percentage energy from total sugars ($p < 0.01$) and gross weekly household income. Boys living in London and the South East had, on average, a lower BMI and those living in Scotland a higher BMI than the overall average (both: $p < 0.05$). Boys living in households with a gross weekly household income of less than £160 had, on average, a lower BMI ($p < 0.05$).

Girls aged 4 to 18 years for whom menarché had occurred had a higher BMI than girls for whom menarché had not occurred ($p < 0.001$) and there was also an inverse relationship between BMI and father's reported height and for those from a manual social class background (both: $p < 0.05$).

For boys and girls aged 4 to 18 years, the characteristics entered in the model accounted for 50% and 49% respectively of the variation in BMI.

As described above, the same variables plus calculated physical activity score were included in a regression analysis, but restricted to those aged 7 to 18 years (Tables 10.33(b) and (e)). For this group of boys and girls there was no significant association between calculated physical activity score and BMI. For boys, this model identified the same significant associations as for all boys aged 4 to 18 years. Additionally this model identified a significant inverse association between BMI and diastolic blood pressure ($p < 0.05$) and boys aged 7 to 18 living in the Northern region had, on average, a lower BMI ($p < 0.05$).

For girls aged 7 to 18 years, this model identified the same significant associations with BMI as for all girls aged 4 to 18 years, with additionally an inverse relationship between BMI and the percentage energy from sugars ($p < 0.05$).

For boys and girls aged 7 to 18 years the characteristics entered in this model accounted for 47% and 41% respectively of the variation in BMI.

The final model, which was for boys aged 10 to 16 years, included blood testosterone tertile which was not significantly associated with BMI (Table 10.33(c)). The model accounted for 37% of the variation in BMI for this group of boys and significant independent associations were found for age ($p < 0.05$), reporting being on a diet to lose weight ($p < 0.001$), systolic blood pressure and average daily energy intake (both: $p < 0.01$). *(Tables 10.33(a) to 10.33(e))*

Characteristics independently associated with waist to hip ratio
After controlling for the effects of the other characteristics entered into the model, for both boys and girls aged 11 to 18 years age was inversely associated with waist to hip ratio (both: $p < 0.05$) and positively

associated with whether the young person reported currently being on a diet to lose weight (boys: $p < 0.001$; girls: $p < 0.05$).

In addition, for boys waist to hip ratio was significantly associated with region, gross weekly household income and whether the young person was living with both parents. For girls aged 11 to 18 years waist to hip ratio was significantly associated with whether menarché had occurred, the social class of the head of household, reporting being a current smoker and father's reported height.

Boys aged 11 to 18 years living in London and the South East had, on average, a lower waist to hip ratio ($p < 0.01$) and those living in Northern England and the Central and South West regions and Wales had a higher waist to hip ratio ($p < 0.01$ and $p < 0.05$ respectively) than the overall average. Boys living in households with two parents and other children had a significantly lower waist to hip ratio than average ($p < 0.05$).

Girls aged 11 to 18 years who had reached menarché had a lower waist to hip ratio than other girls ($p < 0.01$), as did girls from a non-manual social class background ($p < 0.01$), and those who reported being current smokers ($p < 0.05$). There was an inverse relationship between waist to hip ratio and father's reported height ($p < 0.05$) and girls who reported currently being on a diet to lose weight had a significantly greater waist to hip ratio than other girls ($p < 0.05$).

The characteristics entered in this model accounted for 11% of the variation in waist to hip ratio for boys aged 11 to 18 years and 20% of the variation for girls.

The final model which was for boys aged 10 to 16 years included blood testosterone tertile (Table 10.34(b)). None of the variables included in the model was significantly associated with variation in waist to hip ratio for this group of boys and the model accounted for 4% of the variation in the ratio.
(Tables 10.34(a) to 10.34(c))

10.12 Comparisons with other studies
In this section, data on the anthropometric measurements from this Survey are compared with data from the Health Survey for England: The Health of Young People, carried out in 1995-97[1] and the National Study of Health and Growth (NSHG), carried out in 1994[2].

Both the Health Survey and the NDNS used a multi-stage probability sample, with postcode sectors as primary sampling units and the Postcode Address File as the sampling frame for households (see *Chapter 1* and *Appendix D* for further details of the NDNS sample design). For the Health Survey, interview data were obtained from 76%, 81% and 85% of eligible children in sampled households in 1995, 1996 and 1997 respectively. Among co-operating households, child response was around 98% in each year. The NSHG sample was selected via primary schools. Areas were selected by stratified random sampling and schools were then selected within these areas. All children in co-operating schools were measured and weighed unless their parent(s) refused; approximately 95% of children were measured each year.

Data for all three surveys are presented by the young person's age last birthday. Tables showing comparisons between data from the Health Survey and the NDNS relate only to young people living in England.

The NSHG collected data on pupils from all ethnic groups, but for its 1972-94 trend analyses only data for white pupils aged 5 to 10 years were analysed, of whom about 5200 had their height and weight measured in 1994. Comparisons between the NSHG, the Health Survey and the NDNS in this Report relate only to white young people aged 5 to 10 years living in England. In the NSHG 'white' children were those considered white by the fieldworker. In the Health Survey and NDNS, the classification was based on the ethnic group to which the young person or their parent(s) considered they belonged. The combined 1995-97 Health Survey samples included about 5600 such children and the NDNS 666 such children.

The measurement procedures for the three surveys were broadly similar. Measurements were carried out by a school nurse assisted by a trained fieldworker in the NSHG and by a trained interviewer in the Health Survey and NDNS.

In all three surveys, height was measured using a stadiometer with the fieldworker applying traction to the young person's neck to ensure that they were measured to their fullest height. In the NDNS, height was recorded to the nearest millimetre (for protocols for the anthropometric measurements see *Appendix L*). In the NSHG height was recorded to the last complete millimetre, 0.05cm being added to correct the bias. In the Health Survey, height was also recorded in centimetres and millimetres, but if a measurement fell between two millimetres, it was recorded to the nearest even millimetre.

In all three surveys weight was measured using electronic digital scales and recorded to the nearest 100g. Young people were weighed wearing only under-pants in the NSHG, while in both the Health Survey and the NDNS respondents were asked to remove shoes, heavy outer garments such as jackets and cardigans, heavy jewellery, loose change and keys. For the purpose of comparing data from the NDNS and the Health Survey with the NSHG (but not elsewhere in the chapter), weights for the Health Survey and NDNS have been adjusted for clothing weight, giving estimated

unclothed weights comparable with the NSHG data. Adjustments used were those from a previous survey which estimated average clothing weights by age and sex as shown below[17].

Clothing adjustment factors

Age of young person (years)	Sex of young person and clothing weight (kg)	
	Males	Females
5–7	0.64	0.55
8–10	0.76	0.62

The need to adjust for clothing weight is an additional methodological difference that makes it more difficult to make accurate comparisons between the surveys and to detect any possible change with confidence.

10.12.1 Findings

Height
There were no significant differences between the mean heights of young people living in England measured in the NDNS and those of young people of a corresponding age measured in the Health Survey for England.

Table 10.36 shows that for young, white people aged 5 to 10 years living in England mean height was similar in the NDNS, the Health Survey and the NSHG. Mean heights for all white girls and boys at each individual year of age did not vary significantly between the three surveys. *(Tables 10.35 and 10.36)*

Weight
There was no significant difference in the mean weight of boys or girls living in England at each individual year of age measured in the NDNS compared with the Health Survey.

Table 10.38 shows that for young, white people aged 5 to 10 years living in England mean weight was broadly similar in the NDNS, the Health Survey and the NSHG. After adjusting for clothing weight, there was no significant difference in mean weight between the three surveys for all white girls and all white boys at each individual year of age. *(Tables 10.37 and 10.38)*

BMI
Mean BMI was similar for young people living in England measured in the NDNS and the Health Survey. There was no significant difference in mean BMI for boys and girls by individual year of age between those measured in the NDNS and the Health Survey.

Table 10.40 shows that for young, white people aged 5

to 10 years living in England, mean BMI was broadly similar in the NDNS, the Health Survey and the NSHG. After adjusting for clothing weight, there was no significant difference in mean BMI between the three surveys for all white girls and all white boys at each individual year of age.   *(Tables 10.39 and 10.40)*

Mid upper-arm circumference

There were no significant differences in mean mid upper-arm circumferences for young people living in England measured in the NDNS and the Health Survey.
                                                                (Table 10.41)

Comparing anthropometric data from the NDNS, the Health Survey and the NSHG

The comparison of data on selected anthropometric measurements between the NDNS, the Health Survey and the NSHG shows that the three data sets are broadly comparable with no significant differences by sex or age between the three data sets.

Taking into account the small groups created when the NDNS data set is considered by sex and individual year of age, and the fact that in making comparisons with the NSHG it is not possible to control for clothing weight accurately, these findings indicate that the three survey samples are comparable and that the NDNS data constitute a continuation of, rather than a break from, the existing data on the anthropometric measurements of young people.

References and endnotes

[1] Prescott-Clarke P, Primatesta P. Eds. *Health Survey for England. The Health of Young People '95-97. Volume 1: Findings.* TSO (London, 1998).

[2] The National Study of Health and Growth was set up in 1972 to monitor the growth of primary school children. For example, see Chinn S, Price CE, Rona RJ. The need for new reference curves for height. *Arch Dis Childh* 1989; **64**: 1545-1553.

[3] The non-response weights were calculated using age-sex specific response rates for those who consented to the height measurement. There were 4 cases (unweighted) where a height measurement was *not* achieved but a weight measurement *was* achieved; for each of these cases, the age-sex specific weight calculated using the data for height was applied.

[4] Freeman JV, Cole TJ, Chinn S, Jones PRM, White EM, Preece MA. Cross-sectional stature and weight reference curves for the UK, 1990. *Arch Dis Childh* 1995, **73**: 17-24.

[5] Cole TJ, Freeman JV, Preece MA. Body mass index reference curves for the UK, 1990. *Arch Dis Childh* 1995, **73**: 25-29.

[6] Harvey D, Kovar I. Eds. *Child health: a textbook for the DCH.* Second Edition. Churchill Livingstone (Edinburgh, 1991).

[7] Data for plasma testosterone concentration are presented unweighted (see *Section 12.1.2* for further information).

[8] Data have been combined for boys aged 15 and 16 years, since there were only 17 boys aged 16 for whom plasma testosterone concentration was available.

[9] International Obesity Task Force. *Obesity: preventing and managing the global epidemic. Report of WHO consultation on obesity, Geneva, 3-5 June 1998.* WHO (Geneva, 1998).

[10] Rimm EB, Stampfer MJ, Giovannucci E et al. Body size and fat distribution as predictors of heart disease among middle aged and older U.S. men. *Am J Epid* 1995: **141**: 117-127.

[11] Folsom AR, Kaye SA, Sellers TA. et al. Body fat distribution and 5 year risk of death in older women. *J Am Med Assoc,* 1993; **269**: 484-487.

[12] A skewness (*sk*) value of +1.0 represents extreme positive skewness and a value of -1.0 extreme negative skewness Loether HJ, McTavish DG. *Descriptive and inferential statistics: an introduction.* Second Edition. Allyn and Bacon (Massachusetts, 1980).

[13] The procedure was run in SPSS for Windows v9.0. For further details of the general method used and interpretation of results see *Appendix E.*

[14] For example: Tanner JM. Use and abuse of growth standards. In: *Human growth.* Eds. Falkner F, Tanner JM. Second edition. Plenum Press (London, 1986).

[15] Poskitt EME. Which children are at risk of obesity? *Nutr Res* 1993; **13**: Suppl 1: s83-s93.

[16] Hill A. and Roberts J. Body Mass Index: a comparison between self-reported and measured height and weight. *J Pub H Med* 1998; **20**: 206-210.

[17] Cameron N. The growth of London schoolchildren 1904-66: An analysis of secular trend and intra-county variation. *Ann Hum Biol* 1979; **6**: 505-525.

Table 10.1 Mean plasma testosterone concentration by age

Boys aged 10 to 16 years

Age last birthday (years)	Plasma testosterone concentration (nmol/l)			Base
	Mean	Median	sd	
10	2.2	0.9	4.52	*41*
11	4.5	1.2	7.57	*51*
12	9.9	5.5	10.00	*36*
13	15.8	17.0	9.69	*38*
14	20.8	20.6	8.82	*39*
15	25.5	26.4	8.34	*38*
16				*17**
All cases**	13.4	11.4	11.89	*260*

* This age group included 17 boys (unweighted) and means could therefore not be calculated.
**Includes those aged 16 years.

Table 10.2 Plasma testosterone concentration - tertiles by age*

Boys aged 10 to 16 years

Age last birthday (years)	Plasma testosterone concentration – tertiles		
	Bottom	Middle	Top
	%	%	%
10	41	6	1
11	44	11	3
12	10	23	8
13	2	25	16
14	2	17	25
15 and over**	-	17	46
Base = 100%	86	87	87

*The data for plasma testosterone concentration for all boys aged 10 to 16 years were pooled and non-age-specific tertiles were calculated.
** Includes 17 boys aged 16 years

Table 10.3 Percentage of girls for whom menarche had occurred and median age at menarche by age

Girls aged 10 to 18 years co-operating with the self-completion questionnaire

Age last birthday (years)	Percentage of girls for whom menarche had occurred	Age at menarche (years)	Base
	%	Median	
10	4	9.8	*68*
11	11	11.0	*67*
12	44	11.0	*75*
13	62	12.0	*63*
14	86	12.1	*69*
15	92	12.1	*66*
16	96	13.0	*71*
17	98	13.0	*61*
18	100	13.0	*60*
All cases	61	12.1	*600*

Table 10.4 Height of young person by sex and age

Height (cm)	Males aged (years)				All males	Females aged (years)				All females
	4–6	7–10	11–14	15–18		4–6	7–10	11–14	15–18	
	cum %	cum %	cum %	cum %	cum %	cum %	cum %	cum %	cum %	cum %
Less than 100	3	–	–	–	1	4	–	–	–	1
Less than 110	31	–	–	–	7	41	–	–	–	9
Less than 120	81	5	–	–	19	85	6	–	–	20
Less than 130	100	35	0	–	31	98	36	–	–	30
Less than 140		78	8	–	44	100	75	6	–	43
Less than 150		99	35	–	57		98	25	4	55
Less than 160		100	68	2	66		100	73	35	77
Less than 170			92	31	79			97	89	97
Less than 180			99	77	94			100	99	100
Less than 190			100	98	99				100	100
All				100	100					
Base	*212*	*287*	*268*	*223*	*990*	*201*	*251*	*263*	*241*	*956*
Mean (average value)	113	133	155	175	145	112	133	155	162	142
Median value	114	133	154	174	145	111	134	155	163	145
Lower 5.0 percentile	101	120	138	162	108	100	119	140	152	107
Upper 5.0 percentile	126	146	174	188	181	123	148	168	172	168
Standard deviation of the mean	7.2	8.3	10.7	7.6	23.9	7.1	8.8	8.5	6.4	20.4

Table 10.5 Height of young person by sex and age in single years

Height (cm)	4	5	6	7	8	9	10	11	12	13	14	15	16	17	18
Age (in years)	cum %	cum %	cum %	cum %	cum %	cum %	cum %	cum %	cum %	cum %	cum %	cum %	cum %	cum %	cum %
Males															
Less than 100	15	–	–	–	–	–	–	–	–	–	–	–	–	–	–
Less than 110	81	33	3	–	–	–	–	–	–	–	–	–	–	–	–
Less than 120	100	90	65	20	6	–	–	–	–	–	–	–	–	–	–
Less than 130	–	100	100	87	39	16	9	1	–	–	–	–	–	–	–
Less than 140	–	–	–	100	98	79	37	24	2	1	–	–	–	–	–
Less than 150	–	–	–	–	100	97	94	69	37	21	3	–	–	–	–
Less than 160	–	–	–	–	–	100	100	97	82	63	25	7	–	–	–
Less than 170	–	–	–	–	–	–	–	100	98	90	73	48	27	18	7
Less than 180	–	–	–	–	–	–	–	–	100	99	98	89	80	69	62
Less than 190	–	–	–	–	–	–	–	–	–	100	100	99	98	95	100
All	100	100	100	100	100	100	100	100	100	100	100	100	100	100	100
Base	_55_	_70_	_88_	_64_	_81_	_71_	_70_	_82_	_61_	_59_	_66_	_65_	_57_	_52_	_49_
Mean (average value)	106	113	119	124	131	136	141	146	153	157	165	171	175	176	178
Median value	106	112	117	124	132	136	142	146	152	158	165	170	176	175	178
Lower 5.0 percentile	98	103	110	118	120	126	129	135	144	143	153	160	164	165	168
Upper 5.0 percentile	113	122	128	133	140	147	148	159	168	173	178	186	185	191	189
Standard deviation of the mean	4.6	5.3	5.4	4.8	6.3	6.2	6.3	7.6	7.5	9.0	7.6	7.6	6.5	7.6	6.7
Females															
Less than 100	13	4	–	–	–	–	–	–	–	–	–	–	–	–	–
Less than 110	89	42	13	–	–	–	–	–	–	–	–	–	–	–	–
Less than 120	100	97	70	22	4	1	–	–	–	–	–	–	–	–	–
Less than 130	–	98	98	79	47	18	13	–	–	–	–	–	–	–	–
Less than 140	–	100	100	100	91	76	45	22	2	–	–	–	–	–	–
Less than 150	–	–	–	–	100	97	94	58	28	13	5	3	6	2	2
Less than 160	–	–	–	–	–	100	100	95	84	61	51	42	41	27	30
Less than 170	–	–	–	–	–	–	–	100	100	100	88	96	86	90	85
Less than 180	–	–	–	–	–	–	–	–	–	–	100	100	99	98	100
Less than 190	–	–	–	–	–	–	–	–	–	–	–	–	100	100	–
All	100	100	100	100	100	100	100	100	100	100	100	100	100	100	100
Base	_55_	_63_	_83_	_57_	_51_	_76_	_67_	_66_	_76_	_57_	_64_	_63_	_64_	_59_	_55_
Mean (average value)	105	111	117	125	130	136	140	147	154	158	160	161	162	164	163
Median value	104	111	117	124	131	137	141	146	153	159	160	162	162	165	163
Lower 5.0 percentile	99	103	109	114	121	126	126	137	143	145	150	151	150	154	154
Upper 5.0 percentile	111	119	128	136	142	147	150	160	162	169	172	169	175	173	173
Standard deviation of the mean	3.8	5.4	5.6	6.0	6.7	6.5	7.5	7.8	6.3	7.2	6.4	6.3	7.0	6.1	5.8

Table 10.6 Body weight of young person by sex and age

Body weight (kg)	Males aged (years)				All males	Females aged (years)				All females
	4–6	7–10	11–14	15–18		4–6	7–10	11–14	15–18	
	cum %	cum %	cum %	cum %	cum %	cum %	cum %	cum %	cum %	cum %
Less than 17	8	–	–	–	2	15	–	–	–	3
Less than 20	43	2	–	–	9	48	2	–	–	11
Less than 25	85	22	–	–	24	91	18	–	–	24
Less than 30	98	58	3	–	37	98	48	1	–	34
Less than 40	100	91	31	1	54	100	85	26	1	51
Less than 50		98	63	8	66		99	58	18	68
Less than 60		99	88	32	79		100	88	59	86
Less than 70		100	94	66	90			96	82	94
Less than 80			98	82	95			98	95	98
All			100	100	100			100	100	100
Base	*213*	*288*	*268*	*222*	*991*	*202*	*253*	*259*	*241*	*955*
Mean (average value)	21	30	47	68	42	20	32	49	60	41
Median value	21	29	45	65	37	20	31	48	57	39
Lower 5.0 percentile	16	22	32	48	19	16	22	33	45	18
Upper 5.0 percentile	26	39	64	86	71	24	42	61	75	63
Standard deviation of the mean	3.6	7.6	11.8	14.8	20.3	3.5	7.5	11.2	11.8	17.4

Table 10.7 Body weight of young person by sex and age in single years

Body weight (kg)	4	5	6	7	8	9	10	11	12	13	14	15	16	17	18
Age (in years)	cum %	cum %	cum %	cum %	cum %	cum %	cum %	cum %	cum %	cum %	cum %	cum %	cum %	cum %	cum %
Males															
Less than 17	22	5	2	–	–	–	–	–	–	–	–	–	–	–	–
Less than 20	87	47	13	3	3	–	–	–	–	–	–	–	–	–	–
Less than 25	99	85	77	53	26	8	3	–	–	–	–	–	–	–	–
Less than 30	100	98	97	93	68	50	23	10	–	–	–	–	–	–	–
Less than 40		100	100	100	98	93	72	59	32	25	2	2	–	–	–
Less than 50					100	100	93	87	75	60	27	15	3	7	3
Less than 60							96	96	90	91	73	49	28	30	13
Less than 70							99	99	95	97	85	83	65	56	54
Less than 80								100	99	100	96	90	81	82	73
All									100		100	100	100	100	100
Base	*55*	*70*	*88*	*65*	*81*	*72*	*70*	*82*	*61*	*59*	*66*	*64*	*57*	*52*	*49*
Mean (average value)	18	21	23	25	28	31	37	40	46	48	57	62	69	70	72
Median value	18	20	23	25	28	30	35	38	44	48	54	60	64	68	69
Lower 5.0 percentile	15	17	19	21	22	24	27	28	32	34	45	46	51	46	52
Upper 5.0 percentile	23	28	29	32	37	43	56	59	70	66	79	88	94	92	101
Standard deviation of the mean	2.1	3.6	3.1	3.2	4.9	5.7	9.5	9.5	10.3	9.4	11.1	12.9	15.7	14.7	13.8
Females															
Less than 17	35	14	2	–	–	–	–	–	–	–	–	–	–	–	–
Less than 20	77	45	31	8	–	1	–	–	–	–	–	–	–	–	–
Less than 25	98	97	82	47	26	4	3	–	–	–	–	–	–	–	–
Less than 30	100	98	96	82	57	43	19	4	1	–	–	–	–	–	–
Less than 40		100	100	100	94	85	67	62	17	16	8	1	–	2	–
Less than 50					100	98	97	83	68	47	30	24	19	12	14
Less than 60						100	99	100	92	82	75	64	62	59	47
Less than 70							100		97	90	95	86	83	76	80
Less than 80									100	95	98	95	96	94	95
All										100	100	100	100	100	100
Base	*56*	*63*	*83*	*58*	*51*	*76*	*68*	*64*	*76*	*55*	*64*	*63*	*64*	*59*	*55*
Mean (average value)	18	20	22	26	30	33	36	40	48	53	54	58	60	61	61
Median value	18	20	21	25	29	32	36	39	47	51	54	55	59	57	60
Lower 5.0 percentile	15	16	17	19	22	25	26	31	34	37	37	40	47	45	47
Upper 5.0 percentile	23	24	29	34	42	48	49	58	62	75	71	78	77	88	79
Standard deviation of the mean	2.5	2.9	3.7	4.4	6.1	7.0	7.2	8.5	8.7	13.1	9.5	12.0	13.6	13.6	10.6

Table 10.8 BMI of young person by sex and age

BMI (kg/m^2)	Males aged (years)				All males	Females aged (years)				All females
	4–6	7–10	11–14	15–18		4–6	7–10	11–14	15–18	
Mean (average value)	16	17	19	22	19	16	18	20	23	19
Median value	16	16	19	21	18	16	17	20	22	19
Lower 5.0 percentile	14	14	16	17	15	14	14	16	18	15
Upper 5.0 percentile	19	22	26	29	26	19	23	29	30	26
Standard deviation of the mean	1.5	2.6	3.2	3.9	3.7	1.6	2.7	3.7	4.0	4.0
Base	*212*	*287*	*268*	*222*	*989*	*201*	*251*	*260*	*241*	*953*

Table 10.9 BMI of young person by sex and age in single years

BMI (kg/m^2)	Age (in years)														
	4	5	6	7	8	9	10	11	12	13	14	15	16	17	18
Males															
Mean (average value)	16	16	16	16	16	17	19	19	19	19	21	21	22	22	23
Median value	17	16	16	16	16	17	17	18	19	19	20	21	21	22	22
Lower 5.0 percentile	15	14	14	14	14	14	15	15	16	15	17	16	18	17	18
Upper 5.0 percentile	18	21	19	19	21	20	27	26	25	25	28	26	30	29	32
Standard deviation of the mean	1.3	1.8	1.4	1.6	1.9	2.1	3.7	3.4	3.0	3.0	3.1	2.9	4.3	4.3	3.7
Base	*55*	*70*	*87*	*64*	*81*	*72*	*70*	*82*	*61*	*59*	*66*	*64*	*57*	*52*	*49*
Females															
Mean (average value)	16	16	16	16	17	18	19	19	20	21	21	22	23	23	23
Median value	17	16	16	16	17	17	18	18	20	20	21	21	22	22	23
Lower 5.0 percentile	14	14	14	14	14	14	15	15	16	16	17	17	18	18	17
Upper 5.0 percentile	19	19	20	20	21	23	23	27	26	30	28	29	32	33	30
Standard deviation of the mean	1.6	1.5	1.7	2.0	2.2	2.7	2.9	3.3	3.1	4.4	3.5	4.0	4.1	4.4	3.4
Base	*55*	*63*	*83*	*57*	*51*	*76*	*68*	*64*	*76*	*55*	*64*	*63*	*64*	*59*	*55*

Table 10.10   Mid upper-arm circumference of young person by sex and age

Mid upper-arm circumference (cm)	Males aged (years)				All males	Females aged (years)				All females
	4–6	7–10	11–14	15–18		4–6	7–10	11–14	15–18	
	cum %	cum %	cum %	cum %	cum %	cum %	cum %	cum %	cum %	cum %
Less than 16	9	1	–	–	2	7	–	–	–	1
Less than 18	48	18	1	–	16	51	9	–	–	13
Less than 20	85	57	9	0	36	84	36	7	1	30
Less than 22	97	79	33	3	50	95	60	25	6	44
Less than 24	99	90	62	15	64	99	81	46	23	61
Less than 26	100	96	78	37	77	100	94	74	45	78
Less than 28		97	87	63	86		97	89	67	88
Less than 30		99	94	77	92		100	96	81	94
Less than 32		99	98	89	96			98	92	97
Less than 34		100	100	95	99			99	96	99
All				100	100			100	100	100
Base	*207*	*287*	*269*	*222*	*985*	*201*	*253*	*263*	*241*	*958*
Mean (average value)	18	20	24	28	23	18	21	24	27	23
Median value	18	20	23	27	22	18	21	24	26	23
Lower 5.0 percentile	16	17	19	23	16	16	17	20	22	17
Upper 5.0 percentile	21	25	31	34	31	23	26	30	33	30
Standard deviation of the mean	1.9	2.9	3.4	3.6	4.6	2.0	3.0	3.2	3.7	4.4

Table 10.11 Mid upper-arm circumference of young person by sex and age in single years

Mid upper-arm circumference (cm)	Age (in years)														
	4	5	6	7	8	9	10	11	12	13	14	15	16	17	18
	cum %	cum %	cum %	cum %	cum %	cum %	cum %	cum %	cum %	cum %	cum %	cum %	cum %	cum %	cum %
Males															
Less than 16	10	15	6	2	1	3	-	-				-	-	-	-
Less than 18	70	56	35	34	22	15	8	2	-	-	-	-	-	-	-
Less than 20	92	84	83	80	70	49	31	17	12	2	-	1	-	-	-
Less than 22	99	96	97	95	88	76	54	51	38	7	8	6	1	-	3
Less than 24	100	98	100	100	96	90	75	80	63	25	42	24	14	13	5
Less than 26		99			99	95	89	94	79	49	60	50	36	33	27
Less than 28		100			100	97	91	95	86	76	78	81	59	52	47
Less than 30						100	95	98	96	87	88	90	73	74	67
Less than 32							98	99	99	93	93	93	89	87	82
Less than 34							100	100	100	100	100	99	94	91	94
All												100	100	100	100
Base	*53*	*67*	*87*	*65*	*80*	*73*	*69*	*83*	*61*	*58*	*67*	*65*	*57*	*52*	*48*
Mean (average value)	17	18	19	19	20	20	22	22	24	24	26	26	28	28	28
Median value	17	18	19	19	19	20	22	22	23	24	25	26	27	28	28
Lower 5.0 percentile	16	16	16	16	17	17	18	18	19	19	21	22	23	23	24
Upper 5.0 percentile	20	21	22	22	24	27	32	28	30	31	33	33	34	36	34
Standard deviation of the mean	1.6	2.1	1.8	1.7	2.0	2.7	3.7	2.9	3.2	3.1	3.4	3.2	3.8	3.7	3.2
Females															
Less than 16	11	6	6	-	-	-	-	-	-	-	-	-	-	-	-
Less than 18	63	48	48	20	9	9	2	17	4	-	-	-	-	-	-
Less than 20	87	86	81	60	40	35	19	47	18	4	4	7	1	2	1
Less than 22	98	96	89	79	67	59	47	73	41	21	12	28	13	7	7
Less than 24	100	100	98	92	89	82	69	89	78	38	29	57	42	32	17
Less than 26			100	100	99	93	87	98	91	61	61	78	68	47	39
Less than 28					100	96	96	99	98	82	84	83	86	64	55
Less than 30						100	99	100	99	89	95	92	93	78	74
Less than 32							99		99	95	98	95	99	92	90
Less than 34							100		100	100	100	100	100	98	99
All									100	100	100	100	100	100	100
Base	*54*	*64*	*83*	*58*	*51*	*76*	*68*	*65*	*76*	*58*	*64*	*63*	*64*	*59*	*55*
Mean (average value)	18	18	18	20	21	21	23	22	24	25	25	26	27	27	27
Median value	18	18	18	19	20	21	22	22	25	25	25	26	27	26	27
Lower 5.0 percentile	15	16	16	16	17	18	18	19	20	20	20	21	23	21	21
Upper 5.0 percentile	20	22	23	24	25	27	27	27	29	32	31	34	33	34	32
Standard deviation of the mean	1.6	1.8	2.2	2.3	2.3	3.0	3.2	2.5	2.7	3.5	3.1	4.0	3.2	3.9	3.4

Table 10.12 Waist circumference of young person by sex and age

Young people aged 11 to 18 years

Waist circumference (cm)	Males aged (years)		All males	Females aged (years)		All females
	11–14	15–18		11–14	15–18	
	cum %	cum %	cum %	cum %	cum %	cum %
Less than 55	0	–	0	1	–	1
Less than 60	4	–	2	11	2	6
Less than 65	22	5	14	37	14	25
Less than 70	49	13	32	58	38	48
Less than 75	74	34	54	85	65	75
Less than 80	83	58	71	91	82	87
Less than 85	89	73	81	95	88	91
Less than 90	96	85	91	96	94	95
Less than 95	99	91	95	99	97	98
All	100	100	100	100	100	100
Base	*268*	*222*	*490*	*258*	*239*	*497*
Mean (average value)	72	80	76	69	74	71
Median value	70	78	74	68	72	70
Lower 5.0 percentile	60	65	62	58	62	59
Upper 5.0 percentile	89	99	95	87	93	90
Standard deviation of the mean	9.1	10.6	10.7	8.4	9.0	9.0

Table 10.13 Waist circumference of young person by sex and age in single years

Young people aged 11 to 18 years

Waist circumference (cm)	Age (in years)							
	11	12	13	14	15	16	17	18
	cum %	cum %	cum %	cum %	cum %	cum %	cum %	cum %
Males								
Less than 55	1	–	–	–	–	–	–	–
Less than 60	8	1	2	1	–	–	–	–
Less than 65	37	27	18	5	11	–	7	–
Less than 70	70	55	43	26	21	15	11	5
Less than 75	89	77	73	53	45	36	30	23
Less than 80	92	84	84	71	74	63	50	37
Less than 85	94	91	91	80	85	75	67	59
Less than 90	99	100	97	90	91	84	84	77
Less than 95	99		100	96	96	89	89	88
Less than 100	99			97	97	96	95	95
All	100			100	100	100	100	100
Base	*82*	*61*	*58*	*67*	*65*	*57*	*52*	*48*
Mean (average value)	68	71	72	76	77	80	81	83
Median value	66	69	71	74	76	78	80	81
Lower 5.0 percentile	59	61	62	66	63	67	62	71
Upper 5.0 percentile	88	88	89	93	94	96	101	99
Standard deviation of the mean	8.7	8.1	7.6	9.4	9.0	10.9	11.8	9.5
	cum %	cum %	cum %	cum %	cum %	cum %	cum %	cum %
Females								
Less than 55	3	2	–	–	–	–	–	–
Less than 60	24	8	8	5	4	–	2	–
Less than 65	66	23	35	24	16	10	19	10
Less than 70	79	53	55	45	49	29	40	31
Less than 75	87	86	79	86	69	65	63	62
Less than 80	95	92	85	91	81	85	79	84
Less than 85	97	98	89	95	90	88	82	92
Less than 90	100	98	91	97	95	95	90	95
Less than 95		99	99	99	100	97	96	96
Less than 100		100	99	99		99	98	98
All			100	100		100	100	100
Base	*65*	*75*	*55*	*63*	*61*	*64*	*59*	*55*
Mean (average value)	65	70	70	71	73	74	74	74
Median value	63	69	68	71	70	74	71	73
Lower 5.0 percentile	57	60	58	61	61	64	62	62
Upper 5.0 percentile	81	82	93	89	93	90	93	91
Standard deviation of the mean	7.6	7.4	9.7	7.9	8.5	8.3	10.8	8.2

Table 10.14 Hip circumference of young person by sex and age

Young people aged 11 to 18 years

Hip circumference (cm)	Males aged (years)		All males	Females aged (years)		All females
	11–14	15–18		11–14	15–18	
	cum %	cum %	cum %	cum %	cum %	cum %
Less than 70	1	–	1	0	–	0
Less than 75	10	–	5	4	–	2
Less than 80	24	1	12	17	0	9
Less than 85	48	7	28	33	2	18
Less than 90	72	20	46	54	14	34
Less than 95	86	40	63	74	41	58
Less than 100	92	65	79	90	65	77
Less than 105	95	81	88	95	78	87
Less than 110	99	91	95	98	88	93
Less than 115	100	98	99	98	95	97
All		100	100	100	100	100
Base	*268*	*222*	*490*	*258*	*239*	*497*
Mean (average value)	86	97	92	89	98	94
Median value	85	97	91	89	97	93
Lower 5.0 percentile	73	83	75	75	86	77
Upper 5.0 percentile	103	113	110	104	116	111
Standard deviation of the mean	8.9	9.1	10.6	9.4	8.9	10.2

Table 10.15 Hip circumference of young person by sex and age in single years

Young people aged 11 to 18 years

Hip circumference (cm)	Age (in years)							
	11	12	13	14	15	16	17	18
	cum %	cum %	cum %	cum %	cum %	cum %	cum %	cum %
Males								
Less than 70	3	–	–	–	–	–	–	–
Less than 75	18	9	9	1	–	–	–	–
Less than 80	41	30	17	4	2	–	–	–
Less than 85	71	54	34	25	13	3	7	5
Less than 90	94	83	58	50	34	19	10	13
Less than 95	95	87	91	70	59	42	27	26
Less than 100	96	92	94	85	78	68	61	50
Less than 105	97	96	100	88	91	81	75	74
Less than 110	99	98		100	92	88	93	89
Less than 115	99	100			99	97	98	95
All	100				100	100	100	100
Base	*82*	*61*	*58*	*67*	*65*	*57*	*52*	*48*
Mean (average value)	82	85	87	91	94	98	99	100
Median value	82	84	88	90	93	96	97	101
Lower 5.0 percentile	70	74	74	81	83	87	80	85
Upper 5.0 percentile	99	101	101	107	112	113	111	114
Standard deviation of the mean	8.2	8.5	7.3	8.3	8.5	9.7	8.6	8.3
	cum %	cum %	cum %	cum %	cum %	cum %	cum %	cum %
Females								
Less than 70	–	1	–	–	–	–	–	–
Less than 75	11	2	2	–	–	–	–	–
Less than 80	45	13	6	2	1	–	–	–
Less than 85	70	25	23	13	6	–	2	2
Less than 90	87	60	42	24	24	11	11	8
Less than 95	92	80	70	51	52	35	41	36
Less than 100	98	90	87	83	73	71	57	54
Less than 105	100	97	88	95	80	83	77	71
Less than 110		99	94	97	87	92	83	90
Less than 115		100	95	97	93	99	89	99
All			100	100	100	100	100	100
Base	*65*	*75*	*55*	*63*	*61*	*64*	*59*	*55*
Mean (average value)	82	89	92	94	97	98	99	100
Median value	81	88	91	94	94	97	97	99
Lower 5.0 percentile	72	76	79	80	83	87	88	87
Upper 5.0 percentile	98	104	111	109	118	111	118	112
Standard deviation of the mean	7.3	7.7	10.3	7.8	9.5	7.9	10.0	7.9

Table 10.16 Waist to hip ratio of young person by sex and age

Young people aged 11 to 18 years

Waist:hip ratio	Males aged (years)		All males	Females aged (years)		All females
	11–14	15–18		11–14	15–18	
	cum %	cum %	cum %	cum %	cum %	cum %
Less than 0.675		1	0	1	3	2
Less than 0.700	0	1	1	4	14	9
Less than 0.750	3	7	5	36	55	46
Less than 0.800	25	42	33	73	88	80
Less than 0.850	65	72	69	91	96	93
Less than 0.900	91	95	93	98	98	98
Less than 0.950	96	99	98	100	100	100
All	100	100	100			
Base	*268*	*222*	*490*	*258*	*239*	*497*
Mean (average value)	0.83	0.82	0.83	0.77	0.75	0.76
Median value	0.83	0.81	0.82	0.77	0.74	0.75
Lower 5.0 percentile	0.76	0.75	0.75	0.70	0.69	0.69
Upper 5.0 percentile	0.93	0.90	0.92	0.87	0.86	0.87
Standard deviation of the mean	0.051	0.055	0.053	0.052	0.050	0.053

Table 10.17 Waist to hip ratio of young person by sex and age in single years

Young people aged 11 to 18 years

Waist:hip ratio	Age (in years)							
	11	12	13	14	15	16	17	18
	cum %	cum %	cum %	cum %	cum %	cum %	cum %	cum %
Males								
Less than 0.675	–	–	–	–	3	–	–	–
Less than 0.700	–	–	–	1	3	–	–	–
Less than 0.750	3	–	6	5	5	8	9	3
Less than 0.800	26	19	30	30	40	45	46	29
Less than 0.850	59	73	67	65	75	72	75	62
Less than 0.900	89	94	95	91	91	99	91	96
Less than 0.950	95	96	98	97	98	100	98	98
All	100	100	100	100	100		100	100
Base	*82*	*61*	*58*	*67*	*65*	*57*	*52*	*48*
Mean (average value)	0.84	0.83	0.83	0.83	0.82	0.81	0.82	0.83
Median value	0.83	0.83	0.82	0.84	0.81	0.82	0.81	0.82
Lower 5.0 percentile	0.75	0.77	0.74	0.74	0.74	0.75	0.74	0.75
Upper 5.0 percentile	0.96	0.92	0.89	0.93	0.93	0.89	0.92	0.89
Standard deviation of the mean	0.053	0.044	0.051	0.053	0.057	0.051	0.059	0.048
	cum %	cum %	cum %	cum %	cum %	cum %	cum %	cum %
Females								
Less than 0.675	–	–	3	–	1	2	1	8
Less than 0.700	2	4	12	3	15	6	18	18
Less than 0.750	20	27	47	57	49	49	60	70
Less than 0.800	65	63	76	90	91	87	82	89
Less than 0.850	89	85	94	99	97	94	94	95
Less than 0.900	95	97	100	100	99	96	98	96
Less than 0.950	100	99			100	100	100	100
All		100						
Base	*65*	*75*	*55*	*63*	*61*	*64*	*59*	*55*
Mean (average value)	0.79	0.79	0.76	0.75	0.75	0.76	0.75	0.74
Median value	0.78	0.78	0.77	0.74	0.75	0.75	0.74	0.74
Lower 5.0 percentile	0.72	0.70	0.68	0.71	0.69	0.70	0.69	0.67
Upper 5.0 percentile	0.89	0.88	0.88	0.82	0.82	0.87	0.86	0.89
Standard deviation of the mean	0.048	0.059	0.053	0.035	0.044	0.050	0.052	0.055

Table 10.18 Partial correlation coefficient matrix for anthropometric measurements controlling for age of young person by sex and age of young person†

Measurement, age (years) and sex of young person	Standing height Coefficient	Base	Body weight Coefficient	Base	Mid upper-arm circumference Coefficient	Base	Body mass index Coefficient	Base	Waist to hip ratio Coefficient	Base
Standing height										
4–6	1.00	413o	0.75**	212	0.43**	206	0.20**	212	na	
7–10	1.00	538o	0.64**	287	0.37**	286	0.28**	287	na	
11–14	1.00	531o	0.66**	268	0.37**	268	0.25**	268	−0.19**	268
15–18	1.00	464o	0.54**	222	0.32**	221	0.20**	222	0.09	222
All	1.00	1946o	0.52**	989	0.33**	982	0.19**	989	−0.10*	490
Body weight	FEMALES		MALES							
4–6	0.75**	201	1.00	413o	0.77**	206	0.80**	212	na	
7–10	0.67**	251	1.00	538o	0.83**	286	0.91**	287	na	
11–14	0.52**	259	1.00	527o	0.82**	268	0.88**	268	0.17**	268
15–18	0.42**	241	1.00	463o	0.86**	221	0.93**	222	0.44**	221
All	0.47**	952	1.00	1946o	0.81**	983	0.89**	989	0.53**	489
Mid upper-arm circumference			FEMALES		MALES					
4–6	0.46**	200	0.81**	200	1.00	406o	0.76**	206	na	
7–10	0.38**	251	0.87**	251	1.00	537o	0.85**	236	na	
11–14	0.23**	262	0.85**	259	1.00	530o	0.84**	268	0.29**	268
15–18	0.17**	240	0.89**	240	1.00	462o	0.88**	221	0.40**	222
All	0.28**	953	0.85**	953	1.00	1943o	0.85**	981	0.50**	490
Body mass index					FEMALES		MALES			
4–6	0.26**	201	0.83**	201	0.80**	200	1.00	413o	na	
7–10	0.25**	251	0.88**	251	0.90**	251	1.00	538o	na	
11–14	0.12	260	0.91**	259	0.88**	259	1.00	528o	0.35**	268
15–18	0.03	241	0.91**	241	0.90**	240	1.00	463o	0.47**	221
All	0.08*	953	0.88**	953	0.87**	950	1.00	1942o	0.51**	489
Waist to hip ratio							FEMALES		MALES	
4–6	na		na		na		na		na	
7–10	na		na		na		na		na	
11–14	−0.15*	258	0.16**	257	0.25**	258	0.26**	257	1.00	526o
15–18	−0.17**	239	0.24**	239	0.26**	239	0.33**	239	1.00	461o
All	−0.13**	497	0.52**	496	0.48**	497	0.46**	496	1.00	987o

* p < 0.05
** p < 0.01
o All young people
† Coefficients above and below the 'diagonal' are for boys and girls respectively.

363

Table 10.19 Partial correlation coefficient matrix for anthropometric measurements with dietary intakes controlling for age of young person by sex and age of young person

Measurement, sex and age (years) of young person	Dietary intake				Base: total number of young people
	Average daily energy intake (MJ)	Percentage energy from:			
		Total fat	Total carbohydrate	Total sugars	
Correlation coefficients					
Males					
Mid upper-arm circumference					
4–6	0.18*	−0.09	0.15*	0.07	207
7–10	0.22**	−0.12	0.05	0.06	287
11–14	0.11	0.06	−0.07	−0.13*	269
15–18	0.07	0.11	−0.05	−0.11	222
All	0.11**	0.01	−0.01	−0.06	985
Body mass index					
4–6	0.12	−0.14	0.10	0.00	212
7–10	0.16*	−0.12*	0.03	0.02	287
11–14	0.09	0.08	−0.05	−0.10	268
15–18	0.02	0.13	−0.02	−0.07	222
All	0.07*	0.03	−0.02	−0.07*	989
Waist to hip ratio					
4–6	na	na	na	na	na
7–10	na	na	na	na	na
11–14	−0.08	0.04	0.11	0.09	268
15–18	−0.05	−0.07	−0.07	−0.09	222
All	−0.06	0.05	0.01	−0.00	490
Females					
Mid upper-arm circumference					
4–6	0.32**	0.07	−0.04	−0.03	201
7–10	0.21**	−0.03	0.09	0.08	253
11–14	−0.08	−0.17**	−0.08	−0.11	263
15–18	0.09	0.02	0.00	0.00	241
All	0.10**	−0.04	0.02	−0.01	958
Body mass index					
4–6	0.29**	−0.01	−0.09	−0.07	201
7–10	0.21**	−0.06	0.08	0.04	251
11–14	−0.09	−0.21**	−0.04	−0.15*	260
15–18	0.04	0.06	0.03	−0.01	241
All	0.03	−0.06	−0.00	−0.05	953
Waist to hip ratio					
4–6	na	na	na	na	na
7–10	na	na	na	na	na
11–14	−0.07	−0.04	0.04	−0.07	258
15–18	−0.06	0.01	−0.04	−0.08	239
All	0.03	−0.01	0.01	−0.10*	497

* p < 0.05
**p < 0.01
na not applicable

Table 10.20 Anthropometric measurements for young person by region

Measurement	Region															
	Scotland				Northern				Central, South West and Wales				London and the South East			
	Mean	Median	sd	Base	Mean	Median	sd	Base	Mean	Median	sd	Base	Mean	Median	sd	Base
Males																
Body weight (kg)	45	40	21.4	80	42	38	20.6	272	43	37	20.4	342	42	36	19.5	296
Height (cm)	147	147	24.4	80	145	145	23.5	272	145	144	24.1	344	145	145	24.1	295
Mid upper-arm circumference (cm)	22	22	4.6	80	23	22	4.8	269	23	22	4.6	341	22	22	4.5	295
Waist circumference (cm)*	74	71	11.1	35	77	75	11.5	133	76	74	11.0	174	75	74	9.2	148
Hip circumference (cm)*	91	90	11.3	35	91	90	10.6	133	92	90	11.4	174	92	93	9.6	148
BMI (kg/m²)	19	18	4.3	80	19	18	4.0	272	19	18	3.6	342	18	18	3.4	295
Waist to hip ratio*	0.81	0.80	0.053	35	0.84	0.84	0.053	133	0.83	0.82	0.054	174	0.81	0.81	0.047	148
Females																
Body weight (kg)	41	38	18.0	79	41	40	17.2	249	42	40	18.4	342	40	38	16.2	286
Height (cm)	143	148	21.3	79	142	145	20.3	248	142	146	20.6	341	142	144	20.1	287
Mid upper-arm circumference (cm)	22	22	4.4	79	23	23	4.4	249	23	23	4.5	343	22	22	4.0	287
Waist circumference (cm)*	70	71	8.1	41	71	69	9.0	126	73	71	9.9	177	70	70	8.0	153
Hip circumference (cm)*	93	92	9.7	41	93	93	10.1	126	95	94	10.9	177	93	93	9.4	153
BMI (kg/m²)	19	19	3.9	79	19	19	4.0	248	20	19	4.4	340	19	18	3.5	286
Waist to hip ratio*	0.75	0.75	0.044	41	0.76	0.75	0.051	126	0.77	0.76	0.056	177	0.76	0.75	0.051	153

*Young people aged 11 to 18 years.

365

Table 10.21 Anthropometric measurements for young person by social class of head of household

Measurement	Social class of head of household											
	Non-manual				Manual				All**			
	Mean	Median	sd	Base	Mean	Median	sd	Base	Mean	Median	sd	Base
Males												
Body weight (kg)	42	37	20.6	461	43	37	20.2	455	42	37	20.3	990
Height (cm)	145	144	24.1	460	145	145	23.7	456	145	145	23.9	991
Mid upper-arm circumference (cm)	23	22	4.7	459	23	22	4.6	452	23	22	4.6	985
Waist circumference (cm)*	76	74	10.5	218	75	74	10.9	231	76	74	10.7	490
Hip circumference (cm)*	92	92	10.8	218	91	90	10.7	231	92	91	10.6	490
BMI (kg/m^2)	19	18	3.7	460	19	18	3.8	455	19	18	3.7	989
Waist to hip ratio*	0.83	0.82	0.052	218	0.83	0.82	0.054	231	0.83	0.82	0.053	490
Females												
Body weight (kg)	41	40	17.2	438	40	39	16.8	422	41	39	17.4	956
Height (cm)	143	146	20.9	439	141	144	20.4	420	142	145	20.4	955
Mid upper-arm circumference (cm)	23	23	4.2	441	23	22	4.3	421	23	23	4.4	958
Waist circumference (cm)*	71	70	8.1	222	71	70	8.8	222	71	70	9.0	497
Hip circumference (cm)*	95	94	9.9	222	92	92	9.5	222	94	93	10.2	497
BMI (kg/m^2)	19	19	3.8	437	19	18	3.9	420	19	19	4.0	953
Waist to hip ratio*	0.75	0.74	0.048	222	0.77	0.76	0.054	222	0.76	0.75	0.053	497

*Young people aged 11 to 18 years.
**Includes those for whom social class could not be assigned.

Table 10.22 Anthropometric measurements for young person by gross weekly household income

Measurement	Gross weekly household income																			
	Less than £160				£160 to less than £280				£280 to less than £400				£400 to less than £600				£600 and over			
	Mean	Median	sd	Base	Mean	Median	sd	Base	Mean	Median	sd	Base	Mean	Median	sd	Base	Mean	Median	sd	Base
Males																				
Body weight (kg)	36	32	16.6	158	42	37	19.4	181	42	37	19.9	182	44	41	19.7	199	45	40	21.9	235
Height (cm)	137	138	23.1	159	145	145	23.5	181	144	142	24.0	182	149	148	22.9	199	148	147	24.4	234
Mid upper-arm circumference (cm)	21	21	4.0	158	23	22	4.5	179	23	22	4.7	181	23	23	4.6	199	23	23	4.8	233
Waist circumference (cm)*	72	70	8.7	62	76	74	11.1	86	76	74	9.5	85	75	74	10.3	113	77	74	10.7	120
Hip circumference (cm)*	88	86	8.2	62	91	92	10.7	86	92	94	9.6	85	91	89	10.9	113	94	93	11.4	120
BMI (kg/m²)*	18	17	3.1	158	19	18	3.8	181	19	18	3.5	182	19	18	3.5	199	19	18	4.0	234
Waist to hip ratio*	0.82	0.82	0.068	62	0.83	0.83	0.053	86	0.82	0.81	0.050	85	0.83	0.82	0.046	113	0.82	0.82	0.048	120
Females																				
Body weight (kg)	38	34	16.1	156	40	37	18.0	170	39	38	15.9	170	42	42	18.1	215	44	45	17.6	211
Height (cm)	139	142	19.4	156	139	141	20.6	171	140	142	20.1	171	142	149	20.7	215	147	155	20.4	210
Mid upper-arm circumference (cm)	22	22	4.2	155	23	22	4.6	171	22	22	3.9	171	23	23	4.5	216	23	23	4.2	213
Waist circumference (cm)*	71	71	9.2	70	71	69	10.1	82	69	69	7.1	82	72	71	9.5	114	71	71	8.0	127
Hip circumference (cm)*	91	91	10.1	70	93	91	11.8	82	92	92	9.1	82	95	93	9.7	114	95	95	10.1	127
BMI (kg/m²)*	19	18	3.9	156	19	19	4.3	170	19	19	3.4	170	19	19	4.1	215	20	19	3.8	209
Waist to hip ratio*	0.78	0.77	0.050	70	0.77	0.77	0.057	82	0.75	0.75	0.042	82	0.76	0.75	0.050	114	0.75	0.74	0.048	127

*Young people aged 11 to 18 years.

367

Table 10.23 Anthropometric measurements for young person by whether young person's 'parents' were receiving certain benefits

Measurement	Whether receiving benefits							
	Receiving benefits			*Base*	Not receiving benefits			*Base*
	Mean	Median	sd		Mean	Median	sd	
Males								
Body weight (kg)	40	34	18.4	*230*	43	38	20.8	*759*
Height (cm)	142	141	24.1	*232*	147	146	23.8	*758*
Mid upper-arm circumference (cm)	22	21	4.4	*229*	23	22	4.7	*755*
Waist circumference (cm)*	74	73	9.9	*103*	76	74	10.9	*386*
Hip circumference (cm)*	90	89	9.0	*103*	92	92	11.1	*386*
BMI (kg/m^2)	19	18	3.4	*230*	19	18	3.8	*758*
Waist to hip ratio*	0.82	0.82	0.061	*103*	0.83	0.82	0.050	*386*
Females								
Body weight (kg)	38	35	17.1	*241*	42	41	17.4	*714*
Height (cm)	139	141	19.8	*241*	143	149	20.5	*713*
Mid upper-arm circumference (cm)	22	22	4.3	*241*	23	23	4.4	*716*
Waist circumference (cm)*	72	70	10.7	*111*	71	70	8.4	*385*
Hip circumference (cm)*	92	91	11.5	*111*	94	94	9.7	*385*
BMI (kg/m^2)	19	18	4.0	*240*	19	19	4.0	*712*
Waist to hip ratio*	0.78	0.77	0.055	*111*	0.76	0.75	0.051	*385*

*Young people aged 11 to 18 years.

Table 10.24 Anthropometric measurements for boys by plasma testosterone concentration – age-specific tertiles**

Boys aged 10 to 16 years

Measurement	Plasma testosterone concentration–tertiles											
	Bottom				Middle				Top			
	Mean	Median	sd	Base	Mean	Median	sd	Base	Mean	Median	sd	Base
Body weight (kg)	49	46	17.0	88	49	49	13.6	88	50	49	12.7	84
Height (cm)	154	152	14.6	88	157	159	13.7	88	159	161	12.0	84
Mid upper-arm circumference (cm)	24	24	4.0	88	25	24	3.7	88	24	24	3.3	84
Waist circumference (cm)*	74	71	11.6	73	73	72	8.0	74	73	72	7.0	70
Hip circumference (cm)*	88	86	11.7	73	89	88	8.5	74	88	87	8.0	70
BMI (kg/m^2)	20	19	4.2	88	20	19	3.2	88	19	19	2.7	84
Waist to hip ratio*	0.84	0.83	0.053	73	0.82	0.82	0.055	74	0.82	0.83	0.043	70

*Young people aged 11 to 16 years.
**Plasma testosterone concentration tertiles were calculated for boys at each individual year of age. The data for all boys aged 10 to 16 were then pooled to allow the calculation of means, medians and standard deviations.

Table 10.25 Measurements by age and whether menarche had occurred*

Girls aged 12 to 13 years co-operating with the self-completion questionnaire

Measurement and age	Whether menarche had occurred							
	Occurred			*Base*	Not occurred			*Base*
	Mean	Median	sd		Mean	Median	sd	
Height (cm)								
12 years	156	156	6.4	*29*	152	152	5.7	*46*
13 years	159	160	6.9	*35*	156	157	7.2	*22*
Body weight (kg)								
12 years	52	52	7.1	*29*	45	44	8.7	*46*
13 years	57	55	12.6	*33*	46	46	11.4	*22*
Waist to hip ratio								
12 years	0.77	0.76	0.05	*29*	0.80	0.78	0.06	*46*
13 years	0.75	0.74	0.06	*33*	0.78	0.78	0.04	*22*

*Sample sizes for these groups are small (< 50) and estimates should be treated with caution.

Table 10.26 BMI quintile by sex of young person and region

BMI (kg/m²)	Sex of young person and region									
	Males					Females				
	Scotland	Northern	Central, South West and Wales	London and the South East	All males	Scotland	Northern	Central, South West and Wales	London and the South East	All females
	%	%	%	%	%	%	%	%	%	%
Age-sex specific BMI quintile										
Bottom	26	24	14	21	20	22	22	18	20	20
Second	13	17	21	23	20	19	21	22	20	20
Third	15	17	23	20	20	25	16	20	22	20
Fourth	14	24	20	20	20	22	19	18	22	20
Top	32	17	22	16	20	13	23	23	15	20
Base	*80*	*272*	*342*	*295*	*989*	*79*	*248*	*340*	*286*	*953*

Table 10.27 BMI quintile by sex of young person and social class of head of household

BMI (kg/m²)	Sex of young person and social class of head of household					
	Males			Females		
	Non-manual	Manual	All males*	Non-manual	Manual	All females*
	%	%	%	%	%	%
Age-sex specific BMI quintile						
Bottom	21	19	20	18	22	20
Second	20	20	20	20	23	20
Third	22	18	20	23	18	20
Fourth	21	21	20	22	19	20
Top	17	22	20	17	19	20
Base	*460*	*455*	*989*	*437*	*420*	*953*

*Includes those not allocated a social class because their job was inadequately described, they were a member of the armed forces, had never worked or it was not known whether they had ever worked.

Table 10.28 BMI quintile by sex of young person and gross household income

BMI (kg/m²)

	Sex of young person and gross household income											
	Males						Females					
	Less than £160 per week	£160 to less than £280 per week	£280 to less than £400 per week	£400 to less than £600 per week	£600 or more per week	All males*	Less than £160 per week	£160 to less than £280 per week	£280 to less than £400 per week	£400 to less than £600 per week	£600 or more per week	All females*
	%	%	%	%	%	%	%	%	%	%	%	%
Age-sex specific BMI quintile												
Bottom	20	26	15	22	18	20	21	20	20	18	22	20
Second	22	15	21	20	22	20	24	22	21	21	17	20
Third	22	17	20	19	21	20	17	18	17	22	24	20
Fourth	18	20	26	21	20	20	18	18	23	21	20	20
Top	18	21	18	17	20	20	20	22	19	18	17	20
Base	*158*	*181*	*182*	*199*	*234*	*989*	*156*	*170*	*161*	*215*	*209*	*953*

* includes those not answering income question.

371

Table 10.29   BMI quintile by sex of young person and whether young person's 'parents' were receiving certain benefits

BMI (kg/m^2)	Sex of young person and whether 'parents' receiving benefits					
	Males			Females		
	Receiving benefits	Not receiving benefits	All males	Receiving benefits	Not receiving benefits	All females*
	%	%	%	%	%	%
Age-sex specific BMI quintile						
Bottom	20	20	20	21	20	20
Second	19	20	20	24	20	20
Third	21	19	20	18	21	20
Fourth	17	22	20	18	21	20
Top	23	18	20	20	19	20
Base	*230*	*758*	*989*	*240*	*712*	*953*

Table 10.30   BMI quintile by whether menarche had occurred

Girls aged 10 to 18 years co-operating with the self-completion questionnaire

Whether menarche had occurred	Age-sex specific BMI quintile					
	Bottom	Second	Third	Fourth	Top	Total
	%	%	%	%	%	%
Occurred	49	60	68	70	74	64
Not occurred	51	40	32	30	26	36
Base	*107*	*115*	*114*	*116*	*106*	*558*

Table 10.31   BMI quintile by whether young person was dieting to lose weight

Sex and whether dieting to lose weight	Age-sex specific BMI quintile					
	Bottom	Second	Third	Fourth	Top	Total
	%	%	%	%	%	%
Males						
Dieting	–	1	1	2	9	3
Not dieting	100	99	99	98	91	97
Base	*199*	*199*	*196*	*199*	*196*	*989*
Females						
Dieting	1	3	6	8	14	6
Not dieting	99	97	94	92	86	94
Base	*186*	*198*	*189*	*194*	*186*	*953*

Table 10.32   Reported height of young person's parents*

	Mother's height (cm)	Father's height (cm)
Mean	162	177
Median	163	178
Percentiles:		
2.3	150	160
9.0	152	165
25.0	157	173
50.0	163	178
75.0	168	183
91.0	170	188
97.7	175	193
Standard deviation	7.3	8.3
Base	*1920*	*1867*

*Based only on biological parents of the young person

10.33(a) Characteristics found to be independently related to BMI: males aged 4 to 18 years

Characteristic	Unstandardised coefficient (B)	Standard error of B	Standardised regression coefficient (β)	T–value
Constant (natural log (ln) BMI)	2.85	0.25		
Age at measurement of height and weight (years)	0.01	0.00	0.31	7.64***
Systolic blood pressure (mmHg)	0.00	0.00	0.26	7.48***
Diastolic blood pressure (mmHg)				−1.22
Reported dieting to lose weight	0.24	0.03	0.20	7.53***
Average daily total energy intake (MJ)	0.00	0.00	0.16	4.62***
Percentage energy from total fat	0.00	0.00	−0.14	−2.39*
Percentage energy from total sugars	0.00	0.00	−0.12	−3.28**
Percentage energy from total carbohydrate				−1.64
Gross weekly household income				
Less than £160	−0.03	0.01	−0.11	−2.04*
£160–less than £400	0.01	0.01	0.06	1.49
£400 & over	0.01	0.01	0.06	1.53
Region				
Scotland	0.03	0.01	0.10	2.45*
Northern	−0.01	0.01	−0.06	−1.72
Central, South West & Wales	0.00	0.01	0.01	0.22
London & South East	−0.02	0.01	−0.06	−2.41*
Whether living with both parents				
Both parents & other children				−1.89
Both parents & no other children				−1.04
Single parent & other children				0.57
Single parent & no other children				1.33
Social class of head of household				
Non-manual				0.04
Manual				−0.99
Unclassified				0.58
Parents were receiving benefits				0.97
Reported currently smoking				0.90
Average daily alcohol intake (g)				−1.12
Mother's reported height (cm)				−0.23
Father's reported height (cm)				−0.45
Percentage of variance explained		50%		
Number of young people		*767*		

* $p < 0.05$; ** $p < 0.01$; *** $p < 0.001$

10.33(b)   Characteristics found to be independently related to BMI: males aged 7 to 18 years

Characteristic	Unstandardised coefficient (B)	Standard error of B	Standardised regression coefficient (β)	T–value
Constant (natural log (ln) BMI)	2.89	0.31		
Age at measurement of height and weight (years)	0.02	0.00	0.33	6.99***
Reported dieting to lose weight	0.25	0.04	0.22	7.07***
Systolic blood pressure (mmHg)	0.00	0.00	0.27	6.80***
Diastolic blood pressure (mmHg)	0.00	0.00	−0.07	−1.98*
Average daily total energy intake (MJ)	0.00	0.00	0.16	4.29***
Percentage energy from total fat	0.00	0.00	−0.14	−1.95*
Percentage energy from total sugars	0.00	0.00	−0.12	−2.77**
Percentage energy from total carbohydrate				−1.61
Region				
Scotland	0.03	0.02	0.11	2.20*
Northern	−0.02	0.01	−0.09	−2.04*
Central, South West & Wales	0.00	0.01	0.01	0.33
London & South East	−0.02	0.01	−0.05	−1.68
Gross weekly household income				
Less than £160	−0.03	0.02	−0.13	−2.11*
£160–less than £400	0.01	0.01	0.07	1.64
£400 & over	0.02	0.01	0.07	1.53
Calculated activity score				−1.74
Social class of head of household				
Non-manual				0.51
Manual				−0.54
Unclassified				−0.01
Average daily alcohol intake (g)				−1.19
Mother's reported height (cm)				0.75
Father's reported height (cm)				−0.82
Whether living with both parents				
Both parents & other children				−0.92
Both parents & no other children				−1.43
Single parent & other children				0.62
Single parent & no other children				1.02
Parents were receiving benefits				0.89
Reported currently smoking				0.21
Percentage of variance explained	47%			
Number of young people	595			

* p < 0.05; ** p < 0.01; *** p < 0.001

10.33(c) Characteristics found to be independently related to BMI: males aged 10 to 16 years with plasma testosterone concentration

Characteristic	Unstandardised coefficient (B)	Standard error of B	Standardised regression coefficient (β)	T–value
Constant (natural log (ln) BMI)	2.47	0.64		
Age at measurement of height and weight (years)	0.02	0.01	0.21	2.34*
Reported dieting to lose weight	0.47	0.06	0.43	7.49***
Systolic blood pressure (mmHg)	0.00	0.00	0.19	2.69**
Diastolic blood pressure (mmHg)	0.00	0.00	−0.08	−1.24
Average daily total energy intake (MJ)	0.00	0.00	0.22	3.33**
Percentage energy from total fat				−0.36
Percentage energy from total carbohydrate				−0.25
Percentage energy from total sugars				−1.20
Average daily alcohol intake (g)				1.84
Calculated activity score				−1.85
Region				
Scotland				−0.08
Northern				−1.63
Central, South West & Wales				1.76
London & South East				0.13
Social class of head of household				
Non-manual				−0.11
Manual				0.18
Unclassified				−0.04
Mother's reported height (cm)				1.12
Father's reported height (cm)				0.01
Plasma testosterone concentration				
Bottom tertile				−0.39
Middle tertile				0.09
Top tertile				0.35
Whether living with both parents				
Both parents & other children				1.18
Both parents & no other children				0.19
Single parent & other children				−0.33
Single parent & no other children				−0.54
Gross weekly household income				
Less than £160				0.46
£160–less than £400				0.22
£400 & over				−0.82
Parents were receiving benefits				−0.39
Reported currently smoking				−0.31
Percentage of variance explained	37%			
Number of young people	*217*			

* p < 0.05; ** p < 0.01; *** p < 0.001

375

10.33(d)   Characteristics found to be independently related to BMI: females aged 4 to 18 years

Characteristic	Unstandardised coefficient (B)	Standard error of B	Standardised regression coefficient (β)	T–value
Constant (natural log (ln) BMI)	2.98	0.28		
Age at measurement of height and weight (years)	0.01	0.00	0.26	5.16***
Had reached menarche	0.11	0.02	0.28	6.00***
Systolic blood pressure (mmHg)	0.00	0.00	0.23	6.29***
Diastolic blood pressure (mmHg)				−1.60
Average daily total energy intake (MJ)	0.00	0.00	0.08	2.67**
Percentage energy from total fat				−1.92
Percentage energy from total carbohydrate				−1.08
Percentage energy from total sugars				−1.70
Reported dieting to lose weight	0.09	0.02	0.12	4.11***
Social class of head of household				
Non-manual	−0.01	0.01	−0.05	−1.55
Manual	−0.02	0.01	−0.06	−2.04*
Unclassified	0.03	0.01	0.11	2.48*
Mother's reported height (cm)				0.24
Father's reported height (cm)	0.00	0.00	−0.07	−2.41*
Region				
Scotland				−1.19
Northern				0.68
Central, South West & Wales				0.70
London & South East				0.53
Average daily alcohol intake (g)				−1.26
Whether living with both parents				
Both parents & other children				−1.57
Both parents & no other children				−0.89
Single parent & other children				0.32
Single parent & no other children				1.29
Gross weekly household income				
Less than £160				−0.71
£160–less than £400				0.50
£400 & over				
Parents were receiving benefits				−0.78
Reported currently smoking				−1.58
Percentage of variance explained		49%		
Number of young people		*711*		

* p < 0.05; ** p < 0.01; *** p < 0.001

10.33(e) Characteristics found to be independently related to BMI: females aged 7 to 18 years

Characteristic	Unstandardised coefficient (B)	Standard error of B	Standardised regression coefficient (β)	T–value
Constant (natural log (ln) BMI)	2.98	0.35		
Age at measurement of height and weight (years)	0.01	0.00	0.21	3.38***
Had reached menarche	0.11	0.02	0.29	5.08***
Systolic blood pressure (mmHg)	0.00	0.00	0.24	5.56***
Diastolic blood pressure (mmHg)				−1.48
Reported dieting to lose weight	0.09	0.02	0.13	3.73***
Social class of head of household				
Non-manual	−0.01	0.01	−0.05	−1.25
Manual	−0.02	0.01	−0.07	−2.11*
Unclassified	0.03	0.01	0.12	2.34*
Average daily total energy intake (MJ)	0.00	0.00	0.07	1.96*
Percentage energy from total fat				−1.73
Percentage energy from total carbohydrate				−0.97
Percentage energy from total sugars	0.00	0.00	−0.09	−2.01*
Mother's reported height (cm)				0.44
Father's reported height (cm)	0.00	0.00	−0.07	−2.00*
Region				
Scotland				−0.62
Northern				0.56
Central, South West & Wales				0.66
London & South East				−0.20
Average daily alcohol intake (g)				−1.40
Whether living with both parents				
Both parents & other children				−1.22
Both parents & no other children				−1.27
Single parent & other children				0.87
Single parent & no other children				0.93
Gross weekly household income				
Less than £160				−0.71
£160–less than £400				−0.05
£400 & over				0.92
Parents were receiving benefits				−0.77
Reported currently smoking				−1.15
Calculated activity score				0.11
Percentage of variance explained		41%		
Number of young people		*554*		

* p < 0.05; ** p < 0.01; *** p < 0.001

10.34(a) Characteristics found to be independently related to waist to hip ratio: males aged 11 to 18 years

Characteristic	Unstandardised coefficient (B)	Standard error of B	Standardised regression coefficient (β)	T–value
Constant (natural log (ln) waist to hip ratio)	–0.07	0.18		
Age at measurement of waist and hip (years)	0.00	0.00	–0.16	–2.31*
Region				
Scotland	–0.02	0.01	–0.14	–1.69
Northern	0.02	0.01	0.20	2.86**
Central, South West & Wales	0.01	0.01	0.17	2.50*
London & South East	–0.01	0.01	–0.13	–2.64**
Gross weekly household income				
Less than £160	–0.02	0.01	–0.20	–1.92
£160–less than £400	0.01	0.01	0.15	2.05*
£400 & over	0.01	0.01	0.08	1.00
Reported dieting to lose weight	0.07	0.02	0.19	3.77***
Whether living with both parents				
Both parents & other children	–0.01	0.01	–0.13	–2.18*
Both parents & no other children	–0.01	0.01	–0.08	–1.25
Single parent & other children	0.01	0.01	0.07	1.31
Single parent & no other children	0.01	0.01	0.10	0.96
Systolic blood pressure (mmHg)				–1.25
Diastolic blood pressure (mmHg)				0.84
Average daily total energy intake (MJ)				–0.81
Percentage energy from total fat				–0.02
Percentage energy from total carbohydrate				–0.50
Percentage energy from total sugars				0.45
Calculated activity score				–0.25
Social class of head of household				
Non-manual				0.24
Manual				–0.75
Unclassified				0.31
Average daily alcohol intake (g)				0.34
Mother's reported height (cm)				0.34
Father's reported height (cm)				0.06
Parents were receiving benefits				0.94
Reported currently smoking				0.74
Percentage of variance explained		11%		
Number of young people		*378*		

* $p < 0.05$; ** $p < 0.01$; *** $p < 0.001$

10.34(b) Characteristics found to be independently related to waist to hip ratio: males aged 11 to 16 years with plasma testosterone concentration

Characteristic	Unstandardised coefficient (B)	Standard error of B	Standardised regression coefficient (β)	T–value
Constant (natural log (ln) waist to hip ratio)	0.24	0.32		
Age at measurement of waist and hip (years)				−0.71
Calculated activity score				−1.91
Region				
Scotland				−0.94
Northern				1.92
Central, South West & Wales				0.60
London & South East				−0.88
Reported dieting to lose weight				1.24
Systolic blood pressure (mmHg)				−0.80
Diastolic blood pressure (mmHg)				−0.01
Average daily total energy intake (MJ)				−0.84
Percentage energy from total fat				−0.10
Percentage energy from total carbohydrate				−0.61
Percentage energy from total sugars				0.52
Average daily alcohol intake (g)				0.93
Social class of head of household				
Non-manual				−0.81
Manual				−0.99
Unclassified				1.14
Mother's reported height (cm)				0.65
Father's reported height (cm)				−1.51
Plasma testosterone concentration****				
Bottom tertile				0.71
Middle tertile				0.28
Top tertile				−1.07
Whether living with both parents				
Both parents & other children				−0.28
Both parents & no other children				−1.16
Single parent & other children				0.24
Single parent & no other children				0.70
Gross weekly household income				
Less than £160				0.56
£160–less than £400				−0.08
£400 & over				−0.74
Parents were receiving benefits				−0.47
Reported currently smoking				0.91
Percentage of variance explained	4%			
Number of young people	*182*			

* $p < 0.05$; ** $p < 0.01$; *** $p < 0.001$
**** Tertiles were re-calculated for the sample aged 11 to 16 years

10.34(c) Characteristics found to be independently related to waist to hip ratio: females aged 11 to 18 years

Characteristic	Unstandardised coefficient (B)	Standard error of B	Standardised regression coefficient (β)	T–value
Constant (natural log (ln) waist to hip ratio)	0.05	0.18		
Age at measurement of waist and hip (years)	0.00	0.00	−0.16	−2.22*
Had reached menarche	−0.03	0.01	−0.19	−3.05**
Social class of head of household				
Non-manual	−0.02	0.01	−0.16	−2.75**
Manual	0.01	0.01	0.07	1.36
Unclassified	0.01	0.01	0.09	1.10
Reported dieting to lose weight	0.03	0.01	0.13	2.48*
Mother's reported height (cm)				−1.47
Father's reported height (cm)	0.00	0.00	−0.11	−2.16*
Reported currently smoking	−0.02	0.01	−0.11	−2.04*
Region				
Scotland	−0.02	0.01	−0.13	−1.70
Northern	0.01	0.01	0.06	0.90
Central, South West & Wales	0.01	0.01	0.08	1.14
London & South East	0.00	0.01	0.03	0.68
Systolic blood pressure (mmHg)				1.15
Diastolic blood pressure (mmHg)				0.02
Average daily total energy intake (MJ)				−0.38
Percentage energy from total fat				−0.44
Percentage energy from total carbohydrate				0.28
Percentage energy from total sugars				−1.61
Average daily alcohol intake (g)				−0.32
Whether living with both parents				
Both parents & other children				−0.07
Both parents & no other children				0.85
Single parent & other children				−0.02
Single parent & no other children				−0.59
Gross weekly household income				
Less than £160				0.46
£160–less than £400				−0.90
£400 & over				0.11
Parents were receiving benefits				1.32
Calculated activity score				0.44
Percentage of variance explained		20%		
Number of young people		*358*		

* p < 0.05; ** p < 0.01; *** p < 0.001

Table 10.35 Height of young person by sex and age in single years compared with the Health of Young People '95-'97*

Young people living in England

Height (cm)

	Age (in years)														
	4	5	6	7	8	9	10	11	12	13	14	15	16	17	18
Males															
Health Survey 1995-97															
Mean (average value)	105.9	112.2	118.9	125.0	131.1	135.9	141.3	147.3	152.6	159.7	165.6	172.0	175.0	176.0	176.4
Lower 5.0 percentile	98.2	103.9	110.9	116.8	122.2	126.0	130.4	136.0	140.2	145.6	150.6	160.2	162.7	164.6	166.2
Upper 5.0 percentile	113.6	121.2	127.4	133.9	141.2	145.4	151.8	158.6	165.9	175.1	180.0	184.8	186.8	187.0	188.1
Standard error of the mean	0.22	0.25	0.24	0.25	0.26	0.30	0.31	0.33	0.39	0.43	0.45	0.38	0.45	0.46	0.45
Base	*528*	*520*	*527*	*526*	*550*	*476*	*507*	*498*	*498*	*461*	*470*	*451*	*297*	*248*	*234*
NDNS 1997															
Mean (average value)	105.9	113.3	118.4	124.3	130.8	135.9	140.8	146.3	152.9	157.0	165.3	171.6	174.0	176.5	178.1
Lower 5.0 percentile	99.5	105.3	110.0	117.9	119.5	126.3	128.8	134.5	143.5	141.8	152.7	159.9	163.3	164.7	169.7
Upper 5.0 percentile	112.1	122.3	127.8	134.4	139.6	147.5	148.1	159.4	168.1	170.0	177.6	185.8	185.8	191.8	188.9
Standard deviation of the mean	4.56	5.21	5.33	4.96	6.38	6.16	6.24	7.58	7.68	8.43	7.78	7.65	6.75	7.76	6.70
Base	*47*	*59*	*76*	*57*	*73*	*59*	*59*	*73*	*52*	*49*	*61*	*58*	*47*	*48*	*44*
Females															
Health Survey 1995-97															
Mean (average value)	105.5	112.0	118.2	124.1	129.7	135.8	142.0	148.1	153.9	157.9	161.1	162.4	163.8	163.2	163.4
Lower 5.0 percentile	98.3	102.9	108.5	115.4	121.1	125.2	131.9	135.8	142.1	146.4	151.2	151.0	154.1	153.1	153.2
Upper 5.0 percentile	113.0	121.0	126.4	134.6	139.2	147.3	153.2	161.2	164.5	168.7	171.4	172.5	174.2	173.7	173.9
Standard error of the mean	0.21	0.25	0.25	0.28	0.26	0.32	0.31	0.37	0.34	0.34	0.32	0.35	0.34	0.37	0.42
Base	*548*	*534*	*516*	*527*	*549*	*471*	*529*	*476*	*459*	*444*	*477*	*420*	*333*	*305*	*247*
NDNS 1997															
Mean (average value)	104.7	111.0	116.7	125.0	130.7	136.1	139.5	146.7	153.9	157.7	160.7	160.8	162.0	163.5	163.0
Lower 5.0 percentile	99.5	102.7	108.3	114.2	121.4	124.1	125.6	137.0	143.1	144.5	151.0	151.1	149.5	153.7	154.2
Upper 5.0 percentile	110.9	119.1	127.6	136.4	143.9	146.9	149.7	160.4	163.9	168.3	172.9	168.7	174.9	170.3	171.6
Standard deviation of the mean	3.74	5.54	5.73	6.09	6.21	6.61	7.59	7.79	6.19	7.04	6.03	6.18	7.09	5.90	5.50
Base	*44*	*56*	*75*	*50*	*41*	*63*	*61*	*59*	*66*	*48*	*59*	*53*	*59*	*51*	*46*

* Prescott-Clarke P, Primatesta P. Eds. *Health Survey for England. The Health of Young People 95-97. Volume 1: Findings*. TSO (London, 1998).

Table 10.36   Height of white children in the NDNS, the Health of Young People '95-'97* and the NSHG 1994** by sex and age

White young people aged 5 to 10 years living in England

Height (cm)	Age (in years)						
	5	6	7	8	9	10	All
Males							
NSHG 1994							
Mean (average value)	112.8	118.9	124.9	130.6	136.8	141.2	127.0
Standard error of the mean	0.23	0.25	0.24	0.28	0.32	0.32	0.22
Median	112.8	119.2	124.7	130.7	136.3	141.3	127.0
Base	*460*	*443*	*495*	*459*	*386*	*401*	*2644*
Health Survey 1995-97							
Mean (average value)	112.1	118.9	124.9	131.0	135.8	141.4	127.3
Standard error of the mean	0.26	0.25	0.26	0.28	0.31	0.33	0.23
Median	112.0	119.2	125.0	130.6	136.1	141.3	127.5
Base	*461*	*488*	*487*	*489*	*435*	*459*	*2819*
NDNS 1997							
Mean (average value)	113.1	118.3	124.3	130.2	136.3	141.1	126.8
Standard deviation of the mean	5.34	5.29	5.15	6.22	6.18	6.10	11.20
Median	113.4	117.5	123.8	131.4	135.8	142.6	126.5
Base	*55*	*72*	*48*	*67*	*53*	*55*	*350*
Females							
NSHG 1994							
Mean (average value)	111.3	118.3	124.3	129.6	135.5	141.3	126.4
Standard error of the mean	0.25	0.25	0.25	0.31	0.35	0.32	0.23
Median	111.3	118.3	124.0	129.6	135.5	141.0	125.8
Base	*443*	*440*	*455*	*398*	*378*	*434*	*2548*
Health Survey 1995-97							
Mean (average value)	111.7	118.1	124.0	129.8	135.8	142.0	126.8
Standard error of the mean	0.26	0.26	0.29	0.28	0.32	0.32	0.24
Median	111.6	118.2	123.8	129.3	135.5	141.7	126.6
Base	*483*	*464*	*468*	*485*	*427*	*477*	*2804*
NDNS 1997							
Mean (average value)	110.6	116.6	124.8	130.5	136.3	139.4	126.2
Standard deviation of the mean	4.84	5.60	5.92	6.09	6.06	7.63	12.37
Median	111.0	116.0	124.8	131.5	137.0	140.6	125.7
Base	*54*	*66*	*40*	*38*	*55*	*60*	*313*

* Prescott-Clarke P, Primatesta P. Eds. *Health Survey for England. The Health of Young People '95-97. Volume 1: Findings.* TSO (London, 1998).
** The National Study of Health and Growth was set up in 1972 to monitor the growth of primary school children. For example, see Chinn S, Price C.E, Rona R.J. The need for new reference curves for height. *Arch Dis Childh* 1989; **64:** 1545-1553.

Table 10.37 **Body weight of young person by sex and age in single years compared with the Health of Young People '95-'97***

Young people living in England

Body weight (kg)	Age (in years)														
	4	5	6	7	8	9	10	11	12	13	14	15	16	17	18
Males															
Health Survey 1995-97															
Mean (average value)	18.4	20.4	22.9	25.8	29.1	32.0	35.6	40.2	44.8	50.8	56.4	62.9	66.7	70.1	70.5
Lower 5.0 percentile	15.0	16.3	18.0	20.5	22.7	24.0	26.7	29.3	31.0	35.0	39.0	47.1	49.5	52.1	55.5
Upper 5.0 percentile	22.5	25.5	29.1	33.7	39.4	43.9	51.8	55.2	63.1	71.6	79.7	85.6	89.7	95.9	92.1
Standard error of the mean	0.11	0.15	0.16	0.19	0.26	0.30	0.34	0.42	0.50	0.58	0.63	0.62	0.76	0.88	0.81
Base	*532*	*519*	*518*	*526*	*542*	*472*	*503*	*488*	*491*	*457*	*462*	*448*	*288*	*242*	*231*
NDNS 1997															
Mean (average value)	18.4	21.2	23.0	25.0	27.8	31.0	37.1	40.4	45.6	47.9	57.2	63.0	67.5	69.2	71.6
Lower 5.0 percentile	15.6	16.7	19.2	20.5	21.0	22.5	27.0	27.9	32.4	34.0	44.5	46.8	50.5	46.2	54.8
Upper 5.0 percentile	23.5	28.0	28.1	32.6	36.6	39.0	60.7	58.5	66.5	68.0	78.6	89.6	94.0	91.7	90.8
Standard deviation of the mean	2.04	3.43	2.84	3.27	4.62	5.03	9.67	9.73	10.23	9.53	11.32	12.79	15.47	15.31	11.88
Base	*47*	*59*	*77*	*58*	*73*	*59*	*59*	*73*	*52*	*49*	*61*	*57*	*47*	*48*	*44*
Females															
Health Survey 1995-97															
Mean (average value)	18.3	20.4	22.8	25.9	28.8	32.7	37.1	42.4	47.5	51.8	56.7	58.4	60.3	60.2	61.6
Lower 5.0 percentile	14.7	16.2	17.7	19.8	21.7	24.2	27.8	28.9	34.4	38.9	41.3	43.6	46.4	46.5	46.7
Upper 5.0 percentile	23.4	25.5	30.2	37.9	41.0	45.7	52.9	62.3	66.0	70.6	80.3	79.2	79.4	77.2	83.9
Standard error of the mean	0.12	0.15	0.18	0.26	0.27	0.36	0.38	0.51	0.50	0.53	0.59	0.65	0.60	0.60	0.81
Base	*549*	*525*	*508*	*519*	*544*	*466*	*522*	*462*	*448*	*430*	*457*	*410*	*319*	*290*	*237*
NDNS 1997															
Mean (average value)	18.1	20.2	22.0	25.9	29.8	33.6	36.3	40.6	48.8	51.9	54.4	57.3	59.8	59.9	60.6
Lower 5.0 percentile	15.1	15.7	17.3	19.3	23.1	24.2	25.6	30.1	37.0	34.9	38.3	40.0	47.4	44.6	46.3
Upper 5.0 percentile	22.2	24.8	28.5	33.5	42.7	48.1	49.1	59.5	63.2	75.5	65.5	88.1	78.8	79.2	81.6
Standard deviation of the mean	2.51	2.99	3.65	4.39	5.99	7.42	7.33	8.59	8.50	12.91	8.95	12.74	10.71	11.24	10.84
Base	*45*	*56*	*75*	*51*	*41*	*63*	*62*	*57*	*66*	*46*	*59*	*53*	*59*	*51*	*46*

* Prescott-Clarke P. Primatesta P. Eds. *Health Survey for England. The Health of Young People 95-97. Volume 1: Findings.* TSO (London, 1998).

Table 10.38 Body weight† of white children in the NDNS, the Health of Young People '95–'97* and the NSHG 1994 by sex and age**

White young people aged 5 to 10 years living in England

Body weight (kg)	Age (in years)						
	5	6	7	8	9	10	All
Males							
NSHG 1994							
Mean (average value)	19.8	22.1	24.8	27.7	31.4	34.8	26.5
Standard error of the mean	0.14	0.16	0.18	0.22	0.29	0.36	0.14
Median	19.5	21.8	24.3	27.0	30.3	33.2	25.3
Base	*459*	*443*	*492*	*459*	*386*	*404*	*2643*
Health Survey 1995–97							
Mean (average value)	19.7	22.3	25.1	28.4	31.1	34.7	26.9
Standard error of the mean	0.14	0.16	0.20	0.28	0.31	0.35	0.15
Median	19.4	22.0	24.4	27.3	29.8	33.5	25.6
Base	*460*	*479*	*486*	*484*	*432*	*453*	*2794*
NDNS 1997							
Mean (average value)	20.1	22.2	24.6	26.8	30.5	36.8	26.6
Standard deviation of the mean	2.83	2.79	3.20	4.35	5.12	9.90	7.45
Median	19.8	22.1	24.2	26.8	30.0	34.1	25.1
Base	*55*	*73*	*49*	*67*	*53*	*55*	*352*
Females							
NSHG 1994							
Mean (average value)	19.3	22.0	24.9	27.7	31.9	35.5	26.7
Standard error of the mean	0.14	0.17	0.21	0.28	0.37	0.38	0.16
Median	19.1	21.5	24.2	26.8	30.5	34.2	25.1
Base	*445*	*439*	*453*	*397*	*375*	*432*	*2541*
Health Survey 1995–97							
Mean (average value)	19.6	22.2	25.2	28.4	31.9	36.6	27.3
Standard error of the mean	0.14	0.18	0.26	0.29	0.34	0.38	0.16
Median	19.5	21.7	24.1	27.3	30.7	34.9	25.8
Base	*474*	*459*	*461*	*481*	*423*	*472*	*2770*
NDNS 1997							
Mean (average value)	19.4	21.4	25.3	29.0	33.3	35.5	27.3
Standard deviation of the mean	2.52	3.63	3.98	5.57	7.44	7.39	8.24
Median	19.6	20.6	25.0	28.5	32.9	34.0	25.1
Base	*54*	*66*	*41*	*38*	*55*	*60*	*314*

† Weight for the Health Survey and NDNS was adjusted for clothing to obtain unclothed weight; in NSHG informants were weighed wearing underpants.
* Prescott-Clarke P, Primatesta P. Eds. *Health Survey for England. The Health of Young People 95-97. Volume 1: Findings.* TSO (London, 1998).
** The National Study of Health and Growth was set up in 1972 to monitor the growth of primary school children. For example, see Chinn S, Price C.E, Rona R.J. The need for new reference curves for height. *Arch Dis Childh* 1989; **64:** 1545–1553.

Young people living in England

BMI (kg/m²)	Age (in years)														
	4	5	6	7	8	9	10	11	12	13	14	15	16	17	18

Males

Health Survey 1995–97

BMI (kg/m²)	4	5	6	7	8	9	10	11	12	13	14	15	16	17	18
Mean (average value)	16.4	16.2	16.1	16.4	16.8	17.2	17.7	18.4	19.1	19.7	20.4	21.2	21.7	22.6	22.6
Lower 5.0 percentile	14.4	14.2	13.9	14.3	14.2	14.4	14.6	15.0	15.2	15.7	16.3	17.1	17.7	17.9	18.7
Upper 5.0 percentile	19.1	18.5	19.1	19.5	20.7	21.8	23.1	24.0	25.0	25.9	27.0	27.9	28.5	30.6	29.8
Standard error of the mean	0.07	0.08	0.08	0.08	0.11	0.12	0.12	0.14	0.15	0.17	0.18	0.18	0.21	0.26	0.23
Base	*518*	*513*	*515*	*523*	*541*	*472*	*499*	*487*	*489*	*456*	*462*	*446*	*288*	*242*	*231*

NDNS 1997

BMI (kg/m²)	4	5	6	7	8	9	10	11	12	13	14	15	16	17	18
Mean (average value)	16.4	16.4	16.3	16.2	16.2	16.7	18.6	18.7	19.3	19.4	20.8	21.2	22.2	22.2	22.5
Lower 5.0 percentile	14.3	14.4	14.4	13.9	14.0	14.1	15.1	15.2	15.6	14.8	17.1	17.3	17.6	17.0	18.7
Upper 5.0 percentile	19.1	21.0	18.7	18.9	20.4	20.1	29.0	25.6	24.2	25.0	28.2	27.0	29.2	29.4	26.6
Standard deviation of the mean	1.39	1.71	1.32	1.58	1.77	1.67	3.71	3.53	2.83	3.19	3.16	2.87	4.15	4.43	2.86
Base	*47*	*59*	*76*	*57*	*73*	*59*	*59*	*73*	*52*	*49*	*61*	*57*	*47*	*48*	*44*

Females

Health Survey 1995–97

BMI (kg/m²)	4	5	6	7	8	9	10	11	12	13	14	15	16	17	18
Mean (average value)	16.4	16.2	16.2	16.4	17.0	17.6	18.3	19.2	20.0	20.7	21.8	22.1	22.4	22.6	23.0
Lower 5.0 percentile	14.2	14.2	13.7	13.9	13.8	14.3	14.8	14.9	15.6	16.2	16.7	17.4	17.9	18.1	17.9
Upper 5.0 percentile	19.3	19.6	20.4	19.5	22.4	22.9	24.9	26.6	26.7	27.2	29.7	28.9	29.1	29.8	30.2
Standard error of the mean	0.08	0.09	0.09	0.11	0.12	0.14	0.14	0.18	0.17	0.18	0.20	0.20	0.21	0.21	0.30
Base	*541*	*522*	*507*	*517*	*544*	*465*	*522*	*462*	*448*	*429*	*456*	*409*	*318*	*290*	*236*

NDNS 1997

BMI (kg/m²)	4	5	6	7	8	9	10	11	12	13	14	15	16	17	18
Mean (average value)	16.4	16.3	16.1	16.4	17.3	18.0	18.5	18.8	20.5	20.8	21.0	22.1	22.8	22.4	22.8
Lower 5.0 percentile	13.7	14.0	13.8	13.9	14.3	14.3	15.3	15.4	16.3	15.8	16.7	16.1	18.3	17.8	17.3
Upper 5.0 percentile	18.9	18.9	19.6	19.5	21.2	23.0	22.6	27.0	26.3	30.3	26.3	31.8	31.7	30.2	29.9
Standard deviation of the mean	1.66	1.53	1.67	2.02	2.21	2.87	2.92	3.37	3.08	4.55	3.30	4.25	4.14	3.87	3.59
Base	*44*	*56*	*75*	*50*	*41*	*63*	*62*	*57*	*66*	*46*	*59*	*53*	*59*	*51*	*46*

* Prescott-Clarke P. Primatesta P. Eds. *Health Survey for England. The Health of Young People 95–97. Volume 1: Findings.* TSO (London, 1998).

Table 10.40   BMI† of white children in the NDNS, the Health of Young People '95-'97* and the NSHG 1994 by sex and age**

White young people aged 5 to 10 years living in England

BMI (kg/m²)	Age (in years)						
	5	6	7	8	9	10	All
Males							
NSHG 1994							
Mean (average value)	15.5	15.6	15.8	16.2	16.7	17.3	16.1
Standard error of the mean	0.07	0.07	0.08	0.09	0.12	0.13	0.04
Median	15.4	15.4	15.6	15.8	16.3	16.7	15.8
Base	*458*	*443*	*492*	*459*	*386*	*401*	*2639*
Health Survey 1995–97							
Mean (average value)	15.6	15.7	16.0	16.5	16.8	17.3	16.3
Standard error of the mean	0.07	0.08	0.09	0.12	0.12	0.13	0.04
Median	15.4	15.5	15.7	15.9	16.2	16.8	15.8
Base	*455*	*477*	*484*	*483*	*432*	*451*	*2782*
NDNS 1997							
Mean (average value)	15.7	15.8	15.9	15.7	16.3	18.3	16.3
Standard deviation of the mean	1.15	1.32	1.44	1.73	1.74	3.83	2.21
Median	15.5	15.9	15.8	15.4	16.4	17.0	15.9
Base	*55*	*72*	*48*	*67*	*53*	*55*	*350*
Females							
NSHG 1994							
Mean (average value)	15.6	15.6	16.0	16.4	17.2	17.6	16.4
Standard error of the mean	0.07	0.09	0.09	0.12	0.14	0.14	0.05
Median	15.3	15.4	15.7	15.9	16.4	17.0	15.9
Base	*443*	*439*	*453*	*397*	*375*	*432*	*2539*
Health Survey 1995–97							
Mean (average value)	15.7	15.8	16.3	16.8	17.2	18.0	16.6
Standard error of the mean	0.09	0.09	0.12	0.13	0.14	0.15	0.05
Median	15.4	15.5	15.7	16.3	16.8	17.2	16.1
Base	*472*	*458*	*460*	*481*	*422*	*472*	*2765*
NDNS 1997							
Mean (average value)	15.8	15.7	16.1	16.9	17.7	18.2	16.8
Standard deviation of the mean	1.52	1.70	1.79	2.11	2.97	2.97	2.49
Median	15.6	15.6	16.0	16.6	17.2	17.9	16.1
Base	*54*	*66*	*40*	*38*	*55*	*60*	*313*

† Weight for the Health Survey and NDNS was adjusted for clothing to obtain unclothed weight; in NSHG informants were weighed wearing underpants.
* Prescott-Clarke P, Primatesta P. Eds. *Health Survey for England. The Health of Young People 95-97. Volume 1: Findings.* TSO (London, 1998).
** The National Study of Health and Growth was set up in 1972 to monitor the growth of primary school children. For example, see Chinn S, Price C.E, Rona R.J. The need for new reference curves for height. *Arch Dis Childh* 1989; **64:** 1545–1553.

Table 10.41 Mid upper-arm circumference of young person by sex and age in single years compared with the Health of Young People '95–'97*

Young people living in England

Mid upper-arm circumference (cm)	Age (in years)											
	4	5	6	7	8	9	10	11	12	13	14	15
Males												
Health Survey 1995–97												
Mean (average value)	17.8	18.1	18.5	19.2	20.0	20.7	21.6	22.7	23.5	24.3	25.4	26.8
Lower 5.0 percentile	15.5	15.6	15.7	16.5	17.0	17.3	17.8	18.2	19.0	19.4	20.4	22.1
Upper 5.0 percentile	21.1	20.9	22.6	23.1	24.6	25.7	27.5	28.9	30.0	30.7	32.6	33.6
Standard error of the mean	0.08	0.08	0.10	0.10	0.12	0.14	0.14	0.17	0.18	0.18	0.20	0.19
Base	*486*	*481*	*495*	*503*	*510*	*440*	*480*	*450*	*457*	*422*	*418*	*413*
NDNS 1997												
Mean (average value)	17.5	18.2	18.7	18.8	19.4	20.3	22.3	22.4	23.8	24.2	25.6	26.6
Lower 5.0 percentile	15.5	15.6	16.1	16.1	16.9	16.2	17.8	18.2	19.5	19.0	20.7	22.4
Upper 5.0 percentile	20.3	20.9	21.8	22.0	23.3	25.0	31.8	28.5	29.6	30.5	32.5	32.8
Standard deviation of the mean	1.66	1.98	1.63	1.78	1.92	2.52	3.66	2.94	3.06	3.28	3.45	3.17
Base	*45*	*56*	*76*	*58*	*72*	*60*	*58*	*74*	*52*	*48*	*62*	*58*
Females												
Health Survey 1995–97												
Mean (average value)	18.2	18.4	18.9	19.8	20.7	21.7	22.5	23.6	24.4	25.0	26.3	26.5
Lower 5.0 percentile	15.6	15.9	16.0	16.5	17.2	17.8	18.3	19.2	19.6	20.4	21.1	21.9
Upper 5.0 percentile	21.8	21.6	23.1	24.7	25.9	27.3	28.6	30.8	30.9	30.9	34.2	33.9
Standard error of the mean	0.09	0.09	0.11	0.12	0.13	0.15	0.15	0.18	0.18	0.18	0.21	0.21
Base	*510*	*485*	*476*	*497*	*514*	*442*	*488*	*442*	*428*	*408*	*439*	*384*
NDNS 1997												
Mean (average value)	17.7	18.5	18.4	19.7	20.9	21.5	22.6	22.5	24.6	25.0	25.5	26.4
Lower 5.0 percentile	15.3	16.3	15.8	16.3	17.2	17.6	18.3	18.4	20.4	20.1	20.4	20.9
Upper 5.0 percentile	20.1	21.9	23.0	24.4	25.5	28.5	27.3	26.9	29.5	31.6	29.3	38.5
Standard deviation of the mean	1.64	1.72	2.20	2.37	2.33	3.08	3.32	2.54	2.70	3.49	2.96	4.15
Base	*44*	*57*	*75*	*51*	*41*	*63*	*62*	*58*	*66*	*49*	*59*	*53*

* Prescott-Clarke P, Primatesta P. (Eds.) *Health Survey for England. The Health of Young People 95–97. Volume 1: Findings.* TSO (London, 1998).

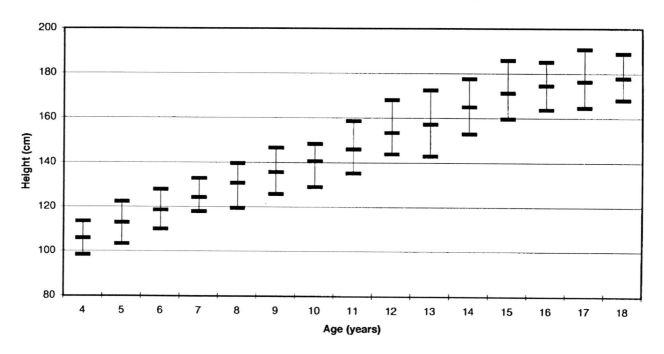

Figure 10.1a Height by age: males - means and lower and upper 5.0 percentiles

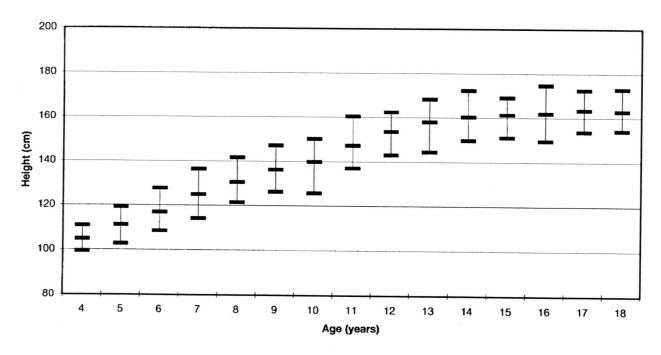

Figure 10.1b Height by age: females - means and lower and upper 5.0 percentiles

Figure 10.2a Weight by age: males - means and lower and upper 5.0 percentiles

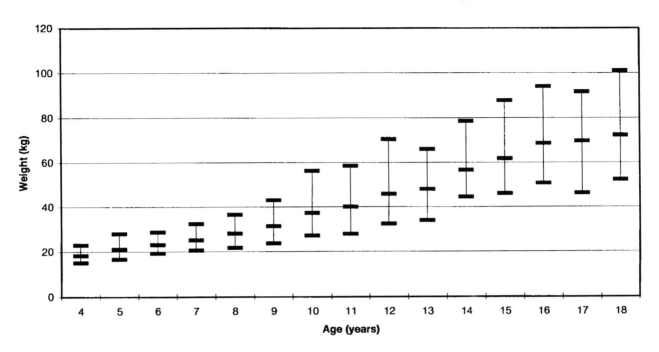

Figure 10.2b Weight by age: females - means and lower and upper 5.0 percentiles

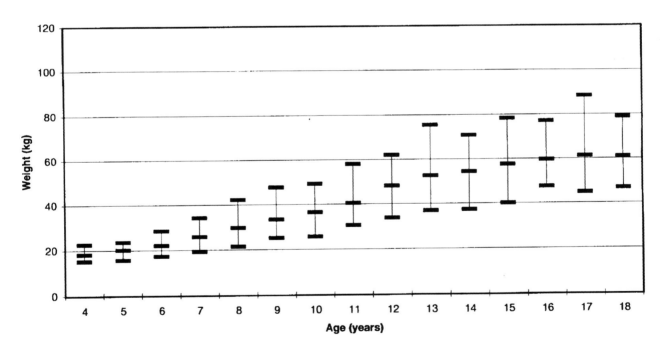

389

Figure 10.3a BMI by age: males - means and lower and upper 5.0 percentiles

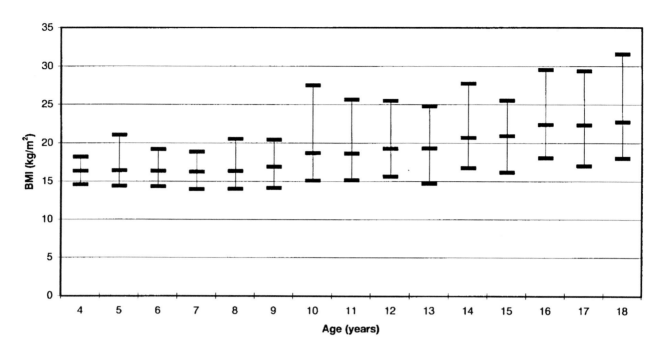

Figure 10.3b BMI by age: females - means and lower and upper 5.0 percentiles

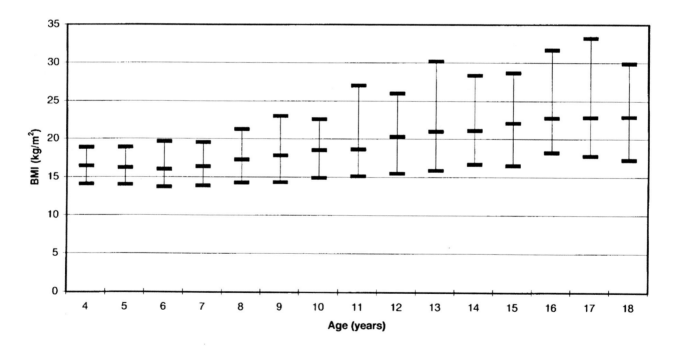

Figure 10.4a Mid upper-arm circumference by age: males - means and lower and upper 5.0 percentiles

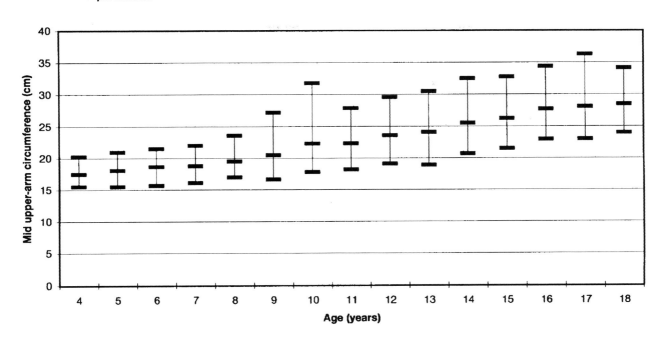

Figure 10.4b Mid upper-arm circumference by age: females - means and lower and upper 5.0 percentiles

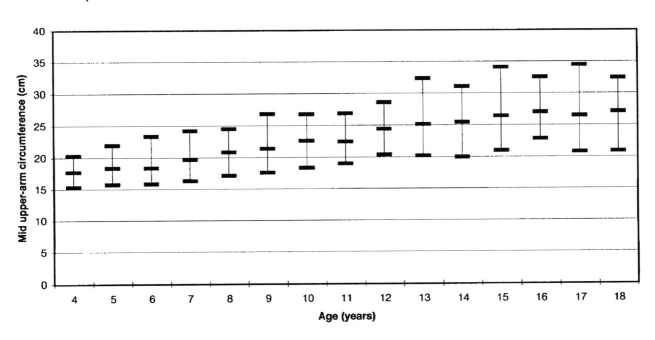

Figure 10.5a Waist circumference by age: males - means and lower and upper 5.0 percentiles

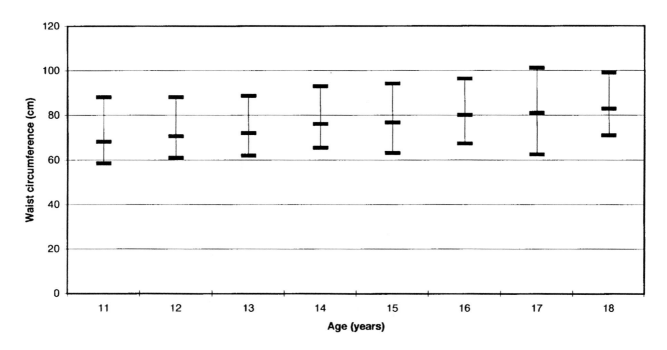

Figure 10.5b Waist circumference by age: females - means and lower and upper 5.0 percentiles

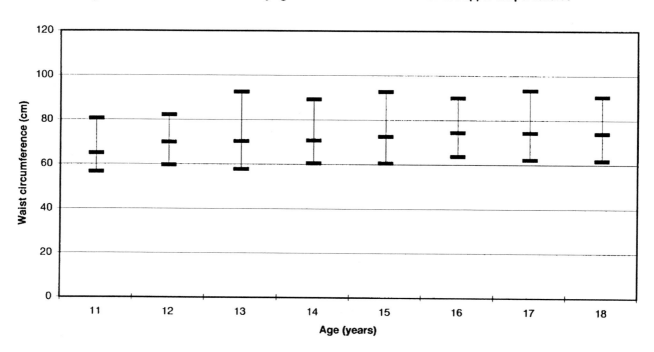

Figure 10.6a Hip circumference by age: males - means and lower and upper 5.0 percentiles

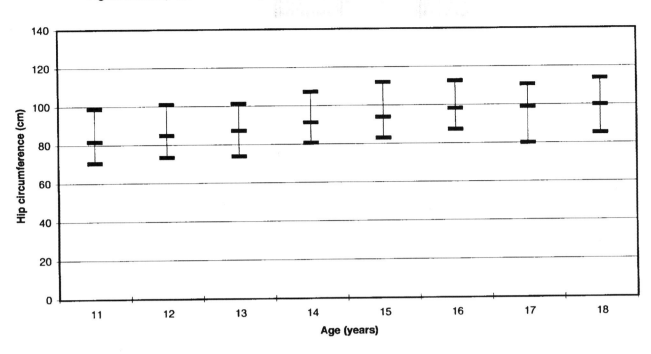

Figure 10.6b Hip circumference by age: females - means and lower and upper 5.0 percentiles

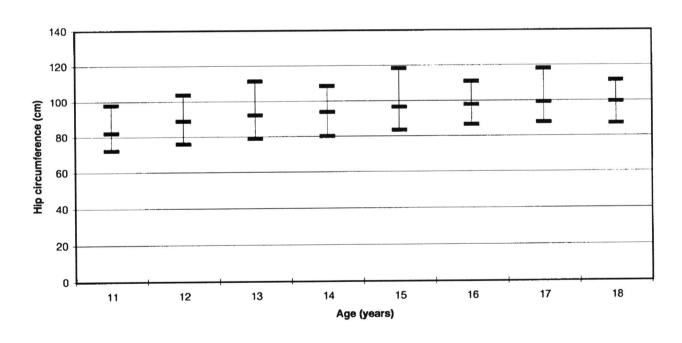

11 Blood pressure

11.1 Introduction

The purpose of making the blood pressure measurements is explained in Chapters 1 and 2 and response rates for the measurements are presented in Chapter 3. Also the equipment and procedures for taking the measurements are fully described in Chapter 2 and in Appendix L.

This chapter presents descriptive data on blood pressures for young people in the survey, and in Section 11.3.3 considers the independent effects on blood pressure of various socio-demographic, behavioural and dietary variables.

11.1.1 Blood pressure measurements used in the analyses

Measurements were only made if signed consent had been obtained both to taking the measurements and to passing the readings to the young person's General Practitioner[1]. If both these consents were obtained and the young person assented to the procedure then three measurements of blood pressure were made at pre-set intervals of one minute (see *Chapter 2*). Since the first measurement might have been artificially high, particularly if the young person was anxious, the first reading from each set of three measurements was excluded and the mean of the subsequent two readings calculated. It is this average value that has been used for analyses and is presented in the tables and charts in this chapter. Where it was possible to take only two blood pressure measurements for a young person, the second reading has been used in the analysis. For seven young people (unweighted) only one cycle of blood pressure measurements was made successfully; these seven cases have been excluded from the analysis. This method of treating and presenting the data has been used in previous NDNS and other surveys, including major national surveys where blood pressure measurements have been made[2,3,4]. It is believed to be more likely to approximate to the participants' usual blood pressure, which in turn is more likely to predict adverse cardiovascular events[5].

Interviewers were encouraged to report any difficulties they had in making the blood pressure measurements or any unusual circumstances; these were recorded on the measurement schedule. In about 5% of cases where at least two successful measurements were made, some difficulty or unusual circumstance was reported[6].

Difficulty in wrapping the blood pressure cuff, either because the young person had a conical-shaped upper arm or the circumference of their arm was larger than could accommodate a cuff of the appropriate width, accounted for about half the difficulties.

Mean arterial pressure has been estimated by adding the level of the diastolic pressure to one third of the difference between the systolic and diastolic blood pressures. This method of deriving mean arterial pressure has been used in the NDNS progamme[2,3]. However the Dinamap automatically provides a figure for mean arterial pressure, and this figure is reported in the Health Survey of Young People[4]. Comparisons of mean arterial pressure for young people in this survey with data from the Health Survey of Young People are therefore based on the Dinamap direct measure. Indications are that the direct measure provided by the Dinamap is higher by an average of about 2mmHg than the calculated value for the young people in this survey.

11.1.2 Interpretation of blood pressure levels

As described in Appendix L the Dinamap 8100 automatic monitor which was used to measure blood pressures in this survey has been validated in several studies, but compared with measurements made using a mercury sphygmomanometer, the Dinamap has been shown to produce higher systolic and lower diastolic blood pressure levels, both in children and in adults[7,8,9,10]. This means that direct comparison between measurements made using the Dinamap monitor and other blood pressure data where measurements have been made using a different instrument, in particular those using an ausculatory method, are inadvisable. However, as noted above, the Dinamap 8100 was used to measure blood pressure in the Health Survey of Young People[4] and given this similarity in methodology, results from the two surveys are compared in Section 11.4.

In interpreting the blood pressure results for the young people in this survey it should also be remembered that these are cross-sectional data, in that the blood pressure was measured at a single point in time, and for children, more so than for adults, blood pressure is likely to be variable over time.

Other studies have shown that blood pressure in children and young people is more strongly associated with age than in adults, and hence the results presented in this Chapter are classified by age[11,12]. However these studies have also shown that blood pressure in children is associated with height and weight, and that ideally when reporting blood pressures for children they should be adjusted for age and height, as has been done for the Health Survey of Young People[4]. The relatively small size of the single-year age and sex groups in this survey (approximately 55 cases per group, unweighted) have not allowed this adjustment for height to be made, and this needs to be borne in mind when interpreting the results.

The available guidelines for blood pressure in children are based on combined data collected from nine studies, using a different methodology and different instruments, a mercury sphygmomanometer, or in the case of infants, Doppler instruments[13]. Hence they are inappropriate for comparisons with data collected using the Dinamap.

11.2 Results

Results are presented for 968 males and 930 females (unweighted numbers) who took part in the survey. Distributions and descriptive statistics are given for measurements of systolic and diastolic pressures and mean arterial pressure by sex and age group and by the main socio-demographic characteristics of the sample. Descriptive statistics are also given for pressures according to whether the young person reported currently smoking cigarettes (young people aged 11 to 18 years only), average daily intake of alcohol, as derived from the 7-day weighed intake dietary record (young people aged 15 to 18 years only), whether the young person reported currently being on a diet to lose weight, and by the reported use of salt in the young person's food at the table and in cooking. In all these tables age groups are shown as for the dietary analysis, that is one three-year age band, 4 to 6 years, and three four-year age bands, 7 to 10 years, 11 to 14 years and 15 to 18 years. In figures which show blood pressures for males and females in the survey, age is shown in single-year age bands. Age has been calculated by subtracting the young person's date of birth from the date when the blood pressure measurements were made, and therefore some young people may be classified in different age bands to those at other stages of the survey.

At the end of this chapter blood pressures measured in this survey are compared with pressures reported in the Health Survey of Young People[4], and for these comparisons age is shown in single-year bands, based on age last birthday. This means that the numbers of males and females in each of the age bands is relatively small, and this needs to be borne in mind when comparing the two sets of data, and determining the significance of any differences.

Systolic blood pressure[14]
Mean systolic blood pressure was 110mmHg for males and 108mmHg for females (p < 0.05). Median values were close to and slightly below mean values, 109mmHg for boys and 107mmHg for girls. For both sexes mean systolic blood pressure increased with increasing age from 102mmHg and 101mmHg for boys and girls aged 4 to 6 years, to 121mmHg and 114mmHg for boys and girls aged 15 to 18 years (p < 0.01).

At the lower 5.0 percentile systolic blood pressure for all age groups of both boys and girls, except the oldest boys, was below 100mmHg, but for both sexes tended to rise with age. For boys aged 15 to 18 years, 5% had a systolic blood pressure at or below 104mmHg. At the upper 5.0 percentile systolic blood pressure ranged from 115mmHg and 116mmHg respectively for boys and girls aged 4 to 6 years, to 138mmHg for boys and 132mmHg for girls aged 15 to 18 years.
(Table 11.1; Figures 11a, 11d and 11e)

Diastolic blood pressure[14]
Mean diastolic blood pressure was 56mmHg for both boys and girls in the survey. For boys, mean diastolic pressure, unlike mean systolic blood pressure, varied very little with age, rising from 55mmHg for boys aged 4 to 6 years to 57mmHg for boys aged 15 to 18 years (ns). However for girls, mean diastolic pressure, like mean systolic pressure, increased significantly with age, from 54mmHg for the youngest girls to 59mmHg for the oldest group of girls (p < 0.01).

Median values were very close to mean values, 55mmHg for boys and 56mmHg for girls. At the lower 5.0 percentile, diastolic pressure for boys varied hardly at all with age and overall was 20% lower than the median value (43mmHg). For girls there was some variation, but the pattern was not consistent. For girls aged 4 to 6 years diastolic blood pressure at the lower 5.0 percentile was 44mmHg and for those aged 15 to 18 years, 48mmHg.

At the upper 5.0 percentile diastolic blood pressure for boys was between 67mmHg and 71mmHg, increasing with age, while for girls diastolic pressures were between 66mmHg and 74mmHg, also increasing as age increased. *(Table 11.2; Figures 11b, 11f and 11g)*

Mean arterial pressure (MAP)[14]
The mean value for mean arterial pressure was 74mmHg for boys and 73mmHg for girls in the survey, and for both sexes increased significantly with age. For boys and girls aged 4 to 6 years mean values for mean arterial pressure were 71mmHg and 70mmHg respectively (ns); among the oldest age group mean values for mean arterial pressure were 78mmHg for boys and 77mmHg for girls (p < 0.01). Median values for mean arterial pressure were almost identical to mean values, 73mmHg for both sexes.

Mean arterial pressures for young people at the lower and upper 5.0 percentiles of the distribution also varied with age. For example, for boys aged 4 to 6 years MAPs were 60mmHg and 82mmHg at the lower and upper 5.0 percentiles, compared with 66mmHg and 93mmHg for boys aged 15 to 18 years.

(Table 11.3; Figures 11c, 11h and 11i)

11.3 Variation in blood pressure

11.3.1 Effects of dietary behaviours on blood pressure

Tables 11.4 and 11.5 show statistics for average systolic, diastolic and mean arterial blood pressures for boys and girls in the survey according to the reported use of salt in their food when cooking, and the reported frequency of salt being added to their food at the table. Information on the use of salt in cooking and at the table was collected during the initial interview, which preceded the 7-day dietary record. Tables showing the use of salt by boys and girls in the four age groups are presented in Chapter 9 (see *Tables 9.19 and 9.20*).

For boys there were no significant differences in mean systolic, diastolic or mean arterial blood pressures associated with whether *salt was usually added to their food in cooking*, although there was a general pattern for blood pressures to be slightly higher for those who had salt added in cooking. At the lower and upper extremes of the distribution, 5.0 and 95.0 percentiles, average pressures differed by up to 3mmHg between boys who had salt generally added to their food in cooking and those for whom salt was not added.

For girls, mean systolic pressure was significantly higher for those who had salt added to their food in cooking, 109mmHg, than for those for whom salt was reported as not being added, 106mmHg (p < 0.01). However, like boys, there were no significant differences in either mean diastolic or mean arterial pressures between the two groups of girls.

A similar pattern was apparent when *the use of salt at the table* was considered. Young people who usually added salt to their food at the table had diastolic and mean arterial blood pressures which were slightly higher than for those who only *occasionally, rarely or never* added salt to their food at the table. For mean systolic pressures the differences between those who usually added salt to their food at the table and those who did so occasionally, rarely or never, reached the level of statistical significance for both boys and girls (p < 0.01).

(Tables 11.4 and 11.5)

Tables 11.6 and 11.7 show mean blood pressures for boys and girls according to whether they reported *dieting to lose weight* at the time of the survey and whether they reported currently *smoking* cigarettes. Both tables are restricted to young people aged 11 to 18 years.

Mean systolic blood pressure for the very few boys who reported dieting to lose weight (19 boys, unweighted) was significantly higher than for boys who were non-dieters, 124mmHg compared with 115mmHg (p < 0.05). For girls however mean systolic pressure was the same for those who reported currently dieting to lose weight and for those who were not dieting, 112mmHg.

For both boys and girls, the group who were dieting to lose weight generally had a somewhat higher mean diastolic and mean arterial blood pressure than non-dieters, but none of the differences was statistically significant.

Boys who were smokers had a significantly higher mean systolic pressure than boys who reported being non-smokers, 120mmHg compared with 114mmHg (p < 0.01). For girls, mean systolic pressure was somewhat higher for those who were smokers, 114mmHg compared with 111mmHg for non-smokers, but the difference did not reach the level of statistical significance (p > 0.05).

Girls who reported being current smokers generally had a somewhat higher mean diastolic pressure than non-smokers and both boys and girls who reported being smokers had a higher mean arterial blood pressure than non-smokers, but none of the differences was statistically significant.

(Tables 11.6 and 11.7)

Table 11.8 shows mean blood pressures for young people in the survey aged 15 to 18 years by their *reported alcohol intake*, that is the average daily intake of alcohol calculated from their entries in the 7-day dietary record. The numbers of young people reporting consuming alcohol were relatively small, and this may account for some of the differences in the data not being statistically significant. However, for boys there was a general pattern for blood pressure, and particularly for diastolic and mean arterial pressure, to be higher for those with the highest levels of alcohol consumption. For example, mean diastolic pressure for those who had intakes of an average of 10g or more of alcohol a day was 60mmHg, compared with 56mmHg for those who had zero alcohol intakes during the 7-day recording period, (medians 61mmHg and 56mmHg) (p < 0.05).

For girls, the data consistently show that the highest mean blood pressures were in those consuming alcohol but less than an average of 3g a day, although it should be noted that this is a very small group of girls. For example, mean systolic pressure in girls aged 15 to 18 years with zero alcohol intake was 113mmHg, in those with intakes up to 3mg alcohol a day, 120mmHg, and in those with intakes of 10g or more a day, 115mmHg (medians 112mmHg, 117mmHg and 117mmHg). This pattern among those who reported consuming the very smallest amounts of alcohol might suggest an under-reporting of alcohol consumption by this particular group.

(Table 11.8)

As Table 11.9 shows, mean blood pressures for young people who reported being *unwell* during the dietary recording period were very similar to mean blood pressures for those who reported not being unwell. There was however a consistent pattern for mean pressures for those whose eating was affected by being unwell to be lower than mean pressures for both those who were not unwell and for those who were unwell but whose eating was not affected. However the differences were relatively small and did not reach statistical significance (p > 0.05). *(Table 11.9)*

11.3.2 Effects of socio-demographic factors on blood pressure

Tables 11.10 to 11.13 show mean blood pressures for boys and girls in the survey according to the main socio-demographic variables, including region, gross weekly household income and household type.

The data show only very small, and non-significant differences (p > 0.05) in mean blood pressures for young people living in different *regions*, from different *social class* backgrounds, according to *gross weekly household income*, and household *benefit status*.

Table 11.14, which shows mean blood pressures by household type, suggests that mean systolic pressures were significantly higher for young people living with both parents and no other children, than for young people living with just one parent or those living with both parents and with other children. For example, mean systolic pressure for boys living with both parents and no other children was 114mmHg, compared with 109mmHg for those living with one parent, and 108mmHg for those living with both parents and other children (p < 0.01). However, as has been noted before, the age composition of the different household types is markedly different. In particular over 50% of the young people living with both parents and no other children were in the top age group, 15 to 18 years, compared with about 15% of those living with both parents and other children (see Table 3.19). Thus the higher mean systolic pressures reported for boys and girls living with both parents and no other children might be accounted for by there being a much larger proportion of the oldest children in the group. *(Tables 11.10 to 11.14)*

11.3.3 Characteristics independently associated with variation in blood pressure

The method

Multiple regression modelling was carried out to find out which combinations of socio-demographic, behavioural and physiological variables were independently associated with blood pressure for young people. Analyses were carried out separately for systolic and diastolic pressures and for boys and girls separately.

Tables 11.15 to 11.18 show the regression coefficients from the regression models for the variables that were entered into the models and found to be significant (p < 0.05, p < 0.01 and p < 0.001).

The technique of multiple regression calculates coefficients based on the number of cases for which there are valid values for all the variables included in the analysis. Among the behavioural variables of interest was physical activity level, as indicated by the calculated activity level score. However this was only derived for young people aged 7 to 18 years who completed a full 7-day physical activity diary, a total of 711 boys and 713 girls; young people aged 4 to 6 years did not keep physical activity diaries (see *Chapter 13*). Additionally for boys, the effect of blood testosterone level on blood pressures was of interest. Blood testosterone concentration was only measured for boys aged 10 to 16 years who provided a blood sample, a total of 260 boys (see *Chapter 12*). Including physical activity score and, in the analysis for boys, blood testosterone level, in a single regression would therefore markedly reduce the number of cases available for analysis. It was therefore decided that a number of separate analyses should be run:

for boys:
- all boys aged 4 to 18 years, *excluding* physical activity score and blood testosterone level – Tables 11.15(a) and 11.17(a);
- all boys aged 7 to 18 years, *including* physical activity score, but *excluding* blood testosterone level – Tables 11.15(b) and 11.17(b);
- all boys aged 10 to 16 years, *including* physical activity score and blood testosterone level – Tables 11.15(c) and 11.17(c);

for girls:
- all girls aged 4 to 18 years, *excluding* physical activity score – Tables 11.16(a) and 11.18(a);
- all girls aged 7 to 18 years, *including* physical activity score – Tables 11.16(b) and 11.18(b)

Except for those analyses that included blood testosterone level the regression analyses were carried out after weighting for differential sampling probabilities and differential non-response. The analyses for boys that included blood testosterone level were not weighted (see *Chapter 12; Section 12.1.2*)[15].

The regression coefficients show the amount by which a factor increased or decreased the blood pressure once all the other factors in the model were taken into account. Thus the coefficients can be used to estimate the blood pressure for young people with particular characteristics by adding the unstandardised coefficients for each relevant characteristic to the constant calculated by the model.

For example, from Table 11.15(a), a male aged 16 years, who currently smoked, was unwell and his eating was affected during the dietary recording period, with a diastolic blood pressure of 56mmHg and a body weight 69.5kg would have a predicted systolic blood pressure of:

$$65.96 + (0.34 \times 16) + 2.96 - 1.94 + (0.46 \times 56) + (0.29 \times 69.5) = 118\text{mmHg}$$

where 65.96 (constant)
 + 0.34 (per year age)
 + 2.96 (current smoker)
 − 1.94 (unwell and eating affected)
 + 0.46 (per mmHg diastolic pressure)
 + 0.29 (per kilo weight)

Findings: systolic blood pressure
It can be seen from Table 11.15(a) that for boys aged 4 to 18 years there were very few significant associations between systolic blood pressure and the socio-demographic variables included in the analyses. Overall for boys the most significant associations with systolic blood pressure were with the physiological measurements included in the analysis, that is with diastolic blood pressure and weight (both: $p < 0.001$). Age was also independently related to systolic blood pressure ($p < 0.05$). Taking account of all other variables in the model, there was a significant inverse association with systolic blood pressure for boys who were unwell during the 7-day dietary recording period and whose eating was affected ($p < 0.05$) and a significant positive relationship with systolic blood pressure for boys who were smokers ($p < 0.05$). Overall being a smoker increased systolic blood pressure in boys aged 4 to 18 years by + 2.96mmHg compared with being a non-smoker.

For girls, as for boys the most significant associations with systolic blood pressure were with diastolic blood pressure and body weight (both: $p < 0.001$) (Table 11.16(a)). There was also a significant inverse relationship for girls living in London and the South East but none of the other socio-demographic, dietary or behavioural variables included in the model was significantly related to systolic blood pressure.

Overall these models accounted for 50% of the variation in systolic blood pressure for boys aged 4 to 18 years and 47% for girls aged 4 to 18 years.

As described above the same variables plus calculated physical activity score were included in a regression analysis but restricted to those aged 7 to 18 years (Tables 11.15(b) and 11.16(b)). For this group of both boys and girls there was no significant association between calculated physical activity score and systolic blood pressure. For boys, this model again identified significant associations with age ($p < 0.01$), diastolic blood pressure and weight (both: $p < 0.001$) and an inverse association for boys who were unwell and their eating affected (($p < 0.01$). For this group of boys being a smoker had no significant effect on systolic blood

pressure. For girls the equivalent model only identified significant relationships with diastolic blood pressure and weight (both: $p < 0.001$). This second model accounted for 48% of the variation in systolic blood pressure for boys aged 7 to 18 years and 45% of the variation in systolic blood pressure for girls.

The final model which was for boys aged 10 to 16 years, included blood testosterone tertile, which was not significantly associated with systolic blood pressure (Table 11.15(c)). The model accounted for 37% of the variation in systolic blood pressure for this group of boys, mainly accounted for by variation in diastolic blood pressure and weight (both: $p < 0.001$).

Findings: diastolic blood pressure
Generally, and for boys in particular, less of the variation in diastolic blood pressure was explained by the variables included in the regression analyses. For boys the models explained between 16% and 18% of the variation in diastolic pressure and for the two groups of girls the models explained 32% and 35% of the variation.

For boys aged 4 to 18 years the strongest relationship was between diastolic pressure and systolic pressure ($p < 0.001$). There were however also significant inverse independent relationships between diastolic blood pressure and weight, with the urinary potassium to creatinine ratio and for those interviewed in Wave 3 of fieldwork, July to September[16], (all: $p < 0.05$). Overall this model accounted for 18% of the variation in diastolic blood pressure (Table 11.17(a)).

The model for boys aged 7 to 18 years, which included calculated physical activity score, accounted for 17% of the variation in diastolic pressure (Table 11.17(b)). As was found overall for all boys there was a significant positive association with systolic pressure ($p < 0.001$) and a significant inverse relationship with weight ($p < 0.05$). None of the other variables included in this model, including the calculated physical activity score was significantly associated with diastolic blood pressure.

The final model for boys, which included only those aged 10 to 16 years for whom plasma testosterone concentration was measured, accounted for 16% of the variation in diastolic blood pressure (Table 11.17(c)). In common with the other two models, diastolic pressure was again found to be positively associated with systolic pressure ($p < 0.001$) and, in this model, with whether the boy's parents were in receipt of benefits ($p < 0.05$). There was no significant association between diastolic blood pressure and body weight for this group of boys.

As Table 11.18(a) shows overall for girls aged 4 to 18 years systolic pressure was significantly and positively associated with diastolic pressure ($p < 0.001$). There were also significant independent associations with fieldwork wave, positively for those interviewed in Wave 1 (January to March) (p < 0.05) and inversely for those interviewed in Wave 3 (July to September) (p < 0.01). Living with one parent and other children, usually adding salt to the food during cooking, and body weight were all independently inversely related to diastolic blood pressure for all girls (weight: p < 0.01; others: p < 0.05). This model accounted for 32% of the variation in diastolic blood pressure for girls aged 4 to 18 years.

In the analysis for girls aged 7 to 18 years which included the calculated physical activity score, the same independent associations were found as in the model for all girls aged 4 to 18 years described above. Calculated physical activity score was not significantly related to diastolic blood pressure and this model accounted for 35% of the variation in diastolic blood pressure for this group of girls.   *(Tables 11.15 to 11.18)*

11.4 Comparisons with other surveys

Tables 11.19 to 11.21 show mean systolic, diastolic and mean arterial pressures for boys and girls who took part in this NDNS of young people and who were living in England and for young people living in England who took part in the Health Survey of Young People[4]. The data are shown for single-year age groups, and for the Health of Young People Survey are combined data from three years, 1995 to 1997. In both surveys age is reported as age last birthday. Mean arterial pressures in Tables 11.21(a) and (b) are reported as direct readings from the Dinamap monitor.

All surveys used the same equipment and protocol for measuring blood pressures and the measurements obtained are reported in the same way, that is as the average value of the 2nd and 3rd readings, or if only two successful measurements were made, reporting the 2nd measurement made.

There were however differences in the survey protocols, which need to be taken into account when comparing the results from the different surveys. As described in Chapter 2 and Appendix L, in this NDNS of young people the blood pressure measurements were made by an interviewer, who had already visited the young person on several occasions, to carry out an initial interview, place and check the 7-day weighed intake dietary record, and make various anthropometric measurements. In the Health Survey of Young People blood pressures were measured by nurses, recruited specially to the survey, and, importantly, the occasion when the blood pressure measurement was made was the first occasion that the young person had met the nurse, who was not accompanied by the interviewer. Moreover in the Health Survey of Young People, at the same visit as measuring blood pressure, and depending on the young person's age, the nurse also measured mid upper-arm circumference (those under age 16 years),

waist and hip circumferences (those aged 16 and over), lung function (those aged 7 and over), obtained a saliva sample (sub-sample of those aged 4 to 17 years), and, if consent was given, attempted to obtain a blood sample (those aged 18 and over). In the NDNS the protocol specified that blood sampling could only take place after the end of the dietary recording period, and after the other anthropometric and physiological measurements, including blood pressure, had been made. This protocol was designed to minimise possible non-response to other aspects of the survey that might be associated with attempting to obtain the blood sample.

Tables 11.19 (a) and (b) show that the mean systolic blood pressure for both boys and girls taking part in the NDNS of young people was lower than the equivalent pressure reported for young people in the Health Survey of Young People. Thus for boys aged 5 to 15 years taking part in this NDNS mean systolic pressure was 107mmHg, compared with 111mmHg reported for boys in the Health Survey (p < 0.01). For girls the equivalent mean systolic pressures from the two surveys are 106mmHg and 111mmHg (p < 0.01). Also, in each single-year age group, the mean value for the average systolic pressure is lower for young people in the NDNS than in the Health Survey. The single year differences were statistically significant as follows: for boys, ages 9, 12 to 14, and 16 years: p < 0.01; ages 5 to 7, 15 and 17 years: p < 0.05; for girls, ages 5, 8 to 16, and 18 years: p < 0.01; age 17 years: p < 0.05.

There was a similar but less marked pattern in the data for diastolic blood pressures, Tables 11.20(a) and (b). Again overall the mean diastolic blood pressure for both boys and girls aged 5 to 15 years taking part in the NDNS was lower than the pressure reported in the Health Survey for young people of the same age; for boys taking part in the NDNS, 55mmHg, compared with 57mmHg reported for boys in the Health Survey, and for girls taking part in the NDNS, 55mmHg, compared with 58mmHg reported for girls in the Health Survey (both sexes: p < 0.01). By single-year age groups differences in mean diastolic pressure were statistically significant as follows: for boys, ages 8, 9, 12, 15, 16 and 18 years: p < 0.01; for girls, ages 5, 8, 10, 12, 13 and 15 years: p < 0.01; ages 9 and 18 years: p < 0.05.

Although the Health Survey data cover a three-year period, two of which were before this NDNS of young people, it is unlikely that the generally lower systolic and diastolic pressures measured in the NDNS represent a real reduction in mean blood pressures over such a relatively short time. Given that the same equipment was used to make the blood pressure measurements, it may be possible that the data from the different surveys illustrate what is frequently referred to as 'the white coat effect' that is a tendency for blood pressure to rise when it is measured by a doctor or nurse[17]. Although the nurses working on the Health Survey did not visit homes in their uniforms, the fact that they were not previously known to the young person may have had the same effect, raising the blood pressure. The finding that the difference between the surveys in mean systolic pressures is greater than the difference for diastolic pressures, which are less labile, supports this explanation.

It is worth noting that this effect is identifiable even though the first reading from three measurements, which is thought likely to be artificially high, was discarded. *(Tables 11.19 to 11.21)*

References and endnotes

1 If the young person was not registered with a General Practitioner then blood pressure measurements were not taken.

2 Gregory J, Foster K, Tyler H, Wiseman M. *The Dietary and Nutritional Survey of British Adults*. HMSO (London, 1990).

3 Finch S, Doyle W, Lowe C, Bates CJ, Prentice A, Smithers G, Clarke PC. *National Diet and Nutrition Survey: people aged 65 years and over. Volume 1: Report of the diet and nutrition survey*. TSO (London, 1998).

4 Prescott–Clarke P, Primatesta P. Eds *Health Survey for England. The Health of Young People '95–97. Volume 1: Findings*. TSO (London, 1998).

5 Petrie JC, O'Brien ET, Littler WA, de Swiet M. Recommendations on blood pressure measurement. *Br Med J* 1986: **293**: 611–615.

6 Where at least two successful measurements were made they have been included in the analyses, even if difficulties were reported.

7 Bolling K. *The Dinamap Calibration Study*. OPCS HMSO (London, 1994).

8 O'Brien E, Fitzgerald D, O'Mally K. Blood pressure measurement: current practice and future trends. *Br Med J* 1985; **290**: 729–734.

9 Weaver MG, Park MK, Lee KH. Differences in Blood Pressure Levels Obtained by Ausculatory and Oscillometric Methods. *Am J Dis Childh* 1990; **144**: 911–914.

10 O'Brien E. Automated blood pressure measurement: state of the market in 1998 and the need for an international validation protocol for blood pressure measuring devices. *Blood Pressure Monitoring* 1998; **3**: 205–211.

11 Kaas Ibsen K. Factors influencing blood pressure in children and adolescents. *Acta Paediatr Scand* 1985; **74**: 416–422.

12 Chen Y, Rennie DC, Reeder BA. Age–related associations between body mass index and blood pressure: The Humboldt Study. *Am J Epidemiol* 1986; **124**: 195–206.

13 National Heart, Lung and Blood Institute, Bethesda, Maryland, US. Report of the Second Task Force on Blood Pressure Control in Children – 1987. *Paediatrics* 1987; **79** (1).

14 Values for systolic, diastolic and mean arterial pressures are *average* values, derived as described in section 11.1.1 of this chapter. Mean values refer to the mean of the average systolic, diastolic or mean arterial pressures as appropriate.

15 The procedure was run in SPSS for Windows v9.0. For further details of the general method used and interpretation of results see Appendix E.

16 See *Appendix U 'Glossary'* for more details of the definition of fieldwork wave.

17 J Larry Hornsby J L (Ed), Mongan PF, A Thomas Tyler, Treiber FA. 'White Coat' Hypertension in Children. *J Fam Pract* 1991; **33**: 617–623.

Table 11.1 Percentage distribution of systolic blood pressure by sex and age of young person

Systolic blood pressure (mmHg)	Males aged (years)				All males	Females aged (years)				All females
	4–6	7–10	11–14	15–18		4–6	7–10	11–14	15–18	
	cum %	cum %	cum %	cum %	cum %	cum %	cum %	cum %	cum %	cum %
Less than 90	5	3	3	-	3	9	6	1	1	4
Less than 100	38	31	15	2	21	46	29	14	8	23
Less than 105	63	52	25	5	35	72	49	32	21	42
Less than 110	81	71	49	18	54	85	70	51	36	59
Less than 115	93	89	69	33	70	95	87	69	53	75
Less than 120	99	95	86	50	82	98	95	84	70	86
All	100	100	100	100	100	100	100	100	100	100
Base	*204*	*280*	*265*	*219*	*968*	*188*	*247*	*259*	*236*	*930*
Mean (average value)	102	104	110	121	110	101	105	110	114	108
Median value	102	105	110	120	109	101	105	110	114	107
Lower 5.0 percentile	90	90	93	104	92	87	90	95	97	91
Upper 5.0 percentile	116	120	126	138	131	115	122	126	132	126
Standard deviation of the mean	8.1	9.0	9.6	10.9	11.9	8.8	9.6	9.6	10.5	10.8

Table 11.2 Percentage distribution of diastolic blood pressure by sex and age of young person

Diastolic blood pressure (mmHg)	Males aged (years)				All males	Females aged (years)				All females
	4–6	7–10	11–14	15–18		4–6	7–10	11–14	15–18	
	cum %	cum %	cum %	cum %	cum %	cum %	cum %	cum %	cum %	cum %
Less than 50	27	25	21	18	23	29	23	21	12	21
Less than 55	49	51	50	41	48	54	50	46	34	46
Less than 60	73	75	70	64	70	76	74	71	61	70
Less than 70	97	98	96	95	96	98	96	97	92	96
All	100	100	100	100	100	100	100	100	100	100
Base	*204*	*280*	*265*	*219*	*968*	*188*	*247*	*259*	*236*	*930*
Mean (average value)	55	55	56	57	56	54	56	56	59	56
Median value	55	55	55	57	55	54	55	56	58	56
Lower 5.0 percentile	43	44	43	44	43	44	45	43	48	45
Upper 5.0 percentile	68	67	69	71	69	66	69	70	74	70
Standard deviation of the mean	8.5	7.5	8.0	8.1	8.0	7.5	7.6	7.8	8.0	8.0

Table 11.3 Percentage distribution of mean arterial blood pressure by sex and age of young person

Mean arterial blood pressure (mmHg)	Males aged (years)				All males	Females aged (years)				All females
	4–6	7–10	11–14	15–18		4–6	7–10	11–14	15–18	
	cum %	cum %	cum %	cum %	cum %	cum %	cum %	cum %	cum %	cum %
Less than 65	23	16	11	3	13	22	16	11	3	12
Less than 70	47	41	27	15	32	54	40	34	18	35
Less than 75	72	70	56	35	58	77	68	57	44	61
Less than 80	88	90	83	63	81	95	89	81	68	83
All	100	100	100	100	100	100	100	100	100	100
Base	*204*	*280*	*265*	*219*	*968*	*188*	*247*	*259*	*236*	*930*
Mean (average value)	71	71	74	78	74	70	72	74	77	73
Median value	71	71	74	78	73	69	72	74	77	73
Lower 5.0 percentile	60	61	61	66	61	60	60	62	66	62
Upper 5.0 percentile	82	82	86	93	87	80	85	88	92	87
Standard deviation of the mean	7.2	6.8	7.2	7.8	7.0	6.8	7.3	7.4	7.8	7.8

Table 11.4 Blood pressure by sex of young person and whether salt was usually used in cooking young person's food*

Blood pressure (mmHg)	Sex of young person and whether salt used in cooking					
	Males		All males	Females		All females
	Salt used in cooking	Salt not used in cooking		Salt used in cooking	Salt not used in cooking	
Systolic pressure (mmHg)						
mean	110	108	110	109	106	108
median	109	108	109	109	105	107
5th percentile	93	91	92	91	91	91
10th percentile	95	94	95	95	94	95
90th percentile	127	125	126	124	119	123
95th percentile	131	129	131	127	123	126
standard deviation of the mean	12.0	11.5	11.9	11.1	9.8	10.8
Diastolic blood pressure (mmHg)						
mean	56	56	56	56	56	56
median	55	55	55	56	56	56
5th percentile	44	43	43	44	46	45
10th percentile	46	45	45	46	48	47
90th percentile	66	66	66	67	66	66
95th percentile	69	68	69	70	70	70
standard deviation of the mean	8.1	7.9	8.0	7.2	7.2	8.0
Mean arterial pressure (mmHg)						
mean	74	73	74	74	73	73
median	74	73	73	74	72	73
5th percentile	62	61	61	61	63	62
10th percentile	64	64	64	63	65	64
90th percentile	84	83	84	84	81	83
95th percentile	88	85	87	89	85	87
standard deviation of the mean	7.9	7.6	7.8	8.2	6.9	7.8
Base = number of young people	*624*	*344*	*968*	*613*	*317*	*930*

Table 11.5 Blood pressure by sex of young person and whether salt was added to young person's food at the table*

Blood pressure (mmHg)	Males		All males	Females		All females
	Salt usually added at table	Occasionally, rarely or never added		Salt usually added at table	Occasionally, rarely or never added	
Systolic pressure (mmHg)						
mean	112	109	110	110	107	108
median	111	108	109	110	107	107
5th percentile	92	92	92	93	90	91
10th percentile	96	95	95	97	94	95
90th percentile	129	125	126	124	122	123
95th percentile	131	130	131	127	126	126
standard deviation of the mean	11.9	11.8	11.9	10.8	10.7	10.8
Diastolic blood pressure (mmHg)						
mean	56	56	56	57	56	56
median	55	55	55	56	56	56
5th percentile	43	44	43	45	45	45
10th percentile	47	45	45	48	47	47
90th percentile	66	66	66	67	66	66
95th percentile	67	69	69	70	70	70
standard deviation of the mean	7.5	8.2	8.0	7.6	8.0	8.0
Mean arterial pressure (mmHg)						
mean	74	73	74	74	73	73
median	75	73	73	74	73	73
5th percentile	62	61	61	62	62	62
10th percentile	65	63	64	65	64	64
90th percentile	84	83	84	83	83	83
95th percentile	86	87	87	87	87	87
standard deviation of the mean	7.2	7.9	7.8	7.5	7.8	7.8
Base = number of young people	214	754	968	183	747	930

* As reported in the dietary interview.

Table 11.6 Blood pressure by sex of young person and whether the young person reported currently dieting to lose weight: young people aged 11 to 18 years only*

Young people aged 11 to 18 years

Blood pressure (mmHg)	Sex of young person and whether dieting to lose weight					
	Males		All males	Females		All females
	Dieting	Not dieting		Dieting	Not dieting	
Systolic pressure (mmHg)						
mean	124	115	115	112	112	112
median	122	114	115	110	112	111
5th percentile	110	97	97	93	96	96
10th percentile	111	101	101	100	100	100
90th percentile	150	131	131	127	125	125
95th percentile	154	133	134	132	128	128
standard deviation of the mean	13.2	11.3	11.5	10.6	10.2	10.2
Diastolic blood pressure (mmHg)						
mean	58	56	56	58	57	57
median	56	56	56	58	57	57
5th percentile	45	44	44	47	45	45
10th percentile	52	46	46	48	48	48
90th percentile	68	66	66	68	69	68
95th percentile	69	70	70	72	71	71
standard deviation of the mean	6.8	8.1	8.1	7.6	8.1	8.1
Mean arterial pressure (mmHg)						
mean	80	76	76	76	75	75
median	80	76	76	74	75	75
5th percentile	68	62	62	62	64	64
10th percentile	72	66	67	66	66	66
90th percentile	93	86	86	87	86	86
95th percentile	95	90	91	90	90	90
standard deviation of the mean	7.0	7.8	7.8	7.6	7.8	7.8
Base = number of young people	*19***	*465*	*465*	*52*	*443*	*495*

* As reported in the dietary interview.
** Small base number; results for this group should therefore be treated with caution.

Table 11.7 Blood pressure by sex of young person and whether young person currently smoked cigarettes: young people aged 11 to 18 years only*

Young people aged 11 to 18 years

Blood pressure (mmHg)	Sex of young person and whether currently smoked cigarettes					
	Males		All males**	Females		All females**
	Smoker	Non-smoker		Smoker	Non-smoker	
Systolic pressure (mmHg)						
mean	120	114	115	114	111	112
median	121	113	115	115	111	111
5th percentile	104	96	97	95	96	96
10th percentile	107	99	101	100	99	100
90th percentile	134	129	131	128	124	125
95th percentile	138	133	134	133	128	128
standard deviation of the mean	10.7	11.4	11.5	11.2	10.0	10.2
Diastolic blood pressure (mmHg)						
mean	56	56	56	58	57	57
median	56	56	56	58	57	57
5th percentile	44	44	44	47	44	46
10th percentile	46	46	46	49	47	48
90th percentile	66	66	66	69	68	68
95th percentile	69	70	70	74	71	71
standard deviation of the mean	7.7	8.2	8.1	7.6	8.2	8.1
Mean arterial pressure (mmHg)						
mean	78	76	76	77	75	75
median	76	75	76	77	75	75
5th percentile	66	62	62	67	63	64
10th percentile	67	66	67	67	66	66
90th percentile	88	85	86	87	86	86
95th percentile	92	90	91	90	89	90
standard deviation of the mean	7.5	7.8	7.8	7.4	7.8	7.8
Base = number of young people	*83*	*397*	*480*	*97*	*392*	*489*

* As reported in the dietary interview.
** Includes those not answering smoking questions.

Table 11.8 Blood pressure by sex of young person and their average daily intake of alcohol during dietary recording period: young people aged 15 to 18 years

Young people aged 15 to 18 years

Blood pressure (mmHg)	Sex of young person and average daily intake of alcohol (g)									
	Males				All males*	Females				All females*
	Nil	Less than 3g	3g to less than 10g	10g or more		Nil	Less than 3g	3g to less than 10g	10g or more	
Systolic pressure (mmHg)										
mean	120	120	122	123	121	113	120	113	115	114
median	120	118	124	125	120	112	117	114	117	114
5th percentile	104	106	108	102	104	97	105	96	100	97
10th percentile	107	109	108	107	107	99	106	99	101	101
90th percentile	133	136	136	137	134	127	137	124	130	127
95th percentile	138	136	137	144	138	133	141	124	130	132
standard deviation of the mean	11.5	10.3	10.2	11.4	10.9	10.7	11.2	9.4	9.8	10.5
Diastolic blood pressure (mmHg)										
mean	56	56	58	60	57	58	63	59	60	59
median	56	56	57	61	57	57	63	59	59	58
5th percentile	43	46	47	50	44	48	52	46	50	48
10th percentile	45	47	48	50	47	49	53	50	50	49
90th percentile	66	68	66	69	67	70	76	67	69	70
95th percentile	69	69	70	71	71	74	86	70	76	74
standard deviation of the mean	8.5	6.7	7.2	6.9	8.1	8.1	9.4	7.0	7.7	8.0
Mean arterial pressure (mmHg)										
mean	77	77	79	81	78	76	82	77	78	77
median	77	76	79	82	78	75	82	77	80	77
5th percentile	65	70	68	67	66	65	72	67	68	66
10th percentile	68	70	70	72	68	67	72	68	69	68
90th percentile	87	86	86	92	88	87	92	84	89	87
95th percentile	95	86	89	92	93	93	104	87	94	92
standard deviation of the mean	8.1	6.2	6.7	7.1	7.7	7.9	9.0	5.9	7.9	7.8
Base = number of young people	96	19**	25**	38	219	120	19**	39	27**	236

* Includes those not completing a 7-day dietary record.
** Small base numbers; results for this group should therefore be treated with caution.

Table 11.9 Blood pressure by sex of young person and whether young person was reported as being unwell during the dietary recording period

Blood pressure (mmHg)	Sex of young person and whether unwell during period							
	Males			All males	Females			All females
	Unwell and eating affected	Unwell and eating not affected	Not unwell		Unwell and eating affected	Unwell and eating not affected	Not unwell	
Systolic pressure (mmHg)								
mean	107	110	110	110	107	107	108	108
median	106	110	109	109	107	108	107	107
5th percentile	89	95	92	92	89	89	92	91
10th percentile	92	98	95	95	94	93	95	95
90th percentile	124	123	127	126	122	122	123	123
95th percentile	126	126	132	131	128	126	126	126
standard deviation of the mean	11.0	9.4	12.3	11.9	10.9	10.7	10.8	10.8
Diastolic blood pressure (mmHg)								
mean	55	56	56	56	55	57	56	56
median	55	56	55	55	56	57	55	56
5th percentile	43	44	43	43	44	47	45	45
10th percentile	45	46	45	45	46	49	47	47
90th percentile	66	66	· 66	66	66	66	67	66
95th percentile	68	71	69	69	69	70	70	70
standard deviation of the mean	8.0	8.4	8.0	8.0	7.8	7.2	8.0	8.0
Mean arterial pressure (mmHg)								
mean	72	74	74	74	73	74	73	73
median	72	74	73	73	72	74	73	73
5th percentile	61	63	61	61	60	62	62	62
10th percentile	63	66	63	64	63	64	64	64
90th percentile	82	82	84	84	82	82	83	83
95th percentile	84	85	87	87	89	86	88	87
standard deviation of the mean	7.4	7.1	7.9	7.8	7.9	7.2	7.9	7.8
Base = number of young people	*92*	*124*	*751*	*968*	*99*	*136*	*695*	*930*

Table 11.10 Blood pressure by sex of young person and region

Blood pressure (mmHg)	Males				All males	Females				All females
	Scotland	Northern	Central, South West & Wales	London & South East		Scotland	Northern	Central, South West & Wales	London & South East	
Systolic pressure (mmHg)										
mean	111	109	110	109	110	109	107	108	107	108
median	110	109	110	108	109	107	107	108	106	107
5th percentile	94	91	91	92	92	91	92	91	91	91
10th percentile	96	95	95	95	95	97	94	95	95	95
90th percentile	126	127	128	126	126	126	123	123	119	123
95th percentile	131	130	131	130	131	131	126	127	124	126
standard deviation of the mean	12.3	11.5	12.0	11.8	11.9	11.8	11.0	11.0	10.0	10.8
Diastolic pressure (mmHg)										
mean	56	56	56	55	56	55	56	57	56	56
median	55	55	56	55	55	54	55	57	56	56
5th percentile	45	44	44	42	43	43	46	45	45	45
10th percentile	48	46	46	45	45	48	47	47	47	47
90th percentile	67	66	66	66	66	66	67	66	66	66
95th percentile	69	68	70	68	69	70	70	69	70	70
standard deviation of the mean	7.6	7.8	8.3	7.9	8.0	7.5	7.8	8.2	7.8	8.0
Mean arterial pressure (mmHg)										
mean	75	74	74	73	74	73	73	74	73	73
median	74	73	74	73	73	71	73	74	72	73
5th percentile	63	62	61	60	61	62	62	61	62	62
10th percentile	66	64	64	63	64	64	64	64	64	64
90th percentile	85	83	84	83	84	87	83	83	82	83
95th percentile	88	85	88	87	87	90	87	87	87	87
standard deviation of the mean	7.7	7.3	8.0	8.0	7.8	8.3	7.8	7.8	7.6	7.8
Base = number of young people	77	265	334	292	968	75	243	332	280	930

Table 11.11 Blood pressure by sex of young person and social class of head of household

Blood pressure (mmHg)	Social class of head of household					
	Males		All males*	Females		All females*
	Non-manual	Manual		Non-manual	Manual	
Systolic pressure (mmHg)						
mean	110	109	110	107	108	108
median	110	109	109	107	107	107
5th percentile	92	91	92	91	92	91
10th percentile	95	95	95	95	95	95
90th percentile	127	126	126	123	121	123
95th percentile	132	131	131	128	124	126
standard deviation of the mean	12.3	11.6	11.9	11.4	9.9	10.8
Diastolic blood pressure (mmHg)						
mean	56	56	56	56	56	56
median	55	56	55	55	56	56
5th percentile	43	43	43	44	45	45
10th percentile	45	45	45	47	47	47
90th percentile	66	66	66	67	66	66
95th percentile	70	69	69	70	69	70
standard deviation of the mean	8.4	7.8	8.0	8.5	7.6	8.0
Mean arterial pressure (mmHg)						
mean	74	73	74	73	73	73
median	73	73	73	72	74	73
5th percentile	61	61	61	61	62	62
10th percentile	63	63	64	63	65	64
90th percentile	85	83	84	84	82	83
95th percentile	90	86	87	89	86	87
standard deviation of the mean	8.2	7.6	7.8	8.4	7.3	7.8
Base = number of young people	*450*	*444*	*968*	*427*	*412*	*930*

* Includes those for whom a social class could not be assigned.

Table 11.12 Blood pressure by sex of young person and gross weekly household income

Blood pressure (mmHg)	Males						Females					
	Less than £160	£160 to less than £280	£280 to less than £400	£400 to less than £600	£600 and over	All males*	Less than £160	£160 to less than £280	£280 to less than £400	£400 to less than £600	£600 and over	All females*
Systolic pressure (mmHg)												
mean	108	109	109	110	111	110	107	108	107	108	108	108
median	108	108	109	109	110	109	107	108	107	108	106	107
5th percentile	92	93	91	91	92	92	90	91	92	89	91	91
10th percentile	96	96	94	95	94	95	96	96	94	94	94	95
90th percentile	121	125	126	127	128	126	120	123	120	123	124	123
95th percentile	125	131	129	131	132	131	122	126	126	128	127	126
standard deviation of the mean	10.8	11.2	11.1	12.4	13.0	11.9	9.8	10.3	10.2	11.4	11.8	10.8
Diastolic blood pressure (mmHg)												
mean	56	56	55	55	56	56	56	56	56	56	56	56
median	56	55	56	55	55	55	55	57	56	56	55	56
5th percentile	44	45	42	43	44	43	45	45	43	45	45	45
10th percentile	46	47	44	45	45	45	47	47	46	46	48	47
90th percentile	67	66	66	64	66	66	66	66	64	67	67	66
95th percentile	69	69	68	69	71	69	70	70	70	69	70	70
standard deviation of the mean	8.3	7.5	8.2	7.9	8.4	8.0	8.0	7.3	8.0	8.4	7.9	8.0
Mean arterial pressure (mmHg)												
mean	74	74	73	73	74	74	73	73	73	73	73	73
median	73	74	73	73	74	73	73	74	73	72	73	73
5th percentile	61	62	61	60	61	61	61	62	61	60	62	62
10th percentile	64	65	63	63	64	64	66	65	63	63	64	64
90th percentile	82	83	84	84	85	84	82	82	81	85	85	83
95th percentile	85	86	86	88	92	87	86	85	86	89	88	87
standard deviation of the mean	7.3	7.0	7.9	8.0	8.5	7.8	7.4	6.9	7.7	8.6	8.3	7.8
Base = number of young people	153	175	179	193	233	968	150	165	158	211	209	930

* Includes those not answering income question.

Table 11.13 Blood pressure by sex of young person and whether young person's 'parents' were receiving certain benefits

Blood pressure (mmHg)	Sex of young person and whether 'parents' receiving benefits					
	Males		All males	Females		All females
	Receiving benefits	Not receiving benefits		Receiving benefits	Not receiving benefits	
Systolic pressure (mmHg)						
mean	109	110	110	108	108	108
median	109	109	109	108	107	107
5th percentile	94	91	92	91	91	91
10th percentile	96	94	95	96	94	95
90th percentile	123	127	126	120	123	123
95th percentile	127	131	131	125	127	126
standard deviation of the mean	10.6	12.3	11.9	9.8	11.1	10.8
Diastolic blood pressure (mmHg)						
mean	56	56	56	56	56	56
median	55	55	55	55	56	56
5th percentile	44	43	43	45	45	45
10th percentile	46	45	45	47	47	47
90th percentile	66	66	66	66	67	66
95th percentile	68	69	69	70	70	70
standard deviation of the mean	7.8	8.1	8.0	7.7	8.0	8.0
Mean arterial pressure (mmHg)						
mean	74	74	74	73	73	73
median	73	74	73	73	73	73
5th percentile	63	61	61	62	61	62
10th percentile	66	63	64	65	64	64
90th percentile	82	84	84	82	83	83
95th percentile	86	87	87	86	88	87
standard deviation of the mean	7.0	8.1	7.8	7.1	8.0	7.8
Base = number of young people	*223*	*744*	*968*	*232*	*697*	*930*

Table 11.14   Blood pressure by sex of young person and whether living with both parents

Blood pressure (mmHg)	Sex of young person and whether living with both parents*							
	Males: living with			All males	Females: living with			All females
	both parents and:		single parent with/out other children		both parents and:		single parent with/out other children	
	other children	no other children			other children	no other children		
Systolic pressure (mmHg)								
mean	108	114	109	110	106	111	108	108
median	108	114	109	109	106	110	107	107
5th percentile	91	95	93	92	90	92	91	91
10th percentile	94	97	96	95	93	97	95	95
90th percentile	123	131	128	126	121	125	125	123
95th percentile	127	133	133	131	125	128	127	126
standard deviation of the mean	11.0	12.6	12.5	11.9	10.5	11.0	11.0	10.8
Diastolic blood pressure (mmHg)								
mean	56	56	56	56	56	58	56	56
median	55	56	55	55	55	58	56	56
5th percentile	43	45	44	43	45	47	44	45
10th percentile	45	46	46	45	46	49	46	47
90th percentile	66	67	66	66	65	68	65	66
95th percentile	68	70	68	69	70	70	70	70
standard deviation of the mean	8.0	7.9	8.1	8.0	7.9	8.1	7.5	7.9
Mean arterial pressure (mmHg)								
mean	73	76	74	74	73	76	73	73
median	73	75	73	73	72	75	73	73
5th percentile	61	62	62	61	61	64	61	62
10th percentile	63	66	64	64	63	66	65	64
90th percentile	83	86	84	84	82	86	82	83
95th percentile	86	90	87	87	87	88	87	87
standard deviation of the mean	7.6	8.0	7.9	7.8	7.7	8.0	7.4	7.8
Base = number of young people	584	192	188	968	543	191	187	930

* Includes 13 young people (unweighted), four boys and nine girls, who were living with others, not parents.

413

Table 11.15(a)   Characteristics independently related to systolic blood pressure: males aged 4 to 18 years

Characteristic	Unstandardised coefficient (B)	Standard error of B	Standardised regression coefficient β	T - value
Constant (systolic blood pressure - mmHg)	65.96	2.63		
Age at time of measurement (years)	0.34	0.16	0.12	2.11*
Diastolic blood pressure (mmHg)	0.46	0.04	0.31	12.09***
Body weight (kg)††	0.29	0.03	0.48	8.70***
Reported currently smoking	2.96	1.20	0.07	2.47*
Whether unwell during dietary recording period				
Not unwell	0.62	0.54	0.03	1.15
Unwell & eating not affected	1.32	0.80	0.05	1.64
Unwell & eating affected	−1.94	0.75	−0.10	−2.58*
Salt usually added to food during cooking				0.53
Salt usually added to food at the table				0.58
Urinary sodium to urinary creatinine ratio				0.82
Urinary potassium to urinary creatinine ratio				0.12
Reported dieting to lose weight				1.05
Average daily alcohol intake (g)				0.04
Fieldwork wave †				
Wave 1				1.22
Wave 2				−1.32
Wave 3				0.72
Wave 4				−0.64
Region				
Scotland				1.19
Northern				−1.32
Central, South West & Wales				0.39
London & South East				−0.96
Social class of head of household				
Non-manual				0.51
Manual				−0.03
Unclassified				−0.33
Gross weekly household income				
Less than £160				0.20
£160 - less than £400				−0.22
£400 & over				−0.09
Parents were receiving benefits				1.77
Whether living with both parents				
Both parents & other children				0.60
Both parents & no other children				−0.52
Single parent & other children				−0.81
Single parent & no other children				0.71
Percentage of variance explained	50%			
Number of young people	*775*			

* p < 0.05; ** p < 0.01; *** p < 0.001
† Wave 1: Jan - March 1997; Wave 2: April - June 1997; Wave 3: July - Sept 1997; Wave 4 Oct - Dec 1997 see also *Glossary*.
†† Height and BMI were highly correlated (collinear) with weight (variance inflation factor > 10). It is difficult to distinguish the effects in a multiple regression of highly correlated characteristics if both are included and the results may be unreliable. One characteristic of a collinear pair must be dropped. Since weight can be modified by an individual while height cannot, height and BMI were dropped from the regression.

Table 11.15(b)   Characteristics independently related to systolic blood pressure: males aged 7 to 18 years

Males aged 7 to 18 who kept a full 7-day physical activity diary

Characteristic	Unstandardised coefficient (B)	Standard error of B	Standardised regression coefficient β	T - value
Constant (systolic blood pressure - mmHg)	68.99	5.77		
Age at time of measurement (years)	0.55	0.21	0.16	2.63**
Diastolic blood pressure (mmHg)	0.48	0.05	0.32	10.42***
Body weight (kg) †	0.28	0.04	0.43	7.58***
Whether unwell during dietary recording period				
Not unwell	0.93	0.64	0.05	1.45
Unwell & eating not affected	1.69	0.96	0.06	1.75
Unwell & eating affected	–2.62	0.90	–0.14	–2.92**
Calculated physical activity score				–1.33
Salt usually added to food during cooking				0.52
Salt usually added to food at the table				0.32
Urinary sodium to urinary creatinine ratio				1.48
Urinary potassium to urinary creatinine ratio				–1.03
Reported dieting to lose weight				1.04
Reported currently smoking				1.90
Average daily alcohol intake (g)				0.12
Fieldwork wave ††				
Wave 1				0.89
Wave 2				–0.78
Wave 3				0.68
Wave 4				–0.53
Region				
Scotland				1.06
Northern				–0.75
Central, South West & Wales				0.61
London & South East				–0.93
Social class of head of household				
Non-manual				0.75
Manual				0.21
Unclassified				–0.62
Gross weekly household income				
Less than £160				0.32
£160 - less than £400				–0.78
£400 & over				0.17
Parents were receiving benefits				1.40
Whether living with both parents				
Both parents & other children				0.42
Both parents & no other children				–0.68
Single parent & other children				–1.25
Single parent & no other children				1.33
Percentage of variance explained	48%			
Number of young people	599			

* p < 0.05; ** p < 0.01; *** p < 0.001
† Height and BMI were highly correlated (collinear) with weight (variance inflation factor > 10). It is difficult to distinguish the effects in a multiple regression of highly correlated characteristics if both are included and the results may be unreliable. One characteristic of a collinear pair must be dropped. Since weight can be modified by an individual while height cannot, height and BMI were dropped from the regression.
†† Wave 1: Jan - March 1997; Wave 2: April - June 1997; Wave 3: July - Sept 1997; Wave 4 Oct - Dec 1997 see also *Glossary*.

Table 11.15(c)   Characteristics independently related to systolic blood pressure: males aged 10 to 16 years

Males aged 10 to 16 who provided a blood sample for analysis of testosterone concentration - unweighted data

Characteristic	Unstandardised coefficient (B)	Standard error of B	Standardised regression coefficient β	T - value
Constant (systolic blood pressure – mmHg)	75.84	11.24		
Age at time of measurement (years)				1.82
Diastolic blood pressure (mmHg)	0.49	0.07	0.38	6.61***
Body weight (kg)†	0.19	0.06	0.29	3.38***
Calculated physical activity score				−1.37
Testosterone concentration - tertile				
Bottom				−0.37
Middle				−1.16
Top				1.36
Salt usually added to food during cooking				−0.42
Salt usually added to food at the table				−1.48
Urinary sodium to urinary creatinine ratio				0.53
Urinary potassium to urinary creatinine ratio				0.06
Reported dieting to lose weight				0.55
Reported currently smoking				−0.68
Average daily alcohol intake (g)				1.30
Fieldwork wave††				
Wave 1				−1.02
Wave 2				0.11
Wave 3				0.71
Wave 4				0.19
Whether unwell during dietary recording period				
Not unwell				0.38
Unwell & eating not affected				0.33
Unwell & eating affected				−0.64
Region				
Scotland				1.25
Northern				−1.42
Central, South West & Wales				0.80
London & South East				−1.44
Social class of head of household				
Non-manual				−0.40
Manual				1.15
Unclassified				−0.48
Gross weekly household income				
Less than £160				1.44
£160 - less than £400				−1.63
£400 & over				−0.70
Parents were receiving benefits				−1.22
Whether living with both parents				
Both parents & other children				−1.81
Both parents & no other children				−1.20
Single parent & other children				0.15
Single parent & no other children				1.71
Percentage of variance explained		37%		
Number of young people		*218*		

* p<0.05; ** p<0.01; *** p<0.001

† Height and BMI were highly correlated (collinear) with weight (variance inflation factor > 10). It is difficult to distinguish the effects in a multiple regression of highly correlated characteristics if both are included and the results may be unreliable. One characteristic of a collinear pair must be dropped. Since weight can be modified by an individual while height cannot, height and BMI were dropped from the regression.

†† Wave 1: Jan - March 1997; Wave 2: April - June 1997; Wave 3: July - Sept 1997; Wave 4 Oct - Dec 1997 see also *Glossary*.

Table 11.16(a)   Characteristics independently related to systolic blood pressure: females aged 4 to 18 years

Characteristic	Unstandardised coefficient (B)	Standard error of B	Standardised regression coefficient β	T - value
Constant (systolic blood pressure – mmHg)	59.4	2.59		
Age at time of measurement (years)				0.02
Diastolic blood pressure (mmHg)	0.62	0.04	0.47	16.44***
Body weight (kg)†	0.29	0.03	0.47	8.30***
Region				
Scotland	1.36	0.82	0.07	1.66
Northern	–0.78	0.53	–0.06	–1.48
Central, South West & Wales	0.49	0.50	0.04	0.98
London & South East	–1.07	0.53	–0.06	–2.02*
Menarche had occurred				–0.91
Salt usually added to food during cooking				1.56
Salt usually added to food at the table				–0.22
Urinary sodium to urinary creatinine ratio				–0.41
Urinary potassium to urinary creatinine ratio				0.57
Reported dieting to lose weight				–1.50
Reported currently smoking				0.08
Average daily alcohol intake (g)				0.06
Fieldwork wave††				
Wave 1				–1.01
Wave 2				0.48
Wave 3				–0.68
Wave 4				1.25
Whether unwell during dietary recording period				
Not unwell				0.33
Unwell & eating not affected				–0.30
Unwell & eating affected				0.07
Social class of head of household				
Non–manual				0.44
Manual				0.31
Unclassified				–0.52
Gross weekly household income				
Less than £160				–1.22
£160 – less than £400				1.60
£400 & over				0.32
Parents were receiving benefits				1.40
Whether living with both parents				
Both parents & other children				1.04
Both parents & no other children				–0.17
Single parent & other children				–1.29
Single parent & no other children				–1.58
Percentage of variance explained	47%			
Number of young people	725			

* p < 0.05; ** p < 0.01; *** p < 0.001
† Height and BMI were highly correlated (collinear) with weight (variance inflation factor > 10). It is difficult to distinguish the effects in a multiple regression of highly correlated characteristics if both are included and the results may be unreliable. One characteristic of a collinear pair must be dropped. Since weight can be modified by an individual while height cannot, height and BMI were dropped from the regression.
†† Wave 1: Jan – March 1997; Wave 2: April – June 1997; Wave 3: July – Sept 1997; Wave 4 Oct – Dec 1997 see also *Glossary*.

Table 11.16(b)   Characteristics independently related to systolic blood pressure: females aged 7 to 18 years

Females aged 7 to 18 who kept a full 7–day physical activity diary

Characteristic	Unstandardised coefficient (B)	Standard error of B	Standardised regression coefficient β	T - value
Constant (systolic blood pressure – mmHg)	57.89	5.70		
Age at time of measurement (years)				−0.34
Diastolic blood pressure (mmHg)	0.66	0.04	0.52	15.75***
Body weight (kg)†	0.27	0.04	0.40	7.41***
Calculated physical activity score				0.20
Menarche had occurred				−0.45
Salt usually added to food during cooking				1.72
Salt usually added to food at the table				0.59
Urinary sodium to urinary creatinine ratio				−0.53
Urinary potassium to urinary creatinine ratio				0.32
Reported dieting to lose weight				−0.95
Reported currently smoking				0.30
Average daily alcohol intake (g)				0.10
Fieldwork wave††				
Wave 1				−1.12
Wave 2				−0.19
Wave 3				0.04
Wave 4				1.28
Whether unwell during dietary recording period				
Not unwell				0.52
Unwell & eating not affected				0.12
Unwell & eating affected				−0.49
Region				
Scotland				1.68
Northern				−1.31
Central, South West & Wales				0.61
London & South East				−1.89
Social class of head of household				
Non–manual				0.50
Manual				0.44
Unclassified				−0.66
Gross weekly household income				
Less than £160				−0.21
£160 – less than £400				0.88
£400 & over				−0.40
Parents were receiving benefits				0.62
Whether living with both parents				
Both parents & other children				1.03
Both parents & no other children				−0.40
Single parent & other children				1.16
Single parent & no other children				−1.34
Percentage of variance explained	45%			
Number of young people	*568*			

* p < 0.05; ** p < 0.01; *** p < 0.001
† Height and BMI were highly correlated (collinear) with weight (variance inflation factor > 10). It is difficult to distinguish the effects in a multiple regression of highly correlated characteristics if both are included and the results may be unreliable. One characteristic of a collinear pair must be dropped. Since weight can be modified by an individual while height cannot, height and BMI were dropped from the regression.
†† Wave 1: Jan – March 1997; Wave 2: April – June 1997; Wave 3: July – Sept 1997; Wave 4 Oct – Dec 1997 see also *Glossary*.

Table 11.17(a) Characteristics independently related to diastolic blood pressure: males aged 4 to 18 years

Characteristic	Unstandardised coefficient (B)	Standard error of B	Standardised regression coefficient β	T - value
Constant (diastolic blood pressure – mmHg)	23.58	3.01		
Age at time of measurement (years)				−1.18
Systolic blood pressure (mmHg)	0.36	0.03	0.52	12.09***
Body weight (kg)†	0.06	0.03	−0.16	−2.09*
Urinary potassium to urinary creatinine ratio	−0.16	0.07	−0.09	−2.24*
Fieldwork wave††				
Wave 1	0.49	0.46	0.04	1.06
Wave 2	0.41	0.46	0.04	0.89
Wave 3	−1.20	0.48	−0.10	−2.50*
Wave 4	0.30	0.46	0.03	0.67
Salt usually added to food during cooking				−1.07
Salt usually added to food at the table				−1.25
Urinary sodium to urinary creatinine ratio				−0.73
Reported dieting to lose weight				−0.19
Reported currently smoking				−1.67
Average daily alcohol intake (g)				1.28
Whether unwell during dietary recording period				
Not unwell				−1.49
Unwell & eating not affected				0.71
Unwell & eating affected				0.31
Region				
Scotland				−0.72
Northern				1.06
Central, South West & Wales				0.56
London & South East				−0.44
Social class of head of household				
Non–manual				−0.16
Manual				−0.22
Unclassified				0.24
Gross weekly household income				
Less than £160				1.25
£160 – less than £400				−0.09
£400 & over				−1.54
Parents were receiving benefits				−0.82
Whether living with both parents				
Both parents & other children				0.90
Both parents & no other children				1.05
Single parent & other children				−0.02
Single parent & no other children				−1.26
Percentage of variance explained	18%			
Number of young people	*775*			

* p<0.05; ** p<0.01; *** p<0.001
† Height and BMI were highly correlated (collinear) with weight (variance inflation factor > 10). It is difficult to distinguish the effects in a multiple regression of highly correlated characteristics if both are included and the results may be unreliable. One characteristic of a collinear pair must be dropped. Since weight can be modified by an individual while height cannot, height and BMI were dropped from the regression.
†† Wave 1: Jan – March 1997; Wave 2: April – June 1997; Wave 3: July – Sept 1997; Wave 4 Oct – Dec 1997 see also *Glossary*.

Table 11.17(b)   Characteristics independently related to diastolic blood pressure: males aged 7 to 18 years

Males aged 7 to 18 who kept a full 7–day physical activity diary

Characteristic	Unstandardised coefficient (B)	Standard error of B	Standardised regression coefficient β	T - value
Constant (diastolic blood pressure – mmHg)	26.42	5.30		
Age at time of measurement (years)				−0.20
Systolic blood pressure (mmHg)	0.34	0.03	0.51	10.42***
Body weight (kg)†	−0.07	0.03	−0.17	−2.25*
Calculated physical activity score				−0.59
Salt usually added to food during cooking				−0.79
Salt usually added to food at the table				−1.49
Urinary sodium to urinary creatinine ratio				−1.13
Urinary potassium to urinary creatinine ratio				−0.98
Reported dieting to lose weight				0.52
Reported currently smoking				−1.61
Average daily alcohol intake (g)				1.28
Fieldwork wave††				
Wave 1				0.85
Wave 2				0.54
Wave 3				−1.56
Wave 4				0.24
Whether unwell during dietary recording period				
Not unwell				−0.16
Unwell & eating not affected				−0.93
Unwell & eating affected				1.11
Region				
Scotland				−0.61
Northern				−0.18
Central, South West & Wales				0.50
London & South East				0.68
Social class of head of household				
Non–manual				−1.12
Manual				0.18
Unclassified				0.64
Gross weekly household income				
Less than £160				0.17
£160 – less than £400				1.01
£400 & over				−0.97
Parents were receiving benefits				−1.06
Whether living with both parents				
Both parents & other children				1.04
Both parents & no other children				0.30
Single parent & other children				0.49
Single parent & no other children				−1.24
Percentage of variance explained		17%		
Number of young people		599		

* $p < 0.05$; ** $p < 0.01$; *** $p < 0.001$

† Height and BMI were highly correlated (collinear) with weight (variance inflation factor > 10). It is difficult to distinguish the effects in a multiple regression of highly correlated characteristics if both are included and the results may be unreliable. One characteristic of a collinear pair must be dropped. Since weight can be modified by an individual while height cannot, height and BMI were dropped from the regression.

†† Wave 1: Jan – March 1997; Wave 2: April – June 1997; Wave 3: July – Sept 1997; Wave 4 Oct – Dec 1997 see also *Glossary*.

Table 11.17(c)   Characteristics independently related to diastolic blood pressure: males aged 10 to 16 years

Males aged 10 to 16 who provided a blood sample for analysis of testosterone concentration – unweighted data

Characteristic	Unstandardised coefficient (B)	Standard error of B	Standardised regression coefficient β	T - value
Constant (diastolic blood pressure – mmHg)	28.13	11.02		
Age at time of measurement (years)				−1.76
Systolic blood pressure (mmHg)	0.39	0.06	0.50	6.61***
Parents' were receiving benefits	4.22	1.20	0.22	2.01*
Body weight (kg)†				−1.92
Calculated physical activity score				−0.25
Testosterone concentration – tertile				
Bottom				−0.74
Middle				0.73
Top				0.22
Salt usually added to food during cooking				0.01
Salt usually added to food at the table				−0.47
Urinary sodium to urinary creatinine ratio				−0.74
Urinary potassium to urinary creatinine ratio				−0.70
Reported dieting to lose weight				1.18
Reported currently smoking				1.67
Average daily alcohol intake (g)				−0.33
Fieldwork wave††				
Wave 1				−0.22
Wave 2				0.74
Wave 3				−0.69
Wave 4				−0.01
Whether unwell during dietary recording period				
Not unwell				−0.47
Unwell & eating not affected				0.57
Unwell & eating affected				−0.28
Region				
Scotland				−1.86
Northern				1.04
Central, South West & Wales				0.64
London & South East				1.48
Social class of head of household				
Non–manual				0.51
Manual				−0.09
Unclassified				−0.27
Gross weekly household income				
Less than £160				−1.37
£160 – less than £400				1.47
£400 & over				0.73
Whether living with both parents				
Both parents & other children				1.90
Both parents & no other children				0.42
Single parent & other children				−0.06
Single parent & no other children				−1.32
Percentage of variance explained	16%			
Number of young people	*218*			

* $p < 0.05$; ** $p < 0.01$; *** $p < 0.001$
† Height and BMI were highly correlated (collinear) with weight (variance inflation factor > 10). It is difficult to distinguish the effects in a multiple regression of highly correlated characteristics if both are included and the results may be unreliable. One characteristic of a collinear pair must be dropped. Since weight can be modified by an individual while height cannot, height and BMI were dropped from the regression.
†† Wave 1: Jan – March 1997; Wave 2: April – June 1997; Wave 3: July – Sept 1997; Wave 4 Oct – Dec 1997 see also *Glossary*.

Table 11.18(a)   Characteristics independently related to diastolic blood pressure: females aged 4 to 18 years

Characteristic	Unstandardised coefficient (B)	Standard error of B	Standardised regression coefficient β	T - value
Constant (diastolic blood pressure – mmHg)	11.57	2.88		
Age at time of measurement (years)				0.46
Systolic blood pressure (mmHg)	0.45	0.03	0.60	16.44***
Body weight (kg)†	–0.10	0.03	–0.21	–3.07**
Salt usually added to food during cooking	–1.30	0.53	–0.08	–2.44*
Fieldwork wave††				
Wave 1	1.12	0.45	0.10	2.48*
Wave 2	0.66	0.44	0.06	1.50
Wave 3	–1.30	0.44	–0.12	–2.97**
Wave 4	–0.47	0.44	–0.04	–1.08
Whether living with both parents				
Both parents & other children	–0.17	0.46	–0.01	–0.38
Both parents & no other children	0.81	0.59	0.05	1.36
Single parent & other children	–1.28	0.65	–0.07	–1.96*
Single parent & no other children	0.64	0.77	0.05	0.84
Menarche had occurred				1.78
Salt usually added to food at the table				0.31
Urinary sodium to urinary creatinine ratio				0.02
Urinary potassium to urinary creatinine ratio				–0.65
Reported dieting to lose weight				–0.17
Reported currently smoking				0.29
Average daily alcohol intake (g)				0.76
Whether unwell during dietary recording period				
Not unwell				
Unwell & eating not affected				–0.44
Unwell & eating affected				1.00
				–0.71
Region				
Scotland				
Northern				–1.44
Central, South West & Wales				0.90
London & South East				–0.17
				1.49
Social class of head of household				
Non–manual				
Manual				0.60
Unclassified				0.38
				–0.68
Gross weekly household income				
Less than £160				
£160 – less than £400				1.59
£400 & over				–0.71
				–1.47
Parents were receiving benefits				–0.50
Percentage of variance explained		32%		
Number of young people		*725*		

* p < 0.05; ** p < 0.01; *** p < 0.001

† Height and BMI were highly correlated (collinear) with weight (variance inflation factor > 10). It is difficult to distinguish the effects in a multiple regression of highly correlated characteristics if both are included and the results may be unreliable. One characteristic of a collinear pair must be dropped. Since weight can be modified by an individual while height cannot, height and BMI were dropped from the regression.

†† Wave 1: Jan – March 1997; Wave 2: April – June 1997; Wave 3: July – Sept 1997; Wave 4 Oct – Dec 1997 see also *Glossary*.

Table 11.18(b) Characteristics independently related to diastolic blood pressure: females aged 7 to 18 years

Females aged 7 to 18 who kept a full 7–day physical activity diary

Characteristic	Unstandardised coefficient (B)	Standard error of B	Standardised regression coefficient β	T - value
Constant (diastolic blood pressure – mmHg)	10.75	5.23		
Age at time of measurement (years)				1.10
Systolic blood pressure (mmHg)	0.47	0.03	0.61	15.75***
Body weight (kg)†	–0.09	0.03	–0.18	–2.89**
Salt usually added to food during cooking	–1.40	0.62	–0.08	–2.27*
Fieldwork wave††				
Wave 1	1.32	0.51	0.11	2.57*
Wave 2	0.72	0.50	0.06	1.46
Wave 3	–1.38	0.50	–0.12	–2.74**
Wave 4	–0.67	0.50	–0.06	–1.33
Whether living with both parents				
Both parents & other children	–0.23	0.50	–0.02	–0.45
Both parents & no other children	0.79	0.64	0.05	1.23
Single parent & other children	–1.50	0.71	–0.08	–2.10*
Single parent & no other children	0.94	0.81	0.07	1.16
Calculated physical activity score				–0.83
Menarche had occurred				1.12
Salt usually added to food at the table				–1.00
Urinary sodium to urinary creatinine ratio				0.06
Urinary potassium to urinary creatinine ratio				–0.24
Reported dieting to lose weight				–0.55
Reported currently smoking				0.07
Average daily alcohol intake (g)				0.50
Whether unwell during dietary recording period				
Not unwell				–0.24
Unwell & eating not affected				0.42
Unwell & eating affected				–0.24
Region				
Scotland				–1.09
Northern				0.63
Central, South West & Wales				–0.43
London & South East				1.48
Social class of head of household				
Non–manual				–0.14
Manual				–0.29
Unclassified				0.29
Gross weekly household income				
Less than £160				0.48
£160 – less than £400				–0.40
£400 & over				–0.29
Parents were receiving benefits				–0.03
Percentage of variance explained	35%			
Number of young people	*568*			

* p < 0.05; ** p < 0.01; *** p < 0.001

† Height and BMI were highly correlated (collinear) with weight (variance inflation factor > 10). It is difficult to distinguish the effects in a multiple regression of highly correlated characteristics if both are included and the results may be unreliable. One characteristic of a collinear pair must be dropped. Since weight can be modified by an individual while height cannot, heeight and BMI were dropped from the regression.

†† Wave 1: Jan – March 1997; Wave 2: April – June 1997; Wave 3: July – Sept 1997; Wave 4 Oct – Dec 1997 see also *Glossary*.

Table 11.19(a)   Systolic blood pressure by sex and age of young person: NDNS young people aged 4 to 18 years

NDNS: young people aged 4 to 18 years living in England

Age last birthday	Systolic blood pressure (mmHg)								Base = number of young people
	Mean	Standard deviation of the mean	Standard error of the mean	Percentiles					
				5th	10th	50th	90th	95th	
Males									
4	101	8.04	1.17	87	89	103	110	113	47
5	101	8.16	1.10	89	91	102	114	115	55
6	103	8.36	0.97	92	93	102	115	117	75
7	103	7.73	1.04	90	93	103	114	117	55
8	104	10.78	1.30	85	91	104	116	123	69
9	104	7.03	0.92	91	94	104	113	114	59
10	107	9.22	1.20	91	95	108	118	123	59
11	109	8.48	1.00	92	95	109	118	120	72
12	108	9.67	1.35	90	96	109	120	127	51
13	109	9.41	1.33	91	94	110	120	124	50
14	114	10.15	1.31	96	102	114	129	130	60
15	117	10.67	1.43	102	105	118	132	137	56
16	120	9.54	1.38	100	106	120	132	136	48
17	122	10.77	1.59	100	107	124	135	138	46
18	124	10.16	1.53	108	111	125	136	138	44
All males aged 5–15	107	10.33	0.21	91	94	108	120	125	661
All males aged 4–18	109	11.68	0.40	91	95	108	126	130	846
Females									
4	99	7.65	1.18	85	90	101	107	115	42
5	98	8.27	1.12	85	87	97	109	111	55
6	103	9.68	1.18	88	91	103	114	117	67
7	106	9.07	1.28	86	95	105	116	119	50
8	103	8.31	1.30	89	93	103	115	117	41
9	105	8.59	1.09	92	94	106	115	124	62
10	105	11.43	1.48	88	90	106	116	126	60
11	109	8.57	1.15	93	97	108	121	123	56
12	107	10.23	1.28	89	93	107	120	125	64
13	110	10.31	1.47	94	96	109	123	128	49
14	110	9.51	1.24	95	96	111	124	127	59
15	111	9.83	1.36	94	97	111	124	127	52
16	114	11.10	1.45	98	101	113	130	137	59
17	115	10.74	1.53	98	100	116	128	133	49
18	113	9.97	1.49	98	100	112	128	130	45
All females aged 5–15	106	10.22	0.21	90	93	106	120	124	615
All females aged 4–18	107	10.76	0.38	91	94	107	122	126	810

Table 11.19(b)   Systolic blood pressure by sex and age of young person: the Health of Young People '95 - 97*

Young people aged 5 to 18 years living in England: 1995 to 1997 data combined

| Age last birthday | Systolic blood pressure (mmHg) | | | | | | | Base = number of young people |
| | Mean | Standard error of the mean | Percentiles | | | | | |
			5th	10th	50th	90th	95th	
Males								
5	104	0.4	91	95	104	115	119	401
6	106	0.4	92	95	106	117	121	445
7	106	0.4	93	95	107	117	120	441
8	107	0.4	92	96	107	119	124	463
9	109	0.4	96	98	109	120	124	409
10	110	0.4	97	100	110	122	125	432
11	111	0.4	98	100	111	123	126	416
12	114	0.5	100	103	114	125	129	418
13	117	0.5	101	105	117	131	134	388
14	120	0.5	105	108	119	133	137	384
15	122	0.5	107	110	122	135	139	382
16	126	0.7	109	112	126	140	144	240
17	128	0.8	109	114	128	142	148	193
18	129	0.8	112	116	129	144	152	184
All males aged 5–15	111	0.2	95	98	111	126	130	4579
Females								
5	104	0.4	91	94	104	116	120	411
6	106	0.5	90	93	105	119	122	415
7	107	0.4	93	96	107	119	125	434
8	109	0.5	93	97	108	122	127	469
9	110	0.5	95	98	110	124	128	406
10	111	0.4	98	100	111	124	127	452
11	114	0.5	98	102	113	128	131	407
12	116	0.5	101	104	115	129	132	399
13	117	0.5	102	105	116	129	133	381
14	117	0.5	102	105	117	132	137	403
15	118	0.6	102	105	117	132	137	349
16	121	0.7	105	108	120	136	141	273
17	121	0.7	105	108	120	134	139	243
18	121	0.8	105	107	121	137	141	188
All females aged 5–15	111	0.2	95	98	111	126	130	4526

* Prescott-Clarke P, Primatesta P. Eds. Health Survey for England. *The Health of Young People '95 - 97*. TSO (London, 1998)

Table 11.20(a)   Diastolic blood pressure by sex and age of young person: NDNS young people 4 to 18 years

NDNS: young people aged 4 to 18 years living in England

Age last birthday	Diastolic blood pressure (mmHg)								Base = number of young people
	Mean	Standard deviation of the mean	Standard error of the mean	Percentiles					
				5th	10th	50th	90th	95th	
Males									
4	55	7.67	0.59	41	43	56	64	65	*47*
5	56	9.02	0.63	44	45	55	67	69	*55*
6	55	8.98	0.54	41	43	55	66	68	*75*
7	56	6.84	0.49	47	47	57	66	68	*55*
8	54	7.60	0.47	42	45	54	65	67	*69*
9	55	7.55	0.51	44	44	54	66	68	*59*
10	56	8.51	0.59	41	44	57	66	67	*59*
11	56	8.64	0.53	43	45	54	67	69	*72*
12	55	7.85	0.58	42	45	55	66	68	*51*
13	56	6.88	0.51	45	47	55	64	68	*50*
14	56	6.74	0.46	45	48	56	65	70	*60*
15	55	8.75	0.55	39	44	56	65	69	*56*
16	55	7.29	0.51	42	44	55	65	66	*48*
17	59	8.44	0.59	45	47	60	70	74	*46*
18	59	7.03	0.53	48	50	60	69	71	*44*
All males aged 5–15	55	8.05	0.16	43	45	55	66	68	*661*
All males aged 4–18	56	8.04	0.14	43	45	56	66	69	*846*
Females									
4	56	7.24	0.58	42	47	58	64	66	*42*
5	53	8.02	0.54	44	45	53	63	66	*55*
6	55	7.16	0.44	45	46	54	65	68	*67*
7	57	7.64	0.55	46	49	56	69	70	*50*
8	54	6.90	0.55	45	47	53	64	65	*41*
9	56	6.15	0.40	47	48	56	63	65	*62*
10	56	8.90	0.58	43	45	57	62	72	*60*
11	57	7.09	0.51	46	47	59	65	70	*56*
12	54	7.01	0.46	42	43	54	63	65	*64*
13	55	6.87	0.52	42	46	53	64	67	*49*
14	58	9.03	0.64	39	48	57	70	76	*59*
15	56	7.01	0.48	45	48	55	68	70	*52*
16	60	7.89	0.50	50	51	59	73	76	*59*
17	60	8.41	0.63	48	51	59	74	76	*49*
18	60	8.24	0.67	47	50	59	73	76	*45*
All females aged 5–15	55	7.60	0.16	44	46	55	65	69	*615*
All females aged 4–18	56	7.91	0.14	45	47	56	66	70	*810*

Table 11.20(b) Diastolic blood pressure by sex and age of young person: the Health of Young People '95–97*

Young people aged 5 to 18 years living in England: 1995 to 1997 data combined

Age last birthday	Diastolic blood pressure (mmHg)								Base = number of young people
	Mean	Standard error of the mean	Percentiles						
			5th	10th	50th	90th	95th		
Males									
5	55	0.4	43	45	55	66	70		401
6	56	0.4	42	46	56	66	70		445
7	56	0.4	43	46	56	66	69		441
8	56	0.4	44	47	56	67	71		463
9	58	0.4	44	48	58	68	71		409
10	57	0.4	45	48	57	68	71		432
11	57	0.4	46	48	57	69	72		416
12	58	0.5	45	47	58	69	71		418
13	57	0.4	45	48	56	68	69		388
14	57	0.5	45	47	57	68	72		384
15	58	0.5	44	47	57	69	74		382
16	58	0.6	45	47	58	71	74		240
17	59	0.7	45	49	59	70	72		193
18	62	0.7	49	53	63	73	78		184
All males aged 5–15	57	0.1	44	47	57	68	71		4579
Females									
5	56	0.4	44	47	56	66	70		411
6	56	0.4	44	45	56	67	70		415
7	57	0.4	45	48	56	67	71		434
8	57	0.4	45	46	57	68	71		469
9	58	0.4	47	49	58	69	71		406
10	58	0.4	45	47	58	69	70		452
11	58	0.4	46	48	58	69	73		407
12	58	0.4	45	48	58	69	72		399
13	58	0.4	46	48	58	68	72		381
14	58	0.5	45	48	58	69	73		403
15	59	0.5	47	50	59	71	75		349
16	61	0.6	47	49	61	72	74		273
17	61	0.5	48	51	61	71	77		243
18	63	0.7	49	51	63	74	77		188
All females aged 5–15	58	0.1	45	48	57	69	72		4526

* Prescott-Clarke P, Primatesta P. Eds. Health Survey for England. *The Health of Young People '95–97*. TSO (London, 1998)

Table 11.21(a)   Mean arterial pressure (from Dinamap) by sex and age of young person: NDNS young people 4 to 18 years

NDNS: young people aged 4 to 18 years living in England

Age last birthday	Mean arterial pressure (mmHg)								Base = number of young people
	Mean	Standard deviation of the mean	Standard error of the mean	Percentiles					
				5th	10th	50th	90th	95th	
Males									
4	73	5.89	0.48	63	64	74	80	81	*45*
5	74	9.08	0.64	60	63	73	85	88	*54*
6	73	8.41	0.50	60	62	73	82	84	*75*
7	73	6.15	0.44	65	65	75	82	83	*55*
8	73	8.56	0.54	57	62	74	84	86	*67*
9	73	7.21	0.48	63	65	73	83	85	*59*
10	75	8.01	0.55	64	64	75	85	89	*59*
11	75	8.77	0.54	62	63	76	86	90	*71*
12	76	8.01	0.60	62	65	77	87	88	*50*
13	77	7.15	0.53	67	67	77	88	89	*50*
14	77	7.32	0.50	64	68	76	88	90	*59*
15	79	8.31	0.53	66	69	79	91	98	*56*
16	79	7.68	0.54	65	69	79	90	95	*48*
17	82	7.17	0.50	69	74	83	92	95	*46*
18	84	8.07	0.60	71	72	85	95	97	*44*
All males aged 5–15	75	8.22	0.17	62	64	75	85	89	*655*
All males aged 4–18	76	8.50	0.15	63	65	76	87	91	*838*
Females									
4	73	6.47	0.52	60	65	75	81	84	*45*
5	69	8.14	0.56	57	58	69	81	84	*54*
6	72	7.81	0.48	60	65	72	82	87	*75*
7	75	7.65	0.55	63	64	75	84	89	*55*
8	72	6.46	0.51	62	65	73	82	85	*67*
9	74	6.66	0.43	64	66	75	83	85	*59*
10	74	10.46	0.68	57	63	75	86	95	*59*
11	76	6.69	0.48	66	67	77	88	89	*71*
12	74	7.05	0.47	65	66	76	84	87	*50*
13	76	8.15	0.62	66	67	74	88	91	*50*
14	79	8.46	0.60	63	71	79	92	94	*59*
15	77	7.41	0.50	65	66	77	88	89	*56*
16	80	8.67	0.55	67	69	79	91	97	*48*
17	81	8.47	0.63	68	72	80	92	95	*46*
18	80	8.47	0.69	66	68	81	92	96	*44*
All females aged 5–15	74	8.21	0.17	61	65	75	85	89	*613*
All females aged 4–18	75	8.52	0.15	63	66	75	87	90	*838*

Table 11.21(b) Mean arterial blood pressure by sex and age of young person: the Health of Young People '95 - 97*

Young people aged 5 to 18 years living in England: 1995 to 1997 data combined

| Age last birthday | Mean arterial pressure (mmHg) | | | | | | | Base = number of young people |
| | Mean | Standard error of the mean | Percentiles | | | | | |
			5th	10th	50th	90th	95th	
Males								
5	75	0.4	62	65	75	84	87	*401*
6	76	0.4	63	67	76	87	89	*445*
7	76	0.4	63	66	77	85	88	*441*
8	76	0.4	64	67	77	86	90	*463*
9	78	0.4	65	68	78	88	92	*409*
10	78	0.4	65	68	78	88	91	*432*
11	78	0.4	67	68	78	89	91	*416*
12	79	0.4	67	70	80	90	94	*418*
13	80	0.4	68	71	80	90	94	*388*
14	81	0.4	69	71	81	92	94	*384*
15	82	0.5	69	72	82	94	96	*382*
16	84	0.6	70	73	83	96	98	*240*
17	85	0.7	70	74	85	96	99	*193*
18	88	0.7	75	77	87	100	103	*184*
All males aged 5 to 15	78	0.1	65	68	78	89	92	*4579*
Females								
5	75	0.4	64	66	75	85	90	*411*
6	76	0.4	62	66	77	87	90	*415*
7	77	0.4	64	67	77	86	91	*434*
8	77	0.4	65	67	78	89	92	*469*
9	79	0.4	68	69	79	90	93	*406*
10	79	0.4	66	69	79	89	92	*452*
11	79	0.4	68	70	79	92	95	*407*
12	80	0.4	69	71	80	92	95	*399*
13	81	0.4	69	71	81	91	93	*381*
14	81	0.5	68	71	81	93	95	*403*
15	82	0.5	70	73	82	93	99	*349*
16	84	0.6	71	74	83	96	99	*273*
17	84	0.5	72	74	83	95	98	*243*
18	85	0.7	70	73	86	98	100	*188*
All females aged 5 to 15	79	0.1	66	69	78	90	93	*4526*

* Prescott-Clarke P, Primatesta P. (Eds) Health Survey for England. *The Health of Young People '95–97*. TSO (London, 1998)

Figure 11a   Mean systolic pressure by age and sex

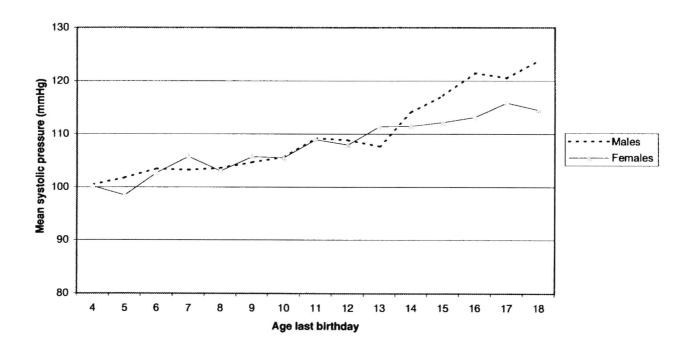

Figure 11b   Mean diastolic blood pressure by age and sex

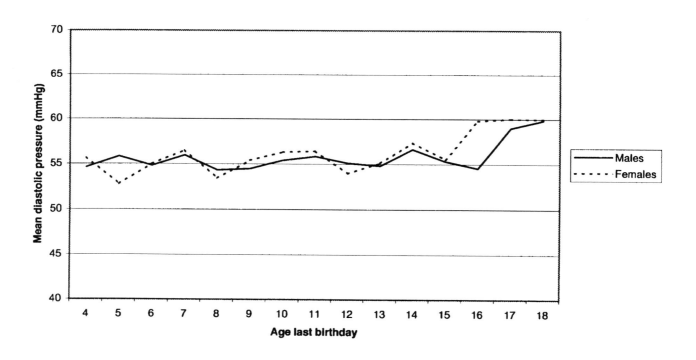

430

Figure 11c   Mean arterial pressure by age and sex

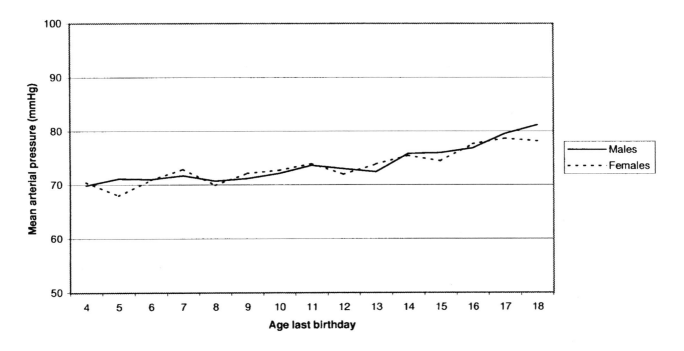

Figure 11d   Mean systolic pressure by age: males

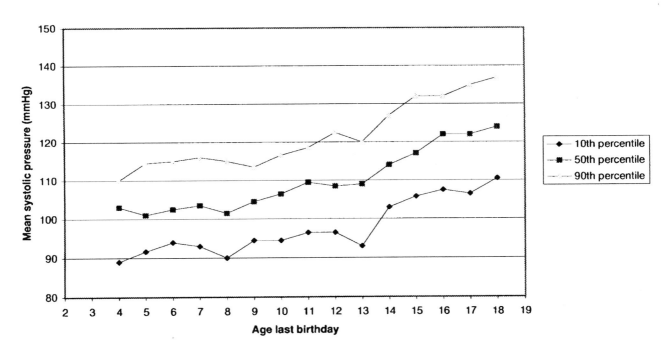

Figure 11e   Mean systolic pressure by age: females

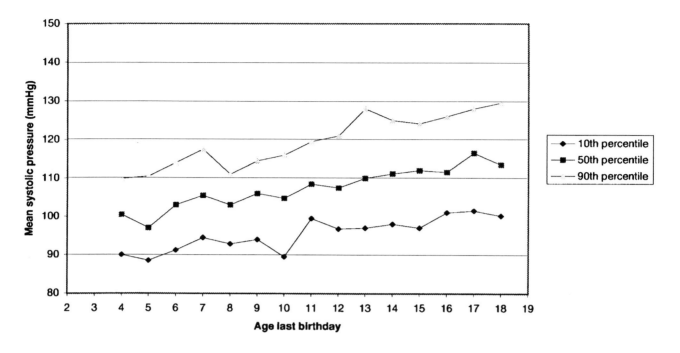

Figure 11f   Mean diastolic pressure by age: males

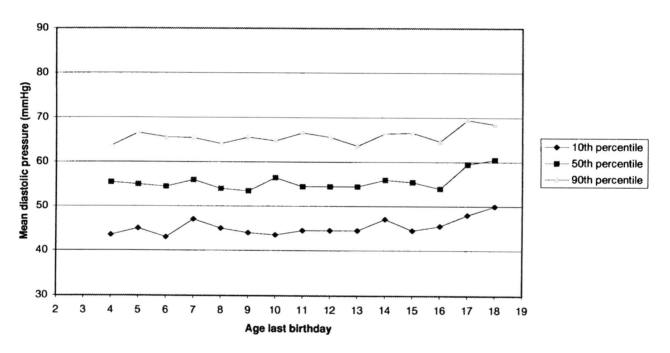

Figure 11g   Mean diastolic pressure by age: females

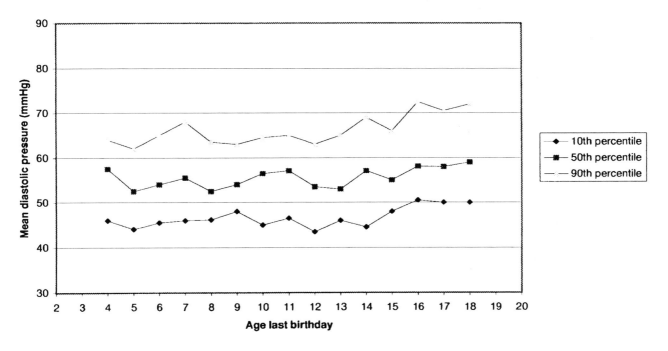

Figure 11h   Mean arterial pressure by age: males

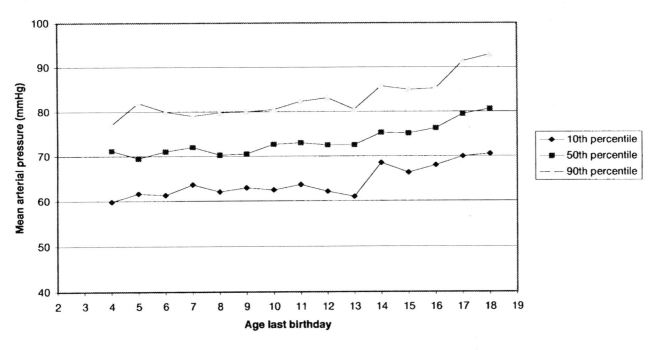

Figure 11i   Mean arterial pressure by age: females

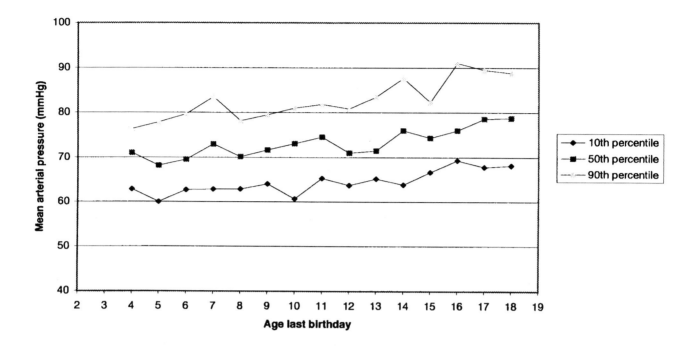

12 Blood analytes and correlations with nutrient intakes

12.1 Introduction

Chapters 1 and 2 of this Report describe the purpose, methodologies and other procedures associated with obtaining venous blood samples from young people taking part in this survey. In Chapter 3 response rates for obtaining the samples are given. In Appendix P further information is given on the procedures for obtaining and processing the samples and in Appendix Q the assay techniques are described and quality assurance data are given. This chapter reports on the results from the analysis of the blood samples.

12.1.1 Obtaining the blood sample

As described in Chapter 2 (see *Section 2.11.4)*, young people consenting to provide a fasting blood sample were asked to comply with an overnight fast before an early morning visit from a phlebotomist, accompanied by an interviewer, to attempt venepuncture. If the young person consented only to a non-fasting blood sample, or if he or she consumed anything on the morning prior to the venepuncture, then the phlebotomist still attempted to obtain a blood sample. Of the 1181 blood samples obtained, 1080 (91%) were achieved after an overnight fast; a further 13 (1%) samples were obtained from young people who consented to providing a non-fasting sample only, and the remaining 88 samples (8%) were obtained from young people who had consented to the fasting procedure, but had eaten or drunk something on the morning before the blood sample was obtained.

The results presented in this chapter are based on the results of the assays of all samples, except for results for plasma retinyl palmitate and plasma triglycerides, where only the results for fasting samples are included (see *Sections 12.4.1* and *12.5.1)*.

As described in Chapter 3, it was not possible to obtain a blood sample from all young people who consented to the procedure. For example, in a small number of cases (55) the phlebotomist was unable to obtain a sample, or sufficient sample to send for analysis, and a few young people withdrew their consent when, or before, the phlebotomist visited.

As described and shown in Appendix P, the analytes were priority ordered to take account of technical constraints and clinical and policy relevance. As also described in Appendix P, the results for some analytes

were routinely reported to the young person and their GP. The need to have certain results available for reporting also, to some extent, determined the order in which the analyses were carried out. Where it was not possible to obtain a sufficient volume of blood, the assays were carried out in the order of priority, and thus not all the assays were carried out on all the samples. The base numbers in the tables of results therefore vary for different analytes (see also *Section 12.1.2* below).

Data are presented giving distributions and descriptive statistics for the blood analytes by age and sex cohorts[1]. For selected analytes, tables are given showing the variation in analyte levels between various subgroups in the sample based on socio-demographic characteristics of the young people and their households. Again for selected analytes, tables are also given showing correlation coefficients between the analyte and the dietary intake of the relevant nutrient[2]. Correlations were run on weighted data, within age groups. Not all tables are commented on in the text.

For convenience of presentation and discussion the analytes are divided into the following main groups:

- haematology, including measures of iron status
- water soluble vitamins and plasma zinc
- fat soluble vitamins and carotenoids
- blood lipids
- other blood analytes, including mineral and trace element indices, nitrogen metabolites and acute phase reactants.

As described in Chapter 2 one of the main reasons for including a venepuncture procedure in the survey was to establish reference ranges for young people in the age range, using modern analytical techniques. Where reference ranges are quoted in the text they generally are for adults; it should therefore not be assumed, *a priori,* that values outside the reference ranges are necessarily abnormal, or that they indicate a risk of dietary inadequacy or pathology in the young people.

12.1.2 Weighting the data

As with data presented elsewhere in this report, the results for each of the blood analytes, except testosterone, plasma urea, plasma creatinine, alkaline phosphatase and erythrocyte glutathione peroxidase have been weighted at case level for both differential non-response and differential sampling probabilities and the tables present the data after weighting, with the unweighted base numbers shown (see *Appendix D*).

Testosterone was assayed only in samples from boys aged 10 to 16 years (260 cases) and the glutathione peroxidase assay was only carried out on samples collected during the last two waves of fieldwork (659 cases). The assays for plasma urea and plasma creatinine and alkaline phosphatase were of lowest priority and could only be carried out if sufficient of the sample remained after all the other, higher priority, analyses had been carried out (see *Appendix Q*). The number of samples available for these three final assays was relatively small, 611, 567 and 619 respectively. The weighting factors that would need to be applied to these relatively small numbers of cases were large and for that reason the results for testosterone, plasma urea, plasma creatinine, alkaline phosphatase and erythrocyte glutathione peroxidase are presented unweighted.

12.2 Haematology, including measures of iron status

12.2.1 The analytes and results

Tables 12.1 to 12.9 show the results for haematology analytes, including serum ferritin, for young people by age and sex. These tables give distributions of analyte levels as well as mean and median levels, and levels at the upper and lower 2.5 percentiles of the distribution.

Haemoglobin concentration (grams /decilitre)
Haemoglobin is the oxygen-carrying, iron-containing molecule in red blood cells. Circulating levels of haemoglobin are indicative of the oxygen-carrying capacity of the blood. A low haemoglobin level can indicate iron deficiency. The WHO lower limits for haemoglobin concentration are 13.0g/dl for adult males and 12.0g/dl for adult females[3]. Concentrations lower than these are indicative of anaemia. The haemoglobin levels of women of childbearing age, and therefore of young girls who have reached menarche, tend to be lower because of menstrual loss. Upper limits of haemoglobin have been set at 18g/dl for adult males and 16.5g/dl for adult women[4]. Ferritin and plasma iron percentage saturation may be used to assess iron overload.

In the NDNS of children aged 1½ to 4½ years the mean haemoglobin concentration for all children providing blood samples was 12.2g/dl[5]. However, about one in twelve children overall, and one in eight children aged between 1½ and 2½ years had a mean haemoglobin concentration below 11.0g/dl, the WHO limit defining anaemia for children aged 6 months to 6 years[3]. There is no limit defining anaemia for children after the age of 6 years or for adolescents[6].

Mean haemoglobin concentration for young people aged 4 to 18 years was 13.5g/dl for boys and significantly lower, 12.9g/dl, for girls (p < 0.01).

For boys, mean concentration increased significantly with age from 12.5g/dl for boys aged 4 to 6 years, to 14.9g/dl for boys aged 15 to 18 years (p < 0.01). In the youngest group of boys, 3%, and in those aged 7 to 10 years, 1% of boys had mean haemoglobin concentration below 11.0g/dl, the WHO limit defining anaemia for children between 6 months and 6 years. Of those aged 15 to 18 years 1% had a haemoglobin concentration below the WHO lower limit for adult males (13.0g/dl).

For girls mean haemoglobin concentration was significantly higher for those aged 7 to 10 years, 12.8g/dl, than for those in the youngest age group, 12.4g/dl (p < 0.05), but in contrast to boys there was no further marked increase in mean concentration with age. In the youngest group of girls, 8%, and in the 7 to 10 year old age group, 4%, had a mean haemoglobin concentration below 11.0g/dl, the WHO lower limit for children between 6 months and 6 years. As noted above the WHO lower limit defining anaemia for adult females, 12.0g/dl, is lower than for adult males, 13.0g/dl. For 9% of the oldest girls haemoglobin concentration was below the adult gender-specific lower limit compared with 1% found for boys aged 15 to 18 years (p < 0.05). *(Table 12.1)*

Mean corpuscular volume (MCV) (femtolitres)
The mean corpuscular volume is a measure of the average size of the red blood cells, and for children usually is between 70fl and 80fl and for adults between 83fl and 101fl[4]. A low MCV (microcytosis) is usually an indication of iron deficiency. High MCV (macrocytosis) is rare in early childhood and may be due to folate or vitamin B_{12} deficiency.

The mean MCV was 87.8fl for boys and 89.0fl for girls (p < 0.05), and for both sexes increased significantly with age (p < 0.01)[7].

In the NDNS of young children aged 1½ to 4½ years, MCV for those aged 3½ to 4½ years was 79.9fl for boys and 80.2fl for girls[5]. In this present survey mean MCV for boys and girls aged 4 to 6 years was 85.1fl and 85.8fl respectively (comparing surveys, both sexes: p < 0.01).

Overall 2.5% of all boys had an MCV at or below 78.9fl, however for those aged 11 to 14 years MCV at the lower 2.5 percentile was 68.6fl, suggesting iron deficiency in some individuals in this group of boys. Overall for girls MCV at the lower 2.5 percentile was 79.8fl. Three per cent of boys aged 11 to 14 years and 2% of girls aged 4 to 6 years, and 7 to 10 years had an MCV below 70.0fl, the lower end of the normal range for children. For girls aged 15 to 18 years 2.5% had an MCV at or above 102.5fl. In the oldest group, 2% of boys and 1% of girls had levels below the lower limit of the normal range for adults. *(Table 12.2)*

Haematocrit (packed cell volume – PCV) (litres/litre fractional volume)
The haematocrit is the proportion of the blood volume taken up by the red cells, and is determined by the cell

size and number. A lower level may indicate abnormal cell development, as shown by abnormally small red blood cells (microcytosis). Cells containing less haemoglobin may also be abnormally pale (hypochromic). Typically, iron deficiency produces a microcytic, hypochromic picture. In adult men haematocrit is usually between 0.40 1/l and 0.50 1/l and between 0.36 1/l and 0.46 1/l in adult women[4]. The normal range for children under 5 years of age is between about 0.33 1/l and 0.40 1/l[8].

Overall mean haematocrit for boys and girls were 0.425 1/l and 0.412 1/l respectively (p < 0.01), and for both sexes increased with age, for example from 0.392 1/l for boys aged 4 to 6 years to 0.468 1/l for boys aged 15 to 18 years (p < 0.01). In the oldest age group, there were no boys, but 1% of girls with haematocrit levels below the lower limit of the usual range for adults, 0.40 1/l for men and 0.36 1/l for women. Overall there were 1% of boys and 2% of girls aged 4 to 6 years with a haematocrit of less than 0.33 1/l, the lower limit for the normal range in pre-school children. *(Table 12.3)*

Mean cell haemoglobin (MCH) (picograms)

This is a measure of the mean weight of haemoglobin in each red blood cell. Cells with low values are termed hypochromic and haemoglobin production is impaired. A low MCH is a feature of iron deficiency, lead poisoning, inherited disorders of haemoglobin synthesis such as thalassaemias and other rarer disorders. In adults MCH is usually between 26.5pg and 31.5pg[4].

Overall mean MCH was 27.9pg for both boys and girls and for both sexes MCH increased significantly with age. Thus for boys and girls aged 4 to 6 years mean MCH was 26.9pg and 27.1pg respectively, increasing to 29.3pg for boys and 28.8pg for girls aged 15 to 18 years (p < 0.01).

At the lower 2.5 percentile of the distribution MCH for boys was between 21.6pg for those aged 11 to 14 years, and 26.1pg for those aged 15 to 18 years, and between 22.8pg for girls aged 7 to 10 years and 25.2pg for girls in the oldest group. In the oldest age group, 3% of boys and 7% of girls had a mean MCH below 26.5pg, the lower limit of the normal range for adults. *(Table 12.4)*

Mean cell haemoglobin concentration (MCHC) (grams/decilitre of red cell intracellular fluid)

This is a measure of the mean haemoglobin concentration in each red blood cell. For adults, if the value is lower than 30g/dl the cells are termed hypochromic, and the normal range is usually between 32g/dl and 36g/dl[4]. For pre-school children the lower limit of the usual range is about 30g/dl.

Overall mean MCHC was 31.8g/dl for boys and significantly lower, 31.4g/dl, for girls (p < 0.01)[7]. For both sexes there was no significant variation with age.

Three percent of boys and 8% of girls had a MCHC of less than 30.0g/dl. There was no clear association with age, but the proportions with a low MCHC, that is less than 30g/dl, varied by age, for boys, from none of those aged 4 to 6 years, to 7% of those aged 11 to 14 years, and for girls, from 6% of those aged 7 to 10 and 15 to 18 years, to 11% of 4 to 6 year-old girls. *(Table 12.5)*

Plasma iron (micromoles/litre)

Although it is normal for plasma iron concentration for an individual to vary throughout the day and between days, a low concentration, below 13μmol/l in adults, is indicative of iron-deficiency, inflammation, infection, surgery and chronic disease. High concentrations are indicative of liver disease, hypoplastic anaemia, ineffective erythropoiesis and iron overload. For younger adult men and women the normal range is between 13μmol/l and 32μmol/l[4].

Mean plasma iron concentration for boys was 13.67μmol/l and for girls 13.06μmol/l. For boys, there was a marked increase in mean levels as age increased, from 12.23μmol/l for boys aged 4 to 6 years, to 15.52μmol/l for boys aged 15 to 18 years (p < 0.01). For girls there was no significant variation in mean plasma iron concentration with age.

Of those aged 15 to18 years, 38% of boys and 55% of girls had plasma iron concentrations below 13.00μmol/l. For boys, the proportion tended to decrease as age increased from 50% of boys aged 4 to 6 years. For girls, the proportions with plasma iron concentrations below 13.00μmol/l varied very little between the age groups. At the lower 2.5 percentile concentrations ranged from 1.97μmol/l and 6.21μmol/l respectively for boys and girls aged 4 to 6 years to 6.54μmol/l for boys and 3.88μmol/l for girls aged 15 to 18 years. *(Table 12.6)*

Total iron-binding capacity (TIBC) (micromoles/litre)

Extracellular iron in the blood is bound to the protein, *transferrin*. The TIBC reflects the amount of transferrin that is available to be bound to iron. The laboratory method measures the amount of iron required to achieve complete saturation of the transferrin. TIBC is raised in iron-deficiency anaemia, but is lowered with infections, malignant disease, renal disease and iron overload[9]. For adults the normal range is 45μmol/l to 70μmol/l[4].

The mean TIBC for boys in the survey was 60.4μmol/l, and significantly higher, 61.8μmol/l for girls (p < 0.05). For girls, mean TIBC increased steadily across the age range, from 60.3μmol/l for girls aged 4 to 6 years, to 64.2μmol/l for girls aged 15 to 18 years (p < 0.05). For boys, TIBC increased from 59.0μmol/l for those aged 4 to 6 years up to 62.3μmol/l for those aged 11 to 14 years (p < 0.05).

Fewer than 2.5% of any age/sex group had TIBC levels

below 45μmol/l, the lower limit of the normal adult range. For girls, the proportions with TIBC at or above 70.0μmol/l increased with age, from 10% and 11% of 4 to 6 and 7 to 10 year olds respectively, to 15% of 11 to 14 year olds and 27% of 15 to 18 year-old girls. For boys the comparable proportions with TIBC at or above 70.0μmol/l for the four age groups, were 2%, 5%, 15% and, in the top age group, 13%. *(Table 12.7)*

Percentage saturation of plasma iron (%)
Transferrin is the circulating transport protein for iron. The percentage of transferrin that is saturated with iron is derived from plasma iron and total iron-binding capacity (TIBC). A decrease in percentage saturation is an indicator of a progressive iron deficiency state with depleted iron stores. When the percentage transferrin saturation drops to a certain level haemoglobin formation is likely to be impaired. For adults this level is usually considered to be 15%[10].

Overall mean plasma iron percentage saturation was 23.0% for boys, increasing significantly with age, from 20.8% for boys aged 4 to 6 years to 26.0% for boys aged 15 to 18 years (p < 0.05). For girls the overall mean was 21.5% (ns) and, unlike boys, varied very little across the age groups.

For boys the proportion with low levels of plasma iron percentage saturation, that is less than 15%, was highest for the youngest age group, 23%, but then fell to 12% for the oldest age group (youngest and oldest age groups: p < 0.01). In contrast, for girls the proportion with levels below 15% was 24% of 4 to 6 year olds and 20% of 11 to 14 year olds (ns), and then increased for the oldest age group to 30% (p < 0.01). *(Table 12.8)*

Serum ferritin (micrograms/litre)
Serum ferritin gives an indication of the level of iron stores as well as being an acute phase reactant that is raised in response to infection or inflammation.

The normal range for serum ferritin is generally taken to be 20μg/l to 300μg/l for adult males and 15μg/l to 150μg/l for adult females[4]. Raised serum ferritin levels should be interpreted with care as they can also result from inflammatory conditions, liver disease or other chronic disorders.

Mean serum ferritin was 39μg/l for boys and 32μg/l for girls (p < 0.05). For boys there was a significant increase in mean concentration as age increased, rising from 31μg/l for boys aged 4 to 6 years to 52μg/l for boys aged 15 to 18 years (p < 0.01). For girls, mean serum ferritin concentration was highest for those aged 7 to 10 years, 38μg/l, with almost no difference between the other age groups.

Serum ferritin concentrations of less than 20μg/l were found for 13% of boys overall, ranging from 18% for the youngest age group to 5% for those aged 15 to 18

years (ns). For girls, 9% of those aged 4 to 6 years had a serum ferritin below 15μg/l, but this proportion increased to 27% for those aged 15 to 18 years (p < 0.01).

At the lower 2.5 percentile of the distribution serum ferritin ranged between 7μg/l and 15μg/l depending on the age and sex of the young person. *(Table 12.9)*

The haematology assay carried out at the Great Ormond Street Hospital routinely produces results for a large number of analytes in addition to those of principal interest in the context of this survey. In particular, the assay reports a number of cell counts, including red and white blood cells, platelets, neutrophils, lymphocytes and monocytes. Table 12.10 shows mean levels for the following other analytes that were routinely produced as part of the haematology assay, and is given without comment:

- blood cell counts:
  red blood cells, red cell distribution width, platelets, mean platelet volume, platelet distribution width, white cells, neutrophils, lymphocytes, monocytes, eosinophils, basophils
- HbF (percentage)
- HbA$_2$ (percentage)

The assays also identified the following numbers of young people with abnormal haemoglobin:

sickle cell trait:	4
sickle cell anaemia:	1
HbD Punjab:	1
HbC trait:	2
beta thalassaemia trait:	2

The survey doctor reported the results of the white cell differential counts and the abnormal haemoglobins to the young person and his or her GP, along with other results, as described in Appendix N. *(Table 12.10)*

12.2.2 Correlation with dietary intakes
Table 12.11 gives correlation coefficients for haemoglobin and serum ferritin concentrations with dietary intakes, from all sources, including supplements, of total iron, haem and non-haem iron, vitamins C and B$_{12}$ and folate.

In interpreting these and other correlations between blood analyte levels and dietary intakes, particularly when correlations do not reach the level of statistical significance, it should be remembered that blood samples could not be taken until after the end of the dietary recording period. While every effort was made to visit the young person as soon as possible, in some cases a period of a week or longer elapsed before a blood sample could be taken.

It should also be noted that where correlations are statistically significant the relationship between the analyte and intake may not necessarily be causal; other factors, in particular the young person's health at the time, may have affected the size of the correlation. Finally, multiple tests for significance can suggest associations or differences which may have arisen by chance.

The table shows that overall for boys haemoglobin concentration was positively correlated with dietary intakes of total, haem and non-haem iron, vitamins C and B_{12}, and folate (all $p < 0.01$). For girls, the correlations were less marked; haemoglobin concentration was positively correlated with intake of haem iron ($p < 0.01$) and to a lesser extent with intakes of total iron, non-haem iron and vitamin C ($p < 0.05$).

For both boys and girls serum ferritin levels were positively correlated with dietary intake of haem iron ($p < 0.01$) and, additionally for boys, but not girls, with intakes of total iron, non-haem iron and folate ($p < 0.05$). *(Table 12.11)*

12.2.3 *Variation in the levels of haematology analytes and measures of iron status*

Results for the main haematology analytes and measures of iron status were examined in relation to various social and demographic characteristics of the young person and their household, in the same way as variation in food and nutrient intakes has been examined.

Generally the associations were statistically weak, not reaching significance level ($p > 0.05$), which may at least be in part due to the relatively small size of some of the subgroups.

From Table 12.13 it can be seen that girls living in London and the South East had a mean serum ferritin concentration which was higher than for girls living elsewhere ($p < 0.05$[11]). There were no other significant haematological differences between the regions for boys or girls.

Table 12.14 shows that for both boys and girls mean levels for most of the haematology analytes were lower for young people living in households where the parents were in receipt of benefits. For boys the differences were statistically significant for both haemoglobin concentration and mean cell haemoglobin (both: $p < 0.05$).

As Table 12.15 shows for most analytes there was a clear pattern of mean analyte levels increasing as total gross weekly household income increased. For boys mean cell haemoglobin was significantly higher for those living in households where the gross weekly household income was £600 or more compared with those where the gross household income was less than £160 a week (boys:

$p < 0.01$; girls: ns). Boys in households with the highest gross weekly income had significantly higher mean levels of mean cell volume, plasma iron % saturation and plasma iron concentration than those from the lowest income households (all: $p < 0.05$). Levels of TIBC and serum ferritin did not show the same association with income; serum ferritin levels for both boys and girls and TIBC for girls showed no consistent association with household income level, but for boys, mean TIBC was significantly higher for those in households where the income was between £280 and less than £400 (compared with those in the lowest and highest income households: $p < 0.05$).

There was no clear or statistically significant association between levels of the haematology analytes and whether the young person had been unwell during the dietary recording period or with the social class of the head of the young person's household. *(Tables 12.12 to 12.16)*

12.3 Water soluble vitamins and plasma zinc

12.3.1 *The analytes and results*

Plasma ascorbate (vitamin C) (micromoles/litre)
Fasting plasma vitamin C concentrations reflect tissue levels, as well as recent dietary intakes of vitamin C, with values of less than $11 \mu mol/l$ indicative of biochemical depletion[12].

Mean plasma vitamin C concentration for boys and girls was similar, $56.4 \mu mol/l$ and $58.8 \mu mol/l$ respectively and for both sexes mean concentration tended to decrease as age increased. For example for 4 to 6 year olds, mean plasma vitamin C concentration was $61.6 \mu mol/l$ for boys and $64.6 \mu mol/l$ for girls, falling to $50.2 \mu mol/l$ and $55.7 \mu mol/l$ for boys and girls aged 15 to 18 years (boys: $p < 0.05$; girls: ns).

No more than 5% of any age/sex group had a plasma vitamin C concentration below $11 \mu mol/l$. Young people at the lower 2.5 percentile of the distribution had plasma vitamin C levels which ranged from only $0.6 \mu mol/l$, for the youngest cohort of boys, to $17.0 \mu mol/l$, for girls aged 11 to 14 years. *(Table 12.17)*

Red cell folate and serum folate (nanomoles/litre)
The term folate includes several derivatives of the parent molecule folic acid (pteroyl monoglutamic acid). Red cell folate is usually a better measure of long-term status because it reflects body stores at the time of red cell synthesis. However fasting serum folate concentration reflects tissue levels, as well as recent dietary intake of folate.

Folate values and normal ranges are assay-method dependent, which makes it difficult to compare values directly between different studies and surveys. The following interpretation of ranges was suggested[13]:

for red cell folate:
  deficient   less than 337nmol/l
  intermediate 337nmol/l – 422nmol/l
  normal   422nmol/l –1463nmol/l
for serum folate:
  deficient   less than 6.3nmol/l
  intermediate 6.3nmol/l – 7.0nmol/l
  normal   7.0nmol/l – 28.1 nmol/l

Based on an older, probably microbiological assay, the normal range for serum folate concentration in adults is usually considered to be between 7nmol/l and 46nmol/l[4]. In adults, red cell folate concentrations below 230nmol/l are considered to be severely deficient, while concentrations between 230nmol/l and 345nmol/l indicate marginal status[14]. Statistically defined upper limits for nutrients such as folate, do not have any well-established or nutritional significance. The normal range of values for these analytes in pre-school age children has not been defined, but the NDNS of young children aged 1½ to 4½ years reported mean concentrations for serum folate for boys and girls aged 3½ to 4½ years of 22.0nmol/l and 20.4nmol/l respectively[5].

The mean concentration of *red cell folate* in the samples provided by boys in the survey was 626nmol/l and for girls 573nmol/l. For both boys and girls the mean level decreased significantly as age increased (both sexes: p < 0.01). For example, for girls aged 4 to 6 years mean red cell folate was 677nmol/l compared with 500nmol/l for girls aged 15 to 18 years.

Levels of less than 350nmol/l were found in 7% of the samples from boys and 9% of the samples from girls (ns), but no more than 1% of any age/sex group had a red cell folate of less than 230nmol/l, showing that severe folate deficiency is negligible in young people. Young people at the lower 2.5 percentile of the distribution had red cell folate levels which ranged from 268nmol/l for girls aged 15 to 18 years to 365 nmol/l for the youngest cohort of girls.

Mean *serum folate* concentration was similar for boys and girls, 21.7nmol/l and 20.6nmol/l respectively, with median values very close to mean levels. One per cent of boys aged 15 to 18 years, and 1% of girls aged 11 to 18 years, had a serum folate concentration below 6.3nmol/l. At the lower 2.5 percentile of the distribution levels ranged between 7.0nmol/l, for girls aged 15 to 18 years, and 13.4nmol/l, for girls aged 4 to 6 years.

Levels of serum folate and red cell folate were strongly positively correlated with each other for both boys and girls in each of the age groups (all: p < 0.01). Coefficients ranged from 0.45 for boys aged 4 to 6 years, to 0.56 for boys aged between 11 and 18 and girls aged 7 to 10 years.   *(Tables 12.18 to 12.20)*

Serum vitamin B$_{12}$ (picomoles/litre)

Serum concentration of vitamin B$_{12}$ is a good indicator of vitamin B$_{12}$ status. Vitamin B$_{12}$, with folate, is required for methyl group transfer during protein metabolism and DNA synthesis. Vitamin B$_{12}$ is also required to maintain the integrity of the nervous system. For adults, the lower level of normality for serum vitamin B$_{12}$ concentration is usually taken as 118pmol/l[4].

There was no significant difference between boys and girls in the mean concentration of serum vitamin B$_{12}$, at 403pmol/l and 395pmol/l respectively. However for both sexes mean levels decreased markedly as age increased, from 525pmol/l and 550pmol/l for boys and girls aged 4 to 6 years, to 277pmol/l and 267pmol/l for those aged 15 to 18 years (both sexes: p < 0.01).

There were no young people in the three youngest age groups with serum vitamin B$_{12}$ levels below 118pmol/l, but 1% of boys and 8% of girls in the oldest group had levels below this, the lower level of normality for adults. Overall, the lower 2.5 percentile for girls was 119pmol/l, but in the oldest cohort of girls the level at the lower 2.5 percentile of the distribution was only 97pmol/l.
                                                                (Table 12.21)

Erythrocyte Transketolase Activation Coefficient (ETKAC)

As with most water-soluble vitamins, there is virtually no recognisable store of non-functional thiamin in the body and the only reserve is that which is functionally bound to enzymes within the tissues. The *erythrocyte transketolase activation coefficient* depends on the reactivation of the cofactor-depleted red cell enzyme transketolase *in vitro*. This index is sensitive to the lower to moderate range of intakes of thiamin. For adults, values above 1.25 are indicative of biochemical thiamin deficiency[10].

Mean ETKAC for both boys and girls was 1.12, and for both sexes the mean ratio increased as age increased (both sexes: p < 0.01). For boys and girls aged 4 to 6 years mean ETKAC was 1.10, rising to 1.13 for those aged 15 to 18 years (p < 0.01).

For boys ETKAC at the upper 2.5 percentile was below 1.25 for each age group. For girls aged 7 to 10 years and 15 to 18 years ETKACs at the upper 2.5 percentile were 1.25 and 1.26 respectively.   *(Table 12.22)*

Erythrocyte Transketolase Basal Activity (ETK-B) (micromoles/gram haemoglobin/min)

Prolonged thiamin deficiency *in vivo* or non-ideal storage conditions for the red cell enzyme *in vitro* can lead to a disproportionate loss of cofactor depleted apoenzyme, presumably to a degraded, non-reactivatable form. For this reason it is recommended that the basal activity, that is the activity without added cofactor, as well as the activation coefficient of erythrocyte transketolase is quoted as two partly independent indices of thiamin status. The basal activity and activation coefficient together are sometimes used to distinguish between acute and chronic thiamin deficiency.

Mean ETK-B was 0.87μmol/g Hb/min for boys and 0.85μmol/g Hb/min for girls. For both sexes the mean level decreased as age increased, from 0.90μmol/g Hb/min for boys and 0.91μmol/g Hb/min for girls aged 4 to 6 years to 0.82μmol/g Hb/min for those aged 15 to 18 years (boys: $p < 0.05$; girls: $p < 0.01$).

At the lower 2.5 percentile of the distribution levels ranged between 0.56μmol/g Hb/min, for girls aged 11 to 14 years, to 0.66μmol/g Hb/min, for boys aged 7 to 10 years.   *(Table 12.23)*

Erythrocyte Glutathione Reductase Activation Coefficient (EGRAC)
The *erythrocyte glutathione reductase activation coefficient* is a measure of red cell enzyme saturation with its riboflavin, vitamin B_2, derived cofactor, flavin adenine dinucleotide, FAD. Riboflavin is needed for the utilisation of energy from food. The coefficient is expressed as the ratio of two activity measures of the enzyme glutathione reductase, with and without the cofactor FAD. The higher the coefficient the lower the saturation *in vitro*. A coefficient of between 1.0 and 1.3 is generally considered to be normal. The test is most sensitive at low levels of riboflavin intake. Like EAATAC, the EGRAC index is highly sensitive to small degrees of cofactor desaturation, and moderately raised values are not associated with known functional abnormality.

The mean EGRAC for boys, 1.42, was significantly lower than the mean ratio for girls, 1.47, ($p < 0.01$), but for both sexes, EGRAC increased significantly as age increased. Thus mean EGRAC was, respectively, 1.36 and 1.38 for boys and girls aged 4 to 6 years, rising to 1.48 and 1.53 for boys and girls aged 15 to 18 years (both sexes: $p < 0.01$).

In Chapter 8 it was shown that 6% of boys in the top two age groups had intakes of riboflavin from food sources which were below the LRNI, as did 22% of girls aged 11 to 14 years and 21% of girls aged 15 to 18 years (see *Table 8.15*). Table 12.24 shows that 75% of boys and 87% of girls aged between 4 and 18 had an EGRAC above 1.30. In the NDNS of pre-school children 29% of boys and 38% of girls aged 3½ to 4½ years were found to have an EGRAC greater than 1.30[5]. As this present survey of young people shows the proportion of boys with an EGRAC greater than 1.30 continues to rise from 59% of boys aged 4 to 6 years, to 78% for boys aged 7 to 10 years ($p < 0.05$), but with no further significant increase for the remaining two upper age groups. For girls however the rise in the proportion with an EGRAC above 1.30 continues throughout the age range, from 75% of 4 to 6 year-old girls to nearly all,

95%, of 15 to 18 year-old girls ($p < 0.01$). It should be noted that the apparently high proportion of 'deficient' values, that is greater than 1.30, is a characteristic of the sensitive assay procedure used. The same procedure was used for the earlier surveys in the NDNS programme, of pre-school children[5] and people aged 65 years and over[15] but differs in detail from the assay procedure used in the 1986/87 Dietary and Nutritional Survey of British Adults[16].   *(Table 12.24)*

Erythrocyte Aspartate Aminotransferase Activation Coefficient (EAATAC)
The *erythrocyte aspartate aminotransferase activation coefficient* is a measure of red cell enzyme saturation with pyridoxal phosphate, vitamin B_6, derived cofactor, and aspartate aminotransferase saturation with pyridoxal phosphate, its vitamin B_6 - derived cofactor. Like other coefficients the test is most sensitive at and below marginal intakes. For adults, values above 2.00 are indicative of biochemical vitamin B_6 deficiency[4].

Mean EAATAC for boys was 1.80, and for girls, 1.79. For boys mean EAATAC tended to rise with age, from 1.75 for those aged 4 to 6 years to 1.82 for those in the two upper age groups ($p < 0.05$). For girls there was no clear association with age. Overall 10% of boys and girls had an EAATAC greater than 2.00, suggesting possible vitamin B_6 deficiency. At the upper 2.5 percentile of the distribution ratios were above 2.00 for all groups, ranging from 2.10, for boys aged 11 to 14 years, to 2.30 for boys aged 4 to 6 years.
                                      (Table 12.25)

Plasma zinc (micromoles/litre)
Zinc is an essential component of a number of enzymes in which it has structural, regulatory or catalytic roles[17]. Zinc deficiency adversely affects cellular immunity at all ages. A low zinc concentration may be due to a number of factors other than simple zinc deficiency, such as low albumin concentration. For adults, zinc deficiency has been defined as a concentration below 10.71μmol/l (below 0.70μg/ml) for a fasting sample, or a concentration below 9.95μmol/l (below 0.65μg/ml) for a non-fasting sample[18].

Overall mean plasma zinc concentration for both boys and girls was 14.6μmol/l. For girls levels tended to decline steadily with increasing age, so that among girls aged 4 to 6 years, mean plasma zinc was 15.1μmol/l, falling to 13.9μmol/l for girls aged 15 to 18 years ($p < 0.01$).

At the lower 2.5 percentile of the distribution plasma zinc concentration ranged between 7.0μmol/l, for boys aged 4 to 6 years, and 12.3μmol/l, for girls aged 4 to 6 years.   *(Table 12.26)*

12.3.2 Correlation with dietary intakes
Table 12.11 and Tables 12.27 to 12.31 show correlation

coefficients for blood analytes for water-soluble vitamins and plasma zinc with dietary intakes, from all sources, of these vitamins and related nutrients.

Plasma vitamin C was strongly and positively correlated with intakes of dietary vitamin C for boys and girls in each of the four age groups ($p < 0.01$); coefficients ranged from 0.28, for boys aged 15 to 18 years, to 0.49, for boys aged 11 to 14 years.

Overall for boys red cell folate concentration correlated positively with intakes of non-haem iron and folate ($p < 0.05$), and more strongly with intakes of vitamins C and B_{12} ($p < 0.01$); intake of haem iron was negatively correlated with red cell folate ($p < 0.01$). For girls the same associations were found (haem iron, vitamin B_{12} and folate: $p < 0.01$; vitamin C: $p < 0.05$), but, in addition, red cell folate was also strongly positively correlated with total iron intake ($p < 0.01$). For boys significant correlations between red cell folate level and dietary intakes of these nutrients were least likely for those aged between 7 and 10 years; for girls similar significant correlations were generally found for each of the four age groups. *(Table 12.11)*

Levels of serum vitamin B_{12} and dietary intakes of this vitamin were strongly and positively correlated for both boys and girls (boys: $p < 0.05$; girls $p < 0.01$).

Table 12.29 shows that ETKAC and dietary intake of thiamin were, as predicted, generally negatively correlated. However the correlation only reached the level of statistical significance for girls overall, (-0.11: $p < 0.05$) and not for individual age groups nor for all boys.

Dietary intake of riboflavin was significantly and negatively correlated with EGRAC for each age/sex group, (all: $p < 0.01$) indicating that EGRAC increased as dietary intake of riboflavin fell. Coefficients ranged between -0.30, for boys aged 7 to 10 years, to -0.49, for girls in the same age group.

Levels of plasma zinc were quite weakly correlated with dietary intake of zinc, but the relationship was somewhat stronger for intake of protein. Thus the only significant correlation between plasma zinc and dietary intake of zinc was for all girls ($+0.15$; $p < 0.01$). For plasma zinc with protein the coefficients were significant for all boys ($+0.11$; $p < 0.05$) and for all girls ($+0.15$; $p < 0.01$) and girls aged 15 to 18 years ($+0.28$; $p < 0.01$). *(Tables 12.27 to 12.31)*

12.3.3 Variation in the levels of water soluble vitamins and plasma zinc

Tables 12.32 to 12.36 show the variation in mean analyte levels for water soluble vitamins and plasma zinc according to various socio-demographic characteristics and whether the young person was unwell during the 7-day dietary recording period.

Generally the differences between the different socio-demographic groups in mean levels for the water soluble vitamins were small, not reaching the level of statistical significance ($p > 0.05$)[11]. However there were some clear trends in the data, with water soluble vitamin status tending to be lower for boys and girls from lower socio-economic backgrounds, and for those living in Scotland and the Northern region.

For vitamin C, mean plasma levels were significantly lower for both boys and girls from households with a gross weekly income of less than £160 and for those whose parents were in receipt of benefits (all: $p < 0.01$). Additionally girls from a manual social class background and those living in the Northern region had a significantly lower mean plasma vitamin C level (social class: $p < 0.01$; region: $p < 0.05$).

Mean levels of serum folate were significantly lower for boys from a manual social class background ($p < 0.05$).

Girls in the Central and South West regions of England and in Wales had a lower mean EAATAC than girls in the Northern region ($p < 0.05$).

There was very little variation in mean levels of plasma zinc for boys or girls associated with any of the socio-demographic characteristics considered, although again the data suggest the mean levels were generally lower for those from lower socio-economic backgrounds. The only difference reaching the level of statistical significance was for boys in the lowest income households, less than £160 a week, whose mean plasma zinc was lower than for boys living in households where the gross weekly household income was £600 or more, 13.68μmol/l compared with 14.83μmol/l ($p < 0.05$).

There were almost no significant differences in blood analytes levels associated with whether the young person was unwell during the dietary recording period. Only for red cell folate was there a significant difference in mean concentration with girls who were unwell and whose eating was affected having a lower mean red cell folate than girls who were not unwell ($p < 0.05$). *(Tables 12.32 to 12.36)*

12.4 Fat soluble vitamins and carotenoids

12.4.1 The analytes and results

Plasma retinol (vitamin A) (micromoles/litre)
Plasma retinol is related to long-term dietary intake of vitamin A. The plasma concentration is homeostatically controlled with little variation either within or between subjects. For adults, concentrations below 0.35μmol/l are considered to be severely deficient and concentrations between 0.35μmol/l and 0.70μmol/l indicate marginal status[10].

Overall mean plasma retinol concentration was

1.29µmol/l for boys and 1.29µmol/l for girls. For both sexes mean values increased as age increased, from 1.12µmol/l and 1.15µmol/l for boys and girls aged 4 to 6 years, to 1.53µmol/l and 1.51µmol/l for boys and girls aged 15 to 18 years (both sexes: p < 0.01).

There were no young people with plasma retinol values of less than 0.35µmol/l and no more than 3% in any age/sex group with levels between 0.35µmol/l and 0.70µmol/l indicating marginal status. *(Table 12.37)*

Plasma retinyl palmitate (micromoles/litre)

Plasma retinyl palmitate is a fatty acid ester of retinol, which is normally present at very low concentrations compared with unesterified retinol, which is associated with retinol-binding protein. Retinyl esters increase considerably if not measured on a fasting sample and peak about 4 to 6 hours after a meal[19]. Results for plasma retinyl palmitate are therefore reported only for fasting blood samples.

Blood samples from 1080 young people (unweighted) were analysed for plasma retinyl palmitate concentration. Of these 990 (92%) were fasting samples, 80 (7%) were from young people who consented to a fasting sample, but had eaten or drunk something shortly before providing a sample, and 10 (1%) were from young people who consented to providing a non-fasting sample. The results for plasma retinyl palmitate concentration are therefore based on results for 990 samples.

Retinyl palmitate may increase considerably in people with very high intakes of the vitamin, and is sometimes used as an indicator of vitamin A overload.

Mean concentration of plasma retinyl palmitate in fasting samples was 0.115µmol/l for boys and 0.111µmol/l for girls. For both sexes, levels tended to decrease as age increased, but the differences were not statistically significant (p > 0.05).

At the upper 2.5 percentile of the distribution values were between 0.208µmol/l and 0.244µmol/l for boys and 0.195µmol/l and 0.259µmol/l for girls respectively. *(Table 12.38)*

Plasma α- and β-carotene and α- and β-cryptoxanthin (micromoles/litre)

These are all carotenoids with vitamin A activity and reflect short to medium term intakes over a wide range. Concentration of carotenoids may be influenced by conversion to vitamin A, the conversion being dependent on vitamin A status and requirements. This may confound comparisons between dietary intakes and blood concentrations.

There were no significant differences (p > 0.05) in mean levels of either α- or β-carotene between boys and girls. Mean α-carotene for boys and girls respectively was

0.044µmol/l and 0.049µmol/l and for β-carotene 0.316µmol/l and 0.312µmol/l.

Mean β-carotene levels decreased significantly with age for both boys and girls, as did mean α-carotene concentration for girls, but not for boys. For example, mean β-carotene for girls aged 4 to 6 years was 0.418µmol/l compared with 0.257µmol/l for girls aged 15 to 18 years (p < 0.01).

At the lower 2.5 percentile of the distribution there was little difference in each age group between boys and girls in α-carotene concentration. However, levels of β-carotene at the lower 2.5 percentile were somewhat higher for boys aged 4 to 6 and 15 to 18 years, 0.141µmol/l and 0.063µmol/l, than levels for girls in the same two age groups, 0.107µmol/l and 0.048µmol/l respectively.

Mean concentrations of both α- and β-cryptoxanthin were not significantly different overall for boys compared with girls (p > 0.05); for α-cryptoxanthin means were 0.061µmol/l and 0.058µmol/l for boys and girls respectively, and for β-cryptoxanthin, 0.165µmol/l and 0.179µmol/l. For both analytes and for both sexes, in particular girls, mean concentrations were highest for those in the youngest age group and lowest for the 15 to 18 year olds. For example, mean concentration for girls aged 4 to 6 years for α-cryptoxanthin was 0.069µmol/l and for β-cryptoxanthin was 0.238µmol/l, compared with 0.053µmol/l and 0.156µmol/l for girls aged 15 to 18 years (both: p < 0.05).

At the lower 2.5 percentile of the distribution there was less variation by age for either boys or girls. Concentrations ranged for α-cryptoxanthin from 0.017µmol/l, for boys aged 15 to 18 years, to 0.022µmol/l, for girls aged 7 to 10 years, and for β-cryptoxanthin from 0.026µmol/l, for girls aged 15 to 18 years, to 0.045µmol/l, for boys aged 7 to 10 years. *(Tables 12.39 to 12.42)*

Plasma lycopene and plasma lutein and zeaxanthin (micromoles/litre)

Lycopene, lutein and zeaxanthin are also carotenoids but with no provitamin A activity. The main sources of dietary lycopene are tomatoes and processed tomato products. Plasma lutein concentration may be a useful marker of green vegetable intake.

Mean plasma lycopene for boys was 0.489µmol/l and for girls, 0.485µmol/l (ns) and for both sexes there was very little variation in mean concentration associated with age. However, at the lower 2.5 percentile of the distribution concentrations were generally lower in each age group for boys than for girls. For example, for boys aged 7 to 10 years, lycopene concentration at the lower 2.5 percentile was 0.083µmol/l, compared with 0.115µmol/l for girls in the same age group, and for those aged 15 to 18 years was 0.112µmol/l for boys compared with 0.180µmol/l for girls.

Mean plasma lutein and zeaxanthin also showed very little variation either by sex or age group. Mean concentrations were 0.324μmol/l for boys and 0.323μmol/l for girls (ns). At the lower 2.5 percentile concentrations ranged between 0.125μmol/l, for girls aged 15 to 18 years, and 0.174μmol/l, for girls aged 11 to 14 years.   *(Tables 12.43 and 12.44)*

Plasma 25-hydroxyvitamin D (nanomoles/litre)
Plasma 25-hydroxyvitamin D (25-OHD) is derived from ergocalciferol and cholecalciferol which is obtained from the diet and from synthesis in the skin of cholecalciferol during ultraviolet irradiation from sunlight. It is a measure of vitamin D status and reflects the availability of vitamin D in the body from both dietary and endogenous sources. Factors influencing exposure to sunlight, such as the time of year, habit of dress and time spent outdoors should therefore be considered when interpreting 25-OHD results. Vitamin D is required for calcium absorption from the intestine as well as for a range of other metabolic processes. The lower level of the normal range for adults for plasma 25-OHD is usually considered to be 25nmol/l.

Mean plasma 25-OHD for boys was 62.0nmol/l and for girls 60.6nmol/l (ns). For both sexes mean concentration decreased significantly as age increased, from 71.8nmol/l and 68.9nmol/l for boys and girls aged 4 to 6 years respectively, to 51.6nmol/l and 53.7nmol/l for boys and girls aged 15 to 18 years ($p < 0.01$).

Median values were lower than mean values for each age and sex group, the difference being most marked for the oldest group of boys.

Three per cent of boys aged 11 to 14 years, and 2% of girls in each of the two top age groups had plasma 25-OHD concentrations of less than 12.0nmol/l. The proportions with concentrations below 25.0nmol/l increased with age for both boys and girls from 3% for boys and 2% for girls aged 4 to 6 years, to 16% for boys aged 15 to 18 years, and 11% for girls aged 11 to 14 years (both sexes: $p < 0.05$). For girls aged 15 to 18 years the proportion was 10%, and for boys aged 11 to 14 years, 11%.

For boys aged 11 to 14 years 2.5% had a plasma 25-OHD concentration at or below 11.8nmol/l; for girls in this age group the level at the 2.5 percentile was 13.5nmol/l. At the upper 2.5 percentile concentrations ranged between 103.5nmol/l, for boys aged 11 to 14 years, and 145.7nmol/l, for boys aged 7 to 10 years.

Seasonal variation in concentration of plasma 25-OHD
Vitamin D synthesised by the skin in the presence of sunlight is an important source and plasma levels of 25-OHD are likely to be higher during the summer months. Plasma 25-OHD concentration was therefore tabulated by the month when the blood sample was taken[20].

Figures 12.1 to 12.3 show variation in mean plasma 25-OHD concentration for boys and girls by when the blood sample was taken. The mean plasma 25-OHD concentration for both boys and girls was higher for those who provided a sample in the summer months, July to September, than for those who gave a sample at other times of the year (both sexes: $p < 0.01$). Mean concentrations were also significantly higher in samples obtained between October and December than those obtained in the following three months (both sexes: $p < 0.01$) and for girls, but not boys, between samples obtained in April to June compared with those obtained between January and March ($p < 0.01$). Twelve per cent of samples from girls taken in January to March, and 14% of samples from boys taken in April to June had a mean plasma 25-OHD concentration of less than 25.0nmol/l.

It was noted above that boys aged 11 to 18 years were most likely to have a poor vitamin D status (less than 25nmol/l). Further analysis (*table not shown*) showed the extent of seasonal variation for this group. From samples obtained in January to March there were 19% of boys in this age group with poor status, from April to June 15%, 6% from July to September and 10% from October to December. From samples for boys aged 15 to 18 years between April and June, nearly one quarter, 23% had 25-OHD below 25nmol/l.
                    (Table 12.45 and Figures 12.1 to 12.3)

Plasma α- and γ-tocopherol (micromoles/litre)[21]
Plasma tocopherol concentration can be used as a measure of vitamin E status. α-tocopherol is the predominant form in human tissues. It has the highest biological activity and is the least resistant to oxidation. Increased concentration of plasma lipids appears to cause tocopherols to partition out of cellular membranes, thus increasing concentrations of tocopherol and resulting in a correlation between tocopherol and total lipid in the blood, particularly with the cholesterol fraction. For this reason plasma tocopherol can be usefully expressed as tocopherol/cholesterol (μmol/μmol) ratio[22], enabling comparisons to be made between age groups with different plasma lipid levels.

For adults plasma tocopherols below 11.6μmol/l, or a tocopherol: cholesterol ratio of below 2.25μmol/mmol, tend to cause red blood cells to haemolyse after exposure to oxidising agents. This is sometimes considered to be an indicator of biochemical deficiency but is not indicative of a clinical deficiency of vitamin E. The COMA Panel on Dietary Reference Values considered a tocopherol: cholesterol ratio of 2.25μmol/mmol to be the lowest satisfactory value for adults[23].

Mean α-tocopherol concentration was 19.8μmol/l for boys and 20.6μmol/l for girls ($p < 0.05$). For both sexes there was a tendency for mean concentration to fall slightly with increasing age, although the differences between the highest and lowest concentrations by age group were not significant (p > 0.05). In the youngest age group, 2% of boys and 3% of girls had values below 11.6μmol/l. In the older age groups no more than 1% of either boys or girls had values below 11.6μmol/l. At the lower 2.5 percentile of the distribution plasma α-tocopherol concentrations ranged between 9.5μmol/l, for girls aged 4 to 6 years, below the lower limit of the normal range for adults, and 13.9μmol/l, for girls aged 7 to 10 years and for boys aged 11 to 14 years.

Mean concentration of γ-tocopherol was 1.48μmol/l for boys and 1.50μmol/l for girls (ns). For boys there was no clear association between mean concentration and age, but for girls levels tended to decline as age increased. Thus for girls aged 4 to 6 years, mean γ-tocopherol concentration was 1.58μmol/l falling to 1.34μmol/l for girls aged 15 to 18 years (p < 0.05).

At the lower 2.5 percentile of the distribution there was little significant or systematic variation by sex or age with plasma γ-tocopherol concentration ranging between 0.56μmol/l, for the oldest group of girls, and 0.70μmol/l, for girls aged 11 to 14 years.

(Tables 12.46 and 12.47)

Overall the mean tocopherol to cholesterol ratio was 5.34μmol/mmol for both boys and girls. For boys, the ratio appeared to increase steadily across the age range, from 5.23μmol/mmol for those aged 4 to 6 years to 5.43μmol/mmol for those aged 15 to 18 years (ns). For girls the mean ratio also appeared to increase with age group up to those aged 11 to 14 years, from 5.26μmol/mmol to 5.43μmol/mmol (ns) and then to decrease for the top age group, girls aged 15 to 18 years, to 5.25μmol/mmol (ns). There were no cases below 2.25μmol/mmol, the lowest satisfactory value for adults, and at the lower 2.5 percentile the ratio ranged between 3.44μmol/mmol, for boys aged 7 to 10 years, and 4.05μmol/mmol, for boys aged 15 to 18 years. At the upper 2.5 percentile the ratio ranged between 7.43μmol/mmol, for boys aged 11 to 14 years, and 8.70μmol/mmol, for girls aged 11 to 14 years.

(Table 12.48)

12.4.2 Correlation with dietary intakes

Table 12.49 shows that overall for both boys and girls concentration of plasma retinol correlated significantly with dietary intakes of both α- and β-carotene (all p < 0.01, except for α-carotene for girls, where p < 0.05). For the youngest age group the coefficients were negative, indicating that plasma vitamin A concentration tended to increase as dietary intake of carotenes decreased (boys: ns; girls: p < 0.05). For all other age/sex groups the correlation coefficients were positive.

Plasma retinol was significantly positively correlated with dietary intake of vitamin A (retinol equivalents) for all boys (p < 0.01) and for boys aged 7 to 10 years (p < 0.05) and 15 to 18 years (p < 0.01). The correlation

was less strong for girls and only reached the level of significance for all girls (p < 0.05). *(Table 12.49)*

Dietary intakes of α-carotene were strongly positively correlated with plasma α-carotene concentration for both sexes (p < 0.01). Generally the coefficients were largest for the younger age groups, and for girls aged 15 to 18 years did not reach the level of statistical significance (boys and girls aged 4 to 14: p < 0.01; boys aged 15 to 18: p < 0.05; girls 15 to 18 years: ns).

Correlations between the plasma concentration and the dietary intake of β-carotene were much weaker; overall the coefficient was +0.09 for both boys and girls (p < 0.05) and within age group only reached the level of statistical significance for boys aged 11 to 14 years (p < 0.05) and for girls aged 7 to 10 years (p < 0.01).

(Tables 12.50 and 12.51)

It has already been shown (*Table 12.45 and Figures 12.1 to 12.3*) that plasma 25-OHD concentration varied significantly according to the time of year when the blood sample was taken. Table 12.52 shows that the correlations between plasma 25-OHD concentration and dietary intake of vitamin D were very weak and did not reach the level of statistical significance for any age/sex group (p > 0.05). *(Table 12.52)*

As Table 12.53 shows correlation coefficients between dietary intakes of vitamin E and plasma α-tocopherol, plasma total tocopherol and the ratio between total tocopherol and cholesterol were generally weak, particularly for boys. For girls, correlations were statistically significant between dietary intake of vitamin E and plasma α-tocopherol for those aged 7 to 10 years (+0.18) and 15 to 18 years (+0.21) and between dietary vitamin E and plasma total tocopherol for those aged 11 to 14 (-0.19) and 15 to 18 years (+0.18) (all: p < 0.05). Overall for boys there was a significant positive correlation between vitamin E intake and the tocopherol to cholesterol ratio (+0.10; p < 0.05). *(Table 12.53)*

12.4.3 Variation in the levels of fat soluble vitamins and carotenoids

Tables 12.54 to 12.58 show variations in mean levels of fat soluble vitamins and carotenoids associated with socio-demographic variables.

As for water soluble vitamins the variation in mean levels of fat soluble vitamins and carotenoids between different socio-demographic groups showed some consistent trends, but the differences between groups were not always statistically significant (p > 0.05) possibly due in part at least to the relatively small size of some of the sub-groups. The data indicate that, with the exception of γ-tocopherol, generally mean levels of fat soluble vitamins and carotenoids, like mean levels of the water soluble vitamins, were lower for the lower socio-economic groups.

Variation in mean levels associated with different levels of gross weekly household income and whether the young person's parents were in receipt of benefits were most marked. Thus for both boys and girls mean levels of α- and β-cryptoxanthin, and α- and β-carotene were significantly lower for those young people from benefit households (boys: all p < 0.05, except α-cryptoxanthin: p < 0.01; girls: all p < 0.01, except α-carotene: p < 0.05). Additionally for boys mean levels of plasma retinol, and for girls, lycopene were also significantly lower for those living in households where the parents were in receipt of benefits (both: p < 0.05).

Mean levels of plasma retinol, α- and β-cryptoxanthin, α- and β-carotene and 25-OHD were significantly lower for girls in households with the lowest gross weekly household income, less than £160, compared with those in households where the gross income was £600 a week or more (β-cryptoxanthin and β-carotene: p < 0.01; retinol, α-cryptoxanthin, α-carotene and 25-OHD: p < 0.05). For boys the only significant differences associated with household income were for mean levels of plasma retinol and α-cryptoxanthin (both: p < 0.05).

For girls mean levels of α-cryptoxanthin were significantly lower for those from manual, rather than a non-manual social class background (p < 0.05).

There were no significant differences in mean levels of either lutein + zeaxanthin or 25-OHD for either boys or girls associated with social class.

Differences in mean levels of fat soluble vitamins and carotenoids by region generally did not reach the level of statistical significance, although the data suggest that young people living in Scotland and the Northern region of England were generally associated with lower mean levels of most of these vitamins and carotenoids than those living in other regions of England and in Wales. For girls mean levels of lutein + zeaxanthin were lower for those living in Scotland and the Northern region and highest for those living in London and the South East, although the differences did not reach the level of statistical significance. Mean levels of 25-OHD were also lowest for boys living in the Northern region, but highest for girls from the same region. Highest mean levels of 25-OHD for boys were for those from the Central and South West regions and Wales, and the lowest mean values were for girls in London and the South East (all: ns).

For boys, those who were unwell at the time of the dietary recording period and whose eating was affected had a significantly higher mean level of γ-tocopherol than those who reported not being unwell (p < 0.05). For girls those who were not unwell had a higher mean α-cryptoxanthin than those who were unwell and whose eating was affected (p < 0.05). Other than these differences there was no consistent pattern in mean levels for the fat soluble vitamins and carotenoids associated with whether the young person had been unwell during the dietary recording period. *(Tables 12.54 to 12.58)*

12.5 Blood lipids

12.5.1 The analytes and results

In adults, circulating levels of total plasma cholesterol and its subfractions are among the predictors of coronary heart disease (CHD)[24]. They vary with age, genetic and environmental influences, including dietary factors, notably the amount of saturated fatty acids in the diet. The absolute risk of CHD increases with age but the interactions of risk factors, including plasma cholesterol, cigarette smoking, high blood pressure and body weight obscure individual relationships with CHD.

High levels of total cholesterol occur in some diseases, for example kidney, liver and thyroid disorders, or in diabetes. The specific genetic condition of familial hypercholesterolaemia, which occurs in homozygous form in about 1 in 500 children, results in very high levels. Other genetic conditions, including heterozygous familial hypercholesterolaemia cause variable elevations in plasma total cholesterol. It is not clear whether cholesterol levels in young people who are not affected by these genetic and clinical disorders predict risk in adult life of cardiovascular disease[24].

Cholesterol circulates in the body bound to a variety of proteins, namely the lipoproteins. Cholesterol bound to low density lipoproteins (*LDL cholesterol*) is the major proportion of total circulating cholesterol. In adults, the risk of CHD is positively correlated with concentrations of both total cholesterol and LDL cholesterol. Cholesterol bound to high density lipoproteins (*HDL cholesterol*) is a smaller proportion of the total and may be inversely related to the development of CHD.

For adults, it is generally accepted that a plasma total cholesterol concentration below 5.2mmol/l represents a desirable level, 5.2mmol/l to 6.4mmol/l mildly elevated, 6.5mmol/l to 7.8mmol moderately elevated and above 7.8mmol/l a severely elevated level[25,26].

Blood samples were collected where possible from fasting young people. Total cholesterol and HDL cholesterol are reported for all young people who provided a blood sample. LDL cholesterol has been calculated by subtraction of HDL cholesterol from total cholesterol, uncorrected for plasma triglycerides; for brevity in this Report the term 'LDL cholesterol' has been used for <u>non-HDL cholesterol</u>. Triglycerides concentration, which is particularly affected by the composition of recently consumed foods, is reported only for young people who provided a fasting blood sample. Blood samples from 956 young people (unweighted) were analysed for plasma triglycerides concentration. Of these 873 (91%) were fasting samples, 73

(8%) were from young people who consented to a fasting sample, but had eaten or drunk something shortly before providing a sample, and ten (1%) were from young people who only consented to providing a non-fasting blood sample. The results for the plasma triglycerides concentrations are therefore based on results for 873 samples.

Plasma cholesterol (millimoles/litre)
Mean *plasma total cholesterol concentration* was 4.03mmol/l for boys and 4.24mmol/l for girls. For girls mean concentration decreased steadily with increasing age, from 4.48mmol/l for girls aged 4 to 6 years, to 4.08mmol/l for girls aged 15 to 18 years, although the differences were not statistically significant (p > 0.05). For boys there was no clear association with age.

Overall 8% of boys and 11% of girls had mean plasma total cholesterol concentration at or above 5.20mmol/l. However more than one in five girls aged 4 to 6 years (22%) had plasma total cholesterol at or above this level.

At the upper 2.5 percentile of the distribution plasma total cholesterol concentration for boys ranged between 5.33mmol/l and 6.03mmol/l (aged 15 to 18 and 7 to 10 years respectively), and for girls between 5.65mmol/l and 6.32mmol/l, again for those aged 15 to 18 and 7 to 10 years respectively.

There was almost no difference in mean *HDL cholesterol* concentration between boys and girls, 1.26mmol/l and 1.27mmol/l respectively, and for both sexes there was no systematic variation with age. However boys aged 15 to 18 years had a significantly lower mean HDL cholesterol concentration than boys in younger age groups. For example, mean HDL cholesterol concentration for boys aged 15 to 18 years was 1.09mmol/l compared with 1.31mmol/l for boys aged 11 to 14 years (p < 0.01).

Table 12.60 shows that overall 2.5% of boys had a HDL cholesterol concentration at or above 1.92mmol/l; for girls, the concentration at the upper 2.5 percentile of the distribution was 2.00mmol/l.

Overall girls had a somewhat higher mean *LDL (non-HDL) cholesterol* concentration than boys, 2.97mmol/l compared with 2.77mmol/l (p < 0.05) and for girls mean concentration declined steadily with increasing age, from 3.25mmol/l for those aged 4 to 6 years to 2.84mmol/l for the oldest group. For boys there was no clear association with age.

At the upper 2.5 percentile of the distribution LDL concentration for boys ranged between 3.88mmol/l (those aged 4 to 6 years) and 4.55mmol/l (those aged 7 to 10 years). For girls LDL concentration at the upper 2.5 percentile was between 4.16mmol/l (those aged 11 to 14 years) and 4.98mmol/l (those aged 4 to 6 years).

Plasma triglycerides (millimoles/litre)
Mean concentration of plasma triglycerides in fasting samples provided by boys was 0.88mmol/l, and for girls, 0.93mmol/l (ns).

As Table 12.62 shows, for both sexes mean concentration increased significantly with increasing age, for boys, from 0.65mmol/l (those aged 4 to 6 years) to 1.13mmol/l (those aged 15 to 18 years), and for girls, from 0.79mmol.l to 1.02mmol/l (bottom and top age groups) (both sexes: p < 0.01).

At the upper 2.5 percentile of the distribution plasma triglycerides concentration was between 1.33mmol/l and 3.13mmol/l for boys and 1.24mmol/l and 2.15mmol/l for girls. Again for both sexes concentrations were lowest in the youngest age group and highest for those aged 15 to 18 years. *(Tables 12.59 to 12.62)*

12.5.2 Correlation with dietary intakes
Table 12.63 shows correlation coefficients for plasma cholesterol concentrations and dietary intakes of fat and fatty acids. Generally the correlations were weak and varied in direction, even within sex and age groups.

For boys there were no statistically significant correlations between plasma total cholesterol and dietary intake of total fat or any of the fatty acids considered. Overall for girls plasma total cholesterol was significantly positively correlated with dietary intake of saturated fatty acids (+ 0.10) and negatively correlated with intake of *cis* n-3 polyunsaturated fatty acids (–0.12) (both: p < 0.05). Additionally for girls aged 4 to 6 years plasma total cholesterol correlated significantly negatively with dietary intake of *cis* monounsaturated fatty acids (–0.22; p < 0.05), and for girls aged 11 to 14 years with dietary intake of both *cis* n-3 and *cis* n-6 polyunsaturated fatty acids (–0.30: p < 0.01 and –0.23: p < 0.05 respectively).

For boys, plasma HDL cholesterol concentration was significantly correlated with dietary intake of total fat, saturated, *trans*, *cis* monounsaturated, *cis* n-6 polyunsaturated fatty acids and dietary cholesterol (all p < 0.01). In each case the correlation coefficients were negative indicating that as dietary intake increased plasma HDL cholesterol concentration decreased.

For girls, dietary intakes of total fat, saturated, *trans* and *cis* monounsaturated fatty acids were significantly correlated with plasma HDL cholesterol concentration (*trans* fatty acids: p < 0.05; others: p < 0.01), and in each case the coefficient was positive. Thus for girls, in contrast to boys, as dietary intake of total fat and these fatty acids increased so did HDL cholesterol concentration.

For girls, plasma LDL cholesterol concentration was significantly negatively correlated with dietary intake of *cis* n-3 polyunsaturated fatty acids for those aged 11 to 14 years (-0.26) and all girls (-0.14) (both: $p < 0.01$), and with dietary intakes of *cis* n-6 polyunsaturated fatty acids for girls aged 11 to 14 years (-0.21) ($p < 0.05$). For boys plasma LDL cholesterol concentration was significantly positively correlated with dietary intake of cholesterol for those aged 4 to 6 years (+0.20) and overall for all boys (+0.10) (both: $p < 0.05$).

Correlation coefficients for plasma total cholesterol concentration with the percentage of food energy derived from dietary intakes of total fat and fatty acids were similarly generally weak and variable in direction (*Table 12.64*). Overall for boys, and for boys aged 7 to 10 and 11 to 14 years there were significant positive correlations between plasma total cholesterol and the percentage of food energy derived from total fat and *cis* monounsaturated fatty acids (all $p < 0.05$, except for correlation for all boys with percent energy from total fat, where $p < 0.01$).

Overall for girls, and for girls aged 11 to 14 years there was a significant negative correlation between plasma total cholesterol concentration and percentage food energy from *cis* n-3 polyunsaturated fatty acids (both: $p < 0.01$).

Additionally overall for both boys and girls, total plasma cholesterol concentration was positively correlated with the percentage food energy from saturated fatty acids (boys: $p < 0.05$; girls: $p < 0.01$).

The relationship between HDL cholesterol concentration and the percentage of energy from total fat and fatty acids was not clear. For boys aged 4 to 6 years there was a negative correlation between HDL cholesterol concentration and percentage of energy from *trans* fatty acids ($p < 0.01$) and a positive correlation with percentage energy from *cis* n-6 polyunsaturated fatty acids ($p < 0.05$). For girls the percentage of energy from saturated fatty acids and HDL cholesterol concentration was negatively correlated for the youngest age group ($p < 0.01$), but positively correlated for those aged 11 to 14 ($p < 0.01$) and overall for all girls ($p < 0.05$).

(Tables 12.63 and 12.64)

12.5.3 Variation in the levels of plasma total and plasma HDL cholesterol

As can be seen from Table 12.65 there was very little variation in either mean plasma total cholesterol or HDL cholesterol concentrations for both boys and girls associated with differences in socio-demographic characteristics. Moreover apparent variations in mean cholesterol concentrations were frequently in different directions for boys and girls.

However, for girls mean HDL cholesterol concentration was significantly higher for those who reported not being unwell during the 7-day dietary recording period

compared with those who reported being unwell and whose eating was affected ($p < 0.05$). The only other statistically significant difference found was for boys, where those living in the Central and South West regions of England and Wales had a higher mean total plasma cholesterol than those living in Scotland ($p < 0.05$). *(Table 12.65)*

12.6 Other blood analytes

12.6.1 The analytes and results

Mineral and trace element indices:

Blood lead (micrograms/decilitre)

Blood lead is an index of the body's lead burden. Lead may be found in the air, water, and the soil, in paint, in some cooking utensils, jewellery and in traditional medicines and cosmetics. The effects of lead poisoning are impairment of mental function, and children, especially very young children, are more susceptible than adults to the effects of lead poisoning.

In both adults and children the successful treatment of lead poisoning involves identification and elimination of the source of lead. In adults this is usually occupational, although it may arise from contaminated food or water or the use of traditional medicines, particularly by some ethnic groups. In very young children it often results from unusual behaviours such as *pica*, that is the consumption of non-food material such as dirt or coal, which may be contaminated with lead.

The most recent data suggest that a threshold cannot be determined for impairment of mental performance in infants and young children, with deleterious effects noted at very low exposure levels.

At present the upper tolerable limit for blood lead is taken as 10µg/dl. Decreased sales of leaded petrol since 1987 have contributed up to a five fold decrease in blood lead levels over the past decade[27]. A child or young person with a blood lead level at or above 10µg/dl is likely therefore to have experienced increased exposure to and uptake of lead, although this level is not necessarily indicative of clinical risk.

Overall mean concentration of blood lead was higher for boys than girls, 2.8µg/dl compared with 2.5µg/dl ($p < 0.05$) and there was also a consistent pattern for boys in each of the four age groups to have a higher mean blood lead concentration than the corresponding group of girls. For example, mean blood lead for boys aged 15 to 18 years was 2.4µg/dl and for girls in the same age group 2.0µg/dl ($p < 0.05$). For both sexes mean blood lead decreased significantly with increasing age (boys: $p < 0.05$; girls: $p < 0.01$). At the upper 2.5 percentile of the distribution the differences in blood lead concentration between boys and girls overall and in each age group were marked. Thus overall 2.5% of boys had a blood lead concentration of 8.0µg/dl or above, while for girls the concentration at the upper 2.5 percentile was 5.8µg/dl. In the youngest age group levels at the upper 2.5 percentile were 9.2µg/dl for boys aged 4 to 6 years compared with 6.6µg/dl for girls in the same age group.

None of the girls, but overall 1% of boys and 2% of boys aged 4 to 6 years had a blood lead concentration at or above 10.0µg/dl[28]. *(Table 12.66)*

Plasma magnesium (millimoles/litre)
Magnesium, like potassium, is widely distributed in the soft tissues of the body and the skeleton. Plasma magnesium concentration is very stable and adaptation to variation in dietary intake is regulated by the kidneys. Low levels of plasma magnesium may be due to long-term dietary deficiency, malabsorption or excessive renal loss. For adults the normal range for plasma magnesium is between 17mg/l and 22mg/l (0.7mmol/l to 1.0mmol/l)[29].

Mean plasma magnesium concentration was higher for boys than girls, 0.94mmol/l compared with 0.91mmol/l (p < 0.01). For boys, mean concentration was very similar for each age group, while for girls those in the youngest age group, 4 to 6 years, had a mean plasma magnesium level higher than those in each of the other three, older age groups, 0.94mmol/l compared with 0.90/0.91mmol/l (p < 0.05).

At the lower 2.5 percentile plasma magnesium concentration for boys was 0.79mmol/l, and again varied very little with age, and for girls, was 0.76mmol/l overall, and ranged between 0.74mmol/l and 0.80mmol/l depending on age group. *(Table 12.67)*

Plasma selenium (micromoles/litre) and erythrocyte glutathione peroxidase activity (GSH-Px) (nanomoles/milligram haemoglobin/minute)
Selenium is an essential trace element. It forms part of the structure of certain proteins, and is essential for the activity of some peroxidase enzymes. Many other aspects of its functions are not yet well understood.

There are well-confirmed pathological syndromes associated with selenium overload as well as with selenium deficiency. However there is increasing evidence that relatively high intakes, within the safe range, may have a protective action against some kinds of cancer[30] and other studies have explored the relationships between selenium status or indicators and functional indicators such as immune cell function[31] or risk of vascular disease[32].

Most studies have reported plasma or serum selenium levels (although this can be affected by acute phase), red cell selenium, or blood glutathione peroxidase (GSH-Px) (functional index)[33].

The list of assays originally specified by the Department of Health from samples provided by young people taking part in this NDNS included the measurement of selenium levels in plasma. Part way through the survey it was decided that, provided sufficient sample was remaining after all other assays had been carried out, it would be useful also to measure GSH-Px, as a functional indicator of selenium status. This latter assay was separately funded by the Department of Health as an additional piece of work and was carried out only on samples collected during the last two waves of the survey. The assay for plasma selenium was carried out at the Trace Element Unit, University of Southampton; GSH-Px determinations were carried out at MRC Dunn Nutrition Unit in Cambridge (now MRC Human Nutrition Research (*see Appendix Q*)). The results of both assays are reported below. As noted above, the results for GSH-Px are presented unweighted (*see Section 12.1.1*).

Subsequently an application was made by the Trace Element Unit at Southampton University, in conjunction with MRC Human Nutrition Research in Cambridge, to the Department of Health, for permission to carry out a further assay of selenium status, red cell selenium, on any residual samples remaining for each of the four waves of the survey. This request was granted and the assay was carried out. The results for red cell selenium are not presented in this Report.

Mean *plasma selenium* concentration for boys and girls was 0.86µmol/l and 0.87µmol/l respectively (ns). The lowest mean levels were in samples from children in the youngest age group, 0.82µmol/l and 0.81µmol/l for boys and girls respectively (ns). Mean plasma selenium for both sexes was higher in the next age group, 0.87µmol/l for boys and 0.90µmol/l for girls, but the difference was only statistically significant for girls (boys: p > 0.05; girls p < 0.01). Highest mean levels were for boys and girls aged 15 to 18 years, 0.89µmol/l for boys and 0.91µmol/l for girls, (differences between youngest and oldest age groups boys: p < 0.05; girls p < 0.01).

At the lower 2.5 percentile of the distribution plasma selenium concentration for boys ranged between 0.58µmol/l, for boys aged 4 to 6 years and 0.64µmol/l, for boys aged 15 to 18 years, and for girls between 0.57µmol/l and 0.65µmol/l, for the youngest and oldest age groups respectively. There were no plasma selenium levels as low as 0.11µmol/l, which would correspond with frank selenium deficiency.
At the upper 2.5 percentile plasma selenium levels for boys were between 1.12µmol/l, for 11 to 14 year olds, and 1.18µmol/l, for 7 to 10 year olds, and for girls between 1.05µmol/l and 1.41µmol/l, for the two youngest age groups respectively.

Mean *GSH-Px* for boys was 90.0nmol/mg Hb/min and for girls, 93.5nmol/mg Hb/min (ns). There was no clear association with age for either sex in mean concentration or in levels at the upper and lower 2.5 percentiles. Mean levels ranged for boys between 88.3nmol/mg Hb/min, for those aged 7 to 10 years, and 92.8nmol/mg Hb/min, for those aged 15 to 18 years (ns). For girls, mean levels ranged between 90.1nmol/mg Hb/min, for those aged 4 to 6 years, and 98.1nmol/mg Hb/min, for those aged 11 to 14 years (ns). At the lower 2.5 percentile GSH-Px ranged between 61.3nmol/mg Hb/min, for girls aged 4 to 6 years, and 69.0nmol/mg Hb/min, for boys aged 4 to 6 years. At the upper 2.5 percentile the levels were between 123.0nmol/mg Hb/min, for boys aged 11 to 14 years, and 167.5nmol/mg Hb/min, for boys aged 4 to 6 years. *(Tables 12.68 and 12.69)*

Red cell superoxide dismutase (nanomoles/min/milligram haemoglobin)

Red cell superoxide dismutase is a copper/zinc enzyme which protects the cell against dangerous levels of superoxide. It can be used as an indirect measure of both copper metabolism and zinc status. If copper levels are low the superoxide activity may be low, exposing tissues to oxidative stress. For adults the normal range is usually considered to be between 1102nmol/mg Hb/min and 1601nmol/mg Hb/min[34].

Overall mean red cell superoxide dismutase was 1168nmol/mg Hb/min for both boys and girls. As Table 12.70 shows, for both sexes mean levels decreased as age increased, for boys from 1211nmol/mg Hb/min for those aged 4 to 6 years to 1096nmol/mg Hb/min for those aged 15 to 18 years ($p < 0.05$), and for girls from 1208nmol/mg Hb/min to 1142nmol/mg Hb/min for those in the same two age groups. The proportion of young people with values below 1100 increased with age for both sexes, from 26% and 27% for boys and girls aged 4 to 6 years respectively, to 58% and 55% for those aged 15 to 18 years (both sexes: $p < 0.01$).

At the lower 2.5 percentile levels ranged, for boys, from 614nmol/mg Hb/min for those aged 11 to 14 years, to 824nmol/mg Hb/min for those aged 4 to 6 years. For girls the range was 684nmol/mg Hb/min, for those aged 11 to 14 years, to 897nmol/mg Hb/min, for those aged 4 to 6 years. At the upper 2.5 percentile levels were between 1623nmol/mg Hb/min for boys aged 7 to 10 years and 2413nmol/mg Hb/min for girls aged 15 to 18 years. *(Table 12.70)*

Nitrogen metabolites
Plasma urea concentration (millimoles/litre) and plasma creatinine concentration (micromoles/litre)
Both plasma urea and plasma creatinine concentrations are indicators of kidney function.

Urea is derived from the liver from amino acids and

therefore from protein, either from dietary protein or protein in the tissues of the body. Its rate of production is accelerated by a high protein diet, by increased catabolism due to starvation, by tissue damage or sepsis. The normal kidney can excrete large amounts of urea and in the presence of normal renal function, only a very high protein diet, sustained for some time or severe tissue damage can increase plasma urea concentrations above the reference range. A slightly elevated plasma urea, certainly above 15mmol/l, can be taken to indicate impaired glomerular function. Low plasma urea, below 3mmol/l, may occasionally occur and may have a variety of causes, including low protein intake or severe liver disease.

For adults the normal range for plasma creatinine concentration is 53μmol/l to 97μmol/l for men and 44μmol/l to 80μmol/l for women[35].

Mean *plasma urea* concentration was significantly higher for boys than girls, 4.7mmol/l and 4.2mmol/l respectively ($p < 0.01$). For both sexes mean levels tended to fall with increasing age; thus for boys mean plasma urea was 5.0mmol/l for those aged 7 to 10 years and 4.5mmol/l for those aged 15 to 18 years ($p < 0.05$). For girls the comparable mean levels were 4.7mmol/l and 4.1mmol/l ($p < 0.05$). Plasma urea concentrations below 3.0mmol/l were recorded overall for 2% of boys and 7% of girls, with somewhat higher proportions in the oldest age groups for both sexes, 4% for boys and 11% for girls. There were no cases where plasma urea concentration was 15.0mmol/l or above.

At the lower 2.5 percentile of the distribution plasma urea concentration was 2.9mmol/l for boys and 2.5mmol/l for girls. At the upper 2.5 percentile concentrations ranged between 5.5mmol/l, for girls aged 11 to 14 years, and 7.7mmol/l, for boys aged 7 to 10 years.

Mean *plasma creatinine* concentration was 55μmol/l for both boys and girls. For both sexes there was a marked increase in mean concentration with age; for those aged 4 to 6 years mean plasma creatinine was 43μmol/l for boys and 39μmol/l for girls, rising to 66μmol/l for boys aged 15 to 18 years and 62μmol/l for girls in the same age group (both sexes: $p < 0.01$). At the lower 2.5 percentile plasma creatinine concentration ranged between 12μmol/l and 36μmol/l for boys, and 27μmol/l and 42μmol/l for girls. For boys, 2.5% had a plasma creatinine concentration at or above 85μmol/l; 2.5% of girls had a plasma creatinine level at or above 78μmol/l. *(Tables 12.71 and 12.72)*

Plasma α₁-antichymotrypsin concentration (grams/litre)
α₁-antichymotrypsin (α₁-ACT) is known as a positive acute phase reactant. It is produced in the liver in response to inflammation. Ferritin is also an acute phase reactant and blood α₁-ACT and ferritin concen-

trations may be raised in response to infection or inflammation (see *Section 12.2.1*). The measurement of α_1-ACT can provide independent evidence of infection or inflammation that can assist in the interpretation of haematology assays, especially plasma ferritin. For adults, the normal upper limit for α_1-ACT is usually considered to be 0.65g/l[36].

Overall mean α_1-ACT was significantly higher for girls, 0.30g/l, than for boys, 0.28g/l ($p < 0.01$). For both sexes mean concentration fell significantly as age increased, from 0.31g/l and 0.35g/l for boys and girls aged 4 to 6 years, to 0.27g/l and 0.28g/l for boys and girls aged 15 to 18 years (both sexes: $p < 0.01$).

At the lower 2.5 percentile of the distribution α_1-ACT for boys was 0.20g/l, and for girls 0.18g/l. At the upper 2.5 percentile of the distribution for boys α_1-ACT concentrations were between 0.39g/l and 0.44g/l, and for girls, between 0.39g/l and 0.63g/l. There were two young people with α_1-ACT concentrations above 0.65g/l (0.67g/l and 0.78g/l).

Table 12.74 shows the correlation coefficients for α_1-ACT with serum ferritin. Significant positive correlations were found overall for both boys and girls (both sexes: $p < 0.01$) and for some age groups. For boys, α_1-ACT was significantly correlated with serum ferritin for each age group except those aged 7 to 10 years (11 to 14 years: $p < 0.01$; 4 to 6 and 15 to 18 years: $p < 0.05$). For girls the correlation coefficients were significant for the two youngest age groups (both: $p < 0.01$).

(Tables 12.73 and 12.74)

Total plasma alkaline phosphatase activity (International Units/litre)

Alkaline phosphatase is an enzyme formed in large amounts by osteoblast cells in bone and in cells lining the biliary tract. High levels are found in the circulation when bone turnover is high, in vitamin D deficiency, in secondary bone cancer and when obstruction occurs in the biliary tract. This assay is identical to that used in the NDNS of persons aged 65 years and over[15], but differs from that used in the earlier survey of adults[16]. The analyte was not measured in blood samples from pre-school children in the NDNS[5]. For adults the normal range for alkaline phosphatase is between 30 IU/l and 135 IU/l; for adolescents and pregnant women the upper limit of the normal range is considered to be 450 IU/l.

Mean total plasma alkaline phosphatase activity was significantly higher for boys, 239 IU/l, than girls, 186 IU/l ($p < 0.01$). For both sexes, mean activity was lowest in the oldest age group, 149 IU/l for boys aged 15 to 18 years and 86 IU/l for girls in the same age group (for both sexes compared with each of the other age groups: $p < 0.01$, except boys youngest compared with oldest age group: $p < 0.05$).

At the upper 2.5 percentile of the distribution activity

levels for boys were highest for those aged 11 to 14 years, 471 IU/l, and for girls, for those aged 11 to 14 years, 435 IU/l. There were nine young people, (1%), six boys and three girls with plasma alkaline phosphatase activity above 450 IU/l.

(Table 12.75)

12.6.2 Variation in the levels of blood lead, plasma selenium and plasma magnesium

As Table 12.76 shows, there was more variation in mean blood lead concentration for boys associated with different socio-demographic characteristics than for girls. In particular boys from households receiving benefits, from households in the lowest income band, and from a manual social class background had a significantly higher mean blood lead than boys in non-benefit households, from households in the highest income band, and from non-manual social class background respectively (social class: $p < 0.01$; others $p < 0.05$). There were no significant differences in mean blood lead for girls associated with these, or any of the other socio-economic characteristics considered ($p > 0.05$).

Although there were no clear patterns of differences in mean plasma selenium concentration associated with differences in socio-demographic characteristics there were some significant differences between mean levels for some groups of both boys and girls. For boys, those living in Scotland had a significantly lower plasma selenium than boys in the Northern region and in London and the South East, and for girls mean plasma selenium was lower for those in the Central and South West regions of England and Wales than for those in London and the South East (all: $p < 0.01$). Boys in households with a gross weekly household income of between £280 and £400, and girls in households with a gross weekly income between £160 and £280 had a significantly lower plasma selenium than boys and girls from household in the highest income groups (both sexes: $p < 0.01$).

There were no significant differences in mean levels of plasma magnesium for either boys or girls associated with differences in the socio-demographic characteristics considered ($p > 0.05$). *(Tables 12.76 and 12.77)*

12.7 Plasma testosterone and stage of sexual development in boys

In boys, testosterone is the hormone most closely related to pubertal development and corresponds to height gain and development of the testes and secondary sex characteristics. Hence, for boys plasma testosterone level can provide a proxy measure whether or not puberty has occurred; this may assist in interpreting variation in levels of other blood analytes, anthropometric measurements and blood pressure. For adult males, a plasma testosterone of between 8nmol/l and 32nmol/l generally indicates that the individual has reached or passed puberty. A lower plasma testosterone

451

concentration indicates the individual is pre-pubertal. Females may have testosterone levels up to 3nmol/l.

Plasma testosterone was measured in blood samples from boys aged 10 to 16 years, a total of 260 samples (unweighted)[37].

Table 12.78 shows mean plasma testosterone concentration for boys, by individual year of age. Mean concentration increased significantly with age (p < 0.01) and, as would be expected, (Table 12.79), the majority, 85%, of those in the bottom tertile were aged 10 or 11 years, while the majority, 71%, of those in the top tertile were aged 14 to 16 years.

In Chapter 10 the relationship between plasma testosterone concentration and anthropometric measurements for boys was discussed (see *Table 10.24*). There were no significant variations in any of the anthropometric measurements with the tertiles of plasma cholesterol concentration.

Table 12.80 shows the variation in mean levels for a number of blood analytes associated with differences in plasma testosterone concentration. Plasma testosterone concentration tertiles were calculated for each individual year of age and then pooled to allow the calculation of means for the other blood analytes. Differences in means between the tertiles and the strength of the linear relationship were tested for statistical significance, after adjusting for age. The table shows means for the blood analytes by testosterone tertile and p values for the differences between the tertile groups and the linear relationship[38].

For a number of blood analytes, including plasma vitamin C and plasma 25-OHD, there was no evidence of a significant relationship. However mean haemoglobin concentration and red blood cell count both increased with increasing testosterone concentration (p < 0.01 and p < 0.05 respectively) and mean levels of haemoglobin were significantly higher for the top tertile compared with the lower and middle tertiles (p < 0.05). For plasma iron and plasma iron % saturation mean levels were significantly lower for the middle tertile of plasma testosterone concentration compared with the top and bottom tertiles (p < 0.01). The same was found for serum ferritin, but differences were less marked (p < 0.05). These effects may be associated with a temporary increase in demand for iron during the middle of the growth spurt, which is matched by an increase in haemoglobin concentration and red blood cell count. Since both blood volume and haemoglobin concentration per unit volume increase this may put a temporary strain on iron stores and supplies.

Plasma HDL cholesterol concentration and plasma total cholesterol concentration decreased with increasing plasma testosterone concentration (both: p < 0.05). This is consistent with the recognised effect of the male hormone on HDL cholesterol concentration.

There was also a significant linear relationship between mean blood lead concentration and plasma testosterone concentration, with mean blood lead decreasing as plasma testosterone increased (p < 0.01). Further analysis showed that this relationship was still statistically significant after controlling for differences in haemoglobin concentration and blood red cell count (p < 0.01).

(Table 12.80)

References and endnotes

[1] Age has been calculated by subtracting the young person's date of birth from the date when the blood sample was obtained, and therefore some young people may be classified in different age bands for different aspects of the survey.

[2] Pearson correlation coefficients were calculated in SPSS. Weighting factors, for non-response and sampling probability, were scaled (normalised) to approximate to the original, unweighted, sample size before running the SPSS procedure on weighted data. Pearson correlation coefficients are robust to departures from normally distributed data, that is skewed data, provided the value of the population coefficient is low, which it is for these data. *See:*
Gayen AK. The distribution of Student's t in random samples of any size drawn from non-normal universes. *Biometrica.* 1949; **36**: 353
Gayen AK. The distribution of the variance ratio in random samples of any size drawn for non-normal universes. *Biometrica.* 1950: **37**: 236
Gayen AK. Significance of difference between the means of two non-random samples. *Biometrica.* 1950: **37**: 399
Gayen AK. The frequency distribution of the product-moment correlation coefficient in random samples of any size drawn for non-normal universes. *Biometrica.* 1951: **38**: 219

[3] World Health Organisation. *Nutritional Anaemias.* Technical Report Series: 503. WHO (Geneva, 1972)

[4] Dacie JV, Lewis SM. *Practical Haematology.* 8th Edition. Churchill Livingstone (Edinburgh, 1995)

[5] Gregory JR, Collins DL, Davies PSW, Hughes JM, Clarke PC. *National Diet and Nutrition Survey: children aged 1½ to 4½ years. Volume 1: Report of the diet and nutrition survey.* HMSO (London,1995)

[6] Normal ranges for reporting haemoglobin results to the young person and their GP (see *Appendix N*) were based on age-related references ranges from Great Ormond Street Hospital, as follows:
aged 4 to less than 7 years – 11.5g/dl to 13.5g/dl
aged 7 to less than 13 years – 11.5g/dl to 15.5g/dl
girls aged 13 years and over – 12g/dl to 16g/dl
boys aged 13 years and over – 13g/dl to 16g/dl

[7] Samples delayed in the post by more than 24 hours have been excluded from the MCV and MCHC results. MCHC is artefactually reduced if the MCV is increased by sample deterioration.

[8] Range established from analysis of samples from children attending the Hospital for Sick Children, Great Ormond Street, London. Personal communication from Dr I Hann.

[9] Worwood M. Iron deficiency anaemias. In: *Practical Haematology.* Eds. Dacie JV, Lewis SM. 8th Edition. Churchill Livingstone (Edinburgh, 1995)

[10] Bates CJ, Thurnham DI, Bingham SA, Margetts BM, Nelson M. Biochemical Markers of Nutrient Intake. In: *Design Concepts in Nutritional Epidemiology.* 2nd Edition. OUP (Oxford, 1997) pp170-240.

[11] All comparisons are based on differences between sub groups with the highest and lowest mean values.

[12] Sauberlich HE. Vitamin C status: methods and findings. *Ann N Y Acad Sci* 1971; **24**: 444-454

[13] Based on an analysis of 170 serum samples and 140 whole blood samples. Abbott Laboratories, Diagnostics Division, IMx system: Folate, Technical Information Leaflet, 1997.

[14] Sauberlich HE, Skala JH, Dowdy RP. *Laboratory tests for the assessment of nutritional status.* CRC Press (Cleveland, Ohio, 1974)

[15] Finch S, Doyle W, Lowe C, Bates CJ, Prentice A, Smithers G, Clarke PC. *National Diet and Nutrition Survey: people aged 65 years and over. Volume 1: Report of the diet and nutrition survey.* TSO (London, 1998)

[16] Gregory J, Foster K, Tyler H, Wiseman M. The Dietary and Nutritional Survey of British Adults. HMSO (London, 1990)

[17] Vallee B, Galdes A. The metalobiochemistry of zinc enzymes. In: Meister A, ed. *Advances in Enzymology.* John Wiley (New York, 1984)

[18] Pilch SM, Senti FR. Eds. Assessment of zinc nutritional status of the US population based on data collected in the 2nd National Health and Examination Survey 1976-80. *LSRO, Fed Am Soc Exp Biol (*Bethesda, Md, 1984)

[19] Personal communication from Professor Elaine Gunter. Centres for Disease Control and Prevention, Atlanta. USA.

[20] Note that the date (month) the blood sample was taken may not correspond to the fieldwork wave as defined as an analysis variable for other tabulations in this Report (see *Glossary* for definition of *Fieldwork wave*).

[21] Results for α and γ-tocopherol are reported unadjusted, for cholesterol and triglycerides respectively. It should be noted that high γ-tocopherol levels may reflect recent dietary intake of foods rich in γ-tocopherol.

[22] That is, the ratio of plasma α-tocopherol plus plasma γ-tocopherol to plasma total cholesterol.

[23] Department of Health. Report on Health and Social Subjects: 41. *Dietary Reference Values for Food Energy and Nutrients for the United Kingdom.* HMSO (London, 1991)

[24] Department of Health. Report on Health and Social Subjects: 46. *Nutritional Aspects of Cardiovascular Disease.* HMSO (London, 1994)

[25] *Handbook of coronary heart disease prevention.* Eds. Lewis B, Assman G, Mancini M, Stein Y. Current Medical Literature. (London, 1989)

[26] US Department of Health and Human Services. *National Cholesterol Education Program. Report of the Expert Panel on detection, evaluation, and treatment of high blood pressure cholesterol in adults.* National Institutes of Health. No 88-2925 (Bethesda, 1988)

[27] Delves HT. Overview of UK and international studies on trends in blood lead, and the use of lead isotope ratios to identify environmental sources. In: *Recent UK Blood Lead Surveys Report R9.* Eds. D Gompertz et al. MRC Institute for the Environment and Health, Southampton (1998) pp 40-52.

[28] Variations in levels of dental caries associated with blood lead concentration are discussed in the report of the oral health component of this survey. See Walker A, Gregory, J, Bradnock G, Nunn J, White D. *National Diet and Nutrition Survey: young people aged 4 to 18 years. Volume 2: Report of the oral health survey.* TSO (London, 2000).

[29] Caroli S et al. The assessment of reference values for elements in human biological tissues and fluids: a systematic review. *Crit Rev Anal Chem* 1994; **24**: 363-398

[30] Spallholz JE. On the nature of selenium toxicity and carcinostatic activity. *Free Rad Biol Med* 1994; **17**: 45-64

[31] Roy M, Kiremidjian-Schumacher L, Wishe HI, Cohen MW, Stotzky G. Supplementation with selenium restores age-related decline in immune cell function. *Proc Soc Exp Biol Med* 1995; **209**: 369-375

[32] Salonen JT, Huttunen JK. Se in cardiovascular diseases. *Ann Clin Res* 1986; **18**: 30-35

[33] Neve J. Methods in determination of selenium status. *J Trace Elem Electrolytes Health Dis* 1991; **5**: 1-17

[34] Randox SOD kit (RANSOD) leaflet, Randox Laboratories Ltd, 55 Diamond Road, Crumlin, Co Antrim, Northern Ireland BT29 4QY.

[35] Henry RJ. *Clinical Chemistry, Principles and Techniques.* 2nd Edition. Harper and Row. (New York, 1974)

[36] Calvin J, Price CP. Measurement of serum α$_1$-antichymotrypsin by immunoturbidimetry. *Ann Clin Biochem* 1986; **213**: 206-209

[37] See *Section 12.1.2* for a note on weighting.

[38] The General Linear Model procedure (GLM) in SPSS was used, on unweighted data. Testosterone concentrations were grouped into tertiles, by ascending value. No age adjustment was made to the tertiles. For the tertile comparison, age, as a continuous variable, was the covariate, and ascending tertile group, as a categorical variable, the fixed factor. For the significance of the linear trend, plasma testosterone concentration, and age, as continuous variables, were the covariates.

Table 12.1 Percentage distribution of haemoglobin concentration by sex and age of young person

Haemoglobin concentration (g/dl)	Males aged (years)					Females aged (years)				
	4–6	7–10	11–14	15–18	All males	4–6	7–10	11–14	15–18	All females
	cum %	cum %	cum %	cum %	cum %	cum %	cum %	cum %	cum %	cum %
Less than 11.0	3	1	2	–	1	8	4	1	2	3
Less than 12.0	32	4	8	–	9	22	16	4	9	12
Less than 12.5	50	25	13	–	19	53	31	15	22	28
Less than 13.0	71	47	30	1	35	73	54	32	40	48
Less than 13.5	89	75	52	6	52	85	74	58	59	68
Less than 14.0	96	90	77	13	67	93	90	79	83	86
Less than 15.0	99	100	95	53	86	100	100	99	99	99
All	100		100	100	100			100	100	100
Base	*86*	*185*	*181*	*164*	*616*	*82*	*143*	*171*	*169*	*565*
Mean	12.5	13.0	13.4	14.9	13.5	12.4	12.8	13.3	13.1	12.9
Median	12.5	13.0	13.4	14.9	13.4	12.4	12.9	13.3	13.2	13.0
Lower 2.5 percentile	10.5	11.5	11.4	13.2	11.4	10.9	10.5	11.7	11.4	10.9
Upper 2.5 percentile	14.0	14.6	15.5	16.8	16.1	14.2	14.4	14.6	14.7	14.6
Standard deviation	0.84	0.76	0.99	0.88	1.25	0.99	0.95	0.86	0.92	0.97

Table 12.2 Percentage distribution of mean corpuscular volume by sex and age of young person

Mean corpuscular volume (fl)	Males aged (years)					Females aged (years)				
	4–6	7–10	11–14	15–18	All males	4–6	7–10	11–14	15–18	All females
	cum %	cum %	cum %	cum %	cum %	cum %	cum %	cum %	cum %	cum %
Less than 70.0	–	–	3	–	1	2	2	–	–	1
Less than 83.0	30	12	13	2	13	17	14	5	1	9
Less than 86.0	59	38	31	8	32	49	39	15	8	26
Less than 89.0	82	80	59	23	60	81	73	38	27	52
Less than 92.0	96	95	85	52	82	96	90	63	49	72
Less than 95.0	99	99	99	78	94	100	96	85	77	88
All	100	100	100	100	100		100	100	100	100
Base	*75*	*149*	*156*	*131*	*511*	*65*	*104*	*136*	*140*	*445*
Mean	85.1	86.7	87.3	91.7	87.8	85.8	86.6	90.3	92.1	89.0
Median	84.8	86.8	88.0	91.7	88.0	86.0	86.6	90.3	92.1	88.8
Lower 2.5 percentile	76.8	81.1	68.6	83.7	78.9	79.8	77.6	80.5	83.6	79.8
Upper 2.5 percentile	93.7	93.9	94.2	99.4	97.5	93.3	96.2	98.6	102.5	99.5
Standard deviation	4.05	3.21	5.33	4.36	4.95	4.01	4.51	4.39	4.64	5.12

Table 12.3 Percentage distribution of haematocrit by sex and age of young person

Haematocrit (l/l)	Males aged (years)					Females aged (years)				
	4–6	7–10	11–14	15–18	All males	4–6	7–10	11–14	15–18	All females
	cum %	cum %	cum %	cum %	cum %	cum %	cum %	cum %	cum %	cum %
Less than 0.330	1	–	–	–	0	2	1	–	–	1
Less than 0.360	13	2	2	–	4	10	4	–	1	3
Less than 0.375	26	8	6	–	9	27	9	2	2	9
Less than 0.400	62	33	18	–	26	61	37	18	23	32
Less than 0.425	86	75	51	7	53	84	81	50	53	65
Less than 0.450	96	97	82	26	74	98	94	83	85	89
Less than 0.475	99	100	97	59	88	100	100	99	99	99
All	100		100	100	100			100	100	100
Base	*75*	*149*	*156*	*131*	*511*	*65*	*104*	*136*	*140*	*445*
Mean	0.392	0.409	0.423	0.468	0.425	0.393	0.405	0.425	0.420	0.412
Median	0.390	0.408	0.424	0.468	0.422	0.388	0.406	0.425	0.422	0.413
Lower 2.5 percentile	0.342	0.360	0.360	0.413	0.358	0.330	0.339	0.378	0.376	0.358
Upper 2.5 percentile	0.451	0.450	0.482	0.531	0.508	0.446	0.461	0.466	0.473	0.466
Standard deviation	0.0278	0.0238	0.0288	0.0285	0.0387	0.0282	0.0290	0.0276	0.0264	0.0302

Table 12.4 Percentage distribution of mean cell haemoglobin by sex and age of young person

Mean cell haemoglobin (pg)	Males aged (years)					Females aged (years)				
	4–6	7–10	11–14	15–18	All males	4–6	7–10	11–14	15–18	All females
	cum %	cum %	cum %	cum %	cum %	cum %	cum %	cum %	cum %	cum %
Less than 26.0	23	7	10	2	9	13	15	7	4	9
Less than 26.5	37	16	15	3	16	25	26	9	7	16
Less than 27.0	53	32	24	5	26	42	40	15	12	26
Less than 28.0	67	70	50	15	49	75	63	37	30	49
Less than 29.0	92	87	78	36	72	89	85	66	52	72
Less than 30.0	98	97	91	67	87	97	95	88	77	89
All	100	100	100	100	100	100	100	100	100	100
Base	*86*	*185*	*181*	*164*	*616*	*82*	*143*	*171*	*169*	*565*
Mean	26.9	27.5	27.7	29.3	27.9	27.1	27.3	28.3	28.8	27.9
Median	26.8	27.5	27.9	29.2	28.0	27.1	27.4	28.3	28.8	28.0
Lower 2.5 percentile	23.7	25.5	21.6	26.1	24.3	24.7	22.8	24.1	25.2	24.6
Upper 2.5 percentile	29.6	30.4	30.5	32.4	31.4	30.2	30.5	31.0	32.6	31.4
Standard deviation	1.46	1.27	2.00	1.62	1.84	1.72	1.97	1.55	1.90	1.93

Table 12.5 Percentage distribution of mean cell haemoglobin concentration by sex and age of young person

Mean cell haemoglobin concentration (g/dl)	Males aged (years)					Females aged (years)				
	4–6	7–10	11–14	15–18	All males	4–6	7–10	11–14	15–18	All females
	cum %	cum %	cum %	cum %	cum %	cum %	cum %	cum %	cum %	cum %
Less than 30.0	–	2	7	3	3	11	6	10	6	8
Less than 30.5	11	6	12	9	9	15	16	19	20	18
Less than 31.0	30	21	25	19	23	26	27	33	30	29
Less than 31.5	50	40	42	32	40	43	44	60	53	51
Less than 32.0	62	56	57	47	55	61	62	72	73	68
Less than 32.5	74	75	73	70	73	74	79	89	90	84
Less than 33.0	82	85	91	84	86	88	92	95	95	93
All	100	100	100	100	100	100	100	100	100	100
Base	*75*	*149*	*156*	*131*	*511*	*65*	*104*	*136*	*140*	*445*
Mean	31.7	31.8	31.7	31.9	31.8	31.5	31.6	31.3	31.3	31.4
Median	31.4	31.7	31.7	32.0	31.7	31.6	31.6	31.3	31.3	31.4
Lower 2.5 percentile	30.0	30.1	29.3	29.8	29.8	29.1	29.3	29.3	29.2	29.2
Upper 2.5 percentile	33.9	34.1	34.0	33.6	33.8	33.5	33.7	33.5	33.3	33.5
Standard deviation	1.05	1.15	1.22	1.03	1.12	1.44	1.15	1.10	0.97	1.16

Table 12.6 Percentage distribution of plasma iron by sex and age of young person

Plasma iron (µmol/l)	Males aged (years)					Females aged (years)				
	4–6	7–10	11–14	15–18	All males	4–6	7–10	11–14	15–18	All females
	cum %	cum %	cum %	cum %	cum %	cum %	cum %	cum %	cum %	cum %
Less than 6.00	13	3	7	2	6	–	4	5	14	6
Less than 8.00	18	12	12	8	12	14	10	9	25	15
Less than 10.00	31	28	22	13	23	31	21	25	33	27
Less than 13.00	50	57	48	38	48	56	51	54	55	54
Less than 16.00	78	75	68	64	71	81	75	74	71	75
Less than 20.00	97	94	89	78	89	93	94	89	88	91
All	100	100	100	100	100	100	100	100	100	100
Base	*64*	*154*	*170*	*152*	*540*	*66*	*121*	*157*	*160*	*504*
Mean	12.23	12.90	13.65	15.52	13.67	12.67	13.18	13.22	13.05	13.06
Median	13.29	12.45	13.23	14.40	13.26	11.90	12.54	12.37	12.31	12.33
Lower 2.5 percentile	1.97	4.99	4.40	6.54	4.14	6.21	5.31	5.73	3.88	5.31
Upper 2.5 percentile	23.60	24.10	23.39	29.89	25.56	23.62	23.70	23.00	28.19	24.57
Standard deviation	5.176	4.549	4.954	5.886	5.300	4.590	4.253	4.474	6.238	4.975

Table 12.7 Percentage distribution of plasma total iron binding capacity by sex and age of young person

Plasma total iron binding capacity (μmol/l)	Males aged (years)					Females aged (years)				
	4–6	7–10	11–14	15–18	All males	4–6	7–10	11–14	15–18	All females
	cum %	cum %	cum %	cum %	cum %	cum %	cum %	cum %	cum %	cum %
Less than 50.0	9	8	3	11	8	1	6	4	5	4
Less than 55.0	27	27	15	24	23	17	26	19	12	18
Less than 60.0	54	51	40	49	48	59	45	44	32	44
Less than 65.0	76	81	65	70	73	75	75	64	59	68
Less than 70.0	98	95	85	87	91	90	89	85	73	84
Less than 75.0	100	98	97	96	98	97	97	96	90	95
All		100	100	100	100	100	100	100	100	100
Base	60	150	166	149	525	61	119	155	159	494
Mean	59.0	59.2	62.3	60.6	60.4	60.3	60.4	61.8	64.2	61.8
Median	58.9	59.4	62.0	60.3	60.2	59.1	60.6	61.3	62.8	60.9
Lower 2.5 percentile	45.9	47.2	49.5	46.3	47.1	50.9	47.4	48.0	46.8	48.5
Upper 2.5 percentile	70.5	70.6	76.9	76.4	74.7	75.0	75.1	76.2	82.3	77.3
Standard deviation	6.40	6.65	7.22	8.19	7.32	6.28	6.81	7.61	9.03	7.75

Table 12.8 Percentage distribution of plasma iron % saturation by sex and age of young person

Plasma iron % saturation (%)	Males aged (years)					Females aged (years)				
	4–6	7–10	11–14	15–18	All males	4–6	7–10	11–14	15–18	All females
	cum %	cum %	cum %	cum %	cum %	cum %	cum %	cum %	cum %	cum %
Less than 10.0	16	1	8	3	6	3	5	5	17	8
Less than 15.0	23	18	19	12	17	24	18	20	30	23
Less than 20.0	43	46	41	29	39	53	49	44	55	50
Less than 25.0	64	64	62	54	61	68	65	71	66	67
Less than 30.0	88	87	83	70	81	86	84	85	85	85
Less than 35.0	93	95	93	84	91	93	94	93	90	92
All	100	100	100	100	100	100	100	100	100	100
Base	60	150	166	149	525	61	119	155	159	494
Mean	20.8	22.3	22.3	26.0	23.0	21.4	22.0	21.7	20.8	21.5
Median	22.6	21.3	22.2	23.8	22.4	19.9	20.8	20.9	18.9	20.1
Lower 2.5 percentile	3.0	10.4	7.2	9.8	6.2	9.4	8.4	7.7	5.6	7.3
Upper 2.5 percentile	42.5	46.1	38.3	52.3	45.8	45.6	39.1	37.0	44.7	41.3
Standard deviation	9.49	8.24	8.31	10.66	9.39	8.38	7.68	7.62	10.45	8.64

Table 12.9 Percentage distribution of serum ferritin by sex and age of young person

Serum ferritin (μg/l)	Males aged (years)					Females aged (years)				
	4–6	7–10	11–14	15–18	All males	4–6	7–10	11–14	15–18	All females
	cum %	cum %	cum %	cum %	cum %	cum %	cum %	cum %	cum %	cum %
Less than 15	11	6	5	2	6	9	2	14	27	14
Less than 20	18	14	17	5	13	26	15	27	36	27
Less than 25	36	33	37	15	30	45	32	40	54	43
Less than 30	64	50	53	27	47	57	46	51	60	54
Less than 40	75	71	70	42	64	76	69	78	82	77
Less than 50	86	88	88	57	79	86	82	87	87	86
Less than 60	87	94	94	69	86	97	89	95	93	93
All	100	100	100	100	100	100	100	100	100	100
Base	69	147	153	131	550	63	99	128	136	426
Mean	31	36	35	52	39	30	38	31	29	32
Median	28	29	28	44	31	27	32	28	23	28
Lower 2.5 percentile	9	9	10	15	11	10	15	8	7	8
Upper 2.5 percentile	73	67	98	156	94	61	112	72	90	84
Standard deviation	16.2	51.1	26.0	34.8	36.5	14.9	24.5	16.3	20.5	20.0

Table 12.10 Mean levels for additional haematology analytes by sex and age of young person

Analyte	Units	4–6 years			7–10 years			11–14 years			15–18 years			All		
		Mean	Median	Std Dev	Mean	Median	Std Dev	Mean	Median	Std Dev	Mean	Median	Std Dev	Mean	Median	Std Dev
Males																
Red blood cell count	$\times 10^{12}$/l	4.63	4.64	0.345	4.73	4.75	0.264	4.85	4.82	0.359	5.09	5.07	0.336	4.84	4.83	0.368
Red cell distribution width	%	14.5	14.5	0.65	14.1	14.1	0.56	14.1	14.0	0.93	14.0	13.9	0.59	14.1	14.1	0.73
Platelet count	$\times 10^9$/l	299	300	53.9	271	259	57.5	261	259	57.0	227	223	49.4	262	259	60.0
Mean platelet volume	fl	6.5	6.6	0.86	6.7	6.7	0.73	7.0	7.1	0.81	7.3	7.3	0.86	6.9	6.9	0.87
Platelet distribution width	%	55.1	55.3	3.17	54.8	54.5	2.94	54.2	53.9	3.16	53.9	53.7	3.55	54.4	54.1	3.24
White cell count	$\times 10^9$/l	6.9	6.4	2.06	6.1	5.8	1.56	5.9	5.6	1.60	6.2	6.1	1.53	6.2	5.9	1.69
Neutrophil count	$\times 10^9$/l	3.1	2.6	1.71	2.7	2.4	1.14	2.5	2.4	1.02	3.1	2.8	1.11	2.8	2.5	1.26
Lymphocyte count	$\times 10^9$/l	2.9	2.8	1.02	2.8	2.6	1.11	2.7	2.5	0.73	2.6	2.5	0.65	2.7	2.6	0.90
Monocyte count	$\times 10^9$/l	0.48	0.44	0.250	0.40	0.38	0.147	0.41	0.38	0.188	0.46	0.44	0.152	0.43	0.40	0.186
Eosinophil count	$\times 10^9$/l	0.35	0.23	0.290	0.35	0.24	0.325	0.30	0.18	0.650	0.23	0.17	0.207	0.30	0.19	0.418
Basophil count	$\times 10^9$/l	0.05	0.04	0.022	0.05	0.04	0.025	0.04	0.03	0.018	0.04	0.04	0.017	0.04	0.04	0.021
HbF*	%	0.6	0.5	0.36	0.6	0.5	0.42	0.7	0.5	1.44	0.5	0.5	0.23	0.6	0.5	0.81
HbA$_2$	%	4.6	3.0	7.27	2.9	2.9	0.22	2.9	2.9	0.43	2.8	2.8	0.24	3.2	2.9	3.17
Females																
Red blood cell count	$\times 10^{12}$/l	4.59	4.58	0.326	4.70	4.71	0.361	4.70	4.69	0.304	4.56	4.54	0.299	4.64	4.64	0.329
Red cell distribution width	%	14.2	14.0	1.04	14.0	13.9	0.83	13.9	13.8	0.62	13.9	14.0	0.68	14.0	13.9	0.79
Platelet count	$\times 10^9$/l	316	313	60.7	282	277	50.9	259	255	50.0	250	242	65.6	273	271	62.1
Mean platelet volume	fl	6.5	6.5	0.83	6.8	6.8	0.72	7.1	7.1	0.85	7.2	7.2	0.88	6.9	6.9	0.86
Platelet distribution width	%	54.1	53.7	2.78	54.2	54.1	3.14	54.2	53.9	3.50	53.5	53.1	3.64	54.0	53.7	3.34
White cell count	$\times 10^9$/l	6.5	6.4	1.43	6.2	6.0	1.58	6.0	5.6	1.65	6.3	6.2	1.51	6.2	6.0	1.57
Neutrophil count	$\times 10^9$/l	2.8	2.7	1.09	2.7	2.4	1.02	2.7	2.4	1.22	3.0	2.8	1.26	2.8	2.5	1.17
Lymphocyte count	$\times 10^9$/l	2.9	2.8	0.72	2.8	2.7	0.82	2.6	2.6	0.68	2.6	2.4	0.73	2.7	2.7	0.75
Monocyte count	$\times 10^9$/l	0.39	0.36	0.124	0.38	0.35	0.133	0.38	0.35	0.161	0.42	0.38	0.159	0.39	0.36	0.148
Eosinophil count	$\times 10^9$/l	0.44	0.32	0.424	0.32	0.21	0.310	0.26	0.15	0.271	0.18	0.13	0.160	0.29	0.17	0.307
Basophil count	$\times 10^9$/l	0.04	0.05	0.019	0.04	0.04	0.032	0.04	0.03	0.016	0.04	0.04	0.017	0.04	0.04	0.022
HbF**	%	0.7	0.6	0.45	0.7	0.5	1.25	0.6	0.5	0.54	0.5	0.5	0.24	0.6	0.5	0.74
HbA$_2$	%	2.9	2.9	0.23	3.5	2.9	7.12	3.1	2.8	3.15	3.0	2.8	2.70	3.1	2.8	4.24

* Includes results for 217 males (unweighted) below the precision of the analytic methodology: 26 results were below 0.1% and 191 results were between 0.1% and 0.5%

** Includes results for 150 females (unweighted) below the precision of the analytic methodology: 15 results were below 0.1% and 135 results were between 0.1% and 0.5%

Table 12.10(cont) Mean levels for additional haematology analytes by sex and age of young person – *base numbers*

Analyte	Sex and age of young person (years)									
	Males					Females				
	4–6	7–10	11–14	15–18	All	4–6	7–10	11–14	15–18	All
Red blood cell count	86	185	181	164	616	82	143	171	169	565
Red cell distibution width	75	149	156	131	511	65	104	136	140	445
Platelet count	75	149	156	131	511	65	104	136	140	445
Mean platelet volume	75	149	156	131	511	65	104	136	140	445
Platelet distribution width	75	149	156	131	511	65	104	136	140	445
White cell count	79	166	172	156	573	77	127	163	156	523
Neutrophil count	75	149	156	131	511	65	104	136	140	445
Lymphocyte count	75	149	156	131	511	65	104	136	140	445
Monocyte count	75	149	156	131	511	65	104	136	140	445
Eosinophil count	75	149	156	131	511	65	104	136	140	445
Basophil count	75	149	155	131	510	65	104	135	140	444
HbF	79	167	171	158	575	77	126	162	156	521
HbA$_2$	78	167	171	159	575	77	126	164	156	523

Table 12.11 Correlation coefficients between blood analytes and dietary intakes by sex and age of young person: haemoglobin, serum ferritin and red cell folate with dietary iron, vitamin C, vitamin B_{12} and folate

	Sex and age of young person									
	Males aged (years)				All males	Females aged (years)				All females
	4–6	7–10	11–14	15–18		4–6	7–10	11–14	15–18	
Haemoglobin with dietary intake of:										
Total iron	0.03	0.06	0.16*	0.15	0.40**	−0.09	0.13	0.06	0.03	0.11*
Haem iron	0.03	0.10	0.07	0.18*	0.40**	−0.07	0.14	0.12	0.16*	0.18**
Non-haem iron	0.02	0.06	0.16	0.14	0.38**	−0.08	0.12	0.06	0.02	0.10*
Vitamin C	0.33**	0.17*	0.11	0.10	0.15**	0.17	0.16	0.00	0.10	0.10*
Vitamin B_{12}	0.17	0.16*	0.14	0.16	0.25**	−0.07	0.10	0.13	0.00	0.02
Folate	0.00	0.06	0.13	0.20*	0.42**	−0.02	0.05	0.01	−0.01	0.08
Serum ferritin with dietary intake of:										
Total iron	0.21	−0.08	0.04	0.13	0.11*	0.03	−0.13	0.19	−0.15	−0.04
Haem iron	0.22*	0.09	0.11	0.14	0.19**	0.12	0.15	0.30**	0.14	0.15**
Non-haem iron	0.20	−0.09	0.03	0.12	0.10*	0.02	−0.14	0.17	−0.16	−0.05
Vitamin C	−0.14	0.00	0.07	−0.01	0.01	0.14	0.01	0.12	0.05	0.06
Vitamin B_{12}	0.01	−0.04	0.03	0.06	0.06	−0.14	−0.16	0.12	0.01	−0.03
Folate	0.06	−0.09	−0.01	0.16	0.12*	0.02	−0.13	0.07	−0.10	−0.06
Red cell folate with dietary intake of:										
Total iron	0.34**	0.06	0.44**	0.29**	0.08	0.46**	0.32**	0.39**	0.30**	0.26**
Haem iron	−0.29**	−0.28**	0.07	−0.03	−0.22**	−0.01	−0.14	−0.09	−0.04	−0.15**
Non-haem iron	0.37**	0.08	0.44**	0.30**	0.10*	0.46**	0.33**	0.39**	0.30**	0.28**
Vitamin C	0.08	0.11	0.21*	0.20*	0.13**	−0.19	0.14	0.15	0.24**	0.10*
Vitamin B_{12}	0.20	0.02	0.34**	0.31**	0.13**	0.11	0.16	0.39**	0.15	0.20**
Folate	0.36**	0.12	0.42**	0.30**	0.09*	0.41**	0.35**	0.41**	0.52**	0.32**
Number of young people										
haemoglobin	*81*	*176*	*166*	*140*	*563*	*76*	*133*	*157*	*156*	*522*
serum ferritin	*65*	*141*	*137*	*110*	*453*	*57*	*93*	*121*	*127*	*398*
red cell folate	*74*	*157*	*157*	*133*	*521*	*71*	*118*	*150*	*146*	*485*

* p < 0.05
** p < 0.01

459

Table 12.12 Haematology analytes by sex of young person and whether unwell during the dietary recording period

Sex of young person and haematology analytes	Units	Whether unwell during period												All			
		Unwell and eating affected				Unwell and eating not affected				Not unwell							
		Mean	Median	Std Dev	Base	Mean	Median	Std Dev	Base	Mean	Median	Std Dev	Base	Mean	Median	Std Dev	Base
Males																	
Haemoglobin concentration	g/dl	13.5	13.5	1.01	53	13.4	13.4	1.24	64	13.5	13.4	1.27	499	13.5	13.4	1.25	616
Mean cell haemoglobin	pg	27.5	27.7	2.08	53	27.6	27.5	1.57	64	28.0	28.0	1.83	499	27.9	28.0	1.84	616
Mean cell haemoglobin concentration	g/dl	31.7	31.7	0.99	43	31.8	31.8	0.97	49	31.8	31.8	1.15	419	31.8	31.7	1.12	511
Mean cell volume	fl	86.6	86.3	5.93	43	87.8	88.0	4.04	49	88.0	88.2	4.94	419	87.8	88.0	4.95	511
Haematocrit	l/l	0.429	0.428	0.0326	43	0.423	0.417	0.0382	49	0.425	0.422	0.0392	419	0.425	0.422	0.0387	511
Serum ferritin	µg/l	45	35	29.8	42	34	28	17.9	47	39	31	38.6	411	39	31	36.5	500
Plasma iron	µmol/l	13.43	12.61	4.272	49	13.43	13.18	5.560	50	13.72	13.30	5.364	441	13.67	13.26	5.300	540
Total iron binding capacity	µmol/l	59.2	58.7	7.45	48	62.7	61.6	8.08	47	60.3	60.2	7.18	430	60.4	60.2	7.32	525
Iron % saturation	%	23.0	22.0	7.71	48	23.1	22.7	9.13	47	23.0	22.4	9.57	430	23.0	22.4	9.39	525
Females																	
Haemoglobin concentration	g/dl	13.0	13.1	0.80	69	12.9	13.0	1.16	64	12.9	13.0	0.97	432	12.9	13.0	0.97	565
Mean cell haemoglobin	pg	28.1	28.0	1.58	69	27.5	27.8	2.95	64	28.0	28.0	1.78	432	27.9	28.0	1.93	565
Mean cell haemoglobin concentration	g/dl	31.6	31.6	1.35	50	31.5	31.6	1.32	50	31.4	31.4	1.10	345	31.4	31.4	1.16	445
Mean cell volume	fl	89.6	88.8	5.24	50	87.7	88.3	6.66	50	89.1	89.0	4.83	345	89.0	88.8	5.12	445
Haematocrit	l/l	0.414	0.413	0.0258	50	0.416	0.415	0.0310	50	0.412	0.413	0.0306	345	0.412	0.413	0.0302	445
Serum ferritin	µg/l	32	28	16.1	46	32	28	21.7	49	31	28	20.2	331	32	28	20.0	426
Plasma iron	µmol/l	12.79	13.03	4.269	62	13.49	11.95	4.838	52	13.04	12.35	5.092	390	13.06	12.33	4.975	504
Total iron binding capacity	µmol/l	61.6	60.8	7.59	60	61.7	60.5	8.63	48	61.8	61.1	7.67	386	61.8	60.9	7.75	494
Iron % saturation	%	20.9	20.0	7.32	60	21.9	20.1	8.77	48	21.5	20.1	8.80	386	21.5	20.1	8.64	494

Table 12.13 Haematology analytes by sex of young person and region

Sex of young person and haematology analytes	Units	Scotland*			Northern			Central, South West & Wales			London & South East			All		
		Mean	Median	Std Dev	Mean	Median	Std Dev	Mean	Median	Std Dev	Mean	Median	Std Dev	Mean	Median	Std Dev
Males																
Haemoglobin concentration	g/dl	13.3	13.4	1.24	13.6	13.5	1.22	13.5	13.4	1.23	13.5	13.3	1.29	13.5	13.4	1.25
Mean cell haemoglobin	pg	28.2	28.1	1.66	27.9	28.1	2.12	27.9	28.0	1.51	27.9	27.8	1.93	27.9	28.0	1.84
Mean cell haemoglobin concentration	g/dl	31.7	31.5	1.12	31.9	31.9	1.20	31.9	31.8	1.03	31.6	31.7	1.14	31.8	31.7	1.12
Mean cell volume	fl	88.9	88.2	4.46	87.6	88.4	5.97	87.4	87.8	4.06	88.3	87.9	5.07	87.8	88.0	4.95
Haematocrit	l/l	0.416	0.416	0.0371	0.428	0.423	0.0389	0.423	0.423	0.0385	0.426	0.421	0.0388	0.425	0.422	0.0387
Serum ferritin	µg/l	44	33	96.3	37	30	31.5	38	31	22.6	40	34	26.7	39	31	36.5
Plasma iron	µmol/l	12.87	13.03	5.038	14.17	13.70	5.205	13.80	13.30	5.183	13.30	12.94	5.520	13.67	13.26	5.300
Total iron binding capacity	µmol/l	60.2	59.3	7.56	61.3	62.3	7.26	60.5	60.3	7.32	59.6	59.4	7.24	60.4	60.2	7.32
Iron % saturation	%	22.1	22.8	9.61	23.8	22.6	8.86	23.0	22.6	8.80	22.7	21.8	10.28	23.0	22.4	9.39
Females																
Haemoglobin concentration	g/dl	12.9	12.7	0.94	12.9	13.0	0.92	13.0	13.0	0.97	13.0	13.1	1.03	12.9	13.0	0.97
Mean cell haemoglobin	pg	27.8	27.4	1.98	27.9	28.1	1.83	28.0	28.0	1.80	27.9	28.0	2.12	27.9	28.0	1.93
Mean cell haemoglobin concentration	g/dl	31.3	31.4	0.96	31.6	31.6	1.05	31.5	31.5	1.18	31.2	31.2	1.20	31.4	31.4	1.16
Mean cell volume	fl	88.9	88.2	4.76	88.8	88.5	4.33	88.6	88.0	5.10	89.6	89.6	5.60	89.0	88.8	5.12
Haematocrit	l/l	0.409	0.404	0.0288	0.411	0.412	0.0273	0.411	0.412	0.0297	0.415	0.419	0.0324	0.412	0.413	0.0302
Serum ferritin	µg/l	24	21	11.9	32	30	14.7	29	23	20.3	35	31	22.7	32	28	20.0
Plasma iron	µmol/l	14.07	11.51	6.629	12.85	12.18	4.965	12.59	12.16	4.402	13.48	13.26	5.027	13.06	12.33	4.975
Total iron binding capacity	µmol/l	62.7	62.4	7.80	61.9	61.3	7.44	61.7	61.0	8.22	61.5	60.5	7.50	61.8	60.9	7.75
Iron % saturation	%	23.1	20.1	11.63	21.3	19.9	8.70	20.7	19.5	8.03	22.1	20.7	8.24	21.5	20.1	8.64

Region spans the Scotland, Northern, Central South West & Wales, and London & South East columns.

* For females in Scotland some base numbers are less than 35 and the results should therefore be treated with caution.

Table 12.13(cont) **Haematology analytes by sex of young person and region:** *base numbers*

Haematology analytes	Sex of young person and region									
	Males					Females				
	Scotland	Northern	Central, South West & Wales	London & South East	All males	Scotland	Northern	Central, South West & Wales	London & South East	All females
Haemoglobin concentration	45	166	225	180	616	35	141	201	188	565
Mean cell haemoglobin	45	166	225	180	616	35	141	201	188	565
Mean cell haemoglobin concentration	39	123	191	158	511	28	91	167	159	445
Mean cell volume	39	123	191	158	511	28	91	167	159	445
Haematocrit	39	123	191	158	511	28	91	167	159	445
Serum ferritin	39	118	187	156	500	27	87	161	151	426
Plasma iron	44	145	187	164	540	32	129	173	170	504
Total iron binding capacity	44	138	181	162	525	32	126	169	167	494
Iron % saturation	44	138	181	162	525	32	126	169	167	494

Table 12.14 Haematology analytes by sex of young person and whether 'parents' were receiving certain benefits

Sex of young person and haematology analytes	Units	Whether 'parents' were receiving benefits								All			
		Receiving benefits				Not receiving benefits							
		Mean	Median	Std Dev	Base	Mean	Median	Std Dev	Base	Mean	Median	Std Dev	Base
Males													
Haemoglobin concentration	g/dl	13.3	13.2	1.20	135	13.6	13.5	1.25	480	13.5	13.4	1.25	616
Mean cell haemoglobin	pg	27.6	27.7	1.95	135	28.1	28.1	1.78	480	27.9	28.0	1.84	616
Mean cell haemoglobin concentration	g/dl	31.8	31.8	1.05	112	31.8	31.7	1.14	399	31.8	31.7	1.12	511
Mean cell volume	fl	87.0	87.6	5.46	112	88.1	88.0	4.75	399	87.8	88.0	4.95	511
Haematocrit	l/l	0.418	0.414	0.0380	112	0.427	0.423	0.0387	399	0.425	0.422	0.0387	511
Serum ferritin	µg/l	38	29	24.5	110	39	32	39.6	390	39	31	36.5	500
Plasma iron	µmol/l	12.53	12.24	5.112	115	14.03	13.36	5.309	425	13.67	13.26	5.300	540
Total iron binding capacity	µmol/l	60.2	60.1	6.40	113	60.4	60.3	7.59	412	60.4	60.2	7.32	525
Iron % saturation	%	21.4	21.3	8.79	113	23.5	22.5	9.51	412	23.0	22.4	9.39	525
Females													
Haemoglobin concentration	g/dl	12.8	12.8	1.13	142	13.0	13.1	0.90	423	12.9	13.0	0.97	565
Mean cell haemoglobin	pg	27.6	27.8	2.10	142	28.1	28.1	1.83	423	27.9	28.0	1.93	565
Mean cell haemoglobin concentration	g/dl	31.5	31.5	1.13	106	31.4	31.4	1.17	339	31.4	31.4	1.16	445
Mean cell volume	fl	88.2	87.8	4.75	106	89.3	88.9	5.23	339	89.0	88.8	5.12	445
Haematocrit	l/l	0.409	0.409	0.0346	106	0.414	0.415	0.0282	339	0.412	0.413	0.0302	445
Serum ferritin	µg/l	32	28	21.0	104	31	28	19.5	322	32	28	20.0	426
Plasma iron	µmol/l	12.50	12.11	4.895	124	13.28	12.66	4.991	380	13.06	12.33	4.975	504
Total iron binding capacity	µmol/l	61.8	61.0	7.27	122	61.8	60.8	7.94	372	61.8	60.9	7.75	494
Iron % saturation	%	20.5	19.3	8.08	122	21.9	20.2	8.82	372	21.5	20.1	8.64	494

Table 12.15 Haematology analytes by sex of young person and gross weekly household income

Sex of young person and haematology analytes	Units	Gross weekly household income																	All		
		Less than £160			£160 to less than £280			£280 to less than £400			£400 to less than £600			£600 and over					
		Mean	Median	Std Dev	Mean	Median	Std Dev	Mean	Median	Std Dev	Mean	Median	Std Dev	Mean	Median	Std Dev	Mean	Median	Std Dev
Males																			
Haemoglobin concentration	g/dl	13.1	13.1	1.07	13.4	13.4	1.30	13.5	13.3	1.44	13.7	13.6	1.15	13.7	13.6	1.19	13.5	13.4	1.25
Mean cell haemoglobin	pg	27.2	27.4	1.95	27.9	28.0	1.77	27.7	27.8	1.99	28.2	28.1	1.55	28.3	28.3	1.77	27.9	28.0	1.84
Mean cell haemoglobin concentration	g/dl	31.6	31.6	1.09	31.8	31.8	1.05	31.6	31.5	1.00	31.8	31.7	1.25	31.9	31.9	1.21	31.8	31.7	1.12
Mean cell volume	fl	85.9	87.1	5.38	88.0	87.8	4.79	87.1	87.9	5.60	88.8	88.7	3.99	88.4	88.1	4.56	87.8	88.0	4.95
Haematocrit	l/l	0.416	0.410	0.0318	0.422	0.423	0.0437	0.425	0.422	0.0443	0.431	0.427	0.0336	0.426	0.424	0.0363	0.425	0.422	0.0387
Serum ferritin	µg/l	39	28	23.9	41	34	58.5	37	28	34.5	36	32	18.9	39	33	25.6	39	31	36.5
Plasma iron	µmol/l	12.03	11.85	4.783	13.67	13.78	5.066	13.76	13.46	5.593	13.41	12.45	5.308	14.72	13.73	5.320	13.67	13.26	5.300
Total iron binding capacity	µmol/l	59.7	59.7	6.58	60.1	60.1	7.00	63.0	62.5	7.34	60.4	60.0	7.41	59.3	58.8	7.74	60.4	60.2	7.32
Iron % saturation	%	21.0	21.2	8.76	22.8	22.5	8.67	22.7	21.4	9.82	22.4	21.1	9.18	25.2	23.8	9.91	23.0	22.4	9.39
Females																			
Haemoglobin concentration	g/dl	12.8	12.9	1.21	12.8	12.8	0.84	12.8	13.0	1.03	13.1	13.2	0.86	13.1	13.1	0.83	12.9	13.0	0.97
Mean cell haemoglobin	pg	27.5	27.7	2.35	27.7	27.8	1.56	28.0	28.2	2.09	28.1	28.2	1.96	28.3	28.1	1.63	27.9	28.0	1.93
Mean cell haemoglobin concentration	g/dl	31.4	31.3	0.98	31.3	31.4	1.10	31.5	31.5	1.48	31.6	31.6	1.23	31.4	31.5	1.00	31.4	31.4	1.16
Mean cell volume	fl	88.3	88.2	4.54	88.7	88.0	4.75	88.7	88.2	5.48	88.9	89.2	5.53	90.1	89.4	5.08	89.0	88.8	5.12
Haematocrit	l/l	0.408	0.409	0.0341	0.410	0.412	0.0273	0.405	0.403	0.0299	0.414	0.415	0.0272	0.419	0.418	0.0273	0.412	0.413	0.0302
Serum ferritin	µg/l	34	29	24.5	32	29	19.6	29	25	18.7	29	25	15.8	34	31	20.1	32	28	20.0
Plasma iron	µmol/l	12.54	12.22	4.837	12.66	12.05	5.235	12.95	12.54	4.890	13.54	13.29	4.423	13.44	12.45	5.424	13.06	12.33	4.975
Total iron binding capacity	µmol/l	62.5	61.6	7.72	62.3	61.5	6.64	61.6	60.8	7.68	62.1	60.4	8.60	60.5	60.1	7.79	61.8	60.9	7.75
Iron % saturation	%	20.4	20.2	8.19	20.3	18.9	8.45	21.5	19.8	8.71	22.4	21.7	7.75	22.6	20.2	9.81	21.5	20.1	8.64

* Includes those not answering income question.

Table 12.15(cont) Haematology analytes by sex of young person and gross weekly household income – *base numbers*

Haematology analytes	Sex of young person and gross weekly household income											
	Males						Females					
	Less than £160	£160 to less than £280	£280 to less than £400	£400 to less than £600	£600 and over	All males	Less than £160	£160 to less than £280	£280 to less than £400	£400 to less than £600	£600 and over	All females
Haemoglobin concentration	89	115	106	133	150	616	89	106	94	123	138	565
Mean cell haemoglobin	89	115	106	133	150	616	89	106	94	123	138	565
Mean cell haemoglobin concentration	75	97	89	106	125	511	65	85	73	91	120	445
Mean cell volume	75	97	89	106	125	511	65	85	73	91	120	445
Haematocrit	75	97	89	106	125	511	65	85	73	91	120	445
Serum ferritin	73	97	88	102	123	500	64	80	71	87	113	426
Plasma iron	76	105	88	115	136	540	77	91	84	115	124	504
Total iron binding capacity	74	104	84	113	130	525	75	88	83	113	123	494
Iron % saturation	74	104	84	113	130	525	75	88	83	113	123	494

* Includes those not answering income question.

Table 12.16 Haematology analytes by sex of young person and social class of head of household

Sex of young person and haematology analytes	Units	Social class of head of household											
		Non-manual				Manual				All*			
		Mean	Median	Std Dev	Base	Mean	Median	Std Dev	Base	Mean	Median	Std Dev	Base
Males													
Haemoglobin													
concentration	g/dl	13.5	13.4	1.18	290	13.6	13.4	1.33	286	13.5	13.4	1.25	616
Mean cell haemoglobin	pg	27.9	27.9	1.83	290	28.0	28.0	1.70	286	27.9	28.0	1.84	616
Mean cell haemoglobin													
concentration	g/dl	31.7	31.7	1.10	246	31.9	31.8	1.14	232	31.8	31.7	1.12	511
Mean cell volume	fl	87.9	88.1	4.84	246	88.0	88.0	4.61	232	87.8	88.0	4.95	511
Haematocrit	l/l	0.424	0.422	0.0370	246	0.426	0.424	0.0409	232	0.425	0.422	0.0387	511
Serum ferritin	µg/l	36	30	23.3	242	42	34	47.4	225	39	31	36.5	500
Plasma iron	µmol/l	14.06	13.30	5.242	258	13.40	13.19	5.343	253	13.67	13.26	5.300	540
Total iron binding capacity	µmol/l	60.7	60.9	7.54	248	60.1	60.1	7.07	248	60.4	60.2	7.32	525
Iron % saturation	%	23.3	22.8	8.98	248	22.9	22.1	9.80	248	23.0	22.4	9.39	525
Females													
Haemoglobin													
concentration	g/dl	13.0	13.0	0.84	258	12.9	13.0	1.04	247	12.9	13.0	0.97	565
Mean cell haemoglobin	pg	28.0	27.9	1.84	258	27.9	28.0	1.85	247	27.9	28.0	1.93	565
Mean cell haemoglobin													
concentration	g/dl	31.5	31.6	1.16	215	31.3	31.3	1.20	187	31.4	31.4	1.16	445
Mean cell volume	fl	89.0	88.7	5.45	215	89.1	89.1	4.85	187	89.0	88.8	5.12	445
Haematocrit	l/l	0.414	0.415	0.0279	215	0.411	0.412	0.0324	187	0.412	0.413	0.0302	445
Serum ferritin	µg/l	31	29	17.8	204	31	26	21.4	179	32	28	20.0	426
Plasma iron	µmol/l	13.20	12.45	5.067	231	12.75	12.05	4.796	222	13.06	12.33	4.975	504
Total iron binding capacity	µmol/l	61.5	60.9	7.72	227	62.4	61.3	7.58	218	61.8	60.9	7.75	494
Iron % saturation	%	22.0	20.2	8.93	227	20.7	19.4	8.03	218	21.5	20.1	8.64	494

* Includes those for whom a social class could not be assigned.

Table 12.17 Percentage distribution of plasma vitamin C by sex and age of young person

Plasma vitamin C (µmol/l)	Males aged (years)					Females aged (years)				
	4–6	7–10	11–14	15–18	All males*	4–6	7–10	11–14	15–18	All females*
	cum %	cum %	cum %	cum %	cum %	cum %	cum %	cum %	cum %	cum %
Less than 11.0	5	2	1	3	3	2	3	1	4	3
Less than 30.0	12	12	15	22	15	8	12	13	17	13
Less than 50.0	26	29	43	44	36	26	33	36	37	33
Less than 60.0	42	45	63	64	54	37	45	53	53	47
Less than 70.0	59	64	74	87	71	56	63	74	72	66
Less than 80.0	77	81	86	96	85	75	77	90	85	82
All	100	100	100	100	100	100	100	100	100	100
Base	73	166	176	152	567	76	133	161	158	528
Mean	61.6	60.1	54.2	50.2	56.4	64.6	60.1	55.7	55.7	58.8
Median	67.2	62.4	52.9	51.6	57.6	67.9	62.1	59.1	56.9	61.5
Lower 2.5 percentile	0.6	13.6	12.6	8.6	8.6	14.3	5.3	17.0	9.7	10.0
Upper 2.5 percentile	99.1	101.7	100.6	92.0	98.2	111.1	97.4	88.9	102.7	98.9
Standard deviation	24.51	22.93	22.08	21.93	23.25	22.87	24.33	20.01	24.02	23.14

*Includes 3 results (unwtd), for 2 males and 1 female, below the precision of the analytic methodology.

Table 12.18 Percentage distribution of red cell folate by sex and age of young person

Red cell folate (nmol/l)	Males aged (years)					Females aged (years)				
	4–6	7–10	11–14	15–18	All males	4–6	7–10	11–14	15–18	All females
	cum %	cum %	cum %	cum %	cum %	cum %	cum %	cum %	cum %	cum %
Less than 230	–	1	1	–	0	–	1	–	1	1
Less than 350	3	4	8	12	7	1	9	11	14	9
Less than 425	6	7	17	30	16	5	20	28	39	25
Less than 500	13	17	37	48	30	17	34	47	58	41
Less than 600	30	40	58	67	51	46	56	65	80	63
Less than 800	60	79	83	90	80	74	86	90	92	87
Less than 1000	89	93	96	96	94	88	94	99	99	95
All	100	100	100	100	100	100	100	100	100	100
Base	79	166	172	156	573	77	125	163	156	521
Mean	736	671	598	540	626	677	604	544	500	573
Median	721	653	556	515	594	618	567	515	474	540
Lower 2.5 percentile	336	322	277	283	283	365	270	288	268	274
Upper 2.5 percentile	1132	1154	1089	1045	1113	1125	1168	942	975	1095
Standard deviation	200.7	199.4	208.6	181.0	209.5	209.3	222.7	174.4	171.3	203.9

Table 12.19 Percentage distribution of serum folate by sex and age of young person

Serum folate (nmol/l)	Males aged (years)					Females aged (years)				
	4–6	7–10	11–14	15–18	All males	4–6	7–10	11–14	15–18	All females
	cum %	cum %	cum %	cum %	cum %	cum %	cum %	cum %	cum %	cum %
Less than 6.3	–	–	–	1	0	–	–	1	1	1
Less than 10.0	3	0	4	10	4	1	11	6	14	9
Less than 15.0	7	12	24	42	22	7	22	30	49	29
Less than 20.0	24	24	49	65	42	22	45	58	71	51
Less than 25.0	48	49	72	87	65	46	65	82	85	71
Less than 30.0	76	76	88	92	84	66	80	91	94	84
Less than 35.0	91	96	98	98	96	92	93	98	97	95
All	100	100	100	100	100	100	100	100	100	100
Base	85	185	181	161	612	82	138	168	169	557
Mean	25.0	24.5	20.8	17.6	21.7	25.8	22.0	19.3	16.9	20.6
Median	25.6	25.2	20.2	17.0	21.8	25.6	20.6	18.4	15.2	19.7
Lower 2.5 percentile	9.1	11.1	9.3	7.7	8.6	13.4	8.4	8.9	7.0	8.4
Upper 2.5 percentile	39.2	37.6	34.9	34.0	36.7	37.2	37.2	34.0	37.3	37.1
Standard deviation	7.25	6.91	7.11	6.98	7.64	6.86	8.50	6.93	7.51	8.16

Table 12.20 Pearson correlation coefficients for serum folate with red cell folate by sex and age of young person

Sex and age of young person	Correlation coefficient	Number of young people
Males aged (years)		
4–6	0.45**	77
7–10	0.48**	166
11–14	0.56**	171
15–18	0.56**	153
All males	0.57**	567
Females aged (years)		
4–6	0.49**	77
7–10	0.56**	124
11–14	0.55**	159
15–18	0.55**	156
All females	0.59**	515

** $p < 0.01$

Table 12.21 Percentage distribution of serum vitamin B_{12} by sex and age of young person*

Serum vitamin B_{12} (pmol/l)	Males aged (years)					Females aged (years)				
	4–6	7–10	11–14	15–18	All males	4–6	7–10	11–14	15–18	All females
	cum %	cum %	cum %	cum %	cum %	cum %	cum %	cum %	cum %	cum %
Less than 100	–	–	–	1	0	–	–	–	3	1
Less than 118	–	–	–	1	0	–	–	–	8	2
Less than 150	–	–	0	8	2	–	–	2	13	4
Less than 250	5	6	21	44	20	3	7	25	48	23
Less than 350	16	28	50	78	45	13	33	57	76	47
Less than 450	35	48	78	96	66	37	57	74	94	68
Less than 550	62	64	91	97	80	56	77	86	97	81
Less than 650	78	86	97	100	91	72	90	95	99	90
All	100	100	100		100	100	100	100	100	100
Base	86	183	179	161	609	82	138	169	169	558
Mean	525	479	367	277	403	550	443	371	267	395
Median	506	462	349	265	367	531	419	316	251	359
Lower 2.5 percentile	229	219	174	127	152	249	188	161	97	119
Upper 2.5 percentile	940	820	665	550	798	966	789	833	581	867
Standard deviation	175.8	176.9	143.3	100.6	177.6	192.9	153.3	175.9	118.9	187.6

* Includes 1 result above the precision of the analytic methodology.

Table 12.22 Percentage distribution of erythrocyte transketolase activation coefficient (ETKAC) by sex and age of young person

ETKAC (ratio)	Males aged (years)					Females aged (years)				
	4–6	7–10	11–14	15–18	All males	4–6	7–10	11–14	15–18	All females
	cum %	cum %	cum %	cum %	cum %	cum %	cum %	cum %	cum %	cum %
Greater than 1.25	1	–	0	–	0	1	2	2	3	2
Greater than 1.20	1	4	3	5	3	2	4	8	9	6
Greater than 1.15	7	17	22	35	21	12	16	28	34	23
Greater than 1.10	51	53	67	77	62	48	55	63	73	60
Greater than 1.05	89	83	90	93	89	82	90	92	92	89
All	100	100	100	100	100	100	100	100	100	100
Base	69	165	175	152	561	76	133	163	162	534
Mean	1.10	1.11	1.12	1.13	1.12	1.10	1.11	1.13	1.13	1.12
Median	1.11	1.11	1.13	1.13	1.12	1.10	1.11	1.13	1.14	1.12
Lower 2.5 percentile	1.03	1.01	1.00	1.00	1.01	1.02	1.02	1.00	1.00	1.01
Upper 2.5 percentile	1.18	1.21	1.21	1.22	1.21	1.19	1.25	1.24	1.26	1.25
Standard deviation	0.043	0.051	0.049	0.053	0.051	0.050	0.052	0.059	0.057	0.056

Table 12.23 Percentage distribution of erythrocyte transketolase basal activity (ETK-B) by sex and age of young person

ETK-B (µmol/g Hb/min)	Males aged (years)					Females aged (years)				
	4–6	7–10	11–14	15–18	All males	4–6	7–10	11–14	15–18	All females
	cum %	cum %	cum %	cum %	cum %	cum %	cum %	cum %	cum %	cum %
Less than 0.60	–	1	2	3	1	1	3	5	6	4
Less than 0.70	8	5	12	16	10	9	7	19	14	12
Less than 0.80	26	23	38	49	34	23	29	44	45	35
Less than 0.90	51	45	71	74	60	42	64	72	73	64
Less than 1.00	84	76	89	91	85	79	87	91	91	87
Less than 1.10	91	94	98	98	95	89	95	97	97	95
All	100	100	100	100	100	100	100	100	100	100
Base	69	165	175	152	561	76	133	163	162	534
Mean	0.90	0.91	0.84	0.82	0.87	0.91	0.86	0.81	0.82	0.85
Median	0.89	0.92	0.83	0.80	0.85	0.92	0.87	0.81	0.82	0.85
Lower 2.5 percentile	0.64	0.66	0.64	0.59	0.61	0.64	0.57	0.56	0.57	0.57
Upper 2.5 percentile	1.38	1.19	1.09	1.08	1.15	1.19	1.20	1.13	1.12	1.15
Standard deviation	0.186	0.139	0.122	0.141	0.152	0.143	0.133	0.143	0.133	0.142

Table 12.24 Percentage distribution of erythrocyte glutathione reductase activation coefficient (EGRAC) by sex and age of young person

EGRAC (ratio)	Males aged (years)					Females aged (years)				
	4–6	7–10	11–14	15–18	All males	4–6	7–10	11–14	15–18	All females
	cum %	cum %	cum %	cum %	cum %	cum %	cum %	cum %	cum %	cum %
Greater than 1.60	2	5	20	23	13	4	16	28	29	20
Greater than 1.50	15	13	32	33	24	15	35	47	51	38
Greater than 1.40	36	35	54	59	46	33	57	70	79	61
Greater than 1.30	59	78	80	80	75	75	85	90	95	87
Greater than 1.20	92	98	96	97	96	98	96	100	98	98
All	100	100	100	100	100	100	100		100	100
Base	72	168	178	154	572	76	133	165	163	537
Mean	1.36	1.38	1.46	1.48	1.42	1.38	1.45	1.51	1.53	1.47
Median	1.32	1.36	1.44	1.45	1.39	1.37	1.44	1.49	1.51	1.45
Lower 2.5 percentile	1.17	1.21	1.17	1.20	1.18	1.21	1.20	1.22	1.21	1.21
Upper 2.5 percentile	1.60	1.67	1.91	1.98	1.91	1.66	1.85	1.95	1.93	1.86
Standard deviation	0.126	0.120	0.184	0.198	0.169	0.116	0.151	0.180	0.177	0.169

Table 12.25 Percentage distribution of erythrocyte aspartate aminotransferase activation coefficient (EAATAC) by sex and age of young person

EAATAC (ratio)	Males aged (years)					Females aged (years)				
	4–6	7–10	11–14	15–18	All males	4–6	7–10	11–14	15–18	All females
	cum %	cum %	cum %	cum %	cum %	cum %	cum %	cum %	cum %	cum %
Greater than 2.00	7	8	11	15	10	6	11	14	8	10
Greater than 1.90	11	25	30	25	24	19	22	29	19	22
Greater than 1.80	27	42	51	50	44	31	46	54	46	45
Greater than 1.70	56	72	75	73	70	49	71	81	67	68
Greater than 1.60	91	89	93	92	91	86	90	97	86	90
Greater than 1.50	98	98	97	97	98	96	96	100	96	97
All	100	100	100	100	100	100	100		100	100
Base	72	168	178	154	572	76	133	165	163	537
Mean	1.75	1.79	1.82	1.82	1.80	1.76	1.79	1.84	1.78	1.79
Median	1.72	1.77	1.81	1.81	1.77	1.70	1.78	1.82	1.79	1.78
Lower 2.5 percentile	1.52	1.51	1.50	1.45	1.51	1.49	1.50	1.57	1.47	1.50
Upper 2.5 percentile	2.30	2.15	2.10	2.17	2.16	2.23	2.11	2.19	2.15	2.15
Standard deviation	0.169	0.153	0.162	0.175	0.166	0.175	0.158	0.151	0.163	0.163

Table 12.26 Percentage distribution of plasma zinc by sex and age of young person

Plasma zinc (μmol/l)	Males aged (years)					Females aged (years)				
	4–6	7–10	11–14	15–18	All males	4–6	7–10	11–14	15–18	All females
	cum %	cum %	cum %	cum %	cum %	cum %	cum %	cum %	cum %	cum %
Less than 10.0	10	1	–	1	2	–	1	1	1	1
Less than 12.0	19	7	11	6	10	–	5	6	18	7
Less than 14.0	34	23	38	37	33	23	28	36	56	36
Less than 16.0	74	72	81	77	76	68	78	79	83	77
Less than 18.0	96	94	97	95	95	94	94	97	96	96
All	100	100	100	100	100	100	100	100	100	100
Base	*38*	*124*	*151*	*134*	*447*	*38*	*97*	*139*	*147*	*421*
Mean	14.2	15.0	14.5	14.7	14.6	15.1	14.7	14.6	13.9	14.6
Median	14.5	14.9	14.5	14.5	14.6	14.9	14.6	14.5	13.6	14.5
Lower 2.5 percentile	7.0	11.6	11.3	11.7	10.4	12.3	11.5	11.1	10.4	11.0
Upper 2.5 percentile	18.5	18.4	18.0	18.9	18.5	18.7	19.2	18.2	18.9	18.7
Standard deviation	2.87	1.76	1.77	1.90	2.09	1.48	1.84	1.86	2.22	1.93

Table 12.27 Correlation coefficients for plasma ascorbate with dietary intake of vitamin C

Blood analyte: Plasma ascorbate	Dietary intake of vitamin C	Number of young people
Males aged (years)		
4–6	0.31**	69
7–10	0.40**	158
11–14	0.49**	160
15–18	0.28**	129
All males	0.35**	516
Females aged (years)		
4–6	0.44**	71
7–10	0.39**	123
11–14	0.41**	149
15–18	0.29**	145
All females	0.33**	488

** p < 0.01

Table 12.28 Correlation coefficients for serum vitamin B_{12} with dietary vitamin B_{12} by sex and age of young person

Blood analyte: serum vitamin B_{12}	Dietary intake of vitamin B_{12}	Number of young people
Males aged (years)		
4–6	0.33**	81
7–10	0.43**	174
11–14	0.09	163
15–18	0.36**	137
All males	0.09*	555
Females aged (years)		
4–6	0.25*	75
7–10	0.31**	128
11–14	0.30**	155
15–18	0.16	156
All females	0.22**	514

*p < 0.05
** p < 0.01

Table 12.29 Correlation coefficients for erythrocyte transketolase activation coefficient (ETKAC) with dietary intake of thiamin

Blood analyte: ETKAC	Dietary intake of thiamin	Number of young people
Males aged (years):		
4–6	0.17	69
7–10	−0.08	158
11–14	−0.03	160
15–18	−0.14	129
All males	0.03	516
Females aged (years)		
4–6	−0.04	71
7–10	−0.10	123
11–14	−0.17	149
15–18	−0.16	145
All females	−0.11*	488

** p < 0.05

Table 12.30 Correlation coefficient for erythrocyte glutathione reductase activation coefficient (EGRAC) with dietary intake of riboflavin

Blood analyte: EGRAC	Dietary intake of riboflavin	Number of young people
Males aged (years):		
4–6	−0.36**	69
7–10	−0.30**	160
11–14	−0.46**	162
15–18	−0.42**	131
All males	−0.32**	522
Females aged (years)		
4–6	−0.33**	71
7–10	−0.49**	123
11–14	−0.37**	152
15–18	−0.36**	150
All females	−0.39**	496

**p < 0.01

Table 12.31 Correlation coefficients for plasma zinc with dietary intakes of zinc and protein

Blood analyte: Plasma zinc	Dietary intake of:		Number of young people
	Zinc	Protein	
Males aged (years):			
4–6	0.01	0.16	36
7–10	0.10	0.10	119
11–14	−0.09	−0.01	135
15–18	0.18	0.11	117
All males	0.09	0.11*	407
Females aged (years)			
4–6	0.22	0.03	34
7–10	0.16	0.16	90
11–14	0.14	0.15	127
15–18	0.18	0.28**	135
All females	0.15**	0.15**	386

* p < 0.05
** p < 0.01

Table 12.32 **Water soluble vitamins and plasma zinc by sex of young person and whether unwell during dietary recording period**

Sex of young person and analytes	Units	Whether unwell during period									All		
		Unwell and eating affected			Unwell and eating not affected			Not unwell					
		Mean	Median	Std Dev	Mean	Median	Std Dev	Mean	Median	Std Dev	Mean	Median	Std Dev
Males													
Plasma ascorbate (vitamin C)*	μmol/l	56.7	53.7	22.56	56.5	53.5	26.46	56.4	58.0	22.86	56.4	57.6	23.22
Red cell folate	nmol/l	607	533	211.4	602	519	267.5	631	601	200.6	626	594	209.5
Serum folate	nmol/l	21.7	21.3	8.00	22.1	21.3	8.18	21.7	21.8	7.53	21.7	21.8	7.64
Serum vitamin B$_{12}$	pmol/l	421	359	186.5	400	404	153.2	402	366	179.8	403	367	177.6
Erythrocyte transketolase activation coefficient	ratio	1.12	1.13	0.061	1.12	1.13	0.041	1.12	1.12	0.051	1.12	1.12	0.051
EGRAC**	ratio	1.39	1.34	0.155	1.48	1.42	0.201	1.42	1.40	0.165	1.42	1.39	0.169
EAATAC***	ratio	1.79	1.74	0.150	1.81	1.77	0.153	1.80	1.78	0.169	1.80	1.77	0.166
Plasma zinc	μmol/l	14.60	14.50	2.023	14.79	14.60	1.959	14.60	14.70	2.113	14.62	14.60	2.092
Females													
Plasma ascorbate (vitamin C)*	μmol/l	57.5	58.9	21.75	59.6	61.3	22.13	58.9	61.9	23.47	58.8	61.5	23.13
Red cell folate	nmol/l	511	515	151.7	557	517	201.1	584	540	209.2	573	540	203.9
Serum folate	nmol/l	19.7	18.6	8.21	19.5	20.2	6.18	20.9	19.7	8.39	20.6	19.7	8.16
Serum vitamin B$_{12}$	pmol/l	426	368	237.2	439	378	220.1	383	357	171.4	395	359	187.6
Erythrocyte transketolase activation coefficient	ratio	1.13	1.13	0.064	1.13	1.12	0.053	1.12	1.11	0.055	1.12	1.12	0.056
EGRAC**	ratio	1.46	1.45	0.151	1.47	1.45	0.181	1.48	1.45	0.170	1.47	1.45	0.169
EAATAC***	ratio	1.82	1.82	0.138	1.80	1.80	0.153	1.79	1.78	0.168	1.79	1.78	0.163
Plasma zinc	μmol/l	14.47	14.40	1.579	14.47	14.60	1.472	14.60	14.60	2.026	14.57	14.50	1.926

* Includes 3 results (unwtd), for 2 males and 1 female, below the precision of the analytic methodology.

** Erythrocyte glutathione reductase activation coefficient.

*** Erythrocyte aspartate aminotransferase activation coefficient.

Table 12.32(cont)   Water soluble vitamins and plasma zinc by sex of young person and whether unwell during dietary recording period: *base numbers*

Analytes	Sex of young person and whether unwell during period							
	Males			All males	Females			All females
	Unwell and eating affected	Unwell and eating not affected	Not unwell		Unwell and eating affected	Unwell and eating not affected	Not unwell	
Plasma ascorbate (vitamin C)*	51	57	459	567	60	61	407	528
Red cell folate	48	57	468	573	61	56	404	521
Serum folate	52	65	495	612	69	64	424	557
Serum vitamin B_{12}	51	65	493	609	69	64	425	558
Erythrocyte transketolase activation coefficient	49	55	457	561	63	62	409	534
EGRAC**	50	56	466	572	63	62	412	537
EAATAC***	50	56	466	572	63	62	412	537
Plasma zinc	42	40	365	447	56	42	323	421

* Includes 3 results (unwtd), for 2 males and 1 female, below the precision of the analytic methodology.
** Erythrocyte glutathione reductase activation coefficient.
*** Erythrocyte aspartate aminotransferase activation coefficient.

Table 12.33 Water soluble vitamins and plasma zinc by sex of young person and region

Sex of young person and analytes	Units	Region												All		
		Scotland#			Northern			Central, South West & Wales			London & South East					
		Mean	Median	Std Dev	Mean	Median	Std Dev	Mean	Median	Std Dev	Mean	Median	Std Dev	Mean	Median	Std Dev
Males																
Plasma ascorbate (vitamin C)*	µmol/l	50.7	49.6	21.28	51.8	53.2	24.61	59.5	60.5	20.53	58.4	59.2	24.26	56.4	57.6	23.22
Red cell folate	nmol/l	565	565	152.1	627	580	213.4	644	621	218.1	619	593	204.8	626.0	594	209.5
Serum folate	nmol/l	21.3	21.6	7.27	20.8	20.7	7.57	22.2	22.7	7.55	22.1	22.0	7.82	21.7	21.8	7.64
Serum vitamin B_{12}	pmol/l	380	344	168.7	409	363	184.2	390	337	169.4	418	396	181.4	403.0	367	177.6
Erythrocyte transketolase activation coefficient	ratio	1.12	1.12	0.052	1.12	1.12	0.050	1.11	1.12	0.051	1.12	1.12	0.051	1.12	1.12	0.051
EGRAC**	ratio	1.42	1.37	0.171	1.42	1.40	0.165	1.42	1.39	0.176	1.42	1.39	0.166	1.42	1.39	0.169
EAATAC***	ratio	1.77	1.75	0.153	1.79	1.76	0.163	1.79	1.77	0.164	1.81	1.79	0.173	1.80	1.77	0.166
Plasma zinc	µmol/l	15.09	14.90	1.861	14.81	14.70	1.745	14.54	14.90	2.138	14.42	14.50	2.312	14.62	14.60	2.092
Females																
Plasma ascorbate (vitamin C)*	µmol/l	59.7	65.7	20.01	52.3	56.8	24.58	61.7	62.1	22.25	61.1	62.9	22.43	58.8	61.5	23.13
Red cell folate	nmol/l	591	544	218.8	558	510	199.8	568	539	202.3	585	553	205.2	573.0	540.0	203.9
Serum folate	nmol/l	19.4	15.2	9.12	19.6	18.8	7.79	21.0	20.2	8.44	21.1	20.9	7.86	20.6	19.7	8.16
Serum vitamin B_{12}	pmol/l	399	395	184.1	368	327	177.7	388	359	177.5	424	373	202.7	395.0	359.0	187.6
Erythrocyte transketolase activation coefficient	ratio	1.12	1.11	0.064	1.12	1.12	0.055	1.12	1.11	0.049	1.12	1.12	0.061	1.12	1.12	0.056
EGRAC**	ratio	1.46	1.41	0.216	1.47	1.45	0.170	1.47	1.45	0.152	1.48	1.45	0.175	1.47	1.45	0.169
EAATAC***	ratio	1.78	1.75	0.138	1.83	1.82	0.171	1.76	1.75	0.149	1.80	1.79	0.169	1.79	1.78	0.163
Plasma zinc	µmol/l	14.45	14.70	1.649	14.66	14.80	2.105	14.55	14.40	1.932	14.55	14.40	1.840	14.57	14.50	1.926

For females in Scotland some base numbers are less than 35 and the results should therefore be treated with caution.
* Includes 3 results (unwtd), for 2 males and 1 female, below the precision of the analytic methodology.
** Erythrocyte glutathione reductase activation coefficient.
*** Erythrocyte aspartate aminotransferase activation coefficient.

Table 12.33(cont) **Water soluble vitamins and plasma zinc by sex of young person and region:** *base numbers*

Analytes	Sex of young person and region											
	Males				All males	Females				All females		
	Scotland	Northern	Central, South West & Wales	London & South East		Scotland	Northern	Central, South West & Wales	London & South East			
Plasma ascorbate (vitamin C)*	45	138	181	170	567	32	133	186	177	528		
Red cell folate	44	150	208	171	573	33	124	186	178	521		
Serum folate	46	165	222	179	612	35	139	198	185	557		
Serum vitamin B$_{12}$	46	164	220	179	609	35	139	197	187	558		
Erythrocyte transketolase activation coefficient	44	149	202	166	561	31	134	191	178	534		
EGRAC**	45	153	204	170	572	32	134	193	178	537		
EAATAC***	45	153	204	170	572	32	134	193	178	537		
Plasma zinc	41	112	155	139	447	28	102	143	148	421		

* Includes 3 results (unwtd), for 2 males and 1 female, below the precision of the analytic methodology.
** Erythrocyte glutathione reductase activation coefficient.
*** Erythrocyte aspartate aminotransferase activation coefficient.

Table 12.34 Water soluble vitamins and plasma zinc by sex of young person and whether 'parents' were receiving certain benefits

Sex of young person and haematology analytes	Units	Whether 'parents' were receiving benefits								All			
		Receiving benefits				Not receiving benefits							
		Mean	Median	Std Dev	Base	Mean	Median	Std Dev	Base	Mean	Median	Std Dev	Base
Males													
Plasma ascorbate (vitamin C)*	µmol/l	49.4	50.7	21.78	123	58.8	60.6	23.23	443	56.4	57.6	23.22	567
Red cell folate	nmol/l	606	574	196.4	126	633	603	213.3	446	626	594	209.5	573
Serum folate	nmol/l	20.6	20.2	7.28	134	22.1	22.2	7.72	477	21.7	21.8	7.64	612
Serum vitamin B$_{12}$	pmol/l	405	389	164.7	134	402	366	181.7	474	403	367	177.6	609
Erythrocyte transketolase activation coefficient	ratio	1.12	1.13	0.048	121	1.12	1.12	0.052	439	1.12	1.12	0.051	561
EGRAC**	ratio	1.44	1.39	0.187	122	1.41	1.39	0.162	449	1.42	1.39	0.169	572
EAATAC***	ratio	1.82	1.78	0.164	122	1.79	1.77	0.167	449	1.80	1.77	0.166	572
Plasma zinc	µmol/l	14.13	14.40	2.440	90	14.76	14.90	1.961	357	14.62	14.60	2.092	447
Females													
Plasma ascorbate (vitamin C)*	µmol/l	52.8	53.6	22.26	132	61.3	64.2	23.04	396	58.8	61.5	23.13	528
Red cell folate	nmol/l	579	542	207.3	130	570	533	202.5	391	573	540	203.9	521
Serum folate	nmol/l	19.9	18.8	7.88	139	20.9	20.2	8.26	418	20.6	19.7	8.16	557
Serum vitamin B$_{12}$	pmol/l	380	357	160.9	139	401	360	197.1	419	395	359	187.6	558
Erythrocyte transketolase activation coefficient	ratio	1.12	1.12	0.052	132	1.12	1.12	0.057	402	1.12	1.12	0.056	534
EGRAC**	ratio	1.48	1.47	0.168	132	1.47	1.45	0.170	405	1.47	1.45	0.169	537
EAATAC***	ratio	1.82	1.78	0.164	122	1.79	1.77	0.167	449	1.80	1.77	0.166	572
Plasma zinc	µmol/l	14.21	14.30	1.649	101	14.71	14.70	2.003	320	14.57	14.50	1.926	421

* Includes 3 results (unwtd), for 2 males and 1 female, below the precision of the analytic methodology.

** Erythrocyte glutathione reductase activation coefficient.

*** Erythrocyte aspartate aminotransferase activation coefficient.

Table 12.35 Water soluble vitamins and plasma zinc by sex of young person and gross weekly household income

Sex of young person and haematology analytes	Units	Gross weekly household income															All†		
		Less than £160			£160 to less than £280			£280 to less than £400			£400 to less than £600			£600 and over					
		Mean	Median	Std Dev	Mean	Median	Std Dev	Mean	Median	Std Dev	Mean	Median	Std Dev	Mean	Median	Std Dev	Mean	Median	Std Dev
Males																			
Plasma ascorbate (vitamin C)*	μmol/l	50.1	50.1	23.13	54.4	52.7	21.42	54.9	57.3	27.74	58.1	58.0	20.73	62.9	63.7	21.54	56.4	57.6	23.22
Red cell folate	nmol/l	637	594	213.0	606	583	181.6	666	601	238.9	593	558	214.0	648	630	196.7	626	594	209.5
Serum folate	nmol/l	21.2	21.1	7.65	21.5	22.4	7.33	22.3	21.3	8.14	20.9	21.1	7.59	23.2	23.7	7.37	21.7	21.8	7.64
Serum vitamin B$_{12}$	pmol/l	416	419	153.5	406	373	169.4	422	361	195.5	377	346	153.0	415	373	201.8	403	367	177.6
Erythrocyte transketolase activation coefficient	ratio	1.12	1.13	0.049	1.12	1.13	0.053	1.12	1.12	0.053	1.11	1.12	0.051	1.12	1.12	0.045	1.12	1.12	0.051
EGRAC**	ratio	1.44	1.39	0.192	1.43	1.40	0.173	1.41	1.40	0.148	1.42	1.40	0.154	1.40	1.37	0.152	1.42	1.39	0.169
EAATAC***	ratio	1.81	1.79	0.165	1.80	1.78	0.181	1.80	1.77	0.161	1.78	1.76	0.137	1.78	1.78	0.171	1.80	1.77	0.166
Plasma zinc	μmol/l	13.68	14.40	2.487	14.46	14.40	2.146	15.14	15.00	1.926	14.84	15.10	2.088	14.83	14.90	1.746	14.62	14.60	2.092
Females																			
Plasma ascorbate (vitamin C)*	μmol/l	52.3	52.4	23.17	54.2	59.1	21.77	55.9	59.7	23.56	62.5	62.7	23.90	67.6	69.9	19.90	58.8	61.5	23.13
Red cell folate	nmol/l	547	519	169.3	601	556	225.1	584	540	219.3	551	515	190.8	577	534	204.9	573	540	203.9
Serum folate	nmol/l	19.5	19.3	7.67	20.4	19.3	7.90	20.9	19.5	8.73	20.8	19.7	7.98	21.0	20.4	8.49	20.6	19.7	8.16
Serum vitamin B$_{12}$	pmol/l	363	332	153.4	395	360	182.5	387	352	186.4	423	385	198.1	395	361	201.0	395	359	187.6
Erythrocyte transketolase activation coefficient	ratio	1.12	1.12	0.054	1.12	1.12	0.050	1.12	1.13	0.063	1.11	1.12	0.055	1.12	1.12	0.059	1.12	1.12	0.056
EGRAC**	ratio	1.50	1.47	0.190	1.48	1.46	0.166	1.47	1.45	0.183	1.46	1.44	0.141	1.47	1.43	0.174	1.47	1.45	0.169
EAATAC***	ratio	1.78	1.78	0.169	1.79	1.78	0.167	1.79	1.77	0.178	1.80	1.79	0.159	1.79	1.79	0.149	1.79	1.78	0.163
Plasma zinc	μmol/l	14.26	14.30	1.819	14.10	14.30	1.761	14.81	14.86	1.716	14.87	14.60	2.085	14.75	15.00	2.034	14.57	14.50	1.926

† Includes those not answering income question.
* Includes 3 results (unwtd), for 2 males and 1 female, below the precision of the analytic methodology.
** Erythrocyte glutathione reductase activation coefficient.
*** Erythrocyte aspartate aminotransferase activation coefficient.

477

Table 12.35(cont) Water soluble vitamins and plasma zinc by sex of young person and gross weekly household income: *base numbers*

Analytes	Sex of young person and gross weekly household income														
	Males					All males†	Females						All females†
	Less than £160	£160 to less than £280	£280 to less than £400	£400 to less than £600	£600 and over		Less than £160	£160 to less than £280	£280 to less than £400	£400 to less than £600	£600 and over	
Plasma ascorbate (vitamin C)*	81	112	97	116	139	567	83	100	86	118	128	528
Red cell folate	84	105	100	123	140	573	80	99	87	111	130	521
Serum folate	88	116	106	131	148	612	88	105	95	120	134	557
Serum vitamin B$_{12}$	87	114	106	133	146	609	88	105	94	120	136	558
Erythrocyte transketolase activation coefficient	78	111	96	118	138	561	83	101	87	120	128	534
EGRAC**	79	113	97	120	141	572	83	101	88	121	129	537
EAATAC***	79	113	97	120	141	572	83	101	88	121	129	537
Plasma zinc	58	92	68	97	118	447	62	74	72	99	103	421

† Includes those not answering income question.
* Includes 3 results (unwtd), for 2 males and 1 female, below the precision of the analytic methodology.
** Erythrocyte glutathione reductase activation coefficient.
*** Erythrocyte aspartate aminotransferase activation coefficient.

Table 12.36 Water soluble vitamins and plasma zinc by sex of young person and social class of head of household

Sex of young person and analytes	Units	Social class of head of household								All*			
		Non-manual				Manual							
		Mean	Median	Std Dev	Base	Mean	Median	Std Dev	Base	Mean	Median	Std Dev	Base
Males													
Plasma ascorbate (vitamin C)**	µmol/l	59.6	62.0	22.87	270	54.5	53.7	22.99	262	56.4	57.6	23.22	567
Red cell folate	nmol/l	655	617	212.7	271	613	585	204.6	263	626	594	209.5	573
Serum folate	nmol/l	23.0	23.6	7.54	286	21.0	21.1	7.64	286	21.7	21.8	7.64	612
Serum vitamin B$_{12}$	pmol/l	409	372	178.0	286	398	360	180.6	284	403	367	177.6	609
Erythrocyte transketolase activation coefficient	ratio	1.11	1.12	0.049	268	1.12	1.13	0.050	259	1.12	1.12	0.051	561
EGRAC***	ratio	1.39	1.36	0.151	274	1.43	1.40	0.176	264	1.42	1.39	0.169	572
EAATAC****	ratio	1.79	1.76	0.175	274	1.79	1.77	0.159	264	1.80	1.77	0.166	572
Plasma zinc	µmol/l	14.80	14.90	1.804	217	14.53	14.50	2.359	204	14.62	14.60	2.092	447
Females													
Plasma ascorbate (vitamin C)**	µmol/l	64.1	67.0	23.50	242	56.1	56.9	20.57	230	58.8	61.5	23.13	528
Red cell folate	nmol/l	588	551	199.7	242	565	524	214.3	226	573	540	203.9	521
Serum folate	nmol/l	21.6	20.9	8.04	252	20.1	19.3	8.13	246	20.6	19.7	8.16	557
Serum vitamin B$_{12}$	pmol/l	407	372	196.5	255	391	356	184.7	244	395	359	187.6	558
Erythrocyte transketolase activation coefficient	ratio	1.12	1.11	0.057	245	1.12	1.12	0.053	233	1.12	1.12	0.056	534
EGRAC***	ratio	1.45	1.42	0.161	246	1.49	1.46	0.177	235	1.47	1.45	0.169	537
EAATAC****	ratio	1.80	1.80	0.168	246	1.77	1.75	0.153	235	1.79	1.78	0.163	537
Plasma zinc	µmol/l	14.83	14.80	2.043	190	14.40	14.50	1.770	187	14.57	14.50	1.926	421

* Includes those for whom a social class could not be assigned.

** Includes 3 results (unwtd), for 2 males and 1 female, below the precision of the analytic methodology.

*** Erythrocyte glutathione reductase activation coefficient.

**** Erythrocyte aspartate aminotransferase activation coefficient.

Table 12.37 Percentage distribution of plasma retinol by sex and age of young person

Plasma retinol (μmol/l)	Males aged (years)					Females aged (years)				
	4–6	7–10	11–14	15–18	All males	4–6	7–10	11–14	15–18	All females
	cum %	cum %	cum %	cum %	cum %	cum %	cum %	cum %	cum %	cum %
Less than 0.35	–	–	–	–	–	–	–	–	–	–
Less than 0.70	2	2	–	–	1	3	2	-	0	1
Less than 1.00	35	18	16	4	17	24	22	10	9	16
Less than 1.20	67	54	43	18	44	57	59	46	23	46
Less than 1.50	91	90	81	54	79	94	87	80	52	78
Less than 2.00	99	98	99	88	96	100	97	98	88	96
All	100	100	100	100	100		100	100	100	100
Base	70	162	174	152	558	71	131	159	161	522
Mean	1.12	1.20	1.27	1.53	1.29	1.15	1.21	1.28	1.51	1.29
Median	1.08	1.16	1.26	1.49	1.24	1.14	1.14	1.24	1.46	1.24
Lower 2.5 percentile	0.65	0.79	0.79	0.93	0.80	0.70	0.85	0.86	0.89	0.84
Upper 2.5 percentile	1.66	1.87	1.90	2.48	2.18	1.60	2.00	1.96	2.38	2.08
Standard deviation	0.254	0.267	0.271	0.392	0.339	0.216	0.282	0.285	0.389	0.331

Table 12.38 Percentage distribution of plasma retinyl palmitate by sex and age of young person (fasting samples only)

Plasma retinyl palmitate (μmol/l)	Males aged (years)					Females aged (years)				
	4–6	7–10	11–14	15–18	All males	4–6	7–10	11–14	15–18	All females
	cum %	cum %	cum %	cum %	cum %	cum %	cum %	cum %	cum %	cum %
Less than 0.050	8	4	13	17	11	8	11	12	10	10
Less than 0.080	22	29	37	37	32	30	29	42	31	33
Less than 0.100	41	44	48	50	46	44	43	57	50	49
Less than 0.150	77	72	78	77	76	73	80	83	75	78
Less than 0.200	94	90	93	91	92	92	96	95	91	94
All	100	100	100	100	100	100	100	100	100	100
Base	60	147	164	144	515	62	114	155	144	475
Mean	0.119	0.122	0.110	0.112	0.115	0.122	0.110	0.102	0.114	0.111
Median	0.113	0.109	0.102	0.099	0.106	0.107	0.106	0.087	0.101	0.101
Lower 2.5 percentile	0.027	0.039	0.034	0.025	0.028	0.034	0.026	0.024	0.036	0.030
Upper 2.5 percentile	0.208	0.244	0.230	0.237	0.225	0.259	0.199	0.195	0.215	0.206
Standard deviation	0.0527	0.0617	0.0629	0.0723	0.0635	0.0657	0.0484	0.0656	0.0551	0.0593

Table 12.39 Percentage distribution of plasma α-carotene by sex and age of young person

Plasma α-carotene (μmol/l)	Males aged (years)					Females aged (years)				
	4–6	7–10	11–14	15–18	All males	4–6	7–10	11–14	15–18	All females
	cum %	cum %	cum %	cum %	cum %	cum %	cum %	cum %	cum %	cum %
Less than 0.010	2	4	2	7	4	3	3	2	3	3
Less than 0.020	15	10	22	28	19	12	11	15	20	15
Less than 0.040	52	43	61	64	55	38	37	54	52	45
Less than 0.060	73	68	83	85	77	60	65	78	80	71
Less than 0.080	88	82	91	94	89	77	87	93	89	87
Less than 0.100	94	90	95	96	94	90	96	96	95	94
All	100	100	100	100	100	100	100	100	100	100
Base	70	162	174	152	558	71	131	159	161	522
Mean	0.048	0.053	0.041	0.036	0.044	0.059	0.051	0.044	0.043	0.049
Median	0.038	0.044	0.032	0.031	0.037	0.051	0.048	0.037	0.038	0.042
Lower 2.5 percentile	0.010	0.007	0.010	0.008	0.008	0.009	0.006	0.011	0.009	0.009
Upper 2.5 percentile	0.132	0.157	0.137	0.106	0.136	0.204	0.110	0.109	0.115	0.131
Standard deviation	0.0336	0.0374	0.0323	0.0252	0.0331	0.0421	0.0293	0.0347	0.0308	0.0346

Table 12.40 Percentage distribution of plasma β-carotene by sex and age of young person

Plasma β-carotene (μmol/l)	Males aged (years)					Females aged (years)				
	4–6	7–10	11–14	15–18	All males	4–6	7–10	11–14	15–18	All females
	cum %	cum %	cum %	cum %	cum %	cum %	cum %	cum %	cum %	cum %
Less than 0.100	2	3	8	17	8	2	3	6	11	6
Less than 0.150	4	7	15	35	16	10	13	19	28	18
Less than 0.250	31	37	49	61	45	32	36	58	59	47
Less than 0.350	49	62	70	80	66	52	65	79	75	68
Less than 0.450	71	74	85	89	80	70	79	89	87	82
Less than 0.550	83	85	93	94	89	76	94	92	96	90
All	100	100	100	100	100	100	100	100	100	100
Base	70	162	174	152	558	71	131	159	161	522
Mean	0.372	0.355	0.297	0.249	0.316	0.418	0.321	0.272	0.257	0.312
Median	0.350	0.303	0.255	0.206	0.266	0.324	0.306	0.227	0.223	0.263
Lower 2.5 percentile	0.141	0.090	0.071	0.063	0.070	0.107	0.094	0.080	0.048	0.080
Upper 2.5 percentile	0.904	0.864	0.730	0.749	0.842	1.107	0.640	0.646	0.601	0.841
Standard deviation	0.1973	0.2082	0.2108	0.1781	0.2048	0.3131	0.1529	0.2370	0.1580	0.2265

Table 12.41 Percentage distribution of plasma α-cryptoxanthin by sex and age of young person

Plasma α-cryptoxanthin (μmol/l)	Males aged (years)					Females aged (years)				
	4–6	7–10	11–14	15–18	All males	4–6	7–10	11–14	15–18	All females
	cum %	cum %	cum %	cum %	cum %	cum %	cum %	cum %	cum %	cum %
Less than 0.020	2	1	3	6	3	1	1	2	3	2
Less than 0.040	20	18	32	41	28	18	27	34	37	30
Less than 0.060	58	52	60	70	60	45	66	65	70	63
Less than 0.080	81	74	75	87	79	71	86	83	86	82
Less than 1.000	87	85	88	94	88	89	94	93	93	93
All	100	100	100	100	100	100	100	100	100	100
Base	70	162	174	152	558	71	131	159	161	522
Mean	0.065	0.067	0.062	0.051	0.061	0.069	0.056	0.057	0.053	0.058
Median	0.054	0.058	0.052	0.045	0.053	0.061	0.052	0.048	0.045	0.052
Lower 2.5 percentile	0.021	0.021	0.018	0.017	0.019	0.021	0.022	0.020	0.019	0.021
Upper 2.5 percentile	0.225	0.170	0.144	0.114	0.154	0.145	0.116	0.149	0.149	0.145
Standard deviation	0.0391	0.0351	0.0431	0.0334	0.0382	0.0330	0.0307	0.0364	0.0288	0.0328

Table 12.42 Percentage distribution of plasma β-cryptoxanthin by sex and age of young person

Plasma β-cryptoxanthin (μmol/l)	Males aged (years)					Females aged (years)				
	4–6	7–10	11–14	15–18	All males	4–6	7–10	11–14	15–18	All females
	cum %	cum %	cum %	cum %	cum %	cum %	cum %	cum %	cum %	cum %
Less than 0.040	3	2	4	7	4	4	2	3	9	5
Less than 0.080	10	20	21	32	21	8	21	23	31	21
Less than 0.120	28	38	49	57	44	28	38	47	52	42
Less than 0.160	53	62	66	74	64	48	56	66	68	60
Less than 0.220	66	75	82	87	78	63	76	80	81	76
Less than 0.280	85	80	90	93	87	69	85	90	87	84
All	100	100	100	100	100	100	100	100	100	100
Base	70	162	174	152	558	71	131	159	161	522
Mean	0.190	0.186	0.159	0.128	0.165	0.238	0.175	0.158	0.156	0.179
Median	0.157	0.139	0.123	0.108	0.130	0.169	0.143	0.128	0.113	0.137
Lower 2.5 percentile	0.035	0.045	0.034	0.029	0.033	0.031	0.041	0.033	0.026	0.031
Upper 2.5 percentile	0.502	0.697	0.465	0.338	0.465	0.828	0.541	0.429	0.524	0.569
Standard deviation	0.1267	0.1764	0.1406	0.0867	0.1398	0.2009	0.1284	0.1201	0.1610	0.1558

Table 12.43 Percentage distribution of plasma lycopene by sex and age of young person

Plasma lycopene (μmol/l)	Males aged (years)					Females aged (years)				
	4–6	7–10	11–14	15–18	All males	4–6	7–10	11–14	15–18	All females
	cum %	cum %	cum %	cum %	cum %	cum %	cum %	cum %	cum %	cum %
Less than 0.125	3	4	3	4	3	7	3	2	–	3
Less than 0.250	16	15	18	11	15	18	12	15	9	13
Less than 0.375	37	36	35	38	36	33	38	41	35	37
Less than 0.500	56	50	58	62	57	47	55	66	60	57
Less than 0.625	69	72	77	74	73	68	79	82	74	76
Less than 0.750	87	83	89	86	86	84	88	91	86	87
All	100	100	100	100	100	100	100	100	100	100
Base	*70*	*162*	*174*	*152*	*558*	*71*	*131*	*159*	*161*	*522*
Mean	0.486	0.516	0.478	0.475	0.489	0.513	0.485	0.449	0.498	0.485
Median	0.455	0.500	0.456	0.447	0.457	0.521	0.460	0.409	0.445	0.447
Lower 2.5 percentile	0.100	0.083	0.114	0.112	0.100	0.107	0.115	0.151	0.180	0.115
Upper 2.5 percentile	0.868	1.187	1.114	0.913	1.023	1.102	1.054	0.940	1.057	1.054
Standard deviation	0.2196	0.2698	0.2321	0.2117	0.2362	0.2608	0.2229	0.2009	0.2292	0.2286

Table 12.44 Percentage distribution of plasma lutein + zeaxanthin by sex and age of young person

Plasma lutein + zeaxanthin (μmol/l)	Males aged (years)					Females aged (years)				
	4–6	7–10	11–14	15–18	All males	4–6	7–10	11–14	15–18	All females
	cum %	cum %	cum %	cum %	cum %	cum %	cum %	cum %	cum %	cum %
Less than 0.150	3	2	2	10	4	3	2	1	6	3
Less than 0.200	12	10	13	26	15	15	13	10	20	14
Less than 0.250	32	22	33	45	33	18	24	32	40	29
Less than 0.300	54	37	49	64	50	33	51	52	61	50
Less than 0.350	67	58	67	80	68	58	67	60	71	64
Less than 0.400	79	72	77	86	78	78	81	74	81	78
Less than 0.450	81	77	85	90	83	85	90	86	90	88
All	100	100	100	100	100	100	100	100	100	100
Base	*70*	*162*	*174*	*152*	*558*	*71*	*131*	*159*	*161*	*522*
Mean	0.329	0.359	0.325	0.282	0.324	0.347	0.321	0.330	0.297	0.323
Median	0.290	0.326	0.301	0.261	0.297	0.339	0.298	0.292	0.267	0.299
Lower 2.5 percentile	0.145	0.158	0.155	0.128	0.138	0.138	0.157	0.174	0.125	0.140
Upper 2.5 percentile	0.615	0.760	0.712	0.526	0.656	0.698	0.604	0.674	0.583	0.644
Standard deviation	0.1336	0.1447	0.1264	0.1156	0.1335	0.1347	0.1099	0.1311	0.1180	0.1243

Table 12.45 Percentage distribution of plasma 25-hydroxyvitamin D by sex and age of young person

Plasma 25-hydroxyvitamin D (nmol/l)	Males aged (years)					Females aged (years)				
	4–6	7–10	11–14	15–18	All males	4–6	7–10	11–14	15–18	All females
	cum %	cum %	cum %	cum %	cum %	cum %	cum %	cum %	cum %	cum %
Less than 12.0	–	–	3	–	1	–	–	2	2	1
Less than 25.0	3	4	11	16	8	2	7	11	10	8
Less than 30.0	3	6	12	25	12	3	8	14	20	12
Less than 40.0	8	8	26	43	22	11	15	30	37	24
Less than 50.0	23	26	40	54	36	25	26	44	49	36
Less than 60.0	34	41	54	65	49	42	45	56	65	52
Less than 70.0	53	53	71	80	65	55	62	77	76	68
Less than 80.0	71	68	84	87	78	70	72	87	84	79
Less than 100.0	85	87	96	93	91	91	89	96	96	93
All	100	100	100	100	100	100	100	100	100	100
Base = 100%	*73*	*167*	*177*	*153*	*570*	*76*	*133*	*164*	*162*	*535*
Mean	71.8	70.1	56.7	51.6	62.0	68.9	66.5	54.4	53.7	60.6
Median	67.6	67.9	55.1	46.1	60.7	63.9	63.2	52.6	50.8	58.1
Lower 2.5 percentile	24.1	19.8	11.8	14.2	15.3	26.2	18.2	13.5	16.9	15.8
Upper 2.5 percentile	140.9	145.7	103.5	122.5	127.7	139.6	129.0	105.4	125.0	127.1
Standard deviation	28.10	27.66	24.05	27.55	28.09	27.54	27.47	23.52	27.77	27.42

Table 12.46 Percentage distribution of plasma α-tocopherol by sex and age of young person

Plasma α-tocopherol (μmol/l)	Males aged (years)					Females aged (years)				
	4–6	7–10	11–14	15–18	All males	4–6	7–10	11–14	15–18	All females
	cum %	cum %	cum %	cum %	cum %	cum %	cum %	cum %	cum %	cum %
Less than 11.6	2	–	1	1	1	3	–	–	1	1
Less than 15.0	9	9	9	12	10	3	4	5	8	5
Less than 18.0	29	25	35	44	33	20	17	23	36	24
Less than 21.0	69	61	68	72	67	45	51	56	68	55
Less than 25.0	94	84	91	90	89	79	85	89	89	86
Less than 30.0	97	98	98	98	98	98	98	98	97	98
All	100	100	100	100	100	100	100	100	100	100
Base	*70*	*162*	*174*	*152*	*558*	*71*	*131*	*159*	*161*	*522*
Mean	19.6	20.5	19.7	19.2	19.8	21.2	21.2	20.5	19.8	20.6
Median	19.6	20.1	19.2	18.7	19.4	21.3	20.9	20.5	19.2	20.5
Lower 2.5 percentile	12.4	13.3	13.9	12.4	13.2	9.5	13.9	13.8	13.5	13.7
Upper 2.5 percentile	30.4	29.2	28.9	28.6	29.0	29.2	29.3	28.4	30.0	29.2
Standard deviation	3.77	4.20	4.02	3.97	4.04	4.26	3.88	3.48	3.97	3.92

Table 12.47 Percentage distribution of plasma γ-tocopherol by sex and age of young person

Plasma γ-tocopherol (μmol/l)	Males aged (years)					Females aged (years)				
	4–6	7–10	11–14	15–18	All males	4–6	7–10	11–14	15–18	All females
	cum %	cum %	cum %	cum %	cum %	cum %	cum %	cum %	cum %	cum %
Less than 0.75	12	4	4	6	6	4	3	4	15	7
Less than 1.00	28	15	16	24	20	18	12	12	34	19
Less than 1.50	70	53	57	66	61	44	54	53	67	55
Less than 2.00	91	80	79	85	83	78	87	81	86	83
Less than 2.50	96	95	91	92	93	97	95	92	97	95
All	100	100	100	100	100	100	100	100	100	100
Base	*70*	*162*	*174*	*152*	*558*	*71*	*131*	*159*	*161*	*522*
Mean	1.31	1.55	1.59	1.42	1.48	1.58	1.53	1.57	1.34	1.50
Median	1.27	1.42	1.40	1.29	1.33	1.52	1.47	1.42	1.21	1.42
Lower 2.5 percentile	0.59	0.64	0.69	0.64	0.61	0.69	0.69	0.70	0.56	0.63
Upper 2.5 percentile	2.66	2.91	3.50	2.73	2.95	2.58	2.90	3.30	2.88	2.93
Standard deviation	0.538	0.606	0.761	0.642	0.655	0.546	0.556	0.668	0.590	0.602

Table 12.48 Percentage distribution of tocopherol to cholesterol ratio* by sex and age of young person

Tocopherol to cholesterol ratio (μmol/mmol)	Males aged (years)					Females aged (years)				
	4–6	7–10	11–14	15–18	All males	4–6	7–10	11–14	15–18	All females
	cum %	cum %	cum %	cum %	cum %	cum %	cum %	cum %	cum %	cum %
Less than 2.25	–	–	–	–	–	–	–	–	–	–
Less than 4.25	17	8	9	4	9	18	9	8	16	12
Less than 5.25	62	59	45	50	53	49	50	54	55	52
Less than 6.25	85	89	84	83	85	87	82	85	87	85
Less than 7.25	96	95	97	95	96	97	95	93	95	95
All	100	100	100	100	100	100	100	100	100	100
Base	*55*	*135*	*163*	*143*	*496*	*49*	*108*	*145*	*155*	*457*
Mean	5.23	5.26	5.38	5.43	5.34	5.26	5.37	5.43	5.25	5.34
Median	5.07	5.13	5.41	5.25	5.21	5.30	5.24	5.14	5.09	5.20
Lower 2.5 percentile	3.76	3.44	3.64	4.05	3.76	3.86	3.78	3.94	3.58	3.78
Upper 2.5 percentile	7.89	7.48	7.43	8.02	7.64	7.70	7.49	8.70	7.96	7.75
Standard deviation	1.02	0.98	0.89	1.05	0.99	0.93	0.95	1.35	1.06	1.10

* α-tocopherol + γ-tocopherol to total cholesterol ratio.

Table 12.49 Correlation coefficients for plasma retinol (vitamin A) with dietary intakes of α-carotene, β-carotene and retinol (vitamin A)

Blood analyte: Plasma retinol (vitamin A)	Dietary intake of:			*Number of young people*
	α-carotene	β-carotene	retinol (vitamin A)	
Males aged (years):				
4–6	–0.02	–0.02	0.10	*67*
7–10	0.15	0.18*	0.17*	*155*
11–14	0.11	0.07	0.12	*158*
15–18	0.08	0.11	0.25**	*130*
All males	0.13**	0.17**	0.21**	*510*
Females aged (years)				
4–6	–0.20*	–0.23*	-0.14	*66*
7–10	0.07	0.15	0.10	*121*
11–14	0.08	0.13	0.07	*146*
15–18	0.12	0.15	0.10	*148*
All females	0.09*	0.15**	0.09*	*481*

*p < 0.05
**p < 0.01

Table 12.50 Correlation coefficients for plasma α-carotene with dietary intake of α-carotene

Blood analyte: Plasma α-carotene	Dietary intake of α-carotene	*Number of young people*
Males aged (years):		
4–6	0.51**	*67*
7–10	0.34**	*155*
11–14	0.49**	*158*
15–18	0.20*	*130*
All males	0.35**	*510*
Females aged (years)		
4–6	0.31**	*66*
7–10	0.46**	*121*
11–14	0.31**	*146*
15–18	0.17	*148*
All females	0.26**	*481*

*p < 0.05
**p < 0.01

Table 12.51 Correlation coefficients for plasma β-carotene with dietary intake of β-carotene

Blood analyte: Plasma β-carotene	Dietary intake of β-carotene	*Number of young people*
Males aged (years):		
4–6	0.17	*67*
7–10	0.08	*155*
11–14	0.19*	*158*
15–18	0.12	*130*
All males	0.09*	*510*
Females aged (years)		
4–6	0.18	*66*
7–10	0.26**	*121*
11–14	0.12	*146*
15–18	0.08	*148*
All females	0.09*	*481*

*p < 0.05
**p < 0.01

Table 12.52 Correlation coefficients for plasma 25-hydroxyvitamin D with dietary intake of vitamin D

Blood analyte: Plasma 25-hydroxy-vitamin D	Dietary intake of vitamin D	*Number of young people*
Males aged (years):		
4–6	–0.01	*70*
7–10	0.06	*159*
11–14	0.11	*161*
15–18	0.07	*130*
All males	0.01	*520*
Females aged (years)		
4–6	0.06	*71*
7–10	0.14	*123*
11–14	0.13	*151*
15–18	–0.03	*149*
All females	0.07	*494*

Table 12.53   Correlation coefficients for dietary intakes of vitamin E with plasma α-tocopherol, plasma total tocopherol and total tocopherol to cholesterol ratio#

Dietary intake of vitamin E	Blood analytes		Number of young people	Total tocopherol to cholesterol ratio#	Number of young people
	plasma α-tocopherol	plasma total tocopherol			
Males aged (years):					
4–6	0.13	0.12	67	0.18	53
7–10	0.01	0.00	155	0.03	129
11–14	−0.02	−0.04	158	0.11	147
15–18	0.09	0.07	130	0.07	122
All males	0.04	0.03	510	0.10*	451
Females aged (years)					
4–6	−0.02	−0.03	66	0.14	45
7–10	0.18*	0.17	121	0.14	99
11–14	−0.16	−0.19*	146	0.06	133
15–18	0.21*	0.18*	148	0.08	143
All females	0.08	0.06	481	0.08	420

the ratio of plasma α-tocopherol plus plasma γ-tocopherol to plasma total cholesterol.
*p < 0.05

Table 12.54 Fat soluble vitamins and carotenoids by sex of young person and whether unwell during dietary recording period

Sex of young person and analytes	Units	Whether unwell during period									All		
		Unwell and eating affected			Unwell and eating not affected			Not unwell					
		Mean	Median	Std Dev	Mean	Median	Std Dev	Mean	Median	Std Dev	Mean	Median	Std Dev
Males													
Plasma retinol (vitamin A)	µmol/l	1.351	1.292	0.3957	1.225	1.208	0.3281	1.291	1.237	0.3326	1.289	1.237	0.3389
Plasma α-tocopherol	µmol/l	20.4	20.2	4.41	20.4	20.5	3.92	19.6	19.3	4.00	19.8	19.4	4.04
Plasma γ-tocopherol	µmol/l	1.82	1.62	0.789	1.50	1.43	0.562	1.44	1.32	0.640	1.48	1.33	0.655
Plasma α-cryptoxanthin	µmol/l	0.059	0.051	0.0338	0.064	0.055	0.0418	0.061	0.052	0.0382	0.061	0.053	0.0382
Plasma β-cryptoxanthin	µmol/l	0.174	0.123	0.2347	0.178	0.123	0.1364	0.162	0.134	0.1265	0.165	0.130	0.1398
Plasma lycopene	µmol/l	0.480	0.440	0.2682	0.513	0.505	0.2133	0.487	0.456	0.2353	0.489	0.457	0.2362
Plasma lutein + zeaxanthin	µmol/l	0.327	0.297	0.1278	0.348	0.325	0.1446	0.321	0.296	0.1325	0.324	0.297	0.1335
Plasma α-carotene	µmol/l	0.040	0.034	0.0289	0.039	0.028	0.0302	0.046	0.037	0.0338	0.044	0.037	0.0331
Plasma β-carotene	µmol/l	0.307	0.244	0.1945	0.269	0.245	0.1510	0.323	0.267	0.2108	0.316	0.266	0.2048
Plasma 25-OHD	nmol/l	69.1	63.7	32.32	57.4	55.9	29.08	61.9	60.5	27.37	62.0	60.7	28.09
Females													
Plasma retinol (vitamin A)	µmol/l	1.332	1.250	0.4211	1.324	1.272	0.2907	1.282	1.225	0.3200	1.292	1.237	0.3307
Plasma α-tocopherol	µmol/l	20.3	19.1	4.22	20.8	21.0	3.08	20.7	20.5	3.98	20.6	20.5	3.92
Plasma γ-tocopherol	µmol/l	1.411	1.330	0.5300	1.588	1.640	0.5604	1.505	1.410	0.6152	1.503	1.420	0.6016
Plasma α-cryptoxanthin	µmol/l	0.048	0.047	0.0180	0.060	0.051	0.0311	0.059	0.053	0.0344	0.058	0.052	0.0328
Plasma β-cryptoxanthin	µmol/l	0.163	0.132	0.1440	0.146	0.129	0.0831	0.186	0.141	0.1641	0.179	0.137	0.1558
Plasma lycopene	µmol/l	0.453	0.423	0.1796	0.455	0.410	0.2144	0.493	0.456	0.2361	0.485	0.447	0.2286
Plasma lutein + zeaxanthin	µmol/l	0.303	0.289	0.1010	0.330	0.291	0.1322	0.324	0.302	0.1261	0.323	0.299	0.1243
Plasma α-carotene	µmol/l	0.041	0.034	0.0286	0.052	0.044	0.0315	0.050	0.043	0.0356	0.049	0.042	0.0346
Plasma β-carotene	µmol/l	0.268	0.220	0.1666	0.313	0.271	0.1631	0.319	0.272	0.2404	0.312	0.263	0.2265
Plasma 25-OHD	nmol/l	66.1	63.3	34.50	51.4	46.6	21.50	61.1	59.1	26.69	60.6	58.1	27.42

Table 12.54(cont) Fat soluble vitamins and carotenoids by sex of young person and whether unwell during dietary recording period: *base numbers*

Analytes	Sex of young person and whether unwell during period							
	Males			All males	Females			All females
	Unwell and eating affected	Unwell and eating not affected	Not unwell		Unwell and eating affected	Unwell and eating not affected	Not unwell	
Plasma retinol (vitamin A)	50	53	455	558	61	57	404	522
Plasma α-tocopherol	50	53	455	558	61	57	404	522
Plasma γ-tocopherol	50	53	455	558	61	57	404	522
Plasma α-cryptoxanthin	50	53	455	558	61	57	404	522
Plasma β-cryptoxanthin	50	53	455	558	61	57	404	522
Plasma lycopene	50	53	455	558	61	57	404	522
Plasma lutein + zeaxanthin	50	53	455	558	61	57	404	522
Plasma α-carotene	50	53	455	558	61	57	404	522
Plasma β-carotene	50	53	455	558	61	57	404	522
Plasma 25-OHD	51	56	463	570	62	61	412	535

Table 12.55 Fat soluble vitamins and carotenoids by sex of young person and region

Sex of young person and analytes	Units	Region													All		
		Scotland*			Northern			Central, South West & Wales			London & South East					
		Mean	Median	Std Dev	Mean	Median	Std Dev	Mean	Median	Std Dev	Mean	Median	Std Dev	Mean	Median	Std Dev
Males																
Plasma retinol (vitamin A)	μmol/l	1.195	1.176	0.2580	1.268	1.235	0.2846	1.321	1.237	0.3703	1.294	1.246	0.3572	1.289	1.237	0.3389
Plasma α-tocopherol	μmol/l	18.6	18.8	2.44	20.0	19.7	3.88	19.9	19.5	4.30	19.8	19.1	4.13	19.8	19.4	4.04
Plasma γ-tocopherol	μmol/l	1.36	1.31	0.446	1.46	1.32	0.637	1.54	1.36	0.744	1.45	1.32	0.601	1.48	1.33	0.655
Plasma α-cryptoxanthin	μmol/l	0.055	0.052	0.0230	0.057	0.052	0.0255	0.064	0.053	0.0433	0.064	0.053	0.0434	0.061	0.053	0.0382
Plasma β-cryptoxanthin	μmol/l	0.142	0.123	0.0863	0.156	0.120	0.1208	0.174	0.139	0.1699	0.168	0.132	0.1277	0.165	0.130	0.1398
Plasma lycopene	μmol/l	0.518	0.547	0.2454	0.457	0.426	0.2322	0.488	0.449	0.2454	0.511	0.480	0.2243	0.489	0.457	0.2362
Plasma lutein + zeaxanthin	μmol/l	0.315	0.299	0.1173	0.314	0.300	0.1145	0.315	0.289	0.1262	0.344	0.306	0.1557	0.324	0.297	0.1335
Plasma α-carotene	μmol/l	0.042	0.038	0.0269	0.044	0.037	0.0295	0.045	0.035	0.0330	0.046	0.034	0.0372	0.044	0.037	0.0331
Plasma β-carotene	μmol/l	0.304	0.263	0.1693	0.288	0.254	0.1659	0.316	0.255	0.2235	0.343	0.287	0.2177	0.316	0.266	0.2048
Plasma 25-OHD	nmol/l	63.0	58.8	24.57	58.5	58.7	23.28	64.2	62.1	29.14	62.6	61.1	31.06	62.0	60.7	28.09
Females																
Plasma retinol (vitamin A)	μmol/l	1.306	1.254	0.3567	1.258	1.175	0.3090	1.303	1.252	0.3481	1.308	1.250	0.3218	1.292	1.237	0.3307
Plasma α-tocopherol	μmol/l	19.9	19.4	4.08	20.6	20.3	4.34	20.6	20.3	3.72	20.8	20.9	3.71	20.6	20.5	3.92
Plasma γ-tocopherol	μmol/l	1.56	1.51	0.643	1.49	1.47	0.523	1.47	1.36	0.622	1.53	1.46	0.630	1.50	1.42	0.602
Plasma α-cryptoxanthin	μmol/l	0.060	0.047	0.0298	0.054	0.050	0.0334	0.056	0.050	0.0296	0.063	0.055	0.0354	0.058	0.052	0.0328
Plasma β-cryptoxanthin	μmol/l	0.206	0.130	0.1749	0.148	0.126	0.1333	0.185	0.134	0.1724	0.192	0.153	0.1466	0.179	0.137	0.1558
Plasma lycopene	μmol/l	0.538	0.512	0.2398	0.490	0.433	0.2340	0.474	0.445	0.2201	0.480	0.433	0.2290	0.485	0.447	0.2286
Plasma lutein + zeaxanthin	μmol/l	0.299	0.274	0.0970	0.302	0.285	0.1042	0.326	0.299	0.1425	0.342	0.325	0.1213	0.323	0.299	0.1243
Plasma α-carotene	μmol/l	0.045	0.045	0.0202	0.049	0.039	0.0389	0.049	0.043	0.0332	0.050	0.041	0.0347	0.049	0.042	0.0346
Plasma β-carotene	μmol/l	0.308	0.282	0.1727	0.306	0.255	0.2499	0.299	0.255	0.2391	0.332	0.281	0.2003	0.312	0.263	0.2265
Plasma 25-OHD	nmol/l	60.7	65.6	23.17	63.5	60.2	29.98	62.4	60.1	26.98	56.0	53.1	25.91	60.6	58.1	27.42

* For females in Scotland base numbers are less than 35 and the results should therefore be treated with caution.

Table 12.55(cont)   Fat soluble vitamins and carotenoids by sex of young person and region: *base numbers*

Analytes	Males				All males	Females				All females
	Scotland	Northern	Central, South West & Wales	London & South East		Scotland	Northern	Central, South West & Wales	London & South East	
Plasma retinol (vitamin A)	45	150	195	168	558	31	132	182	177	522
Plasma α-tocopherol	45	150	195	168	558	31	132	182	177	522
Plasma γ-tocopherol	45	150	195	168	558	31	132	182	177	522
Plasma α-cryptoxanthin	45	150	195	168	558	31	132	182	177	522
Plasma β-cryptoxanthin	45	150	195	168	558	31	132	182	177	522
Plasma lycopene	45	150	195	168	558	31	132	182	177	522
Plasma lutein + zeaxanthin	45	150	195	168	558	31	132	182	177	522
Plasma α-carotene	45	150	195	168	558	31	132	182	177	522
Plasma β-carotene	45	150	195	168	558	31	132	182	177	522
Plasma 25-OHD	45	154	201	170	570	32	134	191	178	535

Table 12.56 Fat soluble vitamins and carotenoids by sex of young person and whether 'parents' were receiving certain benefits

Sex of young person and analytes	Units	Whether 'parents' were receiving benefits								All			
		Receiving benefits				Not receiving benefits							
		Mean	Median	Std Dev	Base	Mean	Median	Std Dev	Base	Mean	Median	Std Dev	Base
Males													
Plasma retinol (vitamin A)	μmol/l	1.197	1.122	0.2952	121	1.318	1.261	0.3447	436	1.289	1.237	0.3389	558
Plasma α-tocopherol	μmol/l	19.1	19.0	3.62	121	20.0	19.4	4.14	436	19.8	19.4	4.04	558
Plasma γ-tocopherol	μmol/l	1.56	1.33	0.710	121	1.45	1.33	0.633	436	1.48	1.33	0.655	558
Plasma α-cryptoxanthin	μmol/l	0.051	0.048	0.0233	121	0.065	0.056	0.0414	436	0.061	0.053	0.0382	558
Plasma β-cryptoxanthin	μmol/l	0.136	0.114	0.0971	121	0.175	0.138	0.1504	436	0.165	0.13	0.1398	558
Plasma lycopene	μmol/l	0.484	0.486	0.2317	121	0.491	0.457	0.2379	436	0.489	0.457	0.2362	558
Plasma lutein + zeaxanthin	μmol/l	0.321	0.289	0.1372	121	0.325	0.301	0.1323	436	0.324	0.297	0.1335	558
Plasma α-carotene	μmol/l	0.037	0.032	0.0272	121	0.047	0.037	0.0346	436	0.044	0.037	0.0331	558
Plasma β-carotene	μmol/l	0.269	0.234	0.1555	121	0.332	0.283	0.2168	436	0.316	0.266	0.2048	558
Plasma 25-OHD	nmol/l	56.8	53.7	28.21	124	63.8	61.5	27.87	445	62.0	60.7	28.09	570
Females													
Plasma retinol (vitamin A)	μmol/l	1.240	1.157	0.3086	129	1.313	1.250	0.3369	393	1.292	1.237	0.3307	522
Plasma α-tocopherol	μmol/l	20.2	20.3	3.43	129	20.8	20.6	4.09	393	20.6	20.5	3.92	522
Plasma γ-tocopherol	μmol/l	1.60	1.52	0.588	129	1.46	1.36	0.603	393	1.50	1.42	0.602	522
Plasma α-cryptoxanthin	μmol/l	0.049	0.044	0.0230	129	0.062	0.055	0.0353	393	0.058	0.052	0.0328	522
Plasma β-cryptoxanthin	μmol/l	0.136	0.115	0.0816	129	0.196	0.145	0.1738	393	0.179	0.137	0.1558	522
Plasma lycopene	μmol/l	0.429	0.396	0.2090	129	0.506	0.475	0.2323	393	0.485	0.447	0.2286	522
Plasma lutein + zeaxanthin	μmol/l	0.315	0.299	0.1134	129	0.325	0.298	0.1282	393	0.323	0.299	0.1243	522
Plasma α-carotene	μmol/l	0.041	0.034	0.0262	129	0.052	0.044	0.0370	393	0.049	0.042	0.0346	522
Plasma β-carotene	μmol/l	0.245	0.217	0.1483	129	0.339	0.297	0.2457	393	0.312	0.26287	0.2265	522
Plasma 25-OHD	nmol/l	56.6	55.7	26.70	132	62.2	59.6	27.55	403	60.6	58.1	27.42	535

Table 12.57 Fat soluble vitamins and carotenoids by sex of young person and gross weekly household income

Sex of young person and analytes	Units	Gross weekly household income																	All		
		Less than £160			£160 to less than £280			£280 to less than £400			£400 to less than £600			£600 and over								
		Mean	Median	Std Dev	Mean	Median	Std Dev	Mean	Median	Std Dev	Mean	Median	Std Dev	Mean	Median	Std Dev	Mean	Median	Std Dev		
Males																					
Plasma retinol (vitamin A)	µmol/l	1.184	1.144	0.2581	1.230	1.190	0.3360	1.316	1.250	0.3463	1.326	1.290	0.3320	1.339	1.251	0.3611	1.289	1.237	0.3389		
Plasma α-tocopherol	µmol/l	19.4	19.4	3.84	20.4	19.9	4.04	19.5	19.2	4.55	19.2	18.6	3.56	20.4	20.1	4.10	19.8	19.4	4.04		
Plasma γ-tocopherol	µmol/l	1.63	1.47	0.788	1.52	1.36	0.625	1.45	1.29	0.596	1.42	1.31	0.566	1.44	1.31	0.690	1.48	1.33	0.655		
Plasma α-cryptoxanthin	µmol/l	0.051	0.048	0.0245	0.065	0.057	0.0446	0.062	0.055	0.0383	0.060	0.052	0.0311	0.068	0.056	0.0438	0.061	0.053	0.0382		
Plasma β-cryptoxanthin	µmol/l	0.149	0.119	0.1132	0.188	0.139	0.1906	0.152	0.129	0.1026	0.175	0.138	0.1392	0.160	0.123	0.1233	0.165	0.130	0.1398		
Plasma lycopene	µmol/l	0.486	0.475	0.2548	0.495	0.488	0.2035	0.495	0.447	0.2467	0.471	0.452	0.2369	0.510	0.472	0.2444	0.489	0.457	0.2362		
Plasma lutein + zeaxanthin	µmol/l	0.322	0.305	0.1190	0.354	0.297	0.1641	0.317	0.297	0.1162	0.311	0.301	0.1213	0.324	0.305	0.1295	0.324	0.297	0.1335		
Plasma α-carotene	µmol/l	0.039	0.035	0.0301	0.044	0.038	0.0316	0.046	0.035	0.0338	0.045	0.036	0.0323	0.049	0.037	0.0373	0.044	0.037	0.0331		
Plasma β-carotene	µmol/l	0.270	0.243	0.1577	0.335	0.269	0.2361	0.330	0.263	0.2003	0.331	0.267	0.2367	0.322	0.285	0.1778	0.316	0.266	0.2048		
Plasma 25-OHD	nmol/l	58.1	50.9	30.57	58.5	55.6	27.89	65.0	63.4	24.91	64.6	61.9	29.15	66.4	63.7	27.31	62.0	60.7	28.09		
Females																					
Plasma retinol (vitamin A)	µmol/l	1.215	1.152	0.2882	1.260	1.231	0.3068	1.290	1.247	0.3283	1.310	1.225	0.3278	1.369	1.324	0.3622	1.292	1.237	0.3307		
Plasma α-tocopherol	µmol/l	20.6	20.7	3.87	20.0	19.5	4.03	20.7	20.4	4.10	20.8	20.7	3.88	21.1	20.6	3.51	20.6	20.5	3.92		
Plasma γ-tocopherol	µmol/l	1.61	1.52	0.642	1.56	1.52	0.631	1.38	1.32	0.559	1.45	1.38	0.518	1.49	1.39	0.520	1.50	1.42	0.602		
Plasma α-cryptoxanthin	µmol/l	0.050	0.046	0.0252	0.052	0.047	0.0260	0.060	0.054	0.0374	0.061	0.055	0.0284	0.067	0.061	0.0406	0.058	0.052	0.0328		
Plasma β-cryptoxanthin	µmol/l	0.136	0.127	0.0741	0.156	0.122	0.1150	0.167	0.129	0.1376	0.200	0.141	0.2077	0.222	0.163	0.1703	0.179	0.137	0.1558		
Plasma lycopene	µmol/l	0.436	0.403	0.2131	0.470	0.400	0.2554	0.488	0.472	0.2224	0.502	0.481	0.2178	0.516	0.475	0.2164	0.485	0.447	0.2286		
Plasma lutein + zeaxanthin	µmol/l	0.334	0.329	0.1354	0.301	0.297	0.1024	0.302	0.287	0.1014	0.333	0.292	0.1451	0.339	0.317	0.1238	0.323	0.299	0.1243		
Plasma α-carotene	µmol/l	0.044	0.036	0.0281	0.043	0.040	0.0322	0.053	0.043	0.0412	0.048	0.041	0.0277	0.058	0.050	0.0403	0.049	0.042	0.0346		
Plasma β-carotene	µmol/l	0.259	0.202	0.1749	0.300	0.231	0.3269	0.308	0.256	0.1913	0.311	0.301	0.1459	0.369	0.327	0.2238	0.312	0.263	0.2265		
Plasma 25-OHD	nmol/l	51.7	51.2	25.54	60.9	57.9	26.64	67.4	66.0	29.39	59.8	55.1	27.96	65.3	62.7	24.79	60.6	58.1	27.42		

* Includes those not answering income question.

Table 12.57(cont) Fat soluble vitamins and carotenoids by sex of young person and gross weekly household income: *base numbers*

Analytes	Males						Females					
	Less than £160	£160 to less than £280	£280 to less than £400	£400 to less than £600	£600 and over	All males*	Less than £160	£160 to less than £280	£280 to less than £400	£400 to less than £600	£600 and over	All females*
Plasma retinol (vitamin A)	78	111	91	117	139	558	81	98	87	115	126	522
Plasma α-tocopherol	78	111	91	117	139	558	81	98	87	115	126	522
Plasma γ-tocopherol	78	111	91	117	139	558	81	98	87	115	126	522
Plasma α-cryptoxanthin	78	111	91	117	139	558	81	98	87	115	126	522
Plasma β-cryptoxanthin	78	111	91	117	139	558	81	98	87	115	126	522
Plasma lycopene	78	111	91	117	139	558	81	98	87	115	126	522
Plasma lutein + zeaxanthin	78	111	91	117	139	558	81	98	87	115	126	522
Plasma α-carotene	78	111	91	117	139	558	81	98	87	115	126	522
Plasma β-carotene	78	111	91	117	139	558	81	98	87	115	126	522
Plasma 25-OHD	80	112	96	119	141	570	83	100	87	121	129	535

* Includes those not answering income question.

Table 12.58 Fat soluble vitamins and carotenoids by sex of young person and social class of head of household

Sex of young person and analytes	Units	Social class of head of household								All*			
		Non-manual				Manual							
		Mean	Median	Std Dev	Base	Mean	Median	Std Dev	Base	Mean	Median	Std Dev	Base
Males													
Plasma retinol (vitamin A)	µmol/l	1.302	1.238	0.3342	264	1.283	1.236	0.3489	260	1.289	1.237	0.3389	558
Plasma α-tocopherol	µmol/l	19.8	19.3	4.01	264	19.9	19.4	4.11	260	19.8	19.4	4.04	558
Plasma γ-tocopherol	µmol/l	1.43	1.33	0.563	264	1.50	1.33	0.724	260	1.48	1.33	0.655	558
Plasma α-cryptoxanthin	µmol/l	0.065	0.055	0.0397	264	0.060	0.052	0.0382	260	0.061	0.053	0.0382	558
Plasma β-cryptoxanthin	µmol/l	0.170	0.141	0.1229	264	0.165	0.122	0.1600	260	0.165	0.130	0.1198	558
Plasma lycopene	µmol/l	0.475	0.441	0.2396	264	0.501	0.480	0.2339	260	0.489	0.457	0.2362	558
Plasma lutein + zeaxanthin	µmol/l	0.322	0.303	0.1249	264	0.325	0.293	0.1389	260	0.324	0.297	0.1335	558
Plasma α-carotene	µmol/l	0.047	0.035	0.0355	264	0.043	0.037	0.0312	260	0.044	0.037	0.0331	558
Plasma β-carotene	µmol/l	0.331	0.285	0.2097	264	0.311	0.255	0.2068	260	0.316	0.266	0.2048	558
Plasma 25-OHD	nmol/l	64.6	61.9	27.61	272	61.9	60.4	27.76	264	62.0	60.7	28.09	570
Females													
Plasma retinol (vitamin A)	µmol/l	1.311	1.229	0.3469	236	1.277	1.240	0.3174	230	1.292	1.237	0.3307	522
Plasma α-tocopherol	µmol/l	21.0	20.9	3.84	236	20.2	19.7	4.08	230	20.6	20.5	3.92	522
Plasma γ-tocopherol	µmol/l	1.51	1.38	0.629	236	1.47	1.44	0.556	230	1.50	1.42	0.602	522
Plasma α-cryptoxanthin	µmol/l	0.064	0.057	0.0390	236	0.055	0.052	0.0260	230	0.058	0.052	0.0328	522
Plasma β-cryptoxanthin	µmol/l	0.201	0.146	0.1728	236	0.171	0.133	0.1519	230	0.179	0.137	0.1558	522
Plasma lycopene	µmol/l	0.498	0.472	0.2122	236	0.467	0.408	0.2442	230	0.485	0.447	0.2286	522
Plasma lutein + zeaxanthin	µmol/l	0.333	0.305	0.1290	236	0.309	0.292	0.1174	230	0.323	0.299	0.1243	522
Plasma α-carotene	µmol/l	0.053	0.045	0.0349	236	0.048	0.041	0.0367	230	0.049	0.042	0.0346	522
Plasma β-carotene	µmol/l	0.340	0.314	0.1932	236	0.296	0.237	0.2666	230	0.312	0.263	0.2265	522
Plasma 25-OHD	nmol/l	62.1	58.2	26.24	246	61.9	60.2	28.12	233	60.6	58.1	27.42	535

* Includes those for whom a social class could not be assigned.

Table 12.59 Percentage distribution of plasma total cholesterol by sex and age of young person

Plasma total cholesterol (mmol/l)	Males aged (years)					Females aged (years)				
	4–6	7–10	11–14	15–18	All males	4–6	7–10	11–14	15–18	All females
	cum %	cum %	cum %	cum %	cum %	cum %	cum %	cum %	cum %	cum %
Less than 3.00	4	3	8	8	6	5	5	4	5	5
Less than 3.50	15	16	29	35	24	14	17	18	20	17
Less than 4.00	55	38	54	60	52	26	40	41	46	39
Less than 4.50	87	67	74	88	79	52	63	69	70	64
Less than 5.20	97	87	91	96	92	78	89	93	94	89
Less than 5.80	98	95	98	99	97	92	96	98	98	96
All	100	100	100	100	100	100	100	100	100	100
Base	*55*	*136*	*164*	*143*	*498*	*51*	*109*	*145*	*155*	*460*
Mean	3.99	4.27	4.01	3.84	4.03	4.48	4.30	4.14	4.08	4.24
Median	3.91	4.17	3.90	3.85	3.96	4.41	4.24	4.16	4.05	4.18
Lower 2.5 percentile	2.98	2.95	2.49	2.77	2.77	1.69	2.88	2.89	2.62	2.62
Upper 2.5 percentile	5.61	6.03	5.67	5.33	5.82	6.30	6.32	5.73	5.65	6.03
Standard deviation	0.642	0.768	0.876	0.662	0.765	0.991	0.978	0.715	0.753	0.875

Table 12.60 Percentage distribution of plasma high density lipoprotein cholesterol by sex and age of young person

Plasma high density lipoprotein cholesterol (mmol/l)	Males aged (years)					Females aged (years)				
	4–6	7–10	11–14	15–18	All males	4–6	7–10	11–14	15–18	All females
	cum %	cum %	cum %	cum %	cum %	cum %	cum %	cum %	cum %	cum %
Less than 1.00	10	9	21	40	20	17	17	17	25	19
Less than 1.20	35	30	39	66	43	54	41	43	52	47
Less than 1.40	72	56	63	90	70	71	60	67	69	67
Less than 1.60	88	79	80	96	86	91	81	84	83	84
All	100	100	100	100	100	100	100	100	100	100
Base	*55*	*136*	*164*	*143*	*498*	*51*	*109*	*145*	*155*	*460*
Mean	1.29	1.37	1.31	1.09	1.26	1.23	1.31	1.29	1.24	1.27
Median	1.31	1.33	1.32	1.08	1.25	1.15	1.27	1.26	1.18	1.24
Lower 2.5 percentile	0.68	0.90	0.71	0.53	0.70	0.67	0.75	0.71	0.75	0.74
Upper 2.5 percentile	1.90	1.88	2.10	1.63	1.92	1.74	2.04	1.97	1.88	2.00
Standard deviation	0.272	0.298	0.362	0.280	0.325	0.262	0.342	0.334	0.329	0.323

Table 12.61 Percentage distribution of plasma low density lipoprotein cholesterol by sex and age of young person*

Plasma low density lipoprotein cholesterol* (mmol/l)	Males aged (years)					Females aged (years)				
	4–6	7–10	11–14	15–18	All males	4–6	7–10	11–14	15–18	All females
	cum %	cum %	cum %	cum %	cum %	cum %	cum %	cum %	cum %	cum %
Less than 2.00	9	10	19	10	12	9	10	7	13	10
Less than 2.70	59	42	52	51	51	32	44	47	42	42
Less than 3.40	87	75	82	85	82	58	68	74	79	70
Less than 4.10	98	92	97	95	95	77	92	97	96	91
All	100	100	100	100	100	100	100	100	100	100
Base	*55*	*136*	*164*	*143*	*498*	*51*	*109*	*145*	*155*	*460*
Mean	2.70	2.90	2.70	2.76	2.77	3.25	2.99	2.85	2.84	2.97
Median	2.57	2.82	2.61	2.69	2.69	3.14	2.84	2.78	2.83	2.87
Lower 2.5 percentile	1.65	1.70	1.57	1.79	1.65	0.59	1.60	1.39	1.55	1.45
Upper 2.5 percentile	3.88	4.55	4.20	4.42	4.45	4.98	4.82	4.16	4.34	4.77
Standard deviation	0.624	0.767	0.765	0.677	0.720	0.993	0.973	0.695	0.757	0.872

* Calculated as non-high density lipoprotein cholesterol (non-HDL).

Table 12.62 Percentage distribution of plasma triglycerides by sex and age of young person (fasting samples only)

Plasma triglycerides (mmol/l)	Males aged (years)					Females aged (years)				
	4–6	7–10	11–14	15–18	All males	4–6	7–10	11–14	15–18	All females
	cum %	cum %	cum %	cum %	cum %	cum %	cum %	cum %	cum %	cum %
Less than 0.50	26	11	11	3	12	4	8	2	2	4
Less than 0.75	79	56	41	25	48	48	35	30	24	33
Less than 1.00	92	84	71	48	72	86	66	64	61	68
Less than 1.50	98	97	93	87	93	100	93	89	91	92
Less than 2.00	100	99	98	95	98		98	97	96	97
All		100	100	100	100		100	100	100	100
Base	*45*	*121*	*155*	*135*	*456*	*43*	*94*	*142*	*138*	*417*
Mean	0.65	0.78	0.89	1.13	0.88	0.79	0.92	0.97	1.02	0.93
Median	0.61	0.70	0.82	1.02	0.78	0.77	0.82	0.88	0.92	0.84
Lower 2.5 percentile	0.31	0.36	0.40	0.44	0.40	0.20	0.41	0.48	0.49	0.44
Upper 2.5 percentile	1.33	1.50	1.88	3.13	1.88	1.24	1.75	2.02	2.15	2.02
Standard deviation	0.238	0.319	0.450	0.704	0.506	0.208	0.353	0.368	0.424	0.364

Table 12.63 Correlation coefficients for blood lipids with dietary intakes: total cholesterol, high density lipoprotein cholesterol, and low density lipoprotein cholesterol# with dietary intakes of total fat, fatty acids and cholesterol

Blood analytes and sex and age of young person	Dietary intake of:							Number of young people
	Total fat	Saturated fatty acids	Trans fatty acids	Cis mono-unsaturated fatty acids	Cis n-3 poly-unsaturated fatty acids	Cis n-6 poly-unsaturated fatty acids	Cholesterol	
Total cholesterol								
Males aged (years)								
4–6	-0.08	-0.09	-0.07	-0.06	-0.17	-0.01	0.16	53
7–10	0.07	0.09	-0.03	0.10	-0.04	-0.02	0.06	130
11–14	0.03	0.03	0.01	0.07	0.01	-0.06	0.00	148
15–18	0.00	-0.03	-0.04	0.01	-0.05	0.04	0.09	122
All males	-0.03	-0.03	-0.05	-0.01	-0.06	-0.06	0.02	453
Females aged (years)								
4–6	-0.13	-0.04	-0.02	-0.22*	-0.16	-0.05	-0.16	47
7–10	0.13	0.15	0.14	0.14	0.04	-0.02	0.10	100
11–14	-0.01	0.11	0.01	-0.02	-0.30**	-0.23*	0.03	133
15–18	0.15	0.14	0.06	0.15	0.04	0.14	0.18	143
All females	0.03	0.10*	0.05	0.01	-0.12*	-0.07	0.04	423
High density lipoprotein cholesterol								
Males aged (years)								
4–6	-0.06	-0.10	-0.24*	-0.06	-0.09	0.15	-0.08	53
7–10	-0.05	-0.04	-0.03	-0.02	0.00	-0.12	-0.06	130
11–14	0.00	0.01	-0.07	0.03	0.06	-0.05	-0.15	148
15–18	0.07	-0.06	-0.15	-0.08	-0.08	0.04	-0.05	122
All males	-0.14**	-0.13**	-0.17**	-0.13**	-0.08	-0.13**	-0.17**	453
Females aged (years)								
4–6	-0.03	-0.11	0.15	-0.02	0.15	0.05	0.01	47
7–10	0.11	0.19*	0.01	0.07	0.06	-0.04	-0.05	100
11–14	0.14	0.20*	0.13	0.14	-0.10	-0.05	0.01	133
15–18	0.21*	0.22*	0.17	0.20*	0.10	0.10	0.13	143
All females	0.15**	0.18**	0.12*	0.14**	0.04	0.02	0.04	423
Low density lipoprotein cholesterol#								
Males aged (years)								
4–6	-0.05	-0.05	0.03	-0.03	-0.13	-0.08	0.20*	53
7–10	0.09	0.10	-0.02	0.11	-0.04	0.02	0.08	130
11–14	0.03	0.03	0.04	0.07	-0.01	-0.05	0.07	148
15–18	0.02	-0.01	0.02	0.04	-0.02	0.03	0.11	122
All males	0.03	0.03	0.02	0.05	-0.03	-0.01	0.10*	453
Females aged (years)								
4–6	-0.12	-0.01	-0.06	-0.21	-0.20	-0.06	-0.16	47
7–10	0.09	0.09	0.15	0.12	0.02	-0.01	0.12	100
11–14	-0.08	0.02	-0.06	-0.09	-0.26**	-0.21*	0.02	133
15–18	0.06	0.05	-0.01	0.07	0.00	0.09	0.12	143
All females	-0.02	0.03	-0.01	-0.04	-0.14**	-0.08	0.03	423

\# calculated as non-high density lipoprotein cholesterol.
* p < 0.05
** p < 0.01

Table 12.64 Correlation coefficients for blood lipids with dietary intakes: total cholesterol and high density lipoprotein cholesterol with percentage of food energy derived from dietary intakes of total fat and fatty acids

Blood analytes and sex and age of young person	Percentage of food energy derived from dietary intake of:						Number of young people
	Total fat	Saturated fatty acids	Trans fatty acids	Cis mono-unsaturated fatty acids	Cis n-3 poly-unsaturated fatty acids	Cis n-6 poly-unsaturated fatty acids	
Total cholesterol							
Males aged (years)							
4–6	−0.04	−0.06	−0.06	0.00	−0.16	0.05	53
7–10	0.18*	0.16	−0.03	0.21*	−0.03	0.00	130
11–14	0.20*	0.17	0.09	0.24*	0.04	−0.02	148
15–18	0.18	0.12	0.02	0.14	−0.02	0.12	122
All males	0.13**	0.11*	0.03	0.14*	−0.04	0.01	453
Females aged (years)							
4–6	−0.08	0.03	0.03	−0.20	−0.13	0.02	47
7–10	−0.01	0.08	0.08	0.02	−0.06	−0.14	100
11–14	0.06	0.22	0.06	0.04	−0.27**	−0.20	133
15–18	0.05	0.07	−0.05	0.03	−0.10	0.01	143
All females	0.01	0.13**	0.04	−0.03	−0.16**	−0.11	423
High density lipoprotein cholesterol							
Males aged (years)							
4–6	−0.09	−0.14	−0.31**	−0.07	−0.10	0.22*	53
7–10	0.01	0.03	0.03	0.03	0.02	−0.12	130
11–14	0.02	0.01	−0.06	0.06	0.07	−0.06	148
15–18	−0.01	0.03	−0.13	−0.04	−0.08	0.04	122
All males	−0.03	0.00	−0.08	−0.03	−0.02	−0.04	453
Females aged (years)							
4–6	−0.15	−0.32**	0.15	−0.08	0.18	0.04	47
7–10	−0.02	0.12	−0.10	−0.07	−0.04	−0.11	100
11–14	0.22*	0.30**	0.17	0.18	−0.09	−0.07	133
15–18	0.06	0.12	0.05	0.04	−0.07	−0.06	143
All females	0.06	0.11*	0.06	0.04	−0.03	−0.06	423

* $p < 0.05$
** $p < 0.01$

Table 12.65 Variation in mean total plasma cholesterol and plasma HDL cholesterol by sex of young person and socio-demographic characteristics

Sex of young person and characteristic	Plasma total cholesterol			Plasma HDL cholesterol			No of young people
	Mean	Median	Std dev	Mean	Median	Std dev	
Males							
Whether unwell during dietary recording period							
unwell &							
eating affected	4.26	4.23	1.036	1.22	1.15	0.360	45
eating not affected	4.13	4.09	0.773	1.20	1.20	0.345	47
not unwell	4.00	3.94	0.727	1.27	1.26	0.319	406
Region							
Scotland	3.82	3.82	0.564	1.25	1.11	0.343	44
Northern	3.97	3.91	0.700	1.23	1.23	0.295	129
Central, South West and Wales	4.13	3.98	0.821	1.32	1.32	0.330	169
London & South East	4.04	4.05	0.781	1.24	1.22	0.334	156
Whether 'parents' receiving benefits							
receiving	3.95	3.91	0.697	1.28	1.30	0.263	102
not receiving	4.06	3.98	0.782	1.26	1.22	0.342	396
Gross weekly household income							
less than £160	3.92	3.93	0.633	1.28	1.30	0.216	65
£160 < £280	4.19	4.00	0.760	1.27	1.31	0.302	102
£280 < £400	3.94	3.82	0.839	1.26	1.23	0.339	81
£400 < £600	3.99	3.85	0.756	1.29	1.24	0.610	107
£600 & over	4.06	4.01	0.788	1.23	1.12	0.353	127
Social class of head of household							
Non-manual	3.99	3.90	0.805	1.28	1.23	0.331	239
Manual	4.11	4.00	0.718	1.25	1.26	0.327	230
All males	4.03	3.96	0.765	1.26	1.25	0.325	498
Females							
Whether unwell during dietary recording period							
unwell &							
eating affected	4.16	4.00	1.107	1.14	1.10	0.322	57
eating not affected	4.21	4.17	0.749	1.24	1.22	0.278	48
not unwell	4.25	4.19	0.849	1.30	1.27	0.323	355
Region							
Scotland*	4.37	4.28	0.862	1.26	1.15	0.321	29
Northern	4.26	4.24	1.107	1.27	1.19	0.295	111
Central, South West and Wales	4.22	4.17	0.781	1.24	1.24	0.308	160
London & South East	4.21	4.18	0.751	1.30	1.27	0.356	460
Whether 'parents' receiving benefits							
receiving	4.16	4.17	0.721	1.29	1.27	0.335	113
not receiving	4.27	4.18	0.926	1.26	1.21	0.318	347
Gross weekly household income							
less than £160	4.21	4.18	0.645	1.32	1.29	0.367	68
£160 < £280	4.10	4.18	0.987	1.26	1.24	0.256	83
£280 < £400	4.30	4.39	1.061	1.22	1.17	0.284	80
£400 < £600	4.33	4.18	0.845	1.25	1.18	0.347	105
£600 & over	4.29	4.18	0.748	1.32	1.32	0.344	113
Social class of head of household							
Non-manual	4.25	4.18	0.765	1.27	1.19	0.342	205
Manual	4.20	4.17	1.021	1.25	1.24	0.295	207
All females	4.24	4.18	0.875	1.27	1.24	0.323	460

* For females in Scotland base numbers are less than 35 and the results should therefore be treated with caution.

Table 12.66 Percentage distribution of blood lead by sex and age of young person

Blood lead (µg/dl)	Males aged (years)					Females aged (years)				
	4–6	7–10	11–14	15–18	All males	4–6	7–10	11–14	15–18	All females
	cum %	cum %	cum %	cum %	cum %	cum %	cum %	cum %	cum %	cum %
Less than 2.0	31	31	29	40	33	33	33	42	57	41
Less than 3.0	61	66	63	76	67	62	67	79	83	73
Less than 4.0	77	85	80	88	83	81	86	89	97	88
Less than 5.0	86	91	91	94	91	89	92	96	99	94
Less than 6.0	87	95	98	99	95	96	97	97	100	98
Less than 10.0	98	99	99	100	99	100	100	100		100
All	100	100	100		100					
Base	*78*	*178*	*176*	*165*	*597*	*78*	*136*	*166*	*166*	*546*
Mean	3.3	2.8	2.8	2.4	2.8	2.9	2.7	2.4	2.0	2.5
Median	2.5	2.4	2.5	2.2	2.3	2.6	2.4	2.2	1.8	2.2
Lower 2.5 percentile	0.9	0.9	0.9	0.8	0.9	1.2	0.9	0.8	0.8	0.8
Upper 2.5 percentile	9.2	6.1	5.8	5.5	8.0	6.6	6.0	6.0	4.1	5.8
Standard deviation	2.26	1.61	1.42	1.26	1.66	1.38	1.47	1.24	0.97	1.32

Table 12.67 Percentage distribution of plasma magnesium by sex and age of young person

Plasma magnesium (mmol/l)	Males aged (years)					Females aged (years)				
	4–6	7–10	11–14	15–18	All males	4–6	7–10	11–14	15–18	All females
	cum %	cum %	cum %	cum %	cum %	cum %	cum %	cum %	cum %	cum %
Less than 0.70	–	–	–	–	–	1	1	–	–	0
Less than 0.80	4	3	4	4	4	2	6	10	8	7
Less than 0.85	17	16	13	18	16	13	18	22	25	20
Less than 0.90	35	38	37	38	37	40	47	49	46	46
Less than 0.95	58	62	63	61	61	54	65	72	70	66
Less than 1.00	74	76	76	80	77	71	84	86	83	82
All	100	100	100	100	100	100	100	100	100	100
Base	*79*	*176*	*176*	*159*	*590*	*77*	*134*	*165*	*166*	*542*
Mean	0.94	0.94	0.94	0.93	0.94	0.94	0.91	0.90	0.91	0.91
Median	0.93	0.92	0.91	0.93	0.92	0.93	0.91	0.90	0.90	0.90
Lower 2.5 percentile	0.76	0.79	0.78	0.79	0.79	0.80	0.74	0.76	0.77	0.76
Upper 2.5 percentile	1.19	1.17	1.20	1.16	1.17	1.17	1.07	1.14	1.10	1.11
Standard deviation	0.101	0.096	0.120	0.093	0.103	0.099	0.093	0.086	0.084	0.091

Table 12.68 Percentage distribution of plasma selenium by sex and age of young person

Plasma selenium (µmol/l)	Males aged (years)					Females aged (years)				
	4–6	7–10	11–14	15–18	All males	4–6	7–10	11–14	15–18	All females
	cum %	cum %	cum %	cum %	cum %	cum %	cum %	cum %	cum %	cum %
Less than 0.50	–	–	–	–	–	2	–	–	–	0
Less than 0.60	5	4	3	1	3	5	2	2	1	2
Less than 0.70	17	10	13	7	12	23	10	17	4	13
Less than 0.80	47	32	37	25	34	48	26	36	21	32
Less than 0.90	72	57	71	51	62	76	54	66	48	60
Less than 1.00	88	80	88	79	84	91	76	84	71	80
All	100	100	100	100	100	100	100	100	100	100
Base	*79*	*176*	*176*	*160*	*591*	*76*	*133*	*166*	*165*	*540*
Mean	0.82	0.87	0.84	0.89	0.86	0.81	0.90	0.85	0.91	0.87
Median	0.80	0.86	0.84	0.89	0.85	0.81	0.88	0.83	0.90	0.86
Lower 2.5 percentile	0.58	0.59	0.59	0.64	0.59	0.57	0.64	0.61	0.65	0.60
Upper 2.5 percentile	1.13	1.18	1.12	1.16	1.17	1.05	1.41	1.17	1.21	1.24
Standard deviation	0.152	0.153	0.146	0.137	0.149	0.146	0.175	0.152	0.142	0.160

Table 12.69   Percentage distribution of erythrocyte glutathione peroxidase by sex and age of young person*

Erythrocyte glutathione peroxidase (nmol/mg Hb/min)	Males aged (years)					Females aged (years)				
	4–6	7–10	11–14	15–18	All males	4–6	7–10	11–14	15–18	All females
	cum %	cum %	cum %	cum %	cum %	cum %	cum %	cum %	cum %	cum %
Less than 50	–	1	–	1	1	–	–	–	–	–
Less than 60	–	1	–	1	1	2	–	–	–	–
Less than 70	5	12	6	7	8	6	5	5	4	5
Less than 80	29	34	34	25	31	28	22	16	27	23
Less than 90	48	58	53	52	54	53	58	39	45	48
All	100	100	100	100	100	100	100	100	100	100
Base	*42*	*106*	*102*	*87*	*337*	*47*	*83*	*93*	*99*	*322*
Mean	91.0	88.3	88.8	92.8	90.0	90.1	90.7	98.1	93.0	93.5
Median	90.0	86.0	88.5	89.0	88.0	85.0	88.0	97.0	91.0	90.0
Lower 2.5 percentile	69.0	62.0	64.0	61.8	63.9	61.3	66.0	64.0	68.0	66.0
Upper 2.5 percentile	167.5	134.0	123.0	162.4	129.6	148.9	148.1	147.0	141.0	142.9
Standard deviation	18.58	17.12	14.70	24.03	18.71	18.78	18.02	20.25	18.66	19.17

* Unweighted data; see text *Section 12.1.2*

Table 12.70   Percentage distribution of red cell superoxide dismutase by sex and age of young person

Red cell superoxide dismutase (nmol/mg Hb/min)	Males aged (years)					Females aged (years)				
	4–6	7–10	11–14	15–18	All males	4–6	7–10	11–14	15–18	All females
	cum %	cum %	cum %	cum %	cum %	cum %	cum %	cum %	cum %	cum %
Less than 800	2	2	10	7	5	-	4	4	4	3
Less than 1000	8	9	25	38	21	14	19	25	29	22
Less than 1100	26	27	38	58	38	27	37	43	55	41
Less than 1200	53	49	60	78	60	60	66	66	72	66
Less than 1300	77	70	78	88	78	73	80	79	85	80
Less than 1500	94	90	94	95	93	92	94	92	96	94
Less than 1602	95	97	96	95	96	94	96	94	97	95
All	100	100	100	100	100	100	100	100	100	100
Base	*72*	*168*	*178*	*154*	*572*	*76*	*133*	*164*	*163*	*536*
Mean	1211	1224	1149	1096	1168	1208	1163	1166	1142	1168
Median	1195	1214	1161	1060	1159	1183	1139	1131	1081	1131
Lower 2.5 percentile	824	755	614	677	689	897	746	684	770	774
Upper 2.5 percentile	1821	1623	1765	1770	1702	1625	1681	1876	2413	1774
Standard deviation	211.9	199.4	268.5	277.9	248.7	215.0	218.3	297.5	325.7	270.7

Table 12.71 Percentage distribution of plasma urea by sex and age of young person*

Plasma urea (mmol/l)	Males aged (years)					Females aged (years)				
	4–6**	7–10	11–14	15–18	All males	4–6**	7–10	11–14	15–18	All females
	cum f	cum %	cum %	cum %	cum %	cum f	cum %	cum %	cum %	cum %
Less than 3.0	[1]	2	1	4	2	[-]	3	6	11	7
Less than 3.5	[2]	5	11	6	8	[2]	11	28	28	23
Less than 4.0	[3]	17	30	23	23	[6]	24	41	47	39
Less than 4.5	[8]	39	52	46	46	[11]	43	66	69	61
Less than 5.5	[12]	66	83	85	78	[18]	79	96	86	88
Less than 15.0	[16]	100	100	100	100	[20]	100	100	100	100
All										
Base	*16*	*87*	*108*	*79*	*290*	*20*	*67*	*116*	*118*	*321*
Mean	4.7	5.0	4.6	4.5	4.7	4.4	4.7	4.1	4.1	4.2
Median	4.6	4.9	4.4	4.5	4.5	4.3	4.6	4.1	4.0	4.1
Lower 2.5 percentile	2.8	3.0	3.0	2.6	2.9	3.0	2.8	2.7	2.0	2.5
Upper 2.5 percentile	6.3	7.7	7.1	6.4	7.1	6.9	6.8	5.5	6.3	6.7
Standard deviation	1.03	1.21	1.07	0.88	1.08	0.91	1.13	0.88	1.09	1.04

* Unweighted data; see text *Section 12.1.2.*
** As the sample size for this age group is small, < 35, estimates should be treated with caution.
[ ] indicates number, not percentage

Table 12.72 Percentage distribution of plasma creatinine by sex and age of young person*

Plasma creatinine (μmol/l)	Males aged (years)					Females aged (years)				
	4–6**	7–10	11–14	15–18	All males	4–6**	7–10	11–14	15–18	All females
	cum f	cum %	cum %	cum %	cum %	cum f	cum %	cum %	cum %	cum %
Less than 40	[5]	20	5	7	12	[9]	12	10	1	10
Less than 50	[10]	52	28	14	34	[19]	47	31	13	32
Less than 60	[13]	96	74	29	70		91	73	42	67
Less than 70	100	100	96	51	86		97	96	74	88
Less than 80			100	86	96		98	99	96	98
All				100	100		100	100	100	100
Base	*13*	*81*	*100*	*70*	*264*	*19*	*64*	*108*	*112*	*303*
Mean	43	47	55	66	55	39	50	53	62	55
Median	42	50	55	69	54	40	51	55	61	55
Lower 2.5 percentile	32	12	36	15	23	27	35	33	42	34
Upper 2.5 percentile	58	62	72	92	85	48	72	71	83	78
Standard deviation	8.2	10.6	9.2	16.8	14.3	6.4	9.4	10.5	10.7	11.8

* Unweighted data; see text *Section 12.1.2.*
** As the sample size for this age group is small, < 35, estimates should be treated with caution.
[ ] indicates number, not percentage.

Table 12.73 Percentage distribution of plasma α₁-antichymotrypsin by sex and age of young person

Plasma α₁-antichymotrypsin (g/l)	Males aged (years)					Females aged (years)				
	4–6	7–10	11–14	15–18	All males	4–6	7–10	11–14	15–18	All females
	cum %	cum %	cum %	cum %	cum %	cum %	cum %	cum %	cum %	cum %
Less than 0.22	–	4	10	12	7	–	10	9	6	7
Less than 0.25	11	21	32	32	25	5	15	25	19	17
Less than 0.30	44	62	71	74	63	33	58	66	61	56
Less than 0.35	75	89	92	94	88	58	85	90	91	83
Less than 0.66	100	100	100	100	100	100	98	100	100	99
All							100			100
Base	*54*	*134*	*156*	*140*	*484*	*44*	*107*	*143*	*151*	*445*
Mean	0.31	0.29	0.27	0.27	0.28	0.35	0.30	0.28	0.28	0.30
Median	0.31	0.28	0.26	0.26	0.28	0.34	0.29	0.27	0.27	0.29
Lower 2.5 percentile	0.23	0.20	0.18	0.20	0.20	0.23	0.18	0.17	0.19	0.18
Upper 2.5 percentile	0.42	0.42	0.44	0.39	0.42	0.63	0.51	0.40	0.39	0.48
Standard deviation	0.057	0.051	0.055	0.056	0.056	0.086	0.088	0.058	0.047	0.075

Table 12.74 Correlation coefficients for serum ferritin with plasma α₁-antichymotrypsin

Serum ferritin	α₁-anti-chymotrypsin	*Number of young people*
Males aged (years):		
4–6	0.29*	*45*
7–10	0.17	*109*
11–14	0.27**	*134*
15–18	0.23*	*113*
All males	0.16**	*401*
Females aged (years)		
4–6	0.59**	*38*
7–10	0.36**	*74*
11–14	0.06	*112*
15–18	0.11	*123*
All females	0.26**	*347*

*p < 0.05
**p < 0.01

Table 12.75 Percentage distribution of total plasma alkaline phosphatase activity by sex and age of young person*

Total plasma alkaline phosphatase activity (IU/l)	Males aged (years)					Females aged (years)				
	4–6**	7–10	11–14	15–18	All males	4–6**	7–10	11–14	15–18	All females
	cum f	cum %	cum %	cum %	cum %	cum f	cum %	cum %	cum %	cum %
Less than 100	[1]	–	1	24	7	[-]	–	5	81	32
Less than 150	[1]	2	5	60	19	[-]	3	26	97	46
Less than 200	[8]	19	14	83	36	[5]	13	44	98	56
Less than 250	[13]	49	34	91	56	[15]	48	57	99	72
Less than 300	[14]	75	59	94	74	[20]	72	73	99	84
All	[17]	100	100	100	100	[21]	100	100	100	100
Base	*17*	*88*	*111*	*80*	*296*	*21*	*67*	*117*	*118*	*323*
Mean	221	258	292	149	239	225	270	232	86	186
Median	203	251	277	132	230	210	252	225	81	170
Lower 2.5 percentile	100	149	126	70	83	184	145	83	43	52
Upper 2.5 percentile	470	394	471	356	449	341	402	435	156	402
Standard deviation	84.3	64.8	92.1	66.6	96.8	37.4	71.8	99.7	33.7	105.4

* Unweighted data; see text *Section 12.1.2.*
** As the sample size for this age group is small, <35, estimates should be treated with caution.
[ ] indicates number, not percentage.

Table 12.76 Variation in mean blood lead by sex of young person and socio-demographic characteristics

Sex of young person and characteristic	Blood lead (μ/dl)			No of young people
	Mean	Median	Std dev	
Males				
Whether unwell during dietary recording period				
unwell &				
eating affected	3.1	2.5	2.34	52
eating not affected	2.9	2.5	1.40	61
not unwell	2.7	2.3	1.60	484
Region				
Scotland	2.6	2.2	1.62	46
Northern	2.9	2.5	1.73	157
Central, South West and Wales	2.8	2.4	1.66	221
London & South East	2.7	2.2	1.61	173
Whether 'parents' receiving benefits				
receiving	3.3	2.7	2.07	129
not receiving	2.6	2.3	1.48	467
Gross weekly household income				
less than £160	3.2	2.9	1.88	84
£160 < £280	3.1	2.6	1.84	115
£280 < £400	2.6	2.3	1.31	103
£400 < £600	2.7	2.3	1.80	128
£600 & over	2.5	2.2	1.34	145
Social class of head of household				
Non-manual	2.5	2.2	1.30	284
Manual	3.1	2.7	1.81	274
All males	2.8	2.3	1.66	597
Females				
Whether unwell during dietary recording period				
unwell &				
eating affected	2.7	2.5	1.41	66
eating not affected	2.6	2.3	1.49	61
not unwell	2.4	2.2	1.27	419
Region				
Scotland*	2.4	1.7	1.94	32
Northern	2.4	2.2	1.12	135
Central, South West and Wales	2.5	2.3	1.32	196
London & South East	2.5	2.3	1.30	183
Whether 'parents' receiving benefits				
receiving	2.5	2.1	1.31	136
not receiving	2.5	2.3	1.32	410
Gross weekly household income				
less than £160	2.5	2.1	1.28	85
£160 < £280	2.4	2.2	1.22	100
£280 < £400	2.8	2.4	1.62	91
£400 < £600	2.3	2.2	1.16	122
£600 & over	2.5	2.4	1.24	133
Social class of head of household				
Non-manual	2.4	2.2	1.15	251
Manual	2.6	2.3	1.47	237
All females	2.5	2.2	1.32	546

* For females in Scotland the base number is less than 35 and the results should therefore be treated with caution.

Table 12.77 Variation in mean plasma selenium and plasma magnesium by sex of young person and socio-demographic characteristics

Sex of young person and characteristic	Plasma selenium (µmol/l)			No of young people	Plasma magnesium (mmol/l)			No of young people
	Mean	Median	Std dev		Mean	Median	Std dev	
Males								
Whether unwell during dietary recording period								
unwell &								
eating affected	0.88	0.85	0.179	52	0.96	0.94	0.091	52
eating not affected	0.86	0.84	0.153	63	0.95	0.94	0.115	63
not unwell	0.86	0.85	0.145	476	0.93	0.92	0.103	475
Region								
Scotland	0.79	0.75	0.123	46	0.92	0.90	0.143	46
Northern	0.88	0.86	0.149	155	0.95	0.94	0.103	154
Central, South West and Wales	0.84	0.83	0.142	217	0.93	0.92	0.103	217
London & South East	0.88	0.86	0.155	173	0.94	0.92	0.091	173
Whether 'parents' receiving benefits								
receiving	0.84	0.82	0.178	127	0.94	0.92	0.113	128
not receiving	0.86	0.85	0.138	463	0.94	0.92	0.100	461
Gross weekly household income								
less than £160	0.85	0.82	0.183	83	0.93	0.92	0.095	85
£160 < £280	0.85	0.85	0.154	114	0.95	0.93	0.125	113
£280 < £400	0.82	0.81	0.139	101	0.92	0.91	0.084	100
£400 < £600	0.85	0.83	0.131	126	0.94	0.93	0.097	125
£600 & over	0.89	0.90	0.129	145	0.94	0.93	0.093	145
Social class of head of household								
Non-manual	0.87	0.86	0.140	279	0.94	0.92	0.098	279
Manual	0.84	0.83	0.143	275	0.94	0.92	0.101	273
All males	0.86	0.85	0.149	591	0.94	0.92	0.103	590
Females								
Whether unwell during dietary recording period								
unwell &								
eating affected	0.87	0.86	0.177	65	0.92	0.90	0.100	65
eating not affected	0.88	0.89	0.170	61	0.94	0.93	0.091	61
not unwell	0.87	0.86	0.156	414	0.91	0.90	0.090	415
Region								
Scotland*	0.85	0.87	0.151	32	0.91	0.91	0.113	32
Northern	0.88	0.86	0.139	132	0.91	0.90	0.087	133
Central, South West and Wales	0.84	0.83	0.149	193	0.92	0.91	0.090	194
London & South East	0.91	0.89	0.181	183	0.92	0.91	0.090	183
Whether 'parents' receiving benefits					542			
receiving	0.85	0.82	0.188	131	0.91	0.91	0.082	133
not receiving	0.88	0.86	0.147	409	0.92	0.90	0.095	409
Gross weekly household income								
less than £160	0.88	0.86	0.223	82	0.92	0.93	0.076	83
£160 < £280	0.81	0.80	0.135	98	0.90	0.89	0.089	99
£280 < £400	0.87	0.86	0.149	90	0.91	0.89	0.096	90
£400 < £600	0.87	0.85	0.131	123	0.94	0.92	0.104	123
£600 & over	0.92	0.91	0.134	132	0.91	0.90	0.083	132
Social class of head of household								
Non-manual	0.88	0.87	0.141	247	0.92	0.91	0.095	248
Manual	0.86	0.84	0.160	236	0.90	0.89	0.088	236
All females	0.87	0.86	0.160	540	0.91	0.90	0.091	542

* For females in Scotland base numbers are less than 35 and the results should therefore be treated with caution.

Table 12.78 Mean plasma testosterone concentration by age

Boys aged 10 to 16 years

Age last birthday (years)	Plasma testosterone concentration (nmol/l)			Base
	Mean	Median	sd	
10	2.2	0.9	4.52	*41*
11	4.5	1.2	7.57	*51*
12	9.9	5.5	10.00	*36*
13	15.8	17.0	9.69	*38*
14	20.8	20.6	8.82	*39*
15	25.5	26.4	8.34	*38*
16	*	*	*	*17**
All cases**	13.4	11.4	11.89	*260*

* This age group included 17 boys (unweighted); summary statistics are therefore unreliable
**Includes those aged 16 years.

Table 12.79 Plasma testosterone concentration – tertiles by age*

Boys aged 10 to 16 years

Age last birthday (years)	Plasma testosterone concentration – tertiles		
	Bottom	Middle	Top
	%	%	%
10	41	6	1
11	44	11	3
12	10	23	8
13	2	25	16
14	2	17	25
15	–	11	32
16	–	6	14
Base	86	87	87

*The data for plasma testosterone concentration for all boys aged 10 to 16 years were pooled and non-age-specific tertiles were calculated.

Table 12.80 Blood analyte levels for boys by plasma testosterone concentration adjusted for age#

Boys aged 10 to 16 years

Blood analyte	Units	Estimated marginal means by plasma testosterone concentration tertiles##			p value – between tertile gps	p value – linear trend	Base
		Bottom	Middle	Top			
Haemoglobin	g/dl	13.5	13.5	13.9	0.026*	0.0004**	*258*
Plasma iron % saturation	%	25.1	20.0	24.5	0.0002**	0.55	*256*
Plasma iron	μmol/l	14.8	12.3	14.8	0.0009**	0.449	*260*
Serum ferritin	μg/l	45.4	32.9	35.1	0.048*	0.06	*217*
Red blood cell count	$\times 10^{12}$/l	4.86	4.85	4.96	0.10	0.01*	*258*
Plasma vitamin C	μmol/l	52.9	52.9	60.8	0.056	0.104	*258*
Plasma 25-hydroxyvitamin D	nmol/l	61.5	58.0	57.7	0.72	0.66	*260*
Plasma total cholesterol	mmol/l	4.20	4.01	3.91	0.25	0.03*	*247*
Plasma high density lipoprotein cholesterol	mmol/l	1.382	1.264	1.195	0.043*	0.016*	*247*
Blood lead	μg/dl	3.10	2.66	2.38	0.059	0.007**	*257*
Plasma α_1-antichymotrypsin	g/dl	0.29	0.28	0.26	0.061	0.011*	*238*
Plasma alkaline phosphatase	IU/l	223	295	289	0.002**	0.177	*158*

\# Unweighted data; see text *Section 12.1.2.*
\#\# Tertiles were calculated for boys at each individual year of age. The data for all boys aged 10 to 16 years were then pooled to allow the calculation of means.
* p < 0.05.
** p < 0.01.

Fig 12.1   Comparison of mean plasma 25-OHD levels by date blood sample taken by sex of young person

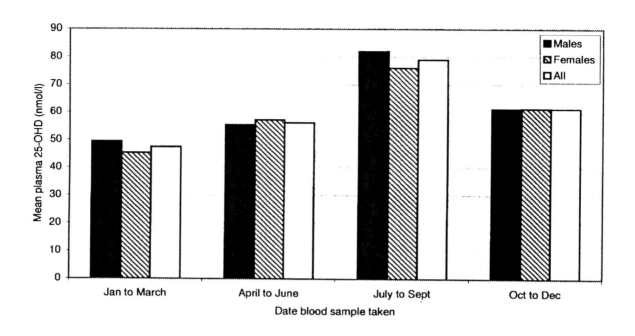

Fig 12.2   Variation in levels of plasma 25-OHD by date blood sample taken – males

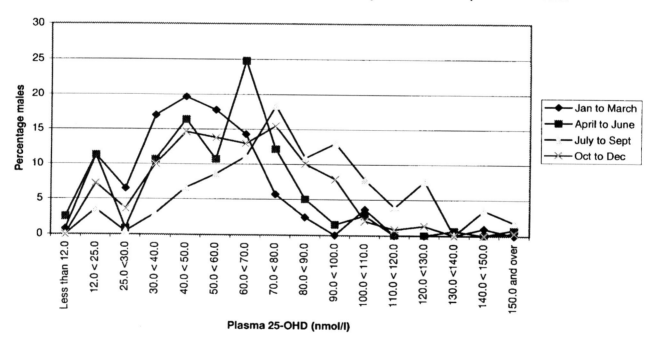

Fig 12.3   Variation in levels of plasma 25-OHD by date blood sample taken – females

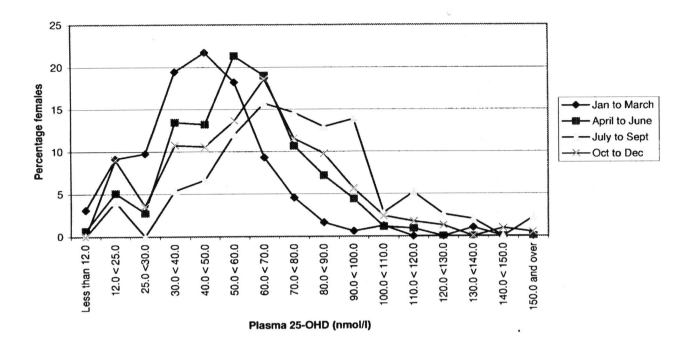

13 Physical activity

13.1 Introduction

Chapter 2 describes the purpose and methodologies for the collection of data on young people's physical activity. This was assessed for young people aged 4 to 6 years using questions asked during the initial dietary interview (see *Appendix K*). For young people aged 7 to 18 years detailed information on their daily activities was collected over the same 7-day period as the dietary record in the 'Diary of Activities and Eating and Drinking Away From Home' (see *Appendix A*). Further information, including the protocol for recording physical activity, is given in Appendix K.

Data are presented on various measures derived from the physical activity data collected for young people aged 7 to 18 years, including a calculated activity score, the total number of activities of at least moderate intensity in which the young person participated during the 7-day recording period and the mean hours spent in all activities of at least moderate intensity per day.

Descriptive statistics are presented for boys and girls separately by age group. Both bivariate and multivariate analyses are presented showing the relationship between the level of physical activity and various sociodemographic, dietary, physiological and behavioural factors.

Comparable data on participation in physical activity from the Health Survey for England[1] are presented for young people aged 7 to 15 years living in England.

13.2 Physical activity for young people in the United Kingdom

Overweight and fatness are increasing among primary school children in Great Britain[2]. Research suggests that these trends may partly be the result of increasingly sedentary lifestyles[3]. One explanation for the possible decrease in the physical activity levels of young people is that children are increasingly travelling to school by car or bus rather than walking or cycling. Data on energy intake and body mass index (BMI) suggest that adolescents in the UK have reduced their energy expenditure in recent years[4]. While young people tend to suffer from very low levels of morbidity and even lower mortality rates, health-compromising behaviours begun in childhood are likely to persist into adulthood leading to an increased risk of chronic disease later in life[5].

The Health Education Authority (HEA) gives the following definitions for physical activity[6].

Physical activity
any bodily movement produced by skeletal muscles that results in energy expenditure.

Exercise
planned, structured and repetitive bodily movement done to improve or maintain one or more components of physical fitness.

Moderate intensity physical activity
activity usually equivalent to brisk walking, which might be expected to leave the participant feeling warm and slightly out of breath.

Vigorous intensity physical activity
activity usually equivalent to at least slow jogging, which might be expected to leave the participant feeling out of breath and sweaty.

Total energy expenditure includes physical activity, resting metabolism, the thermic effect of food and, for children, growth. Ideally energy intakes should approximate requirements. When they are in excess of requirements the surplus will be stored in the body, leading to weight gain.

Data on energy intake given in Chapter 5 show that mean energy intakes were below Estimated Average Requirements (EARs) for each age and sex group (see *Section 5.2*). This disparity may be ascribed to inadequate energy intake, the consistent underestimation of energy intake using the NDNS survey methodology, or an overestimate of energy requirements. The aim of the physical activity component of the survey was to provide an estimate of energy expenditure by young people aged 4 to 18 years, in order to make comparisons with energy intake and measures of body size (BMI, mid upper-arm circumference and waist to hip ratio).

For adults, there are a wealth of data on the health benefits of physical activity and strong international consensus on the amount and type of physical activity that is beneficial to health. However, neither the minimal nor the optimal levels of physical activity for young people have been established. It has been suggested that, in the absence of separate criteria, activity levels known to confer health benefits in adults are also appropriate for children[7].

The levels of activity recommended by the Health Education Authority are based on evidence for current levels of physical activity for young people and are set at a level designed not to discourage young people from attempting to attain them.

Health Education Authority physical activity recommendations for young people

Primary recommendations

All young people should participate in physical activity of at least moderate intensity for *one hour per day*.

Young people who currently do little activity should participate in physical activity of at least moderate intensity for *at least half an hour per day*.

Secondary recommendation

At least twice a week, some of these activities should help to enhance and maintain muscular strength and flexibility and bone health.

Existing evidence suggests that most young people spend 30 minutes or more in activity of at least moderate intensity on most days of the week[7], that boys are more active than girls and that the activity of both declines with age[8]. The decline tends to be steeper in girls than boys and in adolescence compared with earlier stages of childhood[9].

13.3 Outline of methodology

There is no universally accepted 'gold standard' methodology for the assessment of physical activity analogous to the 7-day weighed intake methodology for dietary assessment or the doubly-labelled water method for the assessment of total energy expenditure. Various assessment methods have been validated for use with adults but none for use with children or adolescents.[9]

Studies that rely on self-report methods of data collection tend to conclude that young people engage in relatively high levels of activity, with 60% to 70% of children taking sufficient 'appropriate' physical activity. Studies that apply cardiovascular fitness criteria report much lower levels of activity[7]. However, such studies require observational or cardiovascular data, the collection of which were beyond the scope of this survey. A self-report method was chosen in order to aid compliance, and not to add to the demands of a survey package that was already onerous for participants.

In the design of the methodology for this survey, it was important to take account of the fact that young children's activity can be difficult to quantify, tending to occur in short, intense bursts interspersed with varying intervals of low and moderate intensity activity[10], while older children and teenagers are more likely to engage in structured exercise or sport. The reliability of calculated energy expended in physical activity is reduced when there is frequent change in activity. Data on physical activity was therefore collected using different methods for young children aged 4 to 6 years and for young people aged 7 to 18 years.

Information about the level of physical activity for young people aged 4 to 6 years was assessed using a set of three questions in the initial dietary interview (for more detailed information and the question text see *Appendix K*).

The feasibility study and subsequent qualitative testing prior to the mainstage survey showed that the 7-day diary method was appropriate for the collection of data on physical activity for young people aged 7 to 18 years[11]. In order to collect complete data on physical activity, information on three dimensions of physical activity was required, on duration, intensity and frequency. For young people aged 7 to 18 years, data were collected on each dimension of activity and a calculated activity score derived which can be used as an indicator of energy expended in physical activity.

Activities can be classified by their 'energy cost' measured in metabolic equivalents (METs[12]) into the following intensity levels:

Sleep	=	average 1.0 MET
Very light activity	=	average 1.5 METs (e.g. sitting watching television)
Light activity	=	average 2.5 METs (e.g. table tennis, light household chores)
Moderate activity	=	average 4.0 METs (e.g. badminton, swimming)
Vigorous activity	=	average 6.0 METs (e.g. basketball, disco dancing)
Very vigorous activity	=	average 10.0 METs (e.g. athletics)

The times when the young person went to bed and got up were collected for all young people for each diary day in order to allow the hours of sleep to be calculated[13]. Information was also collected on time spent in very light intensity activities, for example watching TV, playing computer games and listening to music.

In order to collect data on activities of moderate, vigorous and very vigorous intensity, the diary page provided a list of common activities against which the young person could record any time spent that day. Activities on the list included two categories for 'active play', which were designed to collect data for less formal activity. A section was provided for the young person to record activities that were not already listed, with prompts to establish the intensity level involved.

Young people aged 4 to 18 years were asked about their usual method of transport to and from school or work as part of the initial dietary interview. For those who walked or cycled, data were collected on the duration of the journey. If the young person was working part- or full time, the level of physical activity involved and the hours worked per day were collected.

For young people aged 7 to 18 years for whom physical activity data was available, a physical activity score was calculated using data on intensity and duration of activity following the procedure proposed by Blair (1984) for the 7-Day Recall Physical Activity Questionnaire[14]. The advantage of the calculated activity score method is that since light activity is obtained by subtraction from 24 hours, most individuals have to account only for time spent asleep and for relatively brief periods of time engaged in very light, moderate, vigorous and very vigorous activities. The assumption underlying the calculation of the activity score is that most young people spend most of their waking hours in light activity.

For the purposes of the calculated activity score, it was assumed that attending school each day would account for 5½ hours of very light activity. This allowed for that fact that most of the school day would be spent in sedentary activity, while lunch and other break times would be more active.

The score is derived by multiplying the duration of each activity (hours) by the average MET score for the intensity of the activity. For adults, this score is an estimate of energy expenditure while for young people the score can be used only as an indicator of energy expended in physical activity rather than as a direct measure. For further information on the calculation and interpretation of the activity score see Appendix K.

For adults, calculated activity scores of 40 or above indicate a relatively active lifestyle, scores in the mid to high 30s indicate an inactive lifestyle and those in the low 30s indicate a very inactive lifestyle. Previous studies of the physical activity levels of young people have interpreted the calculated activity score as follows [15,16].

40 or over	=	active
37 to < 40	=	moderately active
33 to < 37	=	inactive
< 33	=	very inactive

The categories represent energy expenditures of less than 33 kcal/kg/day (very inactive), between 33 and 36.9 kcal/kg/day (inactive), between 37 and 39.9 kcal/kg/day (moderately active) and 40 kcal/kg/day or more (active). Data from previous studies of physical activity for boys and girls aged 11 to 14 years for which a similar calculated activity score was derived showed that 5% of girls and 24% of boys were active, 16% of girls and 26% of boys were moderately active, 63% of girls and 46% of boys were inactive and 15% of girls and 4% of boys were very inactive[15,16]. However, these studies collected information on light activity and derived time spent in very light activity by subtraction from 24 hours, while conversely this present survey collected time spent in very light activity and derived time spent in light activity by subtraction from 24 hours.

13.4 Findings

The physical activity questions in the initial dietary interview were answered for 188 boys and 176 girls (unweighted) aged 4 to 6 years. Complete 7-day physical activity diaries were obtained from 711 boys and 713 girls (unweighted) aged 7 to 18 years. Overall, data on level of physical activity were available for 87% of boys and 90% of girls in the responding sample.

Tables 13.1 to 13.4 and 13.6 to 13.12 give descriptive statistics for the physical activity data. Figures 13.1(a) and 13.1(b) show the proportion of boys and girls participating in selected activities during the record-keeping period.

Tables 13.5 and 13.13 to 13.26 show the relationships between the measures of physical activity and key socio-demographic, physiological and behavioural characteristics.

13.4.1 Whether the young person was at school or work

Overall, 13% of boys and 15% of girls aged 4 to 18 years were not attending at school or work on any day during the record-keeping period. Of those aged 11 to 14 years, 5% of boys and 4% of girls were working as well as attending school. More than half of both girls and boys aged 15 to 18 years were working during the record-keeping period, including 32% of boys and 25% of girls who were working and attending school. (Table 13.1)

13.4.2 Travel to and from school or work

Table 13.2 shows the usual method of transport to and from school or work for young people aged 4 to 18 years[17]. The method of transport for the journey to and from school or work was recorded separately, but in almost all cases it was the same (table not shown) and the journey to school or work is given in the tables to represent both journeys.

Around half of young people in the two youngest age groups reported walking to school, while just under half travelled by car and between 5% and 7% by bus. By the age of 15 to 18 years, around one third of young people walked to school, another third travelled by bus, and around one quarter travelled by car.

The proportion of young people who walked to work or school decreased significantly with age, for example from 53% for boys aged 4 to 6 years to 39% for boys aged 15 to 18 years (p < 0.05). The proportion of boys cycling to school or work increased with age from 1% for boys aged 7 to 10 years to 6% for boys aged 15 to 18 years (p < 0.05), while overall, a significantly smaller proportion of girls cycled to school or work (p < 0.05) and all were aged 11 to 14 years. For both boys and girls, the proportion travelling by bus increased significantly with age while the proportion travelling by car decreased with age (all: p < 0.01).

Young people who walked or cycled to school or work were asked to estimate the duration of their journey. Table 13.3 gives the mean duration of walk to school or work (the numbers who cycled were too small to allow the calculation of means). There was no difference between boys and girls in mean duration of walk to school or work. The duration of walk to school or work generally increased with age for both boys and girls, with significant differences between young people aged 4 to 10 years and those aged 11 to 18 years (girls aged 7 to 10 years compared with girls aged 11 to 14 years: p < 0.05; others: p < 0.01).

For further analysis of data on young people's method of transport to school or work, see *Sections 13.4.3* and *13.4.4*, where variations in physical activity are shown according to method of transport to school or work.

(Tables 13.2 and 13.3)

13.4.3 Physical activity for young people aged 4 to 6 years

For children aged 4 to 6 years, data on physical activity level were collected using three separate questions in the initial dietary interview, their parents' assessment of their child's current level of activity, and of their level of activity compared with other children of the same sex and compared with other children of the same age.

Table 13.4 gives the distributions for the three questions about level of activity. Overall, 95% of children aged 4 to 6 years were reported to be either fairly active or very active. A significantly greater proportion of boys than girls were reported to be very active, 43% of boys compared with 29% of girls (p < 0.05). This may reflect the fact that parents are more likely to report high levels of activity for boys than for girls[18] rather than a real difference in level of activity by sex.

Just under three quarters of children were reported to have the same level of activity as young people of the same age and sex while less than 5% were reported to be

less active than children of the same age or sex. Compared with young people of the same sex, 18% of boys and 28% of girls were reported to be more active (ns).

(Table 13.4)

Variations in physical activity for young people aged 4 to 6 years

All results reported in this section are significant at least at the p < 0.05 level; separate tables are not shown but the data are summarised in Table 13.5.

A significantly higher proportion of both boys and girls who walked or cycled to school were described as 'very active' compared with young people who mainly travelled to school using other methods of transport (45% compared with 40% for boys; 31% compared with 26% for girls).

Boys were significantly more likely to be described as 'very active' in the fieldwork waves covering the spring and summer months (Wave 2, April to June and Wave 3, July to September) compared with the autumn and winter months (Wave 1, January to March and Wave 4, October to December) (46% and 50% compared with 33% and 44%).

For both boys and girls, the greatest proportions described as 'very active' lived in the Central and South West regions of England and Wales (54% and 36% respectively) while the smallest proportions lived in London and the South East (27% and 19% respectively); there were too few young people living in Scotland for reliable comparisons to be made.

Boys from a manual social class background were significantly more likely than those from a non-manual background to be described as 'very active' (50% compared with 37%), while girls from a manual social class background were significantly less likely than those from a non-manual background to be described as 'very active' (26% compared with 31%). Girls from a manual social class background were more likely than those from a non-manual background to be described as 'fairly inactive' (12% compared with 4%).

Although there was significant variation in the proportions of both boys and girls described as 'fairly inactive', 'fairly active' and 'very active' according to gross weekly household income, the only clear trend was for the proportion of girls described as 'very active', to decrease as income increased, from 37% for girls from households with a gross weekly income of less than £160 to 25% for girls from households with a gross weekly income of £400 or more.

Both boys and girls from households that were in receipt of benefits were significantly more likely than those from households that were not in receipt of benefits to be described as 'very active' (49% compared with 41% and 34% compared with 27% respectively) and significantly less likely to be described as 'fairly active' (48% compared with 55% and 55% compared with 67% respectively).

There were no statistically significant associations between reported level of physical activity and any of the physiological characteristics considered (Body Mass Index – BMI, mid upper-arm circumference and blood pressure) or with intake of energy and selected nutrients[19]. *(Table 13.5)*

13.4.4 Physical activity for young people aged 7 to 18 years

The types of activity in which the young person participated

Figures 13.1(a) and 13.1(b) show the proportion of boys and girls participating in selected activities during the record-keeping period. The activities selected are those reported most frequently.

Overall, the activities in which the highest proportions of boys participated were 'football' (36%), 'walking briskly' (29%), 'playing tag, other chasing games outside' (20%) 'cycling, including doing a paper round on a bike' (17%), 'playing other ball games outside' (12%), 'cleaning your room, gardening or hoovering' (11%) and 'running hard or jogging' (10%). The activities in which the highest proportions of girls participated were 'walking briskly' (41%), 'playing tag, other chasing games outside' (19%) and 'cleaning your room, gardening or hoovering' (18%). The fact that such high proportions of both boys and girls reported 'walking briskly' during the recording period may suggest that every instance of walking was recorded, whether or not it was in fact 'brisk'.

(Figures 13.1(a) and 13.1(b))

Frequency of activity

From the 7-day activity diaries, the frequency of participation in different activities and in activities of different intensity can be estimated. The total number of activities of moderate, vigorous and very vigorous intensity in which young people aged 7 to 18 years participated during the 7-day recording period were calculated. In addition, the numbers of activities of moderate, vigorous and very vigorous intensity were added to give the number of activities of 'at least moderate intensity'. Data are presented for each of these categories (see *Tables 13.6 to 13.8*) although only the results for vigorous, very vigorous and at least moderate intensity activities are reported in the text.

It should be noted that where the young person took part in the same activity more than once on the *same* day, this was recorded as one activity. Also in Tables 13.6 and 13.7 those young people who participated in no activities of moderate intensity may nevertheless have taken part in activities of vigorous or very vigorous intensity during the record-keeping period and vice versa.

Table 13.7 shows that overall 76% of boys and 69% of girls participated in vigorous or very vigorous activity (p < 0.05). Young people aged 15 to 18 years were the least likely and those aged 11 to 14 years were the most likely to have participated in vigorous activity (boys: p < 0.05; girls: p < 0.01).

The data suggest that for boys, the mean number of different activities of vigorous or very vigorous intensity increased between those aged 7 to 10 years and those aged 11 to 14 years and then decreased for the oldest age group (ns). Girls aged 15 to 18 years participated in fewer activities of vigorous or very vigorous intensity than those aged 7 to 14 years, 1.6 per week compared with 2.3 (p < 0.05).

Table 13.8 shows that during the 7-day recording period 96% of boys and 97% of girls took part in activities of at least moderate intensity; for boys this proportion decreased with age (100% of boys aged 7 to 10 years compared with 91% of boys aged 15 to 18 years: p < 0.01). For girls there was no significant difference by age.

In the two youngest age groups and overall, boys participated in significantly more activities of at least moderate intensity than girls, (all: p < 0.01). The mean number of different activities of at least moderate intensity decreased significantly with age for both sexes, for example from 9.4 activities for girls aged 7 to 10 years to 6.7 activities for girls aged 15 to 18 years (both sexes: p < 0.01). *(Tables 13.6 to 13.8)*

Duration of activity

Tables 13.9 to 13.11 give the mean hours spent in activities of different intensity for boys and girls aged 7 to 18 years. As Table 13.10 shows, on average, boys spent 0.4 hours per day and girls 0.3 hours per day in vigorous or very vigorous intensity activities (p < 0.01). For girls, the data suggest that those aged 7 to 14 years spent more time in vigorous and very vigorous intensity activities than those in the oldest age group, although only the difference between those aged 7 to 10 years and those aged 15 to 18 years was statistically significant (p < 0.05). For boys, the data suggest that those aged 11 to 14 years spent the most time in vigorous or very vigorous activities, although the differences did not reach the level of statistical significance.

The HEA primary recommendation for young people is that they should participate in at least one hour of activity of at least moderate intensity per day. Table 13.11 shows that, apart from the oldest age group, boys were significantly more likely than girls to meet the HEA targets for each age group (all: p < 0.01). For boys, 70% of those aged 7 to 10 years participated for one hour or more in at least moderate intensity activity per day; this proportion decreased to 44% for boys aged 15 to 18 years (p < 0.01). For girls, 49% of those aged 7 to 10 years took part for one hour or more in activity of at least moderate intensity per day and this proportion decreased to 31% for girls aged 15 to 18 years (p < 0.01).

The HEA recommendation for less active young people is that they should participate in at least half an hour of at least moderate intensity activity per day. Overall, boys were more likely to achieve this level of activity than girls, with 83% spending half an hour or more per day in activity of at least moderate intensity compared with 73% of girls (p < 0.01).

Boys spent on average 1.4 hours per day engaged in activities of at least moderate intensity, compared with 1.0 hours for girls (p < 0.01). The data suggest that the mean hours spent in at least moderate intensity activity decreased with age for both boys and girls; differences were significant for both boys and girls aged 15 to 18 compared with those aged 7 to 10 and 11 to 14 years (all: p < 0.01). *(Table 13.9 to 13.11)*

The calculated activity score
The derivation of the calculated activity score has been described above (see *Section 13.3* and *Appendix K*). Calculated activity scores ranged between 35 and 61 for young people aged 7 to 18 years (table not shown) suggesting that the calculated activity scores are high and probably represent an over-estimate.

Table 13.12 shows the distribution of the calculated activity score for young people aged 7 to 18 years using the categories in the standard classification. None of the young people aged 7 to 18 years were classified as very inactive (calculated activity less than 33) and less than 6% of each age-sex group were classified as inactive (calculated activity score between 33 and less than 37). Between 11% and 29% were classified as moderately active (calculated activity score between 37 and less than 40), depending on age and sex, but the majority of young people (ranging from 71% to 89%) were classified as active (calculated activity score of 40 or above). Overall, a greater proportion of boys than girls were classified as active, 82% compared with 77% (ns), although this was mainly accounted for by the significantly higher proportion of boys than girls classified as active for those aged 11 to 14 years (89% of boys compared with 76% of girls: p < 0.01).

The distribution of the data shows that, compared with the results from previous studies of physical activity for young people aged 11 to 14 years (see *Section 13.3*), the calculated activity scores derived from the data collected for this survey probably represent an over-estimate. The rounding upwards of time spent in different activities will have contributed to any over-estimate of energy expenditure as represented by the calculated activity score (for further discussion see

Appendix K). Partly due to the likely overestimation of level of physical activity represented by the calculated activity score, the standard classification for the calculated activity score may therefore be inappropriate for the present physical activity data.

The mean calculated activity score was 42 for all girls and 43 for all boys aged 7 to 18 years (p < 0.01). For the two youngest age groups the calculated activity score was higher for boys than for girls (p < 0.01). For both boys and girls, mean calculated activity scores increased with age, for example from a mean of 42 for boys aged 7 to 10 years to a mean of 44 for boys aged 15 to 18 years (p < 0.01). *(Table 13.12)*

Correlations between measures of physical activity
Table 13.13(a) gives a correlation coefficient matrix for the relationships between the various measures of physical activity (base numbers for this table are given in Table 13.13(b)). Individual measures of physical activity tend to be highly correlated with age; *partial correlation coefficients* have therefore been calculated which allow for the effect of age to be controlled. Coefficients are given both for the whole age range and for the four age groups separately, each controlling for age; coefficients above and below the 'diagonals' are for boys and girls respectively. The matrices give partial correlation coefficients and identify the relationships which were statistically significant (p < 0.05 or p < 0.01).

For both boys and girls, the strongest correlations were for the relationship between the total number of different activities of at least moderate intensity and mean hours spent in all activities of at least moderate intensity per day (all: p < 0.01), suggesting that as the number of different activities increased, the amount of time spent in activities increased.

As would be expected, the calculated activity score was positively correlated with the total number of different activities of at least moderate intensity (all: p < 0.01) and mean hours spent in all activities of at least moderate intensity (all: p < 0.01) and negatively correlated with mean hours of sedentary activity per day (all: p < 0.01).

The total number of different activities of at least moderate intensity was negatively correlated with mean hours of sedentary activity for girls aged 7 to 14 years (girls 7 to 10 years: p < 0.01; girls 11 to 14 years: p < 0.05). *(Tables 13.13(a) and 13.13(b))*

Variation in activity for young people aged 7 to 18 years
Tables 13.14 to 13.21 show the relationships between the various measures of activity and key socio-demographic characteristics for young people aged 7 to 18 years; not all the tables are commented on. Mean hours of sedentary activity per day for young people aged 4 to 18 years are discussed in *Section 13.4.5*.

The means for each measure have already been shown to be strongly related to age. It should therefore be borne in mind when considering Tables 13.14 to 13.21 that the variation in activity associated with socio-demographic characteristics may not be significant when the effects of other factors such as age are controlled.

The data suggest that on average young people were most active in the summer fieldwork wave (Wave 3, July to September), less active in the spring wave (Wave 2, April to June) and least active in the autumn and winter waves (Waves 1, January to March and 4, October to December). For example, calculated activity scores increased significantly between Waves 1 and 3 and between Waves 2 and 3 and decreased significantly between Waves 3 and 4 for both boys and girls (for boys all: $p < 0.01$; for girls, Wave 3 compared with Wave 2: $p < 0.05$; others: $p < 0.01$).

There was no significant variation in the measures of physical activity by social class, region, gross weekly household income or being at school or work. For both boys and girls, there was no significant difference in the measures of physical activity according to whether they were well or unwell during the recording period. Boys whose 'parents' were in receipt of benefits had on average lower calculated activity scores than those whose 'parents' were not in receipt of benefits, 42 compared with 43 ($p < 0.05$).

The data suggest that the level of physical activity varied according to whether the young person was living with both parents. However, it should be remembered that the age distribution in the different household types was significantly different (see *Chapter 3, Section 3.3.3*). *(Tables 13.14 to 13.21)*

13.4.5 Mean hours of sedentary activity per day

Information on hours spent in sedentary activity (very light activity) was collected for all young people in the Diary of Activities and Eating and Drinking Away from Home[20]. It should be noted that time spent at school or in a job involving very light intensity activity is not included in this section. Time spent travelling to and from school or work by bus, car or motorcycle is excluded from the total time spent in sedentary activities.

Overall, boys reported spending longer in sedentary activities than girls ($p < 0.05$), although this is mainly due to differences between girls and boys in the first two age groups (4 to 6 years: $p < 0.05$, 7 to 10 years: ns).

Mean hours spent in sedentary activities increased with age, with both boys and girls aged 15 to 18 years spending on average significantly longer in sedentary activities than those aged 4 to 6 years (both sexes: $p < 0.01$).

There was no significant difference in hours of sedentary activity per day according to whether the young person was well or unwell during the recording period, the region in which they lived, gross weekly household income, or, for girls, their social class background. However, boys aged 4 to 18 from a manual social class background spent significantly longer in sedentary activities, 2.8 hours a day, than boys from a non-manual social class background, 2.5 hours a day ($p < 0.05$).

The data suggest that the number of hours spent in sedentary activity were on average higher in the autumn and winter fieldwork waves (Wave 1, January to March and Wave 4, October to December) and lower in the spring and summer fieldwork waves (Wave 2, April to June and Wave 3, July to September), although the only significant differences were between Waves 1 and 3 and between Waves 3 and 4 for boys (both: $p < 0.05$).

Table 13.19 shows that young people from households that were in receipt of benefits spent more time in sedentary activities than those from households that were not in receipt of benefits (both sexes: $p < 0.05$).

Table 13.21 suggests that young people who travelled to school or work by motorcycle, car or bus on average spent less time in sedentary activities than young people who walked or cycled to school or work (boys $p < 0.05$; girls ns). *(Tables 13.14 to 13.22)*

13.5 Correlations with dietary intake

Tables 13.23(a) and 13.23(b) give partial correlation coefficients for the relationships between the measures of physical activity and dietary intake for intakes most likely to be related to energy expenditure, that is average daily energy intake and percentage energy from total fat, total carbohydrate and total sugars (base numbers for these tables are given in Table 13.23(c)). The tables are restricted to young people aged 7 to 18 years who completed a 7-day dietary and physical activity diary.

For boys, associations with average daily energy intake were significant only for those aged 7 to 10 years, correlating significantly and positively with each measure of physical activity except mean hours spent in sedentary activity per day. For girls, average daily energy intake was negatively correlated with mean hours of sedentary activity per day for those aged 7 to 10, and was positively correlated with the total number of activities of at least moderate intensity in which the young person participated during the recording period for all girls aged 7 to 18 years ($p < 0.01$) and for girls aged 7 to 10 years and 11 to 14 years (both: $p < 0.05$).

Percentage energy from total fat was not significantly associated with any measure of physical activity for boys aged 7 to 14 years. For all boys aged 7 to 18 years and boys aged 15 to 18 years, percentage energy from

515

total fat was positively associated with mean hours of sedentary activity per day and negatively associated with the calculated activity score (all: $p < 0.01$).

For girls, percentage energy from total fat was positively correlated with mean hours of sedentary activity per day and negatively correlated with the calculated activity score for those aged 7 to 10 years, 15 to 18 years and for all girls aged 7 to 18 years (calculated activity score for all girls aged 7 to 18 years: $p < 0.01$; others: $p < 0.05$).

Percentage energy from total carbohydrate was not significantly associated with any measure of physical activity for boys aged 7 to 10 years or for all boys aged 7 to 18 years. For boys aged 11 to 14 years, percentage energy from total carbohydrate was negatively correlated with both mean hours spent in all activities of at least moderate intensity per day and the calculated activity score (both: $p < 0.05$). For boys aged 15 to 18 years, percentage energy from total carbohydrate was positively correlated with the total number of activities of at least moderate intensity in which the young person participated during the recording period ($p < 0.05$).

Percentage energy from total sugars was positively associated with the total number of activities of at least moderate intensity in which the young person participated during the recording period for all boys aged 7 to 18 years ($p < 0.05$). The associations between percentage energy from total sugars and the measures of physical activity were most marked for boys aged 7 to 10 years and were absent for boys aged 11 to 18 years.

There were no significant associations between percentage energy from total carbohydrate or percentage energy from total sugars and any of the measures of physical activity for girls. *(Tables 13.23(a) to 13.23(c))*

13.6 Correlations with anthropometric measurements

Tables 13.24(a) and 13.24(b) give partial correlation coefficients for the relationships between the measures of physical activity and anthropometric measures indicating body size.

For all boys aged 7 to 18 years, mean hours of sedentary activity per day was significantly positively correlated with BMI and the total number of activities of at least moderate intensity in which the young person participated during the recording period was negatively associated with waist to hip ratio (both: $p < 0.05$). The associations between the measures of physical activity and the anthropometric measurements were most marked for boys aged 11 to 14 years and absent for boys aged 7 to 10 years and 15 to 18 years.

For girls, there were no significant associations between the measures of physical activity and the anthropo-

metric measurements for those aged 7 to 10 years and 11 to 14 years. For girls aged 15 to 18 years, mean hours spent in all activities of at least moderate intensity per day was negatively associated with BMI while the total number of activities of at least moderate intensity in which the young person participated during the recording period was positively associated with waist to hip ratio (both: $p < 0.05$). For girls aged 7 to 18 years, BMI and mid upper-arm circumference were significantly positively associated with mean hours of sedentary activity and BMI was significantly negatively correlated with the total number of activities of at least moderate intensity and with mean hours spent in all activities of at least moderate intensity (all: $p < 0.05$).
(Tables 13.24(a) and 13.24(b))

13.7 Correlations with blood pressure

Tables 13.25(a) and 13.25(b) give partial correlation coefficients for the relationships between the measures of physical activity and blood pressure.

For all boys aged 7 to 18 years, systolic pressure was significantly positively correlated with mean hours of sedentary activity per day and significantly negatively associated with mean hours spent in all activities of at least moderate intensity per day (both: $p < 0.05$). None of the relationships between the measures of physical activity and diastolic pressure reached the level of statistical significance for all boys aged 7 to 18 years.

Associations between systolic pressure and the measures of physical activity were most marked for boys 11 to 14 years and absent for boys aged 7 to 10 years and 15 to 18 years. Diastolic pressure was significantly negatively associated with mean hours spent in all activities of at least moderate intensity per day for boys aged 7 to 10 years ($p < 0.05$) and for boys aged 15 to 18 years significantly positively associated with mean hours of sedentary activity per day and the total number of activities of at least moderate intensity in which the young person participated during the recording period ($p < 0.05$ and $p < 0.01$ respectively).

For all girls aged 7 to 18 years, systolic pressure was negatively associated with the total number of activities of at least moderate intensity during the 7-day recording period ($p < 0.05$) and the mean hours spent in all activities of at least moderate intensity per day ($p < 0.01$), while diastolic pressure was negatively associated with mean hours spent in all activities of at least moderate intensity per day ($p < 0.05$).

For girls aged 7 to 10 years, systolic pressure was significantly negatively correlated with mean hours spent in all activities of at least moderate intensity per day ($p < 0.05$). There were no significant associations between blood pressure and the measures of physical activity for girls aged 11 to 18 years.
(Tables 13.25(a) and 13.25(b))

13.8 Characteristics found to be independently associated with measures of physical activity

Various socio-demographic characteristics have been shown to be associated with participation in physical activity (see *Section 13.4.4*), but some of these factors are known to be inter-related. This section considers the combined effects of these variables on the measures of physical activity for young people aged 7 to 18 years who completed a 7-day physical activity diary. The technique of multiple regression was used to identify those characteristics with the strongest relationships to the calculated activity score. The tables of results identify those characteristics where the regression coefficients were significantly related to the calculated activity score after controlling the effects of the other characteristics included in the analysis ($p < 0.05$, $p < 0.01$ or $p < 0.001$). Further information on the statistical method is given in Appendix E.

As noted above, for young people there is a strong association between age and the calculated activity score. To control for this effect, age was included in the multiple regression analysis; thus differences in calculated activity score have been tested for significance after taking account of any age variation between groups. There is also a strong association between sex and the calculated activity score; the analysis is therefore presented separately for boys and girls aged 7 to 18 years. Age at menarché is included in the analysis for girls, but plasma testosterone concentration was available only for 260 boys aged 10 to 16 years, for whom a separate analysis is therefore presented.

BMI and waist to hip ratio were correlated with some measures of level of physical activity (see *Tables 13.24(a) and 13.24(b)*); however, waist to hip ratio was only measured for young people aged 11 to 18 years and in order to allow the regression analysis to be carried out for the maximum number of young people, this measure was dropped from the analysis. As body weight, height and BMI are strongly correlated not all of these three variables could be included in the same multiple regression analysis; weight and height were excluded[21].

13.8.1 Findings

This section considers the combined effect of those characteristics found to have significant associations with calculated activity score.

For boys aged 7 to 18 years, (see *Table 13.26(a)*) the independent socio-demographic and behavioural characteristics that contributed significantly to explaining variation in the calculated activity score were, in descending order of predictive value[22], whether the young person was at school or work, fieldwork wave, age, gross weekly household income and whether they were living with both parents. The independent characteristics included in the regression analysis for boys aged 7 to 18 years accounted for 25% of the variation in the calculated activity score.

For boys aged 10 to 16 years for whom plasma testosterone concentration was measured, (see *Table 26(b)*) the independent characteristics that contributed significantly to explaining variation in the calculated activity score were fieldwork wave, the social class of the head of household and average daily alcohol intake. The independent characteristics included in the regression analysis for boys aged 10 to 16 years accounted for 22% of the variation in the calculated activity score.

For girls aged 7 to 18 years, the independent characteristics that contributed significantly to explaining variation in the calculated activity score (see *Table 26(c)*) were age, whether the young person was at school or work, percentage energy from total sugars, fieldwork wave, region and average daily alcohol intake. The independent characteristics included in the regression analysis for girls aged 7 to 18 years accounted for 20% of the variation in the calculated activity score.

For both boys and girls aged 7 to 18 years, the calculated activity score rose significantly with age independently of the other characteristics included in the analysis (boys: $p < 0.05$; girls: $p < 0.001$).

Although the regression coefficients for every category of fieldwork wave and whether the young person was at school or work did not reach the level of statistical significance in each of the three regression analyses, the direction of the relationship between the calculated activity score and each category was the same. The data suggest that young people were more active than average in the summer wave (Wave 3, July to September) and the spring wave (Wave 2, April to June) and less active than average in the autumn and winter waves (Wave 1, January to March and Wave 4, October to December). Young people who were attending school only or school and work were less active than average, while those who attending work only or who were not at school or work were more active than average.

For both girls aged 7 to 18 years and boys aged 10 to 16 years, average daily intake of alcohol was independently positively associated with the calculated activity score, suggesting that the consumption of alcohol may take place jointly with periods of physical activity e.g. dancing at a disco or club. There was also a significant positive relationship between the calculated activity score and percentage energy from sugars for girls. In Chapter 6 it was shown that a significant proportion of total sugars intake was provided by soft drinks suggesting that the more active girls may also have consumed more soft drinks.

For boys aged 7 to 18 years, those from the middle income group were less active than average and those living with a single parent and other children were more active than average (both: p < 0.05). For girls aged 7 to 18 years, those living in the Northern region were significantly less active than average (p < 0.01).

(Tables 13.26(a) to 13.26(c))

13.9 A comparison of data from the NDNS with data from the Health Survey for England

In this section, data on physical activity from this present NDNS are compared with data from the Health Survey for England: The Health of Young People, carried out in 1995 to 1997[1]. Comparable data on participation in physical activity were available for young people aged 7 to 15 years living in England.

There are several important differences between the Health Survey and the NDNS in terms of the data collection method for physical activity, potentially the most significant of which is that, unlike the NDNS, the Health Survey excluded from the analysis activities in which the young person participated as part of the compulsory school curriculum (see *Appendix K* for a detailed discussion of the differences in methodology between the two surveys).

13.9.1 Findings

Level of participation in activity of at least moderate intensity

Table 13.27 suggests that the proportion of both boys and girls who participated in activities of at least moderate intensity was higher at most individual years of age for young people in the NDNS compared with young people of the same age in the Health Survey. However, the differences were only statistically significant for boys aged 7 years and for girls aged 9 years (both: p < 0.05) and these differences may at least partly be explained by the fact that the Health Survey excluded from the analysis activities in which the young person participated as part of the school curriculum.

The number of days on which the young person participated in activity of at least moderate intensity

The number of days on which young people participated in activities of at least moderate intensity were broadly similar for young people in the NDNS and in the Health Survey, with no significant differences by age for either boys or girls between the NDNS and Health Survey data.

Mean number of hours spent in activity of at least moderate intensity

Table 13.27 shows that the mean number of hours which young people participated in activities of at least moderate intensity were broadly similar with no significant differences by age for either boys or girls between the NDNS and Health Survey data.

It can therefore be concluded that, after taking into account differences in the methodologies, data on selected measures of physical activity from this NDNS and the Health Survey are broadly comparable. *(Table 13.27)*

References and endnotes

1. Prescott-Clarke P, Primatesta P. Eds. *Health Survey for England. The Health of Young People '95–97. Volume 1: Findings*. TSO (London, 1998).

2. Chinn S, Rona RJ. Trends in weight-for-height and triceps skinfold thickness for English and Scottish children, 1972–82 and 1982–1990. *Paed Peri Epi* 1994; **8:** 90–106.

3. Riddoch CJ, Boreham CA. The health–related physical activity of children. *Sports Med* 1995; **19:** 86–102.

4. Durnin JVGA. Physical activity levels past and present. *Phys Act and Hlth* pp.20–27. Cambridge University Press (Cambridge, 1992).

5. Riddoch CJ. Relationships between physical activity and physical health in young people. In: Biddle S, Sallis J, Cavill N. Eds. *Young and Active? Young people and health-enhancing physical activity evidence and impli- cations.* pp17–48 HEA (London, 1998).

6. Biddle S, Sallis J, Cavill N. Eds. *Young and Active? Young people and health-enhancing physical activity evidence and implications.* HEA (London, 1998).

7. Armstrong N, Welsman JR. *Young People and Physical Activity.* Oxford University Press (Oxford, 1997).

8. Sallis JF. Epidemiology of physical activity and fitness in children and adolescents. *Crit Rev Food Sci and Nutr* 1993; **33:** 403–408.

9. Melanson EL, Freedson PS. Physical activity assessment: a review of methods. *Crit Rev Food Sci and Nutr* 1996; **36:** 385–396.

10. Bailey RC, Olson J et al. The level and tempo of children's physical activities: an observational study. *Med and Sci in Sports and Exer* 1995; **27:** 1033–1041.

11. Lowe S. *Feasibility study for the National Diet and Nutrition Survey: young people aged 4 to 18 years.* ONS (*In preparation*).

12. A MET is a multiple of the resting rate of oxygen consumption, or the ratio of working metabolic rate to resting metabolic rate (WMR/RMR). One MET represents the resting metabolic rate, so that an individual participating in physical activity at 2 METs is consuming oxygen at twice the resting rate.

13. Time spent sleeping during the day e.g. naps was not collected. This may be of particular importance when looking at data for young people aged 4 to 6 years.

14. Blair SN. How to assess exercise habits and physical fitness. In: Matarazzo JD et al. Eds. *Behavioural Health: A Handbook of Health Enhancement and Disease Prevention.* Wiley & Sons (New York, 1984).

15. Cale L. An assessment of the physical activity levels of adolescent girls implications for physical education. *European Journal of Physical Education* 1996; **1:** 46–55.

16. Cale L, Almond L. The physical activity levels of English adolescent boys. *E J of Phys Ed* 1997; **2:** 74–82.

17. If two methods of transport were used, both were recorded.

18. Sallis J. Self–report measures of children's physical activity. *Jl Sch Hlth* 1991; **61:** 215–219.

19. Physiological characteristics were Body Mass Index, mid upper-arm circumference, systolic and diastolic blood pressure; nutrient intakes were average daily total energy intake and, percentage energy from total fat, total carbohydrate and total sugars.

20. Detailed information about hours spent in different activities was not collected for young people aged 4 to 6 years (see *Appendix K*).

21. For further information on the effect of collinearity in a multiple regression analysis see *Appendix E*.

22. Determined from the size of the standardised regression coefficient (β).

Table 13.1 Whether young person was at school or work during the record–keeping period by sex and age of young person

Physical activity sample

Whether young person was at school or work	Males aged (years)				All males	Females aged (years)				All females
	4–6	7–10	11–14	15–18		4–6	7–10	11–14	15–18	
	%	%	%	%	%	%	%	%	%	%
No school or work	14	13	15	8	13	13	19	14	13	15
School only	86	87	79	38	72	87	81	79	37	71
School and work	–	–	5	32	10	–	0	4	25	8
Work only	–	–	0	23	6	–	–	2	26	7
Base	*188*	*263*	*254*	*194*	*899*	*176*	*236*	*255*	*222*	*889*

Table 13.2 Usual method of transport to and from school or work by age and sex of young person

Interview sample – young people travelling to school or work

Usual method of transport	Males aged (years)				All males	Females aged (years)				All females
	4–6	7–10	11–14	15–18		4–6	7–10	11–14	15–18	
	%	%	%	%	%	%	%	%	%	%
Walk	53	56	43	39	49	50	55	39	33	44
Cycle	–	1	4	6	3	–	–	2	–	1
Motorcycle	–	–	–	1	0	–	–	–	1	0
Car	46	39	25	21	33	44	39	21	25	31
Bus	5	5	27	33	16	6	7	35	38	22
Other	1	1	2	2	1	–	1	5	7	3
*Base**	*211*	*304*	*290*	*242*	*1047*	*211*	*277*	*280*	*245*	*1013*

*Some young people reported usually travelling by two methods and the percentages may therefore add to more than 100%.

Table 13.3 Mean duration of walk to school or work (minutes) by sex and age

Interview sample - young people walking to school or work

Duration of walk to school or work (minutes)	Males aged (years)				All males	Females aged (years)				All females
	4–6	7–10	11–14	15–18		4–6	7–10	11–14	15–18	
Mean (average value)	8.6	8.4	13.1	13.3	10.4	8.5	9.4	12.1	14.2	10.7
Median value	10.0	7.0	10.0	10.0	10.0	7.0	10.0	10.0	12.2	10.0
Standard deviation of the mean	4.76	5.44	8.80	8.01	7.1	5.03	7.05	7.64	9.02	7.4
Base	*111*	*167*	*133*	*80*	*491*	*113*	*154*	*113*	*76*	*456*

Table 13.4 Reported level of activity for young people aged 4 to 6 years by sex

Interview sample - 4 to 6 years only

Reported level of activity	Sex of young person		All
	Male	Female	
	%	%	%
Parent's assessment of young person's current level of activity			
fairly inactive*	3	7	5
fairly active**	53	64	59
very active***	43	29	36
Young person's level of activity compared with boys and girls of the same age			
less active	5	3	4
about the same	69	74	71
more active	26	23	24
Young person's level of activity compared with other children of the same sex			
less active	6	2	4
about the same	76	70	73
more active	18	28	23
Base	*230*	*224*	*454*

* 'Gets little exercise, spends most of their time watching television, looking at books, or sitting playing with toys or games.'
** 'Spends more time in active play or running around than watching television, looking at books, or sitting playing with toys or games.'
*** 'Spends nearly all the time running around or in very active play or games.'

Table 13.5 Summary of variations in reported activity level for young people aged 4 to 6 years by socio-demographic characteristics

Sex	Reported level of physical activity		
	Very active[1]	Fairly active[2]	Fairly inactive[3]
Males	Walking to school or work⊗ > motorcycle, car or bus to school or work** Wave 2 > Wave 4∅** Wave 3 > Waves 1 and 4∅** Central, South West and Wales > London and the South East** and Northern Region* Manual > non-manual** Receiving benefits > not receiving benefits**	Wave 1 > Waves 2, 3 and 4∅** London and the South East > Central, South West and Wales** Non-manual > manual** Not receiving benefits > receiving benefits**	
Females	Walking to school or work⊗ > motorcycle, car or bus to school or work** Central, South West and Wales > London and the South East and Northern Region ** Non-manual > manual ** Gross weekly household income less than £160 > Gross weekly household income £400 or more** Receiving benefits > not receiving benefits**	Motorcycle, car or bus to school or work > walking to school or work⊗** Wave 1 > Waves 2, 3 and 4∅** London and the South East and Northern Region > Central, South West and Wales** Non-manual > manual ** Not receiving benefits > receiving benefits**	Waves 3 and 4 > Waves 1 and 2** London and the South East > Northern Region and Central, South West and Wales** Manual > non-manual **

Note: comparisons show for two groups, that group A was more likely than group B to have reported level of activity. For example, Wave 2 > Wave 4, indicates that those interviewed in Wave 2 were significantly more likely to be (very) active, than those in Wave 4.
* $p < 0.05$
** $p < 0.01$
[1] 'Gets little exercise, spends most of their time watching television, looking at books, or sitting playing with toys or games'.
[2] 'Spends more time in active play or running around than watching television, looking at books, or sitting playing with toys or games'.
[3] 'Spends nearly all the time running around or in very active play or games'.
∅ Wave 1: January to March 1997; Wave 2: April to June 1997; Wave 3: July to September 1997; Wave 4: October to December 1997.
⊗ No young people aged 4 to 6 years cycled to school.

Table 13.6 Total number of activities of moderate intensity during the 7-day recording period by sex and age of young person

Physical activity sample - young people aged 7–18 years

Total number of activities of moderate intensity during the 7-day recording period	Males aged (years)			All males	Females aged (years)			All females
	7–10	11–14	15–18		7–10	11–14	15–18	
	cum %	cum %	cum %	cum %	cum %	cum %	cum %	cum %
No activities of moderate intensity*	1	4	16	7	5	4	9	6
1 or fewer	2	9	22	11	9	9	21	13
2 or fewer	4	13	33	17	13	19	34	22
3 or fewer	10	20	43	24	20	26	40	28
4 or fewer	14	26	54	31	28	37	45	37
5 or fewer	19	32	63	38	36	48	57	47
10 or fewer	56	75	88	73	80	82	90	84
15 or fewer	86	91	97	91	97	96	99	97
20 or fewer	96	98	100	98	99	100	100	100
All	100	100		100	100			
Base	*263*	*254*	*194*	*711*	*236*	*255*	*222*	*713*
Mean (average value)	10.1	7.7	5.1	7.7	7.1	6.5	5.1	6.2
Median value	10.0	7.0	4.0	7.0	7.0	6.0	5.0	6.0
Lower 2.5 percentile	2.0	0.0	0.0	0.0	0.0	0.0	0.0	0.0
Upper 2.5 percentile	22.0	19.0	16.0	19.0	16.0	17.0	14.0	16.0
Standard deviation of the mean	5.13	4.82	4.34	5.21	4.11	4.28	3.94	4.19

* This category includes young people who did not participate in any moderate intensity activity during the recording period. Young people in this category may nevertheless have taken part in a vigorous or very vigorous intensity activity.

Table 13.7 Total number of activities of vigorous or very vigorous intensity during the 7-day recording period by sex and age of young person

Physical activity sample – young people aged 7–18 years

Total number of activities of vigorous or very vigorous intensity during the 7-day recording period	Males aged (years)			All males	Females aged (years)			All females
	7–10	11–14	15–18		7–10	11–14	15–18	
	cum %	cum %	cum %	cum %	cum %	cum %	cum %	cum %
No activities of vigorous intensity*	23	17	32	24	26	22	47	31
1 or fewer	42	34	51	43	46	46	69	54
2 or fewer	56	50	66	57	62	65	79	69
3 or fewer	66	62	75	68	71	77	89	79
4 or fewer	74	70	79	74	84	86	92	87
5 or fewer	83	78	83	81	89	91	94	91
10 or fewer	98	99	98	98	99	99	98	99
15 or fewer	99	100	99	100	100	100	99	100
All	100		100				100	
Base	*263*	*254*	*194*	*711*	*236*	*255*	*222*	*713*
Mean (average value)	2.9	3.2	2.5	2.9	2.3	2.3	1.6	2.1
Median value	2.0	3.0	1.0	2.0	2.0	2.0	1.0	1.0
Lower 2.5 percentile	0.0	0.0	0.0	0.0	0.0	0.0	0.0	0.0
Upper 2.5 percentile	10.0	9.0	9.0	9.0	8.0	9.0	9.0	8.0
Standard deviation of the mean	2.93	2.79	3.12	2.96	2.30	2.38	2.85	2.54

*This category includes young people who did not participate in any vigorous or very vigorous intensity activity during the recording period. Young people in this category may nevertheless have taken part in a moderate intensity activity.

Table 13.8 Total number of activities of at least moderate intensity* during the 7-day recording period by sex and age of young person

Physical activity sample - young people 7 to 18 years

Total number of activities of at least moderate intensity during the 7-day recording period	Males aged (years)			All males	Females aged (years)			All females
	7–10	11–14	15–18		7–10	11–14	15–18	
	cum %	cum %	cum %	cum %	cum %	cum %	cum %	cum %
No activities of at least moderate intensity	0	2	9	4	4	1	5	3
1 or fewer	2	3	12	6	5	3	14	7
2 or fewer	2	6	18	9	8	6	28	14
3 or fewer	6	10	26	14	13	13	34	20
4 or fewer	8	13	37	19	16	22	39	25
5 or fewer	10	15	45	23	22	27	48	32
10 or fewer	36	54	71	53	60	70	83	70
15 or fewer	71	83	91	81	89	89	83	90
20 or fewer	88	93	97	93	98	97	94	97
All	100	100	100	100	100	100	100	100
Base	*263*	*254*	*194*	*711*	*236*	*255*	*222*	*713*
Mean (average value)	13.0	10.9	7.6	10.5	9.4	8.8	6.7	8.3
Median value	12.0	10.0	6.0	10.0	9.0	8.0	6.0	8.0
Lower 2.5 percentile	3.0	1.0	0.0	0.0	0.0	1.0	0.0	0.0
Upper 2.5 percentile	29.0	25.0	22.1	25.0	19.0	21.0	22.0	21.0
Standard deviation of the mean	6.59	5.95	5.87	6.55	4.95	5.15	5.64	5.37

*This category includes activities of moderate, vigorous and very vigorous intensity.

Table 13.9 Mean hours spent in moderate intensity activity per day by sex and age of young person

Physical activity sample - young people aged 7 to 18 years

Hours spent in moderate intensity activity	Males aged (years)			All males	Females aged (years)			All females
	7–10	11–14	15–18		7–10	11–14	15–18	
	cum %	cum %	cum %	cum %	cum %	cum %	cum %	cum %
No time spent in moderate intensity activity*	1	4	16	7	5	4	9	6
Less than half an hour	16	25	48	29	33	37	51	40
Less than one hour	45	52	76	58	70	75	79	75
Less than an hour and a half	68	74	89	77	86	92	92	90
Less than two hours	84	89	95	89	95	97	97	96
All	100	100	100	100	100	100	100	100
Base	263	254	194	711	236	255	222	713
Mean (average value)	1.3	1.1	0.7	1.0	0.8	0.7	0.6	0.7
Median value	1.1	1.0	0.5	0.8	0.7	0.6	0.5	0.6
Lower 2.5 percentile	0.1	0.0	0.0	0.0	0.0	0.0	0.0	0.0
Upper 2.5 percentile	3.6	2.7	2.4	2.9	2.2	2.2	2.1	2.2
Standard deviation of the mean	0.83	0.74	0.63	0.78	0.61	0.56	0.56	0.58

* This category includes young people who did not participate in any moderate intensity activity during the recording period. Young people in this category may nevertheless have taken part in a vigorous or very vigorous intensity activity.

Table 13.10 Mean hours spent in vigorous or very vigorous intensity activity* per day by sex and age of young person

Physical activity sample – young people aged 7 to 18 years

Hours spent in vigorous or very vigorous intensity activity per day	Males aged (years)			All males	Females aged (years)			All females
	7–10	11–14	15–18		7–10	11–14	15–18	
	cum %	cum %	cum %	cum %	cum %	cum %	cum %	cum %
No time spent in vigorous intensity activity**	23	17	32	24	26	22	47	31
Less than half an hour	72	69	73	72	81	80	83	81
Less than one hour	93	89	91	91	98	95	94	96
Less than an hour and a half	97	97	99	97	100	98	98	99
All	100	100	100	100		100	100	100
Base	263	254	194	711	236	255	222	713
Mean (average value)	0.3	0.4	0.3	0.4	0.3	0.3	0.2	0.3
Median value	0.2	0.3	0.2	0.2	0.2	0.2	0.0	0.1
Lower 2.5 percentile	0.0	0.0	0.0	0.0	0.0	0.0	0.0	0.0
Upper 2.5 percentile	1.5	1.6	1.3	1.5	0.9	1.4	1.4	1.2
Standard deviation of the mean	0.4	0.4	0.4	0.4	0.3	0.4	0.4	0.4

* Includes vigorous and very vigorous activity.
** This category includes young people who did not participate in any vigorous or very vigorous intensity activity during the recording period. Young people in this category may nevertheless have taken part in a moderate intensity activity.

Table 13.11   Mean hours spent in activity of at least moderate intensity* per day by sex and age of young person**

Physical activity sample - young people aged 7 to 18 years

Hours spent in activity of at least moderate intensity	Males aged (years)			All males	Females aged (years)			All females
	7–10	11–14	15–18		7–10	11–14	15–18	
	cum %	cum %	cum %	cum %	cum %	cum %	cum %	cum %
No time spent in at least moderate intensity activity	0	2	9	4	4	1	5	3
Less than half an hour*	10	12	29	17	16	24	41	27
Less than one hour**	30	32	56	39	51	56	69	58
Less than an hour and a half	52	55	78	62	75	81	84	80
Less than two hours	73	78	89	80	91	92	92	92
All	100	100	100	100	100	100	100	100
Base	*263*	*254*	*194*	*711*	*236*	*255*	*222*	*713*
Mean (average value)	1.6	1.5	1.0	1.4	1.1	1.0	0.8	1.0
Median value	1.4	1.4	0.9	1.2	1.0	0.9	0.7	0.9
Lower 2.5 percentile	0.1	0.1	0.0	0.0	0.0	0.1	0.0	0.0
Upper 2.5 percentile	4.2	3.7	3.3	3.7	2.6	2.7	2.9	2.7
Standard deviation of the mean	1.00	0.89	0.78	0.93	0.67	0.69	0.74	0.71

* The Health Education Authority recommends that young people who currently do little activity should participate in physical activity of at least moderate intensity for *at least half an hour per day.*
**The Health Education Authority recommends that all other young people should participate in physical activity of at least moderate intensity for *one hour per day.*
***Includes moderate, vigorous and very vigorous activity.

Table 13.12   Calculated activity score by sex and age of young person

Physical activity sample – young people aged 7 to 18 years

Calculated activity score	Males aged (years)			All males	Females aged (years)			All females
	7–10	11–14	15–18		7–10	11–14	15–18	
	cum %	cum %	cum %	cum %	cum %	cum %	cum %	cum %
Less than 33*	–	–	–	–	–	–	–	–
Less than 37**	3	1	4	3	5	1	2	3
Less than 40***	26	11	16	18	29	24	16	23
Less than 42	56	41	33	44	61	56	41	53
Less than 44	80	68	54	68	85	80	67	78
Less than 46	87	84	77	83	96	92	84	91
Less than 48	94	95	84	91	99	98	91	96
All	100	100	100	100	100	100	100	100
Base	*263*	*254*	*194*	*711*	*236*	*255*	*222*	*713*
Mean (average value)	42	43	44	43	41	42	43	42
Median value	42	43	44	43	42	42	43	42
Lower 2.5 percentile	37	38	37	37	36	38	37	37
Upper 2.5 percentile	50	50	53	51	47	48	53	50
Standard deviation of the mean	3.2	3.2	4.0	3.6	2.5	2.6	3.8	3.1

* Less than 33 = very inactive.
** 33 to less than 37 = inactive.
*** 37 to less than 40 = moderately active, 40 and over = active.

Table 13.13(a)   Partial correlation coefficient matrix for measures of physical activity by sex and age of young person*

Physical activity sample – young people aged 7 to 18 years

Measure, age (years) and sex of young person	Mean hours of sedentary activity per day	Total number of activities of at least moderate intensity during the 7–day recording period	Mean hours spent in all activities of at least moderate intensity per day	Calculated activity score
	Coefficient	Coefficient	Coefficient	Coefficient
Mean hours of sedentary activity per day				
Males aged:				
7–10	1.00	−0.12	−0.05	−0.31**
11–14	1.00	−0.03	−0.06	−0.37**
15–18	1.00	0.02	0.01	−0.44**
All males	1.00	−0.03	−0.03	−0.39**
Total number of activities of at least moderate intensity during the 7–day recording period		MALES		
Females aged:	FEMALES		MALES	
7–10	−0.20**	1.00	0.74**	0.55**
11–14	−0.13*	1.00	0.79**	0.54**
15–18	0.11	1.00	0.78**	0.31**
All females	−0.04	1.00	0.77**	0.45**
Mean hours spent in all activities of at least moderate intensity per day				MALES
Females aged:		FEMALES		
7–10	−0.07	0.68**	1.00	0.76**
11–14	−0.10	0.76**	1.00	0.71**
15–18	0.08	0.86**	1.00	0.42**
All females	−0.01	0.78**	1.00	0.62**
Calculated activity score				
Females aged:			FEMALES	
7–10	−0.38**	0.37**	0.62**	1.00
11–14	−0.47**	0.56**	0.67**	1.00
15–18	−0.37**	0.40**	0.52**	1.00
All females	−0.40**	0.42**	0.57**	1.00

* p < 0.05
** p < 0.01
*** Bases are given in Table 13.13(b).

Table 13.13(b) Base numbers for partial correlation coefficients for measures of physical activity by sex and age of young person

Young people aged 7–18 years who kept 7-day physical activity and dietary diaries

Age (years)	Sex of young person		All
	Male	Female	
7–10	263	236	499
11–14	254	255	509
15–18	194	222	416
All aged 7–18	711	713	1424

Table 13.14 Measures of activity for young person by whether young person was reported as being unwell during the dietary recording period

Measures of activity	Whether young person reported as unwell during dietary recording period								
	Unwell and eating affected			Unwell and eating not affected			Not unwell		
	Mean	Median	sd	Mean	Median	sd	Mean	Median	sd
Males aged 4 to 18 years:									
Hours of sedentary activity per day	2.5	2.4	1.46	2.7	2.7	1.38	2.6	2.4	1.45
Males aged 7 to 18 years::									
Total number of activities of at least moderate intensity during the 7-day recording period	1.3	1.4	0.90	1.5	1.4	0.65	1.5	1.4	0.96
Mean hours spent in all activities of at least moderate intensity per day	1.2	1.0	0.93	1.5	1.3	0.90	1.4	1.2	0.94
Calculated activity score	43	42	3.6	43	42	3.0	43	43	3.6
Bases:									
Males aged 4 to 18 years		88			73			738	
Males aged 7 to 18 years		67			60			584	
Females aged 4 to 18 years:									
Hours of sedentary activity per day	2.7	2.4	1.56	2.4	2.0	1.65	2.3	2.1	1.41
Females aged 7 to 18 years:									
Total number of activities of at least moderate intensity during the 7-day recording period	1.0	0.9	0.69	1.2	1.0	0.75	1.2	1.1	0.78
Mean hours spent in all activities of at least moderate intensity per day	0.8	0.7	0.61	0.9	0.8	0.59	1.0	0.9	0.73
Calculated activity score	41	41	2.7	42	42	2.9	42	42	3.1
Bases:									
Females aged 4 to 18 years		96			95			698	
Females aged 7 to 18 years		75			79			559	

Table 13.15 Measures of activity for young person by fieldwork wave

Measures of activity	Fieldwork wave*											
	Wave 1			Wave 2			Wave 3			Wave 4		
	Mean	*Median*	*sd*	*Mean*	*Median*	*sd*	*Mean*	*Median*	*sd*	*Mean*	*Median*	*sd*
Males aged 4 to 18 years:												
Hours of sedentary activity per day	2.8	2.6	1.29	2.4	2.2	1.40	2.4	2.1	1.56	2.8	2.6	1.47
Males aged 7 to 18 years:												
Total number of activities of at least moderate intensity during the 7-day recording period	1.4	1.3	0.79	1.6	1.6	1.09	1.6	1.6	0.94	1.4	1.3	0.87
Mean hours spent in all activities of at least moderate intensity per day	1.2	1.1	0.73	1.4	1.3	1.00	1.6	1.5	1.04	1.2	1.1	0.86
Calculated activity score	42	42	3.2	43	43	3.1	45	44	3.8	42	41	3.4
Bases:												
Males aged 4 to 18 years		198			183			259			259	
Males aged 7 to 18 years		156			139			209			207	
Females aged 4 to 18 years												
Hours of sedentary activity per day	2.6	2.3	1.63	2.3	2.0	1.37	2.3	2.0	1.39	2.4	2.1	1.45
Females aged 7 to 18 years												
Total number of activities of at least moderate intensity during the 7-day recording period	1.1	1.0	0.65	1.4	1.3	0.83	1.2	1.1	0.77	1.1	1.0	0.75
Mean hours spent in all activities of at least moderate intensity per day	0.9	0.8	0.61	1.2	1.0	0.80	1.0	1.0	0.74	0.8	0.7	0.60
Calculated activity score	41	41	2.8	42	42	2.8	43	43	3.3	41	41	3.0
Bases:												
Females aged 4 to 18 years		180			210			260			239	
Females aged 7 to 18 years		145			159			221			188	

* Wave 1: January to March 1997
Wave 2: April to June 1997
Wave 3: July to September 1997
Wave 4: October to December 1997

527

Table 13.16 Measures of activity for young person by region

Measures of activity	Region											
	Scotland			Northern			Central, South West and Wales			London and the South East		
	Mean	Median	sd	Mean	Median	sd	Mean	Median	sd	Mean	Median	sd
Males aged 4 to 18 years: Hours of sedentary activity per day	2.8	2.7	1.54	2.5	2.3	1.38	2.7	2.5	1.41	2.7	2.4	1.51
Males aged 7 to 18 years Total number of activities of at least moderate intensity during the 7-day recording period	1.7	1.6	1.21	1.4	1.4	0.85	1.5	1.3	0.91	1.6	1.6	0.93
Mean hours spent in all activities of at least moderate intensity per day	1.7	1.5	1.14	1.3	1.2	0.89	1.3	1.2	0.91	1.4	1.2	0.92
Calculated activity score	44	43	3.2	43	42	3.9	43	43	3.4	43	43	3.5
Bases:												
Males aged 4 to 18 years		70			255			305			269	
Males aged 7 to 18 years		60			203			246			202	
Females aged 4 to 18 years: Hours of sedentary activity per day	2.4	2.2	1.36	2.4	2.1	1.37	2.4	2.2	1.35	2.4	1.9	1.68
Females aged 7 to 18 years Total number of activities of at least moderate intensity during the 7-day recording period	1.3	1.3	0.61	1.1	1.1	0.71	1.2	1.0	0.86	1.2	1.1	0.75
Mean hours spent in all activities of at least moderate intensity per day	1.1	1.1	0.52	0.9	0.9	0.69	1.0	0.8	0.73	1.0	0.9	0.74
Calculated activity score	42	42	2.5	42	41	3.0	42	42	3.3	42	42	3.0
Bases:												
Females aged 4 to 18 years		72			232			323			262	
Females aged 7 to 18 years		57			186			258			212	

Table 13.17 Measures of activity for young person by social class of head of household

Measures of activity	Social class of head of household								
	Non-manual			Manual			All*		
	Mean	Median	sd	Mean	Median	sd	Mean	Median	sd
Males aged 4 to 18 years:									
Hours of sedentary activity per day	2.5	2.3	1.43	2.8	2.6	1.43	2.6	2.4	1.45
Males aged 7 to 18 years:									
Total number of activities of at least moderate intensity during the 7-day recording period	1.5	1.4	0.91	1.5	1.4	0.94	1.5	1.4	0.94
Mean hours spent in all activities of at least moderate intensity per day	1.3	1.2	0.86	1.4	1.3	0.97	1.4	1.2	0.93
Calculated activity score	43	43	3.5	43	43	3.7	43	43	3.6
Bases:									
Males aged 4 to 18 years		428			413			58	
Males aged 7 to 18 years		335			330			46	
Females aged 4 to 18 years:									
Hours of sedentary activity per day	2.3	1.9	1.49	2.4	2.3	1.38	2.4	2.1	1.46
Females aged 7 to 18 years:									
Total number of activities of at least moderate intensity during the 7-day recording period	1.2	1.1	0.77	1.2	1.0	0.80	1.2	1.1	0.77
Mean hours spent in all activities of at least moderate intensity per day	1.0	0.9	0.70	1.0	0.9	0.75	1.0	0.9	0.71
Calculated activity score	42	42	3.3	42	42	3.1	42	42	3.1
Bases:									
Females aged 4 to 18 years		417			386			86	
Females aged 7 to 18 years		329			311			73	

*Includes those for whom social class could not be assigned.

Table 13.18 Measures of activity for young person by gross weekly household income

Measures of activity	Gross weekly household income														
	Less than £160			£160 to less than £280			£280 to less than £400			£400 to less than £600			£600 and over		
	Mean	Median	sd	Mean	Median	sd	Mean	Median	sd	Mean	Median	sd	Mean	Median	sd
Males aged 4 to 18 years: Hours of sedentary activity per day	3.0	2.7	1.58	2.6	2.5	1.33	2.8	2.6	1.64	2.5	2.4	1.35	2.4	2.2	1.33
Males aged 7 to 18 years: Total number of activities of at least moderate intensity during the 7–day recording period	1.6	1.4	1.11	1.4	1.3	0.95	1.5	1.4	0.94	1.6	1.6	0.87	1.5	1.4	0.88
Mean hours spent in all activities of at least moderate intensity per day	1.5	1.4	1.10	1.3	1.0	0.88	1.4	1.3	0.96	1.4	1.3	0.89	1.3	1.1	0.89
Calculated activity score	43	42	3.8	42	42	3.4	43	42	3.7	44	43	3.3	43	43	3.6
Bases:															
Males aged 4 to 18 years	28			141			165			181			219		
Males aged 7 to 18 years	26			102			128			151			170		
Females aged 4 to 18 years: Hours of sedentary activity per day	2.8	2.6	1.62	2.5	2.3	1.48	2.4	2.3	1.18	2.2	1.9	1.53	2.1	1.8	1.33
Females aged 7 to 18 years: Total number of activities of at least moderate intensity during the 7–day recording period	1.3	1.3	0.72	1.0	0.9	0.72	1.2	1.1	0.72	1.2	1.1	0.80	1.2	1.1	0.70
Mean hours spent in all activities of at least moderate intensity per day	1.1	1.0	0.75	0.9	0.8	0.68	1.0	0.9	0.61	1.0	0.9	0.71	1.0	0.9	0.70
Calculated activity score	41	41	3.0	42	41	2.9	42	42	2.4	43	42	3.4	43	42	3.2
Bases:															
Females aged 4 to 18 years	39			141			151			204			206		
Females aged 7 to 18 years	34			111			121			161			173		

Table 13.19 Measures of activity for young person by whether young person's 'parents' were receiving certain benefits

Measures of activity	Whether receiving benefits					
	Receiving benefits			Not receiving benefits		
	Mean	Median	sd	Mean	Median	sd
Males aged 4 to 18 years:						
Hours of sedentary activity per day	2.9	2.7	1.51	2.5	2.4	1.41
Males aged 7 to 18 years:						
Total number of activities of at least moderate intensity during the 7-day recording period	1.5	1.4	1.02	1.5	1.4	0.91
Mean hours spent in all activities of at least moderate intensity per day	1.4	1.2	0.95	1.3	1.2	0.93
Calculated activity score	42	42	3.3	43	43	3.6
Bases:						
Males aged 4 to 18 years		200			698	
Males aged 7 to 18 years		154			556	
Females aged 4 to 18 years:						
Hours of sedentary activity per day	2.7	2.5	1.62	2.3	2.0	1.38
Females aged 7 to 18 years:						
Total number of activities of at least moderate intensity during the 7-day recording period	1.2	1.1	0.73	1.2	1.1	0.77
Mean hours spent in all activities of at least moderate intensity per day	1.0	1.0	0.69	1.0	0.9	0.71
Calculated activity score	42	41	2.7	42	42	3.2
Bases:						
Females aged 4 to 18 years		212			676	
Females aged 7 to 18 years		170			542	

531

Table 13.20 Measures of activity by whether the young person was living with both parents

Measures of activity	Young person living with:								
	Both parents and other children			Both parents and no other children			Single parent with/out other children		
	Mean	Median	sd	Mean	Median	sd	Mean	Median	sd
Males aged 4 to 18 years:									
Hours of sedentary activity per day	2.5	2.3	1.34	2.9	2.6	1.64	2.7	2.6	1.54
Males aged 7 to 18 years:									
Total number of activities of at least moderate intensity during the 7-day recording period	1.6	1.4	0.91	1.3	1.1	0.92	1.6	1.6	0.99
Mean hours spent in all activities of at least moderate intensity per day	1.4	1.3	0.92	1.2	1.0	0.89	1.4	1.2	1.00
Calculated activity score	43	42	3.2	44	43	4.2	43	43	3.7
Bases:									
Males aged 4 to 18 years		545			183			168	
Males aged 7 to 18 years		414			163			131	
Females aged 4 to 18 years:									
Hours of sedentary activity per day	2.2	2.0	1.38	2.4	2.1	1.33	2.7	2.6	1.59
Females aged 7 to 18 years:									
Total number of activities of at least moderate intensity during the 7-day recording period	1.2	1.1	0.78	1.1	1.0	0.71	1.2	1.1	0.78
Mean hours spent in all activities of at least moderate intensity per day	1.0	0.9	0.71	0.9	0.7	0.75	1.0	1.0	0.67
Calculated activity score	42	42	2.8	43	43	3.8	42	42	2.6
Bases:									
Females aged 4 to 18 years		520			181			179	
Females aged 7 to 18 years		394			162			148	

Table 13.21 Measures of activity for young person by method of transport to school or work

Measures of activity	Method of transport to school or work					
	Walking or cycling			Motorcycle, car, bus or other		
	Mean	Median	sd	Mean	Median	sd
Males aged 4 to 18 years:						
Hours of sedentary activity per day	2.8	2.6	1.52	2.5	2.3	1.35
Males aged 7 to 18 years:						
Total number of activities of at least moderate intensity during the 7-day recording period	1.6	1.6	0.94	1.4	1.3	0.93
Mean hours spent in all activities of at least moderate intensity per day	1.5	1.3	0.94	1.3	1.1	0.92
Calculated activity score	43	42	3.5	43	43	3.6
Bases:						
Males aged 4 to 18 years		439			434	
Males aged 7 to 18 years		349			350	
Females aged 4 to 18 years:						
Hours of sedentary activity per day	2.4	2.2	1.37	2.3	2.0	1.50
Females aged 7 to 18 years:						
Total number of activities of at least moderate intensity during the 7-day recording period	1.3	1.1	0.77	1.2	1.0	0.76
Mean hours spent in all activities of at least moderate intensity per day	1.0	0.9	0.72	0.9	0.9	0.70
Calculated activity score	42	42	2.8	42	42	3.3
Bases:						
Females aged 4 to 18 years		390			474	
Females aged 7 to 18 years		301			398	

Table 13.22 Mean hours spent in sedentary activity* per day by sex and age of young person

Physical activity sample aged 4–18 years

Hours spent in sedentary activity	Males aged (years)				All males	Females aged (years)				All females
	4–6	7–10	11–14	15–18		4–6	7–10	11–14	15–18	
	cum %	cum %	cum %	cum %	cum %	cum %	cum %	cum %	cum %	cum %
More than 4 hours	4	3	7	11	6	1	1	8	10	5
More than 3 hours	10	9	16	22	15	5	7	18	21	13
More than 2 hours	25	27	35	48	34	10	15	35	45	27
More than 1 hour	47	57	68	75	63	31	45	63	70	53
Some sedentary activity	80	88	91	90	88	70	84	89	92	85
All	100	100	100	100	100	100	100	100	100	100
Base	188	263	254	194	899	176	236	255	222	889
Mean (average value)	2.2	2.4	2.7	3.1	2.6	1.7	2.1	2.7	3.0	2.4
Median value	1.9	2.2	2.5	2.9	2.4	1.5	1.9	2.5	2.7	2.1
Lower 2.5 percentile	0.2	0.4	0.5	0.5	0.4	0.1	0.3	0.4	0.5	0.3
Upper 2.5 percentile	5.7	5.6	6.2	7.2	6.0	4.6	4.6	6.3	6.5	6.1
Standard deviation of the mean	1.41	1.22	1.37	1.61	1.45	1.12	1.17	1.54	1.57	1.46

*For each day the young person was asked to estimate the time spent 'watching TV, playing computer games and listening to music'. This table does not include time spent at school or work.

Table 13.23(a) Partial correlation coefficients for measures of physical activity with dietary intakes by age of young person: males

Young people aged 7 to 18 years who kept 7–day physical activity and dietary diaries

Age (years) of young person and measure of physical activity	Dietary intake			
	Average daily total energy intake (MJ)	Percentage energy from:		
		total fat	total carbohydrate	total sugars
Partial correlation coefficients				
Males aged 7 to 10 years:				
Mean hours of sedentary activity per day	−0.04	0.01	0.08	−0.00
Total number of activities of at least moderate intensity during the 7–day recording period	0.32**	0.04	0.09	0.13*
Mean hours spent in all activities of at least moderate intensity per day	0.31**	−0.02	0.10	0.13*
Calculated activity score	0.18**	−0.11	0.06	0.10
Males aged 11 to 14 years:				
Mean hours of sedentary activity per day	−0.04	0.01	0.06	0.01
Total number of activities of at least moderate intensity during the 7–day recording period	0.05	0.03	−0.06	0.02
Mean hours spent in all activities of at least moderate intensity per day	0.11	−0.03	−0.14*	−0.05
Calculated activity score	0.10	−0.02	−0.13*	−0.06
Males aged 15 to 18 years:				
Mean hours of sedentary activity per day	0.02	0.22**	0.08	0.05
Total number of activities of at least moderate intensity during the 7–day recording period	−0.04	−0.08	0.15*	0.12
Mean hours spent in all activities of at least moderate intensity per day	−0.04	−0.07	0.04	0.02
Calculated activity score	0.10	−0.25**	−0.07	−0.03
All males aged 7 to 18 years:				
Mean hours of sedentary activity per day	0.08	0.11**	0.08	0.03
Total number of activities of at least moderate intensity during the 7–day recording period	0.06	0.00	0.06	0.09*
Mean hours spent in all activities of at least moderate intensity per day	−0.01	−0.04	−0.01	0.03
Calculated activity score	−0.06	−0.15**	−0.06	−0.01

* p < 0.05
**p < 0.01

534

Table 13.23(b)   Partial correlation coefficients for measures of physical activity with dietary intakes by age of young person: females

Young people aged 7 to 18 years who kept 7–day physical activity and dietary diaries

Age (years) of young person and measure of physical activity	Dietary intake			
	Average daily total energy intake (MJ)	Percentage energy from:		
		total fat	total carbohydrate	total sugars
Partial correlation coefficients				
Females aged 7 to 10 years:				
Mean hours of sedentary activity per day	−0.15*	0.14*	0.02	−0.07
Total number of activities of at least moderate intensity during the 7–day recording period	0.14*	−0.12	0.04	0.10
Mean hours spent in all activities of at least moderate intensity per day	0.10	−0.03	0.05	0.01
Calculated activity score	0.06	−0.17*	0.06	0.09
Females aged 11 to 14 years:				
Mean hours of sedentary activity per day	−0.00	0.03	0.10	0.02
Total number of activities of at least moderate intensity during the 7–day recording period	0.16*	−0.03	−0.02	0.07
Mean hours spent in all activities of at least moderate intensity per day	0.04	−0.02	0.04	0.10
Calculated activity score	−0.03	−0.07	−0.07	0.05
Females aged 15 to 18 years:				
Mean hours of sedentary activity per day	−0.05	0.15*	−0.01	−0.06
Total number of activities of at least moderate intensity during the 7–day recording period	0.05	0.01	−0.08	−0.02
Mean hours spent in all activities of at least moderate intensity per day	−0.02	−0.01	−0.09	−0.03
Calculated activity score	0.02	−0.14*	−0.06	0.06
All females aged 7 to 18 years:				
Mean hours of sedentary activity per day	−0.05	0.10*	0.04	−0.04
Total number of activities of at least moderate intensity during the 7–day recording period	0.12**	−0.04	−0.01	0.05
Mean hours spent in all activities of at least moderate intensity per day	0.04	−0.02	−0.00	0.03
Calculated activity score	0.01	−0.13**	−0.03	0.06

* p < 0.05
**p < 0.01

Table 13.23(c)   Base numbers for partial correlation coefficients for measures of physical activity with dietary intakes by sex and age of young person

Young people aged 7 to 18 years who kept 7-day physical activity and dietary diaries

Age (years)	Sex of young person		All
	Male	Female	
7 to 10	254	220	474
11 to 14	233	235	468
15 to 18	175	204	379
All aged 7 to 18	662	659	1321

Table 13.24(a)   Partial correlation coefficients for measures of physical activity with anthropometric measurements by age of young person: males

Young people aged 7 to 18 years who kept a 7–day physical activity diary

Age (years) of young person and measure of physical activity	Anthropometric measurements		
	Body mass index	Mid upper–arm circumference	Waist to hip ratio
	Partial correlation coefficients		
Males aged 7 to 10 years:			
Mean hours of sedentary activity per day	0.03	−0.00	na
Total number of activities of at least moderate intensity during the 7–day recording period	−0.01	0.05	na
Mean hours spent in all activities of at least moderate intensity per day	−0.04	0.00	na
Calculated activity score	−0.02	0.01	na
Males aged 11 to 14 years:			
Mean hours of sedentary activity per day	0.17**	0.11	0.06
Total number of activities of at least moderate intensity during the 7–day recording period	−0.08	−0.09	−0.14*
Mean hours spent in all activities of at least moderate intensity per day	−0.13*	−0.13*	−0.16*
Calculated activity score	−0.14*	−0.09	−0.10
Males aged 15 to 18 years:			
Mean hours of sedentary activity per day	0.04	−0.02	−0.06
Total number of activities of at least moderate intensity during the 7–day recording period	0.03	0.04	−0.04
Mean hours spent in all activities of at least moderate intensity per day	0.02	0.05	0.01
Calculated activity score	0.04	0.09	−0.01
All males aged 7 to 18 years:			
Mean hours of sedentary activity per day	0.08*	0.04	−0.01
Total number of activities of at least moderate intensity during the 7–day recording period	−0.02	0.01	−0.11*
Mean hours spent in all activities of at least moderate intensity per day	−0.05	−0.02	−0.07
Calculated activity score	−0.03	0.00	−0.02
Bases: males aged			
7 to 10 years	*264*	*263*	*na*
11 to 14 years	*253*	*253*	*253*
15 to 18 years	*192*	*192*	*192*
All males aged 7 to 18 years	*709*	*708*	*445*

* p < 0.05
**p < 0.01
na not applicable.

Table 13.24(b) Partial correlation coefficients for measures of physical activity with anthropometric measurements by age of young person: females

Young people aged 7 to 18 years who kept a 7–day physical activity diary

Age (years) of young person and measure of physical activity	Anthropometric measurements		
	Body mass index	Mid upper–arm circumference	Waist to hip ratio
	Partial correlation coefficients		
Females aged 7 to 10 years:			
Mean hours of sedentary activity per day	0.02	0.01	na
Total number of activities of at least moderate intensity during the 7–day recording period	−0.06	−0.03	na
Mean hours spent in all activities of at least moderate intensity per day	−0.04	0.02	na
Calculated activity score	−0.03	0.03	na
Females aged 11 to 14 years:			
Mean hours of sedentary activity per day	0.12	0.13	−0.02
Total number of activities of at least moderate intensity during the 7–day recording period	−0.11	−0.08	−0.08
Mean hours spent in all activities of at least moderate intensity per day	−0.07	−0.06	0.02
Calculated activity score	−0.08	−0.08	−0.03
Females aged 15 to 18 years:			
Mean hours of sedentary activity per day	0.06	0.07	0.11
Total number of activities of at least moderate intensity during the 7–day recording period	−0.13	−0.13	0.16*
Mean hours spent in all activities of at least moderate intensity per day	−0.14*	−0.13	0.07
Calculated activity score	−0.04	−0.03	0.04
All females aged 7 to 18 years:			
Mean hours of sedentary activity per day	0.08*	0.09*	0.09
Total number of activities of at least moderate intensity during the 7–day recording period	−0.09*	−0.07	0.04
Mean hours spent in all activities of at least moderate intensity per day	−0.08*	−0.05	0.05
Calculated activity score	−0.05	−0.03	0.03
Bases: females aged			
7 to 10 years	*233*	*234*	*na*
11 to 14 years	*247*	*251*	*246*
15 to 18 years	*220*	*221*	*220*
All females aged 7 to 18 years	*700*	*706*	*466*

* p < 0.05
**p < 0.01
na not applicable.

537

Table 13.25(a)   Partial correlation coefficients for measures of physical activity with blood pressure by age of young person: males

Young people aged 7 to 18 years who kept a 7–day physical activity diary and had blood pressure measured

Age (years) of young person and measure of physical activity	Blood pressure	
	Systolic pressure (mmHg)	Diastolic pressure (mmHg)
	Partial correlation coefficients	
Males aged 7 to 10 years:		
Mean hours of sedentary activity per day	0.05	−0.01
Total number of activities of at least moderate intensity during the 7–day recording period	−0.04	−0.02
Mean hours spent in all activities of at least moderate intensity per day	−0.09	−0.13*
Calculated activity score	−0.03	−0.10
Males aged 11 to 14 years:		
Mean hours of sedentary activity per day	0.18**	0.08
Total number of activities of at least moderate intensity during the 7–day recording period	−0.11	−0.11
Mean hours spent in all activities of at least moderate intensity per day	−0.16*	−0.08
Calculated activity score	−0.21**	−0.08
Males aged 15 to 18 years:		
Mean hours of sedentary activity per day	0.02	0.16*
Total number of activities of at least moderate intensity during the 7–day recording period	0.09	0.17**
Mean hours spent in all activities of at least moderate intensity per day	0.02	0.07
Calculated activity score	0.04	−0.03
All males aged 7 to 18 years:		
Mean hours of sedentary activity per day	0.08*	0.07
Total number of activities of at least moderate intensity during the 7–day recording period	−0.02	0.00
Mean hours spent in all activities of at least moderate intensity per day	−0.09*	−0.06
Calculated activity score	−0.06	−0.05
Bases: males aged		
7 to 10 years	261	
11 to 14 years	252	
15 to 18 years	192	
All males aged 7 to 18 years	705	

* p < 0.05
**p < 0.01

Table 13.25(b)   Partial correlation coefficients for measures of physical activity with blood pressure by age of young person: females

Young people aged 7 to 18 years who kept a 7-day physical activity diary and had blood pressure measured

Age (years) of young person and measure of physical activity	Blood pressure	
	Systolic pressure (mmHg)	Diastolic pressure (mmHg)
	Partial correlation coefficients	
Females aged 7 to 10 years:		
Mean hours of sedentary activity per day	0.08	0.03
Total number of activities of at least moderate intensity during the 7-day recording period	−0.11	−0.07
Mean hours spent in all activities of at least moderate intensity per day	-0.15*	−0.09
Calculated activity score	−0.11	−0.08
Females aged 11 to 14 years:		
Mean hours of sedentary activity per day	0.07	0.09
Total number of activities of at least moderate intensity during the 7-day recording period	−0.08	-0.06
Mean hours spent in all activities of at least moderate intensity per day	−0.12	−0.13
Calculated activity score	−0.05	−0.10
Females aged 15 to 18 years:		
Mean hours of sedentary activity per day	0.01	−0.01
Total number of activities of at least moderate intensity during the 7-day recording period	−0.10	−0.02
Mean hours spent in all activities of at least moderate intensity per day	−0.06	0.00
Calculated activity score	−0.04	−0.01
All females aged 7 to 18 years:		
Mean hours of sedentary activity per day	0.06	0.03
Total number of activities of at least moderate intensity during the 7-day recording period	−0.09*	−0.06
Mean hours spent in all activities of at least moderate intensity per day	−0.10**	−0.08*
Calculated activity score	−0.06	−0.05

Bases: females aged
7 to 10 years	*229*
11 to 14 years	*247*
15 to 18 years	*218*
All females aged 7 to 18 years	*694*

* p < 0.05
**p < 0.01

13.26(a) Characteristics found to be independently related to calculated activity score: males aged 7 to 18 years

Characteristic	Unstandardised coefficient (B)	Standard error of B	Standardised regression coefficient (β)	T–value
Constant (calculated activity score)	52.31	5.85		
Age at physical activity diary (years)	0.15	0.06	0.14	2.45*
Whether at school or work				
School	−1.47	0.26	−0.25	−5.56***
Work	1.54	0.45	0.18	3.44***
School and work	−1.17	0.34	−0.14	−3.42***
No school or work	1.10	0.36	0.13	3.07**
Fieldwork wave†				
Wave 1	−0.53	0.22	−0.11	−2.38*
Wave 2	0.61	0.23	0.12	2.65**
Wave 3	0.77	0.26	0.16	3.03**
Wave 4	−0.85	0.22	−0.17	−3.90***
Whether living with both parents				
Both parents & other children	0.16	0.24	0.03	0.69
Both parents & no other children	−0.17	0.29	−0.02	−0.58
Single parent & other children	0.67	0.34	0.08	1.97*
Single parent & no other children	−0.66	0.40	−0.11	−1.65
Gross weekly household income				
Less than £160	0.33	0.35	0.07	0.94
£160 – less than £400	−0.43	0.20	−0.11	−2.16*
£400 & over	0.10	0.27	0.02	0.39
Average daily total energy intake (MJ)				1.74
Percentage energy from total fat				−1.89
Percentage energy from total carbohydrate				−1.05
Percentage energy from total sugars				0.46
Systolic blood pressure (mmHg)				−1.50
Diastolic blood pressure (mmHg)				−0.48
BMI (kg/m²)††				−0.59
Whether unwell during dietary recording period				
Not unwell				0.28
Unwell & eating not affected				0.13
Unwell & eating affected				−0.35
Region				
Scotland				0.58
Northern				−1.16
Central, South West & Wales				−0.24
London & South East				0.47
Social class of head of household				
Non–manual				−0.79
Manual				0.46
Unclassified				0.24
Parents were receiving benefits				−1.43
Reported currently smoking				−0.37
Reported dieting to lose weight				0.78
Average daily alcohol intake (g)				1.50
Percentage of variance explained	25%			
Number of young people	*630*			

* $p < 0.05$; ** $p < 0.01$; *** $p < 0.001$

† Wave 1: Jan – March 1997; Wave 2: April – June 1997; Wave 3: July – Sept 1997; Wave 4 Oct – Dec 1997 see also *Glossary*

†† Height and BMI were highly correlated (co-linear) with weight (variance inflation factor > 10). It is difficult to distinguish the effects in a multiple regression of highly correlated characteristics if both are included and the results may be unreliable. One characteristic of a co-linear pair must be dropped. Since it is important to investigate the relationship between physical activity and measures of body shape, weight and height were dropped from the regression.

13.26(b) Characteristics found to be independently related to calculated activity score: males aged 10 to 16 years with plasma testosterone concentration

Characteristic	Unstandardised coefficient (B)	Standard error of B	Standardised regression coefficient (β)	T–value
Constant (calculated activity score)	58.77	11.40		
Age at physical activity diary (years)				0.45
Fieldwork wave †				
Wave 1	−0.87	0.40	−0.19	−2.16*
Wave 2	0.60	0.50	0.12	1.19
Wave 3	1.03	0.44	0.24	2.33*
Wave 4	−0.76	0.37	−0.17	−2.07*
Social class of head of household				
Non–manual	−0.70	0.38	−0.13	−1.86
Manual	−0.58	0.38	−0.11	−1.53
Unclassified	1.29	0.58	0.23	2.21*
Average daily alcohol intake (g)	0.02	0.01	0.16	2.32*
Reported dieting to lose weight				1.90
Whether at school or work				
School				−1.65
Work				1.13
School and work				−1.75
No school or work				1.67
Systolic blood pressure (mmHg)				−1.66
Diastolic blood pressure (mmHg)				−0.07
BMI (kg/m^2)††				−1.68
Plasma testosterone concentration				
Bottom tertile				−0.66
Middle tertile				−0.09
Top tertile				0.79
Whether unwell during dietary recording period				
Not unwell				−0.05
Unwell & eating not affected				−0.60
Unwell & eating affected				0.67
Whether living with both parents				
Both parents & other children				0.54
Both parents & no other children				−0.16
Single parent & other children				1.10
Single parent & no other children				−1.15
Region				
Scotland				0.88
Northern				−0.28
Central, South West & Wales				−0.49
London & South East				−0.70
Gross weekly household income				
Less than £160				1.19
£160 – less than £400				−1.32
£400 & over				−0.58
Parents were receiving benefits				−1.55
Reported currently smoking				−0.22
Average daily total energy intake (MJ)				1.50
Percentage energy from total fat				−1.14
Percentage energy from total carbohydrate				−0.71
Percentage energy from total sugars				0.34
Percentage of variance explained		22%		
Number of young people		*224*		

* p < 0.05; ** p < 0.01; *** p < 0.001
† Wave 1: Jan – March 1997; Wave 2: April – June 1997; Wave 3: July – Sept 1997; Wave 4: Oct – Dec 1997 see also *Glossary*
†† Height and BMI were highly correlated (co-linear) with weight (variance inflation factor > 10). It is difficult to distinguish the effects in a multiple regression of highly correlated characteristics if both are included and the results may be unreliable. One characteristic of a co-linear pair must be dropped. Since it is important to investigate the relationship between physical activity and measures of body shape, weight and height were dropped from the regression.

13.26(c)   Characteristics found to be independently related to calculated activity score: females aged 7 to 18 years

Characteristic	Unstandardised coefficient (B)	Standard error of B	Standardised regression coefficient (β)	T–value
Constant (calculated activity score)	37.15	5.20		
Age at physical activity diary (years)	0.24	0.07	0.26	3.42***
Average daily total energy intake (MJ)	0.00	0.00	−0.03	−0.63
Percentage energy from total fat	0.00	0.00	0.03	0.27
Percentage energy from total carbohydrate	0.00	0.00	0.01	0.08
Percentage energy from total sugars	0.00	0.00	0.18	3.29***
Fieldwork wave†				
Wave 1	−0.38	0.22	−0.08	−1.72
Wave 2	0.27	0.21	0.06	1.28
Wave 3	0.61	0.24	0.14	2.60**
Wave 4	−0.50	0.21	−0.11	−2.37*
Whether at school or work				
School	−0.81	0.25	−0.19	−3.29**
Work	0.58	0.36	0.09	1.61
School and work	−0.60	0.32	−0.09	−1.87
No school or work	0.83	0.30	0.13	2.76**
Region				
Scotland	0.34	0.33	0.06	1.02
Northern	−0.54	0.21	−0.14	−2.60**
Central, South West & Wales	0.11	0.20	0.03	0.53
London & South East	0.10	0.21	0.02	0.46
Average daily alcohol intake (g)	0.01	0.00	0.12	2.34*
Whether living with both parents				
Both parents & other children				−0.41
Both parents & no other children				1.68
Single parent & other children				−0.25
Single parent & no other children				−0.86
Systolic blood pressure (mmHg)				0.42
Diastolic blood pressure (mmHg)				−0.71
BMI (kg/m²)††				−0.25
Whether unwell during dietary recording period				
Not unwell				1.54
Unwell & eating not affected				0.23
Unwell & eating affected				−1.32
Social class of head of household				
Non–manual				0.50
Manual				−0.07
Unclassified				−0.32
Gross weekly household income				
Less than £160				0.03
£160 – less than £400				−0.62
£400 & over				0.42
Parents were receiving benefits				−0.23
Reported currently smoking				−1.21
Reported dieting to lose weight				1.59
Monthly periods had started				−1.36
Percentage of variance explained		20%		
Number of young people		*568*		

* p < 0.05; ** p < 0.01; *** p < 0.001
† Wave 1: Jan – March 1997; Wave 2: April – June 1997; Wave 3: July – Sept 1997; Wave 4: Oct – Dec 1997 see also *Glossary*
†† Height and BMI were highly correlated (co-linear) with weight (variance inflation factor > 10). It is difficult to distinguish the effects in a multiple regression of highly correlated characteristics if both are included and the results may be unreliable. One characteristic of a co-linear pair must be dropped. Since it is important to investigate the relationship between physical activity and measures of body shape, weight and height were dropped from the regression.

Table 13.27 Participation in activity of at least moderate intensity by sex and age in single years compared with the Health of Young People '95–'97†

Young people aged 7 to 15 years living in England

Participation in activity	Age (years)								
	7	8	9	10	11	12	13	14	15
Males									
Health Survey 1995–97*									
% who did not participate	9	3	4	3	2	2	2	2	4
% who did participate	91	97	96	97	98	98	98	98	96
Mean number of days***	5.28	5.66	5.92	5.98	5.96	6.02	6.09	6.23	5.95
Standard error of the mean	0.16	0.13	0.13	0.13	0.12	0.12	0.13	0.11	0.14
Mean number of hours***	10.01	10.34	11.43	12.29	10.57	11.41	11.12	10.33	8.53
Standard error of the mean	0.58	0.56	0.67	0.67	0.55	0.61	0.74	0.65	0.58
Base	*265*	*280*	*242*	*246*	*265*	*250*	*198*	*236*	*207*
NDNS 1997**									
% who did not participate	2	–	–	–	2	2	–	–	3
% who did participate	98	100	100	100	98	98	100	100	97
Mean number of days***	6.04	6.04	5.87	6.01	5.67	5.61	5.58	5.51	5.25
Standard deviation of the mean	1.35	1.39	1.38	1.36	1.79	1.41	1.56	1.66	1.89
Mean number of hours***	10.95	11.43	10.21	10.78	9.84	9.56	11.10	10.73	7.86
Standard deviation of the mean	6.43	7.15	5.77	6.86	5.93	4.59	7.77	5.83	4.05
Base	*57*	*74*	*65*	*67*	*77*	*58*	*56*	*63*	*56*
Females									
Health Survey 1995–97*									
% who did not participate	7	5	4	4	3	5	3	4	6
% who did participate	93	95	96	96	97	95	97	96	94
Mean number of days***	5.25	5.29	5.48	5.22	5.34	5.20	5.40	5.36	4.90
Standard error of the mean	0.15	0.15	0.14	0.15	0.15	0.16	0.16	0.15	0.17
Mean number of hours***	8.74	8.07	7.57	7.67	6.69	5.92	5.65	5.61	4.00
Standard error of the mean	0.57	0.48	0.48	0.50	0.50	0.47	0.46	0.48	0.36
Base	*269*	*267*	*252*	*274*	*238*	*220*	*215*	*237*	*207*
NDNS 1997**									
% who did not participate	8	4	–	2	2	1	4	–	4
% who did participate	92	96	100	98	98	99	96	100	96
Mean number of days***	5.23	5.30	5.45	5.02	5.12	4.88	4.90	4.90	4.53
Standard deviation of the mean	2.22	1.93	1.76	1.72	1.65	1.82	1.99	1.78	2.21
Mean number of hours***	7.91	8.67	7.29	7.20	7.49	7.13	7.82	6.13	6.59
Standard deviation of the mean	5.54	5.09	4.37	4.40	4.70	5.45	6.13	3.21	5.71
Base	*59*	*47*	*68*	*62*	*62*	*70*	*59*	*64*	*59*

* Figures based on participation for at least 15 minutes a day.
** Figures based on participation for at least 10 minutes a day.
*** Means based on all informants.
† Prescott-Clarke P, Primatesta P. Eds. *Health Survey for England. The Health of Young People '95–97. Volume 1. Findings.* TSO (London, 1998).

Figure 13.1(a)   Proportion of young people taking part in selected activities during 7-day recording period – males

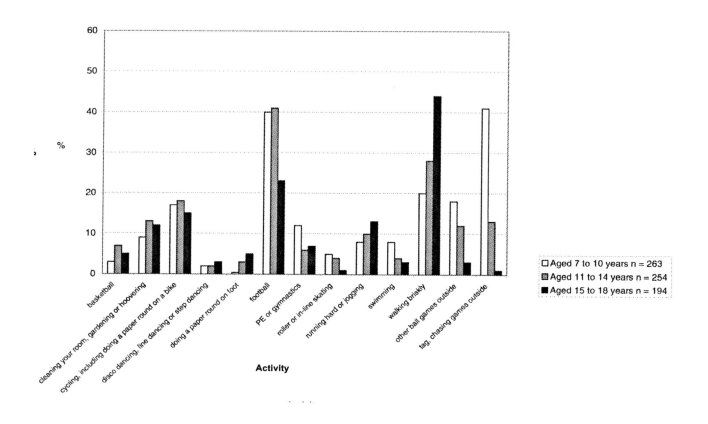

Figure 13.1(b)   Proportion of young people taking part in selected activities during 7-day recording period – females

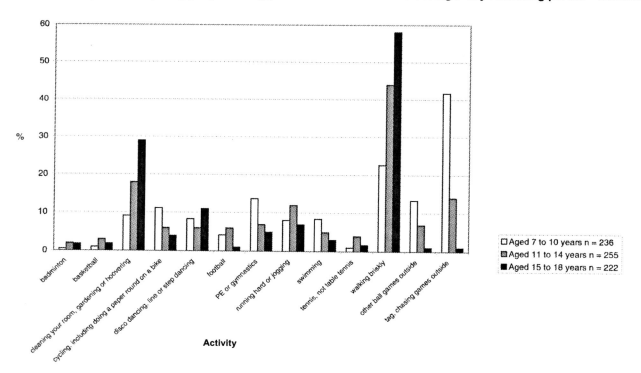

Appendices

Appendix A Fieldwork documents[1]

(see also Appendices B and M)

Sample

Postal sift form
Interviewer sift form (non-responders)
Multi-household selection sheet (example)
Advance letter

Purpose leaflets

General	L1
General – child's version	L2
Physical measurements	L3

Interview

Main interview questionnaire	
Prompt cards	
Dietary interview	A–G
Smoking and drinking self-completion[2]	S2

Dietary survey

Home Record Diary	
Eating and drinking away from home diary, including physical activity diary[3]	
Young person's pocket notebook and diary	P3
How to use the scales for weighing	W1
Check list for recording in the Home Record Diary	W2

Interviewer documents	
Food descriptions prompt card	F1
Eating pattern check sheet	F2
School catering questionnaire	F3
Guide weights card	F5
Dietary assessment schedule	F7
Letter to school re: collecting catering information	F8

Bowel movements

Bowel movements card[4]	B1

Physical measurements

Measurements schedule[5]	M1
Young person's record card[6]	M2

Spot urine sample

Instructions for young person	W3

---

[1] Fieldwork documents for the oral health survey are reproduced as an Appendix to Volume 2 of this report.
[2] Example is for girls aged 10 years and over, which included questions on the contraceptive use and age at menarché.
[3] For those aged 4 to 6 years, diary pages for recording physical activity were omitted.
[4] Bowel movements away from home were recorded in the Eating Away from Home Diary.
[5] Measurements were recorded by the interviewer at the time they were made on this paper document. They were subsequently entered into the CAPI program.
[6] For those aged 4 to 6 years this record card omitted waist and hip circumferences.

Social Survey Division

OFFICE FOR NATIONAL STATISTICS

Tel: 0171 396 2020

Dear Resident(s)

I am writing to ask for your help in planning for a survey to be carried out later this year by this Office for the Department of Health and the Ministry of Agriculture, Fisheries and Food. This survey will find out about the health, eating habits and lifestyles of people in Great Britain.

It is important when we carry out this survey that the people we talk to are representative of the whole country, in terms of their age, gender and where they live, otherwise the findings from the survey will not accurately reflect the circumstances of people in Britain today. Your address is one of 28,000 chosen at random from a complete list of all the addresses in Great Britain, which is compiled by the Post Office.

As we do not have information on the ages of individuals living in these addresses, we need to find this information out in advance of the survey so we are asking for your help in completing the short form on the back of this letter; collecting the information in this way is much cheaper and quicker than asking our interviewers to call at all the addresses. We would like you to list the gender (sex) and date of birth of everyone, including yourself, who usually lives at the address shown on the label at the top of this letter. We do not need to know any names.

In all our surveys we rely on people's voluntary co-operation, which is essential if our work is to be successful. Any information you give will be treated in confidence and the results will not be presented in a way which can be associated with anyone's name or address. No identifiable information will be passed to any other government department, local authorities, members of the public or to the press.

I hope you can spare the time to help us with this survey.

Please return the completed form to us, as soon as possible, in the envelope provided; no stamp is needed. If you have any queries please ring me on the number shown at the top of this letter.

Thank you for your help

Yours faithfully

Sarah Lowe
Research Assistant

If no-one lives permanently at the address on the label at the top of this letter, please tick one of the boxes below and return this form in the envelope provided.

Vacant..........	54	No permanent residents eg holiday home.	56
Used for business purposes only..........	55	Institution, eg hotel, nursing home	57

1 Drummond Gate, London, SW1V 2QQ

Social Survey Division Enquiries (020) 7533 5500   Fax (020) 7533 5300   Visit our website at: http://www.ons.gov.uk

---

Please complete parts 1, 2 and 3 below. At parts 1 and 2 please include everyone, including yourself, who usually lives in your household at the address shown on the label at the top of the letter.

Please also include anyone who usually lives in your household but is temporarily away, for example, because they are in hospital, at school or on holiday. **Exclude** anyone who lives somewhere else permanently.

1. How many people, including yourself, are there in your household living at this address?

Total number of people in the household →

Number

2. For each person in the household, including yourself, please give their gender (sex) and date of birth.

	Gender (sex) Please tick		Date of birth Please write in the day, month and year		
	Male	Female	Day	Month	Year
1					
2					
3					
4					
5					
6					
7					
8					
9					
10					

3. Is any part of the address shown on the label overleaf separately occupied by people not listed above?

Yes   No

Tick one box →

Please return this form as soon as possible in the envelope provided.
Thank you for your help

HC323 4/98

Interviewer sift form (non-responders)

ND NS — NATIONAL DIET AND NUTRITION SURVEY

NATIONAL STATISTICS

B-N1404 (Non-responders and concealed m.h'hlds)

Serial number label

INTERVIEWER SIFT FORM
PLEASE COMPLETE THIS FORM FOR EVERY ADDRESS ON YOUR LIST

RECORD

1 Is this serial number:

a concealed multi-household (with a copy of completed postal sift form)?...... X → Q2
or
a postal sift non-responder (no completed postal sift form)?...... Y

2 Did you find the address?

Yes .... X → Q3
No .... Y → Q7

3 Was the whole address.....

vacant/demolished?.................. 64
business premises?.................. 65
no permanent residents?.................. 66 → END
an institution?.................. 67
an eligible address?.................. X → Q4

4 Is this address occupied by more than one household?

Yes .... X → (a)
No .... Y → Q5

(a) IF YES
PLEASE COMPLETE A MULTI-HOUSEHOLD SELECTION
SHEET AND SELECT HOUSEHOLD

WRITE IN HOUSEHOLD NUMBER SELECTED →

ADDRESS OF SELECTED HOUSEHOLD
Please describe as fully as possible, including flat number.

_____
_____
POSTCODE _____ → Q5

1

ASK

5 How many people are there in your household, living at this address?   WRITE IN NUMBER →

6 **RECORD DETAILS OF THOSE IN THE HOUSEHOLD**

| | Gender (sex) | | Date of birth | | |
	Male	Female	Day	Month	Year
1					
2					
3					
4					
5					
6					
7					
8					
9					
10					

7 **RECORD FINAL OUTCOME**

Full interview 12
Completed, but recall refused (spontaneous)...... 23
Outright refusal 33
Non-contact 41
Could not find address......................... 63

8 PLEASE RECORD THE NUMBER OF CALLS MADE AT THIS ADDRESS
IN THE BOX →

END

RETURN THIS FORM AND COMPLETED MULTI-HOUSEHOLD SELECTION
SHEET, IF USED, IN ENVELOPE PROVIDED, ADDRESSED TO SIU, TITCHFIELD.

2

Multi-household selection sheet (example)

OFFICE FOR NATIONAL STATISTICS

Interviewer's name.................

Office Use ☐

Serial number label

NATIONAL DIET AND NUTRITION SURVEY: YOUNG PEOPLE AGED 4 TO 18 YEARS

Multi-household selection sheet [A]

To be returned to SIU with interviewer sift form

List households

H/hld no. (1)	DESCRIPTION OF HOUSEHOLDS eg location and surnames (2)	No of h/hlds found at address (3)	Interview at household number (4)
1		1	1
2		2	2
3		3	3
4		4	3
5		5	2
6		6	5
7		7	7
8		8	8
9		9	5
10		10	7
11		11	5
12		12	6

IF MORE THAN 12 HOUSEHOLDS PLEASE TURN OVER PAGE →

Procedure:

1 Note down the households on the table above. This must be done systematically. If they are numbered, then list in numerical order, ie flat 1, 2, 3 etc or flat A, B, C etc. Otherwise start at the lowest floor then work and list in clockwise direction.

2 Ring the total number of households found at (3). Read column (4) to identify which household to select for 'interviewing'. Ring the selected household number in column (1).

3 Attach this form to the corresponding interviewer sift form and return to SIU.

FOR USE ONLY ON THE NDNS: YOUNG PERSONS AGED 4 TO 18 YEARS.

NOTE: SELECT ONLY <u>ONE</u> HOUSEHOLD

H/hld no. (1)	DESCRIPTION OF HOUSEHOLDS eg location and surnames (2)	No of h/hlds found at address (3)	Interview at household number (4)
13		13	2
14		14	14
15		15	3
16		16	4
17		17	8
18		18	13
19		19	7
20		20	14
21		21	10
22		22	20
23		23	21
24		24	7
25		25	1
26		26	22
27		27	12
28		28	7
29		29	19
30		30	20

If more than 30 households: ring SIU - 01329 81 3064

Attach this form to the corresponding interviewer sift form and return in the envelope provided, addressed to SIU, Titchfield.

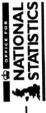

OFFICE FOR
NATIONAL STATISTICS

Social Survey Division

Tel: 0171 533 5387/8

Date as postmark

Dear Resident(s)

YOUNG PERSON'S NUTRITION SURVEY

I am writing to tell you about a survey that this Office, together with the Medical Research Council's Dunn Nutrition Unit, will shortly be carrying out. The main aim of the survey is to find out what young people are eating these days and to relate this to characteristics such as their age, sex, height and weight. The results of the survey will provide a better understanding of the relationship between what young people eat and their health and will help to improve the health of all young people in the future as they grow up.

You will probably remember either filling in a form that we sent you on which you gave information on who lives at your address, or being visited by one of our interviewers. We are now asking one of our interviewers to call on you in the next few weeks to tell you more about the survey and invite your household to take part.

I would like to assure you that any information you or any member of your household gives will be kept in strict confidence by this Office and the Dunn Nutrition Unit. Only ourselves at the Social Survey Division of ONS and the Ministry of Agriculture, Fisheries and Food (MAFF) will see the completed questionnaires, but your name and address will not be given to MAFF, to any other government department, to local authorities, members of the public or to the press. The survey results, which will be published, will not be presented in a form which can be associated with names and addresses; they will be published as tables of results and statistics. The survey is being carried out on behalf of MAFF and the Department of Health (DH).

As in all our surveys we rely on voluntary co-operation; this is essential if our work is to be successful and the results of this survey are to be an accurate account of young people's nutrition in Great Britain today. We have in the past carried out similar nutrition surveys for DH and MAFF, on different age groups in the population, and those who have taken part have found it an interesting experience; I am sure that you will find it interesting and do hope that you will be able to help us.

If you have any questions that you would like to ask before our interviewer calls please contact me on 0171 533 5387/8 (direct line).

Thanking you in anticipation of your help.

Yours faithfully

Jan Gregory
Principal Researcher

1 Drummond Gate, London, SW1V 2QQ
Social Survey Division Enquiries (0171) 533 5500   Fax (0171) 533 5300

551

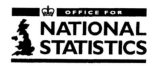

Young people aged 4 to 18 years

This survey is being carried out by the Social Survey Division of the Office for National Statistics in collaboration with the Medical Research Council's Dunn Nutrition Unit in Cambridge, for the Ministry of Agriculture, Fisheries and Food and the Department of Health (in England, Wales and Scotland). This leaflet tells you more about why the survey is being done.

HC48/5 2/97

L1

1. What is it about?

Over the past twenty years or so there has been a considerable increase in the range of foods available in the shops, and for many people, this has meant changes in the kinds of foods they eat.

We have been asked to carry out a large national survey to find out, in detail, about the eating habits of young people in Great Britain. Everyone taking part will be asked to keep a record for 7 days of everything that they eat and drink, while they are at home and when they are out. The survey will also collect information about the young people themselves, not only their age and sex, but also some physical measurements, such as their height and weight, blood pressure and information about their level of physical activity. They will also be asked to provide a small sample of blood and of urine. This information, together with information about the foods they eat and the activities they take part in will provide a better understanding about the important relationship between diet and health in young people.

All the physical measurements will be taken by our interviewers who have been carefully trained, and the blood sample will be taken by qualified people who are particularly skilled in taking blood from young people.

2. Why have we come to your household?

To visit every household in the country would take too long and cost far too much money.

Therefore we selected a sample of addresses from the Postcode Address File and called on them. The Postcode Address File is compiled by the Post Office and lists all the addresses to which mail is sent. We sent a letter to each selected address asking for details of the age and sex of everybody living there. We chose the addresses in a way that gave everyone the same chance of being selected. From the replies we were able to tell which households contained a young person aged 4 to 18, and from those we selected a sample to be interviewed. Your household is one of those chosen to be interviewed.

Some people think either that they or their family are not typical enough to be of any help in the survey or that they are very different from other people and they would distort the survey findings.

The important thing to remember is that the community consists of a great many different types of people and families and we need to represent them all in our survey. We would therefore greatly appreciate it if everyone we approach agrees to take part.

3. Is the survey confidential?

Yes. We take very great care to protect the confidentiality of the information we are given. Access to the completed questionnaires and diaries is restricted to the Social Survey Division of ONS and the Ministry of Agriculture, Fisheries and Food (MAFF). However, the names and addresses of co-operating households will not be released to MAFF, to any other government department, to local authorities, members of the public or the press. The survey results will not be presented in a form which can be associated with names and addresses.

4. Is the survey compulsory?

In all our surveys we rely on voluntary co-operation, which is essential if our work is to be successful.

We give a gift voucher as a small token of our appreciation for keeping the food diary provided the diary is kept for the full number of days.

We hope this leaflet answers some of the questions you might have and that it shows the importance of the survey. The interviewer will leave another leaflet with you which tells you more about the measurements we are making and the blood sample.

Your co-operation is very much appreciated.

If you have any questions, or would like further information, please contact me, Jan Gregory, at:

Social Survey Division
Office for National Statistics
1 Drummond Gate
London SW1V 2QQ

Telephone 0171 533 5387/8

Purpose leaflet (General – Child's version)

Do you have to do it?

No - but I hope you will as it is a very important study. What's more when we tried the survey on some young people earlier in the year they said they enjoyed taking part.

And...when you complete the food diary for us, the interviewer will give you a £5 token which you can spend.

Where can you find out more?

The interviewer will try to answer any questions you or your parent(s) have and has some other information leaflets.

Or, if you like you can write, or speak to me, Jan Gregory, at:

Social Survey Division
Office for National Statistics
1 Drummond Gate
London SW1V 2QQ

Telephone 0171 533 5387/8

Thank you very much for your help.

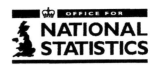

Young people aged 4 to 18 years

Social Survey Division of the Office for National Statistics, and the Medical Research Council's Dunn Nutrition Unit, have been asked by the Ministry of Agriculture, Fisheries and Food and the Department of Health to carry out a survey to find out what young people eat and drink. We would like YOU to take part. Read on to find out more......

L2

HC46/4 2/97

What do we want you to do?

The survey will find out, in great detail, about what young people are eating and drinking these days.

We would like you to help in the survey by keeping a diary for us, writing down everything that you eat and drink at home and when you are away from home. Our interviewer would also like to ask you some questions about yourself and to take some measurements, like your height, weight and blood pressure. If you are willing we would also like you to collect a very small sample of your urine for us - we will provide the container - and allow a qualified and experienced person to come with the interviewer to your home and take a small sample of blood from your arm.

We will try to help you as much as possible. Our interviewer will answer any questions you and your parent(s) have, and visit you from time to time to help you with your diary. You will be able to use the interviewer's computer to answer some of the questions if you like, or you can use pencil and paper if your prefer.

Our interviewer has explained the survey to your parent(s) and got agreement that you can take part.

Why have we come to your address?

By chance... we started by selecting, at random, 28,000 addresses all over Great Britain from a list of all the addresses in the country that the Post Office holds. Then we wrote to them all and asked the people who lived there to tell us the dates of birth of everyone in the household. From these completed forms we could find out which addresses contained young people between the aged of 4 and 18 years. Your address is one of them.

Between now and the end of this year about 2,000 young people like yourself, from all over Great Britain, and all between the ages of 4 and 18 years, will be taking part in this important survey.

You might think either that what you eat is very different from what your friends eat and that including you in the survey would distort the findings - or you might think you are just the same as everyone else and we should find someone who is very different. Neither of these is true - we need to represent all the different types of young people in the country in our survey if it is to give an accurate picture of what young people are eating these days - so we do hope that everyone we ask will agree to take part.

Who will know you've taken part?

We take very great care to protect the confidentiality of the information you give us. No-one in any other government department, in your local authority or the public generally, will know your name and address or be told by us that you have taken part in this survey. When we write a report about the survey, the results will be about young people as a whole; we do not give anyone's name or any other information which could identify an individual.

If you would like to keep your own diary of what you eat when you are not at home private, then our interviewer will give you an envelope that you can keep it in, and it will not be shown to or discussed with anyone else in your home.

553

Purpose leaflet (Physical measurements)

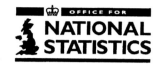

Young people aged 4 to 18 years

This survey is being carried out by the Social Survey Division of the Office for National Statistics in collaboration with the Medical Research Council's Dunn Nutrition Unit in Cambridge, for the Ministry of Agriculture, Fisheries and Food and the Department of Health (in England, Wales and Scotland).

This leaflet tells you more about measurements we are making and the blood and urine samples.

HC45/5 2/97

L3

1. *Height, weight and other measurements*

Obviously what young people eat affects their weight, so we are interested in the weight of the young people in the survey. By itself though, weight is of limited use because taller people will probably weigh more anyway. Hence we need to know about weight in relation to size and the amount of muscle and fat. Therefore we need to measure the young person's height, and the circumference of their arm, and for those aged 11 and over their waist and hip measurements, which are useful indicators of body size.

Very little is known about the range of blood pressures in young people aged between 4 and 18. This survey will provide valuable information on this and allow us to see whether there is any relationship between diet and blood pressure in young people. If you agree, the young person's blood pressure will be measured and the result sent to the young person's GP immediately after the interviewer's visit. Although you can be told the results, the interviewer cannot interpret them for you; your GP would be able to give you more information about the blood pressure result.

2. *Blood sample*

This is a very important aspect of the survey as the analysis of all the blood samples from young people in the survey will tell us a great deal about their health and give us further information on their diet. Providing a blood sample is, of course, voluntary.

A small amount of blood (no more than 15ml) is taken from the young person's arm using new, sterile equipment by a qualified person who is skilled in taking blood from young people in this age range. The blood is sent to laboratories, in Cambridge,

Southampton and Great Ormond Street Children's Hospital in London, for a number of analyses, including measurements of haemoglobin, ferritin and vitamins.

Haemoglobin is the red pigment in the blood which carries oxygen. A low level of haemoglobin in the blood is called anaemia. One reason for a low level of haemoglobin may be a shortage of iron. Ferritin is a measure of the body's iron stores.

If there is any of the blood sample remaining after all the analyses have been carried out we ask for your consent to it being stored for possible further analyses in the future. The sample will not be used now or in the future for viral analyses such as an AIDS test.

With your consent we will let the young person's GP know that they are taking part in the survey and will let you and, with consent, the GP know the results of the blood analyses.

If you consent to the young person's GP receiving results, of either the blood pressure measurement or blood sample analysis, then they may be used by the GP to help him/her monitor the young person's health. The GP may also wish to include the results in any future report about the young person, but they would not be passed on without the GP first obtaining your permission.

3. *Urine sample*

We would like to have a small sample of urine from each young person in the survey. This can be analysed to tell us the level of salt in their diet; this cannot be accurately measured from information in the food diary.

4. *Are the measurements compulsory?*

In all our surveys we rely on voluntary co-operation, which is essential if our work is to be successful. The measurements and the blood and urine samples are a particularly important part of this survey, as from these results we can find out much more about the health of young people than would be possible with just the information about their diet.

5. *Flagging on the NHSCR*

The Department of Health and MAFF would like to be able to know about the health of the young people that take part in this survey as they grow older. We would therefore like your consent to flag the name of the young person on the National Health Service Central Register (NHSCR), so that their health in future years can be monitored.

We hope this leaflet answers some of the questions you might have and that it shows the importance of the survey.

Your co-operation is very much appreciated.

If you have any questions, or would like any further information, please contact me, Jan Gregory, at:

Social Survey Division
Office for National Statistics
1 Drummond Gate
London SW1V 2QQ

Telephone 0171 533 5387/8

Initial dietary interview

COMPLETE FOR EACH YOUNG PERSON

Areacode	Information already entered
Address	Information already entered
Hhld	Information already entered
Wave	Information already entered
IntDate	Enter the date on which first interview started
	_ _ . _ _ . _ _ _ _ (date variable format)

NPerson **All**

ASK OR RECORD

How many people normally live in this household?

1..14

HOUSEHOLD BOX

INFORMATION TO BE COLLECTED FOR EACH PERSON IN THE HOUSEHOLD

Name00..13 **All**

RECORD NAME YOUNG PERSON IS KNOWN BY.
FOR SUBSEQUENT MEMBERS OF HOUSEHOLD RECORD THE NAME OF NEXT HOUSEHOLD MEMBER

Sex00..13 All

CODE SEX OF EACH PERSON IN HOUSEHOLD

Male 1
Female 2

Dob00..13 **For young person only**

Can you tell me *young person's* date of birth?

_ _ . _ _ . _ _ _ _ (date variable format)

Age00..13 All

(Can I just check,) what was ... 's age last birthday?

0..99

Marsta00..13 All aged over 15 years

Are you/is ... married, living together as a couple, single, widowed, divorced or separated?

Married 1
Cohabiting (living together, opposite sex) 2
Single/never been married 3
Widowed 4
Divorced 5
Separated 6
Same sex cohabiting 7

ReltoY00..13 **If NPerson > 1**

What is the relationship of ... to *young person*?

Spouse 1
Cohabitee 2
Son/daughter (incl. adopted) 3
Step-son/daughter 4
Foster child 5
Birth parent 6
Adoptive parent 7
Step-parent 8
Foster parent 9
Parent-in-law 10
Brother/sister (incl. adopted) 11
Step-brother/sister 12
Foster brother/sister 13
Brother/sister-in-law 14
Grandparent 15
Other relative 16
Other non-relative 17

[Hidden variables calculated within program]

If 1 at NPerson - *single-person household, then:*

MaNo **MaNo = 0**
No mother in household
(*MaNo > 0 value = PerNo of Mother*)

PaNo **PaNo = 0**
No father in household
(*PaNo > 0 value = PerNo of Father*)

GaNo	GaNo = 0 No grandparent in household	**ACCOMMODATION**

1. YPInd   **If MaNo = 0 and PaNo = 0 and GaNo = 0**

If NPerson greater than 1 – more than one person in household, then

When did you leave home, move away from your parent's home?

RECORD PERIOD. ENTER IN MONTHS <u>OR</u> YEARS

MaNo   **If code 2 at Sex and codes 6 to 9 at ReltoYP**

0.00..36.00

MaNo = value at NPerson
'Mother figure' in household

a. MYears   CODE WHETHER PERIOD ENTERED AS MONTHS OR YEARS

If (else)

MaNo = 0
No mother in household

Months 1
Years 2

GaNo   **If code 15 at ReltoYP**

2. HOH   **All**

GaNo = value at NPerson
Grandparent in household

ASK OR RECORD

Which member of your household is the head of the household?

If (else)

GaNo = 0
No grandparent in household

1..14

PaNo   **If code 1 at Sex and codes 6 to 9 at ReltoYP**

3. Info   **All**

CODE WHICH MEMBER OF THE HOUSEHOLD IS THE INFORMANT

PaNo = value at NPerson

If (else)

1..14

PaNo = 0
No father in household

4. School   **All**

What does *young person* <u>mainly</u> do?

XMother   **If MaNo ne 0**
XMother = 1

Not yet started school or nursery 1
At school (including nursery) 2

If MaNo = 0
XMother = 0

At college 3
Other training 4
Working 5

XFather   **If PaNo ne 0**
XFather = 1

Unemployed 6
Other (Specify at next question) 7

If PaNo = 0
XFather = 0

a. SOther   **If code 7 at School**

SPECIFY OTHER OCCUPATION

556

5. Coast   **All**

ASK OR RECORD

Do you live within 5 miles of the coast?

Yes 1
No 2

6. Kitchen   **All**

Do you have a kitchen, that is a separate room in which you cook?

Yes 1
No 2

a. ShareKit   If code 1 at Kitchen

Do you share the kitchen with any other household?

Yes 1
No 2

b. Meal   If code 2 at Kitchen

Are you able to cook a hot meal in this accommodation?

Yes 1
No 2

7. CSkill   All

In the last month has *young person* cooked a dish using several different ingredients?

Yes 1
No 2

CONSUMER DURABLES

1.   **All**

Does your household have any of the following items in your (part of the) accommodation?

INCLUDE ITEMS STORED AND UNDER REPAIR

a. Consum1   Refrigerator?

Yes 1
No 2

b. Consum2   Deep freezer or fridge freezer?

Yes 1
No 2

c. Consum3   Microwave oven?

Yes 1
No 2

4. CarVan   **All**

Is there a car or van <u>normally</u> available for use by you or any members of your household?

INCLUDE ANY PROVIDED BY EMPLOYERS IF NORMALLY AVAILABLE FOR PRIVATE USE BY INFORMANT OR MEMBERS OF THE HOUSEHOLD.

EXCLUDE VEHICLES USED SOLELY FOR THE CARRIAGE OF GOODS.

Yes 1
No 2

a. Cars   **If code 1 at CarVan**

Is there one or more than one?

1 1
2 2
3 or more 3

EATING HABITS

1. SchMeal   **If aged under 15 years or codes 2, 3 or 4 at School**

Can I check, when *young person* is at school what type of lunch-time meal is s/he currently having?

PRIORITY CODES 1 AND 2

Free school meal 1
Reduced price or subsidised school meal 2
Paid school meal 3
Packed lunch 4
Other (Specify at next question) 5
No lunch time meal 6

a. SchOth   **If code 5 at SchMeal**

SPECIFY OTHER LUNCH-TIME MEAL

2. WkMeal   **If code 5 at School**

Can I check, when *young person* is at work what type of lunch-time meal does s/he usually have?

CODE ONLY ONE

Packed lunch 1
Meal bought on work premises 2
Meal bought outside work 3
Other (Specify at next question) 4

No lunch-time meal 5

a. WkOther   **If code 4 at WkMeal**

SPECIFY OTHER LUNCH-TIME MEAL

3. Vary   **All**

How would you describe the variety of foods that *young person* generally eats?

Does s/he ....

RUNNING PROMPT

eat most things 1
eat a reasonable variety of things 2
or is s/he a fussy or faddy eater? 3

4. App   **All**

Does *young person* have ....

RUNNING PROMPT

a good appetite 1
an average appetite, or 2
a poor appetite for a young person of his/her age?.. 3

DRINKING

1. Milk   **All**

Nowadays, does *young person* have cow's milk as a drink?

INCLUDE ANY DRINK WHERE MILK IS PRIMARY INGREDIENT E.G. MILKSHAKE, HOT CHOCOLATE MADE WITH MILK (NOT WATER)

Yes 1
No 2

a. MilkA   **If code 2 at Milk**

Has s/he ever had cow's milk as a drink?

Yes 1
No 2

ai. Kind   **If code 1 at Milk or code 1 at MilkA**

What kind of milk does *young person* usually have as a drink these days?

PROMPT AS NECESSARY
CODE ALL THAT APPLY

Whole milk 1
Semi-skimmed milk 2
Skimmed milk 3
Powdered baby milk 4
Soya milk 5
Doesn't have any milk 6
Other (Specify at next question) 7

aii. KindC   **If code 7 at Kind**

SPECIFY THE OTHER KIND(S) OF MILK YOUNG PERSON HAS

2. KindB **All**

What kind of milk does *young person*
usually have on cereal and in
puddings these days?

PROMPT AS NECESSARY
CODE ALL THAT APPLY

Whole milk 1
Semi-skimmed milk 2
Skimmed milk 3
Powdered baby milk 4
Soya milk 5
Doesn't have any milk 6
Other (Specify at next question) 7

a. KindA **If code 7 at KindB**

SPECIFY OTHER KIND(S) OF MILK
YOUNG PERSON HAS

3. Tea **All**

Does *young person* drink tea?

Yes 1
No 2

a. TeaA **If code 1 at Tea**

Does s/he usually take sugar in tea, is it
sweetened with artificial sweetener, or
does s/he drink tea without sugar or
sweetener?

Sugar in tea 1
Artificial sweetener in tea 2
Drinks tea unsweetened 3

b. TeaB **If code 1 at Tea**

On average how many cups per day does
s/he drink?

IF LESS THAN ONE CODE AS 0
IF GREATER THAN 10 CODE AS 11

0..11

4. Herb **All**

May I check, does *young person* drink
herbal teas or herbal drinks?

Yes 1
No 2

a. HerbA **If code 1 at Herb**

On average, how often does s/he drink
herbal teas or have a herbal drink?

More than once a day 1
Once a day 2
Most days 3
At least once a week 4
At least once a month 5
Less than once a month 6

b. HBrand0..5 **If code 1 at Herb**

What brands of herbal tea or herbal
drink is *young person* drinking at the
moment?

RECORD FULL BRAND NAME OF
ALL HERBAL TEAS/DRINKS

c. HType0..5 **If code 1 at Herb**

What flavour is that herbal tea or herbal
drink?

RECORD FLAVOUR FOR EACH
HERBAL TEA/DRINK

d. BRAND If code 1 at Herb
0..05

ENTER BRAND CODE FOR EACH
HERBAL TEA/DRINK

00001..99997

5. Coff **All**

Does *young person* drink coffee?

Yes 1
No 2

a. CoffA **If code 1 at Coff**

Does s/he usually take sugar in coffee, is
it sweetened with an artificial
sweetener, or does s/he drink coffee
without sugar or sweetener?

Sugar in coffee 1
Artificial sweetener in coffee 2
Drinks coffee unsweetened 3

b. CoffB **If code 1 at Coff**

On average how many cups per day does
s/he drink?

IF LESS THAN ONE CODE AS 0

IF GREATER THAN 10 CODE AS 11

0..11

6. Cook   **All**

(Apart from in tea and coffee) do you use artificial sweeteners to sweeten any of *young person's* food, either at the table or in cooking?

Yes 1
No 2

a. CookA   **If code 1 at Cook**

Do you use an artificial sweetener either at the table or in cooking:

..to sweeten stewed or cooked fruit?

Yes used 1
Not used 2

SPONTANEOUS: Not eaten 3

b. CookB   ..to sweeten fresh fruit?

Yes used 1
Not used 2

SPONTANEOUS: Not eaten 3

c. CookC   ..to sweeten breakfast cereals?

Yes used 1
Not used 2

SPONTANEOUS: Not eaten 3

d. CookD   ..to sweeten cakes, biscuits or pastry that are home made?

Yes used 1
Not used 2

SPONTANEOUS: Not eaten 3

e. CookE   ..to sweeten drinks other than tea or coffee?

Yes used 1
Not used 2

SPONTANEOUS: Not eaten 3

f. CookF   ..to sweeten any other food or drink?

Yes used 1
Not used 2

SPONTANEOUS: Not eaten 3

7. Brands0..5   **If code 2 at TeaA or code 2 at CoffA or code 1 at Cook**

FOR EACH ARTIFICIAL SWEETENER USED

What brands of artificial sweetener are you using to sweeten *young person's* food and drinks at the moment?

RECORD FULL NAME OF ALL ARTIFICIAL SWEETENER(S)

a. SType0..5   **If code 2 at TeaA or code 2 at CoffA or code 1 at Cook**

FOR EACH ARTIFICIAL SWEETENER USED

What form does that artificial sweetener take?

Tablet (INCLUDE MINICUBES) 1
Liquid 2
Granulated 3

b. BRAND   **If code 2 at TeaA or**
06..11   **code 2 at CoffA or code 1 at Cook**

FOR EACH ARTIFICIAL SWEETENER USED ENTER THE BRAND CODE FOR THIS PRODUCT

00001..99997

SALT

13. Salt   **All**

Do you usually add salt to *young person's* food during cooking?

Yes, includes sea salt 1
Yes, uses 'Lo-Salt'/ salt alternative (not sea salt) 2
No, does not use salt in cooking 3
Other (Specify at next question) 4

560

a. SaltA	**If code 4 at Salt**	

SPECIFY OTHER SALT ADDED IN COOKING

14. Tabl **All**

<u>At the table</u>, do you or *young person* add salt to his/her food ..

RUNNING PROMPT

usually	1
occasionally	2
rarely	3
or never?	4

a. TablA **If codes 1 to 3 at Tabl**

And can I check, what kind of salt do you add to *young person's* food <u>at the table</u>?

Ordinary salt, including sea salt	1
'Lo-Salt'/ salt alternative (<u>not</u> sea salt)	2
Other (Specify at next question)	3

ai. SaltJ **If code 3 at TablA**

SPECIFY OTHER SALT ADDED AT TABLE

FOOD FREQUENCIES

Intro1 All

I would now like to ask you about a whole range of foods (some of which you may already have told me *young person* doesn't eat). Can you tell me about how often, on average s/he eats these foods? Please choose your answer from this card ..

SHOW CARD A

More than once a day	1
Once a day	2
Most days	3
At least once a week	4
At least once a month	5
Less than once a month	6
Never	7

PROMPT EACH FOOD
FOR SEASONAL FOODS ADD
'..at this time of year'

01 Cereal	Breakfast cereals
02 BiscS1	Biscuits–sweet
03 BiscS2	Biscuits–savoury
04 Cakes	Cakes
05 Yogs	Yogurt (flavoured or plain but not fromage frais), including frozen yogurt and yogurt drinks
06 FromF	Fromage frais, plain or flavoured
07 Cheese	Cheese or cheese spread (not fromage frais)
08 CMilk	Cow's milk (not soya, sheep or goats), including in cooking
09 GMilk	Sheep or goat's milk, including in cooking
10 SMilk	Soya milk, including in cooking
11 IceC	Ice cream (not ice lollies)
12 IceL	Ice lollies
13 Eggs	Eggs, including in home cooking
14 Beef	Beef, including beef products Includes carcass beef purchased raw, cooked and canned beef, corned beef,

	beef in manufactured products e.g. burgers, pies etc. not beef sausages or beef offal.
15 Pork	Pork, including pork products, ham, gammon or bacon. Includes carcass pork purchased raw, cooked pork and pork in manufactured products e.g. pies etc. not pork sausages or offal.
16 Lamb	Lamb or mutton, including products. Includes carcass lamb purchased raw and lamb in manufactured products e.g. pies, etc.–not offal.
17 Chick	Chicken and poultry, including products. Includes purchased raw and in manufactured products e.g. pies, nuggets, burgers, etc.–not offal.
18 Game	Game, including grouse, hare, partridge, pheasant, pigeon, rabbit and venison.
19 Saus	Sausages; English-type requiring cooking. Not continental sausages or vegetarian sausages
20 Liver	Liver and liver products, including liver pate and liver sausage
21 Offal	Other offal e.g. kidney. Any offal except liver
22 OFish	Oily fish (e.g. herring, mackerel, sardines, pilchards, salmon) including products e.g. salmon/smoked mackerel pate
23 SFish	Shellfish e.g. prawns and shrimps
24 Leafy	Leafy green vegetables, including broccoli, greens, spinach. Not cauliflower, courgettes, or leeks
25 SSnack	Savoury snacks including crisps not nuts
26 Nuts	Nuts and nut products: all types of nut; nut roast
27 Juice	Fruit juice; not fruit drinks, squash
28 Carb1	Fizzy drinks; NOT diet/low calorie/no added sugar/sugar free. Exclude mineral water
29 Carb2	Fizzy drinks : diet/low calorie/no added

	sugar/sugar free. Exclude mineral water
30 Conc1	Concentrated fruit drinks: squashes– NOT diet/low calorie/no added sugar/ sugar free
31 Conc2	Concentrated fruit drinks: squashes– diet/low calorie/no added sugar/ sugar free
32 RDF1	Ready to drink fruit drinks: NOT diet/ low calorie/no added sugar/sugar free. Exclude fruit juice
33 RDF2	Ready to drink fruit drinks: diet/low calorie/no added sugar/ sugar free. Exclude fruit juice
34 Choc	Chocolate–confectionery
35 Sweet1	Sugar confectionery
36 Sweet2	Sugar-free confectionery, labelled 'sugar free'
37 SGum	Chewing gum; <u>not</u> sugar-free gum
38 FGum	Sugar-free chewing gum, labelled 'sugar free'

Why01..38   **If code 7 at any item above**

FOR EACH ITEM CODED 7 ASK:

Why does s/he never eat (ITEM NEVER EATEN)?

CODE ALL THAT APPLY

Allergy 1
Religious reasons 2
Health reasons 3
Vegetarian/vegan .4
Doesn't like it 5
Can't afford it 6
Can't get (in this area) 7
Other (Specify at next question) 8

Othe01..38   **If code 8 at Why01..38**

SPECIFY OTHER REASON(S) FOR EACH ITEM NEVER EATEN

AllA01..38   **If code 1 at Why01..38**

AllB01..38 FOR EACH FOOD ITEM WITH ALLERGY ASK:

What form does the allergy take?

CODE ALL THAT APPLY

Hyperactivity/behavioural problems or
changes e.g. tantrums and moods,
aggressive and bad tempered 1
Rash/blotches all over 2
Eczema 3
Asthma/wheeze 4
Upset stomach/diarrhoea/vomiting ...5
Swelling to face/neck/hands 6
Itching (not due to eczema or itchy
eyes) 7
Weight loss/failure to thrive 8
Runny nose/itchy or sore eyes/nasal
symptoms 9
Migraine 10
Other (Specify at next question) 11

Alle201..45 If code 11 at AllA01..38 or AllB01..38

SPECIFY OTHER ALLERGIC
REACTION(S)

AllC01..38 If code 1 at Why01..38

FOR EACH FOOD ITEM WITH
ALLERGY ASK:

Has this allergy been diagnosed by a
doctor?

Yes 1
No 2

Intro2 All

How often, on average, does *young
person* eat each of these foods?

SHOW CARD A

More than once a day 1
Once a day 2
Most days 3
At least once a week 4
At least once a month 5
Less than once a month 6
Never 7

PROMPT EACH FOOD LISTED
FOR SEASONAL FOODS ADD:
'.. at this time of the year'

39 CarotR Raw carrots

40 CarotC Cooked carrots

41 Roots Other root vegetables, apart from carrots
and potatoes e.g. parsnips,
turnips, swedes

42 MushB Mushrooms

43 Apple Apples (fresh)

44 Pear Pears (fresh)

45 Citrus Citrus fruits e.g. oranges, tangerines,
satsumas

46 Toms Fresh tomatoes

47 Cucs Cucumber

Skin01..09 If code ne 7 at any item above

NB **Skin01** applies if **CarotC** ne 7
Skin02 applies if **CarotR** ne 7

FOR EACH ITEM ASK:

Can you tell me whether s/he usually eats
the skin on (FOOD ITEM)?

Yes 1
No 2

Why39..47 If code 7 at any food item above

FOR EACH ITEM CODED 7 ASK:

Why does s/he never eat (ITEM NEVER
EATEN)?

CODE ALL THAT APPLY

Allergy 1
Religious reasons 2
Health reasons 3
Vegetarian/vegan 4
Doesn't like it 5
Can't afford it 6
Can't get (in this area) 7
Other (Specify at next question) 8

Othe39..47 If code 8 at Why39..47

SPECIFY OTHER REASON(S) EACH
ITEM NEVER EATEN

AllA39..47
AllB39..47

If code 1 at Why39..47

FOR EACH FOOD ITEM WITH ALLERGY ASK:

What form does the allergy take?

CODE ALL THAT APPLY

Hyperactivity/behavioural problems or changes e.g. tantrums and moods, aggressive and bad tempered 1
Rash/blotches all over 2
Eczema 3
Asthma/wheeze 4
Upset stomach/diarrhoea/vomiting ... 5
Swelling to face/neck/hands 6
Itching (not due to eczema or itchy eyes) 7
Weight loss/failure to thrive 8
Runny nose/itchy or sore eyes/nasal symptoms 9
Migraine 10
Other (Specify at next question) 11

a. Alle232..40 If code 11 at AllA39..47 or AllB39..47

SPECIFY OTHER ALLERGIC REACTION(S)

AllC39..47 If code 1 at Why39..47

FOR EACH FOOD ITEM WITH ALLERGY ASK:

Has this allergy been diagnosed by a doctor?

Yes 1
No 2

All

ASK FOR EACH FOOD ITEM LISTED BELOW

Does young person eat the skin on (FOOD ITEM) always, sometimes or never?

Always eaten with skin left on 1
Sometimes eaten with skin left on 2
Never eaten with the skin left on 3
Never eaten 4

a. Baked baked or jacket potatoes, cooked without fat

b. BoilNew boiled new potatoes

c. BoilOld boiled old potatoes

d. Roast roast potatoes, cooked in fat

e. Fried fried potatoes or chips

AlRel **All**

(Apart from the foods you have already told me about) are there any (other foods that young person avoids because s/he is allergic to them, or for religious, health or other reasons?

Yes 1
No 2

Which0..4 If code 1 at AlRel

Which food(s) does young person avoid?

SPECIFY ALL OTHER FOODS AVOIDED

Why48..52 If code 1 at AlRel

FOR EACH ITEM AVOIDED ASK:

Why does s/he never eat (ITEM NEVER EATEN)?

CODE ALL THAT APPLY

Allergy 1
Religious reasons 2
Health reasons 3
Vegetarian/vegan 4
Doesn't like it 5
Can't afford it 6
Can't get (in this area) 7
Other (Specify at next question) 8

Othe48..52 If code 8 at Why48..52

SPECIFY OTHER REASON(S) EACH ITEM NEVER EATEN

AllA48..52
AllB48..52

If code 1 at Why48..52

FOR EACH FOOD ITEM WITH ALLERGY ASK:

What form does the allergy take?

CODE ALL THAT APPLY

Hyperactivity/behavioural problems or changes e.g. tantrums and moods, aggressive and bad tempered 1
Rash/blotches all over 2
Eczema 3
Asthma/wheeze 4
Upset stomach/diarrhoea/vomiting ...5
Swelling to face/neck/hands 6
Itching (not due to eczema or itchy eyes) 7
Weight loss/failure to thrive 8
Runny nose/itchy or sore eyes/nasal symptoms 9
Migraine 10
Other (Specify at next question) 11

a. Alle221 0..14

If code 11 at AllA48..52 or AllB48..52

SPECIFY OTHER ALLERGIC REACTION(S)

AllC48..52 **If code 1 at Why48..52**

FOR EACH FOOD ITEM WITH ALLERGY ASK:

Has this allergy been diagnosed by a doctor?

Yes 1
No 2

SLIMMING

Slim **All**

Can I check, is *young person* dieting to lose weight at the moment?

Yes 1
No 2

1. Veg **All**

Can I check, is *young person* a vegetarian or a vegan?

Yes 1
No 2

2. VegA **If code 1 at Veg**

(Apart from foods you have already told me about) what foods does s/he avoid?

CODE ALL THAT APPLY

Red meat 1
White meat 2
Fish 3
Eggs 4
Milk 5
Other dairy products–butter, cheese ...6
All animal products 7
Avoids other food (Specify at next question) 8

a. VegAW **If code 8 at VegA**

SPECIFY OTHER FOOD(S) AVOIDED

3. VegB **If code 1 at Veg**

Why did s/he become a vegetarian/ vegan?

CODE ALL THAT APPLY

Moral or ethical reasons (includes cruelty to animals) 1
Religious reasons 2
Health reasons 3
Preference (doesn't like the taste of meat) 4
Convenience, cost 5
Other (Specify at next question) 6

a. VegBW **If code 6 at VegB**

SPECIFY OTHER REASON(S) FOR VEGETARIANISM

4. VegC **If code 1 at Veg**

Where did s/he get information about a vegetarian/vegan diet?

CODE ALL THAT APPLY

Parents or other relatives 1
Friends 2
Doctor/GP 3
Dietician/nutritionist 4
Vegetarian Society/Vegan Society 5
Newspapers, magazines, books 6
TV / radio 7
Other (Specify at next question) 8

Did not get any information 9

a. VegD   **If code 8 at VegC**

SPECIFY WHERE GOT
INFORMATION

ORGANIC FOODS AND DRINKS

1. Organic   **All**

A lot of shops and supermarkets are
selling foods which are labelled as
'organic' or 'organically grown'. What
do you understand by the term 'organic'
or organically grown?

Grown without pesticides and without
artificial fertilisers 1
Grown without pesticides 2
Grown without artificial fertilisers or
'grown without chemicals 3
Free range 4
A health food–healthier/better for you 5
Something else–including no antibiotics/
hormones, fresh or naturally grown fruit
and veg 6

Don't know, don't understand 7

a. OrgElse   **If code 6 at Organic**

SPECIFY OTHER ANSWER(S) TO
MEANING OF ORGANIC

2. OrgBuy   **All**

Do you buy any 'organic' foods for
young person?

Yes 1
No 2

3   **If code 1 at OrgBuy**

ASK FOR EACH FOOD ITEM
BELOW

Do you buy organic (FOOD ITEM) for
him/her always, sometimes or never?

a. OrgFFrut   ..fresh fruit, including fruit juice..

Always 1
Sometimes 2
Never 3

b. OrgDFrut   ..dried fruit..

Always 1
Sometimes 2
Never 3

c. OrgNut   .. organic nuts..

Always 1
Sometimes 2
Never 3

d. OrgVeg   ..organic vegetables, including celery,
dried beans or lentils..

Always 1
Sometimes 2
Never 3

e. OrgCer   ..organic cereal products, bread, rice,
muesli, pasta etc..

Always 1
Sometimes 2
Never 3

f. OrgMeat   ..organic meat, including chicken..

Always 1
Sometimes 2
Never 3

g. OrgEggs   .. organic eggs (free range)..

Always 1
Sometimes 2
Never 3

h. OrgMilk   ..organic milk..

Always 1
Sometimes 2
Never 3

i. OrgDair   ..organic dairy products (eg yogurt)..

Always 1
Sometimes 2
Never 3

j. OrgSnak   ..organic crisps and savoury snacks..

Always 1
Sometimes 2
Never 3

k. OrgCake   ..organic biscuits and cakes, including cereal crunchy bars..

Always 1
Sometimes 2
Never 3

l. OrgConf   ..organic confectionery..

Always 1
Sometimes 2
Never 3

m. OrgOth   Do you buy anything else that is organic for him/her?

Yes 1
No 2

i. OrgSpec0..2 If code 1 at OrgOth

What else do you buy?

ii. OrgOft0..2 If code 1 at OrgOth

ASK FOR EACH OTHER ORGANIC ITEM BOUGHT

Do you buy (ANSWER AT ORGSPEC) for him/her always or sometimes?

Always 1
Sometimes 2
Never 3

FREE FOODS

1. Hens   **All**

Do you or does anyone in your household keep hens or other animals to provide you with food?

Yes 1
No 2

2. HensA   **If code 1 at Hens**

What kinds of food do these animals provide?

CODE ALL THAT APPLY

Eggs 1
Milk/milk products 2
Meat 3
Honey 4
Other (Specify at next question) 5

a. HensB   **If code 5 at HensA**

SPECIFY OTHER FOOD(S) FROM KEPT ANIMALS

3. Allot   **All**

Do you grow your own fruit and vegetables, either in your garden or on an allotment?

INCLUDE SALAD VEGETABLES AND HERBS GROWN IN THE GARDEN/ALLOTMENT

EXCLUDE HERBS GROWN ON THE WINDOW-LEDGE

EXCLUDE PRODUCE GROWN IN THE GARDEN OF A FRIEND OR RELATIVE

Yes 1
No 2

a. AllotA   **If code 1 at Allot**

Do you grow them without using pesticides?

Yes, all 1
Yes, some 2
No, none 3

567

b. AllotB   **If code 1 at Allot**

Do you grow them without using any
<u>artificial</u> fertilisers?

Yes, all 1
Yes, some 2
No, none 3

4. Free   **All**

Apart from food you grow yourself, does
young person ever eat any 'free
foods' that you have picked, or got
yourself (for example fish, berries,
mushrooms, windfall apples) ?

Yes 1
No 2

a. FreeA   **If code 1 at Free**

What 'free' foods do you eat?

CODE ALL THAT APPLY

Game (rabbit, partridge, pheasant etc.) 1
Venison 2
Berries 3
Other fruit (apples, pears etc.) 4
Fungi (mushrooms) 5
Fish 6
Other (Specify at next question) 7

i. FreeB   **If code 7 at FreeA**

SPECIFY OTHER 'FREE' FOODS

5. Farm   **All**

Do you <u>buy</u> any foods directly from a
farm?

Yes 1
No 2

a. FWhich   **If code 1 at Farm**

What foods do you buy from a farm?

CODE ALL THAT APPLY

Meat 1
Fish 2
Milk 3
Other dairy (yogurt, cheese, butter) ... 4
Eggs 5
Fruit 6
Vegetables 7

Other (Specify at next question) 8

b. FWhichA   **If code 8 at FWhich**

SPECIFY OTHER FOODS BOUGHT
FROM A FARM

STORE CUPBOARD

1.   **All**

Thinking about any food you have in the
house <u>today</u>, which of the
following items do you have here today?

a. Today1   A breakfast cereal?

Yes 1
No 2

b. Today2   Bread, or bread rolls?

Yes 1
No 2

c. Today3   Milk?

Yes 1
No 2

d. Today4   Eggs?

Yes 1
No 2

e. Today5   A tin of baked beans or spaghetti?

Yes 1
No 2

f. Today6   Potatoes?

Yes 1
No 2

g. Today7   Biscuits, of any kind?

Yes 1
No 2

2.   **All**

Thinking now about different foods that
come in cans.
How long, on average, would you keep ...

PROMPT EACH FOOD ITEM

...in an opened can before eating them?

SHOW CARD B

More than a week 1
No more than 4 or 5 days 2
No more than 2 or 3 days 3
No more than 1 day 4
Use on same day 5

SPONTANEOUS: Never stored in
open can 6

SPONTANEOUS: Not eaten/drunk ..7

a. Cans1 Baked beans

b. Cans2 Other canned vegetables

c. Cans3 Spaghetti

d. Cans4 Canned fruit

e. Cans5 Corned beef

f. Cans6 Canned soup

g.Cans7 Canned fish, for example sardines, tuna

FOOD SUPPLEMENTS

1. Fluor **All**

At present are you taking/giving *young person* fluoride tablets or drops?

Yes 1
No 2

a. FName **If code 1 at Fluor**

RECORD FULL NAME OF
FLUORIDE SUPPLEMENT,
INCLUDING BRAND

b. FForm **If code 1 at Fluor**

RECORD FORM

Tablets 1
Capsules 2
Drops 3
Liquid / syrup 4
Powder 5

c. FDose **If code 1 at Fluor**

RECORD DOSE

Dose: no. of tablets, drops, 5 ml spoons

INTERVIEWER OPEN A NOTE IF
NECESSARY

01..10

d. FFreq **If code 1 at Fluor**

RECORD FREQUENCY–NUMBER
OF TIMES AND PERIOD

Once a day 1
Twice a day 2
Three times a day 3
Four times a day 4
Five times a day 5

e. FLicNo **If code 1 at Fluor**

RECORD PRODUCT LICENCE NO.
(IF ANY)

ENTER '0' IF NONE AVAILABLE

............/........... (product licence
variable format)

f. FCat **If code 1 at Fluor**

SYSTEM ENTRY: SUPPLEMENT
CODE FOR FLUORIDE = 1

2. Vita **All**

At present (apart from fluoride tablets/
drops) is *young person* taking any
extra vitamins or minerals as tablets,
pills, powders, syrups or drops?

INCLUDE PRESCRIBED AND NON-
PRESCRIBED SUPPLEMENTS E.G.
CHILDREN'S VITAMIN DROPS,
MULTIVITAMIN TABLETS, IRON
TABLETS.

EXCLUDE DRINKS, YOGURTS OR
FOODS FORTIFIED WITH
VITAMINS

Yes 1
No 2

3. IntroS   **If code 1 at Vita**

ASK RESPONDENT FOR
SUPPLEMENT CONTAINERS

a. Name0..9   **If code 1 at Vita**

RECORD FULL NAME,
INCLUDING BRAND OF EACH
SUPPLEMENT

b. FormIn00..09

If code 1 at Vita

RECORD FORM OF EACH
SUPPLEMENT

Tablets 1
Capsules 2
Drops 3
Liquid / syrup 4
Powder 5

c. VDose0..9   **If code 1 at Vita**

RECORD DOSE TAKEN OF EACH
SUPPLEMENT: NO. OF TABLETS,
DROPS, 5 ml SPOONS

01..10

d. VFreq0..9   **If code 1 at Vita**

CODE FREQUENCY EACH
SUPPLEMENT TAKEN: NO. OF
TIMES AND PERIOD

Once a day 1
Twice a day 2
Three times a day 3
Four times a day 4
Five times a day 5

e. VLicNo0..9   **If code 1 at Vita**

RECORD PRODUCT LICENCE NO.
(IF ANY) OF EACH SUPPLEMENT

ENTER 0 IF NONE AVAILABLE

............./........... (product licence
variable format)

f. Categor0..9   **If code 1 at Vita**

CODE CATEGORY FOR EACH
SUPPLEMENT

Fluoride only 1
Cod liver oil and other fish-based
supplements 2
Evening primrose oil type supplements 3
Vitamin C only 4
Other single vitamins, not vitamin C ..5
Vitamins A, C and D only 6
Vitamins with iron 7
Iron only 8
Multivitamins and multi-minerals 9
Multivitamins, no minerals 10
Minerals only; not fluoride or iron
only 11
Other (Specify at next question) 12

g. Vother0..9   **If code 12 at categor0..9**

SPECIFY OTHER KIND FOR EACH
SUPPLEMENT

4. Herbal   **All**

Does *young person* take any herbal
preparations or other traditional
remedies?

Yes 1
No 2

5. IntroH   **If code 1 at Herbal**

INTERVIEWER: ASK
RESPONDENT FOR HERBAL
REMEDY
CONTAINERS

a. Name10..18 **If code 1 at Herbal**

RECORD FULL NAME OF EACH
HERBAL REMEDY

b. Brand0..9   **If code 1 at Herbal**

RECORD BRAND NAME OF EACH
HERBAL REMEDY

c. Plant0..9   **If code 1 at Herbal**

RECORD MAIN PLANT
INGREDIENT OF EACH HERBAL
REMEDY

d. Strong0..9   **If code 1 at Herbal**

RECORD STRENGTH OF EACH
HERBAL REMEDY
(INCLUDE MG ETC.)

e. Dose0..9   **If code 1 at Herbal**

RECORD DOSE TAKEN OF EACH
HERBAL REMEDY: NO. OF
TABLETS, DROPS, 5 ML SPOONS

01..10

f. Freq0..9   **If code 1 at Herbal**

CODE FREQUENCY EACH
HERBAL REMEDY TAKEN: NO. OF
TIMES AND PERIOD

Once a day 1
Twice a day 2
Three times a day 3
Four times a day 4
Five times a day 5

**g. Formin
10..19**   **If code 1 at Herbal**

CODE FORM OF EACH HERBAL
REMEDY

Form
Tablets 1
Capsules 2
Drops 3
Liquid / Syrup 4
Powder 5

h. LicNo0..9   **If code 1 at Herbal**

RECORD PRODUCT LICENCE NO.
(IF ANY) OF EACH HERBAL
REMEDY

ENTER 0 IF NONE AVAILABLE

............/............ (product licence
variable format)

**YOUNG PERSON'S LEVEL OF
ACTIVITY**

1. Desc   **If young person aged 4 to 6 years**

How would you describe *young person's*
current level of activity?

Fairly Inactive–gets little exercise, spends
most of his/her time watching television,
looking at books, or sitting playing with
toys or games 1
Fairly Active–spends more time in active
play or running around than watching
television, looking at books, or sitting

playing with toys or games 2
Very Active–spends nearly all the time
running around or in very active play
or games 3

2. ASame   **If young person aged 4 to 6 years**

How would you describe *young person's*
level of activity when compared
with boys <u>and</u> girls of the same age?

More active 1
about the same 2
or less active? 3

3. SSame   **If young person aged 4 to 6 years**

How would you describe *young person's*
level of activity when compared
with other children of the same sex?

More active 1
about the same 2
or less active? 3

**YOUNG PERSON'S MEDICAL
HISTORY**

1. Acci   **All**

Has *young person* ever had an accident
which resulted in hospital admission?

Yes 1
No 2

2. Oper   **All**

Has *young person* ever had an operation?

Yes 1
No 2

3. Hosp   **All**

Has *young person* ever stayed in hospital
as an inpatient, overnight or longer?

EXCLUDE PERIOD AFTER BIRTH
UNLESS BABY STAYED IN
HOSPITAL AFTER MOTHER HAD
LEFT

Yes 1
No 2

571

4. Illness   **All**

Does *young person* have any long-standing illness, disability or infirmity? By long-standing I mean anything that has troubled him/her over a period of time or that is likely to affect him/her over a period of time?

Yes 1
No 2

a. LMatter   **If code 1 at Illness**

What is the matter with him/her?

b. LimitAct   **If code 1 at Illness**

Does this illness or disability (do any of these illnesses or disabilities) limit his/her activities in any way?

Yes 1
No 2

5. CutDown   **All**

Now I'd like you to think about the 2 weeks ending yesterday. During those two weeks, did s/he have to cut down on any of the things s/he usually does (about the house/at school/work or in his/her free time) because of *illness* or some other illness or injury?

Yes 1
No 2

a . NDysCutD   **If code 1 at CutDown**

How many days was this in all during these 2 weeks, including Saturdays and Sundays?

1..14

b. CMatter   **If code 1 at CutDown**

What was the matter with him/her?

OCCUPATION: ASKED FOR HEAD OF HOUSEHOLD, MOTHER (if not already asked as HOH) AND YOUNG PERSON (if aged 15 or over and not HOH)

1. WorklWk1   Did *HOH/Mother/Young person* do any paid work last week–that is in the 7 days ending last Sunday–either as an employee or self-employed?

Yes 1
No 2

a. FullPT   **If code 1 at WorklWk1**

Was s/he working full or part time?

Full time 1
Part time 2

b. WorklWk2   **If code 2 at Worklwk1**

Even though s/he wasn't working, did s/he have a job that s/he was away from last week?

HOH and young person
Yes 1
No 2

Mother
Yes, on maternity leave 1
Yes, not on maternity leave 2
No 3

c. WorklWk3   **HOH: if code 2 at Worklwk2**
Mother: if code 3 at Worklwk2
YP: : if code 2 at Worklwk2 and School ne 1 to 3

Last week was s/he ....

CODE FIRST TO APPLY

Waiting to take up a job s/he had already obtained ? 1
Looking for work ? 2
Intending to look for work but prevented by temporary sickness or injury ? (check 28 days or less) 3
Going to school or college full time ? (check 16-49 only) 4
Permanently unable to work because of long-term sickness or disability? (men 16-64; women 16-59 only) 5
Retired? (for women, only if stopped work after age 50) 6
Looking after home or family? 7
Or was s/he doing something else? 8

2. GovSchem During last week, that is the 7 days ending last Sunday was s/he on any of the following government schemes (including those run by Training Enterprise Councils (TEC)–England and Wales and Local Enterprise Companies (LEC)–Scotland)?

INDIVIDUAL PROMPT

Youth Training (YT)? only ask 16-20 yrs 1
Training for work/Employment Training/Employment Action? 2
Community Action? 3
None of these? 4

a. Trn **If codes 1 or 2 at GovSchem**

Last week was s/he ....

CODE FIRST ONE THAT APPLIES

with an employer, or on a project providing work experience or practical training ? 1
or at a college or training course ? 2

TRNCHKA **Variable computed in the CAPI program**

If code 1 at Trn .... TRNCHKA = 1
With an employer/on work experience or practical training

If code 2 at Trn ...... TRNCHKA = 2
At college or training scheme

HOH and YP:
If code 1 at WorklWk1 or code 1 at WorklWk2 or code 3 at GovSchem .... TRNCHKA = 3
Had a job last week

Mother:
If code 1 at WorklWk1 or code 1 or 2 at WorklWk2 or code 3 at GovSchem .... TRNCHKA = 3
Had a job last week

If code 1 at WorklWk3 .... TRNCHKA = 4
Unemployed, waiting to take up a job

If code 2 at WorklWk3 .... TRNCHKA = 5
Unemployed, looking for work

If code 3 at WorklWk3 .... TRNCHKA = 6

Unemployed, prevented by temporary sickness from looking for work

If codes 4 to 8 at WorklWk3 .... TRNCHKA = 7
Other, economically inactive

If na at WorklWk1 ... TRNCHKA = –9
Economic status not known

3. LookWork **If code 6 at TRNCHKA**

Thinking of the 4 weeks ending last Sunday, were you looking for paid work (or a YT/ET etc. place) at any time in those 4 weeks?

Yes 1
No 2

4. AbleStrt **If code 5 or 6 at TRNCHKA**

If a job (or YT/ET etc. place) had been available last week, would s/he have been able to start within 2 weeks?

Yes 1
No 2

5a. UnemWtJ1
If code 4 at TRNCHKA

Apart from the job s/he is waiting to take up, has s/he ever had a paid job or done any paid work?

Yes 1
No 2

b. UnemWtJ2 **W1 and W2: if code 5 or 6 at TRNCHKA**
W3 and W4: if codes 5 to 7 at TRNCHKA

(May I check), has s/he ever had a paid job or done any paid work?

Yes 1
No 2

6. UnempTim **If codes 4 to 6 at TRNCHKA**

How long altogether have you been out of employment but wanting work in this current period of unemployment, that is, since any time you may have spent on a government scheme, such as YT or ET/Training for work ?

PERIOD = UP TO YESTERDAY

Less than a week 1
1 week but less than 1 month 2
1 month but less than 3 months 3
3 months but less than 6 months 4
6 months but less than 12 months 5
12 months but less than 2 years 6
2 years but less than 3 years 7
3 years but less than 5 years 8
5 years or more 9

JOB DETAILS: ASKED FOR HEAD OF HOUSEHOLD, MOTHER (if not already asked as HOH) . Asked for YOUNG PERSON only if Head of own household.

1. Ind

<u>HOH</u>
If (code 1 at WorklWk1) or (code 1 at WorklWk2) or (code 1 at WorklWk3) or (code 1 at UnemWtJ2)

<u>Mother</u>
If (code 1 at WorklWk1) or (code 1 or 2 at WorklWk2) or (code 1 at WorklWk3) or (code 1 at UnemWtJ2)

What did the firm/organisation s/he worked for mainly make or do (at the place where s/he worked)?

DESCRIBE FULLY–PROBE MANUFACTURING OR PROCESSING OR DISTRIBUTION ETC. AND MAIN GOODS PRODUCED, MATERIALS USED, WHOLESALE OR RETAIL ETC.

2. IndT ENTER A TITLE FOR THE INDUSTRY

3. OccT What was his/her (main) job (in the week ending last Sunday)?

ENTER JOB TITLE

4. OccD What did s/he mainly do in his/her job?

CHECK SPECIAL QUALIFICATIONS/TRAINING NEEDED TO DO THE JOB

5. Stat0 -1 Was s/he working as an employee or was s/he self-employed?

Employee 1
Self-employed 2

a. Manage0-1 If code 1 at Stat

Did s/he have any managerial duties, or was s/he supervising any other employees?

Manager 1
Foreman/supervisor 2
Not manager/supervisor 3

b. EmpNo0-1 If code 1 at Stat

How many employees were there at the place where s/he worked?

1-24 1
25 or over 2

c. Solo0-1 If code 2 at Stat

Was s/he working on his/her own or did s/he have employees?

On own/with partner(s) but no employees 1
With employees 2

d. SENo0-1 If code 2 at Solo

How many people did s/he employ at the place where s/he worked?

1-24 1
25 or over 2

OEmpsta0-1 Variable computed in the CAPI program

If code 3 or -8 at Manage 1
Employee (not foreman or manager)

If code 2 at Manage 2
Foreman or supervisor

If code 1 at Solo 3
Self employed–no employees

If code 1 at SeNo 4
Self employed–1 to 24 employees

If code 2 at SeNo 5
Self employed–25 or more employees

If code 1 at Manage and code 1 at EmpNo 6
Manager–1 to 24 employees in establishment

If code 1 at Manage code 2 at EmpNo . 7
Manager–25 or more employees in establishment

574

SOC0-1 Standard Occupational Classification
Job title .... *answer at OccT*
Job description .... *answer at OccD*
Industry .... *answer at IndT*
Employment status .... *Empsta*

Review occupational details and assign
3-digit s.o.c. code

000..999

IEmpSta0-1 Imputed employment status

0..7

SEG0-1 **[Hidden variable calculated within program]**

Socio-economic group

0.0..16.0

SC0-1 **[Hidden variable calculated within program]**

Social class

0.0..6.0

MOTHER'S EDUCATION

1. MAge **if XMother = 1**

How old was *mother* when s/he finished her continuous full-time education?

Not Yet finished 1
14 2
15 3
16 4
17 5
18 6
19 or over 7
No formal education 8

2. MQual **if XMother = 1**

Please look at this card and tell me whether she has any of the qualifications listed. Start at the top of the list and tell me the first one you come to that she has passed

SHOW CARD E

CODE FIRST THAT APPLIES

Degree.................................... 1
Teaching qualifications 2
HNC/HND, BEC/TEC Higher,
BTEC Higher 3
City and Guilds Full Technological
Certificate 4
Nursing qualifications (SRN, SCM,
RGN, RM, RHV, Midwife) 5
'A' levels/SCE Higher 6
ONC/OND/BEC/TEC NOT Higher .. 7
City and Guilds Advanced/Final 8
'O' Level passes (Grade A to C if
after 1975) 9
GCSE (Grades A to C) 10
CSE (Grade 1) 11
SCE Ordinary (Bands A to C) 12
Standard Grade (Levels 1 to 3) 13
SLC Lower 14
SUPE Lower or ordinary 15
School certificate or Matric 16
City and Guilds Craft/Ordinary level 17
CSE Grades 2 to 5 18
GCE 'O' Level (Grades D&E if
after 1975) 19
GCSE (Grades D,E,F,G) 20
SCE Ordinary (Bands D & E) 21
Standard Grade (Level 4, 5) 22
Clerical or commercial qualifications 23
Apprenticeship 24
CSE Ungraded 25
Other qualifications (Specify at next
question) 26
No formal qualifications 27

a. QOthe2 **If code 26 at MQual**

SPECIFY OTHER QUALIFICATION

MOTHER'S AND FATHER'S SMOKING HABITS

1. MCigs **If code 1 at XMother**

Does *mother* smoke cigarettes at all?

Yes 1
No 2

a. MCigsA **If code 1 at MCigs**

About how many cigarettes a day does she usually smoke?

0..97

2. FCigs **If code 1 at XFather**

Does *father* smoke cigarettes at all?
Yes 1

No 2

a. FCigsA   **If code 1 at FCigs**

About how many cigarettes a day does
he usually smoke?

0..97

YOUNG PERSON'S EMPLOYMENT:

1. YPptJob   **If young person is aged 11 to 14 years**

Does *young person* have a part-time job
at the moment?

INCLUDE SATURDAY AND
EVENING JOBS, PAPER ROUNDS,
STACKING SHELVES ETC.

Yes 1
No 2

a. Hours   Waves 1 to 3
**If (code 1 at YPptJob) or (young person is
aged 15 or over and code 1 at WorklWk1)**

Wave 4 only
**If (code 1 at YPptJob) or [young person is
aged 15 or over and (code 1 at WorklWk1)
or (code 1 at WorklWk2)]**

Thinking back over the last 7 days, that
is from last . . . . to yesterday, in
total how many hours did s/he work?

INTERVIEWER: IF AWAY FROM
WORK LAST WEEK ENTER ZERO.

0..100

b. JDesc   Waves 1 to 3
**If (code 1 at YPptJob) or (young person is
aged 15 or over and code 1 at WorklWk1)**

Wave 4 only
**If (code 1 at YPptJob) or [young person is
aged 15 or over and (code 1 at WorklWk1)
or (code 1 at WorklWk2)]**

How would you describe your job .. is it:

SHOW CARD D
INTERVIEWER: DIRECT
QUESTION TO YOUNG PERSON

A job where s/he is sitting or standing for
most of the time, which is not physical or
active 1

a job which is physical and active, but
not so hard as to make him/her puff and
pant and get hot and sweaty for a lot of
the time 2

or a job which is very physical and active
and makes him/her puff and pant and get
hot and sweaty for a lot of the time? ..3

YOUNG PERSON'S EDUCATION

1. YAge   **If young person aged 15 or over and ne
code 2 at School**

How old was *young person* when s/he
finished his/her continuous
full-time education?

Not yet finished 1
14 2
15 3
16 4
17 5
18 6
19 or over 7
No formal education 8

2. YQual   **If young person aged 15 or over**

Please look at this card and tell me
whether *young person* has any of
the qualifications listed. Start at the top
of the list and tell me the first one
you come to that s/he has passed

SHOW CARD E

CODE FIRST THAT APPLIES

Degree 1
Teaching qualifications 2
HNC/HND, BEC/TEC Higher,
BTEC Higher 3
City and Guilds Full Technological
Certificate 4
Nursing qualifications (SRN, SCM,
RGN, RM, RHV, Midwife) 5
'A' levels/SCE Higher 6
ONC/OND/BEC/TEC NOT Higher ..7
City and Guilds Advanced/Final 8

'O' Level passes (Grade A to C if after
1975) 9
GCSE (Grades A to C) 10
CSE (Grade 1) 11
SCE Ordinary (Bands A to C) 12
Standard Grade (Levels 1 to 3) 13
SLC Lower 14
SUPE Lower or ordinary 15
School certificate or Matric 16
City and Guilds Craft/Ordinary level 17
CSE Grades 2 to 5 18
GCE 'O' Level (Grades D&E if after
1975) 19
GCSE (Grades D,E,F,G) 20
SCE Ordinary (Bands D & E) 21
Standard Grade (Level 4, 5) 22
Clerical or commercial qualifications 23
Apprenticeship 24
CSE Ungraded 25
Other qualifications (Specify at next
question) 26
No formal qualifications 27

a. QOthe2   **If code 26 at YQual**

SPECIFY OTHER QUALIFICATION

METHOD OF TRANSPORT

1. TravTo   **If (young person aged 4 to 14 <u>and</u> School
ne 1) <u>or</u> (young person aged 15 or over and
codes 2 to 5 at School)**

How does *young person* <u>usually</u> get to
school/work?

CODE ALL THAT APPLY

Walk 1
Cycle 2
Motorcycle 3
Car 4
Bus 5
Other (specify at next question) 6

a. TravO1   **If code 6 at TravTo**

SPECIFY OTHER WAY TRAVELS
TO SCHOOL

b. Longa   **If code 1 or 2 at TravTo**

How long does it take him/her to walk/
cycle to school/work?

IN MINUTES

0..90

2. TravFr   **If (young person aged 4 to 14 <u>and</u> School
ne 1) <u>or</u> (young person aged 15 or over and
codes 2 to 5 at School)**

How does *young person* <u>usually</u> get
home?

CODE ALL THAT APPLY

Walk 1
Cycle 2
Motorcycle 3
Car 4
Bus 5
Other (Specify at next question) 6

a. TravO2   **If code 6 at TravFr**

SPECIFY OTHER WAY GETS
HOME

b. Longb   **If code 1 or 2 at TravFr**

How long does it take him/her to walk/
cycle home?

IN MINUTES

0..90

**YOUNG PERSON'S ETHNIC
GROUP**

1. Birth   **All**

In which country was *young person* born?

England 1
Scotland 2
Wales 3
N Ireland 4
Outside UK 5

2. EthnGp   **All**

To which of the groups listed on this card
do you consider you / *young person*
belong(s)?

SHOW CARD F

White 1
Black–Caribbean 2
Black–African 3
Black–neither Caribbean nor African .4
Indian 5
Pakistani 6
Bangladeshi 7
Chinese 8
None of these (Include mixed race) ...9

a. EthnOth **If code 9 at EthnGp**

HOW WOULD YOU DESCRIBE THE
RACIAL OR ETHNIC GROUP TO
WHICH YOU/YOUNG PERSON
BELONG(S)?

TENURE

1. OwnHome **All**

Does your household own or rent this
house or flat?

PROMPT AS NECESSARY

Owns–with mortgage /loan 1
Owns–outright 2
Rents–Local Authority/new town 3
Rents–Housing Association 4
Rents–privately unfurnished 5
Rents–privately furnished 6
Rents–from employer 7
Rents–other with payment 8
Rent free 9

HOUSEHOLD INCOME INFORMATION

1. FCredit **All**

Can I just check, are you (and your
partner) currently receiving Family
Credit?

Yes 1
No 2

2. ISupp **All**

And have you (or your partner) drawn
Income Support at any time within
the last 14 days?

Yes 1
No 2

3. ISeek **All**

And have you (or your partner) drawn
(Income related) Job Seeker's
Allowance at any time within the last 14
days?

Yes 1
No 2

4. GIncome **All**

Could you please look at this card and
tell me which group represents the gross
income of the whole household?

Please include income from all sources
before any compulsory deductions such
as income tax, national insurance and
superannuation contributions.

SHOW CARD G

REMIND INFORMANT WHO IS
INCLUDED IN THE HOUSEHOLD

PER WEEK .... PER YEAR

less than £40 .... less than £2,000 .1
£40–less than £80 ... £2,000–less than
     £4,000 2
£80–less than £120 .. £4,000–less than
     £6,000 3
£120–less than £160 £6,000–less than
     £8,000 4
£160–less than £200 £8,000–less than
     £10,000 5
£200–less than £240 £10,000–less than
     £12,000 6
£240–less than £280 £12,000–less than
     £14,000 7
£280–less than £350 £14,000–less than
     £18,000 8
£350–less than £400 £18,000–less than
     £20,000 9
£400–less than £500 £20,000–less than
     £25,000 10
£500–less than £600 £25,000–less than
     £30,000 11
£600 or more .... £30,000 or more 12

Prompt cards

A

1   More than once a day

2   Once a day

3   Most days

4   At least once a week

5   At least once a month

6   Less than once a month

7   Never

B

1   More than a week

2   No more than 4 or 5 days

3   No more than 2 or 3 days

4   No more than one day

5   Use on the same day

Prompt cards – *continued*

C

1   Fairly inactive - gets little exercise, spends most of the time watching television, looking at books, or sitting playing with toys or games.

2   Fairly active - spends more time in active play or running around than watching television, looking at books, or sitting playing with toys or games

3   Very active - spends nearly all the time running around or in very active play or games

D

1   A job where I am sitting or standing for most of the time, which is not physical or active

2   A job which is physical and active, but not so hard as to make me puff and pant and get hot and sweaty for a lot of the time

3   A job which is very physical and active and makes me puff and pant and get hot and sweaty for a lot of time

Prompt cards – *continued*

E

Degree, or degree level qualification

Teaching qualification
HNC/HND, BEC/TEC Higher, BTEC Higher
City and Guilds Full Technological Certificate
Nursing qualifications (SRN, SCM, RGN, RM, RHV, Midwife)

'A' levels/SCE higher
ONC/OND/BEC/TEC not higher
City and Guilds Advanced/Final Level

'O' level passes (Grade A-C if after 1975)
GCSE (grades A-C)
CSE Grade 1
SCE Ordinary (Bands A-C)
Standard Grade (Level 1-3)
SLC Lower
SUPE Lower or Ordinary
School Certificate or Matric
City and Guilds Craft/Ordinary level

CSE Grades 2-5
GCE 'O' level (Grades D & E if after 1975)
GCSE (Grades D, E, F, G)
SCE Ordinary (Bands D & E)
Standard Grade (Level 4, 5)
Clerical or commercial qualifications
Apprenticeships

CSE ungraded
Other qualifications - *please tell the interviewer what*
No qualifications

F

1   White

2   Black - Caribbean

3   Black - African

4   Black - neither Caribbean nor African

5   Indian

6   Pakistani

7   Bangladeshi

8   Chinese

9   None of these; mixed race

G

Gross household income

per week	Group	per year
less than £40	01	less than £2,000
£40 - less than £80	02	£2,000 - less £4,000
£80 - less than £120	03	£4,000 - less £6,000
£120 - less than £160	04	£6,000 - less £8,000
£160 - less than £200	05	£8,000 - less £10,000
£200 - less than £240	06	£10,000 - less £12,000
£240 - less than £280	07	£12,000 - less £14,000
£280 - less than £350	08	£14,000 - less £18,000
£350 - less than £400	09	£18,000 - less £20,000
£400 - less than £500	10	£20,000 - less £25,000
£500 - less than £600	11	£25,000 - less £30,000
£600 or more	12	£30,000 or more

NATIONAL DIET AND NUTRITION SURVEY: YOUNG PEOPLE 4 TO 18 AGED YEARS

Diary pick up interview

1. WhoW   **All**

Who weighed and recorded the food and drink entered in the diary?
Please include all those people who did any weighing and recording.

CODE ALL THAT APPLY

Young person 1
'Mother' figure 2
'Father' figure 3
Brother(s) or sister(s) 4
Other relative in household 5
Nanny or child minder 6
Friend 7
Teacher, dinner lady or play group
helper 8
Other (Specify at next question) 9

a. WWOth1   **If code 9 at WhoW**

SPECIFY OTHER(S) WHO
WEIGHED OR RECORDED

2. WMain   **All**

Who did <u>most</u> of the weighing and recording?

CODE ONLY ONE

Young person 1
'Mother' figure 2
'Father' figure 3
Brother(s) or sister(s) 4
Other relative in household 5
Nanny or child minder 6
Friend 7
Teacher, dinner lady or play group
helper 8
Other (Specify at next question) 9

a. WWOth2   **If code 9 at WMain**

SPECIFY OTHER WHO DID MOST
OF THE WEIGHING OR
RECORDING

3. Offer1   **All**

During the 7 days that you were weighing and recording *young person's* food do you think s/he had more, less or about the same amount of <u>biscuits</u> as usual?

More 1
Less 2
Same 3
Never eats item 4

4. Offer2   **All**

During the 7 days that you were weighing and recording *young person's* food do you think s/he had more, less or about the same amount of <u>sweets</u> as usual?

More 1
Less 2
Same 3
Never eats item 4

5. Offer3   **All**

During the 7 days that you were weighing and recording *young person's* food do you think s/he had more, less or about the same amount of <u>crisps</u> as usual?

More 1
Less 2
Same 3
Never eats item 4

6. Offer4   **All**

During the 7 days that you were weighing and recording *young person's* food do you think s/he had more, less or about the same amount of <u>drinks</u> as usual?

More 1
Less 2
Same 3
Never eats item 4

583

7. Offer5 **All**

During the 7 days that you were weighing and recording *young person's* food do you think s/he had more, less or about the same amount of <u>snacks</u> as usual?

More 1
Less 2
Same 3
Never eats item 4

8. Portion **All**

On the whole, do you think that *young person* had:

RUNNING PROMPT

bigger 1
smaller 2
or the same size portions as usual while you were keeping the diary? 3

9. EatOut **All**

During the 7 days do you think *young person* ate out of the home including at friends, work or school:

RUNNING PROMPT

more often 1
less often 2
or about the same as usual? 3

10. Minder **All**

Did the eating out diary have to be left with someone else, for example a childminder or teacher, for them to record food and drink eaten by *young person*?

Yes 1
No 2

a. ProbM **If code 1 at Minder**

Were there any problems in keeping the eating out diary when *young person* was with someone else?

Yes 1
No 2

i. MindS **If code 1 at ProbM**

What were these problems?

11. BigProb **All**

Did you have any problems with the weighing and recording of what s/he had to eat and drink during the 7-day period?

Yes 1
No 2

a. WhatP **If code 1 at BigProb**

What were these problems?

12. Unwell **All**

(During the past few days/while you were keeping the diary) has *young person* been unwell at all?

Yes 1
No 2

a. Sick0..5 **If code 1 at Unwell ask for each of the following**

0 = Diarrhoea
1 = Sick or vomiting
2 = Cold or flu (include sore throat, runny nose, tonsils with temperature, chest infection, cough, snuffles)
3 = Ear infection
4 = Asthma
5 = Ill in any other way (Specify at next question; include off food; chicken pox; headache; feverish)

Has s/he been ill with (ILLNESS)?

Yes 1
No 2

b. Which100..106 **If code 1 at Sick0**
Which107..113 **If code 1 at Sick1**
Which114..120 **If code 1 at Sick2**
Which121..127 **If code 1 at Sick3**
Which128..134 **If code 1 at Sick4**
Which135..141 **If code 1 at Sick5**

On which day(s) was s/he unwell with (ILLNESS)?

CODE ALL THAT APPLY

Day 1 1
Day 2 2
Day 3 3
Day 4 4
Day 5 5
Day 6 6
Day 7 7

c. Which000..007   **If code 1 at Sick0**
Which008..015   **If code 1 at Sick1**
Which016..023   **If code 1 at Sick2**
Which024..031   **If code 1 at Sick3**
Which032..039   **If code 1 at Sick4**
Which040..047   **If code 1 at Sick5**

On which day(s) did (ILLNESS) affect his/her eating habits?

CODE ALL THAT APPLY

Day 1 1
Day 2 2
Day 3 3
Day 4 4
Day 5 5
Day 6 6
Day 7 7
Did not affect eating habits 8

d. VOther   **If code 1 at Sick5 (ill in any other way)**

SPECIFY OTHER ILLNESS

13. Unusual   **All**

Have there been any (other) unusual circumstances which have affected *young person's* eating habits (during the past few days/while you were keeping the diary)?

Yes 1
No 2

a. UnWhat   **If code 1 at Unusual**

What has been different about *young person's* eating habits over these days?

14. Say   **All**

Is there anything you would like to say about the diary you kept (for *young person*)? (Enter at next question)

Yes 1
No 2

a. SWhat   **If code 1 at Say**

ENTER COMMENTS ABOUT THE DIARY

DIETARY ASSESSMENT SCHEDULE

1. F7Q7   INTERVIEWER: ENTER THE ANSWER TO Q7 ON THE DIETARY ASSESSMENT SCHEDULE (F7)[1]

Overall, how good do you (INTERVIEWER) think the diaries are at reflecting what *young person* ate over the period?

Complete record of items and very few estimated weights 1
Complete record of items and some estimated weights .2
Complete record of items and nearly all estimated weights 3
Some items missing and very few estimated weights .4
Some items missing and some estimated weights 5
Some items missing and nearly all estimated weights .6
Lots of missing items and very few estimated weights .7
Lots of missing items and some estimated weights .8
Lots of missing items and nearly all estimated weights .9

ORAL HEALTH EXAMINATION

1. OConsent   **All**

RECORD

Was consent given to the oral health examination?

Yes 1
No 2

[1]   Only Q7 from the Dietary Assessment Schedule was keyed into the Blaise object: for other questions on this document see Appendix X.

N14/4 /W3

ND NS — NATIONAL DIET AND NUTRITION SURVEY

S2 G:10-18

Serial number label

CONFIDENTIAL

SMOKING AND DRINKING

Most of the questions can be answered by putting a tick in the box next to the answer that applies to you - like this:

Yes [✓ 1]
No [2]

or sometimes you have to write a number in the box, for example:

[2]

Some questions don't apply to everybody. It always tells you by the box which question you should answer next.

1. Do you smoke cigarettes at all nowadays?

Yes [1] ─ Go to Question 2
No [2]

2. Please read all the following statements carefully and tick the box next to the one which best describes you:

I have never smoked [1] ─ Go to Question 3

I have only ever tried smoking once [2]

I used to smoke sometimes but I never smoke a cigarette now [3]

I sometimes smoke cigarettes now but I don't smoke as many as one a week [4] ─ Go to Question 4

I usually smoke between one and six cigarettes a week [5]

I usually smoke more than six cigarettes a week [6]

1

N14/4(S2) MAY'97 V1

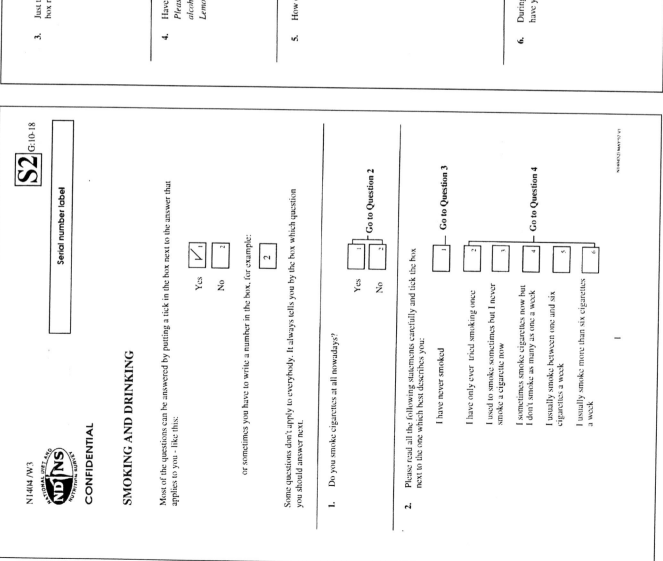

---

3. Just to check, read the statements below carefully and tick the box next to the one which best describes you.

I have never tried smoking a cigarette, not even a puff or two [1]

I did once have a puff or two of a cigarette, but I never smoke now [2]

I do sometimes smoke cigarettes [3] ─ Go to Question 4

4. Have you ever had a proper alcoholic drink - a whole drink, not just a sip? *Please don't count drinks labelled low alcohol but include alcoholic lemonade, alcoholic cola and other alcoholic soft drinks, such as Hooch, Two Dogs and Lemon Head.*

Yes [1] ─ Go to Question 5

No [2] ─ Go to Question 18

5. How often do you **usually** have an alcoholic drink?

Almost every day [1]

About twice a week [2]

About once a week [3]

About once a fortnight [4]

About once a month [5]

Only a few times a year [6] ─ Go to Question 6

I never drink alcohol now [7] ─ Go to Question 18

6. During the **last 7 days**, how much BEER, LAGER AND CIDER have you drunk? *Please don't count drinks labelled low alcohol.*

Have not drunk beer, lager or cider in the last 7 days [1] ─ Go to Question 8

Less than half a pint [2]

Half a pint or more [3] ─ Go to Question 7

2

N14/4(S2) MAY'97 V1

Smoking and drinking self-completion – *continued*

7. Write in the boxes below the number of pints, half pints, large cans, small cans of BEER, LAGER AND CIDER you have drunk in the last 7 days.

   pints (glasses or pint bottles)

   half pints (glasses or small bottles)

   large cans

   small cans

Go to Question 8

8. During the **last 7 days**, how much SHANDY have you drunk?

   Have not drunk shandy in the last 7 days   ☐ 1   **Go to Question 10**

   Less than half a pint   ☐ 2

   Half a pint or more   ☐ 3   **Go to Question 9**

9. Write in the boxes below the number of pints, half pints, large cans, small cans of SHANDY you have drunk in the last 7 days.

   pints

   half pints

   large cans

   small cans

Go to Question 10

---

10. During the **last 7 days**, how much WINE have you drunk?

   Have not drunk wine in the last 7 days   ☐ 1   **Go to Question 12**

   Less than a glass   ☐ 2

   One glass or more   ☐ 3   **Go to Question 11**

11. Write in the box below, the number of glasses of WINE you have drunk in the last 7 days.

   glasses   ☐   **Go to Question 12**

12. During the **last 7 days**, how much MARTINI AND SHERRY have you drunk?

   Have not drunk martini or sherry in the last 7 days   ☐ 1   **Go to Question 14**

   Less than a glass   ☐ 2

   One glass or more   ☐ 3   **Go to Question 13**

13. Write in the box below, the number of glasses of MARTINI OR SHERRY you have drunk in the last 7 days.

   glasses   ☐   **Go to Question 14**

14. During the **last 7 days**, how much SPIRITS (e.g. whisky, vodka, gin) AND LIQUEURS have you drunk?

   By a glass we mean a single pub measure

   Have not drunk spirits or liqueurs in the last 7 days   ☐ 1   **Go to Question 16**

   Less than a glass   ☐ 2

   One glass or more   ☐ 3   **Go to Question 15**

Smoking and drinking self-completion – continued

15. Write in the box below, the number of glasses of SPIRITS (e.g. whisky, vodka, gin) AND LIQUEURS you have drunk in the last 7 days.

glasses ⟶ **Go to Question 16**

16. During the **last 7 days**, how much ALCOHOLIC LEMONADE, ALCOHOLIC COLA or OTHER ALCOHOLIC SOFT DRINKS (e.g. Hooch, Two Dogs, Lemon Head) have you drunk?

Have not drunk alcoholic lemonade, alcoholic cola or other alcoholic soft drinks in the last 7 days [1]

⟶ **Go to Question 18**

Less than a bottle [2]

One bottle or more [3] ⟶ **Go to Question 17**

17. Write in the boxes below the number of bottles and cans of ALCOHOLIC LEMONADE, ALCOHOLIC COLA and OTHER ALCOHOLIC SOFT DRINKS (e.g. Hooch, Two Dogs, Lemon Head) you have drunk in the last 7 days.

bottles

cans ⟶ **Go to Question 18**

The next 3 questions are not about smoking and drinking.

There are two questions about your monthly periods, and one about whether you take the contraceptive pill. They are part of the information we are collecting on your health and growth, and we thought young girls would prefer to answer these questions in private.

18. Have you started having your monthly periods yet?

Yes [1] ⟶ **Go to Question 19**

No [2] ⟶ **Go to Question 20**

19. How old were you when you first started your monthly periods?

Age

years   months

If you cannot remember your age exactly please try to get as close as you can.

20. Are you taking a contraceptive pill?

Yes [1]

⟶ **Go to Question 21**

No [2]

21. **Please check that you have answered all the questions.**

Now please put this form back in the envelope and hand it back to the interviewer.

Thank you for your help.

CONFIDENTIAL

N1404   NATIONAL DIET AND NUTRITION SURVEY: YOUNG PEOPLE AGED 4 -18 YEARS

Serial no. label

Gender
Male   Female

Date of birth

HOME RECORD BOOK

Please record all food and drink
as shown inside.   Thank you.

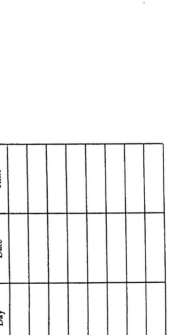

NATIONAL DIET AND NUTRITION SURVEY

Office for National Statistics
Social Survey Division
1 Drummond Gate
London SW1V 2QQ

The interviewer will call again on:

Day	Date	Time

Home Record Diary – continued

YOUR HOME RECORD

MOST OF THE YOUNG PEOPLE IN THIS SURVEY WILL BE KEEPING THEIR OWN HOME RECORD so these instructions are written for them. If you are keeping the record for the young person, or helping them with it, then these instructions still apply, but remember it is only the young person's food and drinks that should be recorded - not your own.

This tells you how we would like you to fill in this record; please read it CAREFULLY before starting the weighing and recording.

The interviewer will go through with you what you need to do before you start and will always help you with any problems you have. If you get stuck, or are unsure what to write down, you should make as many notes as possible on the back of the diary page where there is space for you to do so, and then the interviewer can help sort it out when he or she next calls.

We have also given you a card with some tips on weighing and recording.

Don't forget that when you have completed your food diary for the full 7 days the interviewer will give you a token that you can spend on music or a book.

Describing what you eat and drink: we need to know as much as possible about everything that you eat and drink - you can use as many pages as you like - the interviewer will give you some more if you run out.

Everything you eat or drink needs to be weighed on, or in a container - for example, on a plate, or in a cup, bowl or glass. Each page of the record has lines already printed for your empty plate, cup, glass or bowl. We call these lines the '*empty plate line*'.

Column A: every time you weigh an empty plate, (or cup or other container) you need to fill in the information in column A about what you are weighing on that plate. Write down the weight of the empty plate (or cup etc) and the time of day. Then ring one code to show **where you are going to eat** the food you are going to weigh; ring code 1 if you are going to eat it at home, ring 2 if you are going to eat it at school or college and ring 3 if you are going to eat it somewhere else. Then ring a code to show **who is doing the weighing**; ring 1 if you, the young person, are doing the weighing, and ring 2 if it is someone else.

Now on the lines under the '*empty plate line*' you can tell us all about the food or drink being weighed on that plate or container.

Column B: write down the **brand name** of the food or drink item, giving as much information as possible. This is the name of the company making the product and will be on the wrapper or other packaging - eg Heinz, Cadbury, Walker's etc. Many shops like Tesco and Sainsbury sell their 'own label' brands, such as baked beans, cola, crisps etc, so if it is

an 'own brand' you can write the name of the shop in this column - Tesco (baked beans). Fresh meat and fish, fresh fruit and vegetables and foods that do not come pre-wrapped, like loose cheese and cooked meats, do not have a brand name, so you can leave column B blank.

Column C: write down as full a **description of the item** as possible; use as many lines as you need, but always start a new line for a new item. We need to know the type of food (or drink) and how it was cooked.

For some items we also need to know how many of the item were weighed and served on this plate, for example, 1 can of Diet Pepsi; 2 pork sausages fried in sunflower oil; 2 Shredded Wheat.

For home-made cooked dishes, like Shepherd's pie, or lasagne, weigh the serving on your plate, then on the back of the page, in the space we can give you, write down all the things that went into the recipe with the quantities, for example, 400g minced lean beef, 1 small tin tomatoes, 1lb potatoes etc.

Column D: write down the **weight of each item** of food or drink on this plate or in this cup. The scales only weigh in grams and 'g' for grams is already printed in the column for you, so you only need to write in the number.

Column E: if you do not eat everything that you weighed we need to know the **weight of what is left over**. This might be bones from meat or fish, or stones or peel from fruit or nuts, or just some of the food or drink you did not want. Weigh the same plate with the left overs on it and write in the weight on the '*empty plate line*' in column E. Then put a tick in column E next to every item left on that plate.

Column F: if, after you have weighed something, you spill some of it, someone else eats or drinks some - or your dog eats it - then you will not be able to weigh it as a left over. If this happens try to **estimate** how much you spilt or lost and write it in column F against the food or drink lost. For example, "about half spilt".

Finally in Column G: if the food item is a fresh fruit or vegetable, ring one of the codes in this column to tell us **whether it was home-grown**; ring code 1 if it was home-grown; ring code 2 if it was not home-grown. By home-grown we mean grown in the garden where you live, or in an allotment that your parents have.

There are 6 lines for each plate. If you have more than 6 items on the same plate, then after the 6th item you can put a line through the '*empty plate line*' and carry on using the following lines to tell us about the rest of the items on that plate. Start at a new '*empty plate line*' for the next set of foods or the next drink, as normal.

There is an example on the next page of what a completed page might look like.

Home Record Diary – *continued*

REMEMBER

EACH PAGE SHOULD HAVE:

• date and date
• whether the young person was well or unwell

WHEN RECORDING:

• ALL food should be weighed on a plate and ALL drinks weighed in a container.

• Weigh the empty plate or container first and write the weight on the *'empty plate line'*.

• Complete the information in column A every time you weigh any empty plate or container.

• Start each food item on a new line; you can use more than one line to write the description of the food item.

• Record ALL drinks, including tap water.

• Record ALL vitamin and mineral supplements, including fluoride supplements.

• Record ALL condiments used at the table, apart from salt and pepper, eg tomato sauce, vinegar, mayonnaise.

• Weigh all the leftovers on the plate or in the container, and in column E put a tick against EVERY ITEM left on that plate.

• Show in column F whether any of the original item was lost or spilt and could not be re-weighed. Write an estimate of the amount of food or drink lost.

• Ring one code in column G to show whether fresh fruit and vegetables were home grown.

• Write all home made recipes on the back of the recording page.

PLEASE START A **NEW** PAGE FOR EACH DAY EVEN IF ONLY SOME OF THIS PAGE IS USED.   PLEASE USE A SEPARATE LINE FOR EACH ITEM EATEN OR DRUNK

Today is ......Saturday......day   Recording day: 1 (②) 3 4 5 6 7 (ring one)   Serial number: ____

Today the young person is   (tick one box)   Well ... ✓   Unwell ...

Today's date is: | 2 | 4 | 0 | 2 | 9 | 7 |

A	B BRAND NAME of each item, in full (except for fresh produce)	C FULL DESCRIPTION OF EACH ITEM, including whether fresh, frozen, dried, canned, what flavour, whether sweetened, how cooked, what type of fat food fried in	D Weight of item served (g)	E Any leftovers? Weigh or plate and leftovers (g) then TICK ALL ITEMS LEFT	F Any other losses which could not be weighed? TICK ITEMS AND ESTIMATE HOW MUCH LOST	G If fresh fruit or veg was it home grown? (Ring one) Yes / No	OFFICE USE ONLY Est weight? tick if yes	Food	Brand	Food source
Weight of empty plate? 400g		*EMPTY PLATE · CUP · BOWL · CONTAINER*								
Time eaten? 8.30 am/pm	Kelloggs	Coco - pops	64 g			1 2				
Where eaten? at home ①, at school 2, other place 3	Unigate ①	Whole milk, pasteurised	68 g	442 g ✓		1 2				
	Silver spoon 2	Sugar - granulated	6 g	✓		1 2				
Who weighed? young person ①, other 2	3	1 banana - weighed without its skin	40 g	✓		1 ②				
Weight of empty plate? 220g		*EMPTY PLATE · CUP · BOWL · CONTAINER*								
Time eaten? 9.00 am/pm	Tesco ①	Orange drink, not low calorie	40 g			1 2				
Where eaten? at home ①, at school 2, other place 3	2	Tap water	160 g	g		1 2				
Who weighed? young person ①, other 2	3		g	g		1 2				
Weight of empty plate? 176g	①		g			1 2				
Time eaten? 11.30 am/pm	Hovis ①	4 slices of white bread	144 g	216 g		1 2				
Where eaten? at home ①, at school 2, other place 3	Flora Light ①	Spread	28 g			1 ·2				
	2	English Cheddar cheese	82 g			1 2				
	3	2 sliced tomatoes	134 g	✓		1 ②				
Who weighed? young person ①, other 2	①		g			1 2				

Please use as many pages as you like for each day
Have you included underlined everything eaten and drunk today?
Use the back of this page for any notes, recipes and/or queries

Home Record Diary – *continued*

PLEASE START A **NEW** PAGE FOR EACH DAY EVEN IF ONLY SOME OF THIS PAGE IS USED. PLEASE USE A SEPARATE LINE FOR EACH ITEM EATEN OR DRUNK

Today is .... day   Recording day: 1   2   3   4   5   6   7   Serial number:

(ring one)

Today the young person is

(tick one box)   Well ....

Unwell ....

Today's date is: | 9 | 7 |

A	B BRAND NAME of each item, in full (except for fresh produce)	C FULL DESCRIPTION OF EACH ITEM, including whether fresh, frozen, dried, canned, what flavour, whether sweetened, how cooked, what type of fat food fried in	D Weight of item served (g)	E Any leftovers? Weight of plate and leftovers (g) then TICK ALL ITEMS LEFT	F Any other losses which could not be weighed? TICK ITEMS AND ESTIMATE HOW MUCH LOST	G If fresh fruit or veg. Was it home grown? Yes No *(Ring one)*		OFFICE USE ONLY Est weight? *Tick if yes.*	food	Brand	Food source
Weight of empty plate? .... g	.... g	*EMPTY PLATE - CUP - BOWL - CONTAINER*	.... g	.... g							
Time eaten? am/pm											
Where eaten? at home 1			.... g			1	2				
(ring one) at school 2			.... g			1	2				
other place 3			.... g			1	2				
Who weighed? young person 1			.... g			1	2				
(ring one) other 2			.... g			1	2				
Weight of empty plate? .... g	.... g	*EMPTY PLATE - CUP - BOWL - CONTAINER*	.... g	.... g							
Time eaten? am/pm											
Where eaten? at home 1			.... g			1	2				
(ring one) at school 2			.... g			1	2				
other place 3			.... g			1	2				
Who weighed? young person 1			.... g			1	2				
(ring one) other 2			.... g			1	2				
Weight of empty plate? .... g	.... g	*EMPTY PLATE - CUP - BOWL - CONTAINER*	.... g	.... g							
Time eaten? am/pm											
Where eaten? at home 1			.... g			1	2				
(ring one) at school 2			.... g			1	2				
other place 3			.... g			1	2				
Who weighed? young person 1			.... g			1	2				
(ring one) other 2			.... g			1	2				

Please use as many pages as you like for each day
Have you included underlined everything eaten and drunk today?
Use the back of this page for any notes, recipes and/or queries

Home Record Diary – *continued*

RECIPE INFORMATION

Please use this side of the page to write down the ingredients in any home-made recipe. The ingredients do not have to be weighed separately, but please try to estimate the quantities of each item that were used, including any liquid, for example, in home-made stews, casseroles or soup. For example: 2 onions, 1lb of leeks, 2 large potatoes, ½ pint semi-skimmed milk, 1 pint chicken stock.

Name of the home-made dish:...

When was it eaten? Day:........... **Date:**...........................**Time:**.........am/pm

Quantity of ingredients *please give full details*	Ingredients *please give full details*

Cooking method:

NOTES AND QUERIES

Please use this side of the page for any notes, queries or extra information.

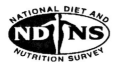

Serial number label

Private and Confidential

Young Person's Diary of Activities ...

 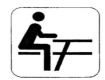

... and Eating and Drinking Away from Home

Name ....

This diary begins on ....(date)   And ends on .... (date)

What time did you go to bed on the last day that you kept the diary?	□□□□

(write in) Hours   Minutes   *(am/pm)*

Record of bowel movements while away from home

Please complete this chart each day recording the number of bowel movements you have while you are away from home. If, on any day, you do not have a bowel movement while you are away from home, then please ring '0' for that day on this chart.

Day of the week - *write in - Tues, Wed, etc*	Number of bowel movements while away from home - *ring next number after each movement*	Day of the week - *write in - Tues, Wed, etc*	Number of bowel movements while away from home - *ring next number after each movement*
1st day is: ....day	0 1 2 3 4 5 6 7	5th day is: ....day	0 1 2 3 4 5 6 7
2nd day is: ....day	0 1 2 3 4 5 6 7	6th day is: ....day	0 1 2 3 4 5 6 7
3rd day is: ....day	0 1 2 3 4 5 6 7	7th, and last day is ....day	0 1 2 3 4 5 6 7
4th day is: ....day	0 1 2 3 4 5 6 7		

Interviewer: check this chart for entries on each of the 7 recording days. Check that they have been copied across onto B1

This is the 5th day of your diary

1 Today is *(ring one)* ⟶ Monday   Tuesday   (Wednesday)   Thursday   Friday   Saturday   Sunday

2 Today's date is: *(write in)* | 1 | 9 | 0 | 2 | 9 | 7 |
   Day   Month   Year

> Please try to record these times to the nearest 10 minutes. Don't forget to say if it was morning (a.m.) or afternoon (p.m.)!

3 What time did you go to bed last night? | 9 | 0 | 0 |
   (write in)   Hours   Minutes   am/pm

4 What time did you get up today? | 8 | 3 | 0 |
   (write in)   Hours   Minutes   am/pm

5 Today were you: at school or college *(ring one)* ⟶ (Yes)   No
   at work? *(ring one)* ⟶ Yes   (No)

> If you did not go to work please leave this question blank

6 If you were at work today, how long did you work today?
   (Please exclude any lunch break) | | | |
   (write in)   Hours   Minutes

7 If you were at school/college or work today, what did you do for lunch?
   (Tick one box)

   took packed lunch from home .... | |
   had school meal, or bought something at school .... | ✓ |
   bought something to eat/drink at work/college .... | |
   came home for lunch .... | |
   bought something outside school/college/work .... | |
   didn't have lunch .... | |

8 How long have you spent watching TV, playing computer games and listening to music today? *(write in)* ⟶ | 2 | 2 | 0 |
   Hours   Minutes

   Do not count any time you spent doing these things while you were at school

> Please try to record this to the nearest 10 minutes

Now please turn over the page and tell us more about what you have been doing today........

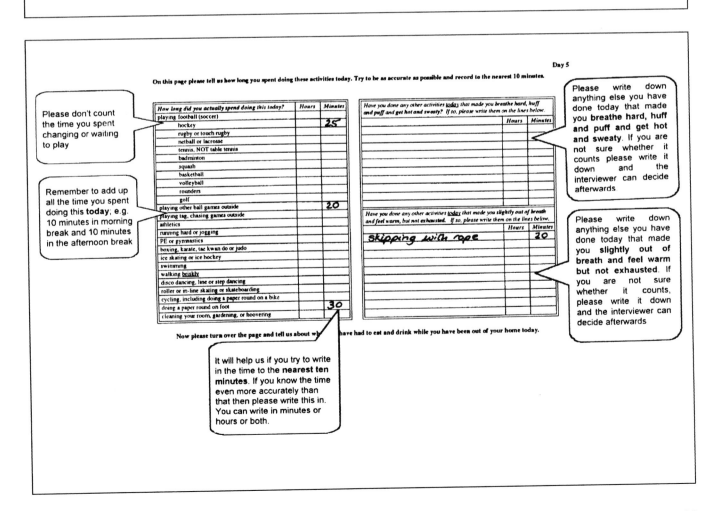

Day 5

On this page please tell us how long you spent doing these activities today. Try to be as accurate as possible and record to the nearest 10 minutes.

> Please don't count the time you spent changing or waiting to play

> Remember to add up all the time you spent doing this today; e.g. 10 minutes in morning break and 10 minutes in the afternoon break

How long did you actually spend doing this today?	Hours	Minutes
playing football (soccer)		
hockey		25
rugby or touch rugby		
netball or lacrosse		
tennis, NOT table tennis		
badminton		
squash		
basketball		
volleyball		
rounders		
golf		
playing other ball games outside		20
playing tag, chasing games outside		
athletics		
running hard or jogging		
PE or gymnastics		
boxing, karate, tae kwan do or judo		
ice skating or ice hockey		
swimming		
walking briskly		
disco dancing, line or step dancing		
roller or in-line skating or skateboarding		
cycling, including doing a paper round on a bike		
doing a paper round on foot		
cleaning your room, gardening, or hoovering		30

Have you done any other activities today that made you breathe hard, huff and puff and get hot and sweaty? If so, please write them on the lines below.	Hours	Minutes

> Please write down anything else you have done today that made you **breathe hard, huff and puff and get hot and sweaty**. If you are not sure whether it counts please write it down and the interviewer can decide afterwards

Have you done any other activities today that made you slightly out of breath and feel warm, but not exhausted. If so, please write them on the lines below.	Hours	Minutes
skipping with rope		20

> Please write down anything else you have done today that made you **slightly out of breath and feel warm but not exhausted**. If you are not sure whether it counts, please write it down and the interviewer can decide afterwards

Now please turn over the page and tell us about what you have had to eat and drink while you have been out of your home today.

> It will help us if you try to write in the time to the **nearest ten minutes**. If you know the time even more accurately than that then please write this in. You can write in minutes or hours or both.

595

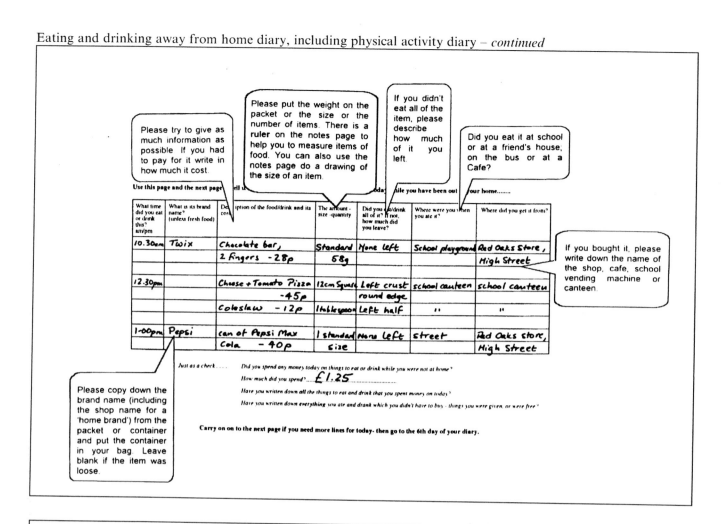

Please try to give as much information as possible. If you had to pay for it write in how much it cost.

Please put the weight on the packet or the size or the number of items. There is a ruler on the notes page to help you to measure items of food. You can also use the notes page do a drawing of the size of an item.

If you didn't eat all of the item, please describe how much of it you left.

Did you eat it at school or at a friend's house; on the bus or at a Cafe?

If you bought it, please write down the name of the shop, cafe, school vending machine or canteen.

Please copy down the brand name (including the shop name for a 'home brand') from the packet or container and put the container in your bag. Leave blank if the item was loose.

Use this page and the next page to tell us ... today ... while you have been out ... your home.......

What time did you eat or drink this? am/pm	What is its brand name? (unless fresh food)	Description of the food/drink and its cost	The amount - size -quantity	Did you eat/drink all of it? If not, how much did you leave?	Where were you when you ate it?	Where did you get it from?
10.30am	Twix	Chocolate bar, 2 fingers - 28p	Standard 58g	None left	School playground	Red Oaks Store, High Street
12.30pm		Cheese + Tomato Pizza -45p	12cm Square	Left crust round edge	school canteen	school canteen
		Coleslaw -12p	1tablespoon	Left half	"	"
1.00pm	Pepsi	can of Pepsi Max Cola - 40p	1 standard size	None left	street	Red Oaks store, High Street

Just as a check . . . . Did you spend any money today on things to eat or drink while you were not at home?

How much did you spend? £1.25 ....

Have you written down all the things to eat and drink that you spent money on today?

Have you written down everything you ate and drank which you didn't have to buy - things you were given, or were free?

Carry on on to the next page if you need more lines for today- then go to the 6th day of your diary.

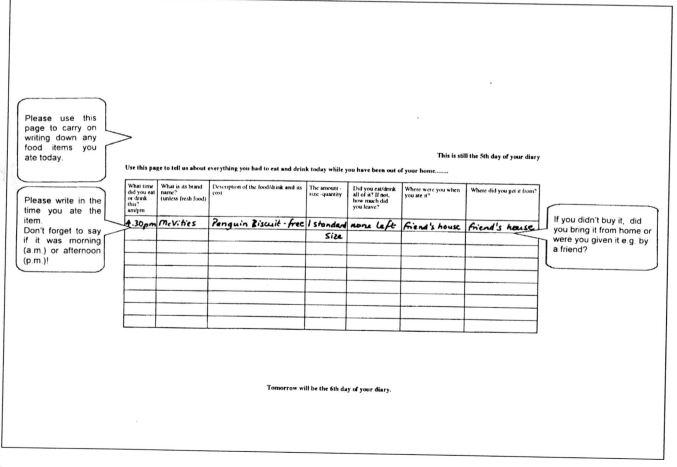

Please use this page to carry on writing down any food items you ate today.

Please write in the time you ate the item. Don't forget to say if it was morning (a.m.) or afternoon (p.m.)!

This is still the 5th day of your diary

Use this page to tell us about everything you had to eat and drink today while you have been out of your home.......

What time did you eat or drink this? am/pm	What is its brand name? (unless fresh food)	Description of the food/drink and its cost	The amount - size -quantity	Did you eat/drink all of it? If not, how much did you leave?	Where were you when you ate it?	Where did you get it from?
4.30pm	McVities	Penguin Biscuit - free	1 standard size	none left	friend's house	friend's house

If you didn't buy it, did you bring it from home or were you given it e.g. by a friend?

Tomorrow will be the 6th day of your diary.

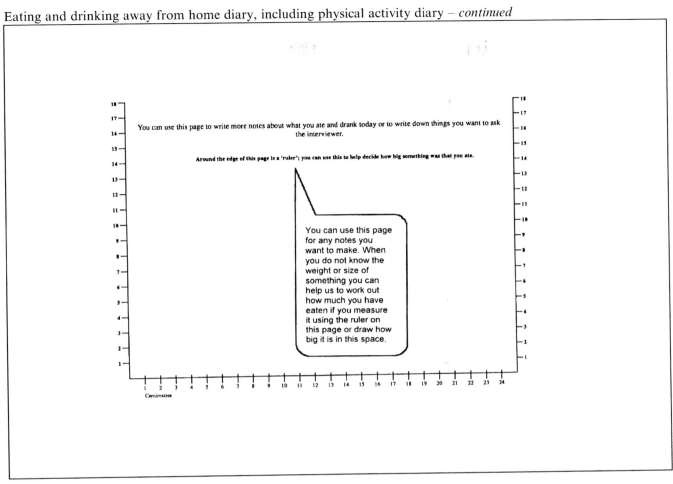

You can use this page to write more notes about what you ate and drank today or to write down things you want to ask the interviewer.

Around the edge of this page is a 'ruler'; you can use this to help decide how big something was that you ate.

You can use this page for any notes you want to make. When you do not know the weight or size of something you can help us to work out how much you have eaten if you measure it using the ruler on this page or draw how big it is in this space.

Centimetres

This is the 1st day of your diary

Serial number label

1   Today is *(ring one)* ——► Monday   Tuesday   Wednesday   Thursday   Friday   Saturday   Sunday

2   Today's date is: *(write in)* | | | | 9 | 7 |
                                            Day   Month   Year

3   What time did you go to bed last night? | | | | |
    (write in)   Hours   Minutes   (am/pm)

4   What time did you get up today? | | | | |
    (write in)   Hours   Minutes   (am/pm)

5   Today were you: at school or college *(ring one)* ——► Yes   No

    at work? *(ring one)* ——► Yes   No

6   If you were at work today, how long did you work today?
    (Please exclude any lunch break)
    | | | | |
    (write in)   Hours   Minutes

7   If you were at school/college or work today, what did you do for lunch?

    (Tick one box)

    took packed lunch from home .... □

    had school meal, or bought something at school .... □

    bought something to eat/drink at work/college .... □

    came home for lunch .... □

    bought something outside school/college/work .... □

    didn't have lunch .... □

8   How long have you spent watching TV, playing computer games and listening to music today? *(write in)* ——► | | | | |
    Hours   Minutes

    Do not count any time you spent doing these things while you were at school

Now please turn over the page and tell us more about what you have been doing today........

© NDNS 1996 V3

Eating and drinking away from home diary, including physical activity diary – *continued*

Day 1

Serial number label

On this page please tell us how long you spent doing these activities today. **Try to be as accurate as possible and record to the nearest 10 minutes.**

How long did you actually spend doing this today?	Hours	Minutes
playing football (soccer)		
hockey		
rugby or touch rugby		
netball or lacrosse		
tennis, NOT table tennis		
badminton		
squash		
basketball		
volleyball		
rounders		
golf		
playing other ball games outside		
playing tag, chasing games outside		
athletics		
running hard or jogging		
PE or gymnastics		
boxing, karate, tae kwan do or judo		
ice skating or ice hockey		
swimming		
walking briskly		
disco dancing, line or step dancing		
roller or in-line skating or skateboarding		
cycling, including doing a paper round on a bike		
doing a paper round on foot		
cleaning your room, gardening, or hoovering		

Have you done any other activities today that made you breathe hard, huff and puff and get hot and sweaty? If so, please write them on the lines below.

	Hours	Minutes

Have you done any other activities today that made you slightly out of breath and feel warm, but not exhausted. If so, please write them on the lines below.

	Hours	Minutes

Now please turn over the page and tell us about what you have had to eat and drink while you have been out of your home today.

This is the 1st day of your diary

Use this page and the next page to tell us about everything you had to eat and drink today while you have been out of your home........

What time did you eat or drink this? am/pm	What is its brand name? (unless fresh food)	Description of the food/drink and its cost	The amount - size -quantity	Did you eat/drink all of it? If not, how much did you leave?	Where were you when you ate it?	Where did you get it from?

Just as a check . . . .   Did you spend any money today on things to eat or drink while you were not at home?

How much did you spend? ....

Have you written down all the things to eat and drink that you spent money on today?

Have you written down everything you ate and drank which you didn't have to buy - things you were given, or were free?

Carry on on to the next page if you need more lines for today- then go to the 2nd day of your diary.

598

Eating and drinking away from home diary, including physical activity diary – *continued*

This is still the 1st day of your diary

Use this page to tell us about everything you had to eat and drink today while you have been out of your home........

What time did you eat or drink this? am/pm	What is its brand name? (unless fresh food)	Description of the food/drink and its cost	The amount - size -quantity	Did you eat/drink all of it? If not, how much did you leave?	Where were you when you ate it?	Where did you get it from?

Tomorrow will be the 2nd day of your diary.

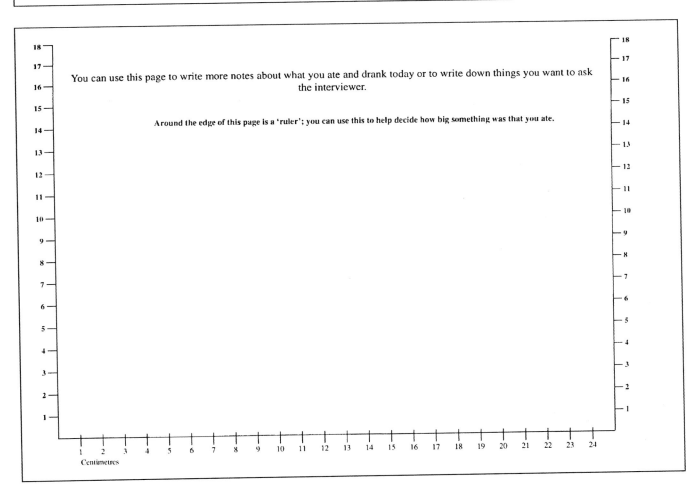

You can use this page to write more notes about what you ate and drank today or to write down things you want to ask the interviewer.

Around the edge of this page is a 'ruler'; you can use this to help decide how big something was that you ate.

Centimetres

P3

ND↑NS
NATIONAL DIET AND
NUTRITION SURVEY

YOUNG PEOPLE AGED 4 TO 18
YEARS

POCKET NOTEBOOK AND DIARY

Private

Recording week:

Social Survey Division
ONS
1Drummond Gate
London SW1V 2QQ

START day......................................

FINISH day.......................................

WHOSE diary...................................

NOTES:

NDNS POCKET NOTEBOOK AND DIARY

This notebook is for you to keep with you when you are not at home. You can make notes in it each day about things you have had to eat and drink while you have been out, and about any physical activities you have done. The headings are just a reminder about some of the details we need, but you can make whatever notes you find useful. **Please remember to copy all the details into your activity and eating and drinking diary at the end of each day.**

Day 1...*day*

Eating and drinking when not at home - *what? - when? - where eaten? - quantity? - cost? - where from?*

Day 7

Activities - *what? - for how long?*

W1

HOW TO USE THE SCALES FOR WEIGHING

Turn the scales on and wait until they show '0 g' on the display. The scales are now ready for use.

Weigh the container that you are going to put the food or drink in and record the weight in the diary.

Leave the container on the scales and press 'ZERO' or 'TARA' (depending on the scales you are using) to set the scales back to '0 g'.

Put your first item of food on the plate on the scales, and write down the weight and description in the diary.

Leave the plate on the scales and press 'ZERO' or 'TARA' again to set the scale back to '0' again.

Repeat the same procedure until you have weighed all the items that are going to be served on the same plate.

Take the plate off the scales.

Press OFF to switch off the scales.

Here is an example of how to weigh a glass of squash and record it in the diary:

- turn on the scales; wait until '0 g' appears;
- weigh the glass; write down the weight;
- press 'ZERO' or 'TARA' to zero the scales and then remove the glass;
- add the squash to the glass, do NOT add the water yet;
- put the glass containing the squash back on the scales;
- write down the weight and description of the squash in the diary;
- press 'ZERO' or 'TARA' to zero the scales and then remove the glass and add the water;
- put the glass and the made-up squash back on the scales;
- write down the weight of the water (and the description - 'tap water') in the diary;
- remove the glass of made-up squash;
- press 'OFF' to switch off the scales.

NOTE: always make sure that the scales show '0 g' BEFORE taking a plate from the scales. When you do this they will show a negative number, for example '-125 g', until you put the plate back on.

W2

CHECK LIST FOR RECORDING IN THE HOME RECORD

EACH PAGE SHOULD HAVE:

- the day and date
- a tick to show whether the young person was well or unwell

WHEN RECORDING:

- start a new page for a new day
- weigh the empty plate or container first
- write down the time the item was eaten, and whether am or pm, in Column A
- start each new food/drink item on a new line; you can use more than one line to describe an item

REMEMBER:

- record all drinks, including tap water, and drinks in bed and during the night
- record all vitamin and mineral supplements, including fluoride supplements
- record all medicines
- record all condiments - sauce, pickle, salad cream etc - used at the table (except salt and pepper)
- for fresh fruit and vegetables ring one code in Column G to show whether or not they were home grown
- weigh the plate with all the leftovers on it and write this in Column E on the *'empty plate line'*
- put a tick in Column E against every item on the plate that was left over
- if anything was lost or spilt and could not be re-weighed put a tick against the item in Column F and describe about how much was lost
- use the back of the diary page to write down recipes, notes and anything you are unsure about

FOOD DESCRIPTIONS PROMPT CARD

Bought form
Fresh
Frozen
Canned
Dried; dehydrated
Ready meal
Smoked; not smoked

Cooking method
Uncooked; raw
Re-hydrated; reconstituted
Boiled; stewed; casseroled
Poached - in milk or water
Steamed
Baked - added fat?- type of fat?
Grilled - added fat? - type of fat?
Roasted - added fat? - type of fat?
Deep fried - type of fat?
Shallow fried - type of fat?
Microwaved - with fat = fried or grilled with fat
Microwaved - with little water = boiled
Dry fried, NO fat = grilled

Leftovers
Meat: fat bones, skin
Fish: bones, skin
Fruit: skin, peel, stones, pips

Coatings
Flour
Batter: egg, flour and milk
Crumb
Egg and crumb

Brand codes
Herbal tea; infant herbal drinks
Bottled water; soft drinks and fruit juices
Artificial sweeteners

Herbal and fruit teas
Herb only; fruit only; herb and fruit mix

Meat preparation
Fat trimmed before cooking or eating?
Fat skimmed from meat dishes?
Lean and fat eaten, or only the lean?

Gravy and sauces
Thickened: with flour, cornflour, Bisto, Gravy Granules
Fat skimmed?
Casseroles: thickened? - fat skimmed?
with vegetables/potatoes?

Pastry
One or two crusts
Type of pastry: shortcrust; flaky; choux; suet
Type of flour: white; wholemeal
Type of fat

Fruit juices
UHT/Longlife/pasteurised/freshly squeezed
Canned?
Sweetened or unsweetened

Soft drinks
Concentrated; ready-to-drink; carbonated
Regular; diet/low calorie/no added sugar/sugar free
Decaffeinated?
Containing fruit juice?
Canned; bottled?
Fortified?

Beverages
Powder made up with milk/water or infusion?
Type of milk

Water - drink on its own or as a diluent?
Tap water
Bottled water - code brand

Artificial sweeteners - code brand
Record and code separately

Fats and oils - refer to checklists
Blended vegetables oil: home fried or takeaway?
Butter: salted or unsalted
Dripping
Lard
Suet - animal or vegetable?
Margarine - hard or soft?
Spread - reduced fat or low fat?
- polyunsaturated?

Dairy products
Full fat or reduced fat?
Milk: skimmed; semi-skimmed; whole; UHT
Yogurt: very low fat; low fat; creamy; UHT;
sweetened with sugar, artificial sweetener
or unsweetened?
fortified/not fortified?
Cheese: full fat or reduced fat

Vegetables and herbs
Home-grown; not home-grown
Carrots: old or new
Potatoes: old or new

Chips
Old/new potatoes: fresh/frozen
Cut: crinkle, straight, fine, thick
Oven ready; fried
Type of fat used

Fruit
Canned in syrup; canned in juice
Fruit only; fruit and juice/syrup
Sweetened with sugar, artificial sweetener,
or unsweetened?
Home-grown; not home-grown
Leftover skin, stones weighed/not weighed

Liquid oral medicine
Sugar free?

Interviewer documents – Eating pattern check sheet

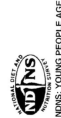

NDNS: YOUNG PEOPLE AGED 4 TO 18 YEARS

EATING PATTERN CHECK SHEET

F2

Serial number label

One sheet must be completed for each young person. Ring code to show number of items eaten each day.

The information for each day must be recorded as soon as the diary pages have been collected, so that any apparently 'missing items' can be probed at the next call; do NOT leave completing this sheet until the diary is complete. Reasons for 'missing items' must be noted on the relevant day page in the diary.

DAY – write in	Drinks			Crisps & savoury snacks			Biscuits & sweets			Supplements, including fluoride			Tick here if note in diary
	Home	School	Other	Home	School	Other	Home	School	Other	Home	School	Other	
...day	1 5	1 5	1 5	1 5	1 5	1 5	1 5	1 5	1 5	1 5	1 5	1 5	5
	2 6	2 6	2 6	2 6	2 6	2 6	2 6	2 6	2 6	2 6	2 6	2 6	6
	3 7	3 7	3 7	3 7	3 7	3 7	3 7	3 7	3 7	3 7	3 7	3 7	7
	4 8	4 8	4 8	4 8	4 8	4 8	4 8	4 8	4 8	4 8	4 8	4 8	8
...day	1 5	1 5	1 5	1 5	1 5	1 5	1 5	1 5	1 5	1 5	1 5	1 5	5
	2 6	2 6	2 6	2 6	2 6	2 6	2 6	2 6	2 6	2 6	2 6	2 6	6
	3 7	3 7	3 7	3 7	3 7	3 7	3 7	3 7	3 7	3 7	3 7	3 7	7
	4 8	4 8	4 8	4 8	4 8	4 8	4 8	4 8	4 8	4 8	4 8	4 8	8
...day	1 5	1 5	1 5	1 5	1 5	1 5	1 5	1 5	1 5	1 5	1 5	1 5	5
	2 6	2 6	2 6	2 6	2 6	2 6	2 6	2 6	2 6	2 6	2 6	2 6	6
	3 7	3 7	3 7	3 7	3 7	3 7	3 7	3 7	3 7	3 7	3 7	3 7	7
	4 8	4 8	4 8	4 8	4 8	4 8	4 8	4 8	4 8	4 8	4 8	4 8	8

Grid for diary days 4 to 7 continues over page →

DAY – write in	Drinks			Crisps & savoury snacks			Biscuits & sweets			Supplements, including fluoride			Tick here if note in diary
	Home	School	Other	Home	School	Other	Home	School	Other	Home	School	Other	
...day	1 5	1 5	1 5	1 5	1 5	1 5	1 5	1 5	1 5	1 5	1 5	1 5	5
	2 6	2 6	2 6	2 6	2 6	2 6	2 6	2 6	2 6	2 6	2 6	2 6	6
	3 7	3 7	3 7	3 7	3 7	3 7	3 7	3 7	3 7	3 7	3 7	3 7	7
	4 8	4 8	4 8	4 8	4 8	4 8	4 8	4 8	4 8	4 8	4 8	4 8	8
...day	1 5	1 5	1 5	1 5	1 5	1 5	1 5	1 5	1 5	1 5	1 5	1 5	5
	2 6	2 6	2 6	2 6	2 6	2 6	2 6	2 6	2 6	2 6	2 6	2 6	6
	3 7	3 7	3 7	3 7	3 7	3 7	3 7	3 7	3 7	3 7	3 7	3 7	7
	4 8	4 8	4 8	4 8	4 8	4 8	4 8	4 8	4 8	4 8	4 8	4 8	8
...day	1 5	1 5	1 5	1 5	1 5	1 5	1 5	1 5	1 5	1 5	1 5	1 5	5
	2 6	2 6	2 6	2 6	2 6	2 6	2 6	2 6	2 6	2 6	2 6	2 6	6
	3 7	3 7	3 7	3 7	3 7	3 7	3 7	3 7	3 7	3 7	3 7	3 7	7
	4 8	4 8	4 8	4 8	4 8	4 8	4 8	4 8	4 8	4 8	4 8	4 8	8
...day	1 5	1 5	1 5	1 5	1 5	1 5	1 5	1 5	1 5	1 5	1 5	1 5	5
	2 6	2 6	2 6	2 6	2 6	2 6	2 6	2 6	2 6	2 6	2 6	2 6	6
	3 7	3 7	3 7	3 7	3 7	3 7	3 7	3 7	3 7	3 7	3 7	3 7	7
	4 8	4 8	4 8	4 8	4 8	4 8	4 8	4 8	4 8	4 8	4 8	4 8	8

Please return the completed sheet, tagged to the front of the Home Record Diary

mealschk.doc:w3

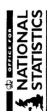

SCHOOL CATERING QUESTIONNAIRE

We would be very grateful if you could provide us with information about catering for

....SCHOOL

This will help us in coding the information on school meals recorded in food diaries kept by young people taking part in the survey. All the information you and the young people provide will be treated in confidence and will not be presented in any way that can be associated with the names or addresses of individuals or schools

Thank you very much for your help

Jan Gregory,
Principal Researcher
ONS
1 Drummond Gate
London SW1V 2QQ
0171 533 5387/8

F3

W4

1

Please answer all the questions and give as much information as possible, including any brand names, a detailed description of the product and the name of the supplier. Please use a separate sheet of paper if you need more space

1 Which oil do you use for deep fat frying?

2 Which oil do you use for all other frying?

3 Which margarine, butter or spread do you use for spreading on sandwiches?

4 Which margarine, butter, spread or other fat, eg suet, do you use for cooking?

5 Which type(s) of milk do you buy?
(tick all that apply)

whole milk

semi-skimmed milk

skimmed milk

dried milk

other *(please describe)*

e.g. soya milk

6 What type(s) of milk do you offer as a drink, and in tea and coffee?

7 What type(s) of cheese do you use in sandwiches and in cooking?

2

W4

8 Which of the following yogurts do you buy?

Tick if bought

creamy yogurts	
low fat yogurts	
very low fat yogurts	
don't buy yogurts	

9 Do you make wholemeal pastry?

Ring one   Yes   No

If yes: what proportion of wholemeal to white flour do you use?

.... wholemeal to

.... white

10 Which of the following types of soft drinks do you serve?

	Diet, low calorie, no added sugar or sugar free	Not diet, low calorie, no added sugar or sugar free
Carbonated soft drinks e.g. lemonade		
Concentrated fruit drinks e.g. squash		
Ready to drink still drinks e.g. Ribena		
Other (please specify)		

10(a) What brand(s) of concentrated fruit drinks/squashes do you serve? Please list the full description from the label.

11 Which of the following types of fruit juices do you serve? *Please tick all that apply*

	Unsweetened	Sweetened
100% pure fruit juice: e.g. apple		
100% pure fruit juice: served diluted e.g. apple		

3

W4

12 How would you usually cook the following foods - grill, oven bake, fry, or cook in some other way?

	Tick method for each food			
	Grill	Oven bake	Fry	Other way (please state what)
Sausages				
Fish				
- in batter				
- plain				
- in breadcrumbs				
Burgers or similar products				
- beef				
- turkey				
- chicken				
- vegetarian				

13 What type(s) of chips do you buy and how do you cook them? (please tick)

	Bought?		Oven Bake	Fry	Other (please say what)
	Yes	No			
Oven chips: standard					
low fat					
Frozen chips: thick cut					
straight cut					
crinkle cut					
fine cut					
French fries					
Pre-fried chips					
Home-made chips: old potatoes					
new potatoes					

4

W4

Interviewer documents – School catering questionnaire – *continued*

14   Apart from potatoes, are vegetables usually bought

Ring one   Fresh   Frozen   Canned

15   Is mashed potato made from

Ring one   Fresh potato   Instant potato

16   Is tinned fruit purchased in syrup or natural juice?

Ring one   Syrup   Natural
                              juice

17   Please describe how much you usually give as one serving of the following foods
     (e.g. ladle, scoop, tablespoon)

        mashed potato   ....

        other vegetables   ....

        gravy   ....

        custard   ....

        other sauce   ....

18   How many boiled or roast potatoes do you normally give in one serving?
     e.g. 2 egg sized potatoes   ....

19   How much meat do you usually give in one serving

        Number of slices?   ....

        Thickness of slices?   ....

        Size of slices? *e.g. 2 x 3 ins*   ....

Thank you for your help. the completed questionnaire will be collected by our
interviewer

5

W4

INTERVIEWER: use this page (both sides) to record answers to probes about specific
items recorded in this young person's Eating Out Diary

6

W4

607

F5

N1404 NDNS: YOUNG PEOPLE AGED 4 TO 18 YEARS

GUIDE WEIGHTS: typical portion sizes for young people

Note: these weights are a guide; reported weights outside these ranges may be correct, but should always have a note to explain the circumstances. You should only use this sheet in the early days of fieldwork. After the first two weeks, you should rely on your own experience. Remember that portion sizes for 18 year olds will be much larger than for 4 year olds.

Approximate conversion factors: grams→ pounds and ounces

454g = 1lb
228g = 8oz
114g = 4oz
60g = 2oz
30g = 1oz

Food	Weight (grams)
Ready Brek, made up	100 - 225
Rice Krispies, 5 -12 tablespoons	20 - 48
Cornflakes/Branflakes 3 - 7 tablespoons	20 - 50
Weetabix, one	20
Bread, one slice, medium-sliced large loaf	36
Bread, without crust, one slice, medium-sliced large loaf	25
Fat spread on a slice of bread	5 - 10
Baked beans canned in tomato sauce, 1 - 5 tablespoons	40 - 200
Fish finger, one	28
Sausage, one	20 - 40
Carrots, boiled	20 - 85
Peas, boiled	30 - 100
Potatoes, mashed or boiled	40 - 220
Chips	40 - 240
Rice, boiled 1-7 tablespoons	40 - 280
Pasta, boiled 1-12 tablespoons	30 - 350

continued over→

Food	Weight (grams)
Yogurt	100 - 150
Fromage frais	40 - 100
Ice cream, 1 scoop	60
Apple, one	65 - 170
Banana, no skin	80 - 120
Digestive biscuit	13 - 18
Sweet or semisweet biscuit eg cream sandwich, Rich Tea	7 - 13
Chocolate coated biscuit, eg Club	20 - 30
Crunchy or chewy cereal bar	25 - 40
Pink wafer biscuit	7
Children's milk chocolate bar, eg Wildlife	22
Square of chocolate, one	7
Finger of Fudge bar	30
Mars bar, standard	65
Crisps, one packet	25 - 30
Cornsnacks, one packet	20 - 25
Glass of wine	125
Can of fizzy drink	330
Carton of drink	200 - 250
Squash concentrate	30 - 50
Mug of tea or coffee	220 - 300
Cup of tea or coffee	150 - 220
Milk in tea or coffee	15 - 50
Sugar in tea or coffee, 1 teaspoon	4 - 6

A: TYPICAL EATING PATTERN

TO BE COMPLETED BEFORE PLACING THE DIETARY RECORD

1 I'd like to ask you about what ...(young person)... usually has to eat at different times of the day, but first I'd like to find out at what times he/she gets up, has breakfast, has lunch and so on.
About what time does ...(young person)... usually...(event)?

Prompt each event for the time on weekdays, on Saturdays and on Sundays. Record approx. times in the grid.

Event	Weekdays	Saturdays	Sundays
get up at:			
have breakfast at:			
have lunch at:			
have tea at:			
have dinner at:			
have supper at:			
go to bed at:			

2 I'd now like to know in general terms what ...(young person)... usually has to eat and drink at these different times. For example, at breakfast does he/she have cereal, or toast, or a cooked breakfast? Some young people do not eat breakfast, so if ...(young person)... does not have anything to eat at a particular time, please tell me.

What does he/she usually have to eat and drink, if anything...

Prompt each event for what is eaten on weekdays, on Saturday and on Sundays. Record a brief description in the grid. Ring code X if nothing eaten.

Event	Weekdays	Saturdays	Sundays
in bed or before breakfast:	Nil.....X	Nil.....X	Nil.....X
for breakfast:	Nil.....X	Nil.....X	Nil.....X

NATIONAL DIET AND NUTRITION SURVEY ND NS

F7

N1404: Dietary assessment schedule

Interviewer's name

Serial number label

This schedule applies if a dietary record is placed:

If dietary record refused, ring code .... [X]

Return this schedule to ONS, Titchfield with all other documents for this serial number

This document contains the following interview schedules

A: TYPICAL EATING PATTERN

  To be asked before placing the 7-day dietary record   pages 1 - 3

B: USUAL FOODS

  To be asked before placing the 7-day dietary record   pages 4 - 6

C: DIETARY RECORD QUALITY ASSESSMENT

  Interviewer assessment to be completed after fully checking and coding the dietary record.   pages 7 - 9

When complete, this schedule should be returned to ONS. Titchfield attached to the front of the Home Record Diary and with all other documents for this serial number

Interviewer documents – Dietary assessment schedule – *continued*

What does he/she usually have to eat or drink:

	Weekdays	Saturdays	Sundays
during the morning before lunch:	Nil.....X	Nil.....X	Nil.....X
for lunch:	Nil.....X	Nil.....X	Nil.....X
during the afternoon:	Nil.....X	Nil.....X	Nil.....X
for tea:	Nil.....X	Nil.....X	Nil.....X
for dinner:	Nil.....X	Nil.....X	Nil.....X
for supper:	Nil.....X	Nil.....X	Nil.....X

What does he/she usually have to eat or drink:

	Weekdays	Saturdays	Sundays
during the evening before going to bed:	Nil.....X	Nil.....X	Nil.....X
in bed, or during the night:	Nil.....X	Nil.....X	Nil.....X

610

Interviewer documents – Dietary assessment schedule – *continued*

B: USUAL FOODS: TO BE COMPLETED BEFORE PLACING THE DIETARY RECORD

Interviewer to ask:

1 Which types of milk do you usually use?
(code all that apply)

full cream; whole milk; silver top - inc homogenized...	1
semi-skimmed; half fat; red and white striped cap on bottles...	2
skimmed; (virtually) fat free; blue and silver cap on bottles...	3
dried or powdered milk; *specify brand*...	4
soya milk, *specify brand*...	5
other type of milk, *specify type and brand*	6

2 Which types of spread do you usually use for bread, toast etc?
Specify full name, including brand

3 Which types of fat or oil do you usually use for cooking - roasting or frying?
Specify full name, including brand

4 What types of soft drinks do you usually have; are they:

RUNNING PROMPT	low calorie/diet drinks...	1
	or standard non-diet drinks?...	2

5 Do you usually buy:
(code all that apply)

INDIVIDUAL PROMPT	fizzy drinks in bottles?...	1
	fizzy drinks in cans? ...	2
SPONTANEOUS	doesn't buy fizzy drinks...	3

6 Which types of bread do you usually have?
(code all that apply)

white...	1
brown or wheatgerm...	2
wholemeal...	3
granary...	4
softgrain - *specify brand*...	5
other type - *specify type and brand*...	6

7 Do you usually buy:

sliced bread...	1
or unsliced loaves?...	2

8 (When you cut it) is your bread usually:

RUNNING PROMPT	thin sliced...	1
	medium sliced...	2
	thick sliced...	3
	or does it vary?...	4

9 What type of fruit juice do you usually have? Is it:
(code all that apply)

RUNNING PROMPT	long life...	1
	pasteurized...	2
	or freshly squeezed?...	3
SPONTANEOUS	doesn't buy fruit juice...	4

Interviewer documents – Dietary assessment schedule – *continued*

10 Do you grow any of your own fruit or **vegetables**?

yes............ 1

no............. 2

C: DIETARY RECORD QUALITY ASSESSMENT: TO BE COMPLETED

BY THE INTERVIEWER AFTER FULLY CHECKING AND CODING THE DIETARY RECORD

1 How often do you think the following items were **omitted** from the <u>Home Record Diary</u>?

	Confectionery and snacks	Full meals	Biscuits and cakes	Drinks
Never	1	1	1	1
Only a couple of times	2	2	2	2
About once a day	3	3	3	3
More often than once a day.	4	4	4	4

2 How often do you think the following items were omitted from the <u>Eating Out Record</u>?

	Confectionery and snacks	Full meals	Biscuits and cakes	Drinks
Never	1	1	1	1
Only a couple of times	2	2	2	2
About once a day	3	3	3	3
More often than once a day.	**4**	**4**	**4**	**4**

3 About what proportion of items in the <u>Home Record Diary</u> do you think were weighed at the time they were eaten?

All or nearly all.................... 1

At least three quarters.......... 2

At least half, but fewer than three quarters 3

Between a quarter and half..... 4

Fewer than a quarter 5

None or almost none 6

612

Interviewer documents – Dietary assessment schedule – *continued*

4   Apart from any things that were missing, how good is the **recording**
    in the <u>Home Record Diary</u> - detail about foods, leftovers etc?

    Very good   1
    Good   2
    Adequate   3
    Poor   4
    Very poor   5

5   And, apart from any things that were missing, how good
    is the **recording** in the <u>Eating Out Record</u> - detail about foods,
    prices, where eaten, leftovers etc?

    Very good   1
    Good   2
    Adequate   3
    Poor   4
    Very poor   5

6   Were there any particular circumstances that affected the young person's
    eating habits during the 7-day dietary recording period?

    Yes........   1   (a)
    No..........   2   Q7

    (a) What was different about the young person's eating
        habits over these days?

Quality assessment

7   Overall, how good do you think the diaries are at reflecting what the
    young person ate over the period?

    Complete record of items <u>and</u>   very few estimated weights....   1
                                            some estimated weights....   2
                                            nearly all estimated weights.... 3

    Some items missing <u>and</u>   very few estimated weights....   4
                                            some estimated weights....   5
                                            nearly all estimated weights.... 6

    Lots of missing items <u>and</u>   very few estimated weights....   7
                                            some estimated weights....   8
                                            nearly all estimated weights.... 9

8   Please use the space below for other comments on the quality of the dietary records

    THIS MUST BE COMPLETED

Quality assessment

613

OFFICE FOR NATIONAL STATISTICS

Social Survey Division

JAN GREGORY
NDNS Project Manager
Social Survey Division: Research
Room D2/23

Tel: **0171 533 5387**
Fax: **0171 533 5300**
Email: jan.gregory@ons.gov.uk

Our ref: B-N1404/W4
Your Ref:

1997

To the Head Teacher

Dear Sir or Madam

National Diet and Nutrition Survey: young people aged 4 to 18 years

Social Survey Division of the Office of National Statistics (ONS) is carrying out this important survey on behalf of the Ministry of Agriculture, Fisheries and Food and the Department of Health. The aim of the survey is to provide information on the diet and nutritional status of young people living in private households in Great Britain, and is part of a programme of surveys which has already covered pre-schoolchildren and elderly persons.

The young people taking part in the survey are asked to keep a diary for 7 days recording, in detail, everything they eat and home and elsewhere. Where the food is provided by the school the young person is generally unable to provide all the information necessary for the coding and nutritional analysis; for example, generally they do not know about portion sizes, cooking methods and types of fats used for cooking and spreading. We are asking the survey interviewer working with the young person and their family to try to find out this information directly from the school.

One of the young people taking part in the survey is a pupil at your school and we would appreciate your co-operation in allowing the interviewer to speak to the catering manager or cook, at a convenient time, when it will cause the minimum inconvenience and disruption.

All our interviewers are employees of ONS and carry an identity card with their name, interviewer number and a photograph.

I have already written to all Directors of Education in areas where we are working informing them of the nature of the survey, and you may have seen something about the survey in the DfEE publication Schools Update. If you would like more information please do not hesitate to ring me.

F8

1 Drummond Gate, London, SW1V 2QQ
Social Survey Division Enquiries (0171) 533 5500 Fax (0171) 533 5300

Thanking you in anticipation of your help.

Yours faithfully

[signature]

JAN GREGORY

Bowel movements card

→ continued from the other side:

Day of the week - write in - Tues, Wed, Thurs, etc	Number of bowel movements at home - ring next number after each movement			Number while not at home - copy total number for the day from the other chart - B2			Total number of bowel movements today - write in
4th day is: ....day	0 4	1 5	2 6	3 7	0 4	1 5	2 6	3 7	Total today: _____
5th day is: ....day	0 4	1 5	2 6	3 7	0 4	1 5	2 6	3 7	Total today: _____
6th day is: ....day	0 4	1 5	2 6	3 7	0 4	1 5	2 6	3 7	Total today: _____
7th, and last day is: ....day	0 4	1 5	2 6	3 7	0 4	1 5	2 6	3 7	Total today: _____

Please hand this chart back to the interviewer
at the end of the 7 days.
Thank you.

Interviewer: check at home and away from home entries.
enter total in Blaise. and return this chart
tagged to front of measurement schedule (M1).

bowelbbv4.doc

YOUNG PEOPLE AGED 4 TO 18 YEARS

Serial number label

Record of bowel movements

We would like to have a record of the number of bowel movements that the young person has on each day that the food diary is kept, starting on the first full day of keeping the food diary - day 1 - and finishing on day 7.

Please keep this chart safely at home. There is another chart on the inside cover of the diary used for recording details of things eaten and drunk while away from home. That chart should be used to record any bowel movements while away from home, for example, while at school or work.

Both charts should be completed each day for the 7 days that the food diary is kept.

At end of each day please write the total number of bowel movements for that day, *number at home plus number away from home*, in the right-hand column of this chart.

If you have any questions, or are not sure how to complete the forms, ask the interviewer who will be pleased to help you.

Thank you.

Day of the week write in - Tues, Wed, Thurs, etc	Number of bowel movements at home - ring next number after each movement			Number while not at home - copy total number for the day from the other chart - B2			Total number of bowel movements today - write in
1st day is: ....day	0 4	1 5	2 6	3 7	0 4	1 5	2 6	3 7	Total today: _____
2nd day is: ....day	0 4	1 5	2 6	3 7	0 4	1 5	2 6	3 7	Total today: _____
3rd day is: ....day	0 4	1 5	2 6	3 7	0 4	1 5	2 6	3 7	Total today: _____

Continues on the other side →

B1

615

N1404/ W3

Serial number label [ ]

MEASUREMENTS SCHEDULE

This schedule contains

A - E: BLOOD PRESSURE AND ANTHROPOMETRIC MEASUREMENTS, including clothing record	pages 2 - 12 pages 19 - 20

All measurements should be recorded on this document at the time they are taken.

F:	**BLOOD SAMPLE RECORD**	pages 13 - 16
G:	**URINE SAMPLE RECORD**	pages 17 - 18
H:	**PRESCRIBED MEDICINES INFORMATION**	pages 21 - 22

The information in this schedule should be subsequently entered in the Blaise questionnaire.

When complete, this schedule should be returned to ONS, Titchfield with all other documents for this serial number

1

BLOOD PRESSURE AND ANTHROPOMETRIC MEASUREMENTS

This page to be completed before returning this schedule.

I:

Measurement	Measurement made?			Tick when entered in Blaise
	DNA	No	Yes	
Blood pressure	9	2	1	
Height		2	1	
Weight		2	1	
Mid-upper arm circumference		2	1	
Waist circumference - applies only if aged 11 years or over	9	2	1	
Hip circumference - applies only if aged 11 years or over	9	2	1	

II: If blood pressure measurement taken:

readings copied onto DNU consent form?   Yes 1

consent form with readings sent to DNU?   Yes 2

2

Measurements schedule – *continued*

A: BLOOD PRESSURE

A1 Blood pressure can only be measured when ALL the following = Yes

Ring code	Yes	No
GP notified of subject's participation in study (Z1)	1	2
Consent to take measurement given (Z3)	1	2
Consent to notify GP of results given (Z3)	1	2

If any of the above = 2, ring code [9] — **Do NOT take BP.**

Introduce

A2 Can I just check, have (you) eaten or drunk anything in the last 30 minutes?

Yes, eaten 1
Yes, drunk something ... 2
No, neither 3

Take three measurements from right arm - if no measurements taken go to A10.

A3 Date of measurement: [ ][ ] [9][7] [ ]
    Day   Month   Year

A4 Time measured - first reading (24 hrs): [ ][ ] Hours Minutes

A5 BP reading:

First reading:
  SYSTOLIC (mmHg) [ ]
  DIASTOLIC (mmHg) [ ]
  MAP (mmHg) [ ]
  PULSE (bpm) [ ]

Second reading:
  SYSTOLIC (mmHg) [ ]
  DIASTOLIC (mmHg) [ ]
  MAP (mmHg) [ ]
  PULSE (bpm) [ ]

Third reading:
  SYSTOLIC (mmHg) [ ]
  DIASTOLIC (mmHg) [ ]
  MAP (mmHg) [ ]
  PULSE (bpm) [ ]

A6 Check: Interviewer code (a) and (b)

(a) Are **all three systolic** readings equal to or above 160mmHg?

Yes .... 1 — **Report results to GP and Dr Jackson**
No .... 2 — (b)

(b) Are **all three diastolic** readings equal to or above 100mmHg?

Yes .... 1 — **Report results to GP and Dr Jackson**
No .... 2 — A7

A7 Cuff size used:

Large adult size 1
Adult size 2
Small adult size 3
Child size 4

A8 Any difficulties in fitting or wrapping cuff?

Yes .... 1 — (a)
No .... 2 — A9

(a) Code difficulties (code all that apply)

Conical shaped arm 1
Obese arm; correct circumference cuff too deep ... 2
Other difficulties with the cuff (specify) ... 3

Measurements schedule – *continued*

A9 Any unusual circumstances?

Yes .... 1 — (a)

No .... 2 — **A10**

(a) **Code unusual circumstances: (code all that apply)**

Young person was upset/anxious/nervous 1

Error 844 -excessive movement 2

Right arm unavailable,taken from left arm 3

Other (specify) 4

A10 If measurement not made: reason (code all that apply)

Attempted,unsuccessful 1

Not attempted, consent withdrawn by young person ... 2

Not attempted, consent withdrawn by 'parent' 3

Equipment failure/unavailable 4

B: **HEIGHT** - if measurement not made go to **B4**

B1 Date of measurement:

		9	7
Day	Month	Year	

B2 **Height:**

1st measurement (cms) →

2nd measurement (cms) →

B3 Any unusual circumstances?

Yes .... 1 — (a)

No .... 2 — **B4**

(a) Code unusual circumstances: (code all that apply)

Affected by hairstyle 1

Wearing turban 2

Posture; back not straight 3

Posture; legs not straight 4

Unable to stand still/unco-operative 5

Other person made measurement 6

Other (specify) 7

Measurements schedule – *continued*

B4 If measurement not made; reason: (code all that apply)

Attempted, but unsuccessful 1
Not attempted, refusal by young person 2
Not attempted, refusal by 'parent' 3
Not attempted, young person chairfast/bedfast 4
Equipment failure/unavailable 5

B5 Ask and record height of 'birth' mother:
(no need to measure)

Not known: **ring code** .... 9 — DNA, go to B6

Height:

☐ . ☐☐ m

☐☐ . ☐ cms

Or

☐ . ☐ feet

☐☐ . ☐ inches

B6 Ask and record height of 'birth' father: (no need to measure)

Not known: **ring code** .... 9 — DNA, go to next measurement

Height:

☐ . ☐☐ m

☐☐ . ☐ cms

Or

☐ . ☐ feet

☐☐ . ☐ inches

C: WEIGHT - if measurement not made go to C6

C1 Date of measurement:

| ☐☐ | ☐ 9 | 7 |
| Day | Month | Year |

C2 Weight:

☐☐ . ☐ 1st measurement (kilograms) ——→

☐☐ . ☐ 2nd measurement (kilograms) ——→

C3 Clothing record

Ask young person to complete the clothing record at the back of this schedule (pages 18/19) and hand back to you. If refused, interviewer to complete.

At home enter information in Blaise document.

Clothing record completed by young person/parent 1
Clothing record refused - interviewer completed 2
No clothing record 3

C4 Ring code if scales placed on: (code all that apply)

Uneven floor 1
Carpet 2

C5 Any unusual circumstances?

Yes .... 1 (a)
No 2 C6

(a) Code unusual circumstances: (code all that apply)

Wearing heavy clothes/shoes 1
Other person did weighing 2
Other (specify) 3
....

Measurements schedule – *continued*

C6 If measurement **not made**; reason: (code all that apply)

Attempted, unsuccessful	1
Not attempted, refusal by young person	2
Not attempted, refusal by 'parent'	3
Not attempted, young person chairfast/bedfast	4
Equipment failure/unavailable	5

D: MID-UPPER ARM CIRCUMFERENCE - if measurement not made go to **D4**

D1 Date of measurement:

Day	Month	Year
	9	7

D2 Circumference

1st measurement (cms) →

2nd measurement (cms) →

D3 Any unusual circumstances?

Yes	1 — (a)
No	2 — **D4**

(a) Code unusual circumstances: **(code all that apply)**

Unco-operative/would not keep still	1
Other person took measurement	2
Left arm unavailable: measured right arm	3
Other (specify)	4

D4 If measurement **not made**; reason: **(code all that apply)**

Attempted, unsuccessful	1
Not attempted, refusal by young person	2
Not attempted, refusal by 'parent'	3

10

Measurements schedule – *continued*

E: WAIST AND HIP CIRCUMFERENCES

Applies if aged 11 and over only

DNA, aged under 11 years; ring code .... 9 → **Go to next measurement**

E1 Date of measurement: – **if measurement not made go to E4**

	9	7	
Day	Month		Year

E2 Circumferences

1st Measurement

Waist ☐☐.☐ cms   **Hip** ☐☐.☐ cms

2nd Measurement

Waist ☐☐.☐ cms   **Hip** ☐☐.☐ cms

E3 Any unusual circumstances?

Yes .... 1 → (a)

No .... 2 → **E4**

(a) Code unusual circumstances: **(code all that apply)**

Clothing thickness different at waist and hips 1

Posture difficulty 2

Unco-operative/would not keep still 3

Other person made measurement 4

(Other (specify)) 5

11

E4 If measurement **not made**; reason: **(code all that apply)**

Attempted, unsuccessful 1

Not attempted, refusal by young person 2

Not attempted, refusal by 'parent' 3

Not attempted, young person chairfast/bedfast 4

12

621

Measurements schedule – *continued*

F: BLOOD SAMPLE RECORD

F1: Interviewer to code:

Consented to fasting sample being attempted .... 1 → F2

Consented to non-fasting sample being attempted .... 2 → (a)

Refused consent to attempt blood sample .... 3 → (b)

(a) Specify reasons for refusal to FASTING sample

(b) Specify reasons for refusal to attempt blood sample

Blood can only be taken if the consent form has been signed and witnessed.

The phlebotomist must be given a copy of the signed and witnessed consent form (Z4) before attempting to take blood.

F2 Date sample attempted

[ ][ ] [ ][9] [9][7]
Day Month Year

F3 Time at start of 'blood visit' (24 hr clock)

[ ][ ] [ ][ ]
Hours Minutes

Phlebotomist will ask the following questions and record on his/her record form; interviewer to record answers below:

F4 **Applies if agreed to fasting sample**

DNA, non-fasting only: **ring code** .... 9 → Go to F5

Did the young person have anything to eat or drink this morning?

Yes .... 1 → (a)

No .... 2 → F5

(a) Specify what eaten/drunk:

F5 Does young person have epilepsy:

Yes .... 1 → Blood must NOT be taken; END

No .... 2 → F6

F6 Has young person ever been told he/she has a clotting or bleeding disorder:

Yes .... 1 → Blood must NOT be taken; END

No .... 2 → F7

F7 Has young person had a blood sample taken in the last 2 years?

Yes .... 1 → (a)

No .... 2 → F8

(a) Was there a problem?

Yes .... 1 → (i)

No .... 2 → F8

(i) Specify problem:

Measurements schedule – *continued*

Outcome:

F8 Number of attempts made (max 2)

Ring number		**(a)**
None	0	**F9**
One	1	
Two	2	

(a) Reason not attempted

No suitable vein	1	**F11**
Young person refused	2	
Young person too upset/nervous	3	
Refusal on behalf of young person	4	

F9 Sample obtained?

Yes	1	**F10**
No	2	**(a)**

(a) Reason attempted, but unsuccessful

Young person's discomfort/distress	1	**F11**
Vein collapsed	2	
Other (specify)	3	

F10 Volume of sample obtained (mls)

(max 15ml) ⟶

F11 Any other problems reported by the phlebotomist?

Yes	1	**(a)**
No	2	**F12**

(a) Specify problems:

15

F12 Any problems or unusual circumstances you (the interviewer) wish to note?

Yes	1	**(a)**
No	2	**F13**

(a) Specify problems:

F13 Was Emla Cream used?

Yes	1	**(a),(b)**
No	2	**F14**

(a) How long was it left on before attempting to take the sample?

[ ] Minutes

(b) Who applied the Emla cream?

Phlebotomist	1
Young person	2
Parent	3
Other (specify)	4

F14 Time at end of blood visit. (24hr clock)

Hours	Minutes

F15 Phlebotomist's name:

....

16

Measurements schedule – *continued*

PART G: URINE SAMPLE RECORD

G1 Interviewer to code:

Agreed to provide a urine sample and sample obtained ..... 1 → G2

Agreed to provide a urine sample and sample **not** obtained . 2 → (a)

Refused to provide a urine sample ..... 3 → (b)

(a) Reason sample not obtained

(b) Reason sample refused

G2 Date urine sample collected
(by young person)

		9	7
	Day	Month	Year

G3 Time sample collected
(by young person) - 24hr clock

Hours	Minutes

G4 Was it an 'early morning' sample - ie first void of the day?

Yes 1

No 2

G5 Approximate time sample posted - 24 hr clock

Hours	Minutes

G6 Were there any problems in collecting the sample?

Yes ..... 1 → (a)

No ..... 2 → G7

(a) Specify problems:

G7 Were there any problems in packing/posting the sample?

Yes ..... 1 → (a)

No ..... 2 → End Urine - Record

(a) Specify problems:

CLOTHING RECORD FOR FEMALES

What people are wearing obviously makes a difference to their weight at the time. To help us allow for this please put a tick by any item of clothing being worn while being weighed. If something is being worn which is not on the list, please tell the interviewer what it is.

Shoes, trainers and jackets are generally the heaviest pieces of clothing, so these items should not be worn while being weighed.

It would also help if any heavy jewellery was taken off for the short time it takes to be weighed, and any keys or money in pockets removed.

Put a tick besides each item being worn eg

Blouse	√
Skirt	√

Items being worn while being weighed	TICK	If more than one is being worn, please write in how many
Vest		
Pair of socks		
Stockings/tights		
Pants/knickers/briefs		
Bra		
Suspender belt		
Petticoat/slip		
Blouse		
T-shirt		
Skirt		
Trousers/Jeans		
Leggings		
Shorts		
Belt		
Dress		
Jumper		
Cardigan		
Something else not on the list - *please tell the interviewer*		

19

CLOTHING RECORD FOR MALES

What people are wearing obviously makes a difference to their weight at the time. To help us allow for this please put a tick by any item of clothing being worn while being weighed. If something is being worn which is not on the list, please tell the interviewer what it is.

Shoes, trainers and jackets are generally the heaviest pieces of clothing, so these items should not be worn while being weighed.

It would also help if any heavy jewellery was taken off for the short time it takes to be weighed, and any keys or money in pockets removed.

Put a tick besides each item being worn eg

Shirt	√
Trousers	√

Items being worn while being weighed	TICK	If more than one is being worn, please write in how many
Vest		
Pair of socks		
Pants/briefs		
T-shirt		
Shirt		
Tie		
Trousers/Jeans		
Shorts		
Belt		
Jumper/Sweatshirt		
Something else not on the list - *please tell the interviewer*		

20

Measurements schedule – *continued*

H: PRESCRIBED MEDICINES - this information is to be collected at the pick-up call at the end of the dietary recording period.

H1 Has the *(young person)* taken any prescribed medicines since the start of the record-keeping period?

If dietary record refused ask:

Is *(young person)* currently taking any prescribed medicines?

Yes .... 1 — H2

No .... 2 — **End of prescribed medicines section**

H2 Interviewer to record details of all prescribed medicines taken during record-keeping period/currently.

Include all prescribed medicines - not just those taken orally: include injections, inhalers, skin preparations etc. Include the oral contraceptive, if taken. Ask to see the medicine container/packet and copy full product name, including brand, and strength if given.

NB Please write in pen (not pencil) and in BLOCK CAPITALS. This information will not be entered by you in Blaise.

Medicine 1:
Name (incl brand)

Strength (if given)

Medicine 2:
Name (incl brand)

Strength (if given)

Medicine 3:
Name (incl brand)

Strength (if given)

Medicine 4:
Name (incl brand)

Strength (if given)

21

Medicine 5:
Name (incl brand)

Strength (if given)

Medicine 6:
Name (incl brand)

Strength (if given)

Medicine 7:
Name (incl brand)

Strength (if given)

Medicine 8:
Name (incl brand)

Strength (if given)

Medicine 9:
Name (incl brand)

Strength (if given)

Medicine 10:
Name (incl brand)

Strength (if given)

Interviewer: after entering the information in this schedule into the Blaise, return the schedule to ONS, Titchfield, with all other documents for this serial number.

22

We would like to thank you, and all the other young people and their families who kindly spared so much of their time to help us with this survey

YOUNG PERSON'S RECORD CARD

This information was collected for the National Diet and Nutrition Survey of Young People aged 4 to 18 years. The survey was carried out by the Social Survey Division of the Office for National Statistics, and is for the Departments of Health and the Ministry of Agriculture, Fisheries and Food

The information from the survey will help in better understanding the relationship between what young people eat and their health, and will help to improve the health of all young people in the future

NAME: ....

DATE: ....

M2

NATIONAL STATISTICS

The results of the survey will be published in Spring 1999. The Report will be available from HMSO. For further information about the survey contact:

Jan Gregory
Social Survey Division, ONS
1 Drummond Gate
London SW1V 2QQ
0171 533 5387/8

These are your measurements:

BLOOD PRESSURE

First reading
Systolic (mmHg)

Second reading
Systolic (mmHg)

Third reading
Systolic (mmHg)

Diastolic (mmHg)

Diastolic (mmHg)

Diastolic (mmHg)

PULSE - beats per minute

First reading

Second reading

Third reading

Interviewer's initials..

HEIGHT .... cm

WEIGHT .... kg

WAIST CIRCUMFERENCE .... cm

HIP CIRCUMFERENCE .... cm

MID UPPER-ARM CIRCUMFERENCE .... cm

The leaflet the interviewer gave you tells you more about all these measurements

627

N1404 NDNS: YOUNG PEOPLE AGED 4 TO 18 YEARS

Metric to imperial weight conversion chart

One pound = 0.454 kilos
One kilo = 2.204 pounds

Kilos	Stones	pounds	Kilos	Stones	pounds	Kilos	Stones	Pounds
10	1	8	30	4	10	50	7	12
11	1	10	31	4	12	51	8	0
12	1	12	32	5	0	52	8	3
13	2	1	33	5	3	53	8	5
14	2	3	34	5	5	54	8	7
15	2	5	35	5	7	55	8	9
16	2	7	36	5	9	56	8	11
17	2	9	37	5	11	57	8	13
18	2	12	38	6	0	58	9	2
19	3	0	39	6	2	59	9	4
20	3	2	40	6	4	60	9	6
21	3	4	41	6	7	61	9	8
22	3	7	42	6	9	62	9	11
23	3	9	43	6	11	63	9	13
24	3	11	44	6	13	64	10	1
25	3	13	45	7	1	65	10	3
26	4	1	46	7	4	66	10	3
27	4	4	47	7	6	67	10	7
28	4	6	48	7	8	68	10	10
29	4	8	49	7	10	69	10	12

metricon doc

The "Salt Check" Urine Sample • • •

It will tell us about the salt in your food, and this in turn can have an effect on your blood pressure, and on whether your heart will remain healthy, as you get older. We can't get this essential information in any other way! We are not testing for drugs or viruses.

First the interviewer will arrange with you a time to pick up the sample, as soon as possible after you have collected it.

We would like it to be an early morning sample, if possible, that is, the first time you pass urine after you get up.

The interviewer will give you the following:

A small disposable pot to collect the urine sample
A plastic syringe (A) with a plastic extension tube (C) and a small push-on cap (B).

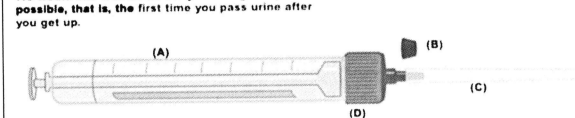

❶ 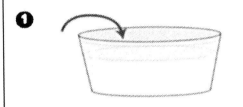 Collect your sample in the disposable pot.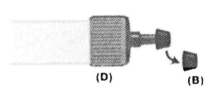

❷ Remove the small push cap (B) from the syringe. DO NOT remove the larger screw-cap (D). There is some "borax" powder in the syringe, to preserve the urine, which will be spilled if you unscrew cap (D). If you make a mistake with this, then mop up the powder carefully with some damp absorbent paper, and throw it away. Ask for another syringe.

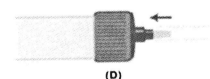

❸ Push the extension tube (C) tightly on the exposed syringe nozzle.

❹ 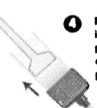 Put the extension tube into the urine in the pot. Pull back the syringe plunger to fill the syringe (DON'T empty and refill it; a single pull on the plunger is enough).

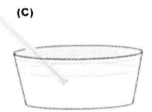

❺ Remove the extension tube and replace the cap (B), pushing it on firmly. You may, if you wish, pull the syringe plunger back until it clicks to a fixed stop-position and then break off the stalk by turning it through a right-angle. (If you are worried about it then leave it to the interviewer to do it).

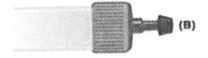

❻ Rinse and throw away the pot and the extension (C) but keep the sample (A) in the syringe, in a cool, dark place, for the interviewer to collect later in the day.

Please Note
1   If you don't understand or have difficulty please ask the interviewer to explain.
2   (Girls) It does not matter if you are having your monthly period, please collect the sample as usual.

THANK YOU!

Appendix B

Example letter as sent to: Directors of Social Services, Chief Constables of Police, Directors of Education, Directors of Public Health and Chief Executives of Health Authorities

Letter to The Director of Social Services

NATIONAL STATISTICS

Social Survey Division

The Director of Social Services

Date as postmark

Dear

National Diet and Nutrition Survey: Young people aged 4 to 18 years

The Social Survey Division of the Office for National Statistics which is the government's survey organization, has been commissioned by the Ministry of Agriculture, Fisheries and Food and the Departments of Health (in England, Wales and Scotland) to carry out a survey to determine the diet and nutritional status of young people aged 4 to 18 years living in private households in Great Britain. This is part of a programme of surveys which has already covered pre-school children and elderly persons.

Because of the nature of the study and its involving young people I am writing to all the Directors of Social Services in the areas where the survey is being carried out. The fieldwork for the survey, which is taking place in 132 areas, will start in January 1997 and continue for 12 months.

Within the area for which you have responsibility, our interviewers will be working as follows:

Overall the survey aims to obtain information for about 2000 young people, about 15 in each area. The sample of addresses for the survey was selected from the Post Office's Postcode Address File and each sampled address was sent a short postal questionnaire to identify those addresses where a young person aged 4 to 18 years was living. Those addresses containing a young person in the eligible age range will be visited by an interviewer who will invite voluntary co-operation. They will be given my name and telephone number to contact for further information.

If co-operation is obtained, the survey starts with a short interview to collect information about the young person and their household and about their general eating habits, physical activities and health. Mothers (or guardians) or the young person themselves, depending on their age, are then asked to keep a detailed diary for seven days weighing and describing every item of food and drink that the young person consumes over the period. A voucher for £5 is given as a token of our appreciation. The interviewer will then seek the young person's

1 Drummond Gate, London, SW1V 2QQ

Social Survey Division Enquiries (020) 7533 5500   Fax (020) 7533 5300   Visit our website at: http://www.ons.gov.uk

co-operation in measuring their blood pressure, height, weight, mid-upper arm circumference, waist and hips and in providing a small sample of urine. Parents will then be invited to consent to allowing a sample of blood to be taken from the young person for analysis. If written witnessed consent is obtained the interviewer will return to the address with the person qualified to take the blood sample. At the end of the survey parents will be invited to co-operate with a further study to find out about their young person's dental habits and condition. This will involve a short interview and a brief dental examination, carried out by a qualified community dentist in the home.

All the interviewers working on the study are employed by the Social Survey Division; all have been trained and are experienced in carrying out surveys on a wide range of topics covering different groups of the population and additionally they will all receive five days of special training for this survey prior to the start of fieldwork. All our interviewers carry identification issued by this Office, and before starting work they will call at the main Police Station(s) covering the sample area to make themselves known to local police. The usual procedure is for their name to be entered in the station 'Day Book'. As the names and addresses of people who take part in any of our surveys are confidential to this Social Survey Division, we are unable to divulge these to the local police or other authorities.

The blood samples are being taken by persons qualified in taking blood, usually a phlebotomist from the local hospital. These personnel have been specially recruited for the study by the Medical Research Council Dunn Nutrition Unit, which is in Cambridge, and which has been contracted to carry out all of the procedures associated with the blood sampling aspects of the survey. These personnel will also receive specialized briefing before the start of fieldwork.

The survey protocol, and in particular the procedures associated with taking the blood sample and blood pressure have been approved by your Local Area National Health Service Ethics Committee. The British Medical Association and the Royal College of Paediatrics and Child Health have been informed of the survey.

I should stress that, as with all the surveys undertaken by this Division, co-operation is voluntary, we rely on people's willingness to take part in order to achieve results which will then be representative of the whole population being studied. In the case of this study, written consent is required for the blood sample from the young person's parent or guardian or from the young person themselves if over the age of 18. It will be made clear to those taking part that they are free to withdraw at any stage.

A pilot survey was conducted earlier this year to test thoroughly the acceptability of the procedures associated with this survey of major importance. All the equipment and instruments being used are of the highest standard to meet the rigorous requirements for quality data demanded by the Ministry of Agriculture, Fisheries and Food and the Departments of Health.

If you would like any further information about the survey, please write to me: Social Survey Division, ONS, 1 Drummond Gate, London SW1P 2QQ or phone 0171 533 5387

I am also writing to Health Authorities, to Directors of Education and of Public Health, and to Chief Constables of Police in the areas to inform them of the survey.

Yours sincerely

Jan Gregory
Principal Social Survey Officer: Project Manager

Appendix C

The feasibility study

Introduction

A feasibility study to test the proposed methodology for the main survey was carried out in 1996 by the Social Survey Division (SSD) of the Office for National Statistics (ONS), the Medical Research Council Dunn Nutrition Unit (DNU) and the Dental Schools at the Universities of Birmingham, Newcastle, Wales and Dundee.

The main aims of the feasibility study were to assess whether the proposed methodologies would provide reliable data on the diets and physical activity of young people in the relevant age range, and whether the proposed measurements and oral health examination were acceptable to respondents and could be carried out effectively. For a sub-group of the study sample, the validity of the dietary recording methodology was tested using the doubly-labelled water methodology to compare energy expenditure against reported energy intake[1]. For the same sub-group the physical activity information collected in the diary was validated by directly measuring the young person's activity level using a motion sensor, the Tritrak monitor.

The main fieldwork for the feasibility study was carried out between February and April 1996. This study identified the need for revisions to and additional fieldwork testing of the dietary and physical activity recording documents, which was completed in October 1996.

The feasibility study covered all of the elements included in the mainstage survey. The design and main findings of the study are summarised here[2].

2   Sample

The feasibility study sample was not designed to be nationally representative but rather aimed to achieve interviews with about 120 young people, both boys and girls, spread across the four age groups and from different social and economic backgrounds. Fieldwork was carried out in six areas selected to cover both rural and urban areas with different socio-economic profiles. Two interviewers worked in each area and used a 'snowballing' method based on an initial list of randomly selected addresses to identify and recruit young people. The postal sift methodology to be used in the mainstage survey was not tested as it had been successfully used on the earlier NDNS survey of children aged 1½ to 4½ years[3]. The design of the feasibility study precluded a test of response.

Initial interviews were achieved with 127 respondents, 66 boys and 61 girls, spread across the four age bands: 4 to 6 years, 7 to 10 years, 11 to 14 years and 15 to 18 years. The 7-day dietary record was completed in 117 cases.

3   Ethical approval and consent protocol

The Dunn Nutrition Unit (DNU) obtained approval for the proposed survey protocol from the LRECs responsible for each survey area.

Some aspects of the survey required that consent was given for the young person's General Practitioner (GP) to be informed: these were the measurement of blood pressure, the blood sample, the doubly-labelled water study and the oral health examination. Individual signed consent was also required for these aspects of the survey. The feasibility study included a test of the procedures for obtaining consent and for notifying the DNU, which was responsible for reporting results from the blood sample and the blood pressure measurement to the young person and their GP. The tested procedures worked effectively but some changes to the design of forms and information leaflets were recommended in order to make them more acceptable to the different age groups involved.

4   Dietary interview

The initial dietary interview, using computer assisted personal interviewing (CAPI), collected basic demographic and socio-economic data as well as information on health, physical activity, typical eating patterns and food preparation. Usually the parent and young person were interviewed together so that questions could be answered by the most appropriate person. A particular focus of the feasibility study was to explore the best way of dealing with questions on potentially sensitive topics and to establish the age from which these questions should be asked. The topics were smoking, consumption of alcohol, use of the contraceptive pill and age at menarché. Two methods of self-completion, either on paper or on the interviewers' laptop computer (CASI), were tested for the questions on smoking and drinking but questions on the other two topics were asked face-to-face during the interview.

The study showed that the interview length was acceptable and the questionnaire successfully obtained the information required. Recommendations for some minor amendments to question design and to instructions were taken forward to the main stage. The questions on potentially sensitive topics were asked successfully but it was recommended that all of the topics should be administered by self-completion, preferably by laptop computer, but with a paper version also available. The study confirmed that it was appropriate to ask questions on smoking and drinking from age seven upwards and questions on use of the contraceptive pill and age at menarché of girls of 10 years and over.

5   The weighed intake dietary record

In order to provide sufficiently detailed information to calculate intakes for a wide range of nutrients, the preferred method of data collection for the young people's survey was a 7-day weighed intake record. This methodology was tested in the feasibility study with particular regard to whether it was suitable for use with all of the age groups and whether the length of the recording period was acceptable, both in terms of response and data quality.

Respondents were asked to keep a weighed record of all food and drink consumed by the young person for seven consecutive days. Interviewers decided who should be the main diary keeper on the basis of the young person's age and ability. The protocol for collecting the detailed dietary information was similar to that used in the NDNS of children aged 1½ to 4½ years[3]. An 'eating out' diary was also provided. This was an A5 version of the main, home record diary, including a scale in centimetres to allow portion sizes to be estimated. Respondents were also asked to keep a record of the number of bowel movements per day during the 7-day dietary record.

After completion, the food intake diaries were initially checked and coded by the interviewers. They were subsequently checked by a qualified nutritionist and coding team at ONS who, in consultation with MAFF, dealt with any coding queries including estimating missing weights using portion size information. Data entry was carried out by ONS using a program incorporating consistency and continuity checks at the point of data entry. A sub-sample of coded diaries was also keyed by a contractor to test whether the information could be fast-keyed and edited by an

organisation that had no prior knowledge of the data.

The study showed that a recording period of 7 days was acceptable to respondents and that young people aged 11 and over were usually able to keep their own diaries. Overall, a third of diaries were mainly completed by the young person and two thirds by a parent. The record of bowel movements was acceptable to respondents and was completed in all but three cases in which the dietary record was obtained.

The nutritionist and interviewers generally found the quality of information in the home record diary to be of an acceptable level. Questions asked when the interviewer collected the diary showed that there were some occasions on which items had not been weighed, for example where the child had helped him or herself to food, but these items had rarely been missed completely. The records of foods eaten out were, however, less complete and there was some concern about data quality. Interviewers found that the young people had generally not taken the eating out diary with them when away from home, and insufficient detail was recorded. Further development work on the methodology for collecting information on foods eaten outside the home was recommended (see *Section 12 below*).

On the basis of the feasibility study findings, minor changes were made to the organisation of the coding lists and documentation. For the main stage it was recommended that keying operations should remain within ONS, with data entry via a program that included consistency and continuity checks.

A short diary pick-up interview was tested and provided useful information to assess whether the diary represented a typical diet. It was recommended that at the main stage respondents should not be asked specifically about the quality of the diary but this should be assessed by the interviewer.

Incentive payments
As on previous NDNS surveys, respondents were given a small sum of money as a token of appreciation for the effort involved in keeping the dietary record. This was in the form of a £5 gift token, given by the interviewer on collection of the completed diary. Interviewers judged that the offer of a token helped in some cases both to encourage initial co-operation and to motivate respondents to complete the diary. The study confirmed that a payment of £5 was an appropriate amount for this age group and that it should be given in the form of a gift token, exchangeable at a national multiple store with a large number of outlets.

6   The physical activity record
The requirement for collecting data on physical activity was to be able reliably to categorise young people into broad bands of activity level (low, medium and high) in

order to investigate the relationship between level of activity and both energy intake and body composition. A 7-day diary of physical activity was tested in the feasibility study, with particular regard to whether the same method of data collection would be suitable for young people throughout the age range.

The young people were asked to keep a record of physical activity for the same 7-day period as the weighed intake dietary record. The diary divided the week into school days and non-school days and each day into broad time periods. Respondents were asked to record the amount of time spent on each of a given list of activities, which included sedentary activities, and to specify any further activities not listed. The diary was intended to be carried by the young person whenever they left the house. Questions about the young person's usual activities were also included as part of the initial interview to help interviewers to check the diaries.

In order to validate the physical activity diaries, an independent measure of activity was obtained for a subset of the sample by use of a Tritrak portable monitor. This small monitor is worn continuously by the respondent, except when in bed, swimming or bathing, and is able to detect and record movement in three dimensions as periods of vigorous, moderate or sedentary activity. The energy expenditure data from the Tritrak could also be compared with energy expenditure data from the doubly-labelled water study.

The feasibility study showed that the young people had difficulties completing the physical activity diary in the form tested. The problems identified included omission of less formal or structured activities, rounding of time periods, probable under-recording of 'other' activities, and double counting where activities in the list were combined in the same time period (for example, time spent watching videos and talking with friends). In addition, the format of the diary was not appropriate for younger children whose activity was mainly unstructured and so did not fit into the listed categories. It was therefore recommended that physical activity information for young people aged 4 to 6 years should be collected in the initial interview.

The information collected in the diaries was analysed by attaching the appropriate MET value (Metabolic Equivalent) to each activity listed and then calculating a daily score for each young person by multiplying the time spent on each activity by its MET score. The average scores across seven days were then used to categorise the young people into broad bands of activity. The results suggested that the methodology might be overestimating the level of activity. Three quarters of the young people reported spending at least 1½ hours per day on moderate or vigorous activity, and the calculated scores placed all of the sampled young people in the most active category.

Although the use of the Tritrak monitor was found to be acceptable to the young people, there were technical difficulties with its use in the context of a private household sample (rather than, for example, in a school-based sample) and the monitor was therefore not considered for use at the main stage.

In response to these results it was recommended that the design of the physical activity diary and recording method should be revised and fieldwork tested before the mainstage survey, and used only for young people aged 7 or over.

7 Anthropometric and blood pressure measurements

The measurements included in the feasibility study were weight, height, mid upper-arm circumference, waist and hip circumferences (for young people aged 11 years and over only) and blood pressure. The protocol required the procedure for each anthropometric measurement and blood pressure to be repeated three times. Most of the equipment used in the feasibility study had been used in previous NDNS surveys and was carried forward to the main stage (for details see *Chapter 2*). For measurement of height, the Digi-Rod stadiometer used in previous surveys was no longer available[4] and was replaced by the Leicester Height Measure, produced for the Child Growth Foundation[5]. Blood pressure was measured using the Dinamap 8100 oscillometric monitor[6], as used on the NDNS of people aged 65 years and over[7] and the latest Health Survey for England[8], and four different cuff sizes were provided.

There was a high level of co-operation with the anthropometric and blood pressure measurements; 90% of the interview sample agreed to the measurements being attempted. Interviewers generally spread the different measurements over a number of visits, particularly for younger children. All of the values recorded were considered to be feasible for the age group covered.

No specific problems were identified with the height and weight measurements. The Leicester Height Measure was both easy to use and acceptable to respondents. It was recommended that longer insertion tapes were required for measuring mid upper-arm circumference for larger young people, and that the tapes could be made easier to read by having black figures on a white background. Some problems were reported in taking accurate measurements of waist and hip circumferences, namely in arranging clothing to obtain the same thickness at the waist and hips. The protocols for the main stage took account of these comments (see *Chapter 2* and *Appendix L*).

Blood pressure measurements were taken successfully although in some cases interviewers had difficulty in wrapping the large cuff. Interviewers recorded any circumstances that may have affected readings. In line with usual practice on NDNS surveys, procedures were established for immediate reporting of abnormal blood pressure readings to the young person's GP and to the survey doctor. In a small number of cases in the feasibility study the criteria for abnormal readings were met and the reporting procedure worked effectively.

8   Blood sample

Phlebotomists with recent paediatric experience took the blood samples. The ONS interviewer accompanied them on their visit to the respondent's household. The procedures for obtaining consent for a sample and the protocol for taking blood, as outlined in Chapter 2, were followed in the feasibility survey. This test was particularly important in assessing the feasibility of taking a fasting sample, which meant taking the blood sample at an early morning visit, before breakfast.

Consent to the blood sample was obtained from 81 (64%) of the young people who took part in the feasibility study; this is a comparable level of response to the NDNS of children aged 1½ to 4½ years[3]. The likelihood of co-operation increased with the age of the child. Agreement to a fasting sample was given in most cases although sometimes not achieved because only one parent knew about the requirement. Overall the procedures worked well. Early morning visits proved to be acceptable to respondents and the requirement for a fasting sample was carried forward to the main stage.

9   Urine sample

The main purpose of a urine sample is to measure the amount of sodium (as salt) in the diet. A sample of urine from a 24-hour collection is generally accepted to be the most reliable way of measuring sodium excretion. However, studies using the PABA marker technique by Williams and Bingham[9] and in the feasibility study for the NDNS of the people aged 65 years and over[10] have shown the difficulties of achieving complete 24-hour samples in different populations. It was acknowledged that the probability of obtaining complete collection for a sample of young people was relatively low so the requirement for the feasibility study was to collect a 'spot' urine sample of approximately 10ml taken from the first void of the day.

The procedures for collection and despatch of the urine samples worked well and were carried forward to the main stage (see *Chapter 2*). Samples were obtained from 114 young people and a sample from the first void of the day was complied with in 90% of cases. In the other 10% of cases the young person had forgotten rather than been unwilling to comply.

10   Oral health survey and examination

The oral health component tested in the feasibility study comprised an examination and a short interview. A dental examiner carried out the oral examination and results and recommendations relating to the clinical aspects of the examination are presented in the companion volume to this Report[11]. A major element tested in the feasibility survey was the use of a Blaise 2.5 laptop computer program into which interviewers entered the oral health examination data.

Response to the oral health component was high; only one young person who had completed a dietary diary refused to take part. The method of recording the examination data on laptop worked effectively and was retained for the main stage. The total length of the oral health visit was, however, considered to be too long, lasting around 30 to 35 minutes. For the mainstage survey it was recommended that the oral health interview (lasting 10 to 15 minutes) should instead be administered at the diary pick-up visit.

11   An assessment of energy expenditure using the doubly-labelled water method

To assess the validity of the dietary data collected by the weighed intake method, each young person in four of the six survey areas was asked to take part in an assessment of energy expenditure using doubly-labelled water.

The doubly-labelled water method is a means of measuring the total energy an individual expends. The respondent is required to drink a glass of water labelled with the stable isotopes deuterium and oxygen-18, and then to collect a small sample of urine each day for the next 10 days. The isotopes used are harmless and occur naturally in all food and drink. By analysing the urine samples it is possible to calculate the amount of energy a person expends over the period of measurement. This estimate of energy output can then be compared with energy input as estimated from the weighed intake dietary record. The precision of the technique when compared with measurements of total energy expenditure using classical indirect calorimetry is better than +/−5% at the Dunn laboratory[12].

Specific consent was required for the young person to take the doubly-labelled water dose. The required dose for each respondent, dependent on the young person's body weight, was prepared in the DNU laboratory but administered by the interviewer. Respondents were required to collect a pre-dose urine sample and then 10 daily samples, at any time other than from the first urine passed in the morning, starting from the dosing day.

Overall the agreement between the estimates for energy expenditure derived from the doubly-labelled water analysis and for energy intake derived from the dietary record was sufficiently good to conclude that the proposed dietary methodology could be used in the mainstage survey. There was, however, evidence of under-reporting among older respondents, particularly girls. This may have been due to the difficulties of collecting adequate information about foods eaten away from home, as mentioned above, and so could be improved by revision of the eating out methodology and by emphasising the importance for interviewers to check diaries and to probe for more information.

12 The second fieldwork test

A second fieldwork test to evaluate changes to the eating out and physical activity recording documents was carried out in October 1996. The feasibility survey had suggested that there was under-recording of food and drink in the eating out diary and that the original diary for physical activity tended to over-estimate activity levels. A qualitative methodology was chosen in order to test respondent's responses to the self-completion diaries and to provide information to enable improved probing techniques. Because qualitative methods are time-consuming for the respondent, the young people were not asked to co-operate with other aspects of the NDNS survey package, including the weighed dietary record.

Interviews were carried out with 16 young people aged between 7 and 18 years; the main feasibility study had shown that a diary method could not be used to collect accurate data on physical activity for 4 to 6 year olds. Each respondent kept the redesigned diaries for eating out and for physical activity for four days, including two weekend days. After two days of record keeping the interviewer checked the diaries and probed each entry in detail with the respondent. After the final two days the young person was asked to take part in a full qualitative interview about the diary design and the process of record keeping.

The further fieldwork test was intended specifically to test the effectiveness of different probing methods for use when checking the eating out diary; one method was based on the young person's spending money and the other on prompts for different times of day. A larger format for the physical activity diary was tested which allowed more space for entries. The diary listed examples of activities under headings for the relevant activity levels (very light, moderate etc.). Respondents were asked to select the activities in which they had taken part and to record the total time spent in the day. Provision was also made to record other moderate or vigorous activities and descriptions were given to help respondents categorise them to the appropriate activity level. Different styles of instruction pages in the two diaries were also tested.

The test showed that the redesigned diaries were acceptable for use in the mainstage survey with some minor changes based on the findings of this study. It was recommended that the eating out and physical activity pages should be combined into one diary to reduce the number of separate documents for the respondent to complete. The test provided helpful information on potential areas of under-recording of eating out and of methods of probing for both diaries. Probing for eating out based on spending money was found not to have any particular advantage over other probing methods that were normally used.

References

[1] Smithers G, Gregory J, Coward WA, Wright A, Elsom R, Wenlock R. British National Diet and Nutrition Survey of young people aged 4 to 18 years: feasibility study of the dietary assessment methodology. Abstracts of the Third International Conference on Dietary Assessment Methods. *Eur J Clin Nutr* 1998; **52**: S2. S76.

[2] Lowe S. *Feasibility study for the National Diet and Nutrition Survey: young people aged 4 to 18 years.* ONS (*In preparation*).

[3] Gregory JR, Collins DL, Davies PSW, Hughes JM, Clarke PC. *National Diet and Nutrition Survey: children aged 1½ to 4½ years. Volume 1: Report of the diet and nutrition survey.* HMSO (London, 1995).

[4] The Digi-Rod was a portable, telescopic stadiometer, with a digital display, modified, to a specification by OPCS (now ONS) from a Rathbone building surveyor's measuring device (no longer available). The modifications were carried out by Glentworth Fabrications Ltd, Molly Millar's Bridge, Molly Millar's Lane, Wokingham, Berkshire, UK.

[5] The Leicester Height Measure is available from the Child Growth Foundation, 2 Mayfield Avenue, Chiswick, London W4 1PW, UK.

[6] The Dinamap Blood Pressure Monitor Model 8100 is available from Critikon Ltd, Monitor House, Unit 3 Cherrywood, Chineham Business Park, Basingstoke, Hampshire RG24 8WF, UK.

[7] Finch S, Doyle W, Lowe C, Bates CJ, Prentice A, Smithers G, Clarke PC. *National Diet and Nutrition Survey: people aged 65 and over. Volume 1: Report of the diet and nutrition survey.* TSO (London, 1998).

[8] Prescott-Clarke P, Primatesta P. Eds. *Health Survey for England 1995.* TSO (London, 1997).

[9] Williams DRR, Bingham SA. Sodium and potassium intakes in a representative population sample: estimation from 24-hour urine collections known to be complete in a Cambridgeshire village. *Br J Nutr* 1986; **55**: 1; 13-22.

[10] Smith P, Lowe C. *National Diet and Nutrition Survey: people aged 55 and over. A report on the feasibility study (January - April 1994).* SCPR (London, 1998).

[11] Walker A, Gregory J, Bradnock G, Nunn J, White D. *National Diet and Nutrition Survey: young people aged 4 to 18 years. Volume 2: Report of the oral health survey.* TSO (London, 2000): Appendix A.

[12] Livingstone MBE, Prentice AM, Strain JJ, Coward WA, Black AE, Barker ME, McKenna PG, Whitehead RG. Accuracy of weighed dietary records in studies of diet and health. *Br Med J* 1990; **300**: 708-712.

Appendix D

Sample design, response and weighting the survey data

1   Sample design - requirements

A representative sample of young people aged between 4 and 18 years living in private households in Great Britain was required.

The sample size needed to be adequate for analysis of the data by sex within four age groups, 4 to 6, 7 to 10, 11 to 14 and 15 to 18 years. These age groups correspond to those used for Dietary Reference Values and it was important that the intakes of energy and nutrients by the young people in the survey could be compared with these values[1]. Apart from the youngest age group, which comprises three single-year birth cohorts, the remaining age groups each comprise four single-year birth cohorts. The requirement was to achieve an approximately equal number of dietary records for the young people in the three top age groups and a proportionately smaller number for the youngest three-year age group. In determining the overall sample size account was taken of the resources required for the survey, particularly the high unit cost of using a weighed intake dietary methodology. The costs associated with using phlebotomists and dental examiners, processing blood samples, obtaining equipment for making measurements of blood pressure and body size, training interviewers and other fieldworkers, and the costs associated with making a relatively large number of calls at each address also needed to be considered in relation to the number of young people who would be invited to take part in the survey.

It was therefore determined that an overall achieved sample of about 1875 dietary records would be required; 500 for each of the four-year age groups and 375 for the youngest group.

Given the comparatively wide age range for the survey it was likely that in many households there would be more than one young person eligible to take part. However the pattern of dietary behaviour within the same household is likely to be more similar than that between different households. Therefore for the same sample size, information on a much greater variety of diets could be collected by selecting only one eligible young person per household. Selecting only one eligible young

person from a household also reduced the burden on the family, which might have affected co-operation and the quality of the data being collected.

2   The sampling frame and sample size

Not all young people aged between 4 and 18 years are attending school; some in the youngest group may not yet be in education and compulsory full-time education finishes at age 16 years. Although in theory it would have been possible to have used schools and school registers as the sampling frame for those in education, supplemented by a sample of those who had not yet started or had left education, it was decided that the sample should be household based. While clustering cases within schools would have reduced costs compared with a household-based sample, the clustering would have had the effect of increasing the sampling error attached to the estimates, since there would be some similarity in diets for the children in the same school who had lunchtime food provided by the school.

The most suitable frame for the sample was therefore the Small Users' File of the Postcode Address File (PAF). A sample of addresses could be selected from this file and then households containing a young person in the eligible age range identified from responses to a postal questionnaire.

In determining the size of the sample to be issued to interviewers in order to achieve approximately 1875 dietary records the following needed to be taken into account:

- the proportion of households in Great Britain containing a young person in the eligible age range; this was estimated to be 28% from General Household Survey data for 1994 and 1995 combined[2];

- response to the postal sift, estimated as 75%;

- the proportion of addresses on the PAF which would be ineligible because they are not private households, have not yet been built or have been demolished - about 12%;

- the proportion of eligible households identified by the postal sift as containing a young person which had moved without trace before the main fieldwork - about 5%;

- response at the interview stage, outright refusals and refusals to keep the dietary record - 25%;

- the need to produce interviewer work quotas of a manageable size - a maximum of 25 addresses.

On this basis it was estimated that a set sample of 20,000 addresses would be required to achieve 1875 dietary records.

Sub-sampling households with only one eligible young person

Selecting only one eligible young person per household meant that the data subsequently needed to be re-weighted, to allow for the fact that, for example from a household with two eligible young people there is a one in two chance of being selected, compared with a one in three chance from a household with three eligible young people and so on. Where there is only one eligible young person in the household then the chances of selection are 100%. To reduce the re-weighting factor that would need to be applied to the data for young people in households where they were the only one eligible, and hence improve the precision of the estimates, it was decided to select young people from only <u>half</u> the households identified as having just a single eligible young person. To ensure that there were sufficient eligible households to allow for this sub-sampling the size of the original set sample for the postal sift needed to be increased to just under 28,000 addresses.

3   Selecting the addresses

To select the sample of addresses for the postal sift a multi-stage random probability design was used, with postal sectors as first stage units.

All postal sectors in England, Wales and mainland Scotland were stratified as follows; by:

- region;
- population density;
- the proportion of heads of household in socio-economic groups 1 to 5 and 13;
- the proportion of households owning a car[3].

These census-derived variables have been found to be the best all-round stratifiers for surveys on health-related topics[4].

A total of 132 postal sectors was systematically selected, the chances of selection being proportional to the size of the sector - the number of postal delivery points.

As in previous surveys in the NDNS series, fieldwork was required to take place over a 12-month period, to cover any seasonality in eating behaviour. For organisational reasons the 12-month fieldwork period was divided into four fieldwork waves each of three months duration. The 132 selected postal sectors were therefore each systematically allocated to one of the four fieldwork waves, ensuring as far as possible a similar regional distribution in each wave. Thus in each wave fieldwork took place in 33 postal sectors.

In each of the 33 postal sectors in each wave, 210 addresses were systematically selected with a random start from the Small Users' File of the PAF.

3.1   Ineligible addresses

The survey was restricted to young people living in private households, therefore anyone living in a residential institution, such as a hospital or care unit was ineligible to take part. The Small User's File of the PAF excludes delivery points receiving more than 25 items of post daily and therefore excludes most large institutions and non-residential addresses, such as businesses. Any other institutions or non-residential addresses in the sample were identified at the sift stage and excluded as ineligible.

3.2   The postal sift form

Approximately five months before the start of each fieldwork wave, each selected address was sent a sift form asking for details of the sex and date of birth of every person living at the household. In order to avoid response bias the accompanying letter did not refer to the eligible age range for the survey or give details of the nature of the survey. A reminder letter was sent two weeks and four weeks after the initial mailing to non-responding addresses. Residual non-responding addresses were called on by an interviewer who attempted to collect the same information as on the postal sift form. Sift procedures were carried out as close as possible to the start of each fieldwork period to minimise losses due to the household moving.

Response to the postal and interviewer sift stages is shown at the end of this Appendix.

3.3   Multi-household addresses

It is not possible from the PAF for England and Wales to identify multi-household addresses; for Scotland the PAF contains a multi-household indicator which is used in the selection of addresses.

In order to identify concealed multi-households in the sample of addresses in England and Wales a question was specifically included on the postal sift form. If the returned sift form indicated that the address contained more than one household then the address was visited by an interviewer who listed all the households at the address and selected one at random, using a random number selection sheet. Interviewers had eight different multi-household random number selection sheets, which were used consecutively to vary the chance of selection of the household relative to the number of households it contained. In this way each household had an equal chance of selection at a multi-household address, with the probability of selecting one household proportional to the number of households at the address. Since addresses containing only one household, which comprised the majority of the sample, had a unitary chance of selection, theoretically, the sample should be re-weighted to adjust for the different probabilities of selection of households. However, as the overall proportion of concealed multi-household addresses is small this was felt to be unnecessary.

Having selected a single household at concealed multi-household addresses, interviewers then recorded details of the sex and date of birth of all household members, as in the postal sift.

4 Selection of eligible young people

Eligibility, being aged between 4 and 18 years, was determined in relation to the mid-point of each fieldwork wave[5]. Households containing an eligible young person were identified from the completed sift forms. If there was more than one eligible young person in the household then one was selected at random. As noted above, to reduce the weighting factors which needed to be applied to allow for the unequal probabilities of selection of one young person from a household containing different numbers of eligible young people, only half the households with just one eligible young person were selected for inclusion in the set sample.

Since each fieldwork wave covered a three-month period, and the mid-point was taken as defining eligibility, dependent on when during the fieldwork period the interview took place, some young people might not have reached their 4th birthday and some might have already passed their 19th birthday. For the purposes of analysis children under 4 years are included in the group with those aged 4 to 6 years; those aged 19 years are included with those aged 15 to 18 years.

Over the four waves a total of 33 households was selected where one of a pair of identical twins was eligible for interview; in these cases the twin to be interviewed was 'identified' by systematically selecting first and second-born twins.

The following were excluded from the sample at the interview stage:

- young people selected for interview but whose date of birth had been wrongly recorded on the sift form and were outside the eligible age range;

- young people away at boarding school, at any other residential educational establishment or resident in any institution, for example in hospital or care, at the time of fieldwork:

- young people living at addresses on foreign defence establishments - for example, US Air-force bases;

- young people subject to Ward of Court Orders and young people being fostered; these were excluded since the family with whom they were living would not have been able to give the necessary consents for the young person to take part in the survey, and in particular to give a blood sample, have their blood pressure measured or have an oral health examination (see *Chapter 2, Section 2.8.2*).

- young girls who were either pregnant or breastfeeding at the time of fieldwork. The diets and physiology of girls who were pregnant or breastfeeding were likely to be so different from those of other girls of the same age, as to possibly distort the results. Since the number of pregnant or breastfeeding girls identified within the overall interview set sample of 2,500 young people would not be adequate for analysis as a single group it was decided that they should be regarded as ineligible for interview.

5 Movers

Normally, in a survey with a random probability design producing a pre-selected sample of individuals, interviewers are asked to attempt to trace and interview any sampled individual who has moved between the time the sample is selected and their calling; the individual currently occupying the original address cannot be substituted for the mover.

In this survey interviewers were instructed to try to find the new address of any sampled young person who had moved between the postal sift stage and their calling at the address. However if the new address was known, then before the interviewer was able to call or the address was re-allocated to another interviewer working in the area, a check needed to be made to establish whether the new address was in an area where approval for the survey to take place had been obtained from the LREC. This checking was carried out by the Dunn Nutrition Unit.

If the new address was not covered by existing LREC approval then it had to be withdrawn from the sample as it was not feasible to approach any more LRECs to obtain approval in the time available.

Addresses withdrawn at the fieldwork stage for this reason are shown in the category of ineligible in the response tables.

641

6 Response to the postal and interviewer sift stages

Figure 1 represents the various stages in identification of households containing an eligible young person. At the postal sift stage households containing an eligible young person were identified from returns from single-household address; multi-household addresses together with non-responding addresses were issued to interviewers.

Response rates for the sift stages are based on the number of private households identified, known as the eligible address sample.

Response to the postal sift stage was 71% and to the interviewer sift, 74%. Overall response was increased by nearly one third from 71% to 92% as a result of the interviewer follow-up sift. One per cent of addresses refused to complete the sift form at the postal sift stage, and 12% refused at the interviewer sift stage. Thus overall 4% of eligible addresses refused to provide the sift information.

Table D1 shows that the total number of households containing an eligible young person was boosted by the interviewer sift stage, from 4643 to 6308; overall 27% of eligible addresses were found to contain a household with a young person in the eligible age range.

Response rates to the sift stages were very similar by wave (*Table D2*).

From the 6308 households containing an eligible young person, 2672 were selected for interview by taking one young person per household from each eligible household (taking only half the households where there was only one young person in the eligible age range), and then sub-sampling to achieve the required number of young people in each of the eight age and sex groups. As the number of 7-day dietary records achieved in Waves 1 and 2 was lower than expected it was decided to increase the number of eligible addresses issued for interview in Waves 3 and 4 in order to achieve approximately the required number of dietary records (*Table D3*).

The 2672 addresses issued for interview are referred to as the interview sample, and is the base for the response calculations given in Chapter 3.

Not all respondents co-operated with all parts of the survey, and Chapter 3 gives response rates for the different parts. The maximum response rate, defined as those agreeing to the initial interview, was 80% (see *Table D3*); 19% of young people refused to take part in any aspect of the survey.

The maximum response rate did not vary significantly by fieldwork wave; the higher number of co-operating

cases in Waves 3 and 4 reflects the increased number of households containing eligible young people issued for interview in these waves.

7 Weighting the survey data

7.1 Weighting for different sampling probabilities

Weighting was needed to compensate for unequal probabilities of selection because, as described above:

only one young person was selected for interview from households containing more than one eligible young person, so in these cases the probability of selection was proportional to the number of eligible young people in the household;

from households containing one eligible young person only half the households were selected;

in the final stage of selection, all the young people selected were sub-sampled to achieve the correct numbers for interview in the four main age groups for boys and girls separately.

Weighting factors based on these sampling probabilities were calculated and each case was assigned the appropriate weight, which has been used in the data analysis.

7.2 Weighting for differential non-response

As is shown in Chapter 3 there was a differential non-response effect, principally a lower response from males in the 15 to 18 year age group; this was most apparent in Scotland. Initial response rates for these older males were lower than for other age and sex groups and this group also had a higher rate of attrition through the different stages of the survey.

Without weighting for this differential response effect, estimates for different groups, for example mean intakes of nutrients in the different social class groups, would be biased estimates, because, in particular, they under-represent the oldest group of males.

The data have therefore been weighted to adjust for differential non-response using weighting factors based on age group and sex within region.

7.3 Effect of non-response weighting

In order to demonstrate the effect of including a weight for non-response, Table D4 shows two sets of values for two variables. The first of each pair of values is weighted to adjust for differential sampling probabilities only and the second weighted for differential sampling probabilities and differential non-response. The figures are presented for the whole sample and by region. Overall, there is little difference between the two sets of figures. With sampling weights only, mean daily intake of total fat was 68.4g and mean systolic blood pressure was 108mmHg. When the cases were weighted using the combined weight for sampling and non-response, their equivalents were 69.0g and 109mmHg respectively.

7.4 Presentation of data in the report

All data presented in the substantive chapters of this report have been weighted using a combined weight based on the weighting factor for differential sampling probabilities and the weighting factor for the differential response. Bases are presented unweighted. Tables in Appendix R show the weighted base numbers by sex for each of the main components of the survey.

References and endnotes

[1] Department of Health. Report on Health and Social Subjects: 41. *Dietary Reference Values for Food Energy and Nutrients for the United Kingdom*. HMSO (London, 1991).

[2] General Household Survey 1994 and 1995 OPCS – *unpublished data*.

[3] 1991 Census data were used.

[4] Elliot D. Optimising sample design for surveys of health and related behaviour and attitudes. *Survey Methodology Bulletin*. Social Survey Division, ONS (1995) **36**: 8-17.

[5] Eligible dates of birth were for each fieldwork wave were as follows:

Wave	Fieldwork dates	Eligible dates of birth
1	1 January - 31 March 1997	15 February 1978 - 14 February 1993
2	1 April - 30 June 1997	16 May 1978 - 15 May 1993
3	1 July - 30 September 1997	16 August 1978 - 15 August 1993
4	1 October - 31 December 1997	16 November 1978 - 15 November 1993

Table D1 Response to the postal and interviewer sift stages

(a) Postal sift

	No.	%
Total sample of addresses	27720	100
Pre-selected multi-household addresses		
– issued to interviewers	659	2
Ineligibles	1459	5
Eligible addresses	25602	100
Refusals	220	1
Non-contacts – re-issued to interviewers	7087	28
Returns:		
multi-household addresses		
– re-issued to interviewers	92	0
single household addresses	18203	71
Single household addresses containing an eligible young person	4643	18

(b) Interviewer sift

	No.	%
Addresses issued to interviewers	7838	100
Ineligibles	1095	14
Eligible addresses	6743	100
Refusals	788	12
Non-contacts	972	14
Returns	4983	74

(c) Overall response to sift stages

	No.	%
Total sample of addresses	27720	100
Ineligibles	2554	9
Total eligible addresses	25166	100
Refusals	1008	4
Non-contacts	972	4
Returns	23186	92
Total households containing an eligible young person	6308	27

Table D2 Response rates for postal and interviewer sift stages (combined) by fieldwork wave*

| | Wave of fieldwork | | | | | | | | | |
| | Wave 1 | | Wave 2 | | Wave 3 | | Wave 4 | | Total | |
	No.	%	No.	%	No.	%	No.	%	No.	%
Total sample of addresses	6930	*100*	6930	*100*	6930	*100*	6930	*100*	27720	*100*
ineligible addresses	677	*10*	650	*9*	640	*9*	587	*8*	2554	*9*
Eligible sample of addresses	6253	*100*	6280	*100*	6290	*100*	6343	*100*	25166	*100*
Refusals	256	*4*	280	*4*	242	*4*	230	*4*	1008	*4*
Non-contacts	259	*4*	304	*5*	226	*4*	183	*3*	972	*4*
Returns:	5738	*92*	5696	*91*	5822	*93*	5930	*93*	23186	*92*
containing an eligible young person	1519	*24*	1590	*25*	1549	*25*	1650	*26*	6308	*25*
no eligible young person	4219	*67*	4106	*65*	4273	*68*	4280	*67*	16878	*67*

* Wave 1: January–March 1997
  Wave 2: April–June 1997
  Wave 3: July–September 1997
  Wave 4: October–December 1997

Table D3 Maximum response rate by fieldwork wave*

| | Wave of fieldwork | | | | | | | | | |
| | Wave 1 | | Wave 2 | | Wave 3 | | Wave 4 | | Total | |
	No.	%	No.	%	No.	%	No.	%	No.	%
Eligible interview sample	557	*100*	573	*100*	779	*100*	763	*100*	2672	*100*
Refusals	6	*1*	3	*1*	5	*1*	12	*2*	26	*1*
Non-contacts	108	*19*	107	*19*	150	*19*	154	*20*	519	*19*
Response to initial interview	443	*80*	463	*81*	624	*80*	597	*78*	2127	*80*

* Wave 1: January–March 1997
  Wave 2: April–June 1997
  Wave 3: July–September 1997
  Wave 4: October–December 1997

Table D4 A comparison of two survey estimates with and without non-response weighting

| Region | Dietary record data | | | Blood pressure | | |
| | Mean daily intake of total fat (g) | | | Mean systolic blood pressure (mmHg) | | |
	Sample weight only	Sample + non-response weight	*Base*	Sample weight only	Sample + non-response weight	*Base*
All	**68.4**	**69.0**	*1701*	**108**	**109**	*1898*
Scotland	67.0	68.0	*137*	110	110	*152*
North	69.7	70.1	*460*	108	108	*508*
C SW & Wales*	68.6	69.2	*606*	109	109	*666*
L & SE**	67.3	68.0	*498*	107	108	*572*
Males	**73.3**	**74.7**	*856*	**109**	**110**	*930*
Scotland	72.4	73.9	*68*	110	111	*75*
North	73.7	74.9	*243*	109	109	*243*
C SW & Wales*	74.0	75.0	*300*	109	110	*332*
L & SE**	72.4	74.2	*245*	108	109	*280*
Females	**63.3**	**63.1**	*845*	**108**	**108**	*968*
Scotland	61.6	61.9	*69*	109	109	*77*
North	65.3	65.0	*217*	108	107	*265*
C SW & Wales*	63.2	63.0	*306*	108	108	*334*
L & SE**	62.0	61.6	*253*	107	107	*292*

* Central and South West regions of England, and Wales.
** London and the South East.

Figure D1

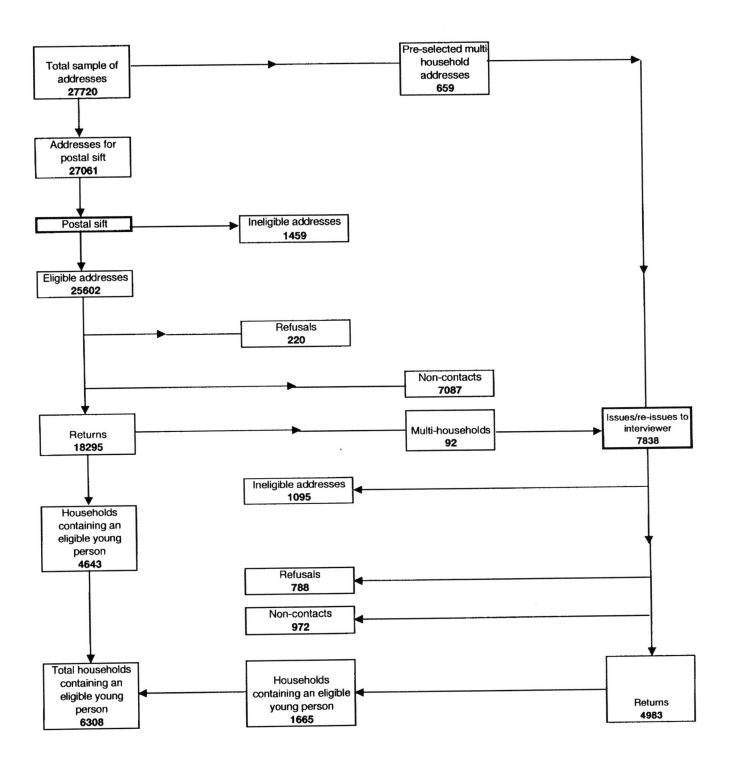

Appendix E

Sampling errors and statistical methods

1 Sampling errors

This section examines the sources of error associated with survey estimates and presents sampling errors of survey estimates, referred to as standard errors, and design factors for a number of key variables shown in this Report. It should be noted that tables showing standard errors in the analysis chapters of this Report have assumed a simple random sample design. In testing for the significance of the differences between two survey estimates, proportions or means, the standard error calculated as for a simple random sample design was multiplied by an assumed, conservative, design factor of 1.5 to allow for the complex sample design.

The estimates presented in the analysis chapters in this Report are based on data weighted to correct both for differential sampling probability and for differential non-response. The sampling errors presented in this appendix were calculated after applying weights for differential sampling probability. The component of the weights which corrects for differential non-response, which is relatively small compared with that which corrects for differential sampling probability, was not applied in order not to inflate the sampling errors by adding further variation to the weights[1].

1.1 The accuracy of survey results

Survey results are subject to various sources of error. The total error in a survey estimate is the difference between the estimate derived from the data collected and the true value for the population. It can be thought of as being comprised of random and systematic errors, and each of these two main types of error can be subdivided into error from a number of different sources.

1.1.1 Random error

Random error is the part of the total error which would be expected to average zero if a number of repeats of the same survey were carried out based on different samples from the same population.

An important component of random error is sampling error, which arises because the estimate is based on a survey rather than a census of the population. The results of this or any other survey would be expected to vary from the true population values. The amount of variation depends on both the size of the sample and the sample design.

Random error may also arise from other sources such as the respondent's interpretation of the questions or from errors associated with taking measurements. As with all surveys caried out by Social Survey Division, considerable efforts were made on this survey to minimise these effects through interviewer and phlebotomist training and through feasibility work; however it is likely some will remain which it is not possible to quantify.

1.1.2 Systematic error

Systematic error, or bias, applies to those sources of error that will not average to zero over a number of repeats of the survey. The category includes, for example, bias due to omission of certain parts of the population from the sampling frame or bias due to interviewer or coder variation. A substantial effort is put into avoiding systematic errors but it is likely that some will remain.

Non-response bias is a systematic error that is of particular concern. It occurs if non-respondents to the survey or to particular elements of the survey differ significantly in some respect from respondents, so that the responding sample is not representative of the total population. Non-response can be minimised by training interviewers in how to deal with potential refusals, and with strategies to minimise non-contacts. However a certain level of non-response is inevitable in any voluntary survey. The resulting bias is, however, dependent not only on the absolute level of non-response but on the extent to which non-respondents differ from respondents in terms of the measures which the survey aims to estimate.

Although respondents were encouraged to take part in all elements of the survey, some refused certain components. Chapter 3 examined the characteristics of groups responding to the different parts of the survey package. The analysis of non-respondents to the postal sift and interviewer follow-up stages showed evidence of some response bias. The lowest response rates for both the initial dietary interview and the dietary record were for boys and girls aged 15 to 18 years. The data for the analysis chapters of the Report were therefore weighted for differential non-response by sex and age within region.

1.2 Standard errors for estimates for the NDNS of young people aged 4 to 18 years

As described in Chapter 1 and Appendix D, this survey used a sample design which involved both clustering and stratification. In considering the reliability of estimates, standard errors calculated on the basis of a simple random sample design will be biased because of the complex sample design.

This dietary survey sample was clustered using postcode sectors as primary sampling units (PSUs). While clustering can increase standard errors, stratification tends to reduce them and is of most advantage where the stratification factor is of relevance to the survey subject matter. The main stratifier used on this survey was Standard Statistical Regions. The PSUs were further stratified by population density, socio-economic group and car ownership.

In a complex sample design the size of the standard error of any estimate depends on how the characteristic of interest is spread within and between PSUs and strata, and this is taken into account in the way data are grouped in order to calculate the standard error.

The formula used to estimate the standard error for this survey's estimates is known as the ratio estimator, and is shown below. The method explicitly allows for the fact that the percentages and means are actually ratios of two survey estimates, both of which are subject to random error.

$$var(r) = \frac{1}{x^2}[var(y) + r^2 var(x) - 2rcov(y,x)]$$

Var (r) is the estimate of the variance of the ratio, *r*, expressed in terms of *var(y)* and *var(x)* which are the estimated variances of *y* and *x*, and *cov(y,x)* which is their estimated covariance. The resulting estimate is only valid if the denominator is not too variable[2]. The method compares the differences between totals for adjacent PSUs (postal sectors) in the characteristic of interest[3]. The characteristic is the numerator, for example the average daily intake of total iron from food sources, and the sample size is the denominator in the ratio estimate[4]. The ordering of PSUs reflects the ranking of postal sectors on the stratifiers used in the sample design.

Tables E1 to E7 give standard errors, taking account of the complex sample design used on this survey, for most of the key variables presented in this report.

For selected nutrients, anthropometric measurements and blood analytes, estimates are shown by age and sex.

Standard errors for estimates of socio-demographic subgroups, such as social class and region, are shown separately for males and females to reflect the way they are presented in the analysis chapters.

1.3 Estimating standard errors for other survey estimates

Although standard errors can be calculated readily by computer, there are practical problems in presenting a large number of survey estimates. One solution is to calculate standard errors for selected variables and, from these, identify design factors appropriate for the specific survey design and for different types of survey variable. The standard error of other survey measures can then be estimated using the approriate design factor together with the sampling error assuming a simple random sample.

1.3.1 The Design Factor (deft)

The effect of a complex sample design can be quantified by comparing the observed variability in the sample with that which would be expected if the survey had used a simple random sample. The most commonly used statistic is the design factor (*deft*) which is calculated as a ratio of the standard error for a survey estimate, allowing for the full complexity of the sample design, to the standard error assuming that the result has come from a simple random sample. The deft can be used as a multiplier to the standard error based on a simple random sample, *se(p)_{srs}*, to give the standard error of the complex design, *se(p)*, by using the following formula:

$$se(p) = deft \ x \ se(p)_{srs}$$

Tables E1 to E7 show defts for certain Dietary Survey measures. The level of deft varies between survey variables reflecting the degree to which the characteristic is clustered within PSUs or is distributed between strata. For a single variable the level of the deft also varies according to the size of the subgroup on which the estimate is based, and on the distribution of the subgroup between PSUs and strata.

The deft values presented here for certain nutrients and main characteristics are for all young people who completed a 7-day dietary record. Defts for blood analytes and physiological measurements are for young people for whom these measures were obtained, and exclude cases where a quality control variable indicated that a particular measurement or result was unreliable (see *Chapters 10 and 12*).

For girls, around 70% of the design factors presented in Tables E1 to E7 are less than 1.2, while for boys 40% are less than 1.2. Design factors of this order are considered to be small and they indicate that the characteristic is not markedly clustered geographically. For girls, 6% of the design factors are greater than 1.5 while for boys 22% are greater than 1.5. The relatively high proportion of design factors above 1.5 for boys is due to the lower response for the oldest age group of boys, particularly for the anthropometric measurements and blood sample.

For socio-demographic characteristics, where geographic clustering would be expected, around two thirds of the design factors are less than 1.2 for both sexes, while 14% of design factors are above 1.5 for boys and none are above 1.5 for girls. *(Tables E1 to E7)*

1.3.2 Testing differences between means and proportions

Standard errors can be used to test whether an observed difference between two proportions or means in the sample is likely to be entirely due to sampling error. An estimate for the standard error of a difference between percentages assuming a simple random sample is:

$$se(p_1-p_2) = \sqrt{[(p_1q_1/n_1) + (p_2q_2/n_2)]}$$

where p_1 and p_2 are the observed percentages for the two subsamples, q_1 and q_2 are respectively *(100-p_1)* and *(100-p_2)*, and n_1 and n_2 are the subsample sizes.

The equivalent formula for the standard error of the difference between the means for subsamples 1 and 2 is:

$$se(diff) = \sqrt{(se_1{}^2 + se_2{}^2)}$$

Allowance for the complex sample design is then made by multiplying the standard error for the difference, from the above formula, by the appropriate value of the deft.

In this report the calculation of the difference between proportions and means assumed a deft of 1.5 across all survey estimates. The calculation of complex sampling errors and design factors for key characteristics show that this was a conservative estimate for some characteristics for some age and sex groups but was an optimistic estimate for other characteristics. Therefore there will be some differences in sample proportions and means which are not commented on in the text but which are significantly different at least at the $p<0.05$ level. Equally, there will be some differences which are described as significant in the text but which are not significantly different when the complex sampling design is taken into account. An indication of the characteristics for which significance tests are likely to provide false-positives or false-negatives can be gained by looking at the size of the defts in the tables in this appendix.

Confidence intervals can be calculated around a survey estimate using the standard error for that estimate. For example, the 95% confidence interval is calculated as 1.96 times the standard error, on either side of the estimated proportion or mean value. At the 95% confidence level, over many repeats of the survey under the same conditions, 95% of these confidence intervals would contain the population estimate. However, when assessing the results of a survey, it is usual to assume that there is only a 5% chance that the true population value will fall outside the 95% confidence interval calculated for the survey estimate.

2 Multiple regression

The substantive chapters of this Report present results from multiple regression analyses. These analyses were carried out in SPSS version 9.0 using the 'enter' method. In each analysis age was always included as an independent variable and the regression analyses were run separately for boys and girls. For each regression the procedure was first run to identify any collinear variables. After excluding one from the pair of any collinear variables the procedure was run again. All the regression analyses were carried out using scaled weights for the dependent variable in the analysis[5,6] and, where necessary, the dependent variable was log transformed.

2.1 The multiple regression analysis method[7]

Most of the tables shown in this Report are based on bivariate analysis. These tables show the relationship between two reported or measured variables, for example, the proportion of young people living in different household types with different average daily intakes of protein. What such tables do not show, however, is how much other factors may interrelate with the independent variable; for example, how much age and sex interrelate with household type to explain variations in intakes.

Figure 1 shows how each of the variables, x_1 and x_2, make an independent contribution to the dependent variable, y, but that there is an area of x_1 that overlaps with x_2. By carrying out a multiple regression analysis the overlap between x_1 and x_2 is eliminated, so that the contribution x_1 makes to y can be measured after controlling for (eliminating) the overlapping contribution of x_2.

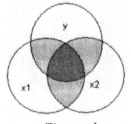

Figure 1

Multiple regression is a multivariate statistical technique that describes the relationship between one survey variable the dependent variable, for example the systolic blood pressure of the young person and several other variables, the independent variables, for example age, sex and whether the young person was living with both parents. For example Table 11.15(a) of the Report shows the results of regression where the dependent variable is the systolic blood pressure for a male aged between 4 and 18 years. The regression calculates a coefficient for each independent variable which quantifies the effect that a change in that variable will have on the predicted systolic blood pressure, leaving all other variables in the regression unchanged (see 2.3 below).

When running regression the interest is in testing whether, for a given model, there is a relationship between the dependent variable and the independent variables in the population. This is done by testing whether the coefficient for the independent variable is equal to zero. A variable is judged to be statistically different from zero if it is significant at the 95% level or above. This means that if there were no relationship in the population between the dependent and the independent variable, there would be a probability of 5% or less that the regression would have estimated a coefficient that was different from zero.

2.1.1 Assumptions for multiple regression analysis

The technique of multiple regression requires a number of conditions of the data to be met or assumed; some are appropriate only to the analysis of particular types of dataset, for example time series, and are not presented here. The assumptions made in respect of the NDNS data for multiple regression analysis were as follows:

- *Linearity and normal distribution*
  The technique of multiple regression calculates coefficients that describe linear relationships between variables and assume that the residuals (the difference between the actual value of the dependent variable and that predicted by the model) are normally distributed. If the residuals are not normally distributed, the significance tests will not be valid. In order to facilitate normally distributed residuals, where the NDNS data for any of the dependent variables included in the analysis were strongly skewed[8] they were transformed by taking the natural log (ln) before being added to the analysis model.

- *That the values for the independent variables in repeated samples are fixed*
  Assumes that if multiple samples are drawn, an independent variable, x, will take the same values in each sample. Chapter 3 shows that for several of the socio-demographic variables used in the multiple regression analysis, the NDNS sample gave comparable results to those found in other surveys.

- *Collinearity (or multicollinearity)*
  The assumption that no two independent variables are close or exact linear combinations of one another. When two variables are strongly positively correlated (collinear), the standard errors will be inflated, making the significance tests misleading. In SPSS, the multiple regression analysis produces a Pearson correlation matrix and two 'collinearity statistics'; the *variance inflation factor* (VIF) and the *tolerance*. The *tolerance* of a variable is $1-R_i^2$ where R_i is the multiple correlation coefficient when the ith independent variable is predicted from the other independent variables. The *VIF* is $1/tolerance$. A value of 10 or more for the *VIF* indicates the presence of significant collinearity between the independent variable against which it appears and one or more of the other independent variables included in the model. The Pearson correlation coefficient matrix gives correlation coefficients for the relationship between each of the independent variables and is used to identify which are strongly correlated.

For each multiple regression analysis carried out, all of the independent variables considered important in explaining the dependent variable were included in an initial regression analysis. The output from this initial analysis identified independent variables with a *VIF* value of greater than 10, and the Pearson correlation matrix was used to show which variables were strongly correlated so that one or more could be excluded from the analysis. The decision which variable(s) to exclude from the regression analysis was made with reference to which might be the more important factor, either in terms of predictive value or in terms of policy relevance.

2.1.2 Preparing variables for multiple regression analysis

In a multiple regression analysis the dependent variable must be continuous and the independent variables either continuous or dichotomous. Independent, categorical variables with more than two categories must be transformed into dichotomous ('dummy') variables before being included in the analysis.

For categorical variables with two categories the two possible 'dummy' variables are complementary, for example, for 'whether the young person was a current smoker' the two possible 'dummy' variables are:

current smoker? yes = 1, no = 0
current smoker? yes = 0, no = 1

The SPSS multiple regression program tests the independent variables for multicollinearity, as described above. Where there is a strong correlation between two variables, the statistics produced by the analysis are not valid and one of the collinear variables must be

650

excluded. However, where there is an *exact* correlation between two variables, for example where two 'dummy' variables are complementary parts of the same variable, SPSS automatically excludes one from the analysis and uses it as the 'reference category'. For a dichotomous variable the regression coefficient gives the expected difference of being in one category (the category that takes the value 1) rather than the other (the category that takes the value 0).

For categorical variables with more than two categories dichotomous 'dummy' variables need to be created. For example, for region, with four categories, four dummy variables need to be created each indicating whether or not the young person lived in one region. Thus the first 'dummy' variable is 'In Scotland' or 'Not in Scotland', the second 'In Northern region' or 'Not Northern region', etc. If all four of the 'dummy' variables for region are included in the analysis, one is automatically treated as the reference category, and the unstandardised coefficients are interpreted with reference to that category. However, to provide correlation coefficients that can be interpreted as deviations from the average effect of all categories, it is necessary to use the 'enter' method for the procedure and to run two versions of each regression analysis.

For example for 'region' in the NDNS dataset two sets of 'dummy' variables were created with one (reference) category coded as –1, and one category excluded:

Set 1:
'Dummy' 1 = (Scotland = 1) (Northern = 0) (C, SW & Wales = 0) (London & South East = –1)
'Dummy' 2 = (Scotland = 0) (Northern = 1) (C, SW & Wales = 0) (London & South East = –1)
'Dummy' 3 = (Scotland = 0) (Northern = 0) (C, SW & Wales = 1) (London & South East = –1)

Set 2:
'Dummy' A = (Scotland = –1) (North = 1) (C, SW & Wales = 0) (London & South East = 0)
'Dummy' B = (Scotland = –1) (North = 0) (C, SW & Wales = 1) (London & South East = 0)
'Dummy' C = (Scotland = –1) (North = 0) (C, SW & Wales = 0) (London & South East = 1)

Note that for the first set the London and South East category is set to –1 and there is no 'dummy' variable for London and the South East. In the second set Scotland is set to –1 and there is no 'dummy' variable for Scotland. Any two categories could have been excluded.

The same procedure was used for all categorical variables for which there were more than two categories, producing two sets of 'dummy' variables that were run in two versions of the same multiple regression analysis. It is only necessary to run the regressions twice, no matter how many categorical variables are included. Where a 'dummy' variable appears in both versions of

the analysis, the coefficients and standard errors are the same and the constant term has increased by the same amount. Having run both versions of the regression analysis, the results can be summarised in a single table.

2.2 The interpretation of statistics produced by multiple regression analysis

The *constant* is the predicted value of the dependent variable when all of the independent variables are held at zero.

The *unstandardised coefficient (B)* quantifies the *effect* that a change in the independent variable will have on the dependent variable, *holding all other variables in the regression analysis constant*. This coefficient should not be used to indicate which independent variable is the best predictor of the dependent variable as the magnitude of the coefficients depends on the units in which the variables are measured.

The *adjusted R^2* is an assessment of the overall fit of the model and is interpreted as the percentage of the variance in the dependent variable that is explained by all of the independent variables included in the regression model. The adjusted R^2 is used in place of the R^2 because the number of variables in the model does not affect it.

The *standardised coefficient (Beta, β)* is standardised for the units of measurement of the independent variable. It shows what the relative effect of each independent variable would be if they were all measured using the same scale. It indicates which independent variable is the best predictor of the dependent variable, with the highest value being the best predictor.

SPSS also gives *t values* and *significance levels* identifying those variables where the regression coefficients are significantly related to the dependent variable after controlling the effects of the other variables included in the analysis. The tables given in this Report show the significance level for each coefficient ($p < 0.05$, $p < 0.01$ or $p < 0.001$[9]). Unstandardised and standardised regression coefficients are only shown in the tables in the Report for variables significantly related to the dependent variable.

2.3 Predicting values from a multiple regression analysis

For categorical variables the coefficients quantify the effect that having a particular characteristic will have on the dependent variable. For a dichotomous variable, the regression coefficient gives the expected difference of being in one category (the category that takes the value 1) rather than the other (the one that takes the value 0). For categorical variables with more than two categories the constant plus the value of the unstandardised coefficient for the independent variable gives the predicted value of the dependent variable for someone with that characteristic, when the values of all the other independent variables in the regression analysis are set to zero.

For continuous variables the value of the coefficient represents the contribution to the dependent variable per unit of the independent variable. For example, for 'weight' this would be per kilogram, if the unit for the variable 'weight' was kilograms, or per gram, if the unit for the variable was grams. The coefficient is multiplied by the value of the continuous variable for which the prediction is being made before being added to the constant. For example if weight = 50kg and the value of the unstandardised coefficient B = 0.45, then (0.45 x 50) is added to the constant.

In Chapter 11, Section 11.3.3 a worked example is given to show how, for boys, systolic blood pressure can be predicted from a multiple regression analysis where age, being a smoker, being unwell, diastolic blood pressure and body weight were all found to be statistically independently related to systolic blood pressure.

References and notes

[1] Weighting for different sampling probabilities results in larger sampling errors than for an equal-probability sample without weights. However, using population totals to control for differential non-response tends to lead to a reduction in the errors. The method used to calculate the sampling errors correctly allows for the inflation in the sampling errors caused by the first type of weighting but, in treating the second type of weighting in the same way as the first, would incorrectly further inflate the estimates. Therefore to avoid over-stating the sampling errors in this way only the first part of the weight has been included in the sampling error calculations.

[2] This variability can be measured by the coefficient of variation of x, denoted by $cv(x)$, which is the standard error of x expressed as a proportion of x

$$cv(x) = \frac{se(x)}{x}$$

It has been suggested that the ratio estimator should not be used if $cv(x)$ is greater than 0.2. The coefficient of variation of x did not exceed 0.2 for any of the estimates presented in this Appendix.

[3] The calculation of standard errors and design factors for this survey used the package STATA. For further details of the method of calculation see: Elliot D. A comparison of software for producing sampling errors on social surveys. *SSD Survey Methodology Bulletin* 1999; **44**: 27-36.

[4] For a survey of this kind the sample size is subject to random fluctuation, both within each PSU and overall. This is because the number of children identified in each PSU is dependent on which households are sampled and there will be differing amounts of non-response. Also some estimates are made for subgroups such as age and sex and there was only a limited amount of control on these sub-sample sizes.

[5] These weights adjusted for differential sampling probability and differential non-response.

[6] Multiple regression analyses for boys, which included plasma testosterone concentration as an independent variable, were run on unweighted data. See *Chapter 11, Section 11.3.3* and *Chapter 12, Section 12.1.2*.

[7] For a more detailed description of multiple regression analysis using SPSS, see Chapter 18, *SPSS for Windows. Base System User's Guide*. SPSS Inc. (Chicago,1993).

[8] A skewness (*sk*) value of + 1.0 represents extreme positive skewness and a value of −1.0 extreme negative skewness. Loether HJ, McTavish DG. *Descriptive and inferential statistics: an introduction*. 2nd Edition. Allyn and Bacon (Massachusetts, 1980).

[9] In the tables presenting results from multiple regression, variables that are significantly different at the 95%, 99% and 99.9% levels are indicated by one, two and three asterisks respectively.

Table E1 True standard errors and design factors for socio-demographic characteristics of the diary sample by sex of young person

Diary sample

Characteristic	Males			Females		
	%(p)	Standard error of p	Design factor	%(p)	Standard error of p	Design factor
Sex	51	1.30	0.76	49	1.30	0.75
Age group						
4–6 years	21	1.25	0.88	21	1.49	1.07
7–10 years	27	1.75	1.10	27	1.28	0.84
11–14 years	26	1.37	0.89	26	1.52	0.96
15–18 years	26	1.28	0.96	26	1.37	0.95
Whether young person was reported as being unwell during the record keeping period						
Unwell, eating affected	10	1.05	1.03	11	1.19	1.13
Unwell, eating unaffected	8	1.20	1.27	9	1.22	1.19
Not unwell	82	1.40	1.06	80	1.79	1.29
Region						
Scotland	8	1.50	1.63	8	0.93	0.97
Northern	28	1.54	0.99	27	1.79	1.17
Central & South West England & Wales	35	1.82	1.12	35	1.86	1.13
London & South East	29	2.10	1.36	29	2.21	1.41
Social class						
Non-manual	47	1.94	1.14	45	2.18	1.27
Manual	45	1.78	1.04	43	2.20	1.29
Unclassified	8	1.54	1.68	12	1.56	1.40
Gross weekly household income						
Less than £160	16	1.50	1.18	17	1.48	1.15
£160 to less than £280	20	1.56	1.13	19	1.57	1.16
£280 to less than £400	18	1.45	1.10	17	1.35	1.05
£400 to less than £600	19	1.58	1.18	22	1.33	0.93
£600 or more	23	1.86	1.29	21	1.38	0.98
Income question refused	3	0.73	1.23	4	0.58	0.88
Whether young person was living with both parents						
Both parents and other children	64	1.30	0.79	60	1.86	1.11
Both parents and no other children	18	1.37	1.06	18	1.41	1.07
Lone parent and other children	12	1.23	1.11	14	1.64	1.37
Lone parent and no other children	6	0.77	0.96	7	0.81	0.93
No parents in household	0	0.14	0.92	1	0.31	1.07
Household receipt of benefits						
Receiving benefits	25	2.20	1.48	26	1.99	1.31
Not receiving benefits	75	2.21	1.49	74	2.06	1.35
Employment status of head of household						
In employment	84	2.01	1.59	80	1.85	1.34
Unemployed	5	1.23	1.61	4	0.75	1.11
Economically inactive	11	1.18	1.11	16	1.70	1.35
Mother's highest educational qualification level						
Above GCE 'A' level	19	1.67	1.20	21	1.72	1.23
GCE 'A' level and equivalent	8	0.85	0.85	8	0.90	1.02
GCSE grades A–C and equivalent	30	1.74	1.13	31	1.64	1.03
GCSE grades D–G and equivalent	15	1.22	0.99	16	1.52	1.20
No qualifications	24	2.19	1.53	22	1.72	1.26
No mother in the household	3	0.37	0.92	2	0.77	1.23
Sample size		856			845	

Table E2(a) True standard errors and design factors for average daily intakes of energy and macronutrients by age of young person: males

Diary sample

Macronutrients	Males aged (years)															
	4–6			7–10			11–14			15–18			All males		
	Mean r	Standard error of r	Design factor	Mean r	Standard error of r	Design factor	Mean r	Standard error of r	Design factor	Mean r	Standard error of r	Design factor	Mean r	Standard error of r	Design factor
Energy (kcal)	1520	27	1.49	1777	26	1.45	1968	36	1.62	2285	42	0.90	1905	20	1.46
Energy (MJ)	6.39	0.11	1.49	7.47	0.11	1.45	8.28	0.15	1.62	9.60	0.18	0.91	8.01	0.08	1.46
Protein (g)	49.0	1.06	1.18	54.8	0.83	1.21	64.0	1.26	1.64	76.5	1.59	1.07	60.6	0.70	1.36
% food energy from protein	12.9	0.13	1.02	12.4	0.11	0.88	13.1	0.19	1.86	13.9	0.19	0.95	13.1	0.09	1.43
Total carbohydrate (g)	209	3.6	1.36	248	3.8	1.47	271	5.2	1.59	301	6.4	0.93	260	2.8	1.49
Total sugars (g)	98	2.5	1.48	115	2.6	1.41	122	3.6	1.61	129	4.6	1.14	117	2.0	1.98
Starch (g)	110	2.0	1.21	133	2.1	1.21	149	2.4	1.21	172	3.3	0.90	143	1.3	0.92
% food energy from total carbohydrate	51.6	0.33	1.16	52.4	0.24	0.90	51.7	0.26	0.77	50.5	0.44	1.04	51.6	0.16	1.10
Alcohol (g)	0.0	0.005	0.84	0.0	0.005	1.46	0.1	0.042	1.39	6.8	1.475	1.08	1.8	0.288	1.07
% energy from alcohol	0.0	0.003	0.86	0.0	0.002	1.37	0.0	0.014	1.45	1.9	0.379	1.13	0.5	0.075	1.11
Total fat(g)	60.1	1.31	1.57	69.8	1.16	1.27	77.2	1.56	1.36	89.0	1.73	0.82	74.7	0.83	1.30
Saturated fatty acids (g)	25.1	0.62	1.53	28.3	0.51	1.23	30.3	0.73	1.59	34.7	0.76	0.86	29.8	0.38	1.53
Cis monounsaturated fatty acids (g)	19.4	0.43	1.52	22.8	0.44	1.39	25.6	0.52	1.24	29.6	0.63	0.92	24.6	0.29	1.32
Cis n-3 polyunsaturated fatty acids (g)	1.29	0.04	1.01	1.58	0.04	1.05	1.95	0.07	0.67	2.19	0.07	0.93	1.77	0.03	0.95
Cis n-6 polyunsaturated fatty acids (g)	8.0	0.21	1.31	9.7	0.23	1.32	11.4	0.26	1.20	13.3	0.32	0.79	10.7	0.13	0.86
Trans fatty acids (g)	2.26	0.06	1.53	2.74	0.07	1.28	2.92	0.08	1.39	3.45	0.10	0.87	2.87	0.04	1.37
Cholesterol (mg)	158	5.5	1.15	181	4.5	1.22	201	6.0	1.36	243	7.1	0.90	198	3.0	1.16
% food energy from total fat	35.5	0.32	1.28	35.2	0.22	0.94	35.2	0.24	0.75	35.9	0.33	0.81	35.4	0.13	0.91
Sample size	*184*			*256*			*237*			*179*			*856*		

654

Table E2(b) True standard errors and design factors for average daily intakes of energy and macronutrients by age of young person: females

Diary sample

| Macronutrients | Females aged (years) | | | | | | | | | | | | | | |
| | 4–6 | | | 7–10 | | | 11–14 | | | 15–18 | | | All females | | |
	Mean r	Standard error of r	Design factor	Mean r	Standard error of r	Design factor	Mean r	Standard error of r	Design factor	Mean r	Standard error of r	Design factor	Mean r	Standard error of r	Design factor
Energy (kcal)	1397	20	0.92	1598	21	1.25	1673	23	0.96	1626	29	0.91	1582	13	1.16
Energy (MJ)	5.87	0.09	0.92	6.72	0.09	1.24	7.03	0.10	0.96	6.82	0.12	0.90	6.65	0.06	1.16
Protein (g)	44.5	0.87	1.02	51.2	0.73	0.97	52.9	1.02	1.48	54.8	1.06	0.92	51.2	0.46	1.00
% food energy from protein	12.7	0.15	1.00	12.8	0.15	1.34	12.7	0.17	1.50	13.9	0.17	0.85	13.1	0.09	1.26
Total carbohydrate (g)	191	3.3	1.15	218	3.1	1.19	228	3.6	1.04	214	3.7	0.75	214	2.1	1.38
Total sugars (g)	95	2.4	1.26	101	2.1	1.05	99	2.5	1.14	92	2.3	0.72	97	1.4	1.35
Starch (g)	96	2.0	1.21	117	1.7	1.06	129	2.0	0.98	122	2.3	0.95	117	1.1	1.00
% food energy from total carbohydrate	51.4	0.45	1.48	51.3	0.28	0.94	51.2	0.38	1.29	50.6	0.39	0.88	51.1	0.18	1.04
Alcohol (g)	0.0	0.006	0.85	0.0	0.010	1.02	0.1	0.068	1.21	3.5	0.504	0.82	0.9	0.125	0.83
% energy from alcohol	0.0	0.003	0.85	0.0	0.004	1.04	0.1	0.026	1.15	1.4	0.201	0.82	0.4	0.050	0.81
Total fat(g)	55.9	1.03	0.96	63.8	1.08	1.34	67.2	1.06	0.89	64.0	1.42	0.95	63.1	0.59	0.98
Saturated fatty acids (g)	23.8	0.49	1.02	25.7	0.48	1.32	26.2	0.43	0.76	24.7	0.61	0.95	25.2	0.26	1.03
Cis monounsaturated fatty acids (g)	17.8	0.32	0.90	20.9	0.38	1.35	22.4	0.39	1.00	20.9	0.47	0.90	20.7	0.20	0.95
Cis n-3 polyunsaturated fatty acids (g)	1.15	0.04	1.05	1.44	0.03	0.87	1.65	0.06	1.52	1.61	0.04	0.94	1.58	0.02	1.03
Cis n-6 polyunsaturated fatty acids (g)	7.2	0.21	1.00	9.0	0.20	1.01	10.2	0.24	1.29	10.2	0.30	1.05	9.3	0.14	1.27
Trans fatty acids (g)	2.09	0.06	1.09	2.48	0.07	1.64	2.48	0.06	0.87	2.34	0.06	0.96	2.36	0.03	1.25
Cholesterol (mg)	156	4.7	1.07	170	4.2	0.87	169	5.0	1.20	177	6.2	1.16	169	2.3	0.91
% food energy from total fat	35.9	0.39	1.38	35.9	0.30	1.13	36.1	0.35	1.25	35.9	0.39	1.00	35.9	0.17	1.04
Sample size	*171*			*226*			*238*			*210*			*845*		

Table E3 True standard errors and design factors for average daily intakes of selected vitamins from food sources by sex and age of young person

Diary sample

Vitamins	Age (years)														
	4–6			7–10			11–14			15–18			All		
	Mean r	Standard error of r	Design factor	Mean r	Standard error of r	Design factor	Mean r	Standard error of r	Design factor	Mean r	Standard error of r	Design factor	Mean r	Standard error of r	Design factor
Males															
Total carotene (µg)	1248	98.5	1.54	1295	71.6	1.31	1396	71.5	1.30	1680	110.2	1.14	1411	36.9	0.98.
Vitamin A (retinol equivalents) (µg)	458	22.4	1.51	505	19.4	1.35	558	41.7	1.41	613	28.3	1.08	537	16.0	1.52
Thiamin (mg)	1.27	0.042	1.35	1.42	0.029	1.45	1.70	0.082	0.94	1.90	0.051	0.89	1.59	0.029	0.97
Riboflavin (mg)	1.56	0.050	1.51	1.62	0.039	1.38	1.73	0.056	1.54	1.92	0.079	1.27	1.71	0.032	1.96
Niacin equivalents (mg)	22.8	0.50	1.01	26.0	0.42	1.37	30.0	0.69	1.65	36.6	0.87	1.13	29.1	0.38	1.56
Vitamin B$_6$ (mg)	1.7	0.04	1.13	1.9	0.04	1.26	2.2	0.05	1.32	2.7	0.08	1.08	2.2	0.03	1.14
Vitamin B$_{12}$ (µg)	4.0	0.15	1.56	3.9	0.11	1.43	4.5	0.20	1.40	5.0	0.17	1.09	4.4	0.09	1.70
Folate (µg)	191	4.9	1.26	212	4.0	1.24	245	6.0	1.35	305	9.6	1.06	240	3.2	1.15
Vitamin C (mg)	67.0	2.80	1.01	72.8	3.29	1.47	76.3	3.50	1.14	83.3	4.29	0.70	75.2	1.88	1.23
Vitamin D (µg)	2.1	0.09	0.89	2.4	0.08	1.31	2.6	0.09	1.21	3.2	0.13	0.98	2.6	0.05	1.08
Vitamin E (mg)	6.6	0.17	1.04	8.1	0.23	1.67	9.1	0.24	1.28	10.3	0.28	0.74	8.6	0.12	1.09
Females															
Total carotene (µg)	1175	59.7	1.14	1304	56.4	1.11	1268	68.5	1.16	1637	138.7	1.08	1354	42.4	1.09
Vitamin A (retinol equivalents) (µg)	449	17.1	1.06	481	19.5	0.94	467	29.0	1.19	545	31.9	0.98	487	15.4	1.48
Thiamin (mg)	1.14	0.039	1.12	1.27	0.026	0.93	1.40	0.053	1.12	1.38	0.052	0.75	1.31	0.018	0.59
Riboflavin (mg)	1.40	0.036	1.08	1.37	0.036	1.26	1.32	0.043	1.40	1.30	0.046	1.02	1.34	0.022	1.43
Niacin equivalents (mg)	20.4	0.41	1.01	23.4	0.40	1.04	24.6	0.51	1.40	25.2	0.54	0.94	23.6	0.24	1.03
Vitamin B$_6$ (mg)	1.5	0.04	1.06	1.7	0.04	1.14	1.9	0.04	1.13	1.8	0.04	0.93	1.8	0.02	1.05
Vitamin B$_{12}$ (µg)	3.6	0.11	0.94	3.5	0.11	1.21	3.2	0.12	1.49	3.4	0.14	1.05	3.4	0.07	1.38
Folate (µg)	169	4.6	1.14	188	4.1	1.27	205	5.2	1.24	210	5.1	0.83	194	2.6	1.19
Vitamin C (mg)	65.2	2.56	1.06	73.5	3.06	1.22	70.8	3.06	1.07	74.0	3.42	0.87	71.2	1.51	1.00
Vitamin D (µg)	1.8	0.07	1.06	2.1	0.08	1.10	2.2	0.08	1.19	2.1	0.08	1.02	2.1	0.04	0.99
Vitamin E (mg)	6.3	0.20	1.07	7.6	0.19	1.03	8.1	0.21	1.26	8.1	0.25	0.98	7.6	0.13	1.42
Sample sizes:															
Males	*184*			*256*			*237*			*179*			*856*		
Females	*171*			*226*			*238*			*210*			*845*		

Table E4 True standard errors and design factors for average daily intakes of selected minerals from food sources by sex and age of young person

Diary sample

Minerals	Age (years) 4–6			7–10			11–14			15–18			All		
	Mean r	Standard error of r	Design factor	Mean r	Standard error of r	Design factor	Mean r	Standard error of r	Design factor	Mean r	Standard error of r	Design factor	Mean r	Standard error of r	Design factor
Males															
Total iron (mg)	8.2	0.20	1.23	9.7	0.17	1.27	10.8	0.22	1.23	12.5	0.32	1.02	10.4	0.12	1.18
Calcium (mg)	706	21.1	1.29	741	16.9	1.40	799	24.3	1.73	878	22.9	0.95	784	12.6	1.83
Phosphorus (mg)	919	20.9	1.33	1008	16.4	1.22	1132	26.1	1.95	1330	26.8	0.98	1105	13.8	1.69
Magnesium (mg)	172	3.9	1.37	194	3.1	1.22	218	4.8	1.58	256	5.8	1.06	212	2.6	1.56
Sodium (mg)	2069	46.7	1.47	2402	43.2	1.41	2683	57.3	1.49	3268	70.4	1.02	2630	32.1	1.43
Chloride (mg)	3105	68.1	1.41	3594	62.2	1.31	4030	85.4	1.53	4938	108.2	1.03	3954	46.2	1.31
Potassium (mg)	1944	41.8	1.32	2136	33.3	1.23	2392	44.4	1.30	2833	67.9	1.11	2343	25.6	1.26
Zinc (mg)	5.5	0.14	1.30	6.1	0.11	1.22	7.1	0.15	1.53	8.7	0.23	1.24	6.9	0.09	1.34
Copper (mg)	0.70	0.021	1.53	0.81	0.014	0.92	0.90	0.021	1.52	1.07	0.025	0.87	0.88	0.011	1.31
Iodine (µg)	156	6.0	1.28	154	4.6	1.52	162	5.3	1.43	181	6.1	1.13	163	3.1	1.74
Manganese (mg)	1.78	0.052	1.32	2.05	0.053	1.43	2.28	0.068	1.50	2.62	0.069	0.83	2.20	0.034	1.42
Females															
Total iron (mg)	7.3	0.18	1.19	8.4	0.15	0.98	8.8	0.20	1.33	8.7	0.21	0.80	8.3	0.10	1.10
Calcium (mg)	657	16.6	0.96	656	13.9	1.13	641	17.2	1.32	653	16.6	0.87	652	8.4	1.16
Phosphorus (mg)	848	16.9	1.03	915	13.8	1.08	932	18.4	1.33	959	18.7	0.88	917	8.8	1.11
Magnesium (mg)	155	3.5	1.26	177	2.9	1.07	182	3.4	1.20	191	4.0	0.93	178	1.9	1.30
Sodium (mg)	1857	36.2	1.10	2155	34.3	1.05	2272	44.9	1.38	2281	42.6	0.86	2156	20.8	1.08
Chloride (mg)	2785	52.5	1.05	3222	49.4	1.02	3403	65.1	1.35	3465	67.6	0.98	3241	31.0	1.10
Potassium (mg)	1774	37.0	1.09	2019	29.4	1.08	2100	41.0	1.37	2162	39.9	0.85	2026	20.4	1.22
Zinc (mg)	4.9	0.11	1.09	5.7	0.09	1.00	5.9	0.12	1.42	6.1	0.15	1.02	5.7	0.06	1.10
Copper (mg)	0.64	0.020	1.48	0.74	0.014	1.03	0.79	0.019	1.39	0.80	0.018	0.76	0.75	0.010	1.23
Iodine (µg)	143	5.5	1.20	131	4.0	1.29	129	5.3	1.65	135	5.1	0.90	134	2.7	1.45
Manganese (mg)	1.56	0.056	1.42	1.85	0.040	0.75	1.96	0.051	1.11	2.04	0.063	0.97	1.87	0.031	1.35
Sample sizes:															
Males	184			256			237			179			856		
Females	171			226			238			210			845		

Table E5 True standard errors and design factors for selected urine analytes by sex and age of young person

Urinary analytes	Age (years)														
	4–6			7–10			11–14			15–18			All		
	Mean r	Standard error of r	Design factor	Mean r	Standard error of r	Design factor	Mean r	Standard error of r	Design factor	Mean r	Standard error of r	Design factor	Mean r	Standard error of r	Design factor
Males															
Urinary sodium (mmol/l)	149.2	4.46	1.13	149.7	3.95	1.36	154.6	4.20	1.11	134.4	4.53	1.19	147.1	2.15	1.19
Urinary potassium (mmol/l)	55.0	2.53	1.22	50.8	2.02	1.20	47.3	1.89	1.25	48.2	2.57	1.07	50.1	0.94	0.84
Urinary creatinine (mmol/l)	9.5	0.45	1.95	10.9	0.35	1.77	13.1	0.35	1.08	17.4	0.72	1.37	12.8	0.21	1.07
Females															
Urinary sodium (mmol/l)	144.4	4.08	0.89	147.6	4.64	1.49	144.9	4.04	1.24	138.5	3.95	0.95	143.9	2.30	1.37
Urinary potassium (mmol/l)	52.1	2.55	1.08	49.6	2.08	1.08	43.4	2.06	1.55	45.8	2.05	1.00	47.5	1.20	1.42
Urinary creatinine (mmol/l)	8.8	0.28	0.99	10.9	0.37	1.47	13.1	0.36	1.02	14.1	0.40	0.87	11.9	0.20	1.19
Sample sizes:															
Males	*199*			*271*			*259*			*202*			*931*		
Females	*181*			*243*			*245*			*229*			*898*		

Table E6 True standard errors and design factors for physiological measurements by sex and age of young person

Physiological measurements	4–6			7–10				11–14				15–18				All				Base
	Mean r	Standard error of r	Design factor	Mean r	Standard error of r	Design factor	Base	Mean r	Standard error of r	Design factor	Base	Mean r	Standard error of r	Design factor	Base	Mean r	Standard error of r	Design factor	Base	
Males																				
Anthropometric measurements																				
Body weight (kg)	21	0.3	1.5	30	0.5	1.5	213	47	0.8	1.2	288	68	1.1	1.2	268	42	0.6	0.9	222	991
Height (cm)	113	0.6	1.6	133	0.5	1.0	212	155	0.5	0.7	287	175	0.5	0.9	268	145	0.7	0.9	223	990
Mid upper-arm circumference (cm)	18	0.1	1.2	20	0.2	1.6	207	24	0.2	1.4	287	28	0.3	1.2	269	23	0.1	1.0	222	965
Waist circumference (cm)*	na	na		na	na	na	na	72	0.7	1.7	na	80	0.8	1.3	268	76	0.5	1.1	222	490
Hip circumference (cm)*	na	na		na	na	na	na	86	0.6	1.4	na	97	0.7	1.4	268	92	0.5	1.0	222	490
BMI (kg/m²)	16	0.1	1.2	17	0.2	1.7	212	19	0.2	1.6	287	22	0.3	1.2	268	19	0.1	1.0	222	989
Waist to hip ratio*	na	na	na	na	na	na	na	0.83	0.004	1.586	na	0.82	0.004	1.304	268	0.83	0.003	1.512	222	490
Blood pressure																				
Systolic pressure (mmHg)	102	0.6	1.1	104	0.6	1.3	204	110	0.6	1.1	280	121	0.9	1.1	265	110	0.4	1.2	219	968
Diastolic pressure (mmHg)	55	0.7	1.1	55	0.5	1.4	204	56	0.6	1.2	280	57	0.7	1.1	265	56	0.3	1.5	219	968
Females																				
Anthropometric measurements																				
Body weight (kg)	20	0.2	0.9	32	0.4	0.9	202	49	0.7	1.0	253	60	0.8	1.2	259	41	0.6	1.0	241	955
Height (cm)	112	0.4	0.7	133	0.5	0.9	201	155	0.7	1.7	251	162	0.4	0.8	263	142	0.7	1.2	241	956
Mid upper-arm circumference (cm)	18	0.1	1.0	21	0.2	0.9	201	24	0.2	0.7	253	27	0.3	1.2	263	23	0.2	1.2	241	958
Waist circumference (cm)*	na	na		na	na	na	na	69	0.5	1.1	na	74	0.6	0.9	258	71	0.4	0.9	239	497
Hip circumference (cm)*	na	na		na	na	na	na	89	0.6	1.1	na	98	0.6	1.0	258	94	0.4	0.8	239	497
BMI (kg/m²)	16	0.1	1.1	18	0.2	0.9	201	20	0.2	0.9	251	23	0.3	1.0	259	19	0.1	0.9	241	953
Waist to hip ratio*	na	na	na	na	na	na	na	0.77	0.004	1.232	na	0.75	0.004	1.124	258	0.76	0.003	1.256	239	497
Blood pressure																				
Systolic pressure (mmHg)	101	0.7	1.1	105	0.7	1.1	188	110	0.7	1.4	247	114	0.9	1.4	259	108	0.5	1.7	236	930
Diastolic pressure (mmHg)	54	0.7	1.3	56	0.7	1.6	188	56	0.6	1.6	247	59	0.6	0.9	259	56	0.3	1.7	236	930

*Young people 11–18 years.
na not applicable

659

Table E7(a) True standard errors and design factors for selected blood analytes by age of young person: males

Blood analytes	Age (years) 4–6				7–10				11–14				15–18				All			
	Mean r	Standard error of r	Design factor	Base	Mean r	Standard error of r	Design factor	Base	Mean r	Standard error of r	Design factor	Base	Mean r	Standard error of r	Design factor	Base	Mean r	Standard error of r	Design factor	Base
Haemoglobin concentration (g/dl)	12.5	0.09	0.92	86	13.0	0.06	1.03	181	13.4	0.09	1.42	185	14.9	0.07	0.98	164	13.5	0.05	0.91	616
Plasma iron (µmol/l)	12.23	0.792	1.52	64	12.90	0.390	1.22	170	13.65	0.406	1.16	154	15.52	0.502	1.05	152	13.67	0.223	0.97	540
Serum ferritin (µg/l)	31	2.1	1.22	69	36	3.7	0.66	153	35	2.2	1.14	147	52	2.5	0.64	131	39	1.6	0.81	550
Plasma vitamin C (µmol/l)	61.6	3.82	1.90	73	60.1	2.31	1.81	176	54.2	1.94	1.40	166	50.2	2.04	1.27	152	56.4	1.33	1.93	567
Red cell folate (nmol/l)	736	24.1	1.19	79	671	18.4	1.49	172	598	15.5	0.97	166	540	16.0	1.19	156	626	9.2	1.14	622
Serum folate (nmol/l)	25.0	0.92	1.42	85	24.5	0.55	1.23	181	20.8	0.59	1.29	185	17.6	0.61	1.15	161	21.7	0.39	1.62	612
Serum vitamin B_{12} (pmol/l)	525	19.9	1.18	86	479	13.8	1.20	179	367	11.3	1.15	183	277	8.6	1.09	161	403	7.9	1.26	609
Erythrocyte transketolase activation coefficient	1.10	0.006	1.52	69	1.11	0.005	1.67	175	1.12	0.004	1.37	165	1.13	0.005	1.53	152	1.12	0.003	1.89	561
Erythrocyte glutathione reductase activation coefficient	1.36	0.018	1.49	72	1.38	0.009	0.97	178	1.46	0.018	1.69	168	1.48	0.019	1.41	154	1.42	0.010	2.15	572
Plasma zinc (µmol/l)	14.2	0.60	1.55	38	15.0	0.18	1.45	151	14.5	0.17	1.36	124	14.7	0.19	1.24	134	14.6	0.12	1.71	447
Plasma retinol (µmol/l)	1.12	0.031	1.04	70	1.20	0.026	1.63	174	1.27	0.025	1.51	162	1.53	0.036	1.22	152	1.29	0.019	1.74	558
Plasma α-carotene (µmol/l)	0.048	0.0036	0.77	70	0.053	0.0034	1.42	174	0.041	0.0023	0.91	162	0.036	0.0019	0.83	152	0.044	0.0015	1.23	558
Plasma α-cryptoxanthin (µmol/l)	0.065	0.0052	1.21	70	0.067	0.0031	1.37	174	0.062	0.0027	0.69	162	0.051	0.0028	1.01	152	0.061	0.0017	1.06	558
Plasma lycopene (µmol/l)	0.486	0.0283	1.21	70	0.516	0.0287	1.91	174	0.478	0.0188	1.20	162	0.475	0.0210	1.43	152	0.489	0.0121	1.46	558
Plasma 25-OHD (nmol/l)	71.8	3.69	1.30	73	70.0	2.52	1.53	177	56.7	2.31	1.70	167	51.6	2.97	1.72	153	62.0	1.81	2.48	570
Plasma α-tocopherol (µmol/l)	19.6	0.45	1.01	70	20.5	0.41	1.69	174	19.7	0.29	0.94	162	19.2	0.43	1.68	152	19.8	0.18	1.17	558
Plasma total cholesterol (mmol/l)	3.99	0.100	1.24	55	4.27	0.072	1.31	164	4.01	0.062	0.84	136	3.84	0.053	0.87	143	4.03	0.031	0.80	498
Plasma high density lipoprotein cholesterol (mmol/l)	1.29	0.036	0.97	55	1.37	0.024	0.92	164	1.31	0.029	1.08	136	1.09	0.028	1.37	143	1.26	0.014	0.93	498
Plasma triglycerides (mmol/l)*	0.65	0.043	1.36	45	0.78	0.029	1.05	155	0.89	0.040	1.26	121	1.13	0.058	0.88	135	0.88	0.027	1.26	456
Blood lead (µg/dl)	3.3	0.31	1.54	78	2.8	0.13	1.26	176	2.8	0.12	1.25	178	2.4	0.10	0.95	165	2.8	0.07	1.21	597
Plasma magnesium (mmol/l)	0.94	0.014	1.58	79	0.94	0.010	1.91	176	0.94	0.011	1.55	176	0.93	0.010	1.85	159	0.94	0.007	2.87	590
Plasma selenium (µmol/l)	0.82	0.022	1.77	79	0.87	0.012	1.24	176	0.84	0.010	0.89	176	0.89	0.010	0.83	160	0.86	0.007	1.19	591
Red cell superoxide dismutase (nmol/mg Hb/min)	1211	28.7	1.31	72	1224	16.8	1.28	178	1149	22.1	1.24	168	1096	22.9	1.04	154	1168	12.8	1.54	572
Plasma α₁-antichymotrypsin (g/l)	0.31	0.009	1.43	34	0.29	0.005	1.38	156	0.27	0.005	1.21	134	0.27	0.006	1.37	140	0.28	0.003	1.55	484

*Fasting cases only

Table E7(b) True standard errors and design factors for selected blood analytes by age of young person: females

Blood analytes	Age (years) 4–6 Mean r	Standard error of r	Design factor	Base	7–10 Mean r	Standard error of r	Design factor	Base	11–14 Mean r	Standard error of r	Design factor	Base	15–18 Mean r	Standard error of r	Design factor	Base	All Mean r	Standard error of r	Design factor	Base
Haemoglobin concentration (g/dl)	12.4	0.13	1.46	82	12.8	0.09	1.19	143	13.3	0.08	1.41	171	13.1	0.08	0.99	169	12.9	0.05	1.64	565
Plasma iron (µmol/l)	12.67	0.552	1.12	66	13.18	0.369	0.87	121	13.22	0.365	1.12	157	13.25	0.442	0.70	160	13.06	0.210	0.87	504
Serum ferritin (µg/l)	30	2.1	1.38	63	38	2.5	0.96	99	31	1.3	0.92	128	29	2.0	1.18	136	32	0.9	0.86	426
Plasma vitamin C (µmol/l)	64.6	3.13	1.49	76	60.1	2.64	1.48	133	55.7	1.80	1.38	161	55.7	2.07	1.05	158	58.8	1.26	1.56	528
Red cell folate (nmol/l)	677	33.6	2.09	77	604	20.0	0.96	125	544	16.0	1.47	163	500	15.0	1.04	156	573	10.8	1.49	521
Serum folate (nmol/l)	25.8	0.94	1.62	82	22.0	0.81	1.19	138	19.3	0.51	0.97	168	16.9	0.55	0.81	169	20.6	0.36	1.07	557
Serum vitamin B₁₂ (pmol/l)	550	21.8	1.08	82	443	13.8	1.08	138	371	15.6	1.42	169	267	8.8	0.81	169	395	8.9	1.28	558
Erythrocyte transketolase activation coefficient	1.10	0.006	0.97	76	1.11	0.004	0.85	133	1.13	0.005	1.38	163	1.13	0.006	1.44	162	1.12	0.003	1.91	534
Erythrocyte glutathione reductase activation coefficient	1.38	0.014	1.13	76	1.45	0.013	0.99	133	1.51	0.014	1.06	165	1.53	0.017	1.31	163	1.47	0.008	1.22	537
Plasma zinc (µmol/l)	15.1	0.22	0.86	38	14.7	0.23	1.39	97	14.6	0.17	1.27	139	13.9	0.20	1.13	147	14.6	0.11	1.39	421
Plasma retinol (µmol/l)	1.15	0.027	1.11	71	1.21	0.025	0.97	131	1.28	0.026	1.45	159	1.51	0.034	1.11	161	1.29	0.018	1.49	522
Plasma α-carotene (µmol/l)	0.059	0.0044	0.81	71	0.051	0.0024	0.84	131	0.044	0.0024	0.74	159	0.043	0.0022	0.70	161	0.049	0.0016	1.12	522
Plasma α-cryptoxanthin (µmol/l)	0.069	0.0040	1.03	71	0.056	0.0027	0.94	131	0.057	0.0030	1.18	159	0.053	0.0025	1.06	161	0.058	0.0016	1.15	522
Plasma lycopene (µmol/l)	0.513	0.0312	1.08	71	0.485	0.0175	0.77	131	0.449	0.0206	1.77	159	0.498	0.0191	0.99	161	0.485	0.0112	1.28	522
Plasma 25-OHD (nmol/l)	68.9	3.38	1.17	76	66.5	2.58	1.11	133	54.4	2.41	1.86	164	53.7	2.46	1.17	162	60.6	1.59	1.81	535
Plasma α-tocopherol (µmol/l)	21.2	0.51	1.08	71	21.2	0.37	1.08	131	20.5	0.30	1.27	159	19.8	0.29	0.75	161	20.6	0.18	1.10	522
Plasma total cholesterol (mmol/l)	4.48	0.148	1.31	51	4.30	0.099	1.06	109	4.14	0.076	1.80	145	4.08	0.059	0.85	155	4.24	0.045	1.33	460
Plasma high density lipoprotein cholesterol (mmol/l)	1.23	0.039	1.13	51	1.31	0.038	1.34	109	1.29	0.027	1.02	145	1.24	0.031	1.20	155	1.27	0.014	0.88	460
Plasma triglycerides (mmol/l)*	0.79	0.030	1.00	43	0.92	0.041	1.19	94	0.97	0.036	1.53	142	1.02	0.038	1.00	138	0.93	0.021	1.34	417
Blood lead (µg/dl)	2.9	0.18	1.42	78	2.7	0.14	1.32	136	2.4	0.11	1.35	166	2.0	0.08	0.92	166	2.5	0.07	1.58	546
Plasma magnesium (mmol/l)	0.94	0.014	1.58	77	0.91	0.009	1.35	134	0.90	0.007	1.26	165	0.91	0.008	1.34	166	0.91	0.006	2.21	542
Plasma selenium (µmol/l)	0.81	0.019	1.26	76	0.90	0.019	1.45	133	0.85	0.013	1.26	166	0.91	0.012	0.99	165	0.87	0.007	1.11	540
Red cell superoxide dismutase (nmol/mg Hb/min)	1208	27.2	1.30	76	1163	18.1	0.87	133	1166	27.6	1.53	164	1142	29.0	1.11	163	1168	13.5	1.23	536
Plasma α₁-antichymotrypsin (g/l)	0.35	0.018	1.89	44	0.30	0.009	1.10	107	0.28	0.006	1.60	143	0.28	0.004	0.96	151	0.30	0.004	1.40	445

* Fasting cases only

Appendix F

Dietary methodology: details of the recording and coding procedures

1 Choice of dietary methodology

For each survey in the NDNS series, the weighed intake methodology has been the preferred method for collecting quantitative information on food and nutrient intakes[1,2]. Compared with other methods, such as 24-hour recall methods and food frequency questionnaires the weighed intake methodology gives more precise estimates of intakes for individuals which can be related to health indices, such as nutritional status measured by blood analytes, as well as allowing distributions of intakes for groups to be calculated. Applied properly, the method avoids recall errors, and for foods eaten at home, minimises the need to estimate quantities consumed[3,4,5].

The weighed intake method gives information on the person's current diet, whereas food frequency questionnaires and recall methods, because they can cover a longer reference period, can provide information on a person's usual diet.

The weighed intake method does of course have disadvantages; it requires a high level of motivation and to some extent greater skill and understanding from respondents than other methods. To apply it properly requires a much greater level of support and assistance from interviewers with the need for frequent and regular calls. Precision scales, which are expensive, are required and together all the above factors make the method resource intensive, and hence costly. In relation to the reliability of the information collected it has been argued that the method can lead to changes in eating habits and under-recording. For each NDNS these issues are tested in feasibility work, before deciding whether the weighed intake is a suitable methodology for the age group being studied. Appendix C describes the feasibility study carried out for this NDNS, including the results of the validation of the dietary intake method using the doubly-labelled water methodology; the conclusion from the feasibility work was that the weighed intake method would be suitable for use in the main stage of this survey of young people[6,7].

2 Recording in the 'Home Record' diary

The 'Home Record' diary was an A3 loose-leaf document designed to collect detailed information on items weighed at home, including items prepared at home, but eaten elsewhere, for example lunches prepared at home and taken to school.

Young people (and other diary keepers) were asked to start a new diary page at the beginning of each day and record the day and date on every page used and to indicate whether the young person was well or unwell on each day; if the young person was unwell for only part of the day then they were coded as being unwell.

Entries made up to midnight on the day the interviewer left the diary were discarded at the analysis stage as the dietary recording period started at midnight and then continued for seven days.

Before weighing each group of food items being served together young people were asked always to weigh the empty plate or container before any item was added. To encourage their weighing an empty container each diary page had pre-printed 'empty plate/container lines' where the weight of the empty plate could be entered. Each 'empty plate line' was followed by lines for information on each item weighed and served on that plate. If there were insufficient lines following an 'empty plate line' for all the items being served together then the young person was told to cross through the next 'empty plate line' and continue with recording the item information on the following lines. Each time a new set of items was weighed, recording started at the next 'empty plate line'. For each set of items weighed together the young person recorded the time the items were eaten, where they were eaten, at home, at school or elsewhere, and who did the weighing, the young person or someone else.

After weighing and recording the weight of the empty container the scales were then set to zero and the first food item put on the plate, weighed and recorded. The scales were then 'zeroed' again and subsequent items added, weighed and recorded in the same way[8]. Each food item was recorded in the diary on a separate line, with a full description including brand information, as shown on the example page of the 'Home Record' diary, reproduced in Appendix A.

Second helpings were weighed and recorded in the same way as the initial serving; the plate, with any items remaining was put on the scales and the scales zeroed. Each second serving of a food was then added to the plate and weighed and recorded separately. These items were then flagged for the attention of the ONS nutritionists who combined the weights of first and second helpings giving an overall weight for each food item consumed.

Items too light to be weighed: for items which were too light to be weighed, for example a very small quantity of instant coffee granules, a description of the quantity was recorded in household measures, for example half a level teaspoon.

Leftovers were also recorded. The individual weighing of leftovers was felt to be too burdensome, and might have led to reduced compliance with keeping the dietary record. Therefore at the end of each eating occasion the plate or container was re-weighed with all the leftover items; the total weight was recorded in the leftover column on the 'empty plate line' with a tick in the leftovers column to indicate each food item that was left. Young people were encouraged also to record additional information on leftovers, for example, that half the mashed potato was left or all the serving of carrots. For foods that have inedible parts such as some meats, fish, fruit and nuts, the young person was asked to note whether the weight of leftovers included the weight of inedible parts, such as bones, peel or shells.

Foods eaten straight from containers: items such as yogurts and desserts eaten straight from the pot were treated in a similar way to leftovers. The full pot was weighed on plate, and after the contents were eaten, the empty pot or pot and any remaining contents were weighed again on the plate.

Spilt or dropped food. If any item was spilt or dropped after weighing, the young person was encouraged wherever possible to recover and re-weigh it on the original plate together with any other leftovers. In some cases this was not possible, for example because the spilt food was eaten by the dog, so an estimate was made of how much of the original item was lost, and recorded in the spillage column of the 'Home Record'.

Recipes for home-made dishes were recorded on the back of the recording sheets in the 'Home Record' diary. Young people were asked to give as much detail as possible about quantities of ingredients used, including liquids added during cooking, and the cooking method used.

Home-grown items: for any fresh fruit or vegetable item recorded in the diary the young person was asked to indicate whether it was home grown, defined as being grown in their own household's garden or allotment.

3 Recording in the 'Eating Out' diary

The 'Eating Out' diary was an A4 document designed for recording information on everything that was eaten or drunk while the young person was away from home, including details of items prepared and weighed at home (and recorded in the 'Home Record' diary) but eaten elsewhere, such as a packed lunch taken to school. For young people aged 7 years and over the 'Eating Out' diary also contained pages for recording details of physical activities over the same 7-day recording period.

For every item eaten away from home the young person was asked to record a full description of the item, including its brand name, together with information on where and when it was eaten, portion size and details of any leftovers. If the item had been bought, then price and place of purchase were required. Prompt questions, designed to improve the completeness of information, asked the young person to record the total amount of money spent on things to eat and drink each day while they were not at home and to check that all the purchased items were recorded. A centimetre rule printed around the edges of the diary pages could be used to measure the size of items, for example a slice of pizza or pie, if the weight was not known.

Interviewers checked the 'Eating Out' diary at each visit and probed for any more information needed to code the food items. At the coding stage interviewers transcribed the entries from the 'Eating Out' diary to the 'Home Record' and split composite items such as sandwiches into their constituent parts (bread, spread and filling). ONS coders and nutritionists carried out a 100% quality check on all the information transcribed from the 'Eating Out' diaries, checking food codes and where necessary estimating gram weights from the quantity described.

3.1 Strategies for obtaining information about items which had not been weighed

Weight information for foods eaten away from home, which could not be weighed, was collected in a variety of ways and added to the record. For items purchased from local shops or cafes, such as cakes, sandwiches and chips, interviewers used the information about price and place of purchase to buy a duplicate item which was either weighed directly or, if it was a composite item, split into its component parts and weighed. Interviewers were also asked to find out further details of foods purchased from takeaway outlets so that they could be correctly coded; for example the type of fat used for frying, and the type of spread used in sandwiches.

For pre-packaged foods eaten outside the home, for example confectionery and soft drinks, weight information was obtained from the packaging. To encourage young people to keep wrappers and cartons they were given plastic bags, which were then returned to the interviewer.

All estimated weights entered by the young person or interviewer were checked by the nutritionists to make sure they were consistent, for example that the weight recorded for a standard chocolate bar corresponded with the weight on the packaging.

Where it was not possible to collect information on the weights of the components of a composite item, individual weights were estimated by the nutritionists using information from *MAFF Food Portion Sizes*[9]. Wherever possible weights allocated were based on similar items recorded elsewhere in the diary that had been weighed, or were allocated to correspond to the general eating habits of the young person over the recording period. This was especially important for items consumed by the younger children, for which the *MAFF Food Portion Sizes* information was not always appropriate.

3.2 Food and drink items provided by the school

If the young person had food or drink items provided by their school (or college), the interviewer invariably needed additional information about the items before they could be transcribed onto pages for coding. Generally the young person did not weigh the items eaten at school, so the interviewer ideally needed either to have weight information from duplicates or to have information on standard portion sizes served at the school. More detail about the items was also frequently required before they could be food and brand coded. Interviewers therefore had to contact the person responsible for food preparation and serving. In most cases this was the school catering manager, but in some schools where food was prepared 'off-premises' an external catering manager as well as at the school had to be contacted.

Directors of Education were asked in the 'letter of information' sent before the start of fieldwork, to provide the name of an individual who would be able to help the interviewer with the detail required, particularly if catering for a number of schools was organised centrally. Despite these efforts collecting information from school caterers proved time consuming and in some cases very difficult, particularly where catering contracts were soon to be re-tendered or renewed.

Feasibility work had shown there was some common information required from schools in nearly every case, and that this could be collected on a short standard questionnaire, which the interviewer could either leave with the catering manager to complete, or could use as an interview document[6]. The catering questionnaire developed for the main stage included questions on the

fats used for frying, types of spread used in sandwiches and baking, types of milk purchased, cooking methods for items such as sausages, burgers, fish, type and method of cooking chips and standard portion sizes for a range of foods. The questionnaire was completed for every young person who had food provided by the school, and additionally the interviewer probed for and recorded further information on specific items recorded in the young person's 'Eating Out' diary. The information was used by the interviewers and subsequently by the ONS nutritionists in checking and coding the young person's 'Eating Out' information.

4 Checks by the interviewer

Interviewers were required to call back to the household approximately 24 hours after placing the diary. Experience on previous surveys has always shown that this call is essential in giving encouragement to continue keeping the record and to help with any problems with the weighing or recording[1,10].

At this call interviewers checked in particular that each food item on a plate was being weighed separately and weights were not being recorded cumulatively, that edible and inedible leftovers were being weighed and recorded correctly, that descriptions of foods consumed were sufficiently detailed, that recipes for home-made items were recorded and that composite items were being split before weighing. To help interviewers identify cumulative weights they were provided with a list of typical portion weights for commonly consumed foods, such as breakfast cereals[11].

Depending on how much support the young person or other record keeper appeared to need interviewers made extra calls throughout the recording period, checking for any obvious difficulties in recording and probing for more details of foods that were inadequately described. At these calls interviewers also checked for items eaten at home and away from home that might have been forgotten, for example drinks taken to bed, or sweets bought on the way home from school. Where necessary a duplicate item was weighed, recorded in the diary and noted as an estimated weight.

5 Eating pattern check sheet

As part of the checking process interviewers completed an eating pattern check sheet for each young person, summarising the number of drinks, crisps and savoury snacks, biscuits and sweets and dietary supplements they had each day. This check sheet was designed to alert the interviewer to marked changes in the dietary record from day to day, such as a decline over time in the number of snacks or drinks being recorded, which could then be checked at the next call.

6 Coding

Interviewers were responsible for coding the food diaries before returning them to ONS. This enabled them readily to identify the level of detail needed for different food items, and probe for missing detail at later visits to the household. At each checking call interviewers took away completed diary pages to be coded; any additional information needed to code the food item was asked for at the next visit.

The first diary returned by each interviewer received a 100% check by ONS nutritionists, which included checks on all aspects of the diary, including coding, recorded weights and descriptions of items consumed. Feedback was given to interviewers on the quality of their coding and probing.

Codes were assigned to identify food items, brand (for selected food types only), and the food source. Any item which could not be coded, for example because it was a new product or a home-made recipe that did not appear in the food code list, was 'flagged' for the attention of the nutritionists at ONS.

ONS nutritionists and coders, advised by MAFF, completed the coding of the diaries and for certain food items carried out a 100% coding check on each item. All food codes were checked for the following items: soft drinks, milk, fat spreads, yogurts, artificial sweeteners, liver and liver products and vitamin and mineral supplements. As a further quality check on food coding, as the food code was keyed into the data entry program the text description of the food item was displayed on the screen so that the code could be visually checked against the diary entry.

6.1   Food code list

MAFF compiled the nutrient databank, details of which are given in Appendix I, and associated food code list which, by the end of the survey, contained over 5000 food codes. A page from the food code list is reproduced in Appendix G. Interviewers were provided with this list, an alphabetical index (paper copy) and an electronic version of the food code list which was loaded onto their laptop computer to help them find particular foods. The code list was regularly updated to take account of new products eaten by the young people that became available during the fieldwork period. A separate list of raw foods not expected to occur in food diaries but used in recipes, for example raw chicken, was also provided for use by the ONS nutritionists.

In order to meet the aims of the survey in providing accurate information on food and nutrient intakes for young people, to relate these to physiological measures and to be able to characterise those young people with nutrient intakes above and below average values it was necessary to collect very detailed information about the items consumed. Only with this detailed information could the correct food code, with its associated nutrient composition data, be assigned to the item consumed. For example, detailed information on the types of fat

spreads used by the young person was needed in order to assign the correct food code according to the different types of fatty acids the spread contained.

In order to code food items to the required level of detail the following types of information were required:

- the form in which the food was bought, for example, whether it was fresh, frozen or canned;

- whether the product was low fat and whether any fat had been trimmed or skimmed from meat or meat dishes;

- the cooking method, for example whether the food item had been boiled, microwaved, baked, grilled, roasted or fried, and if fat was added in cooking the type of fat used;

- whether there were any inedible leftovers, such as bones in meat or fish, or stones in fruit;

- whether a coating was used for fish and meat, and whether sauces and gravies were thickened;

- whether foods had been sweetened and, if so, whether sugar or an artificial sweetener had been used;

- whether soft drinks were low calorie or dec-affeinated; whether they were bottled or canned;

- whether fruit juices were UHT, pasteurised or freshly squeezed;

- whether water was taken as a drink on its own, or used as a diluent;

- whether dairy products were full, or reduced fat;

- details of the type of fat and flour used in home-baked items;

- whether products such as cheese, fish and meat were smoked or not.

Interviewers were provided with a prompt card as an aide-mémoire for the kind of detail needed in order to code different food types.

A number of check lists were prepared for interviewers by ONS and MAFF which helped interviewers correctly code particular food groups which required a lot of detail, for example for soft drinks, fats used for spreading and cooking, and savoury snacks.

The food code list included a number of different codes for tap water, which were assigned according to whether the water was used as a diluent, or drunk as plain water. For example, different codes distinguished tap water used to dilute concentrated low calorie soft drinks, concentrated non-low calorie soft drinks, used to make up instant coffee, used to make up dried milk and used to make up instant beverages such as Horlicks and Ovaltine. Although the nutrient information attached to each food code for tap water is the same, by having different food codes it is possible to determine the total volume of liquids of different types drunk by young people, for example total amounts of diluted soft drinks, instant coffee and plain water.

6.2   Composite and recipe items

Composite items which could be split into their constituent parts
Where foods could be split into their individual components they were weighed, recorded and then coded separately, for example, a cup of tea as tea infusion, milk and sugar; a sandwich as bread, spread and filling(s).

If such composite items had not been split and weighed separately then the interviewer recorded an estimate of the quantity of each of the constituent parts; this could be a relatively standard amount, such as the number of slices of bread, or could involve a description of the quantity or relative proportions of each component, for example the quantity of each vegetable in a mixed salad. Using this information the ONS nutritionists apportioned the total weight between the components of the dish. The components of the composite dish were coded in the normal way.

Recipe items
Diary keepers were asked to record recipes, (ingredients with brand names and their quantities) for most home-made dishes, such as chicken casserole or apple crumble. Where such foods were included in the food code list, they were identified by 'R' preceding the code number; this indicated that their nutrient values were based on standard recipe ingredients. The ONS nutritionists individually checked each recorded recipe and the type and proportions of ingredients used were compared with those of the standard recipe to which the food code referred. If the ingredients differed from the standard recipe in a way that was nutritionally significant the existing food code was not used and a new food code allocated to the item. The appropriate nutrients for the new recipe code were calculated by MAFF and added to the nutrient database.

Where recipe items were eaten away from the home, for example lasagne eaten at a restaurant, and it was not possible to establish details of the ingredients, the standard food code for that item was used. However interviewers were encouraged to collect details of ingredients used in such recipes wherever possible as this information enabled items to be coded appropriately. Codes were also included in the food code list for

menu items purchased from national fast-food chains, for example McDonalds, where data on the nutritional content of the foods are available.

6.3   Brand information
Brand information was recorded for all pre-packaged foods. For some food items, for example, confectionery, biscuits and some breakfast cereals, the brand name was needed in order to code the food item correctly.

Artificial sweeteners, herbal and fruit teas, fruit juices and soft drinks, and bottled water were the only food items to be brand coded. This was necessary to provide accurate information on non-nutrient components such as artificial sweeteners.

6.4   Coding food source
As noted in Chapter 1 there is interest in the contribution made to the total nutrient intake of young people by foods from different sources, in particular comparisons between the contributions made to total intake from different types of lunchtime meal eaten by young people at school or elsewhere, for example food eaten at lunch times at home, food provided by schools, food taken from home, and food purchased outside school, for example, from a 'fast food' outlet, bakers, or chip shop.

It was therefore necessary to 'source' code food items; the source codes identified where the food item was eaten, for example at home, at school or elsewhere, when it was eaten, during school hours or at some other time, and the food provider, home, school, takeaway outlet, or other retail outlet. Food source coding was at plate entry level, rather than at individual food level, and where items on the same plate came from different sources, for example, some items from a 'takeaway' and some from the home food store, the food source code was allocated on the basis of the source of the main food item(s) on the plate.

7   Data entry and editing
Dietary information was keyed by the coding and editing team into an intelligent keying program which incorporated initial edit checks at the point of data entry. At this stage the weight of each food item consumed was automatically calculated by subtracting the weight of any leftovers from the weight of food served; where a combined weight was given for a number of leftover items the total weight of leftovers was divided among the food items indicated as being leftover, usually in proportion to the served weights of those items. The keying program incorporated checks to identify food items where the weight of food consumed was outside a specified range; such cases were individually checked by the nutritionists and any errors corrected.

Checks were run to identify cases where the intake of any nutrient was outside the expected range for normal intakes, although in most cases only a maximum value could be specified; again such cases were individually checked by the ONS nutritionists and any errors corrected. MAFF supplied range information for both food weights and nutrient intakes. Consistency checks between the dietary and questionnaire data were also carried out at this stage.

References and endnotes

[1] Gregory JR, Collins DL, Davies PSW, Hughes JM, Clarke PC. *National Diet and Nutrition Survey: children aged 1½ to 4½ years. Volume 1: Report of the diet and nutrition survey.* HMSO (London, 1995).

[2] Finch S, Doyle W, Lowe C, Bates CJ, Prentice A, Smithers G, Clarke PC. *National Diet and Nutrition Survey: people aged 65 years and over. Volume 1: Report of the diet and nutrition survey.* TSO (London, 1998).

[3] Fehily AM. Epidemiology for nutritionists: four survey methods. *Hum Nutr: App Nutr.* 1983; **37A**; 419–425.

[4] Bingham SA. The Dietary assessment of individuals: methods, accuracy, new techniques and recommendations. *Nutr Abstr Rev.* (series A) 1987; **57**:10; 705–742.

[5] Medical Research Council, Environmental Epidemiology Unit. *The Dietary Assessment of Populations. Southampton 1983.* Southampton (1984) (Conference Proceedings: Scientific Report No 4).

[6] Lowe S. *Feasibility study for the National Diet and Nutrition Survey: young people aged 4 to 18 years.* ONS (*In preparation*).

[7] Smithers G, Gregory J, Coward WA, Wright A, Elsom R, Wenlock R. British National Diet and Nutrition Survey of young people aged 4 to 18 years: feasibility study of the dietary assessment methodology. Abstracts of the Third International Conference on Dietary Assessment Methods. *Eur J Clin Nutr.* 1998; **52**: S2. S76.

[8] Soehnle Quanta and Soehnle Vita scales: these scales have a digital display and tare facility. They are calibrated in units of 1 gram up to 1 kilogram and 2 gram units thereafter.

[9] Ministry of Agriculture, Fisheries and Food. *Food Portion Sizes.* 2nd Ed. HMSO (London, 1993).

[10] Gregory J, Foster K, Tyler H, Wiseman M. *The Dietary and Nutritional Survey of British Adults.* HMSO (London, 1990).

[11] ONS nutritionists had final responsibility for identifying cumulative weights as part of the HQ checking and coding procedures.

Appendix G

Sample page from the food code list

FISH. COATED OR FRIED. FISH PRODUCTS AND FISH DISHES

1405   Cod, no coating, fried in blended vegetable oil

              Coalfish, code as for cod

1406   Cod, no coating, fried in butter

1407   Cod, no coating, fried in dripping

1408   Cod, no coating, fried in lard

1409   Cod, no coating, fried in margarine (NOT polyunsaturated)

1410   Cod, no coating, fried in polyunsaturated margarine or oil

1411   Cod, coated in batter, fried in blended vegetable oil. NOT purchased from takeaway shop

1415   Cod, coated in batter, fried in blended vegetable oil, from takeaway shop

1412   Cod, coated in batter, fried in dripping

1413   Cod, coated in batter, fried in lard

1414   Cod, coated in batter, fried in polyunsaturated oil

1637   Cod, coated in batter, frozen, oven baked or grilled, no added fat

1416   Cod, coated in egg and breadcrumbs, fried in blended vegetable oil

1417   Cod, coated in egg and breadcrumbs, fried in dripping

1418   Cod, coated in egg and breadcrumbs, fried in lard

1419   Cod, coated in egg and breadcrumbs, fried in polyunsaturated oil

9254   Cod, coated in breadcrumbs, frozen, fried in blended vegetable oil

9574   Cod, coated in breadcrumbs, frozen, grilled or baked

8599   Cod, coated in flour, fried in blended vegetable oil

9540   Cod, coated in flour, fried in lard

9613   Cod, coated in flour, fried in olive oil

1539   Dogfish; rock salmon; coated in batter, fried in blended vegetable oil, no bones, or leftover bones weighed. NOT purchased from takeaway shop

1543   Dogfish; rock salmon; coated in batter, fried in blended vegetable oil, purchased from takeaway shop, no bones, or leftover bones weighed

Appendix H

Food types, main and subsidiary food groups[1]

Food types consist of one or more food groups.
Food groups are expressed as integers.
Subsidiary food groups are integers with an alphabetical suffix.

1   Pasta, rice and other miscellaneous cereals

1A	Pasta	all types – dried, fresh and canned; including egg noodles, macaroni cheese, ravioli, canned spaghetti bolognaise
1B	Rice	fried and boiled, savoury rice, egg fried rice, rice flakes, rice flour. (Not rice pudding)
1C	Pizza	all types – thin & crispy, deep pan, French bread
1R	Other cereals	includes flour, bran, oats, dry semolina, papadums, dumplings, Yorkshire pudding

2   White bread

2R	White bread	sliced, unsliced, toast, fried; includes French stick, milk loaf, slimmers, pitta bread, rolls, chappatis, soda bread

3   Wholemeal bread

3R	Wholemeal bread	sliced, unsliced, toast, fried; includes chappatis, pitta bread, rolls, hi-bran bread, wholemeal soda bread

4   Other breads

4A	Softgrain bread	sliced, unsliced, toast, fried, rolls; e.g. Mighty White, Champion, own brands; fortified and not fortified
4R	Other breads	sliced, unsliced, toast, fried; includes brown, granary, high fibre white, rye bread, gluten free, garlic bread, continental breads e.g. ciabatta, oatmeal bread, Vitbe, Hovis, crumpets, English muffins (white & wholemeal), pikelets, brown and granary rolls, bagels, brioche, naan, paratha

5   Wholegrain and high fibre breakfast cereals

5R	Wholegrain and high fibre	all with non-starch polysaccharide (Englyst fibre) breakfast cereals of 4g/100g or more, e.g. All Bran, muesli, Shredded Wheat. Includes porridge & Ready Brek

6	**Other breakfast cereals**	
6R	Other breakfast cereals	all with non-starch polysaccharide (Englyst fibre) of less than 4g/100g, e.g. cornflakes, Coco Pops, Sugar Puffs. Includes Pop Tarts

7	**Biscuits**	
7R	Biscuits	all types, sweet and savoury; includes cream crackers, flapjacks, breadsticks, crispbread, cereal crunchy bars, ice cream cornet

8	**Buns, cakes, pastries and fruit pies**	
8A	Fruit pies	all types, one and two crusts; includes apple strudel, individual fruit pies from takeaways
8R	Buns, cakes and pastries	includes Danish pastries, currant bun, doughnuts, Eccles cakes, Bakewell tarts, jam tarts, scones (sweet and savoury), sponge cakes, fruit cakes, eclairs, currant bread, malt loaf, gateaux, pastry, mince pies, sponge fingers, scotch pancakes, croissants, custard tart, lemon meringue pie

9	**Puddings**	
9A	Cereal-based milk puddings	rice pudding (including canned), custard (not egg custard), Angel Delight, blancmange, confectioners custard, semolina, sweet white sauce
9B	Sponge puddings	steamed, canned, suet pudding, jam roly poly, sponge flan, upside-down pudding
9R	Other cereal-based puddings	includes trifle, fruit fritters, pancakes, crumble, bread pudding, cheesecakes, tiramisu, rum baba, Christmas pudding

Food Type: Cereals and cereal products (Groups 1-9)

10	**Whole milk**	
10R	Whole milk	all types of cow's milk including pasteurised, UHT, sterilised, Channel Island

11	**Semi-skimmed milk**	
11R	Semi-skimmed milk	all types of cow's milk including pasteurised, UHT, sterilised, canned, milk with added vitamins

12	**Skimmed milk**	
12R	Skimmed milk	all types of cow's milk including pasteurised, UHT, sterilised, canned, milk with added vitamins, Vital, Calcia

13	**Other milk and cream**	
13A	Infant formula[2]	
13B	Cream	all types, including imitation cream, aerosol, Dream Topping, Tip Top, creme fraiche
13R	Other milk	includes soya alternative to milk, goats, sheeps, evaporated, condensed, dried milk, milk shake, coffee whitener, buttermilk, flavoured milk drink

14   Cheese

14A   Cottage cheese

includes diet and flavoured

14R   Other cheese

all types, including hard, soft, cream cheese, processed, reduced fat cheeses, vegetarian cheese, cheese spread. (Not fromage frais or Quark)

15   Yogurt, fromage frais and other dairy desserts

15A   Fromage frais

includes fromage frais mousse, Quark

15B   Yogurt

all types including soya, goats, sheeps, yogurt mousse, yogurt drink, frozen yogurt, custard style yogurt, Greek yogurt

15R   Other dairy desserts

includes chocolate and fruit cream desserts, mousse, milk jelly, junket, egg custard, buttermilk desserts, fruit fools, creme caramel

53   Ice cream

53R   Ice cream

all types, including non-dairy, choc ices, ice cream desserts, ice cream containing lollies, milk ice lollies, low fat/low calorie ice cream

Food Type: Milk and milk products (Groups 10-15 & 53)

16   Eggs and egg dishes

16A   Eggs

includes boiled, fried, scrambled, poached, dried, omelettes (sweet and savoury)

16B   Egg dishes

includes quiches, flans, souffles, scotch eggs, eggy bread, apple snow, meringue, pavlova, curried eggs

Food Type: Eggs and egg dishes (Group 16)

17   Butter[3]

17R   Butter

salted and unsalted, butter ghee, spreadable butter

18   Polyunsaturated margarine and oils[3]

18A   Polyunsaturated margarine

margarine claiming to be high in polyunsaturated fatty acids

18B   Polyunsaturated oils

includes corn oil, sunflower oil, solid sunflower oil

19   Low fat spread[3]

19A   Low fat spread polyunsaturated

spreads containing 40% or less fat, claiming to be high in polyunsaturated fatty acids

19R   Other low fat spread polyunsaturated

spreads containing 40% or less fat, not claiming to be high in polyunsaturated fatty acids

20   Margarine and other cooking fats and oils not polyunsaturated[3]

20A   Block margarine

all hard margarine

20B   Soft margarine not polyunsaturated

tub margarine not claiming to be high in polyunsaturated fatty acids

| 20C | Other cooking fats and oils, not polyunsaturated | includes blended vegetable oil, suet, lard, compound cooking fat, dripping, olive oil, rapeseed oil |

21 Reduced fat spread[3]

| 21A | Reduced fat spread, polyunsaturated | spreads containing more than 40% and less than 80% fat, claiming to be high in polyunsaturated fatty acids |
| 21B | Other reduced fat spread | spreads containing more than 40% and less than 80% fat, not claiming to be high in polyunsaturated fatty acids; includes spreads made with olive oil, rapeseed oil or fish oil |

Food Type: Fat spreads (Groups 17-21)

22 Bacon and ham

| 22R | Bacon and ham | including bacon and gammon joints, steaks, chops and rashers; all types of ham, pork shoulder, bacon and cheese grills |

23 Beef, veal and dishes

| 23R | Beef, veal and dishes | includes beef and veal joints, steaks, minced beef, stewing steak, beef stews, casseroles, meat balls, lasagne, chilli con carne, beef curry, bolognaise sauce, shepherds pie, canned beef |

24 Lamb and dishes

| 24R | Lamb and dishes | includes lamb joints, chops, cutlets, fillets, lamb curries, Irish stew, lamb casseroles and stews |

25 Pork and dishes

| 25R | Pork and dishes | includes joints, chops, steaks, belly rashers, pork stews and casseroles, sweet and sour pork, spare ribs, roast roll |

26 Coated chicken and turkey

| 26R | Coated chicken and turkey | chicken and turkey pieces coated in egg and crumb; drumsticks, nuggets, fingers, burgers etc. Includes Kentucky Fried Chicken, chicken Kiev |

27 Chicken and turkey dishes

| 27R | Chicken and turkey dishes | includes roast chicken and turkey, barbecued, fried (no coating), curries, stews, casseroles, chow mein, tandoori, in sauce, spread, chicken/turkey roll |

28 Liver, liver products and dishes

| 28R | Liver, liver products and dishes | includes all types of liver – fried, stewed, braised, grilled; liver casserole, liver sausage, liver pate |

29 Burgers and kebabs

| 29R | Burgers and kebabs | includes beefburgers, hamburgers, cheeseburgers, (with or without roll) doner/shish/kofte kebabs (with or without pitta bread and salad), grillsteaks, steaklets |

30 Sausages

| 30R | Sausages | includes beef, pork, turkey sausages, polony, sausage in batter, saveloy, frankfurters, sausage dishes |

31 Meat pies and pastries

| 31R | Meat pies and pastries | any type of meat; includes chicken/turkey pies, vol-au-vents, beef pies, steak and kidney pudding, pork pies, veal and ham pie, pasties, sausage roll, meat samosas, pancake rolls |

32 Other meat and meat products

| 32R | Other meat and meat products | includes game (e.g. venison, grouse, rabbit, pheasant), duck, goose, all offal (except liver), faggots, black pudding, haggis, haslet, meat paste, tongue, luncheon meats, corned beef, salami, pepperami, meat loaf |

Food Type: Meat and meat products (Groups 22-32)

33 White fish coated and/or fried including fish fingers

| 33R | White fish coated and/or fried including fish fingers | cod, haddock, plaice, etc. fried without coating, or coated in egg and crumb, batter or flour and fried, grilled or baked. Includes fish fingers and fish cakes – fried and grilled, fried cartilaginous fish, scampi, filet-o-fish, cod roe fried, prawn balls, Fish Feasts, fish pancakes |

34 Other white fish, shellfish and fish dishes

| 34A | Other white fish and fish dishes | cod, haddock, plaice etc. poached, steamed, baked, grilled, smoked, dried; includes curried fish, fish in sauce, fish pie, kedgeree |
| 34B | Shellfish | all types including mussels, prawns, crabs, shellfish dishes |

35 Oily fish

| 35R | Oily fish | includes herrings, kippers, mackerel, sprats, eels, herrings roe (baked, fried, grilled), salmon, tuna, sardines, trout, taramasalata, mackerel pate, fish paste |

Food Type: Fish and fish dishes (Groups 33-35)

36 Salad and other raw vegetables

36A	Carrots raw	
36B	Salad and other vegetables (raw)	all types of raw vegetables, including coleslaw, fresh herbs. Not salads made with cooked vegetables or potato salad
36C	Tomatoes (raw)	

37　Vegetables (not raw)

37A	Peas (not raw)	includes canned, dried, mushy, frozen, mange-tout, pease pudding canned
37B	Green beans (not raw)	includes French, runner, green beans; fresh, canned, frozen
37C	Baked beans	canned baked beans in sauce. Includes baked beans with additions e.g. sausages, burgers, pasta
37D	Leafy green vegetables (not raw)	includes broccoli, spinach, cabbage (all types), brussels sprouts; fresh and frozen
37E	Carrots (not raw)	includes fresh, frozen, canned
37F	Tomatoes (not raw)	includes fried, grilled, canned, sun-dried tomatoes
37G	Vegetable dishes (not raw)	includes curries, pulse dishes, casseroles and stews, pies, vegetable lasagne, cauliflower cheese, vegieburgers, bubble and squeak, vegetable samosas, pancake rolls, ratatouille, vegetable fingers etc.
37R	Other vegetables (not raw)	includes lentils, dried beans and pulses, mushrooms, onion, aubergine, parsnips, sweetcorn, peppers, leeks, courgettes, cauliflower, mixed vegetables, TVP/soya mince, quorn, tofu

38　Chips, fried and roast potatoes and potato products

38A	Chips	fresh and frozen, including oven and microwave, French fries
38B	Fried or roast potatoes and fried potato products	roast potato, fried sliced potato with or without batter; fried waffles, croquettes, crunchies, Alphabites, fritters, hash browns
38R	Potato products not fried	croquettes, waffles, fritters, hash browns, Alphabites, Ketchips, grilled or oven baked

39　Other potatoes, potato salads and dishes

39R	Other potatoes, potato salads and dishes	includes boiled, mashed, baked (with or without fat), canned, potato salad, instant potato, potato based curries, cheese and potato pie

42　Crisps and savoury snacks

42R	Crisps and savoury snacks	includes all potato and cereal-based savoury snacks, popcorn (not sweet), Twiglets

Food Type: Vegetables, potatoes & savoury snacks (Groups 36-39, 42)

40　Fruit

40A	Apples and pears not canned	includes raw, baked, stewed (with or without sugar), dried, apple sauce
40B	Citrus fruit not canned	includes oranges, grapefruit, limes, tangerines, ortaniques etc.
40C	Bananas	includes baked bananas, banana chips

40D	Canned fruit in juice	includes canned in water
40E	Canned fruit in syrup	
40R	Other fruit, not canned	includes plums, grapes, apricots (raw and stewed) etc. fruit pie fillings, dried fruit, fruit salad

56 Nuts and Seeds

56R	Nuts and seeds	includes fruit and nut mixes, salted peanuts, peanut butter, tahini, Bombay mix

Food Type: Fruit and nuts (Group 40 & 56)

41 Sugars, preserves and sweet spreads

41A	Sugar	all types, including golden syrup, fructose
41B	Preserves	includes jam, fruit spreads, marmalade, honey, lemon curd
41R	Sweet spreads, fillings, icings	includes ice cream topping sauce, chocolate spread, mincemeat, glace cherries, mixed peel, icing, brandy/rum butter, marzipan

43 Sugar confectionery

43R	Sugar confectionery	includes boiled sweets, gums, pastilles, fudge, chews, mints, rock, liquorice, toffees, chewing gum, sweet popcorn, ice lollies (without ice cream)

44 Chocolate confectionery

44R	Chocolate confectionery	includes chocolate bars, filled bars, assortments

Food type: Sugar, preserves and confectionery (Group 41, 43, 44)

45 Fruit juice

45R	Fruit juice	includes 100% single or mixed fruit juices, vegetable juices, canned, bottled, cartons; carbonated, still, freshly squeezed

57 Soft drinks, not low calorie

57A	Concentrated soft drinks, not low calorie[4]	all types including squashes and cordials
57B	Carbonated soft drinks, not low calorie	all types, including tonic water. Not carbonated mineral water; not alco-pops
57C	Ready to drink soft drinks, not low calorie	all types of still soft drinks, not carbonated

58 Soft drinks, low calorie

58A	Concentrated soft drinks, low calorie[4]	all low calorie, no added sugar, sugar free types

58B	Carbonated soft drinks, low calorie	all low calorie, no added sugar, sugar free types, including slimline tonic water. Not carbonated mineral water
58C	Ready to drink soft drinks, low calorie	all low calorie, no added sugar, sugar free types. Not carbonated

47 Spirits and liqueurs

47A	Liqueurs	includes cream liqueurs, Pernod, Southern Comfort, Tia Maria, Cherry Brandy
47B	Spirits	70% proof spirits – brandy, gin, rum, vodka, whisky

48 Wine

48A	Wine	white, red, sparkling, rosé
48B	Fortified wine	port, sherry, champagne, vermouth
48C	Low alcohol and alcohol free wine	includes fruit juice and wine drinks

49 Beer, lager, cider and perry

49A	Beers and lagers	premium and non premium, stout, strong ale (bottled, draught and canned)
49B	Low alcohol and alcohol-free lager and beer	includes shandy
49C	Cider and perry	includes Babycham
49D	Low alcohol and alcohol-free cider and perry	
49E	Alco-pops	includes alcoholic lemonade

51 Tea, coffee and water

51A	Coffee (made up)	includes instant and leaf bean, decaffeinated, vending machine with whitener, coffee essence
51B	Tea (made up)	infusion, instant, decaffeinated, vending machine with whitener
51C	Herbal tea (made up)	includes fruit teas
51D	Bottled water	includes carbonated and still, herbal tonics, (not sweetened drinks or tonic water)
51R	Tap water	includes tap water as a drink or used as a diluent for powdered beverages only. Includes filtered tap water. Not water as a diluent for concentrated soft drinks, instant coffee or instant tea

Food type: Total drinks[5] (Group 45, 47-49, 51, 57-58)

50   Miscellaneous

50A	Beverages (dry weight)[6]	includes drinking chocolate, cocoa, Ovaltine, Horlicks, malted drinks etc.
50B	Soups	includes homemade, dried, condensed, cartons, canned
50R	Savoury sauces, pickles, gravies, condiments	includes white sauces, cook in sauces, sauce mixes, tomato ketchup, pickles, chutney, stuffing, gravy, mayonnaise, salad cream, dried herbs, spices

52   Commercial toddlers foods and drinks

52A	Commercial toddlers drinks[2]	includes powdered, concentrated and ready-to-drink beverages specifically manufactured for young children
52R	Commercial toddlers foods	includes instant and ready-to-eat foods specifically manufactured for young children

Food type: Miscellaneous (Groups 50 & 52)

54   Dietary supplements

54A	Tablets and capsules	vitamin and mineral tablets and capsules; includes cod liver oil and other oil-based capsules
54B	Oils and syrups	includes cod liver oil etc. (not capsules), malt extract, multivitamin syrups, iron syrups and tonics
54C	Drops and powders	includes cold relief powders with vitamin C, multivitamin drops
54R	Nutritionally complete supplements	liquid or powdered supplement drinks containing protein/fat/carbohydrate plus vitamins/minerals. Includes Complan, Build Up, Fortisip, Ensure, Provide, Fresubin

55   Artificial sweeteners

55R	Artificial sweeteners	includes granulated table top sweeteners, tablet, liquid or mini cube sweeteners

Endnotes

[1] There have been some changes to the structure of the food groups since the last NDNS of people aged 65 years and over. The major changes are as follows:
- New food groups have been created for soft drinks, not low calorie (57) and soft drinks, low calorie (58). New subsidiary groups have been created within these food groups for carbonated, concentrated and ready to drink soft drinks. These new food groups supercede old group 46 – soft drinks.
- A new subsidiary group has been created for alco-pops such as alcoholic lemonade.

[2] Infant formula (13A) and commercial toddlers drinks (52A) were not consumed in this survey, and therefore do not appear in the food consumption tables provided in Chapter 4.

[3] Fats and oils used in cooking are reported with the food they are cooked with.

[4] Concentrated soft drinks reported as made up.

[5] Food type 'drinks' does not include powdered beverages (subsidiary group 50A).

[6] Subsidiary group 50A covers only the dry weight of the powdered beverage. The water or milk used to make up the beverage is reported elsewhere.

Appendix I

The nutrient databank and details of nutrients measured

1 The nutrient databank

Intakes of nutrients were calculated from the records of food consumption using a specially adapted nutrient databank. The nutrient databank originally developed by MAFF for the *Dietary and Nutritional Survey of British Adults*[1], and updated for both the *National Diet and Nutrition Survey: children aged 1½ to 4½ years*[2] and the *National Diet and Nutrition Survey: people aged 65 years and over*[3], was revised for this survey of young people aged 4 to 18 years. Many nutrient values were updated, and some new codes were added to accommodate new products that had become available. The databank now contains nutritional information on over 6000 foods and drinks, including manufactured products, homemade recipe dishes and many types of dietary supplements.

Each food on the databank has values assigned for 55 nutrients and energy. The nutrient values assigned to the foods on the databank are based on McCance and Widdowson's The Composition of Foods[4] and its supplements. The Ministry of Agriculture, Fisheries and Food has an ongoing programme of nutritional analysis of foods. New analytical values for chicken and turkey, pasteurised milk, and some meat products and ready meals were incorporated for this survey. In addition a project was commissioned to obtain up to date nutrient values for some foods commonly consumed by young people aged 4 to 18 years, as identified in the feasibility study for the survey[5]. These included fortified pasta shapes in tomato sauce, low fat processed cheese products, chocolate dairy desserts, and twin pot yogurts. Data obtained from food manufacturers were also used in the databank, as was nutritional information given on labels. Revised coding frames were produced for soft drinks and ice creams which took into account changes in products available and new manufacturers' data. All data were carefully evaluated before being incorporated onto the databank.

In order to calculate the nutrient intakes from the consumption data it is important that there are no missing nutrient values on the databank. For some foods reliable information was not available for all nutrients. Therefore it was sometimes necessary to estimate values for foods for which there were few available data, by referring to similar foods. For homemade dishes and manufactured products for which no data were available, nutrients were calculated from their constituents using a computer recipe program that allows adjustments to be made for weight and vitamin losses in cooking.

During the survey fieldwork period the range of foods included in the databank was extended as new products and recipe dishes with different nutrient contents were consumed. For each new product or recipe dish a decision was made by the survey nutritionists in conjunction with MAFF as to whether it required a new code, based on the nutritional composition compared with that of existing codes and the quantity consumed.

Information on dietary supplements was also included in the nutrient databank. Full details of the brand name, form, strength and quantity of each supplement taken were collected in the dietary record. A supplement was given a new code if it contained different levels of nutrients from existing supplement codes.

Further details of MAFF's nutrient databank have been published[6].

2 Details of nutrients measured and units

Nutrient	Units
water	(g)
sugars	(g) total sugars, expressed as monosaccharide
starch	(g) expressed as monosaccharide
dietary fibre	(g) expressed as modified Southgate method[7]
non-starch polysaccharides	(g) expressed as Englyst method[8]
energy (kJ)	(17 x protein) + (37 x fat) + (16 x carbohydrate) + (29 x alcohol)

energy (kcal)	(4 x protein) + (9 x fat) + (3.75 x carbohydrate) + (7 x alcohol)
protein	(g)
nitrogen	(g)
fat	(g)
carbohydrate	(g) sum of sugars plus starch, expressed as monosaccharide equivalent
alcohol	(g)
sodium	(mg)
potassium	(mg)
calcium	(mg)
magnesium	(mg)
phosphorus	(mg)
iron	(mg)
haem iron	(mg)
non-haem iron	(mg)
copper	(mg)
zinc	(mg)
chloride	(mg)
iodine	(μg)
manganese	(mg)
retinol	(μg) all *trans* retinol equivalents
total carotene	(μg) β-carotene equivalents
α-carotene	(μg)
ß-carotene	(μg)
ß-cryptoxanthin	(μg)
thiamin	(mg)
riboflavin	(mg)
niacin equivalent	(mg) niacin + (tryptophan / 60)
vitamin B_6	(mg)
vitamin B_{12}	(μg)
folate	(μg)
pantothenic acid	(mg)
biotin	(μg)
vitamin C	(mg)
vitamin D	(μg)
vitamin E	(mg) α-tocopherol equivalents

fatty acids

saturated	(g)
cis monounsaturated	(g)
cis n-3 polyunsaturated	(g)
cis n-6 polyunsaturated	(g)
trans fatty acids	(g)

cholesterol	(mg)

sugars

glucose	(g)
sucrose	(g)
fructose	(g)
lactose	(g)
maltose	(g)
other sugars	(g) includes oligosaccharides
non-milk extrinsic sugars	(g) includes all sugars in fruit juices, table sugar, honey, sucrose, glucose and glucose syrups added to food + 50% of the sugars in canned, stewed, dried or preserved fruits[9].
intrinsic and milk sugars	(g) includes all sugars in fresh fruit and vegetables + 50% of the sugars in canned, stewed, dried or preserved fruits + lactose in milk.

References

[1] Gregory J, Foster K, Tyler H, Wiseman M. *The Dietary and Nutritional Survey of British Adults*. HMSO (London, 1990).

[2] Gregory JR, Collins DL, Davies PSW, Hughes JM, Clarke PC. *National Diet and Nutrition Survey: children aged 1½ to 4½ years. Volume 1: Report of the diet and nutrition survey*. HMSO (London, 1995).

[3] Finch S, Doyle W, Lowe C, Bates CJ, Prentice A, Smithers G, Clarke PC. *National Diet and Nutrition Survey: people aged 65 years and over. Volume 1: Report of the diet and nutrition survey*. TSO (London, 1998).

[4] Holland B, Welch AA, Unwin ID, Buss DH, Paul AA, Southgate DAT. *McCance and Widdowson's The Composition of Foods*. 5th edition. Royal Society of Chemistry (Cambridge, 1991).

[5] Lowe S. *Feasibility study for the National Diet and Nutrition Survey: young people aged 4 to 18 years*. ONS (*In preparation*).

[6] Smithers G. MAFF's Nutrient Databank. *Nutr & Fd Science* 1993; **2**: 16-19.

[7] Southgate DAT. Dietary fibre analysis and food sources. *Am J Clin Nutr* 1978; **31**: Suppl S107-110.

[8] Englyst HN and Cummings JH. An improved method for the measurement of dietary fibre as the non-starch polysaccharides in plant foods. *J Assoc Off Anal Chem* 1988; **71**: 808-814.

[9] Buss DH, Lewis J and Smithers G. Non-milk extrinsic sugars. *J Hum Nutr Diet* 1994; **7**: 87.

Appendix J

Under-reporting

1 Introduction

The factors affecting the choice of a 7-day weighed intake dietary record as the dietary methodology used for this survey, together with the advantages and disadvantages associated with this method, are provided in Chapter 2 and Appendix F. As for all dietary assessment methods, this method can underestimate habitual energy intake, which in turn can introduce bias when comparing dietary and nutritional parameters in a population.

Validation of the dietary methodology for this survey was carried out in the feasibility study[1,2]. Energy intake, as estimated from the dietary record, was compared with total energy expenditure as assessed by the doubly-labelled water method. The results showed that under-reporting was a problem in these age groups, particularly in the oldest group of girls. In spite of measures taken in the mainstage survey to help alleviate this, it is considered likely that the estimates of energy intake, particularly for older girls, are underestimates.

This separate analysis has been undertaken to identify and exclude 'under-reporters' and present intakes of energy and selected nutrients for the remaining sample, by age and sex. When considering the results from this analysis it is important to bear in mind the limitations of the methodology used to identify 'under-reporters', and in particular the use of calculated basal metabolic rate (BMR) as opposed to measurement of BMR.

2 Methodology

Cut-off points based on multiples of basal metabolic rate (BMR) have been used to identify and exclude 'under-reporters' for this analysis. This was considered to be the most practically suitable approach.

The use of more sophisticated criteria (using physical activity data to identify discrepancies between reported energy intake and energy expenditure in individuals) was prohibitively complex and beyond the scope of this report, although may form part of further analyses in the future. An alternative approach to the validation of dietary records, that is the use of biological markers (analytes of biological specimens that closely reflect dietary intakes, but which do not rely on food consumption records), was also disregarded. Bingham et al (1995)[3] have concluded that, for most analytes, the weak relationships found with dietary intake limit their use in validating dietary assessment records.

BMR is the energy expenditure of an individual, lying at rest, in a thermoneutral environment and fasted state. BMR can be measured using, for example, whole body calorimetry, or predicted from standard equations using body weight (Schofield et al, 1985[4]). Measurement of BMR did not form part of this survey; hence it was necessary to calculate predicted BMR for this analysis.

Using minimum cut-off points based on multiples of BMR to identify 'under-reporting' uses the principle that an individual of a given sex, age and body weight has a minimum energy intake below which is considered to be an unacceptable representation of habitual intake, and incompatible with long term survival. The following provisional cut-off points, calculated as multiples of BMR, which were proposed by Torun et al[5] (1996) to evaluate dietary surveys among children and adolescents, were used:

Males and females aged 1–5 years:	1.28–1.79 × BMR
Males aged 6–18 years:	1.39–2.24 × BMR
Females aged 6–18 years:	1.30–2.10 × BMR

Those subjects with recorded energy intakes below the lower, and above the upper limits, were classified as 'under-reporters' and 'over-reporters' respectively. Only 'under-reporters' were excluded from this analysis. The percentage of 'over-reporters' was small.

Those subjects who reported that they were dieting (or unwell with eating affected) during the recording period are not excluded from the analysis, as answers to these questions are subjective. In addition, it would be expected that a certain proportion of any population group were dieting or unwell at any particular time and thus exclusion could itself create some bias. However, the proportion of 'under-reporters' who reported that they were either dieting, or unwell with eating affected, has been provided.

Average daily intakes of energy and selected nutrients, including those of particular interest in this age group, and those for which low intakes were reported for a significant proportion of individuals in this survey, were calculated for the remaining sample. These are total fat, saturated fatty acids, total carbohydrate, non-milk extrinsic sugars (NMES), protein, vitamin A (retinol equivalents), riboflavin, folate, calcium, iron, magnesium, potassium and zinc.

3 Results

3.1 Proportion of total diary sample classified as 'under-reporters'

Table J1 provides information on the percentage of those classified as 'over-reporters' and 'under-reporters' in each group, by age and sex. The percentage of young people classified as over-reporting was highest in those aged 4 to 6 years (12% and 10% for boys and girls respectively), and fell to 1% to 2% in the remaining groups, according to age and sex.

The percentage of young people classified as under-reporting increased highly significantly with age for both sexes from 17% and 13% for boys and girls aged 4 to 6 years to 64% and 74% for boys and girls aged 15 to 18 years respectively (p < 0.01)[6].

3.2 Proportion of 'under-reporters' reported to be dieting, or unwell with eating affected

Table J2 shows the proportion of 'under-reporters' who reported that they were currently dieting to lose weight, or were unwell with their eating affected during the dietary record. There was a higher proportion of subjects who reported that they were dieting to lose weight in the 'under-reporting' group compared to the total diary sample in all groups except males aged 7 to 10 years, where the proportions were the same, and girls aged 4 to 6 years where no subjects reported that they were dieting). Similarly, in all age groups the proportion of subjects who reported that they were unwell with their eating affected was higher in the 'under-reporting' group.

3.3 Macronutrient intakes, excluding 'under-reporters'

Average daily intake of energy, total fat, saturated fatty acids, total carbohydrate, NMES and protein by age and sex, after excluding 'under-reporters', is provided in Table J3. Average intake of these nutrients, and intake at the lower 2.5 and upper 97.5 percentile, were equal to or higher in all groups compared to corresponding data for the total diary sample[6].

In line with the age pattern of under-reporting shown in Table J1, the percentage difference in mean daily intake of these nutrients increased with age, particularly for the two oldest age groups. For example, excluding 'under-reporters' increased energy intake by 5% for boys and 4% for girls aged 4 to 6 years (from 6.39MJ to 6.71MJ and 5.87MJ to 6.10MJ respectively), rising to 21% and 28% for boys and girls aged 15 to 18 years (from 9.60MJ to 11.59MJ and from 6.82MJ to 8.75MJ respectively).

Percentage increase in mean daily intake of energy, total fat, saturated fatty acids and total carbohydrate showed a similar trend across all groups, ranging from 4% for those aged 4 to 6 years to 33% for those aged 15 to 18 years. Percentage differences in mean intake were highest for NMES and lowest for protein. For example, excluding 'under-reporters' increased mean intake of NMES by 37% for boys and 47% for girls aged 15 to 18 years (from 97g to 133g in boys, and 66g to 97g in girls). For protein the increases were 13% for boys and 21% for girls aged 15 to 18 years (from 76.5g to 86.4g and from 54.8g to 66.2g respectively).

3.4 Macronutrient intakes as a percentage of food energy

Table J4 shows percentage food energy intake from selected macronutrients by age and sex excluding those classified as 'under-reporters'. Mean intakes for all selected macronutrients as a percentage of food energy, excluding under-reporters, were similar to those presented for the total diary sample, except for NMES in boys aged 11 to 18 years and in girls aged 15 to 18 years. Percentage of food energy from NMES increased from 16.9% to 19.1% for boys aged 11 to 14 years, and from 15.8% to 18.8% for boys aged 15 to 18 years when 'under-reporters' were excluded. For girls aged 15 to 18 years, intake increased from 15.3% to 18.0%. This suggests that those classified as 'under-reporters' in these groups tended to under-report foods that were particularly high in non-milk extrinsic sugars.

3.5 Micronutrient intakes, excluding 'under-reporters'

Table J5 shows average daily intake of vitamin A (retinol equivalents), riboflavin, folate, calcium, iron, magnesium, potassium and zinc by age and sex after excluding 'under-reporters'. Average daily intake of these nutrients and intake at the lower 2.5 percentile, together with those at the upper 97.5 percentile for potassium and zinc, were higher in all groups compared to corresponding data for the total diary sample.

The percentage differences in mean daily intake of riboflavin, calcium, magnesium, and potassium, when 'under-reporters' were excluded, increased steadily with age for both sexes, particularly for the two oldest age groups. Percentage differences in mean intakes of folate for girls, and iron for boys, also increased steadily with age.

Percentage differences in mean daily intake were on the whole highest for the oldest age group when 'under-reporters' were excluded. Mean intakes of riboflavin and calcium for both sexes aged 15 to 18 years, and for iron, magnesium, potassium and zinc for girls, were increased by at least a fifth. In addition, for boys aged 15 to 18 years, mean intake of iron, magnesium and potassium were increased by 15%. Mean intake of vitamin A (retinol equivalents), riboflavin, calcium and magnesium in girls aged 11 to 14 years were increased by at least 15%, and folate in girls aged 15 to 18 years by 19%. Percentage differences in mean intake for all the selected micronutrients ranged from 3% to 9% in the youngest two age groups.

3.6 Intakes of energy and selected nutrients compared with Dietary Reference Values[7]

Energy as a percentage of the estimated average requirement (EAR)

Table J6 provides mean daily energy intake, as a percentage of the EAR, by age and sex after excluding 'under-reporters'. Differences in mean intake as a percentage of EAR between those reported for the total diary sample, and those excluding 'under-reporters', increased steadily with age. Mean intakes were broadly similar to those presented for the total diary sample for the two youngest age groups, with increases of between 3% and 6% of the EAR, depending on age and sex. For those aged 11 to 14 years, mean intake increased from 89% of EAR in both sexes to 102% in boys and 103% in girls. For those aged 15 to 18 years, mean intake increased from 83% to 101% of the EAR in boys and 77% to 99% in girls.

Protein and micronutrient intakes as a percentage of the reference nutrient intake (RNI)

Mean daily intake of protein and selected micronutrients as a percentage of the RNI by age and sex, after excluding 'under-reporters', are shown in Tables J7 and J8. Mean protein intake for both the total diary sample, and after excluding 'under-reporters', was above the RNI for each group. Differences in mean intake of protein as a percentage of the RNI between the total diary sample, and after the exclusion of 'under-reporters', ranged from 7% to 17% for boys and girls aged 4 to 14 years. For boys and girls aged 15 to 18 years, the differences in mean intake of protein as a percentage of the RNI were 18% and 25% (from 139% to 157% and from 121% to 146% of the RNI) respectively.

For each selected micronutrient, and every age and sex group, mean daily intake as a percentage of RNI increased after excluding 'under-reporters'. However mean intakes of some micronutrients remained below the RNI. For the 11 to 14 age group, mean intakes of vitamin A, calcium, magnesium, potassium and zinc for boys and girls, and of iron for girls, remained below the RNI after excluding 'under-reporters' (with intakes ranging from 69% of the RNI for iron in girls, to 98% of the RNI for vitamin A in boys).

For the 15 to 18 year group, mean daily intakes of magnesium and potassium for boys and girls, calcium and iron for girls, and vitamin A for boys remained below the RNI when 'under-reporters' were excluded (with intakes ranging from 73% of the RNI for iron and 99% of the RNI for calcium in girls). For those aged 4 to 10 years, mean intakes of zinc for boys and girls, and of magnesium for girls aged 7 to 10 years remained below the RNI when 'under-reporters' were excluded.

Proportion of subjects with micronutrient intakes below the lower reference nutrient intake (LRNI)

The proportions of subjects with selected micronutrient intakes below the LRNI are provided in Table J9, and are lower in every group after excluding 'under-reporters', compared to the total diary sample. Excluding 'under-reporters' reduced the proportion of subjects with intakes below the LRNI substantially, by up to three-quarters for some nutrients in the older groups. For example, the proportion of subjects with intakes of vitamin A below the LRNI was reduced from 12% to 3% for boys and girls aged 15 to 18 years.

4 Discussion

These findings are consistent with those found in the feasibility study for this survey[1,2], and suggest that there was a high incidence of under-reporting in this sample, particularly in those aged 11 to 18 years.

However, care should be taken when interpreting these data because of the limitations of the methodology used to classify 'under-reporters'. The accuracy of standard equations used for the calculation of predicted BMR has been questioned. Calculated BMR is recognised to be an imperfect estimate of true BMR[5,8]. It has been proposed that the equations tend to overestimate BMR in many populations[9], including children and adolescents[5] leading to an over-estimation of total energy expenditure. This can in turn overestimate the prevalence of under-reporting when BMR cut-off points are used.

The use of BMR cut-off points can not *guarantee* that the remaining data are indeed valid. It can not be assumed that low recorded intakes are attributable solely to inaccurate records, which is what the term 'under-reporting' implies. It has not been possible to account for those who were genuinely 'under-consuming' during the dietary record (in order to facilitate diary recording for example), or those who were under-reporting at higher intakes above the cut-off points. It is also important to consider these findings in context with physical activity data and body weight data; however this is beyond the scope of this report.

The low incidence of under-reporting in those aged 4 to 6 years is comparable to that found in the feasibility study for the National Diet and Nutrition Survey: children aged 1½ to 4½ years[10], where dietary records were validated using the doubly-labelled water method.

This current analysis found that the incidence of over-reporting was highest in this age group. Once again, this may be due in part to the methodology used. Alternatively, this could reflect the under-reporting of leftovers/spillage in this young age group.

After some further analysis comparing those below the BMR cut-off points ('under-reporters') with those above the BMR cut-off points for each group, those girls aged 7 to 18 years and boys aged 11 to 18 years classified as 'under-reporting' were found to have a significantly lower percentage of food energy intake from NMES (all males, and females aged 7 to 10 years: $p < 0.01$; females 11 to 18 years: $p < 0.05$). Females aged 7 to 14 years classified as 'under-reporters' also had a significantly lower percentage of food energy from saturated fatty acids ($p < 0.05$). Males aged 11 to 18 years, and females aged 7 to 10 years and 15 to 18 years who were classified as 'under-reporters', had a significantly higher percentage of food energy from protein (males 15 to 18 years: $p < 0.01$; others: $p < 0.05$).

This suggests that those classified as 'under-reporters' in these groups tended to selectively under-report foods that were high in non-milk extrinsic sugars and high in saturated fatty acids. In addition, initial analysis of 'under-reporting' for the total diary sample, as a function of diary duration, showed that for those aged 11 to 18 years, reported energy intakes were significantly lower towards the end of the recording period compared to those recorded on day one of the dietary record ($p < 0.01$).

References and endnotes

[1] Lowe S. *Feasibility study for the National Diet and Nutrition Survey: young people aged 4 to 18 years:* ONS (*In preparation*).

[2] Smithers G, Gregory J, Coward WA, Wright A, Elsom R, Wenlock R. British National Diet and Nutrition Survey of young people aged 4 to 18 years: feasibility study of the dietary assessment methodology. Abstracts of the Third International Conference on Dietary Assessment Methods. *Eur J Clin Nutr* (1998) **52**: S2. S76.

[3] Bingham SA, Cassidy A, Cole TJ, Welch A, Runswick SA, Black AE, Thurnham D, Bates C, Khaw KT, Key TJA, Day NE. Validation of weighed records and other methods of dietary assessment using the 24 hr urine nitrogen technique and other biological markers. *Br J Nutr* 1995; **73**: 531–550.

[4] Schofield WN, Schofield C, and James WPT. (1985) Basal metabolic rate. *Hum Nutr : Clin Nutr* 39C: (Suppl 1), 1–96.

[5] Torun B, Davies PSW, Livingstone MBE, Paolisso M, Sackett R, Spurr GB. Energy requirements and dietary energy recommendations for children and adolescents 1 to 18 years old. *Euro J Clin Nutr* 1996; **50**: (Suppl 1), S37–S81.

[6] The following positive percentage differences (also referred to as 'increases') in mean daily intakes of selected nutrients, before and after excluding those classified as 'under-reporters', have not been formally tested for statistical significance.

[7] Department of Health. Report on Health and Social Subjects: 41. *Dietary reference values for food energy and nutrients for the United Kingdom.* HMSO. (London, 1991).

[8] Voss S, Kroke A, Klipstein-Grobusch K, Boeing H. Is macronutrient composition of dietary intake data affected by underreporting? Results from the EPIC-Potsdam study. *Euro J Clin Nutr* 1998; **52**: 119-126.

[9] Shetty PS, Henry CJK, Black AE, Prentice AM. Energy requirements of adults: an update on basal metabolic rates (BMRs) and physical activity levels (PALs). *Euro J Clin Nutr* 1996; **50**: suppl. 1, S11-S23.

[10] White AJ, Davies PSW. *Feasibility study for the National Diet and Nutrition Survey of Children Aged 1½ to 4½ Years.* OPCS (London, 1994).

Table J1 Percentage of young people classified as 'over-reporters' and 'under-reporters' by age and sex of young person

	Males aged (years)				Females aged (years)			
	4–6	7–10	11–14	15–18	4–6	7–10	11–14	15–18
Under-reporters (%)	17	29	53	64	13	27	52	74
Over-reporters (%)	12	2	1	1	10	1	2	1
Base	*184*	*256*	*237*	*179*	*171*	*226*	*238*	*210*

Table J2 Percentage of young people who reported currently dieting to lose weight, or unwell with their eating affected, by age and sex of young person, and by whether classified as under-reporters*

	Males aged (years)				Females aged (years)			
	4–6	7–10	11–14	15–18	4–6	7–10	11–14	15–18
Dieting (%)	6 (1)	2 (2)	6 (4)	4 (3)	0 (0)	9 (3)	9 (7)	19 (16)
Unwell with eating affected (%)	19 (8)	19 (12)	13 (9)	10 (9)	29 (13)	14 (8)	18 (12)	12 (11)
Base (under-reporters)	*32*	*75*	*125*	*114*	*22*	*61*	*123*	*155*
Base (total sample)	*184*	*256*	*237*	*179*	*171*	*226*	*238*	*210*

* Values in brackets = total diary sample.

Table J3 Average daily intake of selected macronutrients, by age and sex of young person, excluding those classified as 'under-reporters'*

Macronutrient	Males aged (years)				Females aged (years)			
	4–6	7–10	11–14	15–18	4–6	7–10	11–14	15–18
Energy (MJ)								
Mean	6.71 (6.39)	8.02 (7.47)	9.46 (8.28)	11.59 (9.60)	6.10 (5.87)	7.13 (6.72)	8.14 (7.03)	8.75 (6.82)
Median	6.61 (6.35)	7.85 (7.31)	9.30 (8.32)	11.54 (9.65)	5.97 (5.73)	7.06 (6.72)	8.04 (6.98)	8.68 (6.67)
Lower 2.5 percentile	4.86 (3.54)	6.15 (4.68)	7.41 (4.69)	8.43 (5.57)	4.52 (3.90)	5.46 (4.15)	5.99 (4.08)	6.49 (3.53)
Upper 2.5 percentile	8.77 (8.68)	11.23 (10.50)	13.31 (11.46)	15.82 (13.91)	8.68 (8.58)	9.08 (8.81)	10.74 (10.09)	11.26 (10.08)
Standard deviation	1.08 (1.27)	1.27 (1.49)	1.40 (1.83)	2.04 (2.36)	1.02 (1.15)	0.95 (1.18)	1.16 (1.56)	1.01 (1.75)
Total fat (g)								
Mean	63.1 (60.1)	75.7 (69.8)	88.3 (77.2)	105.9 (89.0)	58.2 (55.9)	68.2 (63.8)	78.3 (67.2)	83.3 (64.0)
Median	61.6 (59.8)	73.9 (68.4)	84.3 (76.7)	106.5 (89.9)	56.4 (54.2)	66.2 (63.4)	79.2 (67.7)	82.0 (64.7)
Lower 2.5 percentile	41.7 (30.9)	51.2 (39.1)	62.1 (41.5)	64.5 (42.8)	38.8 (30.6)	46.7 (36.3)	49.5 (33.4)	54.4 (26.7)
Upper 2.5 percentile	96.1 (95.0)	112.3 (104.8)	142.5 (120.9)	151.4 (134.3)	85.7 (83.5)	91.1 (90.0)	100.7 (99.3)	110.1 (102.6)
Standard deviation	13.20 (14.47)	15.19 (16.95)	19.35 (20.85)	22.43 (24.16)	12.83 (13.76)	11.94 (13.84)	13.69 (17.56)	14.38 (20.14)
Saturated fatty acids (g)								
Mean	26.3 (25.1)	30.7 (28.3)	34.8 (30.3)	42.3 (34.7)	24.9 (23.8)	27.8 (25.7)	31.1 (26.2)	32.8 (24.7)
Median	25.3 (24.0)	30.2 (27.7)	33.6 (30.1)	42.6 (34.4)	23.7 (22.7)	26.9 (25.9)	31.0 (26.2)	32.2 (24.5)
Lower 2.5 percentile	15.3 (13.4)	20.7 (15.5)	25.4 (13.8)	29.6 (16.5)	15.8 (11.2)	17.1 (13.5)	19.7 (11.6)	21.5 (9.4)
Upper 2.5 percentile	40.8 (40.6)	46.6 (42.7)	60.8 (51.0)	59.6 (53.8)	36.1 (35.1)	39.4 (38.3)	43.3 (41.8)	45.6 (41.3)
Standard deviation	6.71 (6.98)	6.71 (7.47)	8.28 (9.04)	8.74 (10.41)	5.99 (6.42)	5.30 (6.27)	6.34 (7.83)	6.37 (8.59)
Total carbohydrate (g)								
Mean	219 (209)	265 (248)	313 (271)	371 (301)	198 (191)	232 (218)	264 (228)	277 (214)
Median	215 (209)	258 (248)	309 (270)	352 (290)	195 (190)	229 (218)	259 (226)	280 (213)
Lower 2.5 percentile	159 (126)	192 (156)	228 (161)	254 (161)	139 (124)	172 (124)	163 (130)	182 (107)
Upper 2.5 percentile	285 (284)	374 (355)	437 (391)	535 (506)	266 (259)	300 (299)	360 (342)	354 (329)
Standard deviation	36 (42)	45 (51)	51 (64)	78 (84)	35 (40)	36 (42)	47 (56)	41 (58)
Non-milk extrinsic sugars (g)								
Mean	71 (66)	90 (83)	112 (90)	133 (97)	69 (66)	79 (72)	90 (73)	97 (66)
Median	71 (64)	87 (80)	109 (87)	135 (89)	67 (65)	78 (70)	89 (72)	98 (63)
Lower 2.5 percentile	35 (26)	33 (32)	49 (33)	50 (24)	25 (19)	36 (29)	29 (23)	35 (17)
Upper 2.5 percentile	115 (115)	150 (147)	188 (177)	261 (224)	117 (116)	135 (133)	156 (151)	168 (144)
Standard deviation	21.5 (23.1)	29.9 (30.8)	34.6 (38.6)	51.0 (49.1)	23.3 (24.2)	24.3 (26.3)	29.9 (31.5)	32.6 (31.7)
Protein (g)								
Mean	51.4 (49.0)	58.6 (54.8)	70.4 (64.0)	86.4 (76.5)	46.0 (44.5)	53.3 (51.2)	59.7 (52.9)	66.2 (54.8)
Median	49.2 (47.9)	58.4 (54.2)	70.6 (64.8)	84.3 (75.5)	43.8 (42.7)	52.8 (50.7)	59.3 (51.7)	63.7 (53.9)
Lower 2.5 percentile	34.1 (25.4)	40.5 (34.5)	46.7 (30.9)	46.7 (45.4)	28.4 (26.3)	35.7 (29.5)	41.2 (26.9)	47.9 (26.4)
Upper 2.5 percentile	76.9 (76.8)	80.6 (79.7)	99.0 (93.9)	154.7 (112.2)	69.3 (66.8)	76.4 (75.2)	82.0 (78.4)	97.5 (87.4)
Standard deviation	12.98 (13.52)	10.83 (12.25)	13.20 (15.36)	20.60 (19.61)	10.70 (11.11)	10.51 (11.08)	10.84 (13.21)	12.21 (15.17)
Base (excluding under-reporters)	*152*	*181*	*112*	*65*	*149*	*165*	*115*	*55*
Base (total sample)	*184*	*256*	*237*	*179*	*171*	*226*	*238*	*210*

* Values in brackets = intakes for total diary sample.

Table J4 Percentage food energy intake from selected macronutrients, by age and sex of young person, excluding those classified as 'under-reporters'*

Percentage food energy from:	Males aged (years)				Females aged (years)			
	4–6	7–10	11–14	15–18	4–6	7–10	11–14	15–18
total fat								
Mean	34.7 (35.5)	34.8 (35.2)	34.4 (35.2)	34.6 (35.9)	35.2 (35.9)	35.3 (35.9)	35.6 (36.1)	35.7 (35.9)
Median	35.0 (35.9)	34.7 (35.2)	34.4 (35.1)	35.2 (36.3)	35.2 (36.0)	35.4 (36.0)	35.9 (36.0)	35.8 (36.6)
Lower 2.5 percentile	27.4 (27.9)	27.8 (28.8)	25.8 (26.0)	27.3 (26.3)	25.1 (26.2)	28.3 (26.6)	26.6 (23.3)	27.2 (22.7)
Upper 2.5 percentile	41.6 (42.5)	42.7 (42.9)	42.1 (43.6)	42.5 (45.3)	43.9 (44.8)	43.6 (44.2)	42.6 (45.2)	44.3 (45.6)
Standard deviation	3.92 (3.90)	3.47 (3.69)	4.36 (4.27)	4.18 (4.68)	4.34 (4.42)	3.79 (4.14)	4.18 (4.98)	4.33 (5.37)
saturated fatty acids								
Mean	14.5 (14.8)	14.1 (14.3)	13.6 (13.8)	13.9 (13.9)	15.1 (15.3)	14.4 (14.5)	14.2 (14.0)	14.0 (13.8)
Median	14.5 (14.9)	14.2 (14.2)	13.6 (13.8)	13.7 (13.9)	14.9 (15.2)	14.3 (14.4)	14.3 (13.9)	13.7 (13.9)
Lower 2.5 percentile	10.2 (10.6)	10.7 (10.5)	10.0 (9.8)	10.6 (9.4)	10.8 (10.4)	10.7 (9.2)	9.7 (9.3)	10.6 (8.8)
Upper 2.5 percentile	19.3 (19.7)	19.0 (19.3)	18.0 (18.6)	16.8 (17.6)	20.8 (21.2)	18.9 (19.2)	17.9 (18.7)	18.0 (19.3)
Standard deviation	2.40 (2.36)	2.01 (2.11)	2.02 (2.19)	1.72 (2.07)	2.45 (2.52)	2.07 (2.29)	2.11 (2.50)	1.97 (2.52)
total carbohydrate								
Mean	52.3 (51.6)	52.8 (52.4)	52.9 (51.7)	52.4 (50.5)	52.1 (51.4)	52.0 (51.3)	51.8 (51.2)	51.3 (50.6)
Median	52.3 (51.6)	52.7 (52.4)	53.1 (51.8)	51.9 (50.1)	52.3 (51.7)	51.5 (50.8)	51.5 (50.7)	51.7 (50.3)
Lower 2.5 percentile	43.7 (43.0)	44.0 (44.2)	44.8 (42.5)	44.1 (39.9)	43.2 (42.1)	43.1 (42.6)	43.9 (42.2)	41.4 (39.9)
Upper 2.5 percentile	59.9 (59.4)	61.2 (60.5)	60.5 (59.8)	61.3 (60.7)	61.2 (60.5)	60.4 (59.9)	61.3 (62.8)	60.8 (64.0)
Standard deviation	4.36 (4.33)	3.92 (4.10)	4.55 (4.57)	5.00 (5.41)	4.85 (5.01)	4.16 (4.32)	4.52 (5.24)	4.68 (5.62)
non-milk extrinsic sugars								
Mean	16.8 (16.2)	18.0 (17.5)	19.1 (16.9)	18.8 (15.8)	18.1 (17.6)	17.8 (16.7)	17.5 (16.2)	18.0 (15.3)
Median	16.4 (16.2)	17.5 (17.0)	18.6 (16.2)	18.5 (15.1)	17.9 (17.2)	17.8 (16.7)	17.2 (16.3)	18.2 (15.0)
Lower 2.5 percentile	9.2 (7.0)	7.0 (6.9)	9.4 (7.1)	8.2 (5.8)	7.6 (7.2)	9.1 (7.4)	7.8 (6.8)	7.7 (5.1)
Upper 2.5 percentile	26.3 (26.1)	31.0 (28.8)	33.4 (31.4)	30.5 (29.9)	29.7 (28.9)	27.6 (26.8)	29.3 (27.1)	29.9 (27.8)
Standard deviation	4.46 (4.80)	5.46 (5.51)	5.39 (5.42)	6.31 (6.02)	5.68 (5.63)	4.81 (4.95)	5.04 (5.45)	5.74 (5.77)
protein								
Mean	13.0 (12.9)	12.5 (12.4)	12.7 (13.1)	13.0 (13.9)	12.8 (12.7)	12.7 (12.8)	12.5 (12.7)	13.1 (13.9)
Median	13.0 (12.9)	12.5 (12.4)	12.7 (13.0)	12.7 (13.6)	12.7 (12.6)	12.7 (12.8)	12.4 (12.5)	12.9 (13.7)
Lower 2.5 percentile	9.7 (9.6)	8.7 (9.0)	8.9 (8.9)	9.5 (9.4)	9.5 (9.4)	9.6 (9.5)	9.2 (9.2)	10.2 (9.9)
Upper 2.5 percentile	16.5 (16.3)	17.3 (17.1)	17.2 (17.6)	19.6 (19.6)	17.0 (17.1)	16.7 (16.7)	17.7 (17.9)	17.6 (18.9)
Standard deviation	1.73 (1.76)	1.84 (1.85)	1.97 (2.20)	2.28 (2.50)	1.96 (1.99)	1.81 (1.90)	1.98 (2.17)	2.02 (2.48)
Base (excluding under-reporters)	*152*	*181*	*112*	*65*	*149*	*165*	*115*	*55*
Base (total sample)	*184*	*256*	*237*	*179*	*171*	*226*	*238*	*210*

* Values in brackets = intakes from total diary sample.

Table J5 Average daily intake of selected micronutrients from all sources, by age and sex of young person, excluding those classified as 'under-reporters'*

Micronutrient	Males aged (years)				Females aged (years)			
	4–6	7–10	11–14	15–18	4–6	7–10	11–14	15–18
Vitamin A (µg) (retinol equivalents)								
Mean	567 (535)	607 (555)	585 (577)	686 (628)	522 (502)	544 (515)	563 (482)	643 (562)
Median	444 (432)	522 (460)	546 (485)	647 (584)	457 (437)	485 (460)	536 (380)	540 (475)
Lower 2.5 percentile	179 (131)	277 (196)	227 (145)	276 (188)	171 (166)	229 (174)	167 (126)	250 (156)
Upper 2.5 percentile	1365 (1314)	1433 (1451)	1202 (1277)	1954 (1579)	1243 (1265)	1359 (1331)	1301 (1296)	1281 (1413)
Standard deviation	323.3 (320.0)	320.1 (340.8)	271.8 (562.5)	361.2 (355.2)	265.9 (268.5)	335.9 (333.3)	264.3 (419.4)	291.7 (463.7)
Riboflavin (mg)								
Mean	1.68 (1.57)	1.75 (1.64)	1.97 (1.74)	2.36 (1.95)	1.49 (1.43)	1.46 (1.38)	1.58 (1.35)	1.64 (1.34)
Median	1.58 (1.50)	1.66 (1.52)	1.94 (1.65)	2.15 (0.86)	1.44 (1.39)	1.41 (1.35)	1.56 (1.31)	1.46 (1.25)
Lower 2.5 percentile	0.77 (0.58)	0.90 (0.80)	0.92 (0.63)	0.99 (0.68)	0.75 (0.62)	0.67 (0.57)	0.58 (0.45)	0.80 (0.39)
Upper 2.5 percentile	3.14 (3.05)	3.08 (2.92)	3.71 (3.49)	5.01 (3.88)	2.56 (2.55)	2.61 (2.62)	2.99 (2.79)	2.96 (3.00)
Standard deviation	0.549 (0.591)	0.606 (0.594)	0.687 (0.706)	0.983 (0.911)	0.459 (0.467)	0.471 (0.498)	0.570 (0.622)	0.591 (0.669)
Folate (µg)								
Mean	204 (192)	224 (213)	269 (247)	352 (309)	176 (171)	198 (190)	238 (210)	256 (215)
Median	194 (185)	213 (203)	258 (234)	318 (284)	166 (162)	192 (187)	223 (200)	243 (197)
Lower 2.5 percentile	106 (93)	138 (123)	138 (114)	162 (130)	103 (89)	119 (93)	126 (90)	144 (88)
Upper 2.5 percentile	352 (350)	373 (373)	417 (405)	712 (615)	324 (317)	335 (341)	399 (398)	434 (402)
Standard deviation	58.0 (61.0)	60.8 (61.1)	80.1 (81.0)	135.8 (123.5)	56.0 (55.6)	52.3 (57.0)	77.9 (83.5)	75.7 (81.9)
Calcium (mg)								
Mean	755 (706)	797 (741)	908 (799)	1057 (878)	691 (657)	703 (656)	759 (641)	793 (653)
Median	690 (666)	769 (700)	892 (781)	1049 (850)	658 (635)	690 (664)	751 (630)	735 (631)
Lower 2.5 percentile	451 (249)	451 (349)	530 (299)	494 (384)	380 (280)	406 (279)	363 (254)	555 (258)
Upper 2.5 percentile	1362 (1303)	1312 (1251)	1498 (1499)	1725 (1474)	1260 (1243)	1090 (1058)	1306 (1200)	1235 (1162)
Standard deviation	239.3 (256.8)	226.3 (234.6)	234.8 (288.4)	289.1 (298.2)	215.5 (219.9)	178.5 (194.2)	227.9 (235.7)	198.7 (242.4)
Iron (mg)								
Mean	8.7 (8.3)	10.4 (9.8)	11.9 (10.8)	14.5 (12.6)	7.7 (7.4)	8.7 (8.5)	10.1 (9.1)	10.9 (8.9)
Median	8.4 (8.0)	10.0 (9.3)	11.7 (10.4)	14.2 (11.7)	7.3 (7.1)	8.5 (8.2)	10.1 (8.6)	10.1 (8.2)
Lower 2.5 percentile	5.0 (4.4)	6.3 (5.7)	6.8 (5.8)	8.4 (6.9)	4.7 (3.9)	5.8 (4.7)	5.7 (4.8)	6.7 (3.9)
Upper 2.5 percentile	14.8 (14.4)	16.5 (15.8)	18.6 (17.6)	24.4 (22.3)	13.6 (11.8)	14.7 (15.0)	17.3 (17.4)	18.8 (17.6)
Standard deviation	2.50 (2.55)	2.72 (2.74)	2.84 (3.15)	4.12 (4.07)	2.17 (2.20)	2.24 (2.42)	2.69 (3.20)	3.15 (3.56)
Magnesium (mg)								
Mean	181 (172)	208 (194)	247 (218)	295 (256)	161 (155)	186 (177)	210 (182)	233 (191)
Median	173 (170)	205 (187)	241 (214)	288 (254)	152 (145)	184 (176)	202 (176)	220 (189)
Lower 2.5 percentile	119 (67)	136 (117)	159 (97)	176 (145)	107 (92)	128 (98)	141 (102)	164 (84)
Upper 2.5 percentile	271 (264)	311 (302)	362 (351)	466 (390)	248 (244)	259 (261)	323 (290)	396 (314)
Standard deviation	41.1 (46.0)	42.5 (46.1)	51.5 (59.8)	69.3 (72.2)	38.6 (39.9)	36.1 (41.0)	43.9 (48.1)	55.4 (57.5)
Potassium (mg)								
Mean	2051 (1944)	2275 (2136)	2682 (2392)	3264 (2833)	1836 (1774)	2124 (2019)	2381 (2100)	2601 (2162)
Median	1988 (1889)	2205 (2086)	2644 (2344)	3153 (2775)	1758 (1661)	2099 (2029)	2367 (2025)	2600 (2148)
Lower 2.5 percentile	1327 (1045)	1518 (1280)	1816 (1201)	1816 (1636)	1127 (1016)	1346 (1098)	1546 (1176)	1753 (1063)
Upper 2.5 percentile	3039 (3019)	3190 (3110)	3933 (3653)	5433 (4416)	2727 (2721)	2839 (2827)	3427 (3159)	3647 (3334)
Standard deviation	452.0 (502.9)	451.0 (488.2)	553.1 (608.2)	926.1 (820.2)	447.0 (458.9)	369.3 (420.2)	477.6 (549.5)	481.0 (592.7)
Zinc (mg)								
Mean	5.9 (5.6)	6.6 (6.1)	7.7 (7.2)	9.6 (8.7)	5.2 (5.0)	5.9 (5.7)	6.7 (5.9)	7.5 (6.1)
Median	5.5 (5.4)	6.4 (6.0)	7.5 (7.0)	9.0 (8.5)	5.1 (4.8)	5.7 (5.6)	6.5 (5.8)	7.1 (6.0)
Lower 2.5 percentile	3.7 (2.5)	4.1 (3.4)	5.0 (3.6)	5.0 (4.6)	2.9 (2.6)	3.8 (3.1)	4.4 (2.6)	4.5 (2.6)
Upper 2.5 percentile	10.4 (10.3)	10.4 (10.3)	12.2 (11.3)	16.9 (15.5)	8.2 (7.9)	9.2 (9.2)	10.0 (9.4)	13.1 (10.7)
Standard deviation	1.75 (1.80)	1.51 (1.60)	1.81 (1.97)	2.83 (2.66)	1.34 (1.39)	1.31 (1.37)	1.46 (1.73)	2.02 (2.02)
Base (excluding under-reporters)	*152*	*181*	*112*	*65*	*149*	*165*	*115*	*55*
Base (total sample)	*184*	*256*	*237*	*179*	*171*	*226*	*238*	*210*

* Values in brackets = intakes for total diary sample.

Table J6 Average daily energy intake (MJ) as a percentage of the estimated average requirement (EAR)*, by age and sex of young person, excluding those classified as 'under-reporters'**

Age and sex of young person	Mean energy intake	EAR	Intake as % EAR	Base
	(MJ)	(MJ)	%	
Males aged (years)				
4–6	6.71 (6.39)	7.16	94 (89)	152 (184)
7–10	8.02 (7.47)	8.24	97 (91)	181 (256)
11–14	9.46 (8.28)	9.27	102 (89)	112 (237)
15–18	11.59 (9.60)	11.51	101 (83)	65 (179)
Females aged (years)				
4–6	6.10 (5.87)	6.46	94 (91)	149 (171)
7–10	7.13 (6.72)	7.28	98 (92)	165 (226)
11–14	8.14 (7.03)	7.92	103 (89)	115 (238)
15–18	8.75 (6.82)	8.83	99 (77)	55 (210)

* Department of Health. Report on Health and Social Subjects: 41. *Dietary Reference Values for Food Energy and Nutrients for the United Kingdom.* HMSO (London, 1991).
** Values in brackets = intakes from total diary sample.

Table J7 Average daily protein intake as a percentage of Reference Nutrient Intake (RNI)*, by age and sex of young person, excluding those classified as 'under-reporters'**

Age and sex of young person	Mean protein intake	RNI	Intake as % RNI	Base
	(g)	(g)	%	
Males aged (years)				
4–6	51.4 (49.0)	19.7	261 (249)	152 (184)
7–10	58.6 (54.8)	28.3	207 (194)	181 (256)
11–14	70.4 (64.0)	42.1	167 (152)	112 (237)
15–18	86.4 (76.5)	55.2	157 (139)	65 (179)
Females aged (years)				
4–6	46.0 (44.5)	19.7	234 (226)	149 (171)
7–10	53.3 (51.2)	28.3	188 (181)	165 (226)
11–14	59.7 (52.9)	41.2	145 (128)	115 (238)
15–18	66.2 (54.8)	45.4	146 (121)	55 (210)

* Department of Health. Report on Health and Social Subjects: 41. *Dietary Reference Values for Food Energy and Nutrients for the United Kingdom.* HMSO (London, 1991).
** Values in brackets = intakes for total diary sample.

Table J8 Average daily intake of selected micronutrients from all sources, as a percentage of Reference Nutrient Intake (RNI)*, by age and sex of young person, excluding those classified as 'under-reporters'**

Micronutrient	Males aged (years)				Females aged (years)			
	4–6	7–10	11–14	15–18	4–6	7–10	11–14	15–18
	%	%	%	%	%	%	%	%
Vitamin A (retinol equivalents) (µg)	142 (134)	121 (111)	98 (96)	98 (90)	131 (126)	109 (103)	94 (80)	107 (94)
Riboflavin (mg)	210 (197)	175 (163)	164 (145)	181 (150)	186 (179)	146 (138)	143 (123)	149 (122)
Folate (µg)	204 (192)	150 (142)	134 (123)	176 (154)	176 (171)	132 (127)	119 (105)	128 (107)
Calcium (mg)	164 (157)	145 (135)	91 (80)	106 (88)	154 (146)	128 (119)	95 (80)	99 (82)
Iron (mg)	143 (136)	120 (112)	105 (96)	129 (111)	125 (121)	100 (97)	69 (61)	73 (60)
Magnesium (mg)	151 (143)	104 (97)	88 (78)	98 (85)	134 (129)	93 (89)	75 (65)	78 (64)
Potassium (mg)	186 (177)	114 (107)	86 (77)	93 (81)	167 (161)	106 (101)	77 (68)	74 (62)
Zinc (mg)	91 (86)	94 (88)	86 (79)	101 (92)	80 (77)	85 (81)	74 (66)	107 (87)
Base (excluding under-reporters)	152	181	112	65	149	165	115	55
Base (total sample)	184	256	237	179	171	226	238	210

* Department of Health. Report on Health and Social Subjects: 41. *Dietary Reference Values for Food Energy and Nutrients for the United Kingdom.* HMSO (London, 1991).
** Values in brackets = intakes for total diary sample.

Table J9 Proportion of subjects with intakes of selected micronutrients, from all sources, below the Lower Reference Nutrient Intake (LRNI)*, by sex and age of young person, excluding those classified as 'under-reporters'**

Micronutrient	Males aged (years)				Females aged (years)			
	4–6	7–10	11–14	15–18	4–6	7–10	11–14	15–18
	%	%	%	%	%	%	%	%
Vitamin A (retinol equivalents) (µg)	4 (8)	2 (9)	5 (12)	3 (12)	5 (6)	6 (9)	6 (20)	3 (12)
Riboflavin (mg)	0 (0)	0 (1)	0 (6)	0 (6)	0 (0)	0 (1)	8 (22)	2 (21)
Folate (µg)	0 (0)	0 (0)	0 (1)	0 (0)	0 (0)	0 (2)	1 (3)	0 (4)
Calcium (mg)	0 (3)	0 (2)	0 (12)	0 (9)	1 (2)	1 (5)	11 (24)	0 (19)
Iron (mg)	0 (0)	0 (1)	0 (3)	0 (2)	0 (1)	0 (3)	22 (44)	12 (48)
Magnesium (mg)	0 (3)	0 (2)	7 (28)	7 (18)	0 (1)	1 (5)	29 (51)	17 (53)
Potassium (mg)	0 (0)	0 (0)	0 (10)	0 (15)	0 (0)	0 (1)	0 (19)	0 (38)
Zinc (mg)	4 (12)	2 (5)	3 (14)	6 (9)	19 (26)	5 (10)	15 (37)	0 (10)
Base (excluding under-reporters)	152	181	112	65	149	165	115	55
Base (total sample)	184	256	237	179	171	226	238	210

* Department of Health. Report on Health and Social Subjects: 41. *Dietary Reference Values for Food Energy and Nutrients for the United Kingdom.* HMSO (London, 1991).
** Values in brackets = intakes for total diary sample.

Appendix K

Physical activity

1 Introduction

This Appendix describes in detail the methodology for collecting information on physical activity for young people aged 4 to 18 years. Details are given of how the activities that young people participated in were coded, of the data editing process and quality checks performed and of the derivation of different measures of physical activity level. Possible sources of both over and under-estimation in activity level are identified and finally differences in the methodology for collecting physical activity information between this survey and the Health Survey for England[1] are described.

2 Data collection methodology

2.1 Overview

Studies that rely on self-report methods of data collection tend to conclude that young people engage in relatively high levels of activity, and studies that apply cardiovascular fitness criteria report much lower levels of activity[2]. Difficulties with self-report measures include the fact that social acceptability may affect the number of activities or the intensity level recorded, for example, research has shown that parents are more likely to report high levels of activity for boys than for girls[3]. Respondents may record the activities in which they usually participate, rather than those in which they did participate during the recording period, feeling that this would be a more accurate reflection of their level of physical activity. Alternatively, teenagers may choose not to record activities that they consider unfashionable.

In the NDNS data on different aspects of physical activity were collected using a different methodology for different age groups. All young people who took part in the survey were asked some physical activity questions as part of the initial dietary interview. However, not all young people aged 4 to 18 years kept a 'Diary of Physical Activity and Eating and Drinking Away from Home'.

For young people aged 4 to 6 years:
- data were collected in the initial dietary interview on:

usual method of transport and duration of journey to and from school;
parent's assessment of current physical activity level;
- data were collected over the 7-day recording period in the 'Diary of Eating and Drinking Away from Home' on:
time spent sleeping per night;
time spent in very light activities per day;
whether the young person was at school each day.

For young people aged 7 to 18 years:
- data were collected in the initial dietary interview on:
usual method of transport and duration of journey to and from school or work;
whether the young person worked full or part-time and the intensity level of their job;
- data were collected over the 7-day recording period in the 'Diary of Physical Activity and Eating and Drinking Away from Home' on:
time spent sleeping per night;
time spent in very light activities per day;
whether the young person was at school or work each day;
time spent at work each day;
time spent in moderate, vigorous and very vigorous intensity activity each day.

2.2 Physical activity information collected for all young people aged 4 to 18 years

2.2.1 Travel to and from work or school

One explanation for the possible decrease in physical activity levels for young people is that children are increasingly travelling to school by car or bus rather than walking or cycling. Young people aged 4 to 18 years were asked about their usual method of transport to and from school or work as part of the initial dietary interview.

*1. How does young person **usually** get to school/work?*

CODE ALL THAT APPLY

- *Walk*
- *Cycle*
- *Motorcycle*
- *Car*
- *Bus*
- *Other (specify at next question)*

If 'Other' at question 1

2. *Specify other way young person travels to school/work*

If 'Walk' or 'Cycle' at question 1

3. *How long does it take him/her to walk/cycle to school/work?*

IN MINUTES

0..90

4. *How does young person* **usually** *get home?*

CODE ALL THAT APPLY

- *Walk*
- *Cycle*
- *Motorcycle*
- *Car*
- *Bus*
- *Other (specify at next question)*

If 'Other' at question 4

5. *Specify other way young person travels home*

If 'Walk' or 'Cycle' at question 4

6. *How long does it take him/her to walk/cycle home?*

IN MINUTES

0..90

In most cases young people used one method of transport, with 2% using more than one method of transport to travel to and from school or work (table not shown). For those who reported walking or cycling, data were collected on the duration of the journey.

2.2.2 Time spent sleeping per night

To allow the hours of sleep to be calculated, all young people aged 4 to 18 years recorded the time they went to bed and got up on each of the 7 recording days. It was assumed that young people would sleep for one unbroken period of time during the day or night and would not take 'naps' at other times during the day. It should be noted that this assumption might not be valid, particularly for younger children.

When the data were keyed the program checked that the 24-hour clock was used.

2.2.3 Time spent in very light activity per day

It is possible that the apparent decrease in physical activity levels among young people is due to their spending more time in very light activities such as watching television, playing computer games, and listening to music rather than participating in physically active games. Information was collected for all young people aged 4 to 18 years on the time they spent in very light activities each day using the following question:

How long had (young person) spent watching TV, playing computer games and listening to music today?

This question was designed to identify time spent in activities in which the young person was mainly seated, that is sedentary activities. The social acceptability of the specified sedentary activities may have resulted in young people or their parent(s) providing an underestimate.

The feasibility study had shown that young people tended to interpret questions literally and to include only those activities mentioned in the question[4]. Therefore at the main stage interviewers were instructed to check with the young person whether they had spent any time in other similar, sedentary activities. However, since the question did not specifically ask about time spent in other, similar, activities, for example 'doing homework', this may also lead to an underestimate of the time spent in very light activity.

2.2.4 Whether the young person was at school or work on each diary day

Information was collected from all young people aged 4 to 18 years for each diary day about whether they were at school or work:

Today were you: at school or college? Yes/no
at work? Yes/no

If you were at work today, how long did you work?

(please exclude any lunch break)

Hours   Minutes

The interviewer checked with the young person that all break times had been excluded from time recorded as being at work.

As part of the initial interview young people with a full or part-time job were asked about the physical intensity of their job. The young person was asked to choose which of the following descriptions best fitted their job:

How would you describe your job .. is it:

- *A job where you are sitting or standing for most of the time, which is not physical or active,*
- *a job which is physical and active, but not so hard as to make you puff and pant and get hot and sweaty for a lot of the time,*
- *or a job which is very physical and active and makes you puff and pant and get hot and sweaty for a lot of the time?*

This question was used to indicate whether the intensity level for the job was very light, light or moderate. In deriving an activity score, time spent working was combined with the intensity information (see *Section 3.1* below).

In deriving the activity score it was also assumed that attending school each day would account for 5 ½ hours of very light activity, that is, that most of the school day would be spent in sedentary activity, while lunch and other break times would be more active.

2.3 Physical activity information collected for young people aged 4 to 6 years

The method of data collection used in the mainstage survey for young people aged 4 to 6 years was decided following the feasibility study and further qualitative testing of the data collection instruments[4]. This earlier work had established that:

- the collection of data on duration, intensity and frequency of activity was not appropriate for young people aged 4 to 6 years;
- parents were unlikely to be able to provide an accurate report of their child's activities for times when their children were not with them, for example, when they were at school;
- parents observed their child interacting with other children and were aware of how their own child's activity level compared with that of children of the same age or sex.

The questions used in the mainstage survey to measure the level of physical activity for young people aged 4 to 6 years were as follows:

1. How would you describe (young person)'s current level of activity?

- *Fairly Inactive – gets little exercise, spends most of his/her time watching television, looking at books, or sitting playing with toys or games*
- *Fairly Active – spends more time in active play or running around than watching television, looking at books, or sitting playing with toys or games*
- *Very Active – spends nearly all the time running around or in very active play or games*

2. How would you describe (young person)'s level of activity when compared with boys and girls of the same age?

- *More active,*
- *about the same,*
- *or less active?*

3. How would you describe (young person)'s level of activity when compared with other children of the same sex?

- *More active,*
- *about the same,*
- *or less active?*

Although these questions ask for the parent(s) assessment of their child's level of physical activity, the answers they gave may also have been affected by their expectations or views, for example, a view that boys are generally more active than girls.

2.4 Physical activity information collected for young people aged 7 to 18 years

The 7-day diary method was used for the collection of data on physical activity for young people aged 7 to 18 years. In order to collect complete data on physical activity, information on three dimensions of physical activity was required; on duration, intensity and frequency. This information was used to calculate an activity score which can be used as an indicator for energy expenditure (see *Section 3.1* below).

2.4.1 Information collected

Information was collected on the time spent being active for a list of prompted moderate, vigorous and very vigorous activities. This list included two categories of 'active play', which were designed to collect data on less formal activity, 'playing other ball games outside', and 'playing tag, chasing games outside'. These activities appeared in the prompted list of activities after ball games such as football and basketball. The interviewer checked for duplicate entries, for example where the same amount of time was recorded against 'playing other ball games outside' and against 'football'. It should be noted, however, that the category 'playing other ball games outside' may give an overestimate if, for example, time spent playing cricket, which is defined as a light intensity activity, is included.

The prompted list of activities included both 'cycling, including doing a paper round on a bike' and 'doing a paper round on foot'. In order to avoid duplicate entries, the interviewer checked that time spent doing a paper round had not been entered against either one of these categories in addition to being recorded against work.

A section was provided for the young person to record activities that were not already listed, with prompts to establish whether they were of vigorous intensity:

*Have you done any other activities today that made you **breathe hard, huff and puff** and **get hot and sweaty**?*

or moderate intensity:

*Have you done any other activities today that made you **slightly out of breath** and feel warm, but **not exhausted**?*

The interviewer was provided with a list of activities by intensity level (given at the end of this Appendix) to assist them in checking that any 'other' activities recorded by the young person had been correctly classified and to delete any activities which were of less than moderate intensity. Interviewers checked for duplicate entries, that is activities recorded in both the prompted list and in the list of 'other activities'.

At each visit interviewers checked the entries in the diary with the young person to probe for any activities that had been overlooked, using specific 'time of day' probes and to collect any additional information needed to code the activities. The interviewer also checked that any time spent in related activity, such as travelling to and from the activity, changing clothes, or taking a break from the activity was not included in the time that was recorded.

2.4.2 Coding the intensity level for physical activities

Data from existing research[5,6], were used to estimate the intensity level for each activity on the prompted list and to develop the Physical Activity Diary Coding Guide for interviewers which is reproduced at the end of this Appendix. Energy expenditure data for many activities have been established, however most through research on adult subjects. Where energy expenditure data for young people were available, these were used. Where only adult data were available, a lower intensity level was generally applied as it was felt that a certain level of skill would be required to expend the same level of energy as an adult for a given activity. Recent studies validating the use of adult classifications in the analysis of data for young people have shown a significant correlation between the activity information derived from four 1-day recall questionnaires and that derived using a heart rate monitoring technique[7].

The interviewer used the coding guide to check that 'other moderate' and 'other vigorous' activities were recorded in the section for the correct intensity level. The intensity level for any 'other' activities not included in the Physical Activity Diary Coding Guide were coded using a compendium of physical activities[8]. The compendium, which gives information for adults, has been shown to compare favourably with classifications established in a previous study of physical activity for young people[5,6].

2.4.3 Editing the data on physical activities

Interviewers entered the physical activity diary data into their laptop computer and internal consistency checks were applied to avoid mis-keying, for example to check that the time spent in all activities did not add up to more than 24 hours.

Subsequent data editing involved further consistency checks and the examination at HQ of some completed activity diaries. Diaries were examined:

- if, for Wave 1 of fieldwork, the case was in the top 10% of the distribution of calculated activity score (see *Section 3.1* below). For Waves 2 to 4 of fieldwork, those cases with a calculated activity score greater than the cut-off point established using the Wave 1 data were examined.
- If the time spent in any 'other' activity was greater than 3 hours.
- If an interviewer had failed to correct an error in the data, all diaries for that interviewer were

manually checked.
- If less than 1 hour or more than 12 hours of sleep were recorded for any day.
- If less than 60 minutes of light activity were calculated for any diary day.
- If the calculated activity score was less than 30. This was used as a default indicator that the interviewer had identified that the time spent in all activities added up to more than 24 hours for an individual day.

In all, 589 (41%) of the 1424 completed diaries were checked, of which just over half were edited. The main problems, in about a quarter of the diaries checked, were the upward rounding of time spent in activities and the incorrect coding of intensity level for 'other' activities.

Generally upward rounding of time could not be changed at the editing stage because the true time spent was unknown. However, it was assumed that breaks and related activity such as time taken changing clothes had been included. Therefore if the time spent on a single activity was greater than 3 hours, the excess above 3 hours was reduced by 50%. For example 5 hours was reduced to 4 hours, 4 hours to 3½ hours etc. Examination of the diaries suggested that very few respondents recorded activities in increments of less than 30 minutes. Assuming that there is no bias in the size of the rounding errors comparisons between sub-groups of the time spent in activities will not be affected.

In the diaries that were checked, 'other' activities that were coded to the wrong intensity level were recoded to the correct level and activities that were not of at least moderate intensity, were deleted. Where possible, 'other' activities were recoded into the prompted list of activities. Most wrongly categorised activities over-estimated the intensity level. In particular older girls were likely to include time spent in light activities, such as walking round the shops, under other moderate or other vigorous activities. After editing the proportion of young people who had participated in an other 'moderate' or other vigorous activity was between 13% and 25%, depending on age and sex. Given that not all the diaries were checked this may mean that any overestimate of physical activity level may be greater for older girls than for other young people.

Duplicate entries were most frequent where time spent at work was entered both for work and either a prompted activity or an 'other' activity, or where time spent in an activity was recorded both for a prompted activity and an 'other' activity. Entries were only edited where duplication was clear and in deciding which entry to delete priority was given firstly to time at work, and then to activities which were on the prompted list.

After editing, 'other' activities, not on the prompted list or deleted, included:

- some sports in which mainly older children participated, for example conditioning exercises (e.g. press-ups), body-building, weight-lifting, rock-climbing;
- less common activities, for example majorettes, scuba diving, shinty;
- DIY, decorating or building work;
- maintenance work for cars or bikes;
- activities connected with army cadets, for example 'field-gun training'.

2.4.4 Data quality

After editing some preliminary analysis was carried to investigate the quality of the final information on activities. Figures 1 and 2 show the mean number of different activities of at least moderate intensity participated in by diary day and day of the week respectively. Figure 1 shows that the mean number of activities recorded decreased over the seven days of record keeping, with the greatest mean number of activities recorded on Day 1 and the fewest recorded on Day 7. Figure 2 shows that on average more activities were recorded from Tuesday to Friday than were recorded from Saturday to Monday.

Although there was no strict placing pattern for the survey practical fieldwork reasons meant that diaries were less likely to be placed on weekend days than on weekdays. Analysis showed that Day 1 of record keeping was most frequently a Wednesday (25%), Tuesday (24%) or Thursday (22%) and least frequently a Saturday (7%), Sunday (3%) or Monday (3%) (table not shown). Figures 1 and 2 therefore suggest either that young people were more active mid-week compared with the weekend or that as the 7-day recording period progressed they tended to omit to record all their activities.   *(Figs K1 and K2)*

3 Derived measures of physical activity

Three measures of level of physical activity were derived from the available data; the mean hours spent in all activities of at least moderate intensity per day, the calculated activity score, and the total number of activities of at least moderate intensity participated in during the 7-day recording period[9]. The first two of these measures are derived in part from information on duration of activity. Any upward rounding of activity time will therefore result in overestimate of energy expenditure as represented by the calculated activity score. However, this may in part be offset by any under-recording of the number of activities participated in.

3.1 Calculating the activity score

Resting metabolism, defined as 1 MET, is approximately equal to an energy expenditure of one kilocalorie (kcal) per kilogram per hour (kcal/kg/hour). For adults an average body weight of 60kg is assumed and therefore for an average adult 1MET is equal to 60kcal/hour or 1kcal/min. For adults METs are therefore taken as numerically equivalent to energy expenditure. For children and young people this equivalence will not hold because of the wide range of body weights and therefore an activity score, based on MET value x time spent should only be used as an indicator of energy expenditure, not actual expenditure.

An example of how the calculated activity score is derived for one day is given below.

3.2 Comparing the derived measures of physical activity

Table K1 shows tertiles for the three derived measures of physical activity. It can be seen that for each indicator a proportion of those in the top tertile is in the bottom tertile of each of the other two measures and vice versa. Thus while all three measures may be used as indicators for physical activity level, each describes a qualitatively different aspect of physical activity. Therefore in the results chapter of this Report (Chapter 13) tables showing variation in physical activity by socio-demographic characteristics give data for all three summary measures of physical activity.   *(Table K1)*

Example of calculated activity score for one day:

Type of activity	Total time spent (hours)	MET value for the type of activity	Activity score
Sleep	9.0	1.0	9.00
Very light activities	7.2	1.5	10.80
Light activities	6.3	2.5	15.75
Moderate activities	1.0	4.0	4.00
Vigorous activities	0.5	6.0	3.00
Very vigorous activities	0.0	10.0	0.00
Total	24.0		42.55

The total for each day is taken and the average daily total energy expenditure calculated.

Table K1 Comparison of physical activity measures

Grouped activity measures	Grouped total number of activities of at least moderate intensity during the 7-day recording period				Grouped mean hours spent in all activities of at least moderate intensity per day			
	Top %	Middle %	Bottom %	Total %	Top %	Middle %	Bottom %	Total %
Tertile of calculated activity score								
Top	17	7	10	33	20	8	6	33
Middle	11	11	11	33	10	14	10	33
Bottom	6	9	19	33	4	12	18	33
Total	33	27	40	100	34	33	34	100
Grouped total number of activities of at least moderate intensity during the 7-day recording period								
Top	33	–	–	33	28	10	2	40
Middle	–	33	–	33	4	15	8	27
Bottom	–	–	33	33	1	9	24	33
Total	33	33	33	100	34	33	34	100

4 The Health Survey for England[1] and the NDNS: physical activity methodologies compared

In the feasibility study for this NDNS, an attempt was made to validate the physical activity data collected by diary methodology with information on physical activity obtained from a three-dimensional motion sensor (Tritrak monitor) worn by the young people. However, there were technical difficulties with its use in the context of a private household sample (rather than, for example, in a school-based sample) and the monitor was therefore not used at the main stage[4].

In the main stage of this NDNS and in the Health Survey, physical activity data were collected by self-report methodology with no attempt to validate against objective measures such as heart rate monitoring. However there are several differences in methodology which should be taken into account when comparing the data:

- the recall period for the Health Survey was longer than for the NDNS. The Health Survey used a 7-day recall while the NDNS used a 7-day diary, which is more likely to equate to a 1-day recall over 7 consecutive days.
- On the Health Survey, if the young person was aged under 13 years, a parent was asked the questions on physical activity. On the NDNS the expectation was that young people aged 11 to 18 years would complete the diary unassisted. For younger respondents it was left to the interviewer to decide whether the parent or young person should be asked to complete the dairy.
- On the Health Survey activities lasting less than 15 minutes were excluded (with the exception of walking where any walk lasting less than 5 minutes was excluded). On the NDNS, activities (including walks) lasting less than 10 minutes were excluded.
- Data on 'at least moderate intensity activity' for

the Health Survey were collected using broader categories than those used for the NDNS; the categories used in the Health Survey were:

> sports and exercise
> active play
> walking
> housework or gardening

- On the Health Survey, data on sedentary activity were collected using a description which included homework and 'playing quietly' in addition to the activities listed in the NDNS description (watching TV, playing computer games and listening to music).
- Activities carried out as part of the school curriculum were excluded in the Health Survey and included in the NDNS. The assumptions underlying this decision for the Health Survey were as follows:

> that on average this would constitute a relatively consistent amount of time and could therefore be discounted;
> that the intention was to survey what children would do of their own accord, not compulsory sports;
> that a large proportion of the Health Survey data was proxy information and would therefore be more accurate if confined to leisure time rather than time spent at school.

The NDNS included all physical activities, whether compulsory or voluntary, in order to allow a valid comparison with the HEA recommendations. Only a small proportion of the NDNS data was proxy information.

References and notes

[1] Prescott-Clarke P, Primatesta P. Eds. *Heath Survey for England. The Health of Young People '95–97. Volume 1: Findings.* TSO (London,1998).

[2] Riddoch CJ, Boreham CA. The health-related physical activity of children. *Sports Medicine* 1995; **19**: 2: 86–102.

[3] Sallis J. Self-report measures of children's physical

activity. *J Sch Hlth* 1991; **61**: *215–219*.

4   For further information see *Appendix C: Feasibility Study* and Lowe S. *Feasibility study for the National Diet and Nutrition Survey: young people 4 to 18 years*. ONS (*In preparation*).

5   Cale L, Almond L. The Physical Activity Levels of English Adolescent Boys. *E J Phys Ed*. 1997; **2**: 74–82.

6   Cale L. An assessment of the physical activity levels of adolescent girls – implications for physical education. *E J Phys Ed*. 1996; **1**: 46–55.

7   Cale L. Self-report measures of children's physical activity: recommendations for the future and a new alternative measure. *H Ed J*. 1994; **53**: 439–453.

8   Ainsworth BE et al. Compendium of physical activities: classification of energy costs of human physical activities. *Med and Sci in Sports Med*. 1993: **25**: 71–79.

9   To allow comparisons between the activity of young people in this present NDNS and the HEA recommendations and with data from the Health Survey for England, the time spent in all activities of moderate, vigorous and very vigorous intensity was combined to give the category 'at least moderate intensity'.

Appendix K   Physical Activity Diary Coding Guide

Note: These codes are a guide to what activities should be coded under which activity level - if an activity is not listed or you are not sure how to code something, **please call research for advice**.

VERY LIGHT ACTIVITIES - AVERAGE 1.5 METS

Card/board games, playing with toys

Using a computer/playing computer games

Drawing/painting

Homework

Listening to music

Playing a musical instrument

Reading for pleasure

Talking with friends

Watching television

Watching videos

LIGHT ACTIVITIES - AVERAGE 2.5 METS

Bowling

Caring for pets

Cricket

Darts

Horseriding

Light household chores, washing up, tidying up etc

Pool, snooker

Shopping

Table tennis

Walking, strolling

Going to a youth club, disco

MODERATE ACTIVITIES - AVERAGE 4.0 METS

Badminton

Cleaning, hoovering, moving furniture

Cycling

Football in the playground

Gardening

Golf

Gymnastics

Hockey

Netball

Playing tag, chasing games in the playground

Playing any other ball game in the playground

Rounders

Swimming

Tennis

Volleyball

Walking briskly

HARD ACTIVITIES - AVERAGE 6.0 METS

Basketball

Disco-dancing

Jogging

Rugby, touch rugby

VERY HARD ACTIVITIES - AVERAGE 10.0 METS

Athletics

Running

Any other activities need to be classified as light, very light, moderate or hard at interviewer's discretion

NOTE:

JOGGING and RUNNING are classified differently:

    JOGGING is a HARD activity;

    RUNNING is a VERY HARD activity.

STROLLING, WALKING and WALKING BRISKLY are classified differently:

    STROLLING, WALKING is a LIGHT activity;

    WALKING BRISKLY is a MODERATE activity.

Figure K1 The mean number of activities of at least moderate intensity in which the young person participated by diary day

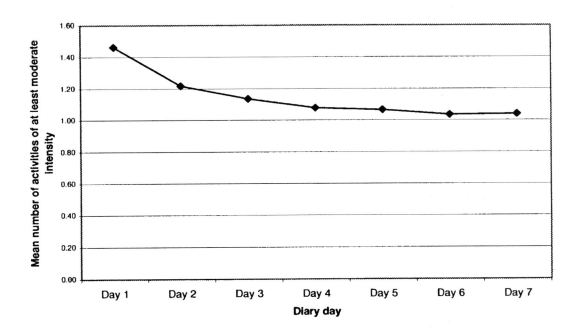

Figure K2 The mean number of activities of at least moderate intensity in which the young person participated by the day of the week

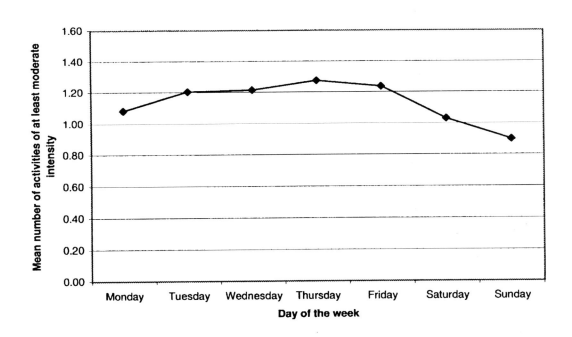

Appendix L

Protocols for anthropometry and blood pressure measurement

1 Stature (height)

Weight was measured using the Leicester Height Measure[1]. This had been tested in the feasibility study[2], and prior to that in a small calibration exercise where measurements taken using the Height Measure were compared with measurements taken using the Digi-Rod, which had been the instrument of choice in the NDNS of young children aged 1½ to 4½ years and the NDNS of persons aged 65 and over[3,4]. It was concluded from the calibration exercise and the feasibility study that the Leicester Height Measure was suitable for use in the main stage of this survey of young people.

The Measure consists of a base plate, four measuring rods, which slot together, two stabilising bars and a head plate, which slides up and down the vertical measuring rods. A frame on the head plate with arrows indicates the point at which the measurement should be read. Each rod is marked in metric (centimetres and millimetres) and imperial (feet and inches) units.

The Measure was constructed and the base plate placed on a hard level surface, uncarpeted where possible, with the two stabilising bars against a vertical surface, such as a wall or door.

The young person was asked to remove their shoes and to wear as few clothes as possible. If the young person's hairstyle was likely to affect their height they were asked to adjust the style. If the hairstyle could not easily be changed for the measurement, for example, the young person had dreadlocks or braids, then the interviewer made a note on the recording document and the measurement was excluded from the survey analysis.

The young person was positioned with their feet together and flat on the base plate of the Measure, their arms loosely at their side, and with their head and back straight and against the vertical measuring rods. The young person's head was correctly positioned in the Frankfort plane[5] by the interviewer and the alignment checked using a card. Once the correct position was achieved the interviewer lowered the head plate until it just touched the top of the young person's head. The interviewer then asked the young person to take a breath and stand as tall as possible, without lifting their heels off the base plate. For the youngest children in the survey the interviewer achieved the necessary stretch by applying gentle traction to the back of the head/neck with his/her hands.

After checking the young person's feet were still flat on the base plate and that the head was still in the correct position the interviewer read the measurement from the vertical rod. Interviewers were instructed that the arrows indicating the point of measurement had to be at eye level, and if necessary they should ask the young person to step off the Measure so that it could be moved and this achieved.

The measurement was recorded by the interviewer in centimetres and millimetres on the measurement schedule, together with an indication of any unusual circumstances which might have affected the measurement.

The complete procedure was then repeated and a second measurement made.

2 Weight

Weight was taken using Soehnle Quantratronic scales, Models 7300 and 7306, calibrated in 100 gram units. The scales were checked for accuracy and calibrated by a specialist contractor prior to the start of fieldwork; during the fieldwork period the batteries were regularly changed[6].

The time of day for taking the measurement was not standardised.

The scale was placed on a hard, level surface. If only a carpeted surface was available then the interviewer noted this.

Since the scales have a memory facility, the previous weight taken needed to be cleared from the scale before each measurement. This was achieved by the interviewer always standing on the scale after every weighing of a young person.

The young person was asked to wear only light clothing while being weighed; heavy items of clothing, including shoes, trainers and jackets and any heavy jewellery, keys and money were removed where possible. A record was made of which items of clothing the young person was wearing while being weighed.

The scale was switched on and when the zero reading was displayed the young person was asked to stand on the scale, with both feet fully on the weighing platform, heels against the back edge, and the arms loosely at the side. While the scale was calculating the weight the young person was instructed to remain still with their head forward facing. Weight was recorded to one tenth of a kilogram (100 grams). The young person was then asked to step off the scale while the interviewer cleared their weight from the scale's memory. The measurement was then repeated.

Any unusual circumstances affecting the weight measurement were noted by the interviewer on the recording document.

3 Mid upper-arm circumference

This measurement was made on the young person's left arm, in two stages. With the left arm bare and at 90° across the body the mid point of the upper arm was located. Using a conventional tape, the distance between the inferior border of the acromion and the tip of the olecranon process was measured, and without removing the tape, the mid point marked on the young person's arm with a dermatological marker pen.

To measure the circumference at the mid point the young person's arm was then positioned loosely at their side. Using an insertion tape of non-stretchable material, the circumference was measured, ensuring that the tape was horizontal, in contact with the arm around the entire circumference and without sufficient tension to compress the tissues of the upper arm[7].

Two measurements were made, each time identifying the mid point of the upper arm. Measurements were recorded to the nearest millimetre.

Any unusual circumstances affecting the measurement were noted by the interviewer on the recording document.

4 Waist and hip circumferences

Waist and hip circumferences were only measured for young people aged 11 to 18 years[8]. Interviewers were instructed not to attempt to measure any young person who was chairbound or bedfast, or had a colostomy or ileostomy.

In preparation for these measurements the young person was asked to wear only light clothing and to have recently emptied their bladder. In particular they were asked to remove any belts or items in pockets that might affect only one of the circumferences and therefore change the ratio between the waist and hip measurements. Young people were also asked to adjust the position of their clothing to try to achieve a similar thickness at both measurement positions.

The waist is defined as the midway point between the iliac crest and the lower rib. The feasibility study found that it was unacceptable both to some interviewers and young people for the interviewer to feel for these bones at the side of the body[2]. At the mainstage survey the point of measurement was therefore located by asking the young person to bend to one side and place their finger at the point where their body bent. They were then asked to straighten, keeping their finger in the same place; this identified the position for the tape for measuring waist circumference.

An insertion tape was passed around the circumference, adjusted and checked for horizontal alignment[9]. Having achieved satisfactory positioning of the tape the interviewer then asked the young person to continue breathing normally (that is, not to hold in the breath) and the measurement was made at the end of a normal expiration.

The hip circumference is defined as being the maximum circumference over the buttocks and below the iliac crest. The insertion tape was passed around the young person's hip area and then adjusted upwards and downwards until the maximum circumference was achieved. After checking the horizontal alignment of the tape and that the young person was not contracting their gluteal muscles the measurement was made.

When making the measurements interviewers were told to kneel or sit at the side of the young person, and to make any adjustments to the tape from the side of the body. Any adjustments needed to the tape at the front or back of the body were made, under instructions from the interviewer, by the young person or their parent.

Interviewers were asked to measure the waist and hip circumference and then to repeat the two measures. Measurements were made and recorded to the nearest millimetre. Any factor which affected the measurements, such as differences in the thickness of clothing at the waist and hip, were recorded on the measurement schedule.

5 Blood pressure

Blood pressure could only be taken if all the following were obtained[10].

- consent to notify the young person's GP of their participation in the survey;

- consent to take the blood pressure measurements;
- signed consent to send a record of the blood pressure measurements to the young person's GP.

Blood pressure was measured using the Dinamap 8100 oscillometric monitor. This device was previously used to measure blood pressure on the NDNS of people aged 65 years and over[4] and the Health Survey for England[11], and was the instrument of choice principally for reasons of methodological comparability between all these surveys, instrument reliability and ease of use. A summary review of studies comparing the Dinamap with other devices, including the standard mercury syphgmomanometer, is given below.

Measurements were made on the young person's right arm. The mid upper-arm circumference was used by the interviewer to decide which cuff size was most appropriate for the young person. Four different sizes were available and each cuff has markings to indicate, whether, after wrapping the cuff around the upper arm, the cuff selected is the appropriate size[12].

The time of day when the measurements were taken was not standardised but interviewers, when arranging an appointment, asked the young person not to eat or drink (or smoke) in the 30 minutes prior to the measurement being made, and to have been sitting quietly for 10 to 15 minutes. Interviewers subsequently checked whether these instructions had been carried out, and, if not and they were not able to reschedule the visit, recorded the relevant details on the measurement schedule.

The young person was asked to remove any jacket, jumper or cardigan they were wearing, and if they were wearing a garment with sleeves, to remove their right arm from the sleeve. If they were unwilling to comply with this and provided their circulation was not impeded, they were asked to roll the sleeve so that it would be above the top edge of the cuff.

The young person was seated so that they were relaxed and had their feet flat to floor. The right arm was rested on a support at a height that brought the antecubital fossa to approximately heart level. The lower edge of the cuff was placed about 2cm above the elbow crease and the arrow marked on the cuff placed over the brachial artery. The cuff was wrapped to a tightness that allowed two fingers to be inserted between it and the young person's arm at the top and bottom edges of the cuff.

The young person was then asked to sit quietly for about 5 minutes before the measurements were taken while the interviewer explained what would happen when the Dinamap was switched on. Three measurements were then taken at one-minute intervals, recording diastolic, systolic and mean arterial blood pressure and pulse rate.

The measurements were recorded on the measurement schedule, with details of any difficulties that might have affected the readings.

Difficulties in wrapping the cuff:

if the young person had a particularly large circumference arm, an appropriate circumference cuff was sometimes too deep for the length of the upper arm. In these circumstances the correct circumference cuff was used with a note made on the measurement schedule.

If the young person's upper arm increased markedly in circumference along its length, it was difficult to fit the cuff evenly and correctly at both its upper and lower edges. In these circumstances a note was made on the measurement schedule.

The three blood pressure readings were recorded on the young person's Record Card for them to keep and the interviewers were instructed not to discuss the readings with the young person or his or her family. If asked, interviewers suggested that the young person should contact his or her GP or the survey doctor for advice and interpretation of the measurements. The blood pressure readings were also recorded on the consent form which was sent to the survey doctor for forwarding to the young person's GP. If all three systolic measurements were equal to or above 160mmHg and/or all three diastolic readings were equal to or above 100mmHg then the interviewer informed the survey doctor by telephone and also directly informed the young person's GP. This was followed by a letter from the survey doctor[13].

Summary of studies comparing the Dinamap with other blood pressure measurement devices[14]

Bolling (1994)[15]: a calibration study carried out for the Department of Health as part of the Health Survey for England.

Concluded that data collected using the Dinamap correlated to a satisfactory degree with data collected using an auscultatory monitor, the mercury sphygmomanometer.

Park and Menard (1987)[16]: compared blood pressure in infants and children (aged 1 month to 16 years), measured using the Dinamap and with measurements using the conventional auscultatory method.

Concluded that the Dinamap correlated better with direct radial artery pressure and produced a smaller mean error. The Dinamap was recommended for use with younger children because it eliminates the difficulties identified when using auscultatory methods in this age group; these difficulties include excessive movement and inaudibility of Korotkoff sounds[17].

O'Brien and Atkins (1997)[18]: compared measurements made using the mercury sphygmomanometer and Dinamap, following the BHS protocol.

Concluded that the Dinamap underestimated systolic blood pressure by 0.71mmHg and diastolic blood pressure by 7.6mmHg. Routine measurements using a Dinamap in clinical practice cannot therefore be compared with those taken using a mercury sphygmomanometer.

Although the mercury sphygmomanometer is relatively cheap, it requires more training to use correctly than an automated device. For epidemiological purposes, automated devices have the advantage that observers need not be highly trained medical or nursing personnel[19]. ONS interviewers are easily able to learn the technique and the risk of observer bias is reduced.

References and endnotes

1. The Leicester Height Measure is available from the Child Growth Foundation, 2 Mayfield Avenue, Chiswick, London W4 1PW, UK.
2. See *Appendix C* and Lowe S. *Feasibility study for the National Diet and Nutrition Survey: young people aged 4 to 18 years*. ONS (*In preparation*).
3. Gregory JR, Collins DL, Davies PSW, Hughes JM, Clarke PC. *National Diet and Nutrition Survey: children aged 1½ to 4½ years. Volume 1: Report of the diet and nutrition survey*. HMSO (London, 1995).
4. Finch S, Doyle W, Lowe C, Bates CJ, Prentice A, Smithers G, Clarke PC. *National Diet and Nutrition Survey: people aged 65 and over. Volume 1: Report of the diet and nutrition survey*. TSO (London, 1998).
5. To achieve the correct Frankfort position, the bottom of the orbital socket should be in a horizontal line with the external auditory meatus.
6. The scales were checked and calibrated by CMS Weighing Equipment Ltd, 18 Camden High Street, London NW1 0JH, UK.
7. Circumference tapes were supplied by the Child Growth Foundation, 2 Mayfield Avenue, Chiswick, London W4 1PW, UK. The Lassoo-o™ circumference tape is manufactured from thin, non-stretch, non-shrink plastic and allows circumferences between 6cm and 70cm to be measured. Interviewers were instructed to replace the tape with a new one if it became creased or otherwise damaged during use.
8. See *Chapter 10, Section 10.7*.
9. Insertion tapes, fitted with a metal buckle and calibrated in centimetres and millimetres, were supplied by CMS Weighing Equipment Ltd, 18 Camden High Street, London NW1 0JH, UK.
10. For full details of the consent procedures see *Chapter 2, Sections 2.8* and *2.9*.
11. Prescott-Clarke P, Primatesta P. Eds. *Health Survey for England 1995*. TSO (London, 1997).
12. Small adult cuff: 17-25cm; standard adult cuff: 23-33cm; large adult cuff: 31-40cm; child size cuff: 10-19cm.
13. See *Chapter 2, Section 2.9* for details of the reporting procedures.
14. More details of these studies are given in the report of the feasibility survey. Lowe S. *Feasibility study for the National Diet and Nutrition Survey: young people aged 4 to 18 years*. ONS (*In preparation*).
15. Bolling K. *The Dinamap 8100 Calibration Study*. HMSO (London, 1994).
16. Park MK, Menard SM. Accuracy of blood pressure measurement by the Dinamap monitor in infants and children. *Pediatrics* 1987; **79**: 907-914.
17. Kirkendall WM, Feinleib M, Freis ED, et al. Recommendation for human blood pressure determination by sphygmomanometers: Subcommittee on the American Heart Association postgraduate education committee. *Circulation* 1980; **62**: 1145A-1155A.
18. O'Brien E, Atkins N. Inaccuracy of the Dinamap 8100 portable monitor. *Lancet* 1997; **349**: 1026.
19. Gillman MW et al. Blood pressure measurement in Childhood Epidemiological Studies. *Circulation* 1995; **92**: 4: 1049-1057.

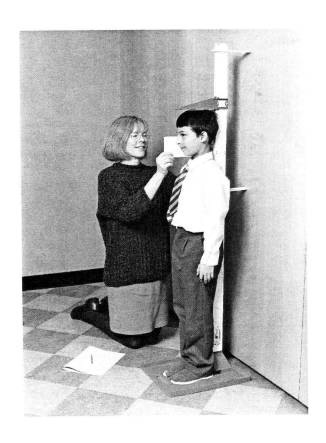

Figure 1   Measurement of height

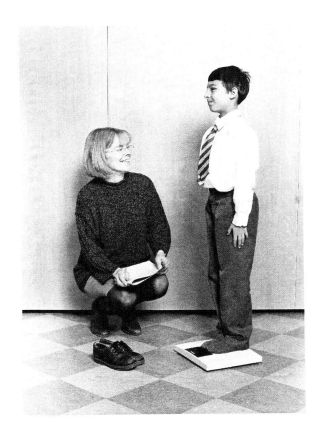

Figure 2   Measurement of weight

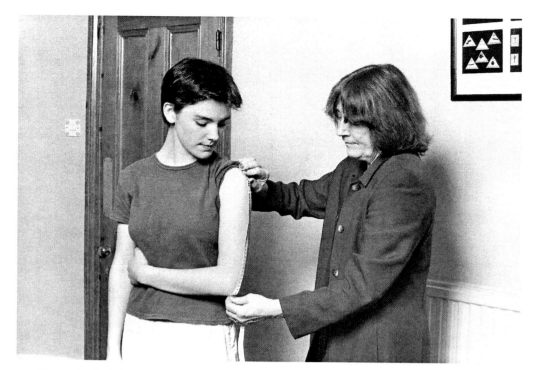

Figure 3(a)   Measurement of mid upper-arm circumference - length of upper arm

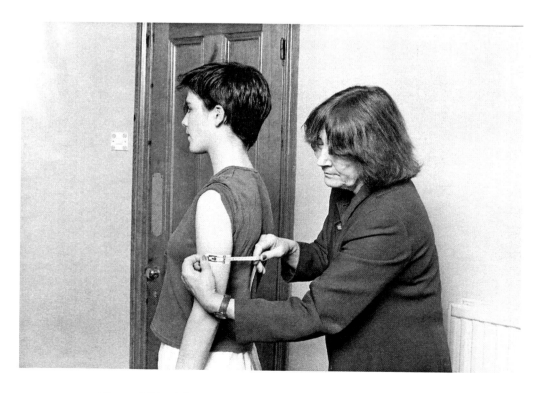

Figure 3(b)   Measurement of mid upper-arm circumference

710

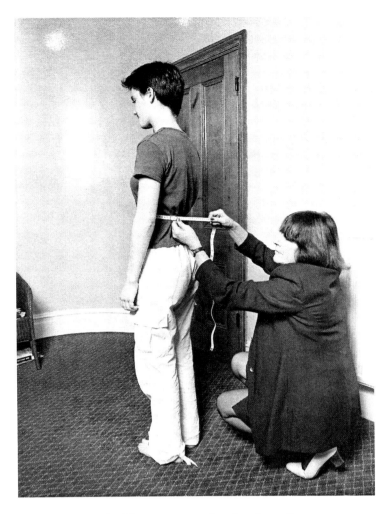

Figure 4   Measurement of waist circumference

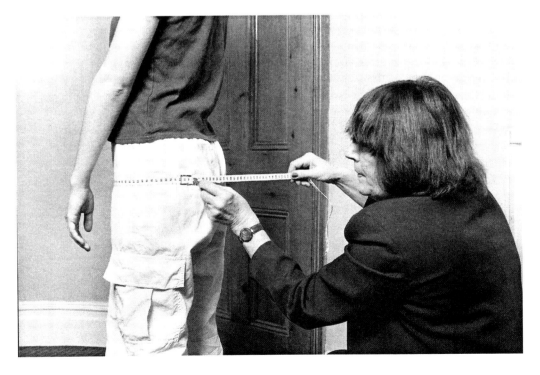

Figure 5   Measurement of hip circumference

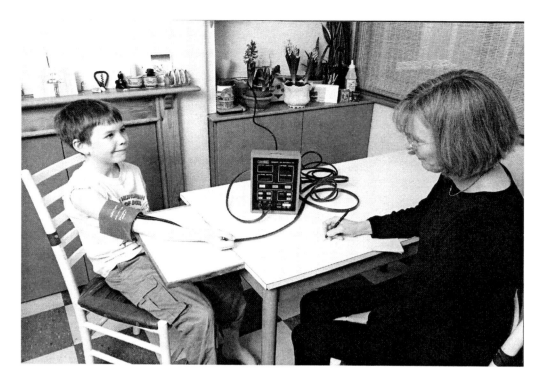

Figure 6   Measurement of blood pressure

Appendix M

Consent forms and information sheets on blood and EMLA cream

Consent forms

GP notification consent form	Z1
GP notification letter	Z2
Blood pressure	Z3
Blood sample	Z4
NHSCR flagging	Z5

Blood sample

Blood sample information leaflet	L4
List of blood analytes	L5
EMLA Cream – information sheet	X1
EMLA Cream screening question	H
EMLA Cream prescription form	X3

GP notification consent form

Tel: 0171 533 5387/8

DUNN NUTRITION UNIT
Tel: 01223 420959

Z1

NATIONAL DIET AND NUTRITION SURVEY: YOUNG PEOPLE AGED 4 TO 18 YEARS
GP NOTIFICATION

Today's date

[ ][ ][ ]

Day   Month   Year

Address label

(if incorrect - use serial number label and write in correct address)

Name of young person: ....
Mr/Mrs/Miss/Ms/Master   First name   Surname   (BLOCK CAPITALS)

Marital status: Single / Married

Gender: Male / Female

Date of birth

[ ][ ][ ]

Day   Month   Year

Age last birthday : [ ] years

Name of parent/ guardian ....
Mr/Mrs/Miss/Ms   First name   Surname   (BLOCK CAPITALS)

Address *(if different from young person's address)* : ....

....   Postcode ....

GP DETAILS:

Name of young person's GP: Dr. .... (BLOCK CAPITALS)

Address of GP: ....

....   Postcode ....

Telephone number (incl. Area Code): ....

Interviewer use only   Ring one code

Consent to notify GP given   1
No GP   2
Consent to notify GP refused   3

Wave 3/4

Copies: GP/ DNU /ONS

GP notification letter

Tel: 0171 533 5387/8

DUNN NUTRITION UNIT
Tel: 01223 420959

Z2

Dear Dr. ....

National Diet and Nutrition Survey: Young People aged 4 -1 8 Years

I am writing to let you know that the young person, whose details are given on the enclosed form, and who is one of your patients, has agreed to take part in the forthcoming National Diet and Nutrition Survey. For young people under the age of 18 years, still living at home, permission to take part in the study will have been given by their parent or legal guardian.

This survey of young people is the third in a programme of surveillance of diet and nutrition which will eventually cover the whole age range of the population. The survey has been commissioned jointly by the Departments of Health and the Ministry of Agriculture, Fisheries and Food and is being carried out by the Office for National Statistics with the Medical Research Council's Dunn Nutrition Unit. The Dental Schools at the Universities of Birmingham and Newcastle are collaborating in those parts of the survey concerned with the oral health of the young people.

The survey will include a random sample of about 2000 young people living in private households in Great Britain. Fieldwork will take place from January to December 1997. I am enclosing a leaflet which has been left with the young person and their family describing the aims and what is involved.

As part of the survey young people are asked to co-operate in providing a blood sample and having their blood pressure measured. The Dunn Nutrition Unit is responsible for all the procedures associated with obtaining and analysing the blood samples. These will be analysed for haemoglobin and ferritin concentrations and for other diet-related analytes. Consent will be sought, depending on the age of the young person, from themselves or their parent/guardian for me to pass on the results of the blood sample analyses and the blood pressure measurement to you at a later date. The subjects are advised that such information becomes part of their medical record and will not be revealed in medical reports by you without their permission.

I can assure you that the protocol for this survey has been examined and approved by the Local Research Ethics Committee of your Area Health Authority, Director for Primary Care or the equivalent in your local Health Authority, Directors of Public Health (CAMO'S in Scotland). The protocol has also been approved by Royal College of Paediatrics and Child Health. Your Chief Constable has also been informed that the survey is taking place, although not all the names of the young people taking part. The procedures included in this survey were all previously used successfully in a recently completed feasibility study.

We have been asked by the Royal College of Paediatrics and Child Health to offer EMLA cream for the venepuncture. We shall request information from the subjects about any anaesthetic allergies. I may contact you if I require any more detailed information. If you know of any relevant information, please contact me via the Survey Office.

I hope that this covering letter provides sufficient explanation for you: should you require any further information please contact Mrs Adrienne Griffin, telephone number 01223 420959, who will be pleased to help you.

Yours sincerely,

Lisa Jackson BSc (Nutrition), MRCGP, DCH
Survey Doctor
enc:

Blood pressure

NATIONAL STATISTICS
OFFICE FOR

Tel: 0171 533 5387/8

DUNN NUTRITION UNIT
Tel: 01223 420959

**NATIONAL DIET AND NUTRITION SURVEY: YOUNG PEOPLE AGED 4 TO 18 YEARS
BLOOD PRESSURE CONSENT FORM**

Serial number label

Name of
young person..   Gender: M / F

Age last birthday ☐

Date of birth

Day	Month	Year

....(BLOCK CAPITALS)

Name of parent/guardian: Mr/Mrs/Miss/Ms...(BLOCK CAPITALS)

I ....
Mr/Mrs/Miss/Ms

- understand that this survey is designed to add to medical knowledge which will help other young people,
- have read the information about the survey, have had time to consider it, and have had the survey explained to me to my satisfaction;
- have been told that I may withdraw my consent to any or all of the survey elements at any time, without needing to give a reason, and without prejudice to further medical treatment;
- have been told that none of the results from the survey will be presented in any way that can be associated with the name and address of anyone in this household;
- have been given a telephone number for further information about the survey, which is 01223 420959 (Dunn Survey Office);

and hereby consent to the Dunn Nutrition Unit informing the above-named young person's GP of their blood pressure measurement.

For young person aged 4 -15 years:
Signature of parent/guardian.   Date................

For young person aged 16 - 17 years:
Signature of young person.   Date................
and, if living at home
Signature of parent/guardian.   Date................

For young person aged 18 years:
*Signature of young
person.*   Date................

PLEASE RECORD BLOOD PRESSURE RESULTS BELOW

BP readings

Systolic (mm Hg)

Diastolic (mm Hg)

1st reading→

2nd reading→

3rd reading→

NATIONAL STATISTICS

NATIONAL DIET AND NUTRITION SURVEY

Z4

Tel: 0171 533 5387/8   DUNN NUTRITION UNIT
Tel: 01223 420959

NATIONAL DIET AND NUTRITION SURVEY: YOUNG PEOPLE AGED 4 TO 18 YEARS

BLOOD SAMPLE CONSENT FORM

Serial number label

Name of young person: ....

Gender: M / F ☐

Age last birthday ☐

Date of birth ☐☐ ☐☐ ☐☐
Day Month Year
(BLOCK CAPITALS)

Name of parent/guardian Mr/Mrs/Miss/Ms .... (BLOCK CAPITALS)

I .... (BLOCK CAPITALS) Mr/Mrs/Miss/Ms

* understand that this survey is designed to add to medical knowledge which will help other young people;

* have read the information about the survey, have had time to consider it, and have had the survey explained to me to my satisfaction;

* have been told that I may withdraw my consent to any or all of the survey elements at any time, without needing to give a reason, and without prejudice to further medical treatment;

* have been told that none of the results from the survey will be presented in any way that can be associated with the name and address of anyone in this household;

* have been given a telephone number for further information about the survey, which is 01223 420959 (Dunn Survey Office);

and hereby consent to the young person taking part in the following aspects of the survey:

(A) For young person aged 4 -15 years:

• providing a blood sample for analyses which are related to nutrition

Signature of
parent/guardian.. Date..................
and
Signature of witness (not
member of Survey Team).. Date..................
(Record details at D below)

• permitting the Dunn Nutrition Unit to inform the young person's GP of the results of the survey

Signature of
parent/guardian.. Date..................

• for any remaining blood to be stored and analysed for analyses related to nutrition in the future

---

Signature of
parent/guardian.. Date..................

(B) For young person aged 16 - 17 years:

• providing a blood sample for analyses which are related to nutrition

Signature of
young person.. Date..................
and, if living at home
Signature of
parent/guardian.. Date..................

Signature of witness (not
member of Survey Team).. Date..................
(Record details at D below)

• permitting the Dunn Nutrition Unit to inform the young person's GP of the results of the survey

Signature of
young person.. Date..................
and, if living at home
Signature of
parent/guardian.. Date..................

• for any remaining blood to be stored and analysed for analyses related to nutrition in the future

Signature of
young person.. Date..................
and, if living at home
Signature of
parent/guardian.. Date..................

(C) For young person aged 18 years:

• providing a blood sample for analyses which are related to nutrition

Signature of
young person..
and
Signature of witness (not
member of Survey Team).. Date..................
(Record details at D below)

• permitting the Dunn Nutrition Unit to inform the young person's GP of the results of the survey

Signature of
young person.. Date..................

• for any remaining blood to be stored and analysed for analyses related to nutrition in the future

Signature of
young person.. Date..................

(D) To be completed for all witnessed signatures:

Name of witness.. (BLOCK CAPITALS)

Address of witness..

.... PostCode..................

NATIONAL STATISTICS

Tel: 0171 533 5387/8

DUNN NUTRITION UNIT
Tel: 01223 420959

NATIONAL DIET AND
NUTRITION SURVEY

Z5

NATIONAL DIET AND NUTRITION SURVEY: YOUNG PEOPLE AGED 4 TO 18 YEARS

CONSENT TO FLAG ON NHSCR

Serial number label

Name of young person, in full .... (BLOCK CAPITALS)

Previous names of young person, in full (if any) .... (BLOCK CAPITALS)

Gender   M / F

Date of birth
Day   Month   Year

National Health Number

Age last birthday

Name of parent/guardian
Mr/Mrs/Miss/Ms ....

I hereby consent to the above-named young person's name being flagged on the NHS Central Register for the purposes of future research.

SIGNATURES

For young person aged 4 -15 years:

Signature of parent/guardian ....
        Date ....

For young person aged 16 - 17 years:

Signature of young person ....
        Date ....

and, if living at home

Signature of parent/guardian ....
        Date ....

For young person aged 18 years:

Signature of young person ....
        Date ....

Copies DNU/SUBJECT/ONS
            Wave 2

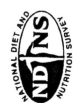

THE BLOOD SAMPLE: WHAT IS IT FOR, AND WHAT WILL HAPPEN?

What is it for?

Everyone's blood is a little bit different. Your blood is a very special part of you, and it can tell us very important things about your health, and about the ways your body benefits from the food you eat.

A blood sample is an important part of the survey. By using modern hospital laboratory methods, we will be able to measure a very wide range of things in your blood. We can look at the blood cells, which carry oxygen and help fight disease, and we can measure fats (like cholesterol); vitamins; important trace minerals; proteins, etc. All these measurements will help add to the information that we will get from the other records of what you eat, and how healthy you are, and all of the measurements will be related to nutrition.

Is it compulsory?

Anyone has the right to refuse. To protect your rights and to ensure that we have your considered opinion, we need to have signed and/or witnessed consent for blood taking from yourself and/or your parent/guardian, depending on how old you are. Even after signing, you can still withdraw your permission, or ask the blood taker to stop at any time.

What will happen?

If you do agree to the blood sample, then the interviewer will arrange for a specially-trained blood-taker, called a "phlebotomist", who works at a nearby hospital, to come with them and take the sample. The interviewer will come with the blood taker to your home; you do not need to go to the hospital or to a doctor.

We would like to take the sample early in the morning, before you have had anything to eat or drink. This is called a "fasting sample", and it gives the very best possible information, especially about the fats in your blood. The blood will be taken from a vein on the inside of your arm, just about where the crease is when you bend your elbow.

Does there need to be more than one needle-prick in my arm?

Almost certainly not. Although the blood-taker will need to fill four different tubes, this can usually be done from one single needle-prick. Experience tells us what size needle is best for each person (the smaller the needle, the less it hurts, but the longer it takes to fill the tubes). The amount of blood that we take is less than one hundredth part of the blood in your body, and is very quickly replaced by new blood. If you would like more information, do talk to the blood-taker about it, and ask him or her to explain it all, beforehand. Very occasionally, if the blood taker cannot fill all four tubes from one needle-prick, you may asked if you are willing for the blood taker to try again on your other arm. As before, you have a perfect right to refuse, if you are at all worried about it.

Will I get any information back about my results?

Yes, those measurements that are most directly related to your health will be sent back to you, and also to your doctor (for his or her records about you), if you agree. Some of these results should reach you (by post) within a few weeks; others will take a few months, because it takes time to gather and analyse all of the survey samples from all over the country.

THANK YOU FOR YOUR CO-OPERATION.

Social Survey Division Office for National Statistics 1 Drummond Gate London SW1V 2QQ
Telephone 0171 533 5387/8

L4

List of blood analytes

NATIONAL DIET AND NUTRITION SURVEY
ND NS

BLOOD ANALYSES FOR YOUNG PEOPLE AGED 4 TO 18 YEARS

The blood sample will be sent to medical laboratories at Great Ormond Street Hospital in London, in Southampton and in Cambridge, for a number of measurements; these include:

FATS: such as cholesterol

PROTEINS: such as alkaline phosphatase, to measure bone health

VITAMINS: including vitamins A, B, C D and E

MINERALS: such as iron, zinc, magnesium and lead

CELLS: red and white blood cells

OTHERS: such as urea, which measures kidney function, and, for boys, testosterone, which measures stage of development.

The blood sample will NOT be used now, or in the future, to look for infections, such as AIDS or Hepatitis.

L5

EMLA Cream – information sheet

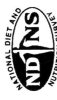

DUNN NUTRITION UNIT
Tel 01223 420959

EMLA CREAM

Everyone who takes part in this survey and agrees to provide a blood sample has the choice of having EMLA CREAM used before the sample is taken.

This leaflet tells you about what the cream does and how it works.

It is important to remember that you do NOT have to have the cream applied; it is up to you to decide.

• *What is Emla Cream?*

It is a white cream, which, when it is put on the skin and left for a while, makes the skin go numb; this means that the slight scratch when the needle pricks the skin is hardly felt.

• *How long does it take to work?*

The cream works best if it is left on the skin for at least an hour, and it needs to be kept covered. This means that you will probably have to get up a bit earlier to have the cream applied before the blood sample is taken. Usually the person who is going to take the blood sample will apply the cream, but it may be possible for you or your parent to be given the cream to apply before the blood taker calls.

Once the blood sample has been taken you can then bath, shower and carry on doing all the things that you would usually do. The effect of the cream will wear off slowly during the day.

• *Can Emla Cream be used on anyone?*

Emla Cream is very safe. People who are allergic or have a bad reaction to local or general anaesthetics are the only ones who should not have Emla Cream applied. If you decide you would like to have the cream applied, the interviewer will check with you that it is safe for you to have the cream, BEFORE it is applied.

We would not apply the cream to any skin which was sore or broken or an area on the skin where there was eczema.

• *Are there any side effects?*

Sometimes the area where the cream has been applied goes white, and on some people the skin goes a bit red. Neither of these effects is serious or harmful and they will wear off as the effect of the cream wears off.

Some people know that they have a allergy to some types of plaster; if you have this, please tell us and we will make sure that the plaster used to cover the blood sample is the right kind for you.

Please remember that you do not have to use Emla Cream. It is your choice. If you have any questions about Emla Cream, or if you are worried about any aspect of the blood sample you can speak to the person who would take the blood sample, before you make up your mind

X1

emlaint/w4

EMLA Cream screening question

H

Emla Cream generally should not be used if a young person has an allergic reaction to anaesthetics.

Please carefully read the question below and tell the interviewer your answer.

Has the young person who will be giving this blood sample ever had a bad reaction to any sort of anaesthetic - that includes:

- a general anaesthetic at the dentist or hospital;

- a local anaesthetic at the doctor, dentist or hospital;

- a local anaesthetic cream bought over the counter at a chemist and applied at home?

If the answer to any one of these is 'Yes', please tell the interviewer about the allergic reaction. The interviewer will check with the Survey Doctor to see whether the young person will be able to have Emla Cream.

Please note that if you wish the young person may still give a blood sample, without the Cream.

EMLA Cream prescription form

DUNN NUTRITION UNIT
Tel: 01223 420969

X3

Prescription for EMLA

PART I
TO BE COMPLETED BY THE INTERVIEWER

Serial Number Label

Name of young person ....

Address: ....
....

Post Code: ....

Date of Birth: Day   Month   Year

The young person and/or parent has confirmed that there is no known allergy to anaesthetics

Signature of Interviewer: .... **Date:**

Name of Interviewer: .... *block capitals*

If in doubt, please contact the Survey Doctor

TO BE COMPLETED BY THE SURVEY DOCTOR

EMLA CREAM 5G

TOPICAL FOR VENEPUNCTURE
DO NOT APPLY TO BROKEN SKIN

Signature of Survey Doctor: .... **Date:**
....

Please detach here after venepuncture

PART 2
TO BE COMPLETED BY PHLEBOTOMIST

EMLA CREAM 5G USED FOR YOUNG PERSON   **X3**

Serial Number Label

Signature of Phlebotomist:........................... Date: ....
Please list any problems encountered in the venepuncture or in the use of EMLA cream below:

Appendix N

Blood and blood pressure results reported to subjects and General Practitioners: normal ranges and copies of letters[1]

The following results were reported to the young person and his or her GP. For each result the normal ranges are shown. Any result for an individual, which was outside the normal range, was indicated by an asterisk in the letter to the young person and GP.

Age (and sex)	Results and normal ranges	
	Blood pressure (mmHg)–all three readings[2]	
	systolic	diastolic
4 yrs to less than 6 yrs	less than 116mmHg	less than 76mmHg
6 yrs to less than 10 yrs	less than 122mmHg	less than 78mmHg
10 yrs to less than 13 yrs	less than 126mmHg	less than 82mmHg
13 yrs to less than 16 yrs	less than 136 mmHg	less than 86mmHg
16 yrs to less than 19 yrs	less than 142mmHg	less than 92mmHg
	Blood haemoglobin (g/dl)	**Blood haematocrit (l/l)**
4 yrs to less than 7 yrs	11.5–13.5g/dl	0.34–0.40l/l
7 yrs to less than 13 yrs	11.5–15.5g/dl	0.35–0.45l/l
girls: 13 yrs and over	12.0–16.0g/dl	0.36–0.46l/l
boys: 13 yrs and over	13.0–16.0g/dl	0.37–0.49l/l
	Mean cell volume (fl)	**Platelet count (x 10^9/l)**
4 yrs and over	75–95fl	150–450 x 10^9/l
	White cell count (x 10^9/l)	**Plasma cholesterol (mmol/l)**
4 yrs and over	4-15 x 10^9/l	less than 6.5mmol/l
	Serum folate (µg/l)[3]	**Serum B$_{12}$ (ng/l)**
less than 12 yrs	greater than 2µg/l	greater than 210ng/l
12 yrs and over	greater than 3µg/l	greater than 150ng/l
	Serum ferritin (µg/l)	
4 yrs to less than 6 yrs	12–200µg/l	
6 yrs to less than 15 yrs	13–200µg/l	
girls: 15 yrs and over	13–200µg/l	
boys: 15 yrs and over	13–300µg/l	
	Plasma iron saturation (%)	
less than 6 yrs	10–50%	
6 yrs to less than 15 yrs	13–50%	
girls: 15 yrs and over	16–60%	
boys: 15 yrs and over	16–50%	
	Plasma 25-hydroxyvitamin D (nmol/l)	**lead (µg/dl)**
4 yrs and over	greater than 12.5nmol/l	less than 10µg/dl

Endnotes

[1] The letters reproduced are those used if the young person was aged 16 years or over and provided a sample of blood for analysis as well as having his or her blood pressure measured. Suitably modified versions of these letters were used if the young person was aged under 16 years (addressed to the parent) and if blood pressure was measured but no blood sample provided.

[2] Reference ranges were based on values reported in: National Heart, Lung and Blood Institute, Bethesda, Maryland, US. Report of the Second Task Force on Blood Pressure Control in Children – 1987. *Paediatrics* 1987; **79**: (1). They were provided for GPs as a guide since the methodologies for this survey and the reported studies differ and hence are not strictly comparable (see *Chapter 11: 11.1.2*).

[3] Reference ranges for serum folate, as µg/l, were supplied by Great Ormond Street Hospital and reported to GPs in these units. In Chapter 11 results for serum folate are shown as nmol/l. For the conversion factor see *Appendix O*.

Dunn Nutrition Centre

patron: **HRH The Princess Royal**

Please reply to:-
Dunn Nutritional Laboratory
Downhams Lane
Milton Road
Cambridge
CB4 1XJ

tel: (01223) 426356
fax: (01223) 426617

NDNS: **Survey Office**

Direct: (01223) 420959

tel/fax: (01223) 423575

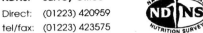

1997

REF: [   ]

Dear [   ]

RE: [   ] [   ] DOB: [   ]

You will recall that the above named individual, who is one of your patients, is participating in the National Diet and Nutrition Survey and has given consent that you should be informed of the results of the blood and blood pressure measurements.

The current results available are enclosed. These have been marked * where values fall outside the attached normal ranges for this age group, and where an abnormality of clinical significance is possible. The young person has been informed of the results, and may contact you to discuss them.

Where no result is given, analysis was not possible due to either an insufficient volume of blood being obtained or technical reasons. Where no abnormality is indicated, the young person has been informed that their results fall within the normal range.

Isolated apparently abnormal blood pressure measurements in young people are unlikely to have clinical significance unless repeated on a number of occasions. The height and weight must be taken into account. Family history may also be relevant in your assessment. If you require references or more detailed information on blood pressure in childhood, please let me know.

To achieve consistent results some analyses are done in batches and hence further blood analyses will be available later. These will include plasma lipids, 25-hydroxy vitamin D, % iron saturation and lead and will also be reported to you.

Should you have any questions regarding the above, or any other matters relating to the survey, please do not hesitate to contact me by pager: Tel: 01426 620185 or alternatively you can contact the Survey Manager, Mrs. Adrienne Griffin, at our office on (01223) 420959.

Yours sincerely,

Dr. Lisa Jackson
Survey Doctor

Medical Research Council and the University of Cambridge

725

Dunn Nutrition Centre

patron: **HRH The Princess Royal**

Please reply to:-
Dunn Nutritional Laboratory
Downhams Lane
Milton Road
Cambridge
CB4 1XJ

tel: (01223) 426356
fax: (01223) 426617

NDNS: Survey Office

Direct: (01223) 420959
tel/fax: (01223) 423575

1997

REF: [ ]

CONFIDENTIAL

Dear [ ]

Re: NDNS: Young People aged 4 - 18 Years

You will doubtless remember taking part recently in the National Diet and Nutrition Survey. As part of the survey, you were kind enough to consent to giving a blood sample and various measurements.

The results which are now available are enclosed. Where none of the results are marked * all the results fall within the normal range for a person of your age. Where no result is given, analysis was not possible due to either an insufficient volume of blood being obtained or technical reasons.

Those results marked with a star (*) may be higher or lower than would be expected for a person of your age. It is possible that these results may be significant for your future health and you may wish to contact your doctor to discuss the results which are marked with *.

One blood pressure which appears unusually high or low is not important unless it is repeated on several occasions. Your doctor can measure it again for you if necessary and will know what is important about you. For example, tall people have higher blood pressures than shorter ones. If you have any worries, the best person to speak to is your doctor.

The survey will obtain some further measurements from the blood sample. We will be sending you a list of these results, for your information, when they are available. However this will take several months, therefore if you are likely to move house, or wish to give an alternative address to which these should be sent (to cover a period of up to 12 months) please could you complete the enclosed form and return it in the reply paid envelope provided.

Thank you for your kind help with the survey.

Yours sincerely,

Dr. Lisa Jackson
Survey Doctor

Medical Research Council and the University of Cambridge

Appendix O

Blood analytes in priority order for analysis, and urine analytes

Analyte	Unit of measurement	Conversion from SI units (factor)	Resulting metric units
Haematology			
Haemoglobin concentration	g/dl	*	
Red blood cell count	$\times 10^{12}$/l	*	
Haematocrit	l/l	*	
Mean cell volume	fl	*	
Mean cell haemoglobin	pg	*	
Mean cell haemoglobin concentration	g/dl	*	
Red cell distribution width	%	n/a	
Platelet count	$\times 10^9$/l	*	
Mean platelet volume	fl	*	
Platelet distribution width	%	n/a	
White cell count	$\times 10^9$/l	*	
Neutrophil count	$\times 10^9$/l	*	
Lymphocyte count	$\times 10^9$/l	*	
Monocyte count	$\times 10^9$/l	*	
Eosinophil count	$\times 10^9$/l	*	
Basophil count	$\times 10^9$/l	*	
Haemoglobin electrophoresis			
HbF	%	n/a	
HbA$_2$	%	n/a	
Serum folate	nmol/l	$\times$ 0.441	µg/l
Red cell folate	nmol/l	$\times$ 0.441	µg/l
Serum vitamin B$_{12}$	pmol/l	$\times$ 1.357	ng/l
Serum ferritin	µg/l	*	
Blood lead	µg/dl	*	
Plasma selenium	µmol/l	$\times$ 0.079	mg/l
Plasma magnesium	mmol/l	$\times$ 24.3	mg/l
Plasma 25-hydroxyvitamin D	nmol/l	$\times$ 0.400	µg/l
Blood lipids			
Plasma total cholesterol	mmol/l	$\times$ 0.387	g/l
Plasma high density lipoprotein cholesterol	mmol/l	$\times$ 0.387	g/l
Non-HDL cholesterol	mmol/l	$\times$ 0.387	g/l
Plasma triglycerides	mmol/l	†	
Plasma iron	µmol/l	$\times$ 55.8	µg/l
Plasma total iron binding capacity	µmol/l	$\times$ 55.8	µg/l
Plasma iron % saturation	%	n/a	
Plasma retinol	µmol/l	$\times$ 0.286	mg/l
Plasma retinyl palmitate	µmol/l	$\times$ 0.525	mg/l
Plasma α-tocopherol	µmol/l	$\times$ 0.552	mg/l
Plasma γ-tocopherol	µmol/l	$\times$ 0.417	mg/l
Plasma α-cryptoxanthin	µmol/l	$\times$ 0.552	mg/l
Plasma ß-cryptoxanthin	µmol/l	$\times$ 0.552	mg/l
Plasma lycopene	µmol/l	$\times$ 0.537	mg/l
Plasma lutein + zeaxanthin	µmol/l	$\times$ 0.569	mg/l
Plasma α-carotene	µmol/l	$\times$ 0.537	mg/l
Plasma ß-carotene	µmol/l	$\times$ 0.537	mg/l
Plasma vitamin C	µmol/l	$\times$ 0.176	mg/l

Analyte	Unit of measurement	Conversion from SI units (factor)	Resulting metric units
Erythrocyte transketolase:			
basal activity	µmol/g Hb/min	*	
activation coefficient	ratio	n/a	
Erythrocyte glutathione reductase			
activation coefficient	ratio	n/a	
Erythrocyte aspartate transaminase			
activation coefficient	ratio	n/a	
Plasma urea	mmol/l	× 60	mg/l
Plasma zinc	µmol/l	× 0.065	mg/l
Plasma testosterone	nmol/l	× 0.289	µg/l
Plasma alkaline phosphatase	IU/l	*	
Plasma alpha$_1$-antichymotrypsin	g/l	*	
Red cell superoxide dismutase	nmol/mg Hb/min	*	
Plasma creatinine	µmol/l	× 0.113	mg/l
Red cell glutathione peroxidase	nmol/mg Hb/min	*	
Urinary analytes			
Urine sodium	mmol/l	× 23	mg/l
Urine potassium	mmol/l	× 39.1	mg/l
Urine creatinine	mmol/l	× 113	mg/l
Urine sodium: creatinine ratio	ratio	n/a	
Urine potassium: creatinine ratio	ratio	n/a	

*   Analyte measured in metric units.

†   Trigylcerides are measured as glycerol; the molecular weight of a glycerol molecule varies with the different fatty acid constituents. Conversion from SI to metric units is not appropriate.

n/a   not applicable.

Appendix P

The blood sample: collecting and processing the blood

This appendix gives further information about the blood sampling procedure including details of the selection and training of the phlebotomists, the fieldwork procedures for obtaining the blood, the local laboratory procedures for processing blood samples, and the system for reporting the clinically-significant results to the young person or their parents or guardians[1] and to the young person's General Practitioners (GPs). All the procedures associated with obtaining and analysing the blood samples were contracted to the Dunn Nutrition Unit (DNU).

All the procedures associated with the blood sample, except for the use of EMLA cream prior to venepuncture, were tested in the feasibility study, and found to be suitable for use in the main stage[2].

Ethics Committee Approvals

The DNU sought approval for the survey procedures from the Local National Health Service Research Ethics Committees (LRECs), covering each of the 132 fieldwork areas. Ethical approval was sought specifically for taking a venepuncture blood sample (15ml max) for nutritional status analyses; storing the residue of blood for further analyses and flagging on the NHS Central Register. However, LREC approval was required for the entire survey package and LRECs considered the adequacy of the procedures adopted for all other survey components as well. All committees approached gave approval, although a small number required some minor alterations to the proposed protocol. The survey protocol was also scrutinised and approved by the Standing Ethics Advisory Committee of the Royal College of Paediatrics and Child Health, which recommended the use of EMLA cream to minimise discomfort. The protocol was also approved by the Ethics Committee of the Dunn Nutrition Unit.

Consent

Signed consent was required for each young person for:
- taking a venous blood sample;
- reporting the clinically significant results to the young person's GP;
- storing any unused sample, for possible nutritional analyses at some time in the future.

The signatures required varied according to the young person's age; for young people aged 4 to 15 years signed consent was sought from a parent or guardian. Young people aged 16 to 18 years were able to sign the form on their own behalf. However, for those aged 16 to 17 years and living with their family, signed consent was also sought from a parent or guardian. Young people and their parents were told that they were free to withdraw their consent to the blood sample at any point, even after the consent form had been signed and young people who did not assent to the procedure had their wishes respected, even if consent had been obtained from a parent or guardian.

To ensure that consent was not obtained under duress, signatures needed to be independently witnessed by someone other than a member of the survey team or the young person's household.

Consents obtained are summarised in Table P1 below:

Table P1 Consent to blood taking by fieldwork wave

	Fieldwork wave								Total	
	1: Jan–March		2: April–June		3: July–Sept		4:Oct–Dec			
	No.	*%*	*No.*	*%*	*No.*	*%*	*No.*	*%*	*No.*	*%*
Consented to blood taking/GP	*258*	*59*	*232*	*51*	*404*	*67*	*328*	*65*	*1222*	*59*
of whom: consented to blood being stored		*99*		*97*		*97*		*98*		*98*
No. young people giving GP details	*435*		*415*		*602*		*568*		*2056*	

The provision of local anaesthetic for venepuncture

EMLA cream (Astra Pharmaceuticals Ltd.), which is a local anaesthetic cream containing lidocaine (lignocaine) and prilocaine, was offered to all respondents who agreed to give a blood sample. EMLA cream is a prescription only medicine, and it was prescribed by the survey doctor using a postal prescription procedure primarily in order to exclude respondents with a known allergy or adverse reaction to related drugs. Any respondent with a known allergy to the components of EMLA was advised by the interviewer, via the survey doctor, not to have EMLA cream applied as a precaution. The interviewer sent an EMLA request form to the survey doctor who signed the 'prescription' having checked that there were no contraindications, and returned it by post to the interviewer. It was then available to the phlebotomist in readiness for the venepuncture procedure. EMLA cream was, if possible, applied over both ante-cubital fossae, covered with a dressing and left for one hour before venepuncture. EMLA was not applied to damaged skin, for example where the young person had eczema. EMLA was applied by either the phlebotomist, a family member or in some cases the young person themselves.

Exclusion from participation in venepuncture

Before venepuncture, questions were asked to ensure exclusion of any respondents with known clotting or bleeding disorders. In view of the existence of two reports of Suspected Adverse Reactions to the Medicine Control Agency (yellow card reports) of generalised seizures associated with EMLA use, young persons known to have generalised tonic-clonic fits were also excluded to minimise the possibility of an adverse reaction.

The use of EMLA is summarised below in Table P2.

Equipment used

The blood samples were collected by the phlebotomist using the Sarstedt Monovette blood-collection system with butterfly or fixed needle, according to preference. The Monovette system of blood collection is an enclosed system which allows the safe, spill-free collection of blood which is critical in the home environment. It can also offer trace element contamination control and is manufactured from plastic which allows the safe transport of the sample, inside an outer container, through the postal system.

The DNU provided each phlebotomist with the following equipment:

Carrying box
Sharp safe box
Tegaderm dressings for use with EMLA cream
Plasters
Tissues
Tourniquet (adjustable)
Stasis pads
Cold box plus two freezer packs
Disposable gloves
Cryo-pen
Milton disinfectant
Steri-swabs
Parcel tape
Pair of scissors
Micropore tape (for butterfly)
Minigrip bags:
biohazard-labelled for contaminated waste NDNS-labelled, to wrap cold packs before freezing and to contain samples within cold box.
Plastic postal containers for blood samples
Stamped, labelled jiffy bag envelopes, addressed to Great Ormond Street (GOS) and Southampton laboratories
Sarstedt monovettes: 2.7 ml EDTA; 1.2 ml serum (beads); 9.0 ml trace element controlled heparin
Sarstedt butterfly needles: 21G and 23G 60mm tube length, 21G 300mm tube length
Sarstedt fixed needles: 21G, 22G
5 ml plain capped tubes, for the plasma after blood separation in the laboratory
EMLA anaesthetic cream for use when prescribed by the survey doctor.

Phlebotomy: training, procedures, instructions, backup

Phlebotomists were employed only if they had recent experience of phlebotomy in young people. Suitable phlebotomists were sought via recommendations from Consultant Haematologists in hospitals in the fieldwork

Table P2   Use of EMLA by fieldwork wave

| | Fieldwork wave | | | | | | | | Total | |
| | 1: Jan–March | | 2: April–June | | 3: July–Sept | | 4:Oct–Dec | | | |
	No.	%	No.	%	No.	%	No.	%	No.	%
No. of samples where EMLA used of which:	55	21	50	23	108	27	81	24	294	25
EMLA applied by phlebotomist		n/a		48		44		41		n/a
No. of blood samples obtained	252		217		392		301		1162	

n/a Information not available.

areas and a written reference was obtained from their current or previous employer to ensure their suitability. Each phlebotomist was provided with specific training on the Sarstedt Monovette system, both at the training courses before each wave of the fieldwork and also, if necessary, by Sarstedt Ltd. The training was provided by the survey doctor and the DNU survey team. The phlebotomists were also provided with a full set of written instructions, record forms, and a checklist reminder of the sequence of the procedures. A total of 79 phlebotomists were employed during the survey.

ONS interviewers were responsible for making the arrangements for the phlebotomy visit to the young person's home, and the phlebotomists were always accompanied in the home by an ONS interviewer. Prior to phlebotomy, the phlebotomist was responsible for contacting the local laboratory to which blood would be taken, to ensure the availability of laboratory staff.

The blood sample was required, wherever possible, to be an early morning 'fasted' sample, to be taken immediately after an overnight fast and before breakfast. The phlebotomist was instructed to check this, and to note any exceptions.

As local laboratory processing facilities were generally not available on Saturdays the samples could only be collected on weekdays from Monday to Thursday inclusive, and not on Bank Holidays.

All sample tubes were labelled with the subject's serial number; these were pre-printed using waterproof ink on adhesive labels designed to withstand moisture and temperatures down to -80°C.

The phlebotomist, carried out the procedures in the following order:

Before visit

- obtain appointment details from interviewer;
- contact local laboratory;
- freeze cold pack;
- prepare necessary blood taking equipment, record forms and postal containers.

At visit
- obtain copy of signed blood sample consent form from interviewer (Z4);
- obtain serial number labels from interviewer;
- ask whether the young person has a clotting or bleeding disorder or if (s)he is epileptic - **IF SO DISCONTINUE VISIT**;
- apply EMLA cream at least 1 hour before venepuncture or check that it has been applied as directed;
- obtain blood sample;
- fill tubes in priority order for GOS, Southampton and local laboratory;
- mix all samples by inversion;
- add serial number label to each tube;
- place blood samples in postal containers and jiffy bags;
- complete postal record forms for GOS and Southampton;
- complete phlebotomist record form.

Immediately after the visit

- post blood samples with record forms to GOS and Southampton;
- post completed phlebotomist record form, consent form copy and EMLA prescription, if any to DNU;
- either take blood sample and contaminated waste to the local laboratory in cold box or inform field lab if no blood sample was obtained.

The approved protocol allowed for two attempts at phlebotomy provided that the young person consented. Phlebotomists were advised on precautions to avoid and deal with any cases of fainting.

The number of bloods obtained are summarised in Table P3 below.

Liaison with, and procedures at, the local hospital laboratories

Several of the required analytes, particularly certain vitamins and vitamin status index analytes, are known to be very labile and therefore need to be stabilised, either by chemical treatment or by low temperature storage or both, at the earliest possible opportunity. This was done at the local laboratories.

Ideally local hospital laboratories needed to be close to the fieldwork areas, accessible by road, have appro-

Table P3   Number of blood samples obtained by fieldwork wave

	Fieldwork wave								Total	
	1: Jan–March		2: April–June		3: July–Sept		4:Oct–Dec			
	No.	*%*	*No.*	*%*	*No.*	*%*	*No.*	*%*	*No.*	*%*
No. of blood samples obtained of which:	252		217		392		301		1162	
fasted samples obtained	240	95	194	89	350	89	279	93	1063	92

priate staff availability, have a refrigerated centrifuge, and storage facilities at $-40°C$ or below. The local laboratories were usually at the hospital where the phlebotomist was based. In a few instances, because of the limited choice of laboratories it was necessary to relax the requirement for a chilled centrifuge, or to accept storage at $-25°C$. A total of 64 local laboratories were used for processing and storing blood samples during the study.

Each local laboratory was provided with the following items:

- written blood-processing instructions and record forms for each subject;

- aliquots of 10% w/v metaphosphoric acid for vitamin C stabilisation, in 2ml pre-labelled and colour-coded screw-cap containers.

The stabilising solutions, frozen in solid CO_2, were delivered from the DNU to the hospital laboratories, and were kept frozen until used.

Immediately upon receiving a young person's heparinised blood samples from the phlebotomist, the analyst was required to:

- transfer an aliquot of the whole blood to an empty container for the glutathione peroxidase assay (Waves 3 and 4 only);
- centrifuge the remaining blood at $4°C$ and then remove the plasma to an empty container;
- transfer an aliquot of plasma to the metaphosphoric acid container, for subsequent vitamin C analysis;
- wash the red cell pellets with normal saline to yield a red cell concentrate depleted of buffy coat;
- label and store all samples in a polythene bag at $-40°C$ or below;
- complete a record form for each sample giving processing dates, times and portions created;
- send the collected samples on dry ice, plus the associated paperwork to the DNU by a road transport carrier. This transfer occurred at the end of each wave of fieldwork and was organised by DNU.

Further subdivision, freezer filing and assay auditing

As soon as the blood sample fractions created at the local laboratory arrived at the DNU they were stored at $-80°C$. Their receipt and subject details were recorded in both a hard copy log book and computer spreadsheet and were cross checked against records of analysis performed by Great Ormond Street and Southampton University Laboratories.

After a single thawing, each plasma sample was further subdivided into discrete sub-samples for assays of:

- 25(OH)-vitamin D and other fat-soluble micronutrients (vitamins A, E and carotenoids);
- iron status;
- lipid profile;
- selected minerals;
- clinical chemistry analytes.

These samples were then filed in the storage freezer strictly in order of receipt. Analysis was conducted in a sequence so as to avoid bunching within the fieldwork areas, during each batch analysis. For each analyte type analytical work was performed in small batches, together with the appropriate quality controls and quality assurance samples. Each assay was performed in duplicate; if agreement between duplicates failed to meet the pre-set criteria for each assay, repeat assays were performed.

Reporting Procedures

Young people and their GP's were informed by letter of the results of a selected number of analytes. This letter also reported the blood pressure measurements for the young person where these had been taken. Letters to respondents listed only results while those sent to the GP had additionally a reference range for each analyte. On request, the survey doctor provided advice to GPs about the need for follow up tests. Any incidental abnormality of potential clinical significance was also separately reported to the GP.

Reference and endnote

[1] The term 'parent or guardian' denotes any person with parental responsibility, and therefore includes, for example, an unmarried father who acquired parental responsibility through the courts.

[2] See Appendix C and Lowe S. *Feasibility study for the National Diet and Nutrition Survey: young people aged 4 to 18 years.* ONS (*In preparation*)

Appendix Q

Methods of blood analysis and quality control

The assays described in 1, 2 and 3 below were conducted at the Department of Haematology, Great Ormond Street Hospital, London. Samples of coagulated and ethylenediaminetetraacetate (EDTA) anticoagulated blood were sent directly to the laboratory by post after their collection throughout fieldwork. Serum samples were obtained by centrifugation of the coagulated blood sample.

The assays described in 4 - 19 below were conducted at the Dunn Nutrition Unit in Cambridge. Samples of lithium heparin anticoagulated blood were collected and stored in a coolbox (at about 4°C) and delivered to a local processing laboratory in the locality of the fieldwork, typically within 5 hours of collection. These local laboratories undertook the processing and initial stabilisation of this blood sample into whole blood, red cells, plasma and metaphosphoric acid stabilised plasma portions. (The metaphosphoric acid had been previously prepared, aliquotted at the Dunn Nutrition Unit, and delivered to each local laboratory). The blood sample subfractions were stored frozen, typically at −40°C, at these laboratories until their removal, on dry ice, to the Dunn Nutrition Unit, Cambridge, where they were stored frozen at −80°C until further subdivided and analysed.

The assays described in 20, 21 and 22 below were conducted at the SAS Trace Element Unit at the University of Southampton. Samples of ethylenediaminetetraacetate (EDTA) anticoagulated blood were sent directly to the laboratory by post after their collection throughout fieldwork. Plasma samples were obtained by centrifugation of the anticoagulated blood sample.

1   Full Blood Count

Full Blood Counts were performed using a Bayer H3 Haematology Analyser. The analyser uses a colorimeter for measuring haemoglobin at wavelength 546nm. From samples of EDTA anticoagulated blood, red cells, white cells and platelets were diluted and hydro-dynamically focused through a flow cell and were counted using light and laser detection systems. The samples were analysed on the day of receipt.

Quality control procedures comprised both internal and external procedures. Daily internal quality control checks were used to establish the running means of the stable red cell indices, mean cell volume (MCV), mean cell haemoglobin (MCH) and mean cell haemoglobin concentration (MCHC) and daily commercial controls (Bayer Testpoint Haematology control) were used to monitor drift in all measured and calculated parameters. External quality assessment schemes included the National External Quality Assessment Scheme (NEQAS) for haematology and External Quality Assessment Scheme (EQAS) for haematology run by Addenbrookes Hospital, Cambridge.

2   Haemoglobin identification

Haemoglobin identification was achieved by separation and quantification using cation exchange high performance liquid chromatography (HPLC). 5µl of EDTA anticoagulated blood was haemolysed and analysed using the Bio-Rad Variant automated analyser. The percentages of each haemoglobin (Hb) type present, normally HbA, HbA_2 and HbF were reported. Where other haemoglobins were found, these were further identified using techniques normally employed for clinical purposes such as electrophoresis, sickle solubility and monoclonal antibodies to haemoglobin. The samples were analysed as soon as possible after receipt.

Quality control procedures comprised both internal and external procedures. Two haemoglobin variant controls with commercially assigned values were included on each run with samples. The NEQAS for haemoglobinopathies provided external control.

3   Serum ferritin, vitamin B_{12}, folate and red cell folate

These assays were performed on the Abbott IMx semi automated analyser which uses Microparticle Enzyme Immunoassay (MEIA) technology. Individual assay kits were used for each of the analytes, but all are based on the same principle. Microparticles coated with analyte specific 'capture' molecules bind to the analyte in the sample. The resulting immune complex binds to a glass fibre matrix. An alkaline phosphatase-labelled conjugate bound to the matrix then reacts with a fluorogenic substrate and the rate of fluorescence development is measured. This is proportional to the concentration of analyte originally present in the sample. Concentrations were determined by comparison with a curve constructed from standards from known concentrations. Samples were analysed as soon as possible after receipt.

Quality control procedures comprised both internal and external procedures. For the serum assays, with each run an internal pooled serum sample was used as a drift control. Drift control for the red cell folate assay was by use of a commercial red blood cell folate control. External quality assessment was by NEQAS for the haematinic assays.

4   Retinol, tocopherols, lutein/zeaxanthin, lycopene, cryptoxanthin, α-carotene and β-carotene in plasma

These determinations were achieved by high performance liquid chromatography using a method derived from that of Thurnham et al[1]. Rapidly-thawed subsamples of plasma (typically 250μl) were extracted with n-heptane in the presence of absolute ethanol, butylated hydroxytoluene (BHT) and α-tocopherol acetate (internal standard). The upper organic phase was evaporated nearly to dryness under vacuum, and was then redissolved in 250μl of the mobile phase, with sonication to achieve dissolution. If necessary a small volume of dichloromethane was added to achieve complete dissolution. 50μl aliquots were then injected onto a 4μ Waters C_{18}, 4.6 x 100mm radial compression cartridge column which was preceded by a 0.5μ reduced stainless steel filter frit, to remove any particles. The mobile phase was acetonitrile, 44%, methanol 44%, dichloromethane 12%, by volume, with added BHT at 10mg/l. The flow rate was 1.5ml/min and the column temperature control jacket was maintained at 25°C. A Waters Millennium-controlled HPLC system, with a model 490E multi-channel ultraviolet (UV)/visible detector, was used. Two wavelength channels, with wavelength switching on both, enabled the internal standard of tocopherol acetate to be used as the sole internal standard on both channels for all the analytes of interest. On channel 1, retinol and retinyl palmitate are estimated at 325nm, and tocopherols at 292nm, at which wavelength the tocopherol acetate is also measured. On channel 2, all the carotenoids are measured at 450nm, with switching to 292nm for the tocopherol acetate standard. Peak area response factors were obtained from semi-pure, commercially available carotenoids, and from retinol, retinyl palmitate, alpha- and gamma-tocopherols. These were then corrected to 100% purity, by means of their HPLC patterns, and from their absolute optical densities and known extinction coefficients.

This procedure was able to separate and quantify all of the following plasma components: retinol and retinyl palmitate at 325nm; alpha- and gamma-tocopherols at 292nm; α- and β-carotenes, lycopene and α- and β-cryptoxanthins at 450nm. Lutein and zeaxanthin eluted as a single peak and were estimated together at 450nm. Run time was 11 minutes, thus permitting a throughput of about five samples per hour. A mixed standard was run at frequent intervals to check the performance characteristics of the column and detectors, the former being replaced when necessary, to ensure adequate peak separation.

Quality control procedures comprised both internal and external procedures including:

- an internal subdivided pool of heparinised human plasma from the Cambridge Blood Transfusion Service, used for long-term drift control and to provide an early warning of any changes in sensitivity of the assay;
- external freeze-dried plasma samples provided by the National Institute of Standards and Technology (NIST) USA which have assigned values for all of the analytes of interest;
- external plasma samples from the UK EQAS scheme for fat-soluble vitamins.

The method used to determine these analytes in plasma samples in this survey was used in the NDNS: children aged 1½ to 4½ years[2] and the NDNS: people aged 65 years and over[3].

5   25-hydroxyvitamin D in plasma

The Incstar (Minnesota, USA) 25(OH)-vitamin D radioimmunoassay (RIA) kit assay was used, which was based on the developmental work of Hollis et al[4]. The antibody to 25(OH)-vitamins D $(D_2 + D_3)$ had been generated in goats by the vitamin D analog, 23,24,25,26,27-pentanor-C(22)-carboxylic acid of vitamin D coupled to bovine serum albumin. Firstly, duplicate extraction of the fat-soluble analyte from the plasma samples and from standards was achieved into pure acetonitrile, precipitating plasma proteins. The extracted 25-hydroxyvitamin D was then diluted with tracer 25-hydroxyvitamin D labelled with ^{125}I. Exposure of this impure mixture to a specific goat antibody against 25-hydroxyvitamin D resulted in specific binding of a proportion of the labelled vitamer, dependent on its concentration. Addition of a second antibody then achieved precipitation. Separation of this precipitated protein-bound fraction was achieved by centrifugation and was followed by gamma-counting of the sedimented fraction.

Quality control procedures comprised both internal and external procedures including:

- an internal subdivided pool of heparinised human plasma from the Cambridge Blood Transfusion Service, used for long-term drift control and to provide an early warning of any changes in sensitivity of the assay;

- a spiked serum with an assigned 25(OH)-vitamin D value, provided with the kit;
- serum with an assigned (Incstar) 25(OH)-vitamin D level, obtained from Bio-Rad Inc;
- samples from the UK EQAS scheme for 25(OH)-vitamin D.

We chose not to use the second high spiked serum that was provided with the kit, because its concentration lay outside the region of good precision of the assay, and it was preferable to dilute any survey samples which fell into this range.

This method was also used to measure 25-hydroxyvitamin D in plasma for the NDNS: children aged 1½ to 4½ years[2] and the NDNS: people aged 65 years and over[3].

6 Erythrocyte transketolase for thiamin status, in washed red blood cells

This assay was based on that of Vuilleumier et al[5]. It depends on the coupling of pyridine nucleotide (NADH) oxidation to glycerol phosphate dehydrogenase, which produces glycerol-3-phosphate after the transketolase-catalysed conversion of ribose-5-phosphate. The rate of oxidation of NADH was monitored at 340nm, on the Cobas Bio analyser. The reaction rate was measured in both the absence and presence of the transketolase enzyme cofactor, thiamine pyrophosphate (cocarboxylase). Thiamin status was measured by both the basal enzyme activity, expressed per unit of haemoglobin in the sample, and by the activation coefficient, which was the ratio of cofactor-stimulated activity to the basal activity without any added cofactor. Haemoglobin was measured separately by the cyanomethaemoglobin procedure.

Quality assurance was achieved with stored red cell preparations from heparinised blood obtained from the Cambridge Blood Transfusion Service and a pooled sample from Tanzanian blood. No commercial materials with assigned values or EQAS were available for this analyte.

7 Erythrocyte glutathione reductase activation coefficient for riboflavin status in washed red cells

This assay has been adapted 'in-house' for use with a Cobas Fara centrifugal analyser from the manual technique developed by Glatzle et al[6]. Washed red cell samples were thawed, diluted in water and buffer, centrifuged and the extract was incubated with and without flavin adenine dinucleotide (FAD). Addition of assay reagents oxidised glutathione and reduced pyridine nucleotide coenzyme took place in the centrifugal analyser, and was followed by a 5 minute measurement of the reaction rate at 340nm and 37°C. The ratio of FAD-stimulated to unstimulated activity is the erythrocyte glutathione reductase activation coefficient (EGRAC) and is a reliable and robust measure of riboflavin status. The initial reactivation of the unsaturated apoenzyme in the sample was carried out for a relatively long period (30 minutes at 37°C), in order to ensure full reactivation of apoenzyme. The assay is conducted at a low final concentration of (FAD) (1.5μm). We have found this to be necessary, in order to eliminate activation coefficients (ratios) less than 1.0, which can result from enzyme inhibition by FAD or its breakdown products, if the final concentration of FAD is too high.

Quality control samples comprised pools of United Kingdom, Gambian and Tanzanian red cell haemolysates, stored in aliquots at −80°C and thawed on the day of analysis. No commercial materials with assigned values or EQAS were available for this analyte.

8 Vitamin C in plasma

The assay was based on the procedure described by Vuilleumier and Keck[7]. The assay is performed on a Roche Cobas Bio centrifugal analyser with fluorescence attachment. It begins with conversion of ascorbic acid in the metaphosphoric acid stabilised plasma sample to dehydroascorbic acid by a specific enzyme, ascorbate oxidase purified from cucumbers, obtained from Sigma, London. This is followed by coupling of the resulting dehydroascorbate with o-phenylene diamine to give a fluorescent quinoxaline. The formation of this quinoxaline is linearly related to the amount of vitamin C in the sample, at least over the range 0-10μg/ml (0-57μmol/l), which is a typical range for vitamin C in plasma, after its pre-storage dilution 1:2 with 10% metaphosphoric acid. The assay was calibrated daily with freshly prepared vitamin C standards. The validity of the fluorimetric assay procedure used was by cross-correlation with HPLC-based assays, and by vitamin C spiking experiments. Preliminary trial runs and literature-assessment verified the stability of the vitamin C under the collection, stabilisation and storage conditions used.

A selection of internal quality controls were included in each run, which comprised aliquots of heparinised plasma spiked with each of three levels of vitamin C and stored at −80°C in metaphosphoric acid. No commercial quality control materials or EQAS were available for this analyte.

9 Alkaline phosphatase in plasma (Roche Unimate 5 ALP IFCC)

This was a Roche kit Cobas Bio assay, run at 37°C. The assay measures the rate of release of the yellow chromophore p-nitrophenol, from the chromogen p-nitrophenyl phosphate, at alkaline pH. The assay was pre-calibrated by the manufacturer using serum with a known alkaline phosphatase activity, which has then been translated into a factor by which the observed change in optical density/min was multiplied to give

IU/l. This calibration factor was further verified using human serum samples with assigned enzyme activity, during each run. The assay is robust and reliable, and the enzyme is reasonably stable in frozen plasma, although there is reputed to be a slow increase in activity with storage. All samples were therefore assayed after the same number of freeze-thaw cycles, and after similar duration of storage.

Quality control procedures comprised both internal and external procedures including heparinised human plasma samples from the Cambridge Blood Transfusion Service and NEQAS.

10 Plasma iron, Total Iron Binding Capacity (TIBC) and iron % saturation (Roche Unimate Iron; Iron binding capacity test)

Measurement of plasma iron by this method depends on the reaction of free ferrous iron with ferrozine, after iron liberation from protein-binding with guanidine, followed by reduction of ferric to ferrous iron with ascorbic acid. The colour was measured on a Cobas Bio analyser at 562nm. The calibrator was a Roche human serum with assigned value.

Quality control procedures comprised both internal and external procedures including heparinised human plasma samples from the Cambridge Blood Transfusion Service, Roche human sera 'N' and 'P' (normal and pathological) at stated, half and quarter dilution and NEQAS for plasma iron.

For assay of TIBC (total iron binding capacity), plasma samples were first mixed with a fixed amount of ferrous chloride in excess of the unsaturated iron-binding capacity. The excess unbound iron was then physically removed by addition of basic magnesium carbonate powder, followed by mixing and centrifugation, leaving only the transferrin-bound iron in solution. This transferrin-bound iron was then measured by the ferrozine reaction in the presence of guanidine giving a direct measure of the total amount of transferrin (iron-binding protein) present in the sample. Percent saturation of transferrin was calculated as 100x [plasma iron/TIBC], both being expressed on a molar basis. Again for this assay the calibrator was a Roche human serum with assigned values.

Quality control procedures comprised internal procedures including heparinised human plasma samples from the Cambridge Blood Transfusion Service and Roche human sera 'N' and 'P' (normal and pathological) at stated and half dilution.

11 Glutathione peroxidase in whole blood (selenium status)

This assay was based on that of Paglia and Valentine[8]. It was further developed into a standardised procedure during an European Community FLAIR Concerted

Action: "Measurement of Micronutrient Absorption and Status"[9]. The assay involves the coupling of glutathione peroxidase-catalysed oxidation of reduced glutathione, in the presence of diothiothreitol, cyanide, ferricyanide and tertiary butyl hydroperoxide, with the glutathione reductase-catalysed reduction of the resulting oxidised glutathione. This results in oxidation of NADPH, measured as a rate reaction at 340nm and 37°C on the Cobas Bio analyser. The samples were diluted with dithioreitol and Drabkins reagent in a two-stage dilution procedure before the assay. Necessary precautions included precise pH control (pH7.0), conservation of reagent stability on ice, and rapid processing of the samples. The enzyme was measured in diluted whole blood and its activity was expressed in nmoles/min/mg haemoglobin, the latter having been measured on separate, but equivalent subsamples of whole blood at Great Ormond Street Haematology Laboratory.

Running quality assurance was achieved with aliquots of heparinised whole blood from the Cambridge Blood Transfusion Service. The enzyme is stable during storage in the frozen state, and the samples were assayed after only a single freeze-thaw cycle after storage. No commercial QC materials or EQAS were available for this analyte.

12 α₁-antichymotrypsin in plasma

Different plasma acute phase proteins respond at different rates following the onset of an inflammatory stimulus[10]. α_1-antichymotrypsin was selected as the most suitable choice of acute phase reactant, with respect to this time course of response as it remains elevated for longer than other acute phase proteins. This Cobas Bio-based nephelometric assay relied on a specific antibody to α_1-antichymotrypsin, raised in rabbits, purchased from Dako and diluted in buffer containing polyethylene glycol. The six-point calibration curve used calibration sera with assigned values. The assay has proved robust and reliable over several years of use at the Dunn Nutrition Unit and samples were analysed after not more than two freeze-thaw cycles. The analyte is stable in frozen plasma, and the assay is highly sensitive, requiring only a few microlitres of sample.

Internal quality control procedures included heparinised human plasma from the Cambridge Blood Transfusion Service and serum samples with assigned values from Dako.

13 Triglycerides (Roche Unimate TRIG), cholesterol (Roche Unimate CHOL) HDL-cholesterol (Roche Unimate CHOL + HDL CHOL) in plasma

The majority of blood samples were collected from the respondents after an overnight fast. These colourimetric assays were performed on the Cobas Fara analyser.

For triglyceride assay, the sample was incubated with a mixture of lipase, glycerokinase, 3-phosphoglycerate dehydrogenase and pyridine nucleotide. The resulting change in optical density at 340nm was a measure of lipid-bound glycerol, and hence of the triglyceride content of the sample. The triglyceride assay was calibrated by use of the Roche human calibrator.

Cholesterol was measured by the oxidation of cholesterol (liberated by cholesterol esterase), by cholesterol oxidase to 7-hydroxy-cholesterol. Hydrogen peroxide thus liberated then reacts with phenol and 4-amino-antipyrine in the presence of peroxidase, to yield a quinoneimine chromophore measurable at 520nm. The cholesterol assay was calibrated by use of the Roche human calibrator.

HDL-cholesterol has been defined as that fraction of total cholesterol which remains in solution after precipitation of LDL and VLDL cholesterol with magnesium chloride plus phosphotungstic acid.

For this assay magnesium/phosphotungstic acid reagent was added to the plasma sample. The sample was then centrifuged, and the clear supernate was assayed by the cholesterol assay described above. The HDL assay was calibrated by the use of Roche P control serum. Studies have shown that this precipitation methodology yields results very similar to those of ultracentrifugal separation, which is the reference method for this assay.

Quality control procedures for all three assays comprised internal procedures including heparinised human plasma samples from the Cambridge Blood Transfusion Service and Roche human sera 'N' and 'P' (normal and pathological) with assigned lipid values. External quality control procedures included NEQAS for cholesterol and triglycerides.

14 Urea in plasma (Roche Unimate 5 UREA)

In this Cobas Bio assay, urea in the samples was degraded to ammonia plus carbon dioxide; the released ammonia converted 2-oxoglutarate to glutamate, which was coupled with the oxidation of NADH, followed at 340nm. The assay used a kinetic rate-measurement and was calibrated by a human Roche serum calibrator of known urea content. Samples of plasma were analysed after not more than two freeze-thaw cycles.

Quality control procedures comprised internal procedures including heparinised human plasma samples from the Cambridge Blood Transfusion Service and Roche human sera 'N' and 'P' (normal and pathological) at stated and half dilution. External quality control procedure was NEQAS for urea.

15 Creatinine in plasma (Roche Unimate 7 CREA)

This Cobas Bio assay is based on the Jaffé reaction (alkaline picrate). It is a rate assay and was calibrated with Roche human serum calibrator of known creatinine concentration. Samples were analysed after not more than two freeze-thaw cycles.

Quality control was achieved with Roche human serum samples with assigned values, and for the running quality assurance human heparinised plasma from the Cambridge Blood Transfusion Service was used. External quality control procedure was NEQAS for creatinine.

16 Plasma zinc (Wako Zinc, Cat. 435-14909)

The Wako Chemicals GmbH, Nauss, Germany 'kit' procedure for plasma zinc was based on the formation of a coloured complex between zinc (released from heparinized plasma by trichloroacetic acid) with '5-Br-PAPS' (2-(5-bromo-2-pyridylazo)-5-(N-propyl-N-sulphopropylamino)-phenol) and salicilylaldoxime. Precautions against sample contamination were taken. The assay was performed on the Cobas Fara centrifugal analyser. This assay has been compared with and validated against a flame atomic absorption assay, by both the kit manufacturer and the Dunn Nutrition Unit, with good inter-method agreement.

Quality control freeze-dried human serum was obtained from Randox Laboratories, and a subdivided heparinised human plasma sample from Cambridge Blood Transfusion Service was used as the internal quality control.

17 Plasma Testosterone

This assay was conducted using the 'Diria-Testok' radioimmunoassay kit manufactured by Sorin using samples of heparinised plasma. The assay is based on the competition of ^{125}I labelled testosterone and the testosterone in standards and unknowns for a fixed number of antibody-binding sites. After incubation and separation with a second antibody, the amount of labelled testosterone bound to the antibody is inversely related to the concentration of testosterone present in the sample. Testosterone concentrations were determined in all available plasma samples from male respondents aged 10 years and over.

Quality Control was achieved by the use of Biorad Lyphochek Immunoassay Plus Control Serum (Level 2) and a subdivided heparinised human plasma sample from Cambridge Blood Transfusion Service.

18 Erythrocyte Superoxide Dismutase (SOD)

The assay is performed using the Randox Ransod Superoxide Dismutase kit for use with the Cobas Fara. The principle of the assay is to add xanthine and xanthine oxidase to standards and samples thus generating superoxide radicals. This mixture is then reacted with 2-(4-iodophenyl)-3-(4-nitrophenol)-5-phenyltetrazolium chloride to form a red formazan dye.

737

As superoxide dismutase breaks down the superoxide radical, the extent of red formazan dye formation monitored at 500nm can be used to quantify the activity of SOD in a sample. The SOD present in a sample is usually expressed as an activity per gram of haemoglobin, the haemoglobin content having been measured by the cyanomethaemoglobin procedure.

Quality control is achieved by the use of Ransod Control provided with the kit at stated, half, quarter and double strength. Running quality assurance was achieved with aliquots of heparinised whole blood from the Cambridge Blood Transfusion Service at stated, half and quarter strength.

19 Erythrocyte aspartate aminotransferase activation coefficient (EAATAC) for vitamin B6 status in washed red cells

This method is based on the procedure described by Vuilleumier et al [5] and uses the Cobas Bio centrifugal autoanalyser to monitor the stimulation of erythrocyte aspartate aminotransferase (EAAT) by pyridoxal-5-phosphate (PLP) at 340nm and 37°C. Washed red cell samples were thawed, diluted in water and buffer, centrifuged, and the extract was incubated with and without PLP. The ratio of PLP-stimulated activity to the basal unstimulated activity is known as EAATAC.

Quality control samples comprised separate pools of United Kingdom, Gambian and Tanzanian red cell haemolysates, stored frozen and thawed on the day of analysis. No commercial QC materials or EQAS were available for this analyte.

20 Magnesium in plasma

Measurements of magnesium in plasma were made by flame atomic absorption spectrometry following a 1 + 100 dilution of 20 μl sample volumes with 2.00 ml of a diluent consisting of 0.1% m/v lanthanum chloride in 1.0% v/v hydrochloric acid. Calibration was effected using aqueous standard solutions which were diluted as for the plasma samples. Instrumental conditions were optimised before analysis at 285.2nm using a stoichiometric air/acetylene flame.

Internal quality controls (IQCs) were three Nycomed materials with target concentrations of 0.50, 0.80 and 1.80 mmol/l. These were analysed at a frequency of not less than one set of three single IQC samples per 10 duplicate test samples. External quality assessment was by participation in schemes organised by Randox Ltd and NEQAS for magnesium.

21 Selenium in plasma

Plasma selenium concentrations were measured by using inductively coupled plasma mass spectrometry (ICP-MS)[11] following 1 + 15 dilutions of 200 μl sample volumes with a diluent which contained 1.0% v/v butan-1-ol, 0.66% m/v Triton X-100, 0.01 M ammonia, 0.0002 M ammoniumdihydrogen ethylenediaminetetraacetic acid and 0.002 M ammoniumdihydrogen phosphate. This diluent destabilised argon-adduct ion species which otherwise would interfere with ICP-MS measurements of selenium and hence allows accurate analyses at ^{78}Se. Matrix-matched standards prepared from bovine serum were used for calibration.

Internal quality control sera were prepared by adding selenium to pools of bovine sera to give increases of 0, 0.40 and 1.60 μmol/l. An additional IQC was provided by using the Seronorm preparation, 311089. The IQCs were analysed at a frequency of not less than one set of four IQCs per 10 duplicate test samples. Participation in quality assessment schemes from Centre du Toxicologie de Quebec and TEQAS provided external quality control.

22 Lead in blood

Measurements of lead in whole blood were made directly with 10μl sample volumes using microsampling flame atomic absorption spectrometry as previously described[12]. This high-throughput technique has been used for almost all major environmental surveys of lead in blood in UK subjects over the past two decades. Calibration is effected by using matrix-matched standards prepared by additions of lead to bovine blood.

Internal quality control blood samples were prepared by adding lead to pools of bovine blood to give target concentrations of 8.7, 16.2 and 31.5 μg/l. These pools of IQC material were also used in previous surveys and allow accurate interpretation of temporal changes in UK blood lead. The IQC samples were analysed at a frequency of not less than one set of three IQCs per six duplicate test samples.

The validity of the blood lead data was established by participation in five external quality assessment schemes two in the UK, two in the USA and one in Canada.

Acknowledgements

We wish to acknowledge the following staff at the Micronutrient Status Laboratory of MRC Human Nutrition Research (formerly of MRC Dunn Nutrition Unit), who were involved the blood and urine analyses: Mr S Austin, Miss K Pearson, Mr R Carter, Miss I Morelli, Miss S Taylor, Mr N Matthews, Mr G Harvey, Miss K Flook and Miss M King; Ms D Muggleston and Mr C Burgess of the Diagnostics Haematology Laboratory, Great Ormond Street Hospital, London; Dr HT Delves, Mrs R Mensikov and Mrs A Clewlow of the SAS Trace Element Unit, Southampton General Hospital.

We would also like to thank Mrs E Moran, Mrs C Allan, Dr TJ Cole, Mrs S Levitt, Mr KC Day and Mr M Garratt at MRC Human Nutrition Research for computing and data handling, advice and data entry, and Ms A Jennings, Mrs J Marshall and Mrs N Macdonald for management of the Survey Office and fieldwork.

We are also indebted to personnel at the following hospitals for their assistance in local sample processing and storage:

Mount Vernon and Watford NHS Trust
King's Mill Centre for Health Care Services NHS Trust, Sutton in Ashfield
Royal Liverpool and Broadgreen University Hospital NHS Trust
South Manchester University Hospitals NHS Trust
Royal Berkshire and Battle Hospitals NHS Trust, Reading
North East Essex Mental Health NHS Trust, Colchester
North Durham Acute Hospitals NHS Trust
Morriston Hospital/Ysbyty Treyforys NHS Trust, Swansea
Glan Hafren NHS Trust, Newport, Gwent
Havering Hospitals NHS Trust, Romford
Royal Surrey County and St. Luke's Hospital NHS Trust, Guildford
Southmead Health Services NHS Trust, Bristol
Glenfield Hospital NHS Trust, Leicester
West Middlesex University Hospital NHS Trust, Isleworth
Victoria Infirmary NHS Trust, Glasgow
Royal United Hospital Bath NHS Trust
St James and Seacroft University Hospitals NHS Trust, Leeds
Barnsley District General Hospital NHS Trust
Dudley Group of Hospitals NHS Trust
Southern General Hospital NHS Trust, Glasgow
Forest Healthcare NHS Trust, Leytonstone, London
Derby City General NHS Trust
Kings Healthcare NHS Trust, London
Walsgrave Hospital NHS Trust, Coventry
Cheviot and Wansbeck NHS Trust, Ashington
Royal Cornwall Hospital NHS Trust, Truro
Oxford Radcliffe Hospitals NHS Trust
Royal Hull Hospitals NHS Trust
Hastings and Rother NHS Trust, St Leonards on Sea
Queen Victoria Hospital NHS Trust, East Grinstead
Taunton and Somerset NHS Trust
Ceredigion and Mid Wales NHS Trust, Aberystwyth
Birmingham Children's Hospital NHS Trust
Monklands and Bellshill Hospital NHS Trust, Aidrie
Burnley Healthcare NHS Trust
Hillingdon Hospital NHS Trust
Queens Medical Centre, Nottingham University NHS Trust
Edinburgh's Sick Children NHS Trust
Chesterfield and North Derbyshire Royal Hospital NHS Trust
Brighton Healthcare NHS Trust
Royal Shrewsbury Hospital NHS Trust

Royal Bournemouth and Christchurch Hospitals NHS Trust
North Hampshire Hospitals NHS Trust, Basingstoke
North Tyneside Healthcare NHS Trust, Tyne and Wear
West Dorset General Hospitals NHS Trust, Dorchester
Countess of Chester Hospital NHS Trust
Angus NHS Trust, Brechin
Mid Kent Healthcare NHS Trust, Maidstone
Northern General Hospital NHS Trust, Sheffield
Southport and Formby NHS Trust
Portsmouth Hospitals NHS Trust
Mid Cheshire Hospitals NHS Trust, Crewe
Worcester Royal Infirmary NHS Trust
Kettering General Hospital NHS Trust
Peterborough Hospital NHS Trust
Redbridge Health Centre NHS Trust, Goodmayes, Essex
Stoke Mandeville Hospital NHS Trust, Aylesbury
Princess Alexandra Hospital NHS Trust, Harlow, Essex
Plymouth Hospitals NHS Trust
Salisbury Healthcare NHS Trust
Swindon and Marlborough NHS Trust
Gwynedd Hospitals NHS Trust, Bangor
University Hospital of Wales Healthcare NHS Trust, Cardiff
Aberdeen Royal Hospitals NHS Trust

References

1   Thurnham DI, Smith E, Flora PS. Concurrent liquid-chromatographic assay of retinol, α-tocopherol, β-carotene, α-carotene, lycopene and β-cryptoxanthin in plasma, with tocopherol acetate as internal standard. *Clin Chem* 1988; **34**: 377-381.

2   Gregory JR, Collins DL, Davies PSW, Hughes JM, Clarke PC. *National Diet and Nutrition Survey: Children aged 1½ to 4½ years. Volume 1: Report of the diet and nutrition survey.* HMSO (London,1995).

3   Finch S, Doyle W, Lowe C, Bates CJ, Prentice A, Smithers G, Clarke PC. *National Diet and Nutrition Survey: people aged 65 years and over. Volume 1: Report of the diet and nutrition survey.* TSO (London, 1998).

4   Hollis BW, Kamerud JQ, Selvaag SR, Lorenz JD, Napoli JL. Determination of vitamin D status by radioimmunoassay with an ^{125}I-labelled tracer. *Clin Chem* 1993; **39**: 529-533.

5   Vuilleumier JP, Keller HE, Keck E: Clinical chemical methods for routine assessment of the vitamin status of populations. Part III. The apoenzyme stimulation tests for vitamins B_1, B_2 and B_6, adapted to the Cobas Bio analyser. *Internat J Vit Nutr Res* 1990; **60**: 126-135.

6   Glatzle D, Korner WF, Christeller S, Wiss O. Method for the detection of a biochemical riboflavin deficiency. Stimulation of $NADPH_2$-dependent glutathione reductase from human erythrocytes by FAD *in vitro*. Investigations on the vitamin B_2 status in healthy people and geriatric patients. *Internat J Vit Nutr Res* 1970; **40**: 166-183.

7   Vuilleumier JP, Keck E. Fluorimetric assay of vitamin C

in biological materials using a centrifugal analyser with fluorescence attachment. *J Micronutrient Anal* 1989; **5**: 25-34.

8 Paglia DE, Valentine WN. Studies on the quantitative and qualitative characterisation of erythrocyte glutathione peroxidase. *J Lab Clin Med* 1967; **70**: 158-169.

9 EC-Food Linked Agro-Industrial Research (EC-FLAIR) Concerted Action No. 10 (Rapporteurs: JL Belsten and AJA Wright). European Community – FLAIR common assay for whole-blood glutathione reductase (GSH-Px); results of an inter-laboratory trial. *Eur J Clin Nutr* 1995; **49**: 921-927.

10 Calvin J, Neale G, Fotherby KJ, Price CP. The relative merits of acute phase proteins in the recognition of inflammatory conditions. *Ann Clin Biochem* 1988; **25**: 60-66.

11 Delves HT, Sieniawska CE. Simple method for the accurate determination of selenium in serum by using inductively coupled plasma mass spectrometry. *J Analyt Atom Spectrom* 1997; **12**: 387-9.

12 Delves HT. A microsampling method for the rapid determination of lead in blood. *Analyst* 1970; **95**: 431-8.

Table Q1   Quality control data for haemoglobin and blood counts

National External Quality Assessment Scheme for haematology*

Analyte**	Result	Mean***	Deviation Index
haemoglobin Hb (g/dl)			
9703 1	135	135.2	−0.12
9703 2	109	109.7	−0.44
9706 1	143	141.5	0.68
9706 2	106	104.9	0.65
9710 1	99	99.2	−0.11
9710 2	143	141.3	0.70
rec cell count RCC (× 10^{12}/l)			
9703 1	4.31	4.393	−1.00
9703 2	3.53	3.589	−0.88
9706 1	4.70	4.674	0.33
9706 2	3.50	3.536	−0.60
9710 1	3.25	3.277	−0.46
9710 2	4.65	4.711	−0.73
PCV (l/l)			
9703 1	0.377	0.3821	−0.54
9703 2	0.310	0.3129	−0.37
9706 1	0.432	0.4278	0.40
9706 2	0.298	0.2991	−0.15
9710 1	0.283	0.2811	0.26
9710 2	0.417	0.4173	−0.03
mean cell volume MCV (fl)			
9703 1	87.5	87.01	0.35
9703 2	87.8	91.84	0.44
9706 1	92.0	91.56	0.28
9706 2	85.0	84.61	0.27
9710 1	87.2	85.80	0.85
9710 2	89.8	88.59	0.72
mean cell haemoglobin MCH (pg)			
9703 1	31.3	30.81	0.65
9703 2	30.9	30.63	0.37
9706 1	30.4	30.27	0.20
9706 2	30.2	29.67	0.81
9710 1	30.5	30.30	0.27
9710 2	30.8	30.02	1.02
mean cell haemoglobin concentration MCHC (%)			
9703 1	35.8	35.50	0.38
9703 2	35.2	35.09	0.11
9706 1	33.0	33.05	−0.06
9706 2	35.5	35.06	0.46
9710 1	34.9	35.30	−0.37
9710 2	34.3	33.92	0.36
white cell count WCC (x10^{9}/l)			
9703 1	5.9	5.66	0.59
9703 2	5.0	4.83	0.51
9706 1	7.5	6.83	1.29
9706 2	4.4	3.94	1.54
9710 1	5.1	4.74	5.10
9710 2	6.9	6.44	6.90
platelet count PLT (x10^{9}/l)			
9703 1	188	192.0	−0.47
9703 2	199	202.0	−0.34
9706 1	186	201.5	−1.75
9706 2	216	235.6	−1.89
9710 1	186	194.0	−1.08
9710 2	149	149.0	−0.10

*NEQAS samples were analysed throughout the survey.
**Data are given for two samples at three timepoints in the survey.
***The mean indicates the mean value calculated for participating laboratories using a particular type of analytical technique.

Table Q2 Quality control data for red cell and serum folate, plasma ferritin and plasma vitamin B_{12}

National External Quality Assessment Scheme for haematinics*

Analyte**	Result	Mean***	Deviation Index
Red cell folate ($\mu g/l$)			
9702	256	237	0.53
9706	135	172	−1.42
9710	205	234	−0.83
Ferritin ($\mu g/l$)			
9702 1	66	66.5	−0.07
9702 2	76	77.9	−0.24
9706 1	39	35.1	1.12
9706 2	43	39.0	1.02
9710 1	19	20.4	−0.67
9710 2	65	71.0	−0.85
Vitamin B_{12} (ng/l)			
9702 1	418	419	−0.01
9702 2	165	166	−0.08
9706 1	238	236	0.07
9706 2	462	459	0.07
9710 1	450	446	0.09
9710 2	256	221	1.60
Serum folate ($\mu g/l$)			
9702 1	7.1	6.5	0.93
9702 2	3.5	3.8	−0.69
9706 1	4.7	5.6	−1.64
9706 2	4.8	5.9	−1.82
9710 1	11.9	11.7	0.13
9710 2	3.2	3.6	−1.19

*NEQAS samples were analysed throughout the survey.
**Data are given for one or two samples at three timepoints in the survey.
***The mean indicates the mean value calculated for participating laboratories using a particular type of analytical technique.

Table Q3 Quality control data for abnormal haemoglobins

National External Quality Assessment Scheme for haemoglobin types*

		Haemoglobin F (%)			Haemoglobin A_2 (%)		
		Results obtained at GOS	Median results of all other participating labs***	Reported range	Results obtained at GOS	Median results of all other participating labs***	Reported Range
9701 1	**	<0.5	0.50	0–1.3	2.8	2.7	2.0–3.4
9701 2	**	2.1	1.80	0.47–3.1	5.6	5.4	3.8–7.0
9701 3	**	<0.5	0.30	0–11.07			
9703 1	**	<0.5	0.50	0–10.7			
9703 2	**	0.4	0.45	0–46.7			
9703 3	**	0.5	0.50	0–5.9	5.2	4.9	1.7–9.5
9704 1	**	<0.5	0.40	0–1.0	6.5	5.8	4.1–7.8
9704 2	**			2.5	2.5	2.3	1.6–3.0
9704 3	**	1.7	0.40	0–4.3			

*NEQAS samples were analysed throughout the survey.
**Data are given for three samples at three timepoints in the survey.
***The median indicates the median value calculated for participating laboratories using a particular type of analytical technique.

742

Table Q4 Quality control data for magnesium

Sample	Target (mmol/l)	Observed (mmol/l) Mean	sd	n
Nycomed Internal quality control:				
Low	0.5	0.53	0.03	168
Medium	0.8	0.84	0.04	168
High	1.8	1.81	0.03	161
National External Quality Assessment Scheme:				
558	1.22	1.34		
559	0.58	0.62		
562	1.14	1.17		
565	1.11	1.16		
566	1.45	1.52		
567	1.56	1.57		
Randox External Quality Assessment:				
16.15	0.93	0.98		
17.03	0.92	0.91		
17.05	1.00	1.01		
17.07	1.01	1.02		
17.09	1.72	1.76		
17.11	0.72	0.72		
17.15	1.36	1.43		
17.17	0.72	0.76		

Table Q5: Quality control data for selenium

Internal Quality Control	Target (μmol/l)	Observed (μmol/l) Mean	sd	n
L1	0.30	0.29	0.030	43
L2	0.77	0.69	0.006	43
L3	1.32	1.30	0.060	43
L4	1.84	1.87	0.090	42
Seronorm	1.06	0.99	0.060	43

Table Q6 Quality control data for lead

Internal Quality Control	Target (μmol/l)	Observed (μmol/l) Mean	sd	n
Low	8.7	8.5	0.7	197
Medium	16.2	15.9	0.7	198
High	31.5	31.5	1.1	197

Table Q7 Quality control data for iron and Total Iron Binding Capacity

Test (units)	Wave*	In-house Control Mean	sd	n	% CV	Roche N Mean	sd	n	Target range	Roche P Mean	sd	n	Target range
Iron (μmol/l)**	1	13.69	0.98	15	7.15	17.73	0.22	15	17.2 (15.5-18.9)	43.28	0.40	15	43.2 (38.9-47.5)
	2	13.55	0.72	13	5.31	17.68	0.49	13	17.2 (15.5-18.9)	43.51	1.41	13	43.2 (38.9-47.5)
	3	13.49	0.51	25	3.75	17.07	0.51		17.2 (15.5-18.9)	42.44	0.66	25	43.2 (38.9-47.5)
	4	13.72	0.28	19	1.03	17.46	0.26		17.2 (15.5-18.9)	42.78	0.38	19	43.2 (38.9-47.5)
TIBC(μmol/l)	1	49.29	1.79	11	3.6	63.41	1.82	11	58.6 (51.0-66.2)	48.28	1.52	11	47.1 (42.1-52.1)
	2	49.56	1.37	10	2.8	64.09	1.8	10	58.6 (51.0-66.2)	50.55	2.14	10	47.1 (42.1-52.1)
	3	47.49	1.30	21	2.7	63.11	2.53	21	58.6 (51.0-66.2)	49.40	2.84	21	47.1 (42.1-52.1)
	4	48.30	1.57	18	3.2	62.73	1.96	18	58.6 (51.0-66.2)	48.68	1.04	18	47.1 (42.1-52.1)

*Fieldwork wave 1: Jan–March 1997
2: April–June 1997
3: July–Sept 1997
4: Oct–Dec 1997
**For iron, in addition to the results obtained on undiluted samples given in the table, some values were also obtained on 1:2 and 1:4 dilutions of one Roche N Control Serum in order to check linearity for a wide range of sample concentrations.
Participation in the NEQAS scheme for iron for 47 samples yielded a mean deviation index of 0.45 for sample concentrations between 11.22 and 35.89μmol/l.

Table Q8 Quality control data for Vitamin A, E and carotenoids

Test	Wave*	In-house Control				NIST (all waves)**		NEQAS (all waves)**	
		Mean	sd	% CV	n	Mean DI	DI Range	Mean DI	DI Range
Retinol (μmol/l)	1	1.297	0.032	2.47	21	−0.56	−1.54 to 0.22		
	2	1.341	0.069	5.15	18			−0.9	−2.06 to −0.11
	3	1.362	0.018	1.32	34				
	4	1.341	0.021	1.57	31				
β-carotene (μmol/l)	1	0.283	0.014	4.89	21	−0.5	−1.1 to −0.19	−0.12	−1.00 to +0.82
	2	0.287	0.013	4.43	18				
	3	0.290	0.010	3.52	34				
	4	0.279	0.008	2.98	31				
α-carotene (μmol/l)	1	0.036	0.004	11.11	21	−0.73	−1.38 to −0.38		
	2	0.036	0.003	8.33	18				
	3	0.032	0.003	9.38	34				
	4	0.039	0.004	10.26	31				
α-cryptoxanthin (μmol/l)	1	0.099	0.004	3.59	21				
	2	0.098	0.004	4.45	18				
	3	0.103	0.004	3.54	34				
	4	0.098	0.003	3.20	31				
β-cryptoxanthin (μmol/l)	1	0.279	0.007	2.51	21	0	−0.42 to +0.44		
	2	0.268	0.006	2.24	18				
	3	0.286	0.005	1.75	34				
	4	0.276	0.010	3.62	31				
Lutein/Zeaxanthin (μmol/l)	1	0.267	0.009	3.37	21	−0.54	−1.28 to −0.25		
	2	0.289	0.010	3.46	18				
	3	0.288	0.008	2.78	34				
	4	0.273	0.010	3.66	31				
Lycopene (μmol/l)	1	0.354	0.015	4.24	21	0.09	−1.33 to +1.18		
	2	0.348	0.018	5.17	18				
	3	0.356	0.015	4.21	34				
	4	0.343	0.011	3.21	31				
α-tocopherol (μmol/l)	1	21.235	0.395	1.86	21	0.35	−0.26 to +0.88	0.71	−0.16 to +2.12
	2	21.930	0.361	1.65	18				
	3	22.109	0.426	1.93	34				
	4	21.393	0.435	2.03	31				
γ-tocopherol (μmol/l)	1	1.527	0.044	2.88	21	−0.44	−1.00 to +0.21		
	2	1.530	0.031	2.03	18				
	3	1.560	0.021	1.35	34				
	4	1.536	0.019	1.24	31				
Retinyl palmitate (μmol/l)	1	0.088	0.012	13.64	21	0.96	−0.66 to +1.87		
	2	0.079	0.005	6.33	18				
	3	0.088	0.007	7.95	34				
	4	0.083	0.007	8.43	31				

*Fieldwork wave 1 Jan–March 1997
2 April–June 1997
3 July–Sept 1997
4 Oct–Dec 1997
**NIST and NEQAS data are given for the entire survey duration.

Table Q9   Quality control data for 25-hydroxyvitamin D

Test (units)	Wave*	In-house Control				Kit Control**				BioRad Lyphochek Control**			
		Mean	sd	*n*	% CV	Mean	sd	*n*	Target range	Mean	sd	*n*	Target
25OH Vit D (nmol/l)	1	59.5	12.56	*38*	21.11	43.5	5.82	*20*	19.5-47.0	61.1	10.04	*27*	70.3(44.8-95.8)
						33.8	5.16	*7*	22.3-53.8				
	2	51.8	7.96	*38*	15.38	38.5	7.74	*25*	22.3-53.9	62.9	9.34	*26*	70.3(44.8-95.8)
	3	55.4	10.14	*72*	18.30	39.6	9.62	*10*	22.3-53.9	62.5	9.43	*36*	70.3(44.8-95.8)
						41.5	5.89	*26*	23.3-56.3				
	4	58.3	10.51	*82*	18.01	40.3	5.96	*41*	23.3-56.4	66.2	13.59	*41*	70.3(44.8-95.8)

*Fieldwork wave 1: Jan–March 1997
2: April–June 1997
3: July–Sept 1997
4: Oct–Dec 1997
**Both the kit and the BioRad Lyphochek control had assigned target ranges based on the Incstar assay kit. In addition a UK EQAS scheme run by Mr G Carter (Endocrine Laboratory, Charing Cross Hospital Fulham Palace Road, London W6 8RS) provided 20 samples for inter-laboratory quality assurance comparisons during the survey period. When compared, analysis of these samples yielded a mean deviation of 0.02 for sample concentrations between 12.9-81.4 nM.

Table Q10   Quality control data for Erythrocyte Glutathione Reductase Activation Coefficient, Erythrocyte Asparate Aminotransferase Activation Coefficient, and Erythrocyte Transketolase Activity and Activation Coefficient

Test	Wave*	In-house controls – UK				In-house control – Gambian				In-house control – Tanzanian			
		Mean	sd	*n*	% CV	Mean	sd	*n*	% CV	Mean	sd	*n*	% CV
EGRAC (Ratio)	1	1.32	0.015	*6*	1.10	1.71	0.03	*6*	1.5	2.98	0.06	*6*	1.90
	2	1.32	0.009	*6*	0.70	1.75	0.02	*6*	1.3	3.00	0.09	*6*	2.90
	3	1.30	0.010	*9*	0.70	1.72	0.01	*9*	0.9	2.92	0.06	*9*	2.20
	4	1.30	0.021	*9*	1.70	1.72	0.02	*6*	1.2	2.98	0.06	*4*	2.00
EAATAC (Ratio)	1	1.74	0.020	*53*	1.28	2.42	0.04	*10*	1.69	1.95	0.04	*10*	2.07
	2	1.75	0.030	*47*	1.94	2.45	0.08	*9*	3.27	2.00	0.04	*6*	1.95
	3	1.72	0.030	*82*	1.90	2.40	0.08	*12*	3.15	1.93	0.03	*13*	1.78
	4	1.74	0.030	*75*	1.61	2.45	0.09	*11*	3.58	1.96	0.04	*12*	1.87
ETK-basal activity (μmol/g Hb/min)	1	0.772	0.052	*49*	6.7	0.626	0.038	10	6.1				
	2	0.771	0.034	*46*	4.5	0.592	0.022	12	3.8				
	3	0.777	0.042	*79*	5.4	0.620	0.048	17	7.8				
	4	0.806	0.043	*73*	5.3	0.630	0.056	18	8.9				
ETKAC (Ratio)	1	1.13	0.03	*49*	2.90	1.21	0.08	10	6.43				
	2	1.11	0.05	*46*	4.76	1.29	0.05	12	3.74				
	3	1.12	0.03	*79*	2.49	1.28	0.06	17	4.35				
	4	1.10	0.05	*73*	4.47	1.25	0.10	18	8.18				

*Fieldwork wave 1 Jan–March 1997
2 April–June 1997
3 July–Sept 1997
4 Oct–Dec 1997

Table Q11 Quality control data for triglycerides, total cholesterol and HDL-cholesterol

Test (units)	Wave*	In-house Control				Roche N**				Roche P**			
		Mean	sd	n	% CV	Mean	sd	n	Target range	Mean	sd	n	Target range
Trigylcerides (mmol/l)	1	0.93	0.03	11	2.93	0.97	0.01	8	0.49 (0.44-0.54)	4.55	0.04	4	4.76 (4.28-5.24)
	2	0.96	0.03	15	2.69	0.97	0.02	11	0.49 (0.44-0.54)	4.66	0.04	2	4.76 (4.28-5.24)
	3	0.94	0.03	19	3.42	0.95	0.02	14	0.49 (0.44-0.54)	4.50	0.03	4	4.76 (4.28-5.24)
	4	0.96	0.03	79	3.63	0.97	0.02	59	0.49 (0.44-0.54)	4.55	0.06	18	4.76 (4.28-5.24)
Total cholesterol (mmol/l)	1	4.44	0.09	11	2.14	4.31	0.09	11	4.25 (3.83-4.67)	2.96	0.06	8	3.06 (2.75-3.37)
	2	4.44	0.08	16	1.86	4.30	0.07	16	4.25 (3.83-4.67)	2.95	0.06	9	3.06 (2.75-3.37)
	3	4.31	0.10	18	2.20	4.19	0.08	18	4.25 (3.83-4.67)	2.87	0.06	10	3.06 (2.75-3.37)
	4	4.38	0.06	15	1.40	4.25	0.04	15	4.25 (3.83-4.67)	2.89	0.06	8	3.06 (2.75-3.37)
HDL-cholesterol (mmol/l)	1	1.28	0.06	12	4.97	0.85	0.05	12	0.85 (0.73-0.95)				
	2	1.28	0.05	14	3.69	0.83	0.05	14	0.85 (0.73-0.95)				
	3	1.27	0.06	18	4.44	0.81	0.04	18	0.85 (0.73-0.95)				
	4	1.28	0.07	15	5.43	0.80	0.05	15	0.85 (0.73-0.95)				

*Fieldwork wave 1 Jan–March 1997
　　　　　　　2 April–June 1997
　　　　　　　3 July–Sept 1997
　　　　　　　4 Oct–Dec 1997
**NEQAS participation yielded mean deviation indices for triglycerides of −0.39 (concentration range 0.55-1.50 mmol/l) and for total cholesterol −0.31 (concentration range 1.82-5.81), for 47 samples respectively. Values not available for HDL-cholesterol. Roche P control used at double concentration for the triglyceride assays.

Table Q12 Quality control data for plasma creatinine and plasma urea

Test (units)	Wave*	In-house Control				Roche N				Roche P			
		Mean	sd	n	% CV	Mean	sd	n	Target range	Mean	sd	n	Target range
Plasma creatinine** (µmol/l)	1	76.67	3.53	10	4.61	100.29	2.99	10	98.6 (88.7-108.6)	482.33	12.17	9	449 (404.7-495.2)
	2	73.10	2.61	7	3.57	101.66	2.56	7	98.6 (88.7-108.6)	470.51	9.06	7	449 (404.7-495.2)
	3	73.38	2.01	14	2.74	99.80	2.44	14	98.6 (88.7-108.6)	477.87	14.43	14	449 (404.7-495.2)
	4	72.03	3.91	9	5.43	102.75	3.20	10	98.6 (88.7-108.6)	492.31	22.11	10	449 (404.7-495.2)
Plasma urea*** (mmol/l)	1	5.84	0.13	5	2.3	6.79	0.14	5	5.73 (5.16-6.30)	18.81	0.39	4	19 (17.1-20.9)
	2	6.04	0.22	8	3.6	5.82	0.21	8	5.73 (5.16-6.30)	19.78	0.73	8	19 (17.1-20.9)
	3	5.61	0.34	14	6.1	5.52	0.22	14	5.73 (5.16-6.30)	18.72	0.47	14	19 (17.1-20.9)
	4	5.82	0.36	12	6.3	5.7	0.24	12	5.73 (5.16-6.30)	18.77	0.44	12	19 (17.1-20.9)

*Fieldwork wave 1 Jan–March 1997
　　　　　　　2 April–June 1997
　　　　　　　3 July–Sept 1997
　　　　　　　4 Oct–Dec 1997
**For plasma creatinine, NEQAS participation for 40 samples yielded a mean deviation of −1.21 with a concentration range for samples of 59.20-65.3 µmol/l.
***For plasma urea, NEQAS participation for 37 samples yielded a mean deviation index of −0.13 with a concentration range of 3.2-25.92 mmol/l.

Table Q13 Quality control data for alkaline phosphatase and α_1-antichymotrypsin

Test (units)	Wave*	In-house Control				Roche N				Roche P			
		Mean	sd	n	% CV	Mean	sd	n	Target range	Mean	sd	n	Target range
Alkaline phosphatase** (IU/l)	1	69.7	1.65	7	2.4	70.20	1.31	7	69:5 (61-78)	308.74	1.59	4	301 (265-337)
	2	71.79	2.47	7	3.4	69.75	1.76	7	69.5 (61-78)	307.30	3.64	7	301 (265-337)
	3	70.30	4.17	12	5.9	69.55	1.00	12	69.5 (61-78)	307.65	12.10	12	301 (265-337)
	4	72.33	4.27	10	5.9	70.66	1.11	10	69.5 (61-78)	309.26	5.27	10	301 (265-337)
α_1-antichymotrypsin (g/l)	1	0.27	0.01	5.07	9	0.26	0.02	9	0.25 (0.23–0.28)	0.97	0.05	5	0.99 (0.89–1.09)
	2	0.27	0.01	3.27	13	0.26	0.01	13	0.25 (0.23–0.28)	1.01	0.03	7	0.99 (0.89–1.09)
	3	0.27	0.01	4.44	20	0.27	0.01	20	0.25 (0.23–0.28)	1.01	0.04	12	0.99 (0.89–1.09)
	4	0.24	0.02	10.07	9	0.24	0.02	9	0.25 (0.23–0.28)	0.86	0.03	5	0.99 (0.89–1.09)

*Fieldwork wave 1 Jan–March 1997
　　　　　　　2 April–June 1997
　　　　　　　3 July–Sept 1997
　　　　　　　4 Oct–Dec 1997
**For alkaline phosphatase, NEQAS participation for 37 samples yielded a mean deviation index 0.95 for concentrations ranging from 74.6 – 87.8 IU/l.

Table Q14 Quality control data for zinc

| Test (units) | Wave | In-house Control | | | | Roche N** | | | |
		Mean	sd	n	% CV	Mean	sd	n	Target range
Zinc	1	23.97	0.83	17	3.46	25.01	0.68	17	25.8 (22.3–29.3)
(μmol/l)	2	23.32	1.43	13	6.14	25.27	0.17	13	25.8 (22.3–29.3)
	3	24.10	0.57	29	2.37	26.43	0.29	29	25.8 (22.3–29.3)
	4	24.19	0.97	25	0.97	25.91	0.25	25	25.8 (22.3–29.3)

*Fieldwork wave 1: Jan–March 1997
              2: April–June 1997
              3: July–Sept 1997
              4: Oct–Dec 1997
**For zinc, NEQAS participation yielded a mean deviation index of 0.96, for a concentration range of 2.22 –34.31 μmol/l for 68 samples.

Table Q15 Quality control data for testosterone

| Test (units) | Wave* | In-house Control | | | | BioRad Lyphochek Control Level 2 | | | |
		Mean	sd	n	% CV	Mean	sd	n	Target range
Testosterone	1	3.96	0.14	10	3.48	6.64	0.22	6	7.3(5.5-9.1)
(nmol/l)	2	3.80	0.07	5	1.88	6.59	0.35	4	7.3(5.5-9.1)
	3	3.79	0.31	9	8.05	6.50	0.43	6	7.3(5.5-9.1)
	4	3.35	0.13	8	3.84	6.03	0.21	6	7.3(5.5-9.1)

*Fieldwork wave 1: Jan–March 1997
              2: April–June 1997
              3: July–Sept 1997
              4: Oct–Dec 1997

Table Q16 Quality control data for superoxide dismutase

| Test (units) | Wave* | In-house Control | | | | Ransod Control | | | |
		Mean	sd	n	% CV	Mean	sd	n	Target
SOD	1	253.86	10.66	14	4.2	212.21	7.51	14	203 (172-234)
(nmol/mg Hb/min)	2	260.32	7.43	12	2.9	215.29	6.95	12	204 (172-234)
	3	251.69	8.12	21	3.2	208.60	6.26	21	205 (172-234)
	4	253.51	7.03	21	2.8	212.51	6.60	21	206 (172-234)

*Fieldwork wave 1: Jan–March 1997
              2: April–June 1997
              3: July–Sept 1997
              4: Oct–Dec 1997

Table Q17 Quality control data for vitamin C

| Test (units) | Wave* | In-house Control | | | |
		Mean	sd	n	% CV
Vit C	1	4.2	0.56	8	13.51
(μmol/l)	2	2.8	0.41	15	14.59
	3	3.1	0.80	17	25.71
	4	2.3	0.47	13	20.21

*Fieldwork wave 1: Jan–March 1997
              2: April–June 1997
              3: July–Sept 1997
              4: Oct–Dec 1997

Appendix R

Weighted base numbers

Table R1   Weighted base numbers: dietary interview, 7-day dietary record and 7-day physical activity diary samples, by sex of young person*

	Interview	7-day weighed intake dietary record	7-day physical activity record
Age			
Males aged			
4–6	854	1134	n/a
7–10	1134	912	959
11–14	1083	870	917
15–18	1072	861	912
All males	4143	3331	2788
Females aged			
4–6	813	656	n/a
7–10	1078	866	915
11–14	1024	821	867
15–18	1017	816	853
All females	3932	3159	2635
Whether unwell during dietary period			
Males			
Unwell and eating affected	347	324	258
Unwell and eating not affected	846	264	228
Not unwell	2946	2743	2302
Females			
Unwell and eating affected	356	334	256
Unwell and eating not affected	834	309	287
Not unwell	2743	2516	2092
Region			
Males			
Scotland	346	267	231
Northern	1119	926	785
Central, South West and Wales	1465	1175	971
London and South East	1241	963	801
Females			
Scotland	331	256	213
Northern	1066	878	744
Central, South West and Wales	1386	1110	919
London and South East	1150	914	759
Whether 'parents' receiving benefits**			
Males			
Receiving benefits	1105	818	645
Not receiving benefits	3035	2507	2138
Females			
Receiving benefits	1111	833	712
Not receiving benefits	2809	2319	1916
Gross weekly household income**			
Males			
Less than £160	701	547	399
£160–less than £280	819	669	570
£280–less than £400	741	600	499
£400–less than £600	801	636	565
£600 and over	881	765	644
Females			
Less than £160	683	528	455
£160–less than £280	735	598	481
£280–less than £400	677	535	418
£400–less than £600	861	705	573
£600 and over	778	676	585
Social class of head of household***			
Males			
Non-manual	1829	1562	1288
Manual	1912	1510	1295
Females			
Non-manual	1706	1424	1156
Manual	1739	1352	1134

Table R1 continued

	Interview	7-day weighed intake dietary record	7-day physical activity record
Household type			
Males			
Living with both parents			
and other children	2546	2083	1663
and no other children	775	648	624
Single parent with/without other children	801	590	489
Others	21	9	11
Females			
Living with both parents			
and other children	2328	1889	1490
and no other children	713	582	531
Single parent with/without other children	851	664	583
Others	41	23	30

* Total number of males and females may vary due to rounding in weighting (and no answers).
** Excludes those not answering.
*** Excludes those for whom a social class could not be assigned.
n/a Not applicable; physical activity diaries were not collected for young people aged 4 to 6 years.

Table R2 Weighted base numbers: anthropometry and blood pressure by sex of young person*

	Height and BMI	Weight	Mid upper-arm circumference	Waist, hip and waist to hip ratio	Blood pressure
Age					
Males aged					
4–6	782	786	754	n/a	763
7–10	1040	1047	1041	n/a	1009
11–14	993	993	998	993	972
15–18	979	975	975	975	961
All males	3794	3801	3768	1968	3705
Females aged					
4–6	744	747	744	n/a	728
7–10	987	994	994	n/a	959
11–14	938	923	939	916	918
15–18	928	928	924	912	905
All females	3597	3592	3601	1828	3510
Whether unwell during dietary period					
Males					
Unwell and eating affected	341	341	341	154	337
Unwell and eating not affected	514	522	515	273	478
Not unwell	2934	2934	2909	1541	2885
Females					
Unwell and eating affected	356	356	356	200	359
Unwell and eating not affected	533	533	523	257	500
Not unwell	2708	2704	2723	1370	2653
Region					
Males					
Scotland	317	317	317	168	306
Northern	1041	1041	1030	538	1017
Central, South West and Wales	1329	1339	1317	694	1294
London and South East	1107	1104	1105	567	1088
Females					
Scotland	303	303	303	160	287
Northern	987	984	987	495	965
Central, South West and Wales	1254	1250	1259	651	1227
London and South East	1052	1055	1051	522	1033
Whether 'parents' receiving benefits**					
Males					
Receiving benefits	981	992	970	461	955
Not receiving benefits	2808	2804	2794	1502	2746
Females					
Receiving benefits	1013	1013	1008	466	967
Not receiving benefits	2576	2572	2586	1354	2537
Gross weekly household income**					
Males					
Less than £160	621	627	624	252	610
£160–less than £280	773	773	754	400	741
£280–less than £400	690	690	688	342	675
£400–less than £600	716	716	712	427	693
£600 and over	850	846	842	445	842
Females					
Less than £160	623	623	616	281	595
£160–less than £280	695	698	698	334	677
£280–less than £400	605	602	602	273	595
£400–less than £600	790	790	796	404	780
£600 and over	730	726	737	430	728

Table R2 continued

	Height and BMI	Weight	Mid upper-arm circumference	Waist, hip and waist to hip ratio	Blood pressure
Social class of head of household*					
Males					
Non-manual	1708	1704	1700	851	1667
Manual	1753	1760	1734	924	1708
Females					
Non-manual	1582	1584	1589	772	1552
Manual	1578	1572	1575	822	1546
Household type					
Males					
Living with both parents					
and other children	2345	2346	2321	1033	2279
and no other children	716	716	712	566	704
Single parent with/without	714	721	717	351	704
other children					
Others	18	18	18	18	18
Females					
Living with both parents					
and other children	2145	2149	2147	899	2095
and no other children	648	641	648	485	644
Single parent with/without	774	774	776	414	743
other children					
Others	30	30	30	30	30

* Total number of males and females may vary due to rounding in weighting (and no answers).
** Excludes those not answering.
*** Excludes those for whom a social class could not be assigned.
n/a Not applicable; waist and hip circumferences were not measured for young people aged 4 to 10 years.

Table R3 Weighted base numbers: urine and blood samples by sex of young person*

	Urine sample	Blood sample**				
		haemoglobin	plasma α-carotene	plasma total cholesterol	plasma zinc	plasma selenium
Age						
Males aged						
4–6	744	424	434	388	348	457
7–10	985	632	578	512	463	604
11–14	935	617	550	488	443	574
15–18	910	622	541	485	438	567
All males	3574	2295	2103	1873	1692	2202
Females aged						
4–6	696	406	415	370	333	435
7–10	928	592	548	487	439	575
11–14	882	568	523	462	418	546
15–18	883	593	514	459	414	537
All females	3389	2159	2000	1778	1604	2093
Whether unwell during dietary period						
Males						
Unwell and eating affected	319	185	177	153	154	187
Unwell and eating not affected	426	252	209	173	141	238
Not unwell	2829	1858	1718	1546	1397	1776
Females						
Unwell and eating affected	347	259	230	212	215	247
Unwell and eating not affected	436	236	210	175	147	224
Not unwell	2605	1664	1560	1392	1241	1623
Region						
Males						
Scotland	287	155	151	146	139	152
Northern	985	623	568	484	436	579
Central, South West and Wales	1270	808	715	631	560	773
London and South East	1033	709	670	611	557	696
Females						
Scotland	278	139	144	140	135	146
Northern	922	567	539	461	414	551
Central, South West and Wales	1201	765	679	595	527	736
London and South East	988	688	638	583	527	660
Whether 'parents' receiving benefits*						
Males						
Receiving benefits	926	565	528	428	374	528
Not receiving benefits	2644	1726	1572	1444	1318	1669
Females						
Receiving benefits	927	633	565	498	436	591
Not receiving benefits	2454	1526	1435	1281	1167	1501
Gross weekly household income*						
Males						
Less than £160	579	346	321	259	236	320
£160–less than £280	725	483	477	432	388	485
£280–less than £400	671	400	335	301	254	383
£400–less than £600	656	457	399	375	337	427
£600 and over	809	526	494	448	430	512
Females						
Less than £160	594	364	332	288	260	343
£160–less than £280	639	463	427	382	321	438
£280–less than £400	550	356	336	300	276	350
£400–less than £600	770	454	430	405	376	464
£600 and over	700	472	426	373	340	449
Social class of head of household**						
Males						
Non-manual	1601	1045	969	888	818	1010
Manual	1654	1073	984	862	777	1028
Females						
Non-manual	1478	934	857	763	723	907
Manual	1484	938	883	791	682	913

	Urine sample	Blood sample**				
		haemoglobin	plasma α-carotene	plasma total cholesterol	plasma zinc	plasma selenium
Household type						
Males						
Living with both parents						
and other children	2218	1458	1330	1216	1089	1387
and no other children	663	432	385	350	328	413
Single parent with/without						
other children	675	389	377	294	270	386
Others	18	16	12	11	5	15
Females						
Living with both parents						
and other children	2025	1272	1209	1093	979	1276
and no other children	602	383	354	310	265	364
Single parent with/without						
other children	731	476	415	355	340	429
Others	30	27	23	21	20	23

* Total number of males and females may vary due to rounding in weighting (and no answers).
** Blood analytes shown are those used to derive weighting factors for groups of analytes with similar numbers of reported results.
*** Excludes those not answering.
**** Excludes those for whom a social class could not be assigned.

Weights for blood analytes

Weights were derived for five groups of blood analytes. The groupings were based on similar numbers of reported results for different analytes.

The five groups were as follows

Group 1: Non-response weight based on number of haemoglobin results

Applies to:

    haemoglobin
    red blood cell count
    haematocrit
    mean cell volume
    mean cell haemoglobin
    mean cell haemoglobin concentration
    red cell distribution width
    mean platelet volume
    platelet distribution width
    white cell count
    neutrophil count
    lymphocyte count
    monocyte count
    eosinophil count
    basophil count
    HbF
    HbA_2
    serum folate
    red cell folate
    serum vitamin B_{12}
    serum ferritin

Group 2: Non-response weight based on number of results for plasma α-carotene

Applies to:

    plasma retinol
    plasma retinyl palmitate
    α- and γ-tocopherol
    plasma lycopene
    plasma lutein + zeaxanthin
    α- and β-cryptoxanthin

    plasma vitamin C
    ETK-B
    ETKAC
    plasma iron
    total iron-binding capacity
    plasma iron % saturation

Group 3: Non-response weight based on number of results for plasma total cholesterol

Applies to:

    plasma total cholesterol
    HDL cholesterol
    LDL cholesterol
    plasma triglycerides
    plasma $α_1$- antichymotrypsin

Group 4: Non-response weight based on number of results for plasma selenium

Applies to:

    plasma selenium
    plasma magnesium
    plasma 25-hydroxyvitamin D
    EGRAC
    EAATAC
    red cell superoxide dismutase

Group 5: Non-response weight based on number of results for plasma zinc

Applies to plasma zinc only.

Results are reported unweighted for the following analytes (see *Chapter 12; Section 12.1.2*):

    plasma urea
    plasma creatinine
    plasma testosterone
    plasma alkaline phosphatase
    erythrocyte glutathione peroxidase

Appendix S

Urine collection, transport and analysis procedures, and quality control data

Collection and transport

A single early morning urine sample was collected for sodium, potassium and creatinine assays. Where possible, and in the majority of cases, this was from the first void after rising.

Each young person who agreed to collect this sample was provided with a clean disposable plastic container for the initial sample collection, a 10ml plastic syringe 'monovette' containing 100 mg boric acid preservative[1] and a simple set of instructions for filling the syringe, which they did themselves. The interviewer carried out the subsequent procedures by appointment, later the same morning. The filled syringe was labelled with the serial number using a cryo-label and date of collection was added using a cryo-pen. Information about time and date of sample collection and posting time was recorded on a standard form which was included with the sample in the postal package. The syringe was placed inside a screw-capped plastic postal container with an absorbent liner in case of leakage. The sample and the completed record form, were sent by first class post to the MRC Dunn Nutrition Unit in a pre-labelled pre-stamped Jiffy bag. Where possible, collections were avoided on Fridays and weekends to ensure that nearly all of the samples would arrive during working hours. On arrival, they were immediately logged and cross-checked, and were then stored at $-40°C$ until analysed.

Analysis Procedures
Sodium and potassium

This assay measures both analytes simultaneously, and was performed by flame photometry with an 'Instrumentation Laboratory' photometer, calibrated by a lithium nitrate internal calibrant of known concentration. QC material was Randox QC urine with assigned values for sodium and potassium, which was measured at normal strength, double strength and at half strength, to check linearity. Quality assurance used an in-house human urine sample and NEQAS was available. The concentration of each alkali metal was expressed as a molar ratio to creatinine, measured as described below. These analytes are stable and were thus unaffected by the duration of storage.

Creatinine (Roche Unimate CREA)

This Cobas Bio assay is based on the Jaffé reaction (alkaline picrate). It is a rate assay and was calibrated with Roche serum calibrator of known concentration. A 1:10 dilution was necessary, and a Randox Urine Control with an assigned value was used for quality control. Linearity was checked with double and half concentrations of the QC materials.

Endnote

[1] Sarstedt Ltd, 68 Boston Road, Beaumont Leys, Leicester LE4 1AW, cat. 10.253: 'Urine Monovette with Stabiliser'.

Table S1   Quality control data for urine alkali metals and creatinine

Test	Fieldwork wave*	In-house control				Randox control**			
		Mean	SD	CV (%)***	n	Target	Observed mean	SD	n
Urine sodium (mM)	1	67.6	0.7	1.01	18	63.7 (54.1-73.3)	64.3	1.2	18
	2	67.6	1.9	2.75	15	63.7 (54.1-73.3)	62.9	2.4	15
	3	67.3	2.1	3.10	19	63.7 (54.1-73.3)	62.3	1.9	20
	4	67.4	0.5	0.69	22	63.7 (54.1-73.3)	63.1	1.4	22
Urine potassium (mM)	1	61.9	0.5	0.87	18	41.4 (35.2-47.6)	41.3	0.8	17
	2	61.6	1.7	2.75	15	41.4 (35.2-47.6)	39.9	1.5	15
	3	61.3	1.9	3.02	19	41.4 (35.2-47.6)	39.6	1.2	20
	4	61.5	0.3	0.42	22	41.4 (35.2-47.6)	40.0	0.9	22
Urine creatinine (μM)	1	7590	178	2.35	20	6800 (5870-7820)	6424	102	20
	2	7896	733	9.29	19	6800 (5870-7820)	6760	289	17
	3	7778	730	9.39	20	6800 (5870-7820)	6597	279	21
	4	7866	278	3.53	29	6800 (5870-7820)	6500	137	29

*Wave 1:   Jan–March 1997
Wave 2:   April–June 1997
Wave 3:   July–Sept 1997
Wave 4:   Oct–Dec 1997
**For all 3 urinary analytes the external control was obtained from Randox (Randox U) with assigned values.
***The % drift across the entire survey dataset, for the 2 controls respectively, was < 1% and < 1% for sodium, 1% and 4% for potassium, and < 1% and 6% for creatinine. 1:2 dilution and 2x concentration of the Randox U control yielded values between 103 and 119% of the predicted values for sodium (n = 56); 102-107% for potassium (n = 57), and 98-105% for creatinine (n = 93).

Appendix T:

Units of measurement used in the Report

Units of energy

kcal   kilocalorie; 1000 calories. A unit used to measure the energy value of food.

kJ   kiloJoule; 10^3 or 1000 Joules. A unit used to measure the energy value of food. 1kcal = 4.184kJ

MJ   megaJoule; 10^6 or 1000,000 joules. A unit used to measure the energy value of food.

Units of length

cm   centimetre; one-hundredth of 1 metre

m   metre; 100 centimetres

mm   millimetre; one-thousandth of 1 metre

Units of volume

dl   decilitre; one-tenth of 1 litre

fl   femtolitre; 1 litre $\times 10^{-15}$

l   litre; 1000 millilitres

l/l   litre per litre (ratio)

ml   millilitre; 10^{-3} litre; one-thousandth of 1 litre

Units of weight

g   gram

kg   kilogram, 1000 grams

mg   milligram, 10^{-3} grams; one-thousandth of 1 gram

mmol   millimol; the atomic or molecular weight of an element or compound in grams $\times 10^{-3}$

µg   microgram; 10^{-6} grams; one-millionth of 1 gram

µmol   micromol; the atomic or molecular weight of an element or compound in grams $\times 10^{-6}$

ng   nanogram; 10^{-9} grams; one-thousand-millionth of 1 gram

nmol   nanomol; the atomic or molecular weight of an element or compound in grams $\times 10^{-9}$

pg   picogram; 10^{-12} grams; one-million-millionth of 1 gram

pmol   picomol; the atomic or molecular weight of an element or compound in grams $\times 10^{-12}$

Appendix U

Glossary of abbreviations, terms and survey definitions

25-OHD	See *plasma 25-hydroxyvitamin D*
α_1-ACT	α_1-antichymotrypsin
Activity score	See *Blair score; calculated activity score*
Benefits (receiving)	Receipt of Income Support, Family Credit or Job Seeker's Allowance by the young person's mother and/or her husband/partner in the 14 days prior to the date of interview.
Biological parent	The term used to describe those who are biologically the parents of the young person, that is, not adoptive, step or foster parents or cohabiting partners not genetically related to the young person.
Blair score; calculated activity score	An indicator of energy expenditure, based on the MET value for an activity and the time spent on that activity.
BMI	see *Body Mass Index*
BMR	Basal Metabolic Rate, a measure of the energy needed per day to maintain vital functions which sustain life.
Body Mass Index	A measure of body fatness which standardises weight for height: calculated as [weight (kg)/height(m)^2]. Also known as the Quetelet Index.
CHD	Coronary heart disease
COMA	The Committee on Medical Aspects of Food and Nutrition Policy
CSE	Certificate of Secondary Education
Cum %	Cumulative percentage (of a distribution)
CV	Coefficient of variation
Deft	Design factor; see *Notes* and *Appendix E*
DH	The Department of Health
Diary sample	Young people for whom a seven-day dietary record was obtained.
dna	does not apply
DNU	Medical Research Council Dunn Nutrition Unit, Cambridge. See also *HNR*

DRV	Dietary Reference Value. The term used to cover LRNI, EAR, RNI and safe intake. (See Department of Health. Report on Health and Social Subjects: 41. *Dietary Reference Values for Food Energy and Nutrients for the United Kingdom.* HMSO (London, 1991))
EAATAC	The erythrocyte aspartate aminotransferase activation coefficient
EAR	The Estimated Average Requirement of a group of people for energy or protein or a vitamin or a mineral. About half will usually need more than the EAR, and half less.
Employment status	Whether at the time of interview the individual was working, unemployed, or economically inactive.
Economically inactive	Those neither working nor unemployed as defined by the International Labour Organisation (ILO) definition (see *Unemployed)*; includes full-time students, the retired, individuals who were looking after the home or family and those permanently unable to work due to ill health or disability.
EGRAC	The erythrocyte glutathione reductase activation coefficient
EMLA cream	A topical local anaesthetic cream applied to the arm of some young people at the site of the venepuncture.
EQA(S)	External quality assurance (scheme)
ETKAC	The erythrocyte transketolase activation coefficient
ETK-B	The erythrocyte transketolase basal activity
Extrinsic sugars	Any sugar which is not contained within the cell walls of a food. Examples are the sugars in honey, table sugar and lactose in milk and milk products.
FAD	Flavin adenine dinucleotide
Fieldwork wave	see *Wave*
Frankfort plane	The desired position for the young person's head when measuring standing height.
FSA	Food Standards Agency
GCE	General Certificate of Education
GCSE	General Certificate of Secondary Education
GHS	The General Household Survey; a continuous, multi-purpose household survey, carried out by the Social Survey Division of ONS on behalf of a number of government departments.
GSH-Px	The erythrocyte glutathione peroxidase activity
GP	General Practitioner
HDL cholesterol	High density lipoprotein cholesterol
HEA	Health Education Authority, now the Health Development Agency.

Head of household	The head of household is defined as follows:

a) in a household containing only a husband, wife and children under age 16 years (and boarders), the husband is always the head of household.

b) in a cohabiting household the male partner is always the head of household.

c) when the household comprises other relatives and/or unrelated persons the owner, or the person legally responsible for the accommodation, is always the head of the household.

In cases where more than one person has equal claim, the following rules apply:

i) where they are of the same sex, the oldest is always the head of household

ii) where they are of different sex the male is always the head of household.

Highest educational activity score

Based on the highest educational qualification obtained, grouped as follows:

Above GCE 'A' level
Degree (or degree level qualification)
Teaching qualification
HNC/HND, BEC/TEC Higher, BTEC
City and Guilds Full Technological Certificate
Nursing qualifications (SRN, SCM, RGN, RM RHV, Midwife)

GCE 'A' level and equivalent
GCE 'A' level/SCE higher
ONC/OND/BEC/TEC not higher

GCE 'O' level and equivalent
GCE 'O' level passes (Grades A-C if after 1975)
CSE (Grades A-C)
CSE (Grade 1)
SCE Ordinary (Bands A-C)
Standard Grade (Levels 1-3)
SLC Lower
SUPE Lower or Ordinary School Certificate or Matriculation
City and Guilds Craft/Ordinary Level

CSE and equivalent
CSE Grades 2-5, and ungraded
GCE 'O' level (Grades D and E if after 1975)
GCSE (Grades D-G)
SCE Ordinary (Bands D and E)
Standard Grade (Levels 4 and 5)
Clerical or commercial qualifications
Apprenticeship
Other qualifications

None
No educational qualifications

The qualification levels do not in all cases correspond to those used in statistics published by the Department of Education.

HNR   Medical Research Council Human Nutrition Research, Cambridge, (formerly part of the Dunn Nutrition Unit).

HOH   see *Head of household*

Household	The standard definition used in most surveys carried out by the Social Survey Division, ONS, and comparable with the 1991 Census definition of a household was used in this survey. A household is defined as a single person or group of people who have the accommodation as their only or main residence and who either share one main meal a day or share the living accommodation. (See McCrossan E. *A Handbook for interviewers*. HMSO: London 1991)
Household type	Classificatory variable based on whether the young person was living with one or both parents and with or without other children. See also *Two-parent household*.
HSE	The Health Survey for England
Income	Respondents were asked to give the usual gross weekly or annual income of their household from all sources before tax and other deductions by choosing one of 12 income groups from a show card (see *Appendix A*).
Intrinsic sugars	Any sugar which is contained within the cell wall of a food.
IQA	Internal quality assurance (see also EQAS, NEQAS)
lc	low calorie
LDL cholesterol	Low density lipoprotein cholesterol. LDL cholesterol was not measured in this survey. Total plasma cholesterol minus HDL cholesterol is taken as approximation of LDL cholesterol, uncorrected for triglycerides. For brevity, the term LDL cholesterol is used for non-HDL cholesterol.
LREC	Local (NHS) Research Ethics Committee
LRNI	The Lower Reference Nutrient Intake for protein or a vitamin or a mineral. An amount of the nutrient that is enough for only the few people in the group who have low needs.
MAFF	The Ministry of Agriculture, Fisheries and Food
Manual social class	Young people living in households where the head of household was in an occupation ascribed to *Social Classes III manual, IV or V*.
MAP	Mean arterial pressure – see *Chapter 11*
Mean	The average value
MET	Metabolic equivalent. For adults metabolic equivalents are taken as numerically equivalent to energy expenditure. For an average adult 1MET is equal to 60kcal/ hour or 1kcal/min.
MCH	Mean cell haemoglobin
MCHC	Mean cell haemoglobin concentration
MCV	Mean corpuscular volume
Median	*see* Quantiles
Menarche	The onset of menstruation in girls.
MRC	The Medical Research Council
MUAC	Mid upper-arm circumference

na	not available, not applicable.
NDNS	The National Diet and Nutrition Survey
NEQAS	The National External Quality Assurance Scheme
NFS	National Food Survey
NHS	National Health Service
nlc	not low calorie
NMES	see *Non-milk extrinsic sugars*
No.	Number (of cases)
Non-manual social classes	Young people living in households where the head of household was in an occupation ascribed to *Social Classes I, II or III non-manual*.
Non-milk extrinsic sugars	Extrinsic sugars, except lactose in milk and milk products
NSP	Non-starch polysaccharides. A precisely measurable component of foods. A measure of 'dietary fibre'.
ONS	Office for National Statistics
PAF	Postcode Address File; the sampling frame for the survey
Percentiles	see *Quantiles*
Physical activity sample	Those for whom a seven-day physical activity diary was obtained.
Plasma 25-hydroxyvitamin D; plasma 25-OHD	Plasma vitamin D
PSU	Primary Sampling Unit; for this survey, postcode sectors.
PUFA	Polyunsaturated fatty acid
QA (QC)	Quality assurance/Quality control
Quantiles	The quantiles of a distribution divide it into equal parts. The median of a distribution divides it into two equal parts, such that half the cases in the distribution fall, or have a value, above the median, and the other half fall, or have a value below the median.
Quetelet Index	see *Body Mass Index*
Region	Based on the Standard regions and grouped as follows:

Scotland

Northern
North
Yorkshire and Humberside
North West

Central, South West and Wales
East Midlands
West Midlands
East Anglia

South West
Wales
London and South East
London
South East

The regions of England are as constituted after local government reorganisation on 1 April 1974. The regions as defined in terms of counties are listed in Chapter 3.

Responding sample	Respondents who co-operated with any part of the survey.
RNI	The Reference Nutrient Intake for protein or a vitamin or a mineral. An amount of the nutrient that is enough, or more than enough, for about 97% of the people in a group. If average intake of a group is at the RNI, then the risk of deficiency in the group is small.
SD/Std Dev	Standard deviation. An index of variability which is calculated as the square root of the variance and is expressed in the same units used to calculate the *mean*.
se	Standard error. An indication of the reliability of an estimate of a population parameter, which is calculated by dividing the *standard deviation* of the estimate by the square root of the sample size.
SI units	Système Internationale d'Unitès (International System of Units)
Social Class	Based on the Registrar General's Standard Occupational Classification, Volume 3. HMSO (London, 1991). Social class was ascribed on the basis of the occupation of the head of household. The classification used in the tables is as follows:

Descriptive description	Social class
Non-manual	
Professional and intermediate	I and II
Skilled occupations, non manual	III non-manual
Manual	
Skilled occupations, manual	III manual
Partly-skilled and unskilled occupations	IV and V

SSD	The Social Survey Division, of the Office for National Statistics.
Tertile	See *Quantiles*
TIBC	Total iron-binding capacity
Two-parent household	Households where the young person was living with two adults who were married or cohabiting, one or both of whom was the young person's parent, step parent or foster parent, or if none of these was present, a grandparent.
Unemployed	International Labour Organisation (ILO) definition: those who were not in employment and were available to start work within two weeks and had either looked for work in the last four weeks, or were waiting to start a new job.
Wave; Fieldwork wave	The 3-month period in which fieldwork was carried out.

Wave 1: January to March 1997
Wave 2: April to June 1997
Wave 3: July to September 1997
Wave 4: October to December 1997

766

Because in some cases fieldwork extended beyond the end of the three-month fieldwork wave or cases were re-allocated to another fieldwork wave, cases have been allocated to a wave for analysis purposes as follows. Any case started more than 4 weeks after the end of the official fieldwork wave has been allocated to the actual quarter in which it was started. For example, all cases allocated to Wave 1 and started January to April appear as Wave 1 cases. Any case allocated to Wave 1 and started in May or later appears in a subsequent wave; for example a case allocated to Wave 1 which started in May appears in the tables under Wave 2. All cases in Wave 4 (October to December 1997) had been started by the end of January 1998. Note that in relation to the results for plasma 25-hydroxyvitamin D, the analyses relate to the exact date the blood sample was taken (see *Chapter 12*).

WHO   World Health Organisation

Working   In paid work, as an employee or self employed, at any time in the 7 days prior to the interview or not working in the 7 days prior to interview but with a job to return to, including, for women, being on maternity leave.

Appendix V

The oral health survey

1   Introduction

The oral health survey was conducted as the final component of the diet and nutrition survey. A full description of the conduct of the survey and the results form Volume 2 of this Report[1]. The oral health component comprised an interview in the home followed at a later date by a home oral health examination conducted by a dentist specially trained for the survey. It was carried out by the Social Survey Division of the Office for National Statistics in collaboration with the Dental Schools at the Universities of Birmingham, Newcastle, Dundee and Wales.

2   Other surveys of oral health of young people

There are two major series of surveys relating to the oral health of young people.

- The surveys of Children's Dental Health[2,3,4] have been conducted every ten years since 1973 on behalf of the United Kingdom Health Departments. The 1993 survey comprised a dental examination of around 17000 children aged 5 to 15 years and a postal interview with around 5500 parents of children who had been examined aged 5, 8, 12 and 15 years.

- The surveys co-ordinated by the British Association for the Study of Community Dentistry[5] have taken place every year since the mid 1980's and comprise a dental examination of between 120,000 and 180,000 young people from one of three age groups (5 years, 12 years and 14 years).

Neither of these series collect detailed information on diet or nutrition so the linking of the diet and nutrition survey with an oral health survey provides a unique opportunity to look at the relationship between oral health and diet and nutrition in a nationally representative sample of young people.

3   The objectives for the oral health survey

The oral health component of the NDNS had five main objectives:

- To establish, by clinical examination, the oral health status of young people aged 4 to 18 years.

- To investigate, through an interview, dietary and other behaviour affecting the mouth and teeth.

- To enable oral health status to be correlated with data on food and nutrient intake and nutritional status.

- To assess the impact of diet and nutritional status upon oral disease.

- To monitor the extent to which oral health targets set by Government are being met and to assist in the development of policies to achieve the targets in the document 'An Oral Health Strategy for England'[6].

This survey also provided an opportunity to monitor changes in the oral health of the population based on a comparison with the results of the 1993 survey of Children's Dental Health[4], although slight differences in methodology meant that only broad comparisons were possible.

Feasibility work carried out in February to April 1996 tested all the elements of the NDNS including the oral health survey and made recommendations for revisions for the main stage. Further details of the design and results of the feasibility study are given in Appendices A and F of the report of the oral health survey.

4   The conduct of the oral health survey

The sample design for the oral health survey was dependent on the needs of the dietary survey and is described in Chapter 1 and Appendix D of this Report.

It has been noted in Chapter 1 that while the aim was to achieve co-operation with all the various elements, the survey design allowed for a young person to participate in some elements only. All respondents took part in the initial face-to-face interview and all those who took part in the oral health examination had already completed an oral health interview. However, not all those who took part in the oral health interview or examination had completed a weighed intake dietary record.

The conduct of the oral health survey was designed to maximise response to this part of the survey, to minimise the time and expenses of the dental examiners and not to affect participation in the dietary aspects of the NDNS. Respondents were asked to take part in the oral health interview after they had completed all aspects of the dietary survey to avoid any effect such participation may have had on dietary behaviour and reporting. Once the oral health interview was completed, respondents were then asked if they would participate in a home dental examination to be carried out at a later date. The interviewer returned with the dental examiner who carried out the oral health examination.

During the fieldwork period a total of 67 interviewers and 65 dental examiners worked on the survey. Full details of the training received by the interviewers can be found in Chapter 1. All interviewers were trained to act as dental recorders for the oral health examination and some attended the training sessions for the dental examiners.

The dental examiners were recruited mainly from the Community Dental Service and Health Authorities of the NHS. All had experience of working with children and most had experience of working on other epidemiological surveys such as those described in Section 2. The dental examiners attended a three-day training course to introduce them to the survey criteria for the oral health examination, to practise the conduct of the examination and to standardise techniques and assessments. For the final day of the training period the examiners were joined by one of the interviewers with whom they would be working. The training sessions were organised by members of the dental team from the collaborating dental schools.

5   The oral health interview

The oral health questionnaire was developed from questionnaires used in the NDNS of children aged 1½ to 4½ years[7] and the survey of Children's Dental Health[4]. It was tested during the feasibility study and amended.

The interview included questions on:

- visiting the dentist and treatment history;
- dental hygiene;
- views on the causes and prevention of dental disease;
- advice received about preventing dental disease;
- aspects of dietary behaviour relating to dental health such as the type of drinks at night and whether drinks are made to last;
- orthodontic treatment;

- satisfaction with appearance of teeth;
- specific health conditions that are thought to be related to dental health.

As was the case for the dietary interview, depending on the age of the young person, the oral health interview was conducted either with a parent, usually the mother, or was conducted jointly with the parent and young person. Some questions relating to views and opinions were specifically asked of young people aged 11 to 18 years or 15 to 18 years. For young people who had left the parental home the interview was conducted with the young person alone.

6   The oral health examination

The criteria for the oral health examination and the conduct of the examination were based on those used in the survey of Children's Dental Health[4]. Amendments were made following the feasibility study.

The oral health examination included:

- identification of which teeth were present;
- the condition of the teeth;
- the presence of sealants;
- an assessment of erosion (the non-carious loss of tooth substance caused by chemical action on the teeth);
- trauma of upper and lower incisors;
- enamel opacities and hypoplasia;
- the presence of plaque and calculus;
- whether the gums were healthy and, for those aged 15 to 18 years, the presence of bleeding or pocketing of the gums.

7   The response

Of the 2672 young people selected to take part in the NDNS, 2127 completed the initial dietary interview and 73% (1943 young people) took part in the oral health interview; 1726 young people participated in the oral health examination representing 89% of those who took part in the oral health interview and 65% of those who were originally selected. Response is covered in more detail in Chapter 2 of the report of the oral health survey and Chapter 3 and Appendix D of this Report.

8   Ethical approval and consent procedures

The conduct of the oral health survey was included in the protocol submitted for ethical approval (see *Chapter 2* of this Report). As explained in Chapter 2, one of the measurements of possible clinical significance included in the survey was the identification of 'serious oral pathology' during the oral health examination, so it was necessary to obtain consent from the subject for their GP (general medical practitioner) to be informed of any such finding by the Dunn Nutrition Unit, and consequently for them to agree for their details, name, address, date of birth and gender, to be passed to the Dunn Nutrition Unit. Full details of the general procedure can be found in Chapter 2. In the case of the identification of serious oral pathology, the survey dentist was to be informed. However, in the event, no such pathology was found.

9 The contents of the report

The report of the oral health survey[1] presents data from the oral health component of the NDNS of young people aged 4 to 18 years.

Chapter 1 gives an introduction to the background and methodologies used.

Chapter 2 gives response data for the various elements in the survey and describes the characteristics of the responding sample.

In the subsequent chapters of the report, the data presented are based on the samples of young people co-operating with the relevant aspect of the survey rather than those who completed all elements.

The substantive results from the survey are presented in Chapters 3 to 8. Chapters 3, 4 and 5 present the data relating to oral health and diet for different socio-demographic groups - for example, by age group, region, social class of head of household and household type (with whom the young person was living).

Chapter 3 presents information relating to the oral health status of young people. The data in this chapter come from the oral health examination and cover the topics shown in Section 6.

Chapter 4 looks at those aspects of dietary behaviour, consumption and the intake of nutrients which may be related to oral health status. Data are presented on the consumption of selected sugary or acidic foods, the intake of sugars and behaviour relating to drinking. The data are drawn from the weighed intake dietary record, the dietary interview and the oral health interview.

Chapter 5 covers reported socio-dental behaviour, views and opinions taken from the oral health interview. The chapter includes information about respondents' views on what could cause or prevent decay; advice on these matters; dental hygiene; visiting the dentist and past treatment history; orthodontic treatment and satisfaction with the appearance of the teeth.

Chapters 6, 7 and 8 investigate the relationships between the different aspects covered in Chapters 3 to 5. Chapter 6 describes the relationship between diet and oral health and Chapter 7 that between socio-dental behaviour and oral health. Both these chapters present cross-tabulations of these data. In Chapter 8 the results of various multivariate analyses are presented looking at the overall relationships between oral health, socio-demographic factors, socio-dental behaviour and diet.

The appendices include a description of the feasibility study (Appendix A); a summary of the dietary survey report (Appendix B); a description of the weighting procedures used (Appendix C); the fieldwork documents (Appendix D); the criteria for the dental examination, the training of the examiners and their names (Appendices E, F and G); a comparison of the oral health data with data from the NDNS of pre-school children[7] and the Children's Dental Health survey[4] (Appendix H); technical appendices describing sampling errors and the multivariate techniques used (Appendices I and J) and a list of the units of measurement together with glossary of terms (Appendices K and L).

References and endnotes

1 Walker A, Gregory J, Bradnock G, Nunn J, White D. *National Diet and Nutrition Survey: young people aged 4 to 18 years. Volume 2: Report of the oral health survey.* TSO (London, 2000)

2 Todd JE. *Children's Dental Health in England and Wales 1973.* HMSO (London, 1975)

3 Todd JE, Dodd T. *Children's Dental Health in the United Kingdom 1983.* HMSO (London, 1985)

4 O'Brien M. *Children's Dental Health in the United Kingdom 1993.* HMSO (London, 1994)

5 Pitts NB and Palmer J. The dental caries experience of 5-, 12-, and 14 year old children in Great Britain. Surveys co-ordinated by the British Association for the Study of Community Dentistry in 1991/2, 1992/3 and 1990/1. *Community Dental Health 1994;* 11: 42-52.

6 Department of Health *An Oral Health Strategy for England.* Department of Health (London, 1994)

7 Hinds K, Gregory JR. *National Diet and Nutrition Survey: children aged 1½ to 4½ years. Volume 2: Report of the dental survey.* HMSO (London, 1995)

Appendix W

Department of Health 1983 Survey of the Diets of British Schoolchildren[1]

The last national survey of the diets of British children was conducted in 1983. The survey aimed to monitor the effect of the 1980 Education Act which released Local Authorities from the requirement to ensure that meals provided by schools in England and Wales conformed with prescribed nutritional standards. The survey was designed to examine the contribution of school meals to the overall diet of British school-children.

The survey was carried out in schools between January and June 1983 and covered two age groups, 10 to 11 year olds and 14 to 15 year olds. A 7-day weighed dietary record was kept by participants and their heights and weights were measured. Energy and nutrient intakes were calculated as were the contributions of different food categories to these intakes. The results were analysed by social class, region, family composition and type of lunch. There were no blood or urine samples taken and the survey did not include any oral health examination. Physical activity was not assessed.

The sample

Sampling in England and Wales and for Scottish primary schoolchildren was based on a multi-stage design to select areas, then eligible schools and finally children in the specified groups. Eight secondary schools were selected from a list of all Scottish secondary schools with probability proportionate to the number of children aged 12 to 15 years. After participating schools were identified and recruited, the parents of all selected children were first contacted by letter to give the opportunity for withdrawal from the study.

In planning the survey there was an interest in the nutrition of children from less advantaged homes. To ensure a large enough subsample within the survey population for separate analysis, the selection procedure was designed to ensure more of these children. Overall completed records were achieved for 1686 boys and 1610 girls (3296 total). Results were weighted to take account of the over selection of the less-advantaged group when presenting results for the survey population

Socio-economic status of families in sample

	Socio-economic status of families	
	10/11 year olds	14/15 year olds
	%	%
One-parent families	12	16
Two-parent families		
Social Class (father working)		
I	6	6
II	23	17
IIInm	10	8
IIIm	22	22
IV + V	12	15
Unemployed	11	11
Father not working		
Long-term sick	1.5	2.5
Other	1.5	1.5

as a whole. The weighted response rate achieved was 75.2%.

Dietary measurements

Children and their parents were then asked to record everything the child ate for the next seven days, using scales which were supplied. The children used note-books to record food eaten outside the home and arrangements were made to have record books and scales available at school canteens.

Intakes were calculated for the following nutrients using the most up-to-date food composition data available; energy, fat, carbohydrate (as monosaccharides), protein, calcium, iron, thiamin, riboflavin, nicotinic acid, nicotinic acid equivalent, retinol, carotene, retinol equivalent, vitamin D and pyridoxine (vitamin B_6).

Anthropometry

The heights and weights of children were measured. The survey used methods developed by the Office of Population Censuses and Surveys (OPCS) in its Survey of Adult Heights and Weights[2].

Children were weighed using the SOEHNLE digital personal weighing scale which has an electronic digital readout and is calibrated in units of 200g up to 135 kg. Shoes and heavier outer garments were removed prior to measurement, but although the child was asked to indicate the clothing he/she was still wearing, no allowance was made for the weight of that clothing in the results.

Children's heights were measured using the OPCS portable stadiometer. Fieldworkers were trained to use a standard method which included ensuring that the head was positioned in the Frankfort Plane position.

Results

Foods consumed

The main sources of dietary energy in the diets of British schoolchildren were bread, chips, milk, biscuits, meat products, cake and puddings. Almost all children in the survey recorded consumption of chips, crisps, cakes and biscuits. Boys recorded more chips consumed than girls along with more milk, breakfast cereals and baked beans; girls recorded more fruit consumed and more girls drank fruit juice than boys. Yogurt, fizzy drinks and sweets were more popular among younger children. Older children recorded consumption of more tea and coffee.

Scottish primary school children appeared to have a distinctive dietary pattern. They recorded higher median consumption of beef, soups, milk, cheese, sausages, chocolates and sweets and lower median consumption of cakes, biscuits, puddings, potatoes and, in particular, of vegetables of all kinds than children in the other regions of Great Britain.

Chips and milk were the two major items in the diets which varied most with social class and other socio-economic variables. Higher median chip consumption was recorded among Social Classes IV and V, children with unemployed fathers, children from families receiving Supplementary Benefit, children taking school meals and those older children who ate out of school at cafes etc. Conversely, median milk consumption was lower among most of these groups.

Heights and weights

Nearly all children were, on average, above the fiftieth centile of standards for both height and weight standards. They also had average Body Mass Indices (BMI) above those calculated from the fiftieth standard centiles.

Among the younger children, those from families with fathers who were unemployed were significantly shorter than those from families in Social Classes I, II and III non-manual. Younger girls with unemployed fathers were also significantly shorter than those in Social Class IV.

The younger children and older boys from families in receipt of supplementary benefit were significantly shorter than those from families not receiving benefits.

At least 5% of girls aged 14 to 15 years were dieting to lose weight.

Nutrient intakes

Differences between energy and nutrient intakes of groups of children reflected the median consumption of chips and milk.

Average energy intakes were about 90% of the existing Recommended Daily Amounts (RDA). There was no evidence to suggest that these intakes were inadequate.

The average proportion of energy from fat ranged from 37.4% to 38.7% across the different age and sex groups and 75% of children had intakes of fat over the level of 35% of their energy recommended by the COMA Panel on Diet and Cardiovascular Disease[3]. Milk and cheese were the two major contributors to these fat intakes.

Nutrient intakes were compared with the Recommended Daily Amounts (RDA) set by COMA in 1979[4]. These RDA are estimated so that the requirements of almost all members of a group of healthy people are met. In practice, if the average intake of a nutrient is at or above the RDA, it can be assumed that the requirements of almost all individuals have been met. While in any group there may be individuals with nutrient intakes below the RDA, this does not necessarily imply dietary deficiency, which can be established only by clinical and biochemical tests of nutritional status.

Average and median nutrient intakes were above the RDA in all age and sex groups for protein, thiamin, nicotinic acid equivalent and vitamin C.

Both mean and median iron intakes of girls were below the RDA. The clinical significance of these iron intakes is not clear without further studies of iron status.

Both the mean and median intakes of riboflavin of the older girls were below the RDA. These girls obtained less of their riboflavin from milk and breakfast cereals which are major sources of this vitamin.

Nearly 60% of older girls had calcium intakes below the RDA. These girls consumed less milk, bread and other cereals which are the main dietary source of calcium.

Scottish primary schoolchildren had lower average intakes of vitamin C, ß-carotene and retinol equivalents than children in the Great Britain sample[5], reflecting lower consumption of carrots and vegetables.

School meals and the diet

Dietary patterns of foods consumed were to some extent dependent on the provision from school meals. Older children obtained over half the chips that they ate in the survey week from school meals, both free and paid for. Younger children obtained over half the buns and pastries they ate from those sources. However, the total average daily intakes of energy and nutrients did not vary with the kind of meal eaten at weekday lunchtimes.

There were no significant differences between the average energy or nutrient intakes of children taking school meals from outlets offering a free choice cafeteria style service and those obtaining a fixed price fixed menu school meal. When school meals were eaten, they contributed on average between 30% and 43% of average daily energy intakes.

Older children, especially girls, who ate out of school at places such as cafes, take-away or 'fast food' outlets chose meals which were low in many nutrients, particularly iron. Their average daily nutrient intakes were not made up to the levels of intake of the rest of the population by the meals they consumed at other times during the week. The overall nutritional quality of their diets was the poorest of any group surveyed.

The school meal was an important contributor of food energy to the diets of older children.

References and endnotes

1. Department of Health. Report on Health and Social Subjects: 36. *The Diets of British Schoolchildren*. HMSO (London, 1989).

2. Knight I, Eldridge J. *The heights and weights of adults in Great Britain: report of a survey carried out on behalf of the Department of Health and Social Security covering adults aged 16-64*. HMSO (London, 1984).

3. Department of Health and Social Security. Report on Health and Social Subjects: 28. *Diet and Cardiovascular Disease*. HMSO (London, 1984).

4. Department of Health and Social Security. Report on Health and Social Subjects: 15. *Recommended Daily Amounts of Food Energy and Nutrients for Groups of People in the United Kingdom*. HMSO (London, 1979).

5. There was a separate, enhanced sample of Scottish primary schoolchildren (aged 10 and 11 years). These were included in the GB sample, weighted to their proportionate share of the total sample.

Appendix X

School meals

This Appendix describes the preliminary analyses of the 7-day weighed dietary intake records for those young people who took school meals during the dietary recording period and presents some data on the biochemical analytes for these respondents. These analyses were designed for, and carried out specifically in order to inform the preparation by Government of draft Regulations on National Nutritional Standards for School Lunches[1]. They are therefore limited in their coverage of age groups and the scope of the foods which contribute to the diets of schoolchildren, to their school meals and their nutrient contents. The range of biochemical analytes is also restricted to haematology and blood cholesterol levels.

1 Definitions, assumptions and methodology

In all the analyses reported here, the 'school meal' has been defined as any food obtained on the school premises and consumed between the hours of 1200 and 1359. It excludes food brought from home to eat at school, for example packed lunches, and food purchased off the school premises. It includes drinks and other items purchased from tuck shops, vending machines, etc at lunchtime.

This definition was adopted in order to be consistent with that used in the 1983 Department of Health Survey of British Schoolchildren[2].

Data were analysed on two different bases. Young people aged 4 to 10 years and 11 to 18 years were included if they took a school meal on at least three days during the 7-day recording period, a total of 487 individuals. Some children may have habitually taken school meals but were not recorded as doing so because they took part in the survey during school holidays. The numbers in each age group who were deemed, on the receipt of benefits, to be entitled to free school meals are shown below[3].

Entitlement to free school meals

Age (years)	Yes, entitled	No, not entitled	Total
4–10	67	185	252
11–18	54	181	235
All	121	366	487

A further set of analyses was carried out which included 4 to 10 year olds only who consumed a school meal on at least one day of their 7-day weighed dietary record. There were 340 children aged 4 to 10 years in this group. These analyses also used a stricter definition for school meals. Savoury snacks and confectionery items were excluded from the definition of a school meal and meals which comprised solely of biscuits, cakes, soft drinks, tea, coffee, alcohol or water were also excluded from the analyses.

2 Results

2.1 Food consumption

The Government's proposed Regulations on National Nutritional Standards for School Lunches will specify food-based standards derived from the *Balance of Good Health*[4] (BGH). Table X1 shows the composition of school meals consumed by those children aged 4 to 10 years who took school meals on any day of the 7-day recording period, using the categories defined in BGH. The table also shows the composition of the daily diet in terms of these categories for all the children aged 4 to 10 years who completed a 7-day weighed dietary record. School meals provide a greater percentage of starchy foods and protein-rich foods than the daily diet but a lower percentage of milk and dairy foods and fatty/sugary foods. However, neither school meals nor the overall daily diet come close to satisfying the BGH requirements that at least 30% of foods should comprise fruit and vegetables and that no more than 10% should comprise fatty/sugary foods.

Table X2 shows the contribution by weight of both free and paid for school meals to the total consumption of selected foods on any days school meals were taken for young people aged 4 to 10 and 11 to 18 years who took school meals on at least three days during the recording period. This excludes all weekend days. Among the younger age group, school meals provided more than half of the total consumption of puddings (including milk and sponge puddings and crumbles), fish and fish products, vegetables, chips and 'other' potatoes. They also provided over one third of the amount of meat and meat products consumed. Among the older age group, school meals provided over half the total consumption of chips and about one third of vegetables and fish and fish products. For young people who had free school meals, these tended to provide a higher proportion of the total consumption of puddings, 'other' potatoes, fruit and ice cream than paid for school meals, but the differences were not statistically significant.

2.2 Nutrient intakes

Table X3 shows average daily intake of selected nutrients by 4 to 10 year olds who took one or more free or paid for school meals during the 7-day recording period and for those who had no school meals. The statistical significance of differences is also shown.[5] Those who took no school meal had significantly lower fat, fibre (NSP) and protein intakes than those obtaining a free school meal and significantly higher non-milk extrinsic sugars and vitamin C intakes. They also had significantly lower energy, fat, fibre (NSP), protein, calcium and vitamin A intakes than those paying for a school meal.

Table X4 shows the average daily intakes of energy and selected nutrients provided for the two age groups by school meals, both free and paid for, where school meals were taken on at least three days. In both age groups, children who had a free school meal tended to obtain more energy and nutrients from their school meal.

Table X5 shows the percentage contribution of school meals to average daily intakes of energy and nutrients for those who took school meals for at least three days. In both age groups, children receiving free school meals obtained a higher proportion of their daily energy and nutrient intakes from school meals than children having paid school meals. Further analyses (*not shown*) indicated that 19% of 4 to 10 year olds and 41% of 11 to 18 year olds receiving free school meals derived less than 30% of their total daily energy intake from school meals. Of those who paid for school meals, 37% of the younger group and 48% of the older group derived less than 30% of the daily total energy intake from school meals.

Table X6 shows the average contribution of main food groups to the average intakes of energy and nutrients from all school meals taken by 4 to 10 year olds. This shows that two food groups, chips, and buns, cakes and pastries are the major dietary components. Buns, cakes and pastries contributed 30% of non-milk extrinsic sugars and between 13% and 15% of intakes of energy, fat, saturated fat, carbohydrate, iron and vitamin A. Chips provided 20% of vitamin C intakes and 11% to 15% of energy, fatty acids, carbohydrate, fibre (NSP) and folate intakes. Meat pies and pastries also provided 7% of saturated fatty acids intakes.

2.3 Biochemical analytes

Table X7 shows the mean levels of blood analytes for different age groups for young people who had no school meal, a free meal and a paid for meal. There was no general trend and no significant differences between young people who received free school meals and those who paid for their school meal. There were also no significant differences for 4 to 10 year olds between those who had no school meal and those that did. However, for 11 to 18 year olds, those who had no school meals had significantly higher haemoglobin and haematocrit levels than those that did. Serum ferritin levels were also significantly higher for those who had no school meal than those who paid for a school meal.

References and endnotes

[1] Department for Education and Employment. *Draft Regulations and Guidance for Nutritional Standards for School Lunches* DfEE (London, 1999).

[2] Department of Health. *The Diets of British Schoolchildren.* HMSO (London, 1989).

[3] All the data in this Appendix are unweighted numbers of cases (ie actual numbers). Cases have not been weighted to correct for differential sampling probability or non response.

[4] Health Education Authority. *The Balance of Good Health.* HEA (London, 1996).

[5] In this Appendix, differences between proportions and means have been tested for statistical significance assuming a simple random sample design with no allowance for any design effects.

Table X1 Composition of a typical school meal (including and excluding drinks/soup) and of the total daily diet of 4 to 10 year olds in terms of 'Balance of Good Health' food types.

Those aged 4 to 10 years who consumed one or more school meals*

Foods	Composition of typical school meal				Composition of daily diet	
	Including drinks		Excluding drinks		Including drinks	
	%	Mass (g)	%	Mass (g)	%	Mass
Fruit & veg	9	42	13	37	11	—
Starchy	24	107	36	107	16	—
Protein-rich	15	68	23	68	9	—
Milk & dairy	12	52	11	32	17	—
Fatty/sugary	19	85	16	49	25	—

*Base = 340

Table X2 Percentage contribution of school meals to total consumption of selected food groups

Those who consumed school meals on at least three days

Food groups	Young people aged (years)			
	4–10		11–18	
	Free school meals	Paid school meals	Free school meals	Paid school meals
	% contribution to total consumption*			
Cereals & cereal products	22	22	17	21
Puddings	71	60	54	36
Milk & milk products	11	10	17	7
Ice cream	42	32	29	9
Eggs & egg dishes	29	23	12	12
Fat spreads	14	12	18	29
Meat & meat products	36	38	25	26
Fish & fish products	56	49	29	32
Vegetables (excl. potatoes)	56	48	31	31
Chips	48	55	53	55
Other potatoes	62	62	41	30
Fruit	23	25	25	14
Soft drinks	10	15	36	31
Sugar, preserves, snacks & confectionery	10	6	15	21
Base	*67*	*185*	*54*	*181*

* Total consumption is based on days when a school meal was consumed.

Table X3 Differences in total daily intake of nutrients among different groups of young people aged 4-10 years defined in terms of school-meal habits and entitlement

Young people aged 4 to 10 years who consumed one or more school meals

Nutrients	Group mean intakes			Significance of between-group differences		
	Type of school meal being taken			Pairs of school meal types being compared		
	Free	Paid	None	Free v Paid	Free v None	Paid v None
Energy (kcal)	1639	1621	1573	NS	NS	*
Fat (g)	66.7	65	61.6	NS	**	**
Saturated fat (g)	25.9	26.6	25.7	NS	NS	NS
Carbohydrate (g)	220	220	219	NS	NS	NS
Non-milk extrinsic sugars (g)	65.3	71.7	75.1	*	**	***
Non-starch polysaccharides (g)	10.1	9.9	9.0	NS	**	***
Protein (g)	53.3	52.6	49.3	NS	**	***
Iron (mg)	8.7	8.6	8.6	NS	NS	NS
Calcium (mg)	673	729	692	**	NS	*
Vitamin A (µg)	540	574	500	NS	NS	**
Folate (mg)	202	198	190	NS	NS	NS
Vitamin C (µg)	62.4	79	77.3	***	***	NS

NS No significant difference
* p < 0.05
**p < 0.01
*** p < 0.001

Table X4 Average daily intake of energy and selected nutrients from school meals

Young people who consumed school meals on at least three days.

Nutrients	Age of young person (years) and type of school meal taken							
	4–10				11–18			
	Free school meal		Paid school meal		Free school meal		Paid school meal	
	av. daily intake	se	av. daily intake	se	av. daily intake	se	av. daily intake	se
Energy (kcal)	619	18.2	527	13.1	599	25.3	544	14.4
Total fat (g)	27.9	0.82	23.8	0.67	26.7	1.4	24.6	0.82
Saturated fatty acids (g)	9.4	0.38	8.3	0.25	9.2	0.57	8.3	0.31
% energy from fat	40.5	0.50	40	0.54	40.9	1.11	39.8	0.65
% energy from saturated fatty acids	13.6	0.34	14.2	0.31	13.6	0.55	13.7	0.38
Non-milk extrinsic sugars (g)	19.3	1.21	16.3	0.68	23.7	1.86	23	1.13
Fibre (NSP) (g)	4.2	0.17	3.5	0.11	3.5	0.19	3.2	0.13
Iron (mg)	2.6	0.09	2.2	0.07	2.2	0.11	2.1	0.06
Calcium (mg)	215	10.5	199	7.05	197	17.6	178	7.5
Vitamin C (mg)	23.8	1.78	21.2	1.15	24	2.33	20.3	1.88
Folate (µg)	64	2.4	54	1.6	56	3.2	49	1.9
Base	*67*		*185*		*54*		*181*	

Table X5 Percentage contribution of school meals–total daily energy and nutrient intakes*

Young people who consumed a school meal on at least three days

Nutrients	Age of young person (years) and type of school meal taken							
	4–10				11–18			
	Free school meal		Paid school meal		Free school meal		Paid school meal	
	% contribution– total intake	se	% contribution– total intake	se	% contribution– total intake	se	% contribution– total intake	se
Energy (kcal)	37	0.93	32	0.69	32	1.34	30	0.80
Total fat (g)	41	1.21	36	0.86	36	1.63	33	1.02
Saturated fatty acids (g)	36	1.33	31	0.86	33	1.77	30	1.08
Non-milk extrinsic sugars (g)	32	1.86	24	0.95	32	2.52	27	1.31
Fibre (NSP) (g)	40	1.25	35	0.95	34	1.79	23	1.05
Iron (mg)	30	0.98	26	0.74	25	1.35	23	0.78
Calcium (mg)	31	1.23	27	0.93	31	2.13	26	0.97
Vitamin C (mg)	39	2.16	29	1.29	39	2.84	28	1.48
Folate (µg)	32	1.11	27	0.74	29	1.52	23	0.89
Base	*67*		*185*		*54*		*181*	

* Total intake based on days when a school meal was consumed.

Table X6   Main food groups contributing to the intake of the 12 key nutrients from school meals by 4 to10 year olds

Nutrients	Average intake from school meals*	Main sources	Average contribution	% contribution
Energy (kcal)	555	Buns, cakes & pastries	72	13
		Chips	59	11
		Cereal-based milk puddings	26	5
		White fish, coated or fried, including fish fingers	24	4
		Other potatoes, potato salads & dishes	24	4
		Meat pies & pastries	23	4
		Biscuits	21	4
		Pizza	20	4
		Sausages	20	4
		Coated chicken & turkey	20	4
Fat (g)	25	Buns, cakes & pastries	3.3	13
		Chips	3.1	12
		Meat pies & pastries	1.6	6
		Sausages	1.5	6
		Pizza	1.2	5
		Coated chicken & turkey	1.2	5
		White fish, coated or fried, including fish fingers	1.2	5
Saturated fat (g)	8.6	Buns, cakes & pastries	1.2	13
		Meat pies & pastries	0.6	7
		Sausages	0.6	6
		Pizza	0.5	6
		Cereal-based milk puddings	0.5	5
		Biscuits	0.4	5
Carbohydrate (g)	68.4	Buns, cakes & pastries	10.2	15
		Chips	7.3	11
		Other potatoes, potato salads & dishes	4.9	7
		Cereal-based milk puddings	4.2	6
		White bread	3.3	5
Non-milk extrinsic sugars (g)	17.1	Buns, cakes & pastries	5.2	30
		Other puddings	1.4	8
		Cereal-based milk puddings	1.4	8
		Sponge puddings	1.2	7
		Concentrated soft drinks, not diet	1.0	6
		Biscuits	0.9	6
Non-starch polysaccharides (g)	3.7	Chips	0.5	14
		Baked beans	0.5	13
		Other potatoes, potato salads & dishes	0.4	10
		Buns, cakes & pastries	0.3	7
		Fried or roast potatoes & fried potato products	0.2	6
		Peas, not raw	0.2	6
Protein (g)	18.4	White fish, coated or fried, including fish fingers	1.5	8
		Coated chicken & turkey	1.2	7
		Buns, cakes & pastries	1.1	6
		Sausages	1.0	5
		Cereal-based milk puddings	0.9	5
		Chicken & turkey dishes	0.9	5
		Chips	0.9	5
		Pizza	0.8	5
Iron (mg)	2.3	Buns, cakes & pastries	0.3	13
		Baked beans	0.2	8
		Chips	0.2	7
		White bread	0.1	5
		Other potatoes, potato salads & dishes	0.1	5
Calcium (mg)	210	Cereal-based milk puddings	32	15
		Pizza	19	9
		Whole milk	17	8
		Buns, cakes & pastries	16	8
		White fish, coated or fried, including fish fingers	13	6
		Cheese	12	6
Vitamin A (µg)	207	Carrots, not raw	66	32
		Buns, cakes & pastries	26	13
		Pizza	9	4
		Sponge puddings	8	4
		Cereal-based milk puddings	7	3
		Biscuits	6	3
		Cheese	6	3

781

Table X6 Continued

Nutrients	Average intake from school meals*	Main sources	Average contribution	% contribution
Folate (µg)	56.7	Chips	8.3	15
		Other potatoes, potato salads & dishes	6.1	11
		Baked beans	4.4	8
		Buns, cakes & pastries	3.7	7
		Fried or roast potatoes & fried potato products	3.5	6
Vitamin C (mg)	21.8	Chips	4.3	20
		Other potatoes, potato salads & dishes	2.8	13
		Fried or roast potatoes & fried potato products	1.9	8
		Ready to drink soft drinks, not diet	1.7	8
		Concentrated soft drinks, not diet	1.4	6
		Fruit juice	1.4	6

*Results are averages across all qualifying school meals taken by 4 to 10 year olds
Savoury snacks & confectionery are excluded.

Table X7   Mean levels of six blood analytes for different groups of young people defined by age, type of school meal and entitlement to free meals

Young people who consumed a school meal on at least one day

Blood analyte	Age of young person (years) and type of school meal								
	4–10			11–18					
	Free	Paid	None	Free	Paid	None	Free v Paid	Free v None	Paid v None
Haemoglobin (g/dl)	12.6	12.8	12.8	13.4	13.5	13.8	NS	*	*
Haematocrit	0.395	0.404	0.403	0.421	0.427	0.437	NS	**	**
Serum ferritin (µg/l)	32	34	39	34	29	41	NS	NS	***
Plasma total cholesterol (mmol/l)	4.42	4.25	4.23	4.08	4.10	4.00	NS	NS	NS
Plasma high density lipoprotein cholesterol (mmol/l)	1.38	1.28	1.33	1.32	1.25	1.23	NS	NS	NS
Plasma low density lipoprotein cholesterol (mmol/l)	3.03	2.97	2.89	2.76	2.85	2.77	NS	NS	NS

NS No significant difference
* $p < 0.05$
**$p < 0.01$
***$p < 0.001$

Appendix Y

List of tables

4: Types and quantities of foods consumed

Tables

784

5: Energy intakes

Tables

Figures

6: Protein, carbohydrate and alcohol intake

Tables

8: Vitamins

Tables

9: Minerals

Tables

790

10: Anthropometry

Tables

11: Blood pressure

12: Blood analytes and correlations with nutrient intakes

Figures

13: Physical activity